Therapeutic Exercise for Musculoskeletal Injuries

Second Edition

Athletic Training Education Series

Peggy A. Houglum, PhD, PT, ATC

Duquesne University

David H. Perrin, PhD, ATC

Series Editor
University of North Carolina at Greensboro

Human Kinetics

Library of Congress Cataloging-in-Publication Data

Houglum, Peggy A., 1948-
   Therapeutic exercise for musculoskeletal injuries / Peggy A. Houglum.-- 2nd ed.
      p. ; cm. -- (Athletic training education series)
   Rev. ed. of: Therapeutic exercise for athletic injuries. c2001.
   Includes bibliographical references and index.
   ISBN 0-7360-5136-8 (hard cover)
  1. Sports injuries--Exercise therapy. 2. Musculoskeletal system--Wounds and injuries--Exercise therapy.
      [DNLM: 1. Athletic Injuries--therapy. 2. Exercise Therapy--methods. 3. Musculoskeletal System--injuries. 4. Sports Medicine--methods. QT 261 H838t 2005] I. Houglum, Peggy A., 1948- Therapeutic exercise for athletic injuries. II. Title. III. Series.
   RD97.H6843 2005
   615.8'2--dc22

ISBN: 0-7360-5136-8

2004024358

Permission notices for material reprinted in this book from other sources can be found on pages xvii-xviii.

This book is a revised edition of Therapeutic Exercise for Athletic Injuries, published in 2001 by Human Kinetics.
The Web addresses cited in this text were current as of October 6, 2004, unless otherwise noted.

Acquisitions Editor: Loarn D. Robertson, PhD
Series Developmental Editor: Elaine Mustain
Developmental Editor: Renee Thomas Pyrtel
Assistant Editors: Ann M. Augspurger and Bethany J. Bentley
Copyeditors: Joyce Sexton and Karen Bojda
Proofreader: Joanna Hatzopoulos Portman
Indexer: Marie Rizzo
Permission Manager: Dalene Reeder
Graphic Designer: Fred Starbird
Graphic Artist: Angela K. Snyder
Photo Manager: Kareema McLendon
Cover Designer: Keith Blomberg
Photographer (cover): Tom Roberts
Photographers (interior): All photos by Tom Roberts unless otherwise noted. Figures 6.17, 16.19, 16.64-16.73, 16.83, and 16.85 by Kelly J. Huff. Photos on pages 67, 89, 125, 155, 199, 327, 479, 557, 647, 689, 745, 821, and 893, © Human Kinetics.
Models: Tracy Beltran, Michael A. Curtis, Rosemary Dent, Tori Depp, Kate Fenner, Koren Forster, James Grimes, Taeyou Jung, Chelsea Kane, Jessica Kane, Kristi LaVanti, Ian McLeod, Susan Saliba, Fred Thomas, Tamara C. Valovich, and Lorraine Vizzuso
Art Managers: Kelly Hendren and Kareema McLendon
Illustrators: Argosy, Angela K. Snyder, and Dawn Sills
Printer: Edwards Brothers, Inc.

Printed in the United States of America

10 9 8 7 6 5 4 3 2 1

Human Kinetics
Web site: www.HumanKinetics.com

United States: Human Kinetics
P.O. Box 5076
Champaign, IL 61825-5076
800-747-4457
e-mail: humank@hkusa.com

Canada: Human Kinetics
475 Devonshire Road Unit 100
Windsor, ON N8Y 2L5
800-465-7301 (in Canada only)
e-mail: orders@hkcanada.com

Europe: Human Kinetics
107 Bradford Road
Stanningley
Leeds LS28 6AT, United Kingdom
+44 (0) 113 255 5665
e-mail: hk@hkeurope.com

Australia: Human Kinetics
57A Price Avenue
Lower Mitcham, South Australia 5062
08 8277 1555
e-mail: liaw@hkaustralia.com

New Zealand: Human Kinetics
Division of Sports Distributors NZ Ltd.
P.O. Box 300 226 Albany
North Shore City
Auckland
0064 9 448 1207
e-mail: blairc@hknewz.com

To

Dan, Becki, Andy, Michelle, Samuel, Cate,

Michael, Emilie, Matthew, Kamryn, Benjamin,

Tony, Amanda,

Misti, and Casie,

you have already impacted so many.

May your lives be as rich in the joy, love, and fulfillment with which

I have been blessed.

Contents

Preface   xi
Acknowledgments   xiv
Introduction to the Athletic Training Education Series   xv
Credits   xvii

Part I   BASIC CONCEPTS 1

Chapter 1   Concepts of Rehabilitation 3

The Rehabilitation Team 4
Interacting With Team Members 7
Qualities of Professionalism 9
Components of a Rehabilitation Program ... 13
Basic Components of Therapeutic Exercise ... 21
Return-to-Competition Criteria 23
Psychological Considerations 23
Learning Aids 26

Chapter 2   Concepts of Healing 29

Primary and Secondary Healing 37
Healing Phases 37
Growth Factors 44
Healing of Specific Tissues 46
Tensile Strength During Healing 51
Factors That Affect Healing 52
The Role of Therapeutic Exercise in Healing ... 58
Learning Aids 60

Chapter 3   Concepts in Physics 65

Force 66
Newton's Laws of Motion 67
Center of Gravity 68
Stability and Fixation 70
Body Levers 72
Levers and Force 75
Physiological Muscle Advantages 76
Other Concepts in Physics 78
Learning Aids 82

Chapter **4** **Examination and Assessment** **87**

Examination: Making a Profile 89
Assessment: Planning for Action 99
Keeping Rehabilitation Records 102
Learning Aids 116

Part **II** **THERAPEUTIC EXERCISE PARAMETERS AND TECHNIQUES** **121**

Chapter **5** **Range of Motion and Flexibility** **123**

Defining Flexibility and Range of Motion 124
Connective-Tissue Composition 124
Effects of Immobilization on Connective Tissue 125
Effects of Remobilization on Connective Tissue 128
Mechanical Properties and Tissue Behavior
  in Range of Motion 128
Neuromuscular Influences on Range of Motion 132
Determining Normal Range of Motion 134
Measuring Range of Motion 134
Terminology in Goniometry 140
Stretching Techniques 141
Exercise Progression 147
Special Considerations 148
Learning Aids 149

Chapter **6** **Manual Therapy Techniques** **153**

Critical Analysis 155
Massage 155
Myofascial Release 158
Myofascial Trigger Points 165
Muscle Energy 170
Joint Mobilization 173
Neural Mobilization 183
Learning Aids 193

Chapter **7** **Muscle Strength and Endurance** **197**

Muscle Structure and Function 199
Neuromuscular Physiology 205
Fast- and Slow-Twitch Fibers 210
Muscle Strength, Power, and Endurance 211

Force Production 214
Types of Muscle Activity 217
Open and Closed Kinetic Chain Activity 219
Evaluating Muscle Strength 221
Gradations of Muscle Activity 230
Strength Equipment 231
Proprioceptive Neuromuscular Facilitation 242
Strengthening Principles 248
Exercise Progression 252
Learning Aids 254

Chapter **8   The ABCs of Proprioception** **259**

Neurophysiology of Proprioception 261
Central Nervous System Proprioceptor Sites 263
Balance 264
Coordination 266
Agility 268
Therapeutic Exercise for Proprioception 269
Learning Aids 273

Chapter **9   Plyometrics** **275**

Neuromuscular Principles 277
Plyometric Force Production 278
Plyometric Exercise Phases 279
Preplyometric Considerations 280
Plyometric Program Design 281
Plyometric Program Considerations 283
Precautions and Contraindications 285
Equipment 285
Lower-Extremity Plyometrics 288
Upper-Extremity and Trunk Plyometrics 296
Learning Aids 298

Chapter **10   Functional Exercise** **301**

Definitions, Foundations, and Goals 303
Contributions to Therapeutic Exercise 303
Basic Functional Activities 305
Advanced Functional Activities 306
Advanced Functional Exercise Progression 306
Precautions 308

Functional Evaluation 309
A Lower-Extremity Functional Progression 310
An Upper-Extremity Functional Progression 315
Returning the Patient to Full Participation 319
Learning Aids 320

Part **III** **GENERAL THERAPEUTIC EXERCISE APPLICATIONS** **323**

Chapter **11** **Posture and Body Mechanics** **325**

Posture 326
Muscle Imbalances 337
Body Mechanics 340
Body-Awareness Programs 345
Learning Aids 351

Chapter **12** **Ambulation and Ambulation Aids** **355**

Normal Gait 356
Pathological Gait 375
Normal Running Gait 377
Mechanics of Ambulation with Assistive Devices . . . 381
Learning Aids 387

Chapter **13** **Aquatic Therapeutic Exercise** **391**

Physical Properties and Principles of Water 393
Equipment 396
Indications, Advantages, Precautions, and
    Contraindications 400
Aquatic Therapeutic Exercise Principles and Guidelines . 402
Deep-Water Exercise 404
Aquatic Therapeutic Exercises 405
Learning Aids 421

Chapter **14** **Swiss Balls and Foam Rollers** **425**

Swiss Balls 426
Swiss-Ball Exercises 430
Foam Rollers 444
Foam-Roller Exercises 445
Learning Aids 453

Chapter **15 Therapeutic Exercise for Tendinitis** **457**

Terminology 458
Tendon Structure 458
Etiology 459
Tendon Response 460
General Treatment 461
Specific Treatment 462
Examples of Tendinitis Cases 464
Learning Aids 466

Part **IV SPECIFIC APPLICATIONS** **469**

Chapter **16 Spine and Sacroiliac** **477**

General Rehabilitation Considerations 479
Rehabilitation Techniques 480
Special Rehabilitation Applications 525
Learning Aids 550

Chapter **17 Shoulder and Arm** **555**

Mechanics of Overhead Sport Activities 557
General Rehabilitation Considerations 564
Rehabilitation Techniques 568
Flexibility Exercises 588
Strengthening Exercises 599
Stabilization Exercises 611
Plyometric Exercises 619
Functional Activities 624
Special Rehabilitation Applications 624
Learning Aids 639

Chapter **18 Elbow and Forearm** **645**

General Rehabilitation Considerations 646
Rehabilitation Techniques 649
Joint Mobilization 658
Flexibility Exercises 662
Strengthening Exercises 667
Functional Activities 672
Special Rehabilitation Applications 673
Learning Aids 683

Chapter **19** **Wrist and Hand** **687**

General Rehabilitation Considerations 689
Soft-Tissue Mobilization 698
Joint Mobilization 704
Flexibility Exercises 711
Strengthening Exercises 715
Plyometric Exercises 725
Functional Activities 725
Special Rehabilitation Applications 726
Learning Aids 738

Chapter **20** **Foot, Ankle, and Leg** **743**

General Rehabilitation Considerations 744
Common Structural Deformities 749
Orthotic Treatment for Foot Deformities 753
Determining Proper Footwear for Patients 758
Soft-Tissue Mobilization 763
Deep-Tissue Massage 774
Joint Mobilization 774
Flexibility Exercises 779
Strengthening Exercises 784
Proprioception Exercises 789
Functional Exercises 795
Special Rehabilitation Applications 795
Learning Aids 813

Chapter **21** **Knee and Thigh** **819**

General Rehabilitation Considerations 821
Soft-Tissue Mobilization 830
Joint Mobilization 838
Flexibility Exercises 842
Strengthening Exercises 848
Proprioception Exercises 858
Functional Exercises 859
Special Rehabilitation Applications 860
Learning Aids 884

Chapter **22** **Hip** **891**

General Rehabilitation Considerations 893
Soft-Tissue Mobilization 897

Joint Mobilization 904
Flexibility Exercises 908
Strengthening Exercises 916
Proprioception Exercises 926
Functional Exercises 926
Special Rehabilitation Applications 926
Learning Aids 936

Glossary   939
Bibliography   959
Index   975
About the Author   1005

Preface

When Dave Perrin invited me to write the first edition of this textbook, it wasn't the first time someone had broached the topic with me. It was, however, the first time I took the task to heart and decided to pursue the idea. Several years before Dave made his invitation, Pete Koehneke had approached me with the idea. At that time there was no textbook on rehabilitation of athletic injuries. By the time I began writing the first edition, there had been textbooks written or edited on the subject. Why, then, did I decide to write the book?

The answer is complex. Although several textbooks are now in print on the topic of athletic rehabilitation, prior to the publication of the first edition of *Therapeutic Exercise for Musculoskeletal Injuries* (formerly *Therapeutic Exercise for Athletic Injuries*), none satisfied the needs of the clinician beyond the technical level. Instructors across the country had repeatedly told me that they did not use a textbook because those available were either incomplete or did not meet their needs. Others had told me that they used more than one text because there was no single textbook that addressed all of their course's content. And over the past 15 years, a number of advances and revolutionary changes have occurred in how musculoskeletal injuries are rehabilitated. The advancement of surgical techniques has been accompanied by a concomitant advancement of rehabilitation techniques. The rehabilitation process is constantly evolving and becomes more sophisticated with changes in surgical techniques, equipment development, and newly acquired knowledge of human physiology.

Overall, the problem was that other textbooks available were for technicians. They addressed how to perform rehabilitation techniques, but they did not tell what occurs physiologically, why applications are important, and how treatments are effective. Rehabilitation clinicians and those who rehabilitate musculoskeletal injuries are allied health medical professionals who are obligated to understand the therapeutic exercise and rehabilitation techniques used by the individuals they treat. This textbook differs significantly from other rehabilitation textbooks because it deals with information vital to these concepts. The reader is guided through a progression of information designed to reveal the whys, hows, whens, and whats of rehabilitation and thus develop the essential building blocks to provide the clinician with the skills to safely and successfully rehabilitate injured individuals.

STRUCTURE AND ORGANIZATION OF THERAPEUTIC EXERCISE FOR MUSCULOSKELETAL INJURIES

This text is divided into four parts. Each successive part builds on the information presented in previous parts. Part I deals with the basic concepts: what is important in a therapeutic exercise program, what factors affect it, the team members involved, and the components involved. It also addresses what happens physiologically to the injury site and emotionally to the individual following an injury, physics principles, assessment techniques, and record keeping.

Part II presents specific techniques—including manual therapy, concepts involving range of motion, strength, proprioception, and functional activities—to serve as a foundation for parts III and IV. Reporting tools for findings and progressions are also discussed. These techniques are the cornerstone of the establishment, progression, and conclusion of a therapeutic exercise program for musculoskeletal injuries.

Part III contains information on general therapeutic exercise application. These chapters cover topics such as posture evaluation, gait analysis, aquatic exercises, Swiss ball and foam roller exercises, and tendinitis treatment strategies. These techniques are all used throughout a treatment program and can be applied to many different body segments. This material is used as building blocks for the last section of the book, part IV, which deals with specific application to each body segment of the techniques discussed in parts I, II, and III. Specific rehabilitation techniques and progressions are presented for each area of the body, with special attention to common problems or unique programs that a body segment requires.

TERMINOLOGY

As allied health professionals, we should be familiar with terms commonly used to identify, treat, and manage musculoskeletal injuries. Though our patients may often be athletes, industrial workers, or computer programmers, as long as a person is under medical care, that individual is considered a patient first. Therefore, individuals needing rehabilitation are referred to as *patients*. The job title of the allied health professional who provides rehabilitative care could be *certified athletic trainer, occupational therapist, physical therapist, or recreational therapist,* but since this textbook deals with rehabilitation generally and therapeutic exercises specifically, the individual who offers this treatment is referred to as a *rehabilitation clinician* or *clinician*.

Treatment is offered in a *clinic*. The clinic can be an athletic training room, an outpatient clinic, a conditioning facility, an industrial clinic; as long as the individual offering therapeutic exercise rehabilitation is an allied health professional and the individual receiving that service is a patient, the facility is a clinic.

NEW TO THIS EDITION

The second edition of *Therapeutic Exercise for Musculoskeletal Injuries* has a few updates, additions, and clarifications from the first edition. Some of the additions are minor, and others are more substantial. The minor additions include some updated perspectives and additional information on rehabilitation programs and techniques for injuries and body segments in chapters 16 through 22. One of the more substantial additions is a clarification of PNF methods in chapter 7 (see "Muscle Structure and Function"). The theory of PNF and its techniques can be confusing, so I've attempted to convert some of the language to a more simple and easy to understand version. Chapter 7 also contains a more extensive chart of manual muscle testing grading. In the first edition, I mentioned the plus and minus system of muscle grading, but didn't elaborate on their descriptions. The new table provides definitions and indications of the grade levels of where the plus and minus system is most appropriate.

I've also added an introductory section in chapter 11 (see "Posture and Body Mechanics"). Since Pilates is becoming more popular both in the sports medicine and orthopedic world and with the public, I have introduced the concepts of Pilates and provided an example as was done with the Feldenkrais Method and the Alexander Technique in the same chapter of the first edition. I have also listed sources through which the reader may obtain additional information on Pilates.

A small but important modification has been made to chapter 16, where I've explained how to instruct a patient in finding and achieving a pelvic neutral position. Probably the largest addition of this edition is also in chapter 16, in the section on the sacroiliac joint and muscle energy. Part of this expanded section includes information on how to examine an SI joint and how to interpret the findings to determine the most appropriate treatment. The new accompanying photos and tables should assist the reader in understanding this text information. With a better understanding of the SI joint and its dysfunctions, the muscle energy treatments presented in the first edition and kept intact for the second edition will carry more meaning for the reader. A more extensive inclusion of pelvic stability exercises is also included in chapter 16.

At the end of each chapter there are lab activities that utilize the information from the chapter for either practice of the techniques presented as well as problem solving activities that simulate clinical activities relative to the chapter's topic. They may be used as laboratory course exercises or as a practical review. The practical scenarios at the beginning of each chapter and the critical thinking questions at the end of each chapter remain as a learning tool for the student. The goal of these activity inserts is to assist the student in putting the chapter's information into clinical and applicable relevance. Sometimes it is difficult for an individual without prior experience to understand the applicability of a topic; these situations and questions are designed to encourage the discovery of how and why the information presented is significant.

PURPOSE OF THERAPEUTIC EXERCISE FOR MUSCULOSKELETAL INJURIES

This text is a compilation of over 30 years of experience in athletic training facilities, orthopedic and physical therapy clinics, hospitals, and sports medicine clinics, and it provides what I believe is comprehensive information on therapeutic exercise for musculoskeletal injuries. It is meant to be an educational tool for the entry-level student as well as a reference text for the practicing rehabilitation clinician. It is meant to offer established and new information and to challenge both the neophyte and experienced rehabilitation clinician to provide a new level of insight and information about therapeutic exercise and our allied health professions.

This text does *not* provide a cookbook approach to therapeutic exercise. However, it does provide the knowledge and tools you will need to develop the skills to determine what to use for each patient you encounter. It provides the instruments you will need for deciding the best course of action, the knowledge of why you are using it, what to expect when you use a technique, the dangers and advantages of applications, proper progressions, and how to apply the knowledge and techniques to specific injuries. Whereas each patient is different and responds differently to injury and treatment, it is neither fair to the patient nor realistic for you to believe that a cookbook approach would be helpful to the patient or to you as the person delivering care for that patient. The best course of action for you as a rehabilitation clinician is to provide the best therapeutic exercise program you can with your knowledge, skills, understanding, and appreciation of the whats, whys, and hows of therapeutic exercise. If you possess these attributes, you won't need or want a cookbook. This text provides you with the tools for developing your own therapeutic exercise programs for your patients. It is your responsibility to use those tools and your own imagination to provide a sound therapeutic exercise program that is fun for you and your patient.

Acknowledgments

Since the first edition's release, several instructors and students, most of whom I did not know, have spontaneously offered their enthusiasm for the text. Others have additionally provided me constructive feedback. I am truly grateful to each of them. I am particularly appreciative of all the students who have communicated with me since they are the ones for whom the book is designed. I am especially thankful to Christopher Schneider, an undergraduate student at the time of his correspondence, whose letter was simultaneously unique and gratifying.

My gratitude also extends to Tracy Beltran. She willingly volunteered to serve as model for the new photographs in this edition. Not knowing what she was getting into and the individuals with whom she had to work, she remained a professional in attitude and response and was wonderful to work with throughout the photo shoot.

Two people to whom I am indebted gave their time willingly and without hesitation when I needed their expertise: Kris Boyle-Walker, MPT, ATC; and Ingrid Provident, EdD, OTR. I am fortunate to call them friends and just as fortunate to have their expertise so willingly provided to me. Kris may laugh at my panicked calls of distress, but I remember when I used to know more than she did. The contributions of both Kris and Ingrid have made this text better than it would have otherwise been.

The Human Kinetics staff once again demonstrated expertise and friendliness that exceeded expectations. Kelly Huff is a true professional photographer, and I was fortunate to have him working with me on this second edition. Renee Thomas Pyrtel, my developmental editor, redefined patience; her guidance, and yes, patience, with me were to a degree that authors dream of. Have no doubt, she kept me on task, but the finesse with which she operated was remarkable. Loarn Robertson, acquisitions editor, reinvigorated the vision of this text and the others in the series and provided me with support, enthusiasm, and honesty throughout the project. HK should be proud of them; I know I am.

Finally, I must acknowledge my family, friends, and Duquesne University colleagues, each of whom, without their knowing it, continually serve as my pillar and inspiration. It is their generous sharing and giving of themselves that makes me a better person.

Introduction to the Athletic Training Education Series

The five textbooks of the Athletic Training Education Series—*Introduction to Athletic Training*, *Examination of Musculoskeletal Injuries* (formerly *Assessment of Athletic Injuries*), *Therapeutic Exercise for Musculoskeletal Injuries* (formerly *Therapeutic Exercise for Athletic Injuries*), *Therapeutic Modalities for Musculoskeletal Injuries* (formerly *Therapeutic Modalities for Athletic Injuries*), and *Management Strategies in Athletic Training*—were written for athletic training students and as a reference for practicing certified athletic trainers. Other allied health care professionals, such as physical therapists, physician's assistants, and occupational therapists, will also find these texts to be an invaluable resource in the prevention, examination, treatment, and rehabilitation of injuries to physically active people.

The rapidly evolving profession of athletic training necessitates a continual updating of the educational resources available to educators, students, and practitioners. The authors of the five new editions in the series have made key improvements and have added important information. *Introduction to Athletic Training* includes a revised and simplified chapter on pharmacology. A new part I in *Examination of Musculoskeletal Injuries* makes this text one of the most comprehensive presentations of the foundational techniques for each assessment tool used in injury examination. Updated information on proprioceptive neuromuscular facilitation and sacroiliac joint evaluation and treatment is included in *Therapeutic Exercise for Musculoskeletal Injuries*, and a section on Pilates has been added. In *Therapeutic Modalities for Musculoskeletal Injuries*, a new chapter on evidence-based practice has been added, and the FDA's approval of laser treatment for selected injuries has led to a new chapter on this topic. Finally, the impact of the Health Insurance Portability and Accountability Act and the appropriate medical coverage model of the National Athletic Trainers' Association (NATA) are now addressed in *Management Strategies in Athletic Training*.

The Athletic Training Education Series offers a coordinated approach to the process of preparing students for the NATA Board of Certification examination. If you are a student of athletic training, you must master the material in each of the content areas delineated in the NATA publication *Competencies in Athletic Training*. The Athletic Training Education Series addresses these competencies comprehensively and sequentially while avoiding unnecessary duplication.

The series covers the educational content areas developed by the Education Council of the National Athletic Trainers' Association for accredited curriculum development. These content areas and the texts that address each content area are as follows:

- Risk management and injury prevention (*Introduction* and *Management Strategies*)
- Pathology of injury and illnesses (*Introduction*, *Examination*, *Therapeutic Exercise*, and *Therapeutic Modalities*)
- Assessment and evaluation (*Examination* and *Therapeutic Exercise*)
- Acute care of injury and illness (*Introduction*, *Examination*, and *Management Strategies*)
- Pharmacology (*Introduction* and *Therapeutic Modalities*)
- Therapeutic exercise (*Therapeutic Exercise*)
- General medical conditions and disabilities (*Introduction* and *Examination*)
- Nutritional aspects of injury and illness (*Introduction*)
- Psychosocial intervention and referral (*Introduction*, *Therapeutic Modalities*, and *Therapeutic Exercise*)
- Health care administration (*Management Strategies*)
- Professional development and responsibilities (*Introduction* and *Management Strategies*)

The authors for this series—Craig Denegar, Susan Hillman, Peggy Houglum, Richard Ray, Ethan Saliba, Susan Saliba, Sandra Shultz, and I—are eight certified athletic trainers and physical therapists with well over a century of collective experience as clinicians, educators, and leaders in the athletic training profession. The clinical experience of the authors spans virtually every setting in which athletic trainers practice, including the high school, sports medicine clinic, college, professional sport, hospital, and industrial settings. The professional positions of the authors include undergraduate and graduate curriculum director, head athletic trainer, professor, clinic director, and researcher. The authors have chaired or served on the NATA's most important committees, including the Professional Education Committee, the Education Task Force, Education Council, Research Committee of the Research and Education Foundation, Journal Committee, Appropriate Medical Coverage for Intercollegiate Athletics Task Force, and Continuing Education Committee.

This series is the most progressive collection of texts and related instructional materials currently available to athletic training students and educators. Several elements are present in all the books in the series:

- Chapter objectives and summaries are tied to one another so that students will know and achieve their learning goals.
- Chapter-opening scenarios illustrate the importance and relevance of the chapter content.
- Cross-referencing among texts offers a complete education on the subject.
- Thorough reference lists allow for further reading and research.

To enhance instruction, each text includes an instructor guide and test bank. *Therapeutic Exercise for Musculoskeletal Injuries*, *Therapeutic Modalities for Musculoskeletal Injuries*, and *Examination of Musculoskeletal Injuries* each includes a presentation package. Presentation packages (formerly known as graphics packages) are usually in Microsoft PowerPoint format and delivered via CD-ROM. They contain selected illustrations, photos, and tables from the text. Instructors can use them to enhance lectures and demonstration sessions. Other features vary from book to book, depending on the subject matter; but all include various aids for assimilation and review of information, extensive illustrations, and material to help students apply the facts in the text to real-world situations.

Beyond the introductory text by Hillman, the order in which the books should be used is determined by the philosophy of each curriculum director. In any case, each book can stand alone so that a curriculum director does not need to revamp an entire curriculum to use one or more parts of the series.

When I entered the profession of athletic training over 25 years ago, one text—*Prevention and Care of Athletic Injuries* by Klafs and Arnheim—covered nearly all the subject matter required for passing the NATA Board of Certification examination and practice as an entry-level athletic trainer. Since that time we have witnessed an amazing expansion of the information and skills one must master to practice athletic training, along with an equally impressive growth of practice settings in which athletic trainers work. You will find these updated editions of the Athletic Training Education Series textbooks to be invaluable resources as you prepare for a career as a certified athletic trainer, and you will find them to be useful references in your professional practice.

David H. Perrin, PhD, ATC
Series Editor

Credits

Figure 1.1 Reprinted, by permission, from J.M. Binkley et al., 1999, "The Lower Extremity Functional Scale (LEFS): Scale development, measurement properties, and clinical application," *Physical Therapy* 79(4): 383.

Figure 2.4 Adapted, by permission, from W.B. Leadbetter, 1994, Soft tissue athletic injury. In *Sports injuries: Mechanisms, prevention, treatment*, edited by F.H. Fu and D.A. Stone (Baltimore: Williams & Wilkins), 765. Copyright 1994 by Lippincott Williams & Wilkins.

Table 2.9 Adapted, by permission, from J.E. Houglum, 1998, "Pharmacologic considerations in the treatment of injured athletes with nonsteroidal anti-inflammatory drugs," *Journal of Athletic Training* 33: 259–263.

Figures 3.10, 3.11, and 3.12 Adapted, by permission, from R. Groves and D.N. Camaione, 1983, *Concepts in kinesiology* (Philadelphia: W.B. Saunders).

Figure 5.1 Adapted, by permission, from S.L.-Y. Woo et al., "Connective tissue response to immobility," *Arthritis and Rheumatism* 18: 257–264.

Figures 5.2, 5.3, 5.4, 5.5, 5.6, 5.7, and 5.10 Figures from "Functional properties of collagenous tissue," by A. Viidik in *International Review of Connective Tissue Research* Volume 6, copyright © 1973 by Academic Press, reproduced by permission of the publisher.

Figure 5.8 Reprinted, by permission, D.L. Butler et al., "Biomechanics of ligaments and tendons," *Exercise and Sport Sciences Reviews* 6: 125–281.

Figure 5.9 Adapted, by permission, from N. Bogduk and L.T. Twomey, 1987, *Clinical anatomy of the lumbar spine* (New York: Churchill Livingstone).

Figure 5.11 Adapted from *Neurosciences for allied health therapies*, D. R. Brown, Copyright (1980), with permission from Elsevier.

Figure 6.15 Adapted, by permission, from D.G. Simons, J.G. Travell, and L.S. Simons, 1999, *Travell & Simons' myofascial pain and dysfunction: The trigger point manual*, Vol. 1, 2nd ed. (Baltimore: Williams & Wilkins).

Figure 6.25 Adapted, by permission, from G. Maitland, 1991, *Peripheral manipulation*, 3rd ed. (Woburn, MA: Butterworth-Heinemann).

Figures 7.7 and 7.13 Adapted, by permission, from National Strength and Conditioning Association, 2000, *Essentials of strength training and conditioning*, 2nd ed., edited by T.R. Baechle and R.W. Earle (Champaign, IL: Human Kinetics), 6 and 17.

Figure 7.14 Reprinted, by permission, from J.H. Wilmore and D.L. Costill, 1999, *Physiology of sport and exercise*, 2nd ed. (Champaign, IL: Human Kinetics), 39.

Table 7.1 Adapted, by permission, from R.M. Enoka, 1995, "Morphological features and activation patterns of motor units," *Journal of Clinical Neurophysiology* 12(6):538–559.

Figures 7.23 and 9.1 Adapted, by permission, from P.-O. Åstrand and K. Rodahl, 1986, *Textbook of work physiology*, 3rd ed. (New York: McGraw-Hill). Copyright 1986 by P.-O. Åstrand.

Figure 11.20 Reprinted, by permission, from J.K. Richardson and Z.A. Iglarsh, 1994, *Clinical orthopaedic physical therapy* (Philadelphia: Saunders).

Figure 11.22, b and c Reprinted, by permission, from J.K. Richardson and Z.A. Iglarsh, 1994, *Clinical orthopaedic physical therapy* (Philadelphia: W.B. Saunders).

Chapter 11 sidebar "An Example of the Feldenkrais Method" from *Mindful Spontaneity: Lessons in the Feldenkrais Method* by Ruthy Alon, copyright 1990. Reprinted with permission of North Atlantic Books.

Chapter 11 sidebar "An Alexander Technique Experiment" from *The Alexander Technique* by Wilfred Barlow. Copyright © 1973 by Wilfred Barlow. Reprinted by permission of Alfred A. Knopf, a Division of Random House, Inc.

Figure 12.9 Adapted, by permission, from M.P. Murray, A.B. Drought, and R.C. Kory, 1964, "Walking patterns of normal men," *Journal of Bone and Joint Surgery* 46-A:335–360, fig. 10.

Figure 12.16 Adapted, by permission, from Perry, J., *Gait analysis: Normal and pathological function*, 1992, with permission from SLACK Incorporated.

Figure 12.18 Adapted from D.E. Klopsteg and P.D. Wilson, 1954, *Human limbs and their substitutes* (New York: McGraw-Hill). Courtesy of the National Academy of Sciences, Washington, DC.

Figures 12.19 and 12.22 Adapted, by permission, from S. Ounpuu, 1994, "The biomechanics of walking and running," *Clinics in Sports Medicine* 13: 843–862.

Figure 12.20 Adapted, by permission, from K.R. Williams, 1985, "The biomechanics of running," In *Exercise and sport sciences reviews*, vol. 13, edited by R.L. Terjung (Baltimore: Williams & Wilkins), 389–441.

Figures 12.21 and 12.23 Adapted, by permission, from R.A. Mann, and J. Hagy, 1980, "Biomechanics of walking, running, and sprinting," *American Journal of Sports Medicine* 8: 345–350.

Figures 13.1, 13.2, and 13.3 From A. Bates and N. Hanson, 1996, *Aquatic exercise therapy.* (Philadelphia: W.B. Saunders).

Figure 13.4 Adapted, by permission, from R.A. Harrison, M. Hillman, and S. Bulstrode, 1992, "Loading of the lower limb when walking partially immersed: Implications for clinical practice," *Physiotherapy* 78 (3): 164–167.

Tables 15.1 and 15.2 Adapted, by permission, from S. Curwin and W.D. Stanish, 1984, *Tendinitis: Its etiology and treatment* (Lexington, MA: Heath). Courtesy of Dr. William D. Stanish, Halifax, Nova Scotia.

Figures 16.1a and 16.6a Adapted, by permission, from D.G. Simons, J.G. Travell, and L.S. Simons, 1999, *Travell & Simons' myofascial pain and dysfunction: The trigger point manual*, Vol. 1, 2nd ed. (Baltimore: Williams & Wilkins). Copyright 1999 by Lippincott Williams & Wilkins.

Figure 17.1 Reprinted, by permission, from F.W. Jobe, and B. Ling, 1986, The shoulder in sports. In *The shoulder: Surgical and non-surgical management*, 2nd ed., edited by M. Post (Philadelphia: Lippincott, Williams, and Wilkins).

Table 17.1 Adapted, by permission, from J.P. Bradley, and J.E. Tibone, 1991, "Electromyographic analysis of muscle action about the shoulder," *Clinics in Sports Medicine* 10: 789–805.

Figure 17.5 Adapted, by permission, from M. Pink, J. Perry, A.A. Browne, M.L. Scovazzo, and J. Kerrigan, 1991, "The normal shoulder during freestyle swimming. An electromyographic and cinematographic analysis of twelve muscles," *American Journal of Sports Medicine* 19: 570; 574.

Figure 19.1 Reprinted, by permission, from E.E. Fess, and C.A. Philips, 1987, *Hand splinting: Principles and methods*, 2nd ed. (St. Louis: Mosby).

Table 19.1 Adapted, by permission, from J.H. Boyes, 1970, *Bunnell's surgery of the hand* (Philadelphia: Lippincott). Copyright 1970 by Lippincott Williams & Wilkins.

Table 19.2 Reprinted, by permission, from R.B. Evans, and W.E. Burkhalter, 1986, "A study of the dynamic anatomy of extensor tendons and implications for treatment," *Journal of Hand Surgery (Am)* 11: 774–779.

Figure 19.3b Adapted, by permission, from H.E. Leinert, S. Schepel, and T. Gill, 1981, "Flexor tendon zones," *Surgical Clinics of North America* 61: 267–286.

Figure 19.4b Adapted, by permission, from American Society for Surgery of the Hand, 1983, Classifications of flexor tendon zones. In *The hand examination and diagnosis*, 2nd ed. (Philadelphia: Churchill Livingstone).

Figure 20.17 Reprinted, by permission, from C. Frey, April 1998, "Common shoe lacing patterns." Retrieved August 28, 2000 from the World Wide Web: www.wcsportsmed.com/lacing.htm. Copyright 1998 by Carol Frey, MD.

Chapter 20 side bar Patient Evaluation Form (2000) courtesy of Biomechanical Services, 1050 Central Ave., Suite D, Brea, CA 92821.

Figure 21.1 From J. Goodfellow, D.S. Hungerford, and M. Zindel, 1976, "Patellofemoral joint mechanics and pathology: 1. Functional anatomy of the patellofemoral joint," *Journal of Bone and Joint Surgery (Br)* 58: 287–290.

Figure 21.3 Adapted, by permission, from B.D. Beynnon et al., 1995, "Anterior cruciate ligament strain behavior during rehabilitation exercises in vivo," *American Journal of Sports Medicine* 23: 24–34.

Figure 21.4 Adapted, by permission, from L.A. Steinkamp, M.F. Dillingham, M.D. Markel, J.A. Hill, and K.R. Kaufman, 1993, "Biomechanical considerations in patellofemoral joint rehabilitation," *American Journal of Sports Medicine* 21: 438–444.

I

Basic Concepts

I keep six honest serving men
(They taught me all I knew)
Their names are What and Why and When
And How and Where and Who.

Rudyard Kipling, *The Elephant Child*

What, *why, when, how, where,* and *who* are questions that are continually asked in medicine. Knowing the answers to them is not always easy or even possible. Understanding them can be even more difficult. Attempting to know and understand the answers, however, is the goal of allied health professionals. Knowing and understanding these whats, whys, whens, hows, wheres, and whos of allied health define the differences between technicians and professionals.

It is one thing to merely do something, and another to understand why something is done. To be a true allied health professional, you must not only know how to perform the techniques and skills that are a part of the profession, but even more important, you must have the knowledge to appreciate why a technique or skill is used and understand the impact of their application. The challenge does not lie in applying a weight to an ankle but in knowing *why* it is done, *when* it should be done, and *what* impact this action has on the body. In a speech delivered in 1985, Diane Ravitch said, "The person who knows 'how' will always have a job. The person who knows 'why' will always be his boss." The technician knows how; the allied health professional knows why. A technician can apply the technique, but a professional knows, appreciates, and understands the technique.

To develop as a professional and gain this knowledge, appreciation, and understanding of therapeutic exercise, you must first establish a foundation. Once this foundation is established, the larger concepts of therapeutic exercise can be addressed.

The fundamentals on which therapeutic exercise is formulated include factors such as interpersonal relationships; ethical, moral, and legal considerations; principles, goals, and objectives of rehabilitation; psychological factors affecting the program progression and success; and the basic components necessary to a successful program. These factors are building blocks for therapeutic exercise and are covered in **chapter 1**. Unfortunately, they are often omitted from therapeutic exercise programs but nevertheless play important roles in the overall rehabilitation process.

In **chapter 2** you are introduced to what happens within the body when an injury occurs. Initiating an activity before healing tissue is able to tolerate the stress can be very detrimental, so understanding the healing process is vital to appreciating the impact of therapeutic exercise during healing. You must be continually aware of the timing of the healing progression during your administration of the rehabilitation program if the program is to be successful.

There are many different ways therapeutic exercises can be applied to the body. Simply changing a patient's position from sidelying to supine can significantly change the stress of an exercise and therefore the effect of that exercise. In **chapter 3** you are introduced to forces that are applied to the body and how they can be changed. Understanding basic physics principles that directly apply to a therapeutic exercise program is fundamental to establishing a sound, beneficial program for the physically active.

How do you know whether what you are doing is working? How do you judge whether your efforts are producing the desired effect? One of the most important ways to answer these questions is to assess the results of your treatments. Even before you can determine what treatment techniques you should use, you must examine the patient. In **chapter 4** the aspects and techniques of evaluation and examination that will guide your decisions for a treatment program are presented. Recording these findings is a part of the evaluation and examination process and is also addressed.

Once these foundations have been established, we can move on to other factors that are critical to a total rehabilitation program. Specifically, we explore in detail techniques and applications for therapeutic exercise. First, however, as you read through part I, think of individuals you have observed or in whose rehabilitation process you have been involved. You will begin to realize that these foundational concepts do indeed play a vital role on a daily basis for any rehabilitation clinician. An understanding and appreciation of these basic concepts is imperative if you are to create and administer a successful rehabilitation program.

Concepts of Rehabilitation

Objectives

After completing this chapter, you should be able to do the following:

1. Identify rehabilitation team members and their roles.

2. Discuss the qualities of professionalism in rehabilitation.

3. Discuss the principles, goals, and objectives of rehabilitation.

4. Describe the relationship among goals, progression, and examination.

5. Outline the importance of outcomes-based rehabilitation.

6. Outline the basic components of a therapeutic exercise program and their interrelationship.

7. Identify the stages of grief and the rehabilitation clinician's role in assisting the patient through these stages.

P am Lee had been in her first athletic training position for three weeks. She felt good about her position as assistant certified athletic trainer at the Division I university and was excited about being the athletic department's first rehabilitation coordinator. Until now, the certified athletic trainers had delivered rehabilitation to patients in a haphazard, inconsistent manner, but it was Pam's task to organize and ensure consistent, efficient, and cooperative rehabilitation programs for all the patients.

Coincidentally, the athletic department also hired a new orthopedic surgeon, Dr. Roberts, as the team physician. Dr. Roberts came to the university with extensive experience at another school where there was good communication and cooperation between the doctor's office and the athletic training staff. Pam looked forward to establishing a good relationship with Dr. Roberts.

Pam's first real challenge came early in the football season when the first-string tight end, Bob "Fastgun" Gullaver, underwent a surgical reconstruction of his anterior cruciate ligament (ACL). Bob was a promising athlete whose football future depended on good rehabilitation of the knee. Pam felt a lot of pressure and mistrust from the coaching staff, Bob's parents, and Bob himself. Pam wasn't sure whether these anxious feelings were because of the injury, the history of the department's care of these types of injuries, or her own limited experience. Pam felt the best way to gain their trust was to handle Bob's case well. Pam knew she must do a good job not only of rehabilitating Bob's knee, but also of communicating with all the people involved.

■ **Learning without thought is useless; thought without learning is dangerous.**

Confucius, *Analects*

The preceding quote by Confucius reminds us of the important relationship between education and critical judgment. A professional should think and analyze throughout the rehabilitation process. Thinking is based on knowledge and sound reasoning. The knowledge you need for making good judgments is in this book. This chapter will provide you with an understanding of the basics of rehabilitation: professional interaction with others, the goals and objectives of rehabilitation, and the components of a good rehabilitation program. Although this chapter includes varied topics, they all form the foundation for the therapeutic exercise program that a clinician provides a patient. To provide a program that works and is successful, you must understand who affects the process and what determines the patient's successful rehabilitation outcome.

THE REHABILITATION TEAM

▶ The primary rehabilitation team members are the patient, rehabilitation clinician, rehabilitation student, physician, patient's family, coach (if the patient is an athlete), and additional medical and allied health personnel. Secondary members include others who play a less significant or less direct part in the patient's rehabilitation. The rehabilitation clinician plays a central role as coordinator of the rehabilitation team.

The injured individual is part of the rehabilitation team. Without the patient, there would be no need for the team. Once the individual becomes injured that person becomes a patient who is cared for by the rehabilitation team. Physicians and allied health personnel, including rehabilitation clinicians, use common medical terminology to communicate. An individual who receives medical care is referred to as a patient. The term *patient* is used in this text when referring to the person receiving treatment and care from a clinician, physician, or other rehabilitation team member. The clinician, physician, parents, and additional medical and allied health personnel are the rest of the members of the primary team. If the patient is an athlete—as often those with musculoskeletal injuries are—then the athletic training student, parents, and coach will also be part of the team. In addition, there can be other team members who play an indirect, or secondary, role. These people do not usually affect the rehabilitation process directly but may have some impact on its ultimate result. These members may include athletic administrators, sport team members, equipment managers, orthotists, pharmacists, nutritionists, teachers, and attorneys.

Primary and Secondary Rehabilitation Team Members

Primary Team Members

- Rehabilitation clinician
- Physician
- Patient
- Orthopedist
- Podiatrist
- Ophthalmologist
- Psychologist or counselor
- Physical therapist

Additional Primary Team Members for Athletes

- Allied health student
- Parents or spouse
- Coach
- School nurse

Secondary Team Members

- Emergency medical technicians
- Orthotist
- Pharmacist
- Kinesiologist
- Exercise physiologist
- Nutritionist
- Attorney
- Supervisor
- Peers

Secondary Team Members for Athletes

- Sport team members
- Equipment manager
- Teachers
- Athletic administrator

Rehabilitation clinician

A rehabilitation clinician is a medical professional who rehabilitates musculoskeletal injuries. In the course of a day's work, the clinician may wear several hats. When dealing with patients who require rehabilitation before returning to full participation in physical activity or sports, the clinician wears the hat of a rehabilitation clinician. This role is different from the role played during the immediate care and treatment of musculoskeletal injuries at the time of their occurrence. As we will discuss, the rehabilitation clinician role requires many professional and interpersonal skills.

At the center of the rehabilitation team, regardless of who or how many people make up the team, is the rehabilitation clinician. As the individual who has daily contact with the patient and often is the only one who has contact with all the other involved parties, the clinician is the coordinator and leader of the rehabilitation team.

Interpersonal Skills

As a vital rehabilitation team member, the rehabilitation clinician must possess good interpersonal skills. Besides being dedicated to the rehabilitation process, the clinician must be competent and energetic, for the rehabilitation process can be very challenging and lengthy. The rehabilitation clinician's interest in the program and empathy for what the patient is enduring has a profound impact on the patient. The rehabilitation clinician must act professionally toward all rehabilitation team members. Your consideration, respect for others, confidence, honesty, and sincerity inspire the patient to comply with the rehabilitation program you provide and reassure parents, physicians, and other team members that you possess the knowledge, ability, and skill required to be the coordinator for their rehabilitation team.

Additional information on management and interaction with others can be found in *Management Strategies in Athletic Training, Third Edition* (Ray 2005).

The rehabilitation clinician also needs good active listening skills. Being an active listener means being involved in the conversation, participating appropriately, and understanding what the other person is saying. These qualities can be reflected by simply paraphrasing to the other person what he or she has just said. This technique imparts to the other person that you are listening and also helps you to understand clearly what is being said.

Record Keeping

One role of the rehabilitation clinician is to keep accurate records regarding the injury, evaluation, rehabilitation treatment, and response to treatment. Summaries, written or verbal, are communicated to the physician. Record keeping is a part of the process until the patient returns to competition or normal activity. Record keeping is discussed in more detail in chapter 4.

Educating Others

As rehab team coordinator, educating the patient, family members, and coach or employer is an important task of the rehabilitation clinician. Understanding the injury, the healing process, and the expected rehabilitation response is important to these individuals. Education prepares the patient for the rehabilitation procedure and prevents surprises. If the patient knows what to expect, he or she has less fear and will be more compliant with the rehabilitation program. Family members' fears are calmed with education. If family members are informed, they are also more willing and able to assist the clinician in helping the patient achieve a successful rehabilitation outcome. Finally, educating the coach provides the coach with a better understanding of what the patient is going through and an appreciation of the time it may take to complete the rehabilitation process.

Allied Health Students

Allied health students are in the unique position of acting as the rehabilitation specialist for a patient but not having the independence of a certified clinician. They operate under the guidance of their approved clinical instructor (ACI). They must be aware of their own limitations and not hesitate to consult the clinician whenever they feel they need advice or assistance.

Physician

As the medical chief of the team, the physician diagnoses the patient's injury, determines the course of treatment, oversees the rehabilitation program, and determines when the patient is ready to resume sports participation or normal activity. The physician and rehabilitation clinician must cooperate and have respect for and confidence in one another. Each should understand the other's role and appreciate the importance of good communication for a successful rehabilitation outcome.

Efforts to plan ahead, communicate, and work together to establish protocols and systems of rehabilitation treatment help to minimize conflicts. It is important for physicians and rehabilitation clinicians to know and understand each other's rehabilitation philosophies and preferred methods of treatment before a rehab program begins. It is not unusual for rehabilitation clinicians and physicians to differ in their perspectives, but it is important for them to reach an understanding and develop a common ground so that they can respect their differences and work with each other in achieving what they both ultimately want: the successful rehabilitation of a patient's injuries.

It is the responsibility of the physician to educate the rehabilitation staff, patient, and family members as the need arises. Communication is the key for everyone to have a good understanding of the injury and the recovery course to be taken.

Family

Family members are important rehabilitation team members. When a patient lives at home, the family members play a vital role because they can assist the patient in complying with the home rehabilitation program. If you are dealing with an athlete at the collegiate level, the patient may not live at home, so family members have a less significant role in assisting with compliance, but they are frequently involved with more serious injuries. More often than not, the rehabilitation clinician maintains the most frequent contact with the family.

Coach/Supervisor

Dealing with a coach obviously only applies if the patient is an athlete. If the patient is an employee, the supervisor takes on the role of "coach." But as a coworker of the clinician, the coach relies on the clinician for information on the current status of the injured athlete. The coach plays an important role on the rehabilitation team regarding the injured athlete's restrictions on participation in practice and competition, through communication with the rehabilitation clinician. If participation is restricted, the coach can help the injured individual continue to feel he or she is part of the team by including the patient in practices, team meetings, and strategy sessions and having the patient assist with sideline activities.

Patient

The patient should inform the rehabilitation clinician of any injury he or she sustains and seek treatment as soon as possible following injury. Delay in treatment can often mean needless prolongation of an injury and can retard or prevent the individual's return to full function.

When an injury occurs, it is important that the patient maintain good nutrition to enhance the healing process. Patients must take responsibility for their rehabilitation program's success by adhering to the recommendations of the physician and rehabilitation clinician. Performing the home treatment regimen provided by the clinician is crucial to the overall success of the rehabilitation program.

Other Team Members

Occasionally, other medical and paramedical professionals are included on the rehabilitation team. They are often called on as consultants by the primary or team physician when their special expertise is indicated to enhance the rehabilitation process. Examples of some ancillary team members include podiatrists, orthopedists, ophthalmologists, psychologists, physical therapists, and emergency medical technicians. Rehabilitation techniques that have been used to treat the patient, peers, the plan for care, and the response to treatment may be among the information that is conveyed by the rehabilitation clinician to the consulting medical professional.

Other peripheral team members may include attorneys, school administrators, sports teammates, and other nonmedical team members. Which of these team members is involved varies according to the specific situation and circumstances. Attorneys may be involved in cases of negligence; school administrators may be active in a variety of situations, such as when rules and regulations require reassessment or when there is a conflict among involved parties; sports teammates or peers can play an important support role for the patient. The level of involvement of these team members varies greatly. When these team members do play a role, the rehabilitation clinician should be aware of this and interact with them appropriately.

INTERACTING WITH TEAM MEMBERS

▶ Courteous, professional, accurate, and appropriate communication among all rehabilitation team members is essential for a successful rehabilitation program.

Now that you have an awareness of the roles of each of the rehabilitation team members, the importance of good interaction among these members becomes apparent. Also apparent is why the rehabilitation clinician is the coordinator for this team. The rehabilitation clinician is easily accessed by the other team members, has daily contact with the patient, has a good understanding of the injury and the healing process, guides the patient along in the rehabilitation program, sees the response to treatment, and knows the expected progression of rehabilitation.

The rehabilitation clinician is the center of the communication process. The clinician communicates with the patient, the parents or spouse, the coach or supervisor, the physician, the ancillary medical personnel, and the specialists. Each of these rehabilitation team members may speak with another, but the clinician has contact with all of them.

With this position comes responsibility. The rehabilitation clinician must be sure any information conveyed is accurate and not a guess. Saying "I don't know" generates more respect than guessing the correct response. "I don't know" accompanied by "but I'll find out and get back to you" is even more appreciated.

Communicating With the Patient

Being responsible in communication also means knowing when to say something, when to withhold information, and how to communicate effectively and appropriately. When an patient has just been injured and feels distraught, it is not the time to explain in detail the process that will occur during rehabilitation. Using big words and medical terminology is not practical when speaking with most patients or family members, especially if they are upset. In a good situation a person normally does not absorb more than seven new items of information. In a stressful situation the ability to understand or retain unfamiliar information is even less. Using good judgment about what to say and when to say it is a skill that is developed with practice by having sensitivity and observing others who are good at it. Be patient with yourself as you develop this skill. Contemplate what you will say before you say it, and put yourself in the place of the patient or family member with whom you are talking. Ask yourself how you would like to be addressed at that time, what information you would want or be able to comprehend without any medical knowledge, and then proceed to listen and observe that person's responses as carefully as you listen to your own words to him or her.

You should communicate with the patient with sincere compassion, understanding of the individual situation, and confidence in your own knowledge of injuries and rehabilitation. It is important to instill in the patient confidence in your ability to treat the injury. This is done by providing the patient with the information he or she seeks about the extent of the injury, the time it will take to heal, and the treatment plan. As mentioned, not all of this information should be provided at once or at the time of injury. Your best judgment about when to provide this information is important in establishing confidence and trust.

Communicating With the Physician

You should not hesitate to contact the physician regarding the patient's injury or response to treatment. Communication between the rehabilitation clinician and the physician is important to the outcome of rehabilitation. Both must be aware of the seriousness and extent of the injury, the patient's response to the injury and treatment, and his or her compliance with the rehabilitation program. Both must also agree with the treatment course and appreciate and respect each other's contributions to the rehabilitation process. This is accomplished by communicating and establishing a rapport with each other. Rehabilitation clinicians communicate with physicians by telephone, through e-mail, in person, and through written reports. Telephone and face-to-face, informal conversations are ways to understand general philosophies and develop rapport. Written and verbal patient reports are also vital to an ongoing professional relationship between the physician and the rehabilitation clinician.

Communicating With Family Members

Depending on the situation, communication with the patient's family varies considerably. At the high school level, parents commonly are intimately involved with the injured youth's recovery process from the start. Communicating with family members at the time of injury is important because it is an opportunity for the rehabilitation clinician to establish a rapport with the family if one has not been established already. It also will reassure parents and calm their fears about serious or lasting results of their son's or daughter's injury. When a patient lives at home, you can inform his or her parents or spouse of home activities that can expedite the rehabilitation program.

When the patient does not live at home, family members do not play as important a role in the rehabilitation program. Occasionally, however, when the patient's injury is more serious and the rehabilitation process is longer and more complicated, family involvement may be more direct. For example, if the patient is to have surgery, he or she may choose to go home for the surgery or following surgery. In other situations—with an injured collegiate athlete, for example—patients may return home at the end of the school year when their rehab program is not yet concluded. In these situations the family may be requested to assist with the rehabilitation program or consult with a local facility to continue the rehabilitation process you have started.

Communicating With the Coach/Supervisor

When a coach or supervisor has confidence and trust in the rehabilitation clinician, cooperation in restricting the patient's workouts is more likely. Impressing upon the coach or supervisor the extent of the patient's injury, the limitations placed on the injured part, and the importance of his or her involvement in the rehabilitation process helps to ensure the success of the rehabilitation program.

Communicating With Secondary Team Members

When a patient is referred to other medical specialists, input from the rehabilitation clinician is appreciated. It provides the specialist with information regarding the patient's injury in the event that the rehabilitation clinician has witnessed the injury. It also provides the specialist with insight regarding the rehabilitation program thus far and the patient's responses to it. The rehabilitation clinician can also assist in and compliment the specialist's course of treatment.

Like all primary rehabilitation team members, secondary team members' communication with other team members should be honest, constructive, and professional. The ultimate goal of all team members should be to assist in whatever way appropriate for their position within the team to provide the patient with satisfactory and successful rehabilitation. Acting responsibly by performing their roles unselfishly, appropriately, and cooperatively ensures that this goal is achieved.

Cautions On Communication

With the recent advance of the Health Insurance Portability Accountability Act (HIPAA), the rehabilitation clinician is under legal obligation when it comes to what information regarding a patient's injury can be provided to whom. An initial segment of HIPAA requirements was instituted in 2003. The regulation impacts several aspects of health care, including the right to privacy regarding health, illness, and injury. Not all rehabilitation clinicians are directly affected by this law; the extent to which it affects communication depends on the type of health care environment of the facility and whether billing is involved. I recommend you seek additional information in the Richard Ray text, *Management Strategies in Athletic Training*, third edition (2005). The government Web site regarding HIPAA is <http://www.hhs.gov/ocr/hipaa/>. Specific information, requirements, and regulations can be found at that Web site.

QUALITIES OF PROFESSIONALISM

Being a professional means looking and acting like one. A true professional gives something back to the profession by being an active member of professional associations and organizations (for example, the National Athletic Trainers' Association or NATA), and making a positive contribution.

Being a professional also means adhering to the legal standards determined by the state's regulating body and if applicable to you, complying with the ethical standards established by your professional organization. Awareness of these professional standards is the responsibility of every individual who considers himself or herself a rehabilitation clinician.

▶ Rehabilitation clinicians demonstrate their professionalism by maintaining a professional appearance and demeanor, continuing their education within the profession, contributing to the profession by being active in professional associations and organizations, and adhering to legal and ethical standards.

Using your knowledge to provide the patient with the best care possible is an undisputed precept of the profession. This means taking the responsibility to learn current information and practices in the profession and delivering only the care you feel confident in providing.

The years you spend in college to attain a degree and become a rehabilitation clinician provide you with a base upon which you will mold your career within the profession. There are more specialized techniques, more complicated information, and more sophisticated treatment application methods that will become available to you as you continue beyond your entry-level education in rehabilitation. Attending postgraduate seminars, participating in professional meetings, and reading professional publications to learn current information regarding rehabilitation and other topics within the profession are means by which professionals keep up to date.

It is your responsibility to yourself and to the patients you treat to be aware of the new and ever-evolving methods of treatment and rehabilitation. Medical science is continually advancing, and research is continually being conducted around the world to lead us to better understanding of treatment methods. As a professional, you have an ethical and moral responsibility to provide the best care you can to a patient. Participating in different types of continuing education to optimize your allied health knowledge, techniques, and skills is an important aspect of fulfilling that responsibility.

Treating the patient with concern, respect, and a consistently professional attitude is vital. This attitude establishes the patient's confidence in your ability to give quality care and guide the patient to a successful rehabilitation outcome.

Looking Like a Professional

Dressing appropriately and being neatly groomed when working as a rehabilitation clinician reflect not only your attitude toward yourself, but also your pride in being an allied health professional. If you dress professionally and are neat, clean, and well groomed, you present an appearance that encourages confidence and respect from others. If you are to be taken seriously, you should look like a professional.

Acting Like a Professional

Showing respect and consideration for others, colleagues or patients, is part of acting like a professional. Acting professionally also involves being sensitive to the privacy of the patients you treat. Privacy is important when taking a patient's medical history or exposing a body part in the clinic. Acting professionally means being morally and legally responsible and conducting yourself in a manner that reflects well on your medical profession.

Qualities of Professionalism

- Looking professional
- Acting professionally
- Being professional

Being a Professional

Being a professional goes beyond looking and acting like one. A true professional also attends professional meetings and becomes active in professional associations. The needs of professionals are met through the profession's association. The association's needs are met through the active participation of its members. It should be the professional responsibility of each clinician to contribute at the local, state, regional, district, or national level to make the association effective and provide vitality to the profession. A professional cannot stand alone, and a profession needs the energy and dedication of its members to play a viable and convincing role in the medical arena today.

The certified athletic trainers' professional association is NATA. If you plan to work with athletes and are not yet a member, I encourage you to ask your athletic training curriculum program director for information regarding student membership in NATA or to contact the NATA office directly to obtain a student membership application.

NATA National Contact Information

Phone: 800-TRY-NATA
Fax: 214-637-2206
Membership e-mail: NataMIS@aol.com
Web site: http://www.nata.org

Ethical and Legal Standards

As allied health professionals, rehabilitation clinicians have a responsibility to themselves, to their profession, to their employers, and to the patients they rehabilitate to act in a consistently professional manner, including following ethical and legal guidelines.

In today's medical environment the legal aspects of athletic training have become more important than in years past. Ethics, however, has always been an important part of this profession. NATA scripted its *Code of Ethics* in its very early days. The founders of NATA realized the importance of providing guidelines for standards of behavior and ensuring high-quality, principled care for patients by certified athletic trainers. The NATA *Code of Ethics* has since been revised to keep in stride with current issues, but the primary precepts have remained the same. Even if you do not work with or do not plan to work with patients, I suggest that you obtain a copy of this document and familiarize yourself with it.

Ethics Guideline Resource

Code of Ethics
National Athletic Trainers' Association
2952 Stemmons Freeway
Dallas, TX 75247

Some of the topics presented here lie in the legal arena, some in the ethical arena, and some in both. These subjects are important enough in the rehabilitation of patients that you should spend a little time understanding them.

State Regulations

Each state has different legal guidelines. The majority of states now have some type of regulation in the form of licensure, certification, registration, or exemption that determines the legal parameters within which a rehabilitation clinician must operate. It is your responsibility to know and operate within the regulations of the state in which you practice.

Consent

Rehabilitation clinicians use their professional skills, knowledge, and best judgment to decide the course of rehabilitation for a patient. Sometimes the patient may not wish to follow the course of treatment that the clinician has proposed. The patient may refuse to perform a specific activity. Although you may attempt to convince the patient that the activity is appropriate for a variety of reasons, you must remember that if the patient refuses to perform the activity you request, you cannot force the patient to do it. For example, if a gymnast who suffered an ankle sprain refuses to do the non-weight-bearing pool therapy that you recommend, you would probably attempt to make her understand why you want her to go into the water. Regardless of the reasons, if she continues to refuse, you cannot force her into the pool. It is up to you to find an alternative program for her. Likewise, if you want a basketball player with a subluxating shoulder to start doing medicine-ball work, but he refuses because he lacks confidence that his shoulder could tolerate the exercise, the same policy would apply. You would attempt to explain why this is an important activity and reassure him that you would not have him do it until you thought the shoulder was ready. If he still refuses, you must use a different type of exercise that would be less threatening to him yet still accomplish the same goal. You can attempt to reintroduce the activity later in the program, once the patient's confidence has improved and he is less likely to object.

In other words, the patient always has the last say on what is or is not done with his or her body. The patient gives consent for treatment by performing what is requested during the rehabilitation program, but the patient always has the right to say no. The patient's consent is assumed to be given in the treatment process until it is taken away. As a rehabilitation clinician, you must always respect the patient's right to consent to or refuse treatment. Generally, your knowledge, skill, and past experiences with the patient give the patient the confidence and trust in you to ultimately comply with your rehabilitation procedures. Occasionally, however, perhaps because the patient lacks confidence in himself or herself, has too much pain, or does not feel comfortable with the activity, he or she refuses to perform it. In those cases, you must respect the patient's refusal and remember that, even though you may disagree, it is the patient who has the final control. Your best defense against this situation is to possess the knowledge to create an appropriate rehabilitation program, self-confidence in your knowledge and mastery as an allied health professional, and an ability to create the same confidence in your patients.

Touch

Rehabilitation is a touching profession. We palpate injuries on a daily basis, feel for spasm and temperature, and touch painful and swollen areas routinely. For this reason, touch becomes something we often do not think about, but we must be continually sensitive to the patient's perception of our touch.

Touching a patient should always be purposeful, with a specific reason and goal in mind. For example, if you touch the thigh of a patient who has received a contusion to the quadriceps, the pressure applied and area palpated should be appropriate.

Touching is an integral and necessary part of a rehabilitation clinician's duties, but you must be acutely aware that a patient may not be accustomed to the intimacy of touch in this context. Presenting yourself in a professional manner, being deliberate in how you touch, demonstrating respect for the patient, and having sensitivity for the patient's situation help to reassure the patient and permit you to perform your tasks appropriately.

If you are unsure of how a patient will respond to your touch, it is best to have another professional present. In today's litigious environment, touch—even when it is purely professional and necessary—can be questioned. If you work with athletes, you will find that most injured athletes are treated in an athletic training clinic where other people are around. However, if you find yourself in an isolated situation or when you feel that questions may potentially arise later, you should take precautions, such as having another professional or someone else present, keeping the treatment room door open, or providing the treatment in a common room where others are present. It is often wise to listen to your instincts; if you have an uneasy feeling about a situation, be cautious.

COMPONENTS OF A REHABILITATION PROGRAM

▶ A rehabilitation program should be designed with seven essential principles, two main objectives, and individual long- and short-term goals in mind. The overall program and individual exercises should progress safely and effectively. Rehabilitation clinicians should know how to assess the patient's status and evaluate the program's outcomes.

This section deals with the general principles, objectives, and goals of an musculoskeletal rehabilitation program. An overview of the components of a rehabilitation program is presented. We also take a brief look at assessing the patient's status, evaluating program progression, and measuring the outcomes of the program.

Rehabilitation Principles, Objectives, and Goals

The principles of rehabilitation are used to achieve the goals and objectives of a therapeutic exercise program. The ultimate design of each therapeutic exercise program is based on these principles, goals, and objectives of rehabilitation. The principles and objectives are constants in a therapeutic exercise program. The goals are established for each individual patient in each situation.

Principles

There are seven principles of rehabilitation. Principles are the foundation upon which rehabilitation is based. This mnemonic may assist you in remembering the principles of rehabilitation: ATC IS IT.

Principles of Rehabilitation

Avoid aggravation
Timing
Compliance
Individualization
Specific sequencing
Intensity
Total patient

A: Avoid Aggravation

It is important not to aggravate the injury during the rehabilitation process. Therapeutic exercise, if administered incorrectly or without good judgment, has the potential to make the injury worse. A prime rule was put forth by Hippocrates when he said, "As to diseases, make a habit of two things: to help, or at least to do no harm." This precaution serves rehabilitation clinicians as well.

Rehabilitating the injured individual in a continually progressive manner without aggravating the injury is a primary concern throughout the therapeutic exercise program. Knowledge of how the body responds to injury, aptitude in determining which exercises to use, good judgment in deciding when the program should progress, and skill in observing the patient's response are needed to recognize when and how far to advance the therapeutic exercise program without aggravating the injury.

T: Timing

The therapeutic exercise portion of the rehabilitation program should begin as soon as possible without aggravating the injury. The sooner the patient can begin the exercise portion of the rehabilitation program, the sooner he or she can return to full activity. Following injury, rest is sometimes necessary. Studies have demonstrated, however, that too much rest is actually detrimental to recovery. Appell (1990) reported the significance of inactivity when he estimated that during the first week of immobilization, 3% to 4% of an individual's strength is lost each day. This strength is not recovered in the equivalent amount of time, but takes much longer (Staron et al. 1991). In chapter 2 we investigate the deleterious effects of prolonged rest and immobilization.

Some studies indicate that the rate of recovery is much slower than the rate at which strength is lost. This finding emphasizes the importance of beginning a therapeutic exercise program as soon as is safely possible. The longer the initiation of therapeutic exercises is delayed, the longer the recovery process will take. For example, if a patient is out for two days with an injury, it may take a week for full recovery to occur. If a patient is put on rest for four days, it may take perhaps as long as three weeks to return to normal activity or competition.

C: Compliance

Without a compliant patient, the rehabilitation program will not be successful. To ensure compliance, it is important to inform the patient of the content of the program and the expected course of rehabilitation. The patient will be more compliant when he or she is better aware of the program to be followed, the work he or she will have to do, and what the whole rehabilitation process entails.

Often an injured individual feels powerless after suffering an injury. That feeling of powerlessness can prevent a successful return to sport participation or normal activity. Knowledge empowers the patient. Empowerment engenders compliance. Compliance leads to success.

Compliance includes several elements. Compliance means that the program is carried out consistently, allowing progressive recovery and improvement. Compliance means that the patient performs whatever exercises or tasks the rehabilitation clinician has instructed the patient to perform outside of the clinic. Compliance means that the patient attends treatment sessions consistently and during those sessions performs whatever activities are included in the program to the best of his or her ability.

I: Individualization

Each person responds differently to an injury and to the subsequent rehabilitation program. Expecting a patient to progress in a program the same way as the last patient you had with a similar injury will prove to be frustrating for both you and the patient. It is no more realistic to compare one patient to another than it is for a parent to compare one child to its sibling. It is first necessary to recognize that each person is different. It is also important to realize that even though an injury may seem the same in type and severity as another, undetectable differences can change an individual's response to the injury. Individual physiological and chemical differences profoundly affect a patient's specific responses to an injury. Several other nonphysical variables can influence the recovery of the patient, including the outside support the patient has from friends, teammates, and family; the patient's psychological makeup and response to the injury; the degree and types of outside pressures the patient may feel to return to competition; and the goals and rewards the patient may want to achieve.

It is your responsibility to understand that these differences exist, be aware of the patient's responses to the injury and rehabilitation program, and design the therapeutic exercise program accordingly to guide the patient through the rehabilitation program as effectively, safely, and efficiently as you can.

S: Specific Sequencing

A specific sequence of events should be followed in a therapeutic exercise program. This specific sequence is determined by the body's physiological healing response. This topic is covered later in this chapter in the section "Basic Components of Therapeutic Exercise."

I: Intensity

The intensity level of the therapeutic exercise program must challenge the patient and the injured area, but at the same time the intensity must not aggravate the injury. Knowing when to increase intensity without overtaxing the injury requires observation of the patient's response and knowledge of the healing process. The healing process is covered in chapter 2.

For you to use the correct exercise intensity in the therapeutic exercise program, knowledge of the progression of exercises and the amount of stress that each exercise imposes is also important. Along with this knowledge, you should have an imagination. This is important because if an exercise is too severe or too easy for the patient to perform, modifying it can permit the right intensity for the patient to progress appropriately. Sometimes all it takes is a slight modification, and other times the modification is more complex. For example, if a patient finds it easy to balance on one leg, having the patient perform the same activity on an unstable surface such as a mini-trampoline makes it more difficult. If doing this exercise on the floor is too easy but doing it on the trampoline is too difficult, you can have the patient perform the exercise on the floor but with eyes closed. Using your imagination and resourcefulness is especially vital if you have a limited equipment budget.

If you combine your knowledge and imagination, you can design a therapeutic exercise program that is challenging and provides the correct intensity level for achieving the goals that have been established. Being imaginative also makes the therapeutic exercise program more interesting for both you and the patient. Making the program interesting enhances the patient's desire to comply and therefore increases the likelihood of a successful outcome.

T: Total Patient

You must consider the total patient in the rehabilitation process. It is important for the injured person to stay finely tuned in the unaffected areas of his or her body. This means keeping the cardiovascular system at a pre-injury level and maintaining range of motion, strength, coordination, and muscle endurance of the uninjured limbs and joints. When a patient is injured, the whole body must be the focus of the rehabilitation program, not just the injured area. Remembering that the total patient must be ready for return to normal activity or competition and providing the patient with a program to keep the uninvolved areas in peak condition, not just rehabilitating the injured area, better prepares the patient physically and psychologically when the injured area is completely rehabilitated.

Objectives

There are two basic objectives for any therapeutic exercise program. The first is related directly to the principle just discussed of treating the total patient. This objective is to prevent deconditioning of uninjured areas. The second objective is to rehabilitate the injured part in a safe, efficient, and effective manner.

Prevent Deconditioning

Preventing deconditioning includes providing exercises for the cardiovascular system, the uninvolved areas of the injured extremity or segment, and the uninvolved extremities. For example, if the patient has a knee injury preventing weight bearing on that leg, the patient can maintain cardiovascular conditioning by performing pool exercises or working out on an upper-body ergometer. The patient can also maintain good strength and range of motion of the trunk, upper body, and uninvolved lower extremity by using weights and other exercises for these segments. Exercises for the involved extremity's hip and ankle can also be used to prevent deconditioning of those areas without applying undue stress to the injured knee.

Similarly, another patient who has suffered a left shoulder injury can exercise the left elbow, wrist, and hand. Even after surgery and immobilization a patient may be able to perform some wrist and hand exercises to help maintain that part's strength and range of motion.

Because of the nature of the injury or the medical restrictions involved, it may sometimes take some imagination on your part to develop exercises that challenge the uninjured parts while not harming the injured area, but it is important for you to design programs with the objective of maintaining current conditioning levels as much as possible.

Rehabilitate the Injured Part

Good knowledge of the injury, healing process, and methods of rehabilitation is paramount in achieving the objective of rehabilitating the injured part. You must use good judgment along with this knowledge to enable the patient to progress safely and effectively through the therapeutic exercise program.

Therapeutic exercise can be used effectively to enhance and promote recovery, but it can also be harmful and ineffective if used incorrectly. It is your responsibility to know the appropriate use of this highly effective yet potentially dangerous therapy.

Rehabilitation Objectives

1. Prevent deconditioning.

2. Rehabilitate the injured part.

Goals

Goals are results one strives to achieve. In therapeutic exercise the ultimate goal is the return of the patient to his or her former activity. That return, however, should be safe yet quick, effective yet efficient, and pursued in an aggressive yet guarded manner. This means that you must work diligently with all the tools available to you to enhance the healing of the injury, restore the deficient parameters that have been lost because of the injury, and regain the patient's self-confidence to permit him or her to return with at least the same level of competence as before the injury. This is done in the minimum amount of time that allows the healing process to occur and also provides enough time to rehabilitate the injured area without undue time lost away from the sport or activity.

There is often a fine line between going too slowly and advancing too quickly. The program should stress the patient just enough to provide gains, not losses, with regular progression. The following image might help you to grasp this concept: Each day it is your responsibility to push the patient up a hill to its peak (applying enough stress to gain as much as possible in an exercise session) without pushing so far that the patient goes over the top and down the other side (applying so much stress that it causes deleterious effects).

Objective and Measurable Goals

Goals should be objective and measurable whenever possible. Goals are occasionally subjective; for example, pain is subjective. However, some objectivity is possible in measuring pain by asking the patient to rate his or her pain on a 10-point scale. Other parameters such as girth, range of motion, and strength can be measured as objective and more concrete goals.

It is necessary to record these measurements at various stages in the therapeutic exercise program, most obviously at the beginning and conclusion of the program. Throughout the program, the patient is reassessed routinely as well. Any changes should be recorded. This is important in assisting you and the patient to identify improvements. This record can also help you more easily notice when changes do not occur as frequently as expected and decide what specific modifications are needed in the program.

Short- and Long-Term Goals

When an injury is severe enough to restrict sport participation or normal activity for at least a month, both long-term and short-term goals should be set. A long-term goal is the final, desired outcome of a therapeutic exercise program. For example, returning the patient to a former level of athletic competition would be a long-term goal. Specifically, this involves returning the patient to normal levels of all parameters that allow full return to sport participation, including flexibility, strength, endurance, coordination, and skill execution. Definitive levels of these parameters are different for each patient and depend on the patient's sport, specific position, age, skill level, and level of participation. These parameters are discussed in more detail later in this chapter in the section "Basic Components of Therapeutic Exercise."

Short-term goals provide both you and the patient with objective aims to guide you toward the long-term goals. Both short-term and long-term goals are specific as to objective measures of what is to be accomplished by the patient within what time frame, and under what conditions. Short-term goals are established weekly or biweekly and depend on the patient's response to the injury and ability to progress, the stage of the rehabilitation process, and the severity of the injury. A short-term goal may be to reduce edema by 1 cm and increase range of motion by 15° in one week. Other short-term goals may be to increase strength by half a grade (the scoring system for muscle strength is discussed in chapter 7), reduce pain to 3 on a scale of 0 to 10, and ambulate with one crutch in 5 days.

Short-term goals are important because they give the patient something concrete to work toward and the psychological boost to achieve them. Looking at long-term goals can be overwhelming, but focusing on short-term goals gives the patient direction and establishes a logical progression for the rehabilitation process.

Short-term goals should be reasonable and attainable yet challenging for the patient. They should be realistic to allow the patient to achieve them within the time established without irritating the injury or frustrating the patient. Establishing realistic goals takes skill, knowledge, practice, and judgment on your part. You must also be aware of additional factors that may affect the patient's ability to achieve these goals, such as the patient's personality and how he or she responds to injury, challenges, and discipline; outside pressures such as from income or scholarships, family, supervisor or coach, and friends; the patient's other activities, including recreational activities, work, and school; the severity, type, and healing process of the injury; and the level of dysfunction involved.

Sample Goals

These are examples of long- and short-term goals that could be set for a patient with a shoulder injury.

Long-term goal:
The patient will have full strength in all rotator cuff muscles at the conclusion of the rehabilitation program.

Short-term goal:
Two weeks from today's treatment session, the patient will have 4/5 strength in the subscapularis, 3+/5 strength in the teres minor and infraspinatus, and 3/5 strength in the supraspinatus (using the scoring system discussed in chapter 7 in which 5 = full strength and 0 = complete loss of voluntary contraction).

An alternate short-term goal:
Two weeks from today's treatment session, the patient will increase strength in each rotator cuff muscle by 1/2 grade from today's evaluation scores.

All injuries involve precautions and contraindications. Complications can occur regardless of the quality of care provided. You must establish goals and place demands on the patient with these factors in mind.

Examination and Assessment

Rehabilitation clinicians continually examine and assess injuries, from the time the injury occurs to the time the patient is ready to return to sport participation or normal activity. Therapeutic exercise programs are one area in which clinicians make frequent assessments.

The only way to establish goals is to examine the patient and make an assessment of the patient's current condition. How much swelling is present? How much range of motion is lost? What is the status of the injured area's strength? These and other questions are assessed on the first day of rehabilitation. They are also reexamined regularly throughout the rehabilitation treatment.

To create short- and long-term goals, you must first establish the current status of the deficient parameters. Then you decide what realistic short-term goals the patient can achieve in a specific amount of time. Once those goals are achieved, you once again perform an examination and make an assessment to decide new and appropriate short-term goals.

You must continually examine and assess the patient's condition to provide the patient with an accurate therapeutic exercise program with appropriate goals. Since examination is performed frequently and throughout the rehab process, it will be covered in more depth in chapter 4.

Progression

A good therapeutic exercise program progresses in a challenging yet safe manner. Accurate examination and assessment of the patient's response to the exercises and treatment is necessary for this to occur. The progression should be in accordance with the severity of the injury, the type of injury, and the patient's response to the injury and treatment. A good progression challenges the patient without causing deleterious effects such as increased pain or swelling or decreased ability to perform.

Exercise Progression

One aspect of progression is the type of exercise. For example, a strength progression may advance from isometrics to isotonics to isokinetics to plyometrics. The patient begins with a level that is challenging but not irritating to the injury, which is determined, in part, by the severity of the injury and the rehabilitation clinician's assessment of the patient's current ability. A patient with a mild ankle sprain who is ambulating without crutches may be able to forgo isometrics and begin isotonic and weight-bearing resistive exercises. However, a patient with profound swelling who is on crutches may be able to tolerate only non-weight-bearing range-of-motion and isometric exercises.

Program Progression

Another level of progression involves the program itself: A program should be designed to emphasize different types of goals as it progresses. Keep in mind that you cannot expect a patient to perform advanced skill drills before flexibility and strength have been achieved, and that full strength cannot be achieved until flexibility is restored. This is discussed in the section "Basic Components of Therapeutic Exercise" later in this chapter.

Outcomes-Based Rehabilitation

Today's buzz word in medicine is *outcomes*. Outcomes are important to the understanding, use, and justification of programs used to treat patients. The outcome of a treatment program is often assessed using a tool that has been devised for measuring the patient's response and satisfaction following a treatment that is given for a specific injury or condition. The outcome tool is most often a questionnaire that is given before the start of the program, sometime during its course, and at its conclusion. Questions often relate to the patient's condition before and after treatment and to the patient's perception of different aspects of the treatment, including quality of care, professional attitudes, and effectiveness of the program in achieving goals. Input from the clinician providing the treatment program is also obtained. Final results are then compiled and statistically analyzed to provide a variety of information to today's medical providers, patients, and payers. Figure 1.1 shows the Lower Extremity Functional Scale (LEFS), an example of a specific outcomes questionnaire.

Outcomes tools are divided into two categories—a general health status measurement tool and a region-specific measurement tool. A generic status measurement tool is used to assess a patient's physical, social, and emotional health and is used for a variety of illnesses and treatment environments. The gold standard for the generic health status tool is the SF-36, originally advanced by John E. Ware, Jr. (Ware and Sherbourne 1992; Ware et al. 1995). Although it has been demonstrated to be a reliable and valid tool, it is time consuming to administer and

Lower-Extremity Functional Scale

We are interested in knowing whether you are having any difficulty at all with the activities listed below *because of your lower limb* problem for which you are currently seeking attention. Please provide an answer for each activity.

Today, *do you* or *would you* have any difficulty at all with:

Activities	Extreme Difficulty or Unable to Perform Activity	Quite a Bit of Difficulty	Moderate Difficulty	A Little Bit of Difficulty	No Difficulty
a. Any of your usual work, housework, or school activities	0	1	2	3	4
b. Your usual hobbies, recreational or sporting activities	0	1	2	3	4
c. Getting into or out of the bath	0	1	2	3	4
d. Walking between rooms	0	1	2	3	4
e. Putting on your shoes or socks	0	1	2	3	4
f. Squatting	0	1	2	3	4
g. Lifting an object, like a bag of groceries, from the floor	0	1	2	3	4
h. Performing light activities around your home	0	1	2	3	4
i. Performing heavy activities around your home	0	1	2	3	4
j. Getting into or out of a car	0	1	2	3	4
k. Walking 2 blocks	0	1	2	3	4
l. Walking a mile	0	1	2	3	4
m. Going up or down 10 stairs (about 1 flight of stairs)	0	1	2	3	4
n. Standing for 1 hour	0	1	2	3	4
o. Sitting for 1 hour	0	1	2	3	4
p. Running on even ground	0	1	2	3	4
q. Running on uneven ground	0	1	2	3	4
r. Making sharp turns while running fast	0	1	2	3	4
s. Hopping	0	1	2	3	4
t. Rolling over in bed	0	1	2	3	4

Column Totals:
(Circle one number on each line)
Error (single measure) ± 5 scale points; MDC: 9 scale points; MCID: 9 scale points

Figure 1.1   Sample outcomes assessment tool.

Reprinted by permission from J.M. Binkley et al. 1999.

was not designed as a tool with which to make treatment decisions for individual patients (Binkley et al. 1999). A variety of condition-specific outcomes tools have been developed in an attempt to more accurately examine and assess items that are related to the specific injury or illness and will reveal changes with treatment applications. For example, a commonly used condition-specific outcomes tool that examines changes in back pain is the Roland-Morris Questionnaire (Stratford et al. 1998).

Some of the problems that are recognized in selecting an assessment tool that restricts the reliability of one tool to assess treatment effects for different conditions include the difficulty in using a tool's scale for different injuries, the shortcomings a tool has in its application to specific individuals, and the clinician's lack of confidence in the meaningfulness of the scores (Binkley et al. 1999). For example, a condition-specific tool that is designed to measure patellofemoral injury treatment outcomes may not be considered a reliable tool to measure outcomes of treatment for a shoulder dislocation, or a tool designed to measure treatment outcomes on a high school athlete may not be applicable to measuring treatment outcomes on a middle-aged laborer.

Outcomes are important in many fields of medicine. They are used in physicians' offices, outpatient clinics, and hospitals. They are used to modify treatment, justify treatment, evaluate the effectiveness of protocols, judge the appropriateness of treatment responses, and assist in authorization of payment. An outcomes assessment tool can be provided by an outside agency, which analyzes the results from many different treatment providers around the country, or it can be devised and analyzed by a single facility.

A couple of the more commonly used outcome research tools used today in rehabilitation are the Functional Independence Measure (FIM) (Keith et al. 1987), a tool used primarily for inpatient rehabilitation facilities, and Focus on Therapeutic Outcomes (FOTO), a tool for outpatient rehabilitation facilities. The following resources are also used in assessment of outcomes.

Outcomes Resources

Guide for the Uniform Data Set for Medical Rehabilitation (Adult FIM), version 4.0. 1993. Buffalo, NY: University of New York at Buffalo/UB Foundation Activities.

Lewis, C., and T. McNerney. 1994. *The functional tool box.* Washington, DC: Learn.

McDowell, I., and C. Newell. 1996. *Measuring health.* 2nd ed. New York: Oxford University Press.

Medical Outcomes Trust approved instruments. 1996. *Medical Outcomes Trust Bulletin* 4(1).

Scientific advisory committee instrument review criteria. 1995. *Medical Outcomes Trust Bulletin* 3(Sept.).

Different users of an assessment tool evaluate outcomes differently, depending on their perspective. For example, an insurance company may use outcomes research results to decide what is usual and customary for expected duration and treatment cost of a specific injury. A patient may use them to see whether the treatment program met his or her needs. Health care providers may look at the outcomes study results to assess whether the programs being used to treat specific injuries and individual patients in their facility are effective, cost efficient, and achieve the goals of the professional administering the treatment. There are occasions, however, when outcomes assessments are used incorrectly to generalize results to a larger population or different situation. Inappropriate inferences should be avoided, for they are misleading, unfair, and erroneous.

Because it is imperative for a rehabilitation clinician to be as effective and efficient as possible in treating patients and returning them to sport participation or normal activity, clinicians are inherently concerned with outcomes. Outcomes assessments may not be as critical, however, for clinicians who practice in an athletic training facility or industrial setting as for those who practice in other settings, such as orthopedic clinics or hospitals. However, as systems of allied health care and payment continue to change, all rehabilitation clinicians will eventually be compelled to deal with outcomes assessments more formally than is currently typical.

BASIC COMPONENTS OF THERAPEUTIC EXERCISE

▶ Therapeutic exercise must address the following physiological parameters in proper order: first, flexibility and range of motion, then muscular strength and endurance, and finally, proprioception and coordination.

In the total rehabilitation program, there are two basic elements, therapeutic modalities and therapeutic exercise. Modalities are used to treat and resolve those effects first seen in injury: spasm, pain and edema. Although modalities are an essential component of a rehabilitation program, they will not be presented in detail in this text; please refer to the Craig Denegar text, *Therapeutic Modalities for Musculoskeletal Injuries, Second Edition* (2005) for detailed information on modalities. Therapeutic exercise (therex) is an essential and critical factor in returning the patient to sport participation or normal activity. If the therapeutic exercise program is to be effective, however, specific parameters must be addressed sequentially. Each of these parameters must be restored to at least pre-injury levels if the patient is to safely resume full sports participation or normal activity. These parameters in their proper sequence are

1. flexibility and range of motion,
2. strength and muscle endurance, and
3. proprioception, coordination, and agility.

Each of these parameters is based on the previous ones, much like a pyramid, stones placed one on the other, layer by layer until the structure is complete. This concept will become clearer as we discuss each parameter.

Flexibility and Range of Motion

There is a technical difference between flexibility and range of motion, but in functional terms the difference is nominal. The term flexibility is often used when referring to the mobility of muscles and the length to which they can extend. If a muscle is immobilized for a period of time, it tends to lose its flexibility, or degree of mobility. If stretching exercises are incorporated as part of a routine conditioning program, the muscle tends to maintain its flexibility or length. Inflexibility usually means that a muscle, not a joint, has limited mobility.

Range of motion, however, refers to the amount of movement possible at a joint. For example, the normal range of motion for shoulder abduction is 170°. Range of motion is affected by the flexibility of the muscles and muscle groups surrounding the joint. If a muscle lacks flexibility, the joint may not have full range of motion. Range of motion is also affected by other factors such as mobility of the joint capsule and ligaments, fascial restraints, and regional scar tissue.

Range of motion is also affected by strength. For example, if a patient does not have the strength to lift the arm fully against gravity, active shoulder range of motion will not reach 170°. This is one reason why active and passive range-of-motion measurements are usually different from each other, passive range of motion being greater than active. Active and passive ranges of motion are discussed in chapter 5.

Because of their close clinical relationship, the terms *range of motion* and *flexibility* are often used interchangeably. We will treat these terms as synonyms throughout the text, but keep in mind that technical differences do exist between them.

A properly designed therapeutic exercise portion of a rehabilitation program places a priority on regaining lost range of motion and flexibility first. Achieving flexibility early in the therapeutic exercise program is necessary because of two important reasons. First, the other parameters are based on the flexibility of the affected area. To make this point clear, consider how handicapped a hurdler would be if the hamstrings were inflexible. The patient's strength and timing would be of little importance if the flexibility necessary to extend the leg over the hurdle was lacking. Using an upper extremity example, a baseball pitcher with less than full shoulder range of motion is at a distinct disadvantage. Lacking full shoulder motion, the pitcher lacks power and is at risk for injury, regardless of strength, endurance, or timing.

The second reason to emphasize regaining range of motion first in the therapeutic exercise program is the impact of the healing process (discussed in chapter 2). As injured tissue heals, scar tissue is laid down. As scar tissue matures, it contracts. This is important in eventually minimizing the size of the scar, but it also can be detrimental because as the tissue contracts, it pulls on surrounding tissue, causing in loss of motion, especially if the scar crosses a joint.

During healing there is a window of opportunity during which scar tissue mobility can be influenced and changed. Once that time frame has passed, the likelihood of successfully achieving full range of motion is diminished considerably. If efforts are not made during the remodeling phase, when the newly formed scar tissue is most easily influenced, attempts to improve range of motion will be very difficult and frustrating at best and futile at worst. Although restoration of other parameters is also sought during the first stage of therapy, flexibility must be the primary emphasis.

Strength and Muscular Endurance

As the patient progresses, achieving normal strength and muscular endurance becomes the priority. With any injury some strength is lost. The amount of strength and muscular endurance lost depends on the area injured, the extent of the injury, and the amount of time the patient has been disabled by the injury.

Figure 1.2 Gymnast in iron-cross position.
© Empics

Muscular strength refers to the maximum force that a muscle or a muscle group can exert. It is most often measured by determining the amount of weight that the muscle or group can lift in one repetition. **Muscular endurance** is the muscle's ability to sustain a sub-maximal force in either a static activity or a repetitive activity over a period of time. An example of muscular endurance in a static activity is the length of time a gymnast can maintain an iron-cross position on the rings (see figure 1.2). A runner in a marathon and a starting pitcher are examples of patients performing repetitive activities that require muscular endurance.

Of all the parameters achieved during therapeutic exercise, strength is probably most obvious and most frequently sought following an injury. It is obvious because it is easily understood that a weightlifter cannot return to competition following a sprain until full knee strength is achieved. It is just as obvious that a wrestler must have normal shoulder strength to return to competition after suffering a dislocation.

The need for muscular endurance and the relationship between muscular strength and endurance are sometimes not considered, however. If a baseball pitcher has good rotator cuff strength but no endurance beyond 10 repetitions, how is he going to manage pitching more than a couple of innings in a game? If a basketball center can leg press 225 kg (496 lb) but can last only five repetitions, will she be able to recover rebounds for an entire game?

Muscular strength and endurance are two dimensions within a continuum of muscle resistance. They also affect each other. When strength improves, there are also gains in endurance, and vice versa. This is an important factor to remember in establishing a therapeutic exercise program for patients. For example, if a patient is attempting to recover from patellofemoral pain syndrome, the patient may not be able to tolerate heavy weights to achieve the strength you would like to see. Exercises for endurance may be more tolerable and will still produce gains in strength until the patient becomes strong enough to tolerate higher resistance. Essential concepts of muscle strength and endurance are presented in chapter 7.

Proprioception, Coordination, and Agility

Proprioception, coordination, and agility are often omitted in a therex program. It is too often assumed that because range of motion and strength are restored, the patient is ready to resume full sport participation or normal activity. This is not the case at all. Impaired balance, proprioception, or coordination—either from injury to the structures controlling these parameters or from lack of practice in a specific skill—increases risk of injury.

A variety of factors affect a patient's proprioception, coordination, and agility. A number of factors in turn are affected by these elements, including muscular power, skill execution, and performance. (The factors that affect and are affected by proprioception, coordination, and agility are discussed later in chapter 8.) To develop appropriate proprioception and coordination skills, enough flexibility and strength must first be achieved. Coordination and agility are based on the patient's having enough flexibility to perform the skill through an appropriate range of motion and enough strength, endurance, and power to perform it repeatedly, rapidly, and correctly. This is the reason that proprioception, coordination, and agility are the last parameters to focus on: they need the foundations of good flexibility, strength, and endurance to be optimal.

Although not all allied health professionals emphasize this parameter, a total rehabilitation program must include the recovery of proprioception, coordination, and agility. Consider a tennis player who has suffered a back injury that has kept him out of competition for two months. The timing of his serve, the coordination of his response to his opponent's serve, and the agility of his feet in sudden lateral movements on the court may all be impaired. Simple exercises for proprioception are introduced early in the therapeutic exercise program, but proprioception, coordination, and agility are not emphasized until after strength and range of motion are achieved. Development of execution skills is the last step before a patient's return to full sport participation. Accurate execution of functional and sport-specific skills requires attainment of all parameters.

The final stage of emphasis on coordination and proprioception evolves into the execution of normal drills that mimic the patient's actual activities. Functional activities, the final step before returning to competition, involve execution of these sport-specific activities. In this final stage the patient regains the confidence necessary to perform at his or her prior activity level. When the patient can perform well and with confidence, the rehabilitation clinician can be assured that the goal of fully rehabilitating the patient has been achieved.

RETURN-TO-COMPETITION CRITERIA

▶ The physician determines when a patient is ready to return to competition based on the information provided by the rehabilitation clinician about the patient's status.

If you work with athletes, returning to competition is nearly always the goal of the therapeutic exercise program. By the time the patient is ready to return to full sport participation, you have fully examined and assessed the injured area, the patient's ability to withstand the demands of the sport, and the patient's readiness to return to competition. Full readiness to resume sport participation means that the injured area has no pain, swelling, or atrophy and has full range of motion, flexibility, strength, and endurance and that the patient can perform the sport skills and coordination tasks at an appropriate functional level.

You and the patient must remember that the physician has the final word on when the patient is able to return to competition. It is through your communication with the physician regarding the patient's response to treatment, the patient's ability to perform activities required in the sport, and the injured area's status that the physician can make that determination.

PSYCHOLOGICAL CONSIDERATIONS

Many psychological factors have a direct and sometimes profound influence on the overall results of the rehabilitation program. The rehabilitation clinician must be aware of these factors not only to be able to promote optimal results of the therapeutic exercise program, but also to encourage and provide needed support to the patient.

Stages of Grief

Kubler-Ross (1969) outlined stages of grief that people go through when confronted by the knowledge of their own death or that of a loved one. Although it has never been measured or conclusively proven, others (Peterson 1986; Rotella 1985) have suggested that patients who have experienced a disabling injury that keeps them out of competition also go through this process. Since anecdotal reports indicate injured athletes go through this process, it will be explained here. Kubler-Ross's stages of grief are denial, anger, depression, and acceptance.

▶ A patient may go through four stages of grieving: denial, anger, depression, and acceptance. To ensure compliance with the therapeutic exercise program, the rehabilitation clinician must recognize the importance of the patient's psychological state, communicate effectively, educate, provide support, set goals cooperatively, establish rapport, and make the program interesting.

1. **Denial.** At first, the patient doesn't believe that the injury is severe and feels that he or she will return to competition in a day or two.

2. **Anger.** As the reality of the severity and consequences of the injury sets in and the patient is forced to see the difficulty he or she is having in recovery, the patient expresses anger as a release of the genuine feelings of frustration and helplessness. This anger is often directed at whom ever is present. It is helpful to remember that during this phase the patient is angry because of the injury and the situation he or she is in, not because of any action or words of those who are around. Attempts to calm, rationalize with, or help the patient see what is really happening are often futile at this point. The patient wants only to express this anger and does not want to be told why he or she should not be angry or that things will get better.

During this stage, you should attempt to prevent the injury from becoming aggravated by any harmful activities the patient may attempt. You should also be a sounding board for the patient, letting the patient express the feelings of frustration and anger at the loss of the ability to perform and the loss of power over the situation.

3. **Depression.** As the patient begins to realize the reality of the situation, depression is the next stage. The patient's self-worth declines during this time. The patient feels he or she has no physical or emotional control. Not participating with the team can cause feelings of isolation, further adding to self-doubt and low self-esteem. Hope is questionable at best because the patient sees no good results forthcoming.

It is during this phase that rehabilitation becomes the most difficult for both you and the patient. It becomes difficult for the patient to comply with the rehabilitation program. The patient may not attend scheduled treatment sessions or may not fully participate in them.

4. **Acceptance.** In this final phase the patient begins the battle of fighting the physical limitations and psychological downswing experienced during the previous stages.

Progression Through the Stages

Throughout the grieving process there are no abrupt changes; rather, the patient goes through gradual transitions, and fluctuation between stages can occur. For example, a patient who has entered the depression phase may swing back into the anger phase in the beginning but later return to the depression phase. As the patient progresses through depression, he or she displays less and less anger. As the patient enters the acceptance phase, he or she may regress to depression before finally accepting the situation.

You must be aware that these swings occur and are natural. Seeing these stages on a continuum from the extreme ends of denial and acceptance, each phase overlapping with the adjacent one, may help you in dealing with the patient as he or she goes through these stages.

When a patient is unable to advance through the grieving process smoothly, or if you are concerned about the patient's emotional condition, it is your responsibility to support the patient and encourage him or her to seek additional psychological support from a counselor, psychologist, psychiatrist, or other psychological professional. You should never hesitate to refer a patient to an appropriate specialist.

The Rehabilitation Clinician's Role in Psychological Recovery

Supporting the patient in psychological recovery is vital to achieving goals of therapeutic exercise and rehabilitation programs. The rehabilitation clinician is crucial to this process because of the role he or she plays in the patient's response to injury and commitment to the rehabilitation program. A survey of certified athletic trainers (Fisher, Mullins, and Frey 1993) revealed the most important variables influenced by certified athletic trainers in patients' compliance with rehabilitation programs. At the top of the list is education and communication. Whether you work with athletes or other populations prone to musculoskeletal injuries, if you educate the patient about the type and extent of the injury, inform him or her about the rehabilitation process, and communicate with him or her in a respectful, open, and honest manner, the patient will exhibit better compliance.

Communication

Using good communication skills throughout the rehabilitation process is important. Being a good and an active listener is a communication skill that every clinician should possess. Repeating the patient's uncertainties, worries, and goals is an active listening skill that demonstrates to the patient your interest and concern. Making good eye contact is a simple yet important part of communication. Being aware of the environment and realizing whether it is conducive to good listening and communication are also necessary. Simply being at the same eye level, instead of standing and looking down at the patient, encourages communication.

As discussed earlier in the section "Communicating with the Patient," appropriate communication incorporates good judgment and interpersonal skills. Being timely with explanations and knowing how much to explain is often vital to patient acceptance. The information you provide the patient educates him or her, enhances compliance with your treatment program, and gives him or her hope for a foreseeable end to the injury and return to competition or normal activity.

Communication includes providing the patient with written and oral instructions and demonstration of any home exercises or activities. Having written descriptions of exercises along with illustrations or photos ensures optimal patient compliance with a home program.

Offering encouragement for the patient's physical efforts throughout the therapeutic exercise program positively impacts the patient's psychological response. Encouragement also improves compliance. When someone of authority and expertise whom the patient respects offers support and encouragement, the patient's performance and compliance are enhanced.

Goal Setting With the Patient

Goal setting is important in facilitating patient compliance and enhancing a positive attitude. The patient's assistance in setting goals offers two benefits: the patient feels he or she has some control over the situation, and working together to establish goals ensures mutual understanding of and agreement on those goals. It is natural for a patient to feel a loss of power or control when injured. Thus, regaining control is important.

You and the patient should have the same goals. If one has a goal that conflicts with the other's goals, failure is certain. You and the patient should understand each other's goals, agree with them, and work together to achieve them. For example, if an injured alpine skier has no desire to return to skiing but instead wants to become a recreational cyclist, while your goal is to have the patient return to the slopes, you will be frustrated when the patient does not work as hard as you would like, and the patient will be frustrated that you are making her work harder than necessary to achieve her goal.

Monitoring the patient's progress, using goals, recording objective changes, and setting new and more challenging goals are all methods of providing the patient with additional incentives to adhere to the therapeutic exercise program. The patient may be able to feel some benefits from the program, but providing him or her with more objective, concrete measurements enhances his or her willingness and motivation to continue the rehabilitation program.

Supporting the Patient

Depending on the environment, the members of the patient's support system may vary. The rehabilitation clinician is central to this support system, however, and acts as the coordinator of the patient's support system to assist him or her in a successful outcome. Support team members can assist the patient with home exercises, provide encouragement, and share with the clinician observations or concerns noted outside the treatment environment.

Establishing Rapport with the Patient

Treating a patient on a frequent, if not daily, basis, the rehabilitation clinician develops a rapport with the patient. This rapport results from their interaction, mutual respect, and desire to achieve the same goals. Establishing rapport can be a challenge when patients are hard to manage or have difficult personalities. In these cases it is the clinician's responsibility to put aside his or her own prejudices and feelings and act in a professional manner. Fortunately, however, this type of uncomfortable situation is rare. Normally, the challenge of the situation and the common bond between the patient and clinician facilitate an easily established rapport. The patient is more compliant and willing to perform any activity requested when this rapport exists.

Making the Program Interesting

Personalizing the program, making its goals challenging yet achievable, and using your imagination to make it interesting are important to overall success and the patient's compliance. The therapeutic exercise program can be a treatment of drudgery or stimulation for both the patient and you. It is up to you to see to it that it is the latter if your common goals are to be achieved.

SUMMARY

1. Identify rehabilitation team members and their roles.

    A rehabilitation team consists of individuals who are closely related to the rehabilitation program or who have peripheral roles. Some of these individuals are the patient, rehabiliatioan clinician, physician, family members, allied healthcare students, coach or supervisor, team members or peers, and specialists.

2. Discuss the qualities of professionalism in athletic training.

    The rehabilitation clinician is an allied health care provider who is responsible for looking, acting, and being professional. Being a professional means acting as a responsible clinician and contributing within the professional organization. Being a professional carries with it the responsibility of continuing to learn new techniques and applications that are pertinent to the profession. It also means always treating others in a respectful and courteous manner.

3. Discuss the principles, goals, and objectives of rehabilitation.

    The mnemonic ATC IS IT can help you remember the principles of rehabilitation. The objectives of any therapeutic exercise program are to prevent deconditioning of the unaffected areas, including the cardiovascular system, and to rehabilitate the injured area safely, efficiently, and successfully.

    The goals established for each patient are based on achieving these objectives and are divided into short-term and long-term goals. The long-term goal is to restore the patient to at least former levels of function to permit the patient to return to sport participation or normal activity. Short-term goals are used when the patient has a more severe injury and cannot participate in sports or normal activities for a while.

    To achieve these goals and objectives, you must be sensitive to the patient and what the patient is going through psychologically.

4. Describe the relationship between goals, progression, and examination.

    Short-term goals are based on measures as objective as possible, recorded to see the patient's progress, and changed when the patient achieves them until the final long-term goals are achieved. You must continually assess the patient's and the injured area's response to treatment. Using objective measures in this assessment and recording the results help the patient and you to realize the changes that are the product of the rehabilitation program and to know how the program should progress.

5. Outline the importance of outcomes-based rehabilitation.

   Outcome assessment investigates whether a program that you design for a patient produces the expected response and whether the program meets expectations and goals.

6. Outline the basic components of a therapeutic exercise program and their interrelationships.

   A rehabilitation program must progress in a sequential manner, since each parameter builds upon the components of the prior parameter so that a patient can ultimately return to full participation or normal activity. The sequential parameters include flexibility and range of motion; strength and muscle endurance; proprioception, coordination, and agility, leading to full functional activity.

7. Identify the stages of grief and the rehabilitation clinician's role in assisting the patient through the stages.

   Although it has not been clearly demonstrated that an injured individual follows the four stages of grief, they follow this sequence: denial, anger, depression, and acceptance. To ensure the patient's compliance with the therapeutic exercise program, the rehabilitation clinician must recognize the importance of the patient's psychological state, communicate effectively, educate, provide support, set goals cooperatively, establish rapport, and make the program interesting.

CRITICAL THINKING QUESTIONS

1. How would you handle a situation in which a certified athletic trainer with whom you work did not properly complete the requirements established by the NATA Board of Certification (NATABOC) to sit for the certification examination but was able to get his or her supervising certified athletic trainer to sign off on the required documents anyway? Would you report him or her to the NATABOC, discuss it with him or her or your supervisor, or ignore it?

2. If you were treating a patient whose injury was severe enough to doubt whether he or she would return to full sport participation at the preinjury level, how would you deal with the questions the patient would have regarding long-term goals? Would you tell the patient in the beginning that returning to his or her prior level of participation was questionable? Would you let the patient discover the reality him- or herself? Would you ease the patient into that reality?

LAB ACTIVITIES

1. Go to the NATA Web site at www.nata.org and perform the following functions:
   a. Identify the different membership categories.
   b. Calculate what your dues would be for national and state membership.
   c. Identify each of the districts and the states within each district.
   d. If your district has a Web site, identify its address.
   e. If your state has a Web site, identify its address.
   f. Locate information at each Web site that is of personal interest to you and indicate what that piece of information is.

2. Role play a situation where you and your lab partner are the clinician and a patient. The patient is going through the grieving phases following a severe and debilitating injury. Act out how the patient may express himself or herself at each of the different grieving stages and how the clinician should respond to each of those stages.

3. Role play a situation where one person is the athletic trainer and the other person is the injured athlete's coach. The coach wants to have the athlete ready to play by the weekend, but the athletic trainer knows that will not be possible. Act out how an athletic trainer should approach the coach so the coach is able to understand and accept that the athlete's injury will not allow the athlete to participate by the weekend.

REFERENCES

Appell, H.J. 1990. Muscular atrophy following immobilization: A review. *Sports Medicine* 10:42–58.

Binkley, J.M., Stratford, P.W., Lott, S.A., Riddle, D.L., and North American Orthopaedic Rehabilitation Research Network. 1999. The Lower Extremity Functional Scale (LEFS): Scale development, measurement properties, and clinical application. *Physical Therapy*, 79:371–383.

Fisher, A.C., Mullins, S.A., and P.A. Frye. 1993. Athletic trainers' attitudes and judgments of injured athletes' rehabilitation adherence. *Journal of Athletic Training* 28:43–47.

Keith, R.H., Granter, C.V., Hamilton, B.B., and F.S. Sherwin. 1987. The functional independence measure: A new tool for rehabilitation. In *Advances in clinical rehabilitation*, ed. M.G. Eisenberg and R.C. Grzesink. New York: Springer.

Kubler-Ross, E. 1969. *On death and dying.* New York: Macmillan.

Peterson, P. 1986. The grief response and injury. *Athletic Training* 21:312–314.

Ray, R. 2005. *Management strategies in athletic training.* 3rd ed. Champaign, IL: Human Kinetics.

Rotella, R.J. 1985. The psychological care of the patient. In *Sports psychology: Psychological consideration in maximizing sport performance.* Ann Arbor, MI: McNaughton and Gun.

Staron, R.S., Leonardi, M.J., Karapondo, D.L., Malicky, E.S., Falkel, J.E., Hagerman, F.C., and R.S. Kikada. 1991. Strength and skeletal muscle adaptations in heavy-resistance-trained women after detraining and retraining. *Journal of Applied Physiology* 70:631–640.

Stratford, P.W., Binkley, J.M., Riddle, D.L., and G.H. Guyatt. 1998. Sensitivity to change on the Roland-Morris Pain Questionnaire: Part 1. *Physical Therapy.* 78:1186–1196.

Ware, J.E., Jr., Kosinski, M., Bayliss, M.S., McHorney, C.A., Rogers, W.H., and A. Raczek. 1995. Comparisons of methods for the scoring and statistical analysis of the SF-36 health profile and summary measures: Summary of results from the Medical Outcomes Study. *Medical Care.* 33: AS264–279.

Ware, J.E., Jr. and C.D. Sherbourne. 1992. The MOS 36-Item Short Form Health Survey (SF-36), I: Conceptual framework and item selection. *Medical Care.* 30:473–483.

2

Concepts of Healing

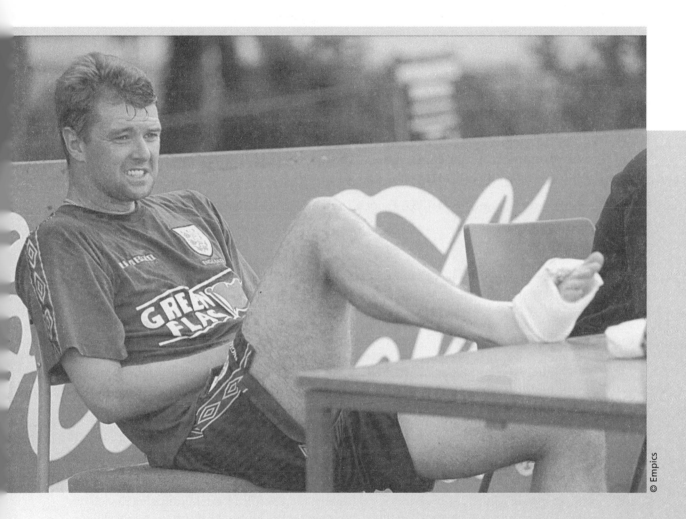

© Empics

Objectives

After completing this chapter, you should be able to do the following:

1. Explain the differences between primary and secondary healing.

2. Identify the healing phases.

3. Describe the primary processes of each healing phase.

4. Discuss the causes for the signs of inflammation.

5. Explain the role of growth factors in healing.

6. Discuss the differences between acute and chronic inflammation.

7. Discuss healing characteristics of specific tissues.

8. Identify the relevance of tensile strength.

9. Discuss factors that can modify the healing process.

10. Explain the role NSAIDs play in inflammation.

11. Discuss the timing of treatment with the various stages of healing.

aniel Edwards has been assigned to work with gymnast Becki Gumble, who underwent an Achilles tendon repair 7 days ago and is now in the clinic for her first day of rehabilitation. Daniel's knowledge of healing allows him to judge where in the healing process such an injury should be and what rehabilitation techniques can be safely applied to the Achilles tendon at this time. He understands the tendon's tensile strength and the precautions that apply for repairs such as Becki's. He also understands the status of the healing connective tissue and the processes that are now under way.

However, Daniel suspects that Becki has poor eating habits. Before applying rehabilitation techniques, Daniel decides to discuss the importance of proper nutrition and the role proteins, vitamins, and minerals play in tissue healing.

■ **Perfection does not exist. To understand this is the triumph of human intelligence; to expect to possess it is the most dangerous kind of madness.**

Alfred de Musset, 1810-1857, French romantic poet, dramatist, and fiction writer

Understanding the healing process, like de Musset's understanding of perfection, is an intellectual triumph. Knowing as much as you can about healing process is important in developing a safe and effective therapeutic exercise program. Performing an exercise before the injured area is ready to tolerate that level of stress can impede healing and cause additional injury. As a professional who rehabilitates musculoskeletal injuries, you have a duty to understand healing and realize the impact of the therex techniques you apply. There are many aspects to healing that are still unknown, even to experts. What is presented here is the most current information we have on the body's response to injury and the process it undergoes in an effort to return to normal.

It is common knowledge that an injury produces a scar when healing. Although there are occasions when the body actually replaces damaged tissue with normal tissue, more frequently in musculoskeletal injuries, scar tissue is the end result of the healing process. This chapter provides an elementary focus on the essential elements of the healing process involved in scar tissue formation following musculoskeletal injuries.

In spite of all that has been written on healing, there is still a lot of information that eludes us. The information presented in this chapter has resulted from the research of a great many people. I have attempted to simplify this complex topic and to present what rehabilitation clinicians should know to safely apply therapeutic exercise and rehabilitation techniques to injured individuals.

This chapter introduces many terms that may be new and unfamiliar to you. To assist you in becoming familiar with these terms, table 2.1 defines the terms that appear in green in this chapter and indicates their most common function or their significance in the healing process.

Table 2.1
Terminology of Wound Healing

Term	Definition	Significance/Function
acetylcholine	A neurotransmitter at the neuro-muscular junction of striated muscles.	Causes vasodilation.
adrenaline	See *epinephrine.*	
angiogenesis	Formation of blood vessels.	Provides for subsequent scar tissue formation and normal healing events that follow.
arachidonic acid	An unsaturated essential fatty acid.	A precursor in the production of leukotrienes, prostaglandins, and thrombaxanes.
basophil	See *granular leukocyte.*	
bradykinin	A local tissue hormone that is activated by the interaction of proteases with the Hageman factor.	A very potent local vasodilator. It increases vascular permeability and stimulates local pain receptors.
callus	Fibrous matrix formed at a bone fracture site.	Immobilizes the bone fragments and serves as the foundation for eventual bone replacement.
chemotactic factor	A chemical gradient. Also referred to as a chemotactin or chemo-attractant.	See *chemotactin.*
chemotactin	An agent that facilitates chemotaxis.	Must be present and function properly to promote the healing process.
chemotaxis	Movement or orientation of cells in response to a chemical stimulus after an injury, which occurs through a complex and not totally understood processes.	Cells either become oriented along a chemical concentration gradient or move in the direction of that gradient. For example, chemicals attract platelets, red blood cells, and PMNs into an injured area.
collagen	Major type of protein in the body. There are five types: I is most abundant, high in tensile strength, and found in dermis, fascia, and bone. II is found in cartilage. III is found in embryonic connective tissue. IV and V are found in basement membranes.	Forms inelastic bundles to provide structure, integrity, and tensile strength to tissues.
collagenase	An enzyme produced by newly formed epithelial cells and fibroblasts.	Involved in degradation of collagen during tissue repair. Important in controlling collagen content in a wound.
complement system	Various proteins found in serum.	Act as chemotactic factors for neutrophils and phagocytes.
drug interaction	When one drug enhances or reduces the effectiveness of other drugs also being taken.	It is important to know what drugs an individual takes so that they are not rendered harmful or ineffective by each other.
duration of drug action	Amount of time the blood level of the drug is above the level needed to obtain a minimum therapeutic effect.	Determined by the drug's half-life.

(continued)

Table 2.1
(continued)

Term	Definition	Significance/Function
elastin	An essential protein of connective-tissue elastic structures. Arranged in a wavy orientation.	Its wavy arrangement allows tissue to change shape with stress and resume normal conditions after stress removal. It plays an as yet unknown role in the remodeling phase.
endothelial cells	Large, flat cells that line blood and lymphatic vessels.	Are restored during angiogenesis.
Endothelial leukocytes	Large white blood cells that circulate in the bloodstream and tissues.	Act as phagocytes to remove debris from an injured area.
eosinophil	See *granular leukocyte*.	
epinephrine	A hormone. Also called adrenaline.	A potent stimulator of the sympathetic nervous system and a powerful vasopressor. Increases blood pressure, stimulates the heart muscle, accelerates heart rate, increases cardiac output, and increases metabolic activities such as glycogenolysis and glucose release.
erythrocyte	An element of blood. Also known as red blood cell or corpuscle.	Used for oxygen transport.
extracellular matrix	The basic material from which tissue develops. Produced by fibroblasts in wounds. Composed of fibers and ground substance.	Serves as a foundation on which new tissue is cast.
exudate	Material that escapes from blood vessels following an injury. Contains high concentrations of protein, cells, and other materials from injured cells.	As PMNs die and decompose, exudate may resemble pus although no infection is present.
factor XII	See *Hageman factor*.	
fibrin	Insoluble fibrous protein formed by fibrinogen.	Important in clotting.
fibrinogen	A globulin present in plasma.	Converts to fibrin to form a plug at the injury site.
fibrinolysin	An enzyme in plasma released in later healing.	Converts fibrin into a soluble substance to unplug lymphatics system at injury site.
fibroblast	A connective tissue cell that differentiates into chondroblasts, osteoblasts, and collagenoblasts.	Forms the fibrous tissues that support and bind a variety of tissues.
fibrocyte	An inactive fibroblast. See *fibroblast*.	
fibronectin	An adhesive glycoprotein found in most body tissues and serum. Fibronectin is plentiful in early granulation tissue formation but gradually disappears during the remodeling phase.	Cross-links to collagen in connective tissue, thereby playing a role in the adhesion of fibroblasts to fibrin. Also involved in the collection of platelets in an injured area and the enhancement of myofibroblast activity.

Term	Definition	Significance/Function
glycoprotein	Protein–carbohydrate compounds. Elements of ground substance. Includes fibronectin.	Probably cross-links with collagen so tissue is able to withstand pressure.
Glycosaminoglycan (GAG)	Compounds occurring mostly in proteoglycans. Nonfibrous elements of ground substance in the extracellular matrix. Examples: hyaluronic acid, proteoglycans.	Different GAGs have different functions: stimulating fibroblast proliferation, promoting collagen synthesis and maturation, contributing to tissue resilience, and regulating cell function.
granuloma	Hard mass of fibrous tissue.	Occurs in chronic inflammatory conditions when the body produces collagen around a foreign substance to protect itself from that substance.
granular leukocytes	White blood cells, which are divided into three groups of polymorphonuclear leukocytes: neutrophils, eosinophils, and basophils.	Among their functions, they are chemotactic and phagocytic and release histamine and serotonin to produce vasoactive reactions following injury.
granulation tissue	Newly formed vascular tissue that is produced during wound healing. Consists of fibroblasts, macrophages, and neovascular cells within a connective tissue matrix of collagen, hyaluronic acid, and fibronectin. Has the appearance of small, red, velvety nodular masses seen in new tissue.	Eventually forms the scar of the wound.
ground substance	Gel-like material in which connective tissue cells and fibers are imbedded. Part of the connective tissue or extracellular matrix.	Reduces friction between the connective tissue fibers when forces are applied to the structure. Adds to the area's density.
growth factor	Components released by platelets and macrophages. Also referred to as growth hormone factor.	Performs numerous complex roles, the stimulation of reepithelialization, and is chemotactic for macrophages, monocytes, and neutrophils. Its role is not thoroughly understood, but it is believed to play an important role throughout tissue repair.
Hageman factor	An enzyme present in the blood.	Initiates the blood coagulation process following trauma by converting prothrombin to thrombin.
half-life	Amount of time it takes for the level of a drug in the blood-stream to diminish by one half.	Determines the frequency with which a medication is taken.
histamine	A local tissue hormone released by mast cells and granulocytes.	Increases vascular permeability to proteins and fibronectin.
hyaluronic acid	A major component of early granulation tissue. Greatest amounts are seen in a wound during the first 4-5 days. See also *glycosaminoglycan (GAG)*.	Promotes cell movement and migration during repair. Stimulates fibroblast proliferation. Produces edema by absorbing large amounts of water to increase fibroblast migration.

(continued)

Table 2.1
(continued)

Term	Definition	Significance/Function
kallikrein	A proteolytic enzyme found in blood plasma, lymph, and other exocrine secretions. Activated by the Hageman factor.	Forms kinins and activates plasminogen, a precursor of plasmin. Increases vascular permeability and vasodilation.
kinin	A generic term for polypeptides that are related to bradykinin. A potent local tissue hormone found in injured tissue, released from plasma proteins. Examples: bradykinin, kallidin.	Mediates the classic signs of inflammation. Acts like histamine and serotonin on the microvascular system in the early inflammation phase to cause increased microvascular permeability.
leukocytes	White blood cells or corpuscles. Different types include polymorphonuclear leukocytes and mononuclear cells.	Have phagocytic properties to remove debris from an injury site.
leukotriene	Compound formed from arachidonic acid.	Regulates inflammatory reactions. Some stimulate the movements of leukocytes into the area.
lipid	A heterogeneous group of fats and fatlike substances, including fatty acids and steroids.	Serves as a source of fuel and is important to the structure and makeup of cells.
lymphocytes	Nonphagocytic leukocytes found in blood and lymph.	Serve in the body's immune system by producing antibodies.
macrophages	Mononuclear phagocytes that arise from stem cells in bone marrow.	Considered one of the regulators of the repair process. Serve to phagocytize injury areas of debris, kill microorganisms, and secrete substances into an injury site, including items such as enzymes, fibronectin, and coagulation factors. Play role in keeping the inflammatory process localized; enhance collagen deposition and fibroblast proliferation.
mast cells	Connective tissue cells. Also referred to as mastocytes and labrocytes.	Store and produce various mediators of inflammation. Through their release of histamine, enzymes, and other mediators, mast cells increase local blood flow, attract immune cells, stimulate cell production of fibroblasts and endothelial cells, and promote and control remodeling of extracellular matrix.
matrix	Substance of a tissue. Can refer to intracellular or extracellular structure.	Forms the basis from which a structure develops.
monocytes	Mononuclear phagocytic leukocytes. Formed in the bone marrow and transported to tissues to become macrophages.	Remove debris from an injury site.
mononuclear phagocytes	Cells with only one nucleus, capable of ingesting particulate matter, i.e., monocytes.	Ingest microorganisms and remove debris from an injury site.

Term	Definition	Significance/Function
myoblast	A cell formed from myogenic cells in muscle.	Forms myotubes, which eventually evolve into muscle fiber.
myofibroblasts	Fibroblasts that have a combination of the ultrastructural features of a fibroblast and the qualities of a smooth muscle cell.	Responsible for wound contraction.
myogenic cells	Cells arising from muscle that later become myoblasts.	See *myoblast*.
neurotransmitters	Hormones such as norepinephrine, epinephrine, and acetylcholine, which are found in capillary, arteriole, and artery walls.	Released at the injury site to enhance platelet and leukocyte adherence to the vessel surface.
neutrophil	See *polymorphonuclear leukocyte*.	
norepinephrine	A hormone.	Acts as a powerful vasoconstrictor at the immediate onset of injury. It may last from a few seconds to a few minutes.
osteoblasts	Osteogenic cells from periosteum.	Lay down the callus of fractured bone. Convert later to chondrocytes.
osteoclasts	Large multinuclear cells.	Resorb dead, necrotic bone tissue.
osteocytes	Cells characteristic of adult bone.	Maintain new bone mineralization.
platelet-derived growth factor (PDGF)	Substance found in platelets.	Essential for the growth of connective tissue cells. Stimulates the migration of polymorphonuclear leukocytes.
PGE1	See *prostaglandin*.	Increases vascular permeability by causing vasodilation.
PGE2	See *prostaglandin*.	Is chemotactic to attract leukocytes to the area.
phagocyte	See *mononuclear phagocyte* and *polymorphonuclear leukocyte (PMN)*.	
phospholipids	Lipids that contain phosphoric acid. Found in all cells and in layers of plasma membranes.	Stimulate the clotting mechanism.
plasmin	An enzyme that occurs in plasma as plasminogen. It is activated by kallikrein and other activators.	Converts fibrin to soluble substances.
Plasminogen activator	See *fibrinolysin*.	
platelets	Irregular cell fragments found in blood.	The first cells seen at an injury site and considered one of the regulatory cells of healing. Releases growth factors. Forms a plug at the injury to stop bleeding.
primary intension	Healing that occurs with minor wounds or surgical wounds.	Re-epithelialization closes the wound within 48 hr. Scarring is minimal when healing by primary intention occurs.

(continued)

Table 2.1
(continued)

Term	Definition	Significance/Function
polymorphonuclear leukocyte (PMN)	A type of white blood cell with more than one nucleus. One of the granular leukocytes. Also referred to as neutrophil.	Chemotactic and phagocytic in the healing process.
prostaglandin (PG)	Hormone formed primarily from arachidonic acid as a result of cell membrane damage. Its release requires the Complement System and follows kinin formation. Specific PG compounds are designated by adding a letter, A through I, and a subscript number, 1 through 3, to designate the number of hydrocarbon bonds. Examples: PGE_1 and PGE_2.	Mediates cell migration during inflammation and modulates serotonin and histamine. Some PGs increase pain sensitivity, induce fever, and suppress lymphocyte transformation, thereby inhibiting the inflammatory reaction. Mediates myofibroblasts, initiates early phases of injury repair, and plays a role in later stages of inflammation.
protease	An enzyme.	Acts as a catalyst to split interior peptide bonds in protein. Activates kallikrein to release bradykinin, ultimately causing increased vascular permeability and an increase in concentration of proteins and cells in the wound spaces.
proteoglycan	Substance found in tissues, including synovial fluid and connective tissue matrix. Proteoglycan solutions are very viscous lubricants and are sulfated GAGs. See also *glycosaminoglycan*.	Provides a resilient matrix to inhibit cell migration. Regulates cell function and proliferation, and regulates collagen fibrillogenesis.
reticulin	Collagen-like fiber. Some consider it type III collagen fiber.	Forms the early framework for collagen deposition in a wound.
satellite cells	Cells present in muscle.	Regenerate new muscle tissue.
secondary intention	Healing that occurs in large wounds associated with soft-tissue loss. The wound heals with granulation tissue from the bottom and sides of the wound. Epithelial tissue does not form until granulation tissue has filled the wound.	Larger scar formation occurs with healing by secondary intention. Wound contraction is evident with this healing.
serotonin	A hormone released by mast cells and platelets.	Produces vasoconstriction in small vessels after norepinephrine activity is complete; occurs only when blood-vessel endothelial walls are damaged. In later phases, initiates reactions leading to collagen cross-linking. Also involved in granuloma formation.
steady state of a drug	Occurs when the average level of drug remains constant in the blood, and the amount of drug leaving the body is equal to the amount being absorbed.	On average, occurs after 5 doses; equals the drug's half-life.
tenocyte	Tendon cell.	Converts to fibroblasts during healing of tendons.

Term	Definition	Significance/Function
tensile strength	Maximal amount of stress or force that a structure is able to withstand before tissue failure occurs.	Varies as tissue healing occurs; must be taken into account when determining appropriate stress application during rehabilitation.
thrombin	An enzyme.	Converts fibrinogen to fibrin to form a fibrin plug early in the inflammation phase. In later inflammation, it stimulates fibronectin production and fibroblast proliferation.
thromboxane	A compound that is produced by platelets and is unstable. Its half-life is 30 s. Related to prostaglandins.	Acts as a vasoconstrictor and is a potent inducer of platelet aggregation.

PRIMARY AND SECONDARY HEALING

▶ Healing by primary intention occurs through a bridge of tissue when the wound separation is small. Healing by secondary intention occurs by filling in the wound with new tissue from the sides and bottom when the separation is large.

When an injury occurs, the healing process that follows depends on the extent of the injury and the approximation of the wound site's stump ends. If the separation of tissue is small, a bridge of cells binds the ends together. This is called healing by **primary intention**. This type of healing commonly occurs in minor wounds. It is also seen in surgical incisions where the stump ends are sutured together.

In more severe wounds where the stump ends are farther apart and cannot be bridged, the wound heals by producing tissue from the bottom and sides of the wound to fill in the space created by the wound. This is called healing by **secondary intention**. This may occur in second-degree sprains where ligament tissue is torn and not surgically repaired. Healing by secondary intention usually takes longer and results in a larger scar.

HEALING PHASES

▶ The three phases of healing are inflammation, proliferation, and remodeling. During inflammation, the injury is contained and stabilized and debris is removed. During proliferation, fibroblasts, myofibroblasts, and collagen peak to begin granulation tissue formation and angiogenesis. During remodeling, wound contraction is well under way, and type III collagen is converted to type I collagen to stabilize and restore the injury site.

Whether the body heals by secondary or primary intention, the process through which it proceeds is consistent and predictable in normal situations. We do not entirely understand the process, but we can determine the outcomes of each phase.

Healing is a continuum of changing events. To understand and clarify this process, researchers and clinicians divide the events into three different phases. Keep in mind, however, that as far as the body is concerned, the process is continuous, without clear-cut delineations. The body merely continues the process until the end is reached. The three phases designated by researchers and clinicians are

1. inflammation phase,
2. proliferation, or fibroplastic phase, and
3. remodeling, or maturation phase.

Inflammation Phase

When an injury occurs, the body attempts to stabilize the injured site by rushing chemicals and cells into the area. These extremely complex processes take three to five days to complete. A simplified version of these processes is summarized in figure 2.1. The body is extremely busy during this phase in its attempt to protect the site and begin the return to status quo as well as possible.

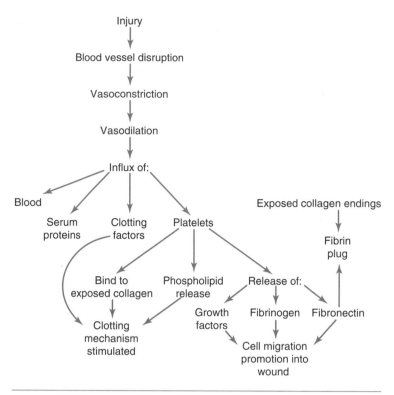

Figure 2.1   Immediate injury response.

Inflammation often has negative connotations. In reality, it is an important and necessary step in the healing process. Without inflammation, the body would be unable to complete the healing process. If inflammation did not occur, proliferation, maturation, and final resolution would not take place. The wound would remain unhealed. Inflammation becomes deleterious when it is prolonged, extending beyond the normal healing time.

The goal of rehabilitation clinicians is to allow inflammation to happen but to minimize it. This is accomplished at the time of injury by applying initial first aid: ice, compression, elevation, and rest.

As the injury's status changes in the first few days, the rehabilitation clinician minimizes inflammation and encourages healing to continue along its normal path by using various treatment modalities that are discussed in the Athletic Training Education Series text *Therapeutic Modalities for Athletic Injuries, Second Edition* (Denegar, Saliba, and Saliba, 2005).

To make appropriate decisions about when to employ modalities and therapeutic exercise techniques, the rehabilitation clinician must first understand the events that occur in the healing process. Let us examine the series of events involved in this first phase of healing.

Vasoconstriction and Vasodilation

When an injury occurs, blood and lymph vessel walls suffer damage. The immediate local vasoconstriction that occurs in the small vessels is followed quickly by vasodilation. You may have observed this reaction if you have suffered a laceration. At first there is no bleeding, but within a few seconds the wound starts to bleed.

Cellular Reactions

It is at this moment of injury that the inflammation phase begins. The vasodilation causes the release of blood and blood products into the injured site, including blood **platelets** and serum proteins as noted in figure 2.2a. As these products accumulate in the injury, chemicals are released, and other cells are attracted into the area. Platelets release **phospholipids**, which stimulate the clotting mechanism to stop the bleeding. Platelets also bind to the **collagen** fiber stumps that were exposed by the injury. Platelets release other important substances, such as **fibronectin**, **growth factors**, and **fibrinogen** (Koopman 1995). Each of these substances is important in the healing process.

Fibronectin binds together **fibrin** and collagen. Fibronectin and fibrin bind together in a cross-link arrangement with the exposed collagen ends to form a latticelike complex, which acts as a plug to stop the bleeding. This plug is temporary and fairly fragile, but in these early hours it provides the wound's only **tensile strength** (Martinez-Hernandez and Amenta 1990). As healing progresses, this plug is replaced by type III collagen.

In addition to blood vessels, the more fragile lymph vessels are also damaged at the time of injury. Leakage from these vessels is also halted by the formation of the fibrin plug. Once fluid accumulates in the extracellular spaces, as it does during an injury, the only way it is removed is through the lymph system. Unfortunately, because the lymph vessels are plugged by the fibrin plug to stop leakage, their ability to remove the extra fluid from the area is

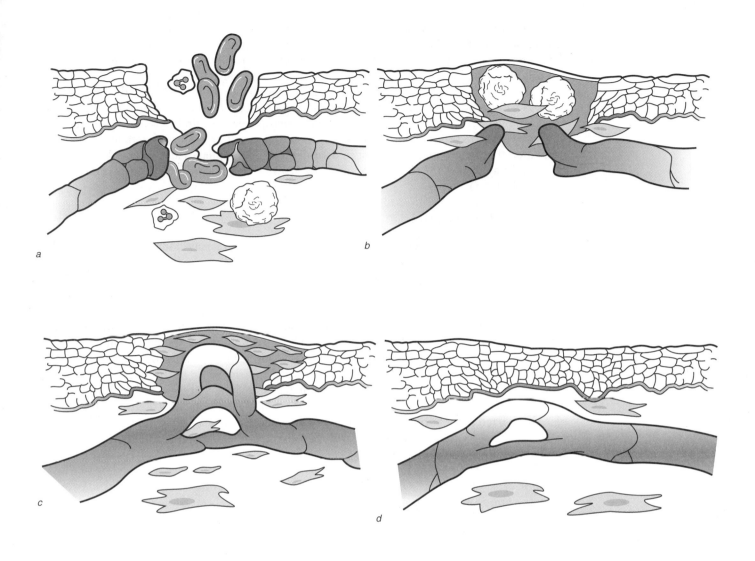

Figure 2.2 Epidermal wound healing. (*a*) Release of blood and blood products at time of injury. (*b*) Macrophages and fibroblasts in the area with capillary buds apparent. (*c*) Angiogenesis has caused anastamosis with new capillary growth. Fibroblasts are present in large numbers. (*d*) Reepitheliazation has occurred. Regression of earlier established capillaries is noted.

compromised. Later, the area becomes stable, and **fibrinolysin** is released. Fibrinolysin is an enzyme that converts fibrin from an insoluble to a soluble protein to promote absorption of the fibrin plug and allow the lymph vessels to perform their normal function, draining the area of edema (excess fluid).

Within the first few hours of injury, the body attempts to remove debris from the site. This process is started by **neutrophils**, or **polymorphonuclear leukocytes (PMNs)**, within 5 to 6 h of injury. The inflammation phase is named after these cells. Neutrophils are the most plentiful white blood cells in the body and migrate into the wound in great numbers, but their presence is short-lived. Other white blood cells in the granular leukocyte family include eosinophils and basophils.

The cells that replace the neutrophils are the **mononuclear phagocytes: monocytes** and **macrophages**. These become the predominant cells at the injury site within 24 to 48 h.

Both the PMNs and the macrophages act as **phagocytes** to remove debris and dead tissue from the area. As the inflammatory process proceeds, an inflammatory **exudate** is formed and consists of fluid escaping from the local vessels, dead tissue from the injury, and dying

PMNs. Inflammatory exudate is commonly whitish and differs from the exudate seen in an infection, which is called pus and contains bacteria. Although normally produced exudate is often referred to as pus, Peacock (1984, p. 2) feels that this is a misnomer and prefers to refer to this uninfected substance as *cell aggregation centers*, not pus.

Debridement (removal of debris) is necessary for healing to continue. Before the subsequent phases can occur, the injury site must be cleared of excess fluid and other waste materials that have accumulated. For this reason alone, macrophages are vital to the healing process, but they perform other important functions as well. Once in the injury site, they recruit and activate other macrophages to assist in debridement. Macrophages also release growth factors and may trigger the termination of tissue growth when the healing process is complete (DiPietro 1995).

Chemical Reactions

There is an intimate interaction between cells and chemicals throughout healing. Some cells stimulate the production of chemicals, and certain chemicals at the injury site stimulate the arrival or production of specific cells in the area. This process of attraction or stimulation is called chemotaxis.

A good example of chemotaxis is the series of events that causes vascular permeability. Vascular permeability is a crucial event in the early inflammation phase. It allows cells and chemicals that normally remain in the bloodstream to enter the injury site and perform their functions to ultimately heal the injured tissue and return the area to as close to normal as possible. Vascular permeability is initially caused by histamine in the area. Histamine is released by cells that enter the area, such as platelets, PMNs, and mast cells. Histamine is chemotactic for leukocytes, or white blood cells, causing them to enter the area. Histamine is a short-lived, local hormone whose function of vascular permeability is continued by serotonin and kinins that also enter the area. Serotonin is released by mast cells and platelets, and kinins are released by plasma.

The presence of kinins in the injury site is short term, but they are followed by prostaglandin (PG) formation. Once kinins are released and a Complement System is formed from serum proteins, PGs are discharged by cells that have been damaged. There are two PGs that are most evident and perform important functions: PGE_1 and PGE_2. The function of PGE_1 is to continue the vascular permeability in the local area. PGE_2 attracts leukocytes to the site. As healing progresses, they both appear to stimulate repair of the damaged area and permit advancement to the proliferative phase. They also seem to have a role in continuing inflammation at the same time (Salter et al. 1980). It is these compounds that are affected by anti-inflammatory drugs, discussed later in this chapter.

During all of this activity, additional chemical reactions are also occurring. Hageman factor, sometimes referred to as factor XII, is produced in the area. It acts to stimulate production of the enzyme kallikrein, which increases vascular permeability and vasodilation (Peacock 1984, p. 4).

Signs of Inflammation

Many complex events go on during the inflammation phase. The injured area undergoes intense activity during this time. We see evidence of the degree of activity as common signs of inflammation, including localized redness, edema, pain, increased temperature, and loss of normal function. Redness, increased local temperature, and edema are caused by the leakage of fluid, cells, and chemicals in the area because of the local vasodilation and increased vascular permeability. The increase in local cellular and chemical activity increases local temperature. Histamine and other released hormones and vasodilation cause redness. Edema is the result of increased substances in the area and blockage of lymph vessels whose normal responsibility of drainage is restricted by the newly formed fibrin plug. The chemical substances that are released at the site, such as histamine, prostaglandins, and bradykinin (Christie 1991; Kibler 1990), make the local nerve endings hypersensitive and irritable, causing pain. Pressure from edema on nerve endings also causes pain. Pain causes a withdrawal reflex, which reduces the function of surrounding structures, limiting the individual's normal functional ability. Direct damage to tissues also prevents them from functioning normally (Kibler 1990).

Proliferation Phase

There is an overlap of phases as the injury site heals. Figure 2.3 demonstrates that there is no clear-cut delineation between one phase and another. Rather, as the body steadily accomplishes the tasks in one phase, the next phase evolves.

Although many cells and chemicals are involved during the inflammation phase, the macrophages are most responsible for removing debris from the area. Once this task is accomplished, the next step in the healing process is the development and growth of new blood vessels and granulation tissue. This transition from debridement to angiogenesis and granulation tissue formation marks the beginning of the proliferation phase. Angiogenesis occurs at a rapid rate during this phase. This is important, for scar tissue formation requires vascular production and supply if subsequent events of healing are to follow.

The cells largely responsible for production of this new growth are fibroblasts. Fibroblasts are seen in greatly increased numbers three to five days following injury. Their increased numbers along with a decrease to minimal or nonexistent levels of PMNs are the hallmarks of the wound site's transition from inflammation to proliferation. Other activities that indicate that the injury has started transition into the proliferation phase include a significant increase in extracellular collagen production, increased proteoglycans, and epithelial cell mitosis (cell division). The duration of the proliferation phase depends on factors such as the size and site of the injury and the tissue type involved. Generally, the phase is thought to last two to four weeks (Peacock 1984, p. 13).

As is true during the inflammation phase, during the proliferation phase there is an interactive response among cells and chemicals in the area. Growth factors, for example, enter into the area through the chemotaxis produced by platelets and macrophages. In turn, these growth factors are responsible for the local migration and proliferation of fibroblasts, myofibroblasts, and endothelial cells.

The migration of fibroblasts is important during proliferation because these cells are primarily responsible for the development of new capillaries and the extracellular matrix. Fibroblasts produce substances that will eventually make up the matrix. These substances, which include collagen, proteoglycans, and elastin, are required for ultimate scar tissue formation and maturation (Kirsner and Eaglstein 1993).

Granulation tissue is the combination of the matrix and newly formed capillary buds. Granulation tissue is typically a bright, beefy red color. This is because the new capillary buds make up a significant part of the granulation tissue. Endothelial cells, the most important cell in the formation of these capillaries, contain a plasminogen activator. The plasminogen activator breaks down and removes the fibrin network that was formed during the inflammation phase so that lymphatic flow can be restored to remove local excess fluid.

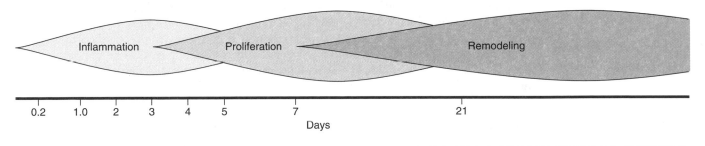

Figure 2.3 Tissue healing phases. Note the overlap of these phases.

The matrix has two components: fibrous and nonfibrous elements. The nonfibrous element is called **ground substance**. This is a gel-like substance composed of **glycosaminoglycan (GAG)**, proteoglycans, and **glycoproteins**. The ground substance fills in the spaces between the fibrous elements of the matrix and reduces friction between the fibers when stress is applied to the tissue.

Fibrous elements of the matrix include collagen, **reticulin**, and **elastin**. Collagen and reticulin are inelastic while elastin has elastic qualities. The combination of these types of fibers provides tensile strength and some resilience to stresses applied to the tissue.

During the proliferation phase, in the first five to seven days following injury, the fibroblasts produce these elements of the extracellular matrix. They form ground substance and rapidly lay down collagen. The activity during this phase is the result of new capillary growth by the fibroblasts. Epithelial advancement is followed by capillary growth across the granulating wound. As the epithelium progresses across the wound, epithelial cells and fibroblasts stimulated by the epithelial cells both release **collagenase**. Collagenase is an enzyme that prevents overproduction of collagen in the wound. This is an important process in normal tissue healing. An example of uncontrolled collagen production is keloid formations (excessive scar-tissue formations), a condition sometimes seen in dermal injuries.

Collagen produced in these early days of healing is type III collagen. It is seen as early as 48 to 72 h after the injury occurs (Kirsner and Eaglstein 1993). The fiber structure of type III collagen is weak and thin. Although it is relatively weak, it is the substance that provides the wound's primary tensile strength in the early stages of healing. Type III collagen is laid down in a haphazard manner, without organized arrangement, further reducing its strength. It is later replaced by type I collagen, a stronger and more durable collagen.

Tensile strength is directly related to the amount, type, and arrangement of collagen. By day 7 there is a significant amount of collagen in the area. By day 12 the immature type III collagen begins to be replaced by the stronger type I collagen. Both these occurrences add significant strength to the injury site.

While these processes are going on, a GAG known as **hyaluronic acid**, a part of the extracellular matrix, draws water into the area. This provides additional room for the proliferating fibroblasts in the wound site.

External signs of this phase demonstrate this ongoing activity. The combination of increased capillaries and additional water volume accounts for the redness and swelling in the area. Pressure-sensitive nerve endings cause the site to be sensitive to pressure just as the tension-sensitive nerve endings make the area painful when it is stretched.

Remodeling Phase

Some of the activities that begin during the proliferation phase continue during the remodeling phase. One example of this is wound contraction. Myofibroblasts are responsible for this activity. They have been observed in wounds by the fifth day and have been seen later than two months after the injury (Betz et al. 1992). Some of the fibroblasts convert to myofibroblasts to contract the wound's size. The entire mechanism is very complex and yet to be fully understood.

Wound contraction makes the scar smaller. This is advantageous, but it can be detrimental in situations in which joints are affected. If an injury occurs at or near a joint, scar tissue contraction and adhesions can cause a loss of motion at that joint. Indirect effects of wound contraction may occur if the wound is large and affects adjacent areas. The importance of preventing the adverse effects of scar tissue contraction is discussed later in this chapter in the section "The Role of Therapeutic Exercise in Healing."

Another activity that begins during the proliferation phase and continues into the remodeling phase is collagen transition. As type I collagen is synthesized, type III collagen is destroyed. When the construction rate equals the destruction rate, the healing process evolves to the final and longest phase, remodeling. This phase is generally thought to be about 12 months long, but may range from 6 months to 18 months (Connolly 1988).

A number of activities diminish as the area becomes more stable and more permanent in its cellular and structural arrangement. The large number of capillaries that were produced during the proliferation phase to promote tissue growth is no longer needed and begins to recede. The extra capillaries will eventually disappear entirely (Peacock 1984, p. 13). Glycoproteins, GAGs, and the cells responsible for them—fibroblasts—in the extracellular matrix decrease significantly. Myofibroblasts also diminish.

With these cellular changes, visible changes can also be observed. These include the loss of the scar's red color with progressive change to white and eventually more normal skin tones. With the loss of extracellular matrix substances, swelling is diminished. Wound sensitivity is also lessened.

As collagen is converted to predominantly type I, it becomes more insoluble and less resistant to destruction. As fluid is reduced in the area, the collagen fibers can produce more cross-links with each other, further strengthening the scar's structure. This collagen cross-linking becomes the primary source of the scar's tensile strength.

The maturation of the wound's collagen structure and arrangement is the primary activity during the remodeling phase, hence its name. Collagen strength is enhanced by the arrangement of collagen fibers. When collagen fibers are aligned in an organized, parallel fashion, collagen can form the greatest number of cross-links and thereby possess optimal strength. The greatest degree of function and mobility is also provided when collagen has this organized arrangement (Peacock 1984, p. 188). Properly applied external forces enhance it.

Phases of Healing

Here is a summary of the three phases of healing, when they occur, their characteristics, and the goals during each phase.

Phase	Duration	Characteristics	Goal
Inflammation	Up to about 5 d	At onset of injury area is warm, red, swollen, and tender.	Stabilize and contain area of injury.
Proliferation	Up to about 21 d	Scar tissue is red and larger than normal because of edema.	Dispose of dead tissue, mobilize fibroblasts, and restore circulation.
Remodeling	Up to 1 y	Water content of the scar is reduced; vascularity and redness are reduced; scar-tissue density increases.	Stabilize and reestablish the area.

Table 2.2 summarizes in chronological order the phases of healing and identifies the primary activities and their time line.

GROWTH FACTORS

▶Growth factors assist healing by causing cell proliferation and attracting fibroblasts, macrophages, and other cells needed for healing.

Growth factors are proteins that serve many functions. They interact with each other and other substances to promote the healing process. Their role is complex and not yet fully understood. One reason their function is difficult to understand is that their action in vitro is different than in vivo, so what is observed in the laboratory is not necessarily what occurs in the body. Another clouding factor is that what they are seen doing in laboratory animals is not necessarily what occurs in humans.

Specific growth factors perform specific tasks that affect specific cells to speed and enhance the healing process. Growth factors are named for the target cell they affect, their source, or their behavior. For example, the growth factor affecting the epidermis is called epidermal growth factor (EGF), the growth factor derived from platelets is called **platelet-derived**

Table 2.2
Chronology of Wound Healing

Phase	Time	Activity	Purpose/Result
Inflammation	1 d	Neutrophil migration	Fight contamination. Release growth factors and biologically reactive substances.
Inflammation	1 d	Fibrin bridge creation	Area is red, warm, swollen, tender to touch.
Inflammation	1-2 d	→ Monocyte migration	Phagocytose bacteria
Inflammation	2 d	Angiogenesis	Ingrowing fibroblasts
Inflammation	2-3 d	Fibroblasts produce type III collagen	
Proliferation	3-4 d	→ Rapid increase in fibroblasts Increased epithelial cell mitosis Increased synthesis of extracellular collagen Increased proteoglycans	
Proliferation	5 d	→ Myofibroblast production	Wound contraction
Proliferation	5-7 d	Collagen synthesis very active	
Remodeling	5-9 d	Reduction in fibroblasts Reduction in macrophages Reduction in wound vascularity → Reduction in fibronectin in proportion to the amount of type I collagen formed	Less redness
Remodeling	10 d	Wound contraction	
Remodeling	12 d	→ Type III collagen converting to type I	
Remodeling	6-18 wk	→ Reduction in capillaries	Reduced fluid content, increased scar density
Remodeling	6-18 mo	Completion of all healing	

→ = key activities of each phase.

growth factor (PDGF), and transforming growth factors (TGFs) transform substances. Many of these growth factors work together to cause desired results in healing. Some of them are chemotactic, and others stimulate cell production.

Growth factors play a role in several key activities of healing. They control the migration and proliferation of cells vital to wound healing, including fibroblasts, macrophages, epithelial cells, and endothelial cells. Some growth factors are important in the early hours of inflammation, acting as stimulators of vasoconstriction and vasodilation. Growth factors also affect the formation of the fibrin plug. Others play roles in controlling macrophages and prevent phagocytization of healthy cells. In the proliferation phase, some growth factors assist and coordinate the capillary endothelial production. A number of growth factors are responsible for angiogenesis, granulation tissue, and collagen production. Growth factors in the remodeling phase stimulate the degradation of type III collagen and the synthesis of type I collagen.

A few growth factors stand out as primary players in healing and are worth identifying. One group is the EGFs. They stimulate production of a number of cells, including epithelial cells, endothelial cells, and fibroblasts. EGFs also draw epithelial cells into the damaged area and stimulate fibroblasts to produce GAG.

Another important group of growth factors is the fibroblast growth factors (FGF). They are believed to be primarily responsible for formation of the new vascular and granulation tissue following injury. They promote angiogenesis by stimulating fibroblasts and capillary endothelial cell proliferation. They also stimulate production of chondrocytes (cartilage cells), keratinocytes (keratin-producing epidermal cells), and myoblasts.

The PDGF group is a family of growth factors that facilitate production of collagenase by stimulating fibroblast activity. The PDGFs are particularly active during the remodeling phase, when they prepare the extracellular matrix. They are produced by a variety of cells, including macrophages, fibroblasts, epithelial cells, and vascular endothelial cells.

The primary TGF in wound healing is TGF-beta. This growth factor has a number of responsibilities. It is involved in stimulating extracellular matrix production and coordinating the process of neovascularization (angiogeneisis). TGF-beta also coordinates other growth factors to regulate the healing process.

Keep in mind that many other growth factors play roles in wound healing. As mentioned, their function is not entirely understood, but their presence is vital if healing is to occur. Table 2.3 summarizes the most common growth factors in the healing process.

Table 2.3

Common Growth Factors in Healing

Growth factor	Source	Target	Cell proliferation and chemotactic activity
EGF	Epithelial cells Macrophages Platelets	Fibroblasts Epithelial cells	Re-epithelialization Angiogenesis Collagenase activity
FGF	Macrophages Endothelial cells	Fibroblasts Endothelial cells	Angiogenesis Granulation tissue
PDGF	Platelets Macrophages Endothelial cells Epithelial cells	Fibroblasts	Fibroblast production Deposition of extracellular matrix
TGF	Macrophages Platelets Epithelium	Endothelial cells Fibroblasts Epithelial cells	Deposition of extracellular matrix Inhibition of epidermal proliferation

Chronic Inflammation

Normal healing of tissue occurs in the sequence just described. Occasionally, the injury does not progress along this process as it should. It gets stuck in the inflammation phase and is unable to proceed in healing. This condition is referred to as *chronic inflammation.* Recall that in acute inflammation, the large number of granular leukocytes that initially invades the area is replaced with mononuclear phagocytes. The cells are transformed into larger macrophages and giant cells to debride the area. As the area is cleared of waste and foreign matter, these cells diminish in number, but in chronic inflammations they persist at the site.

The continued presence of macrophages and giant cells is a key characteristic of chronic inflammation. The granular leukocytes have not been successful in fully debriding these areas, so the mononuclear phagocytes persist to rid the area of unwelcome substances. Their proliferation continues as long as these irritating substances prevail at the injury site.

In open wounds the persistence of foreign substances, such as bacteria, causes continued inflammation. If an insoluble, nonphagotizable foreign substance, such as a sand grain or unabsorbed extracellular blood, is the cause of chronic inflammation, the area's response is the formation of a granuloma. The macrophages become chemotactic for fibroblasts to invade the area. The foreign substance becomes surrounded by the collagen that these fibroblasts produce to isolate the substance and form a granuloma.

It has been shown that chronic wounds have deficient growth factor levels (Hom 1995). The introduction of growth factors such as PDGF, TGF-beta, and others has improved healing. According to Hom, studies have also revealed that protease occurs at higher levels in chronic wounds. Protease degrades growth factors to prevent their presence in the wound. The studies that have investigated chronic wounds and growth factors have looked at several different effects, causes, and preventions and have all come up with one conclusion: Growth factors are necessary for proper healing, and when they are not present, healing is impaired or prevented.

Although not technically a chronic wound condition, overuse injuries are frequently so classified. Overuse and overloading activities lead to cumulative trauma that exceeds the area's stress resistance. This is actually a continual re-injury, not a chronic wound. Overuse and overloading conditions are discussed in chapter 15.

HEALING OF SPECIFIC TISSUES

▶Although all tissues follow the same general steps in healing, the course of healing in different tissues, such as ligaments, tendons, muscles, cartilage, and bone—varies and involves events specific to the tissue.

Specific types and compositions of tissue show some variations in the healing sequence, although each tissue proceeds from inflammation to remodeling generally following the time line. Given structural, cellular, and chemical differences, however, it is not reasonable to expect muscle tissue, for example, to proceed along the exact recovery time line that bone or ligament follows. Let's take a look at some of the differences in tissues that we commonly see traumatized in musculoskeletal injuries.

Ligaments

When a ligament is torn, frayed stump ends are present where the ligament has been separated. The ligament undergoes the expected inflammation process, including local edema formation. The injured ligament stumps become surrounded with fluid, causing the ends to become friable, or easily crumbled. Vascular permeability increases and permits the normal inflammatory products, including PMNs and lymphocytes, to invade the area. Erythrocytes and other cells accumulate to fill the gap between the stump ends. Within the first day, macrophages and monocytes enter the area to begin debridement. Table 2.4 summarizes the time line of ligamentous tissue healing.

Within 48 to 72 h after the injury, the proliferation phase begins with extracellular matrix development and proceeds through production of collagen and ground substance by the fibroblasts. This phase continues for up to six weeks (Andriacchi et al. 1988). Other routine processes occur during this phase, including capillary-bud formation that eventually joins

Table 2.4
Ligament Healing Time Line

Time	Activity
First few hours	The injury site fills with erythrocytes, leukocytes, and lymphocytes. The ligament stumps become progressively more friable with the accumulation of serous fluid in the area.
24 h	Monocytes and macrophages infiltrate the area. Fibroblasts begin to appear and eventually become significant in number.
48-72 h	Fibroblasts produce the extracellular matrix.
1-2 wk	Fibrocytes and macrophages are numerous. Random collagen fibers and abundant ground substance are seen. Fragile vascular granulation tissue is seen at the injury site. The extracellular matrix continues to be synthesized by fibroblasts. Macrophages, mast cells, and fibroblasts continue to predominate. Vascular buds appear in the wound to communicate with existing capillaries. Elastin is seen in the area.
2 d-6 wk	Proliferation phase occurs, during which cellular and matrix structures replace the blood clot formed during inflammation.
6 wk-12 mo	Macrophages and fibroblasts diminish.
Up to 12 mo	Collagen concentration stabilizes with type I collagen replacing type III and collagen cross-links increasing in number. Ligament becomes more normal.
40-50 wk	Near-normal tensile strength is restored.

with existing vessels. Phagocytosis also continues during this time. The quantity of collagen being synthesized is greater than the amount being degraded, so there is an increase in net collagen during this time.

Several weeks later the remodeling phase is heralded by the conversion of type III collagen to type I collagen and an increase in the number of collagen cross-links. There is also a reduction of edema, fibroblasts, and macrophages, and the area takes on a more normal appearance. This final stage may take one year or more to complete.

Tendons

As with ligaments, the tendon inflammatory phase is approximately three days long (Gelberman, Banes, and Goldberg 1988). Tendons have support from local structures that aid in the initial healing process. These structures include the periosteum of underlying bone, the synovial sheath, the epitenon, and the endotenon. They provide the vascular supply and fibroblasts that are needed for healing. The epitenon and endotenon provide macrophage-like cells and fibroblasts to begin debridement. Table 2.5 summarizes the tendon healing time line.

Within the first week, collagen synthesis begins and continues at a rapid rate for the first four weeks (Gelberman, Banes, and Goldberg 1988). During the second week, the collagen starts to become more organized, so by the end of the second week the cells are beginning to align themselves in the direction of stress. Collagen synthesis continues until day 35 (Peacock 1984, p. 319). Granulation tissue produced by fibroblasts migrating from surrounding connective tissue and from the tendon sheath is also seen in rapidly forming quantities. By day 28 collagen and active fibroblasts producing the collagen are clearly aligned along the tendon's long axis. This assists the remaining collagen to form in a proper orientation.

During the first three weeks, the area undergoes a significant revascularization. Because of this restoration of blood supply, it is possible to begin mobilization of a surgically repaired tendon by day 21. Immobilization prior to this time is important to allow reconstruction and restoration of local circulation because circulation is so vital to the tendon's successful recovery and function. Thus, immobilization is necessary not for the tendon to reconnect, but for the blood supply to be restored.

Table 2.5
Tendon Healing Time Line

Time	Activity
First 3 days	Cells that originate from extrinsic peritendinous tissue and from intrinsic tissue from the epitenon and endotenon are active.
5 d	Wound gap is filled by phagocytes.
1 wk	Collagen synthesis is initiated, with new collagen fibers placed in a random and disorganized way.
10 d	Collagen synthesis is maximal.
3 wk	The endotenon provides significant fibroblast proliferation in the injury site. Significant revascularization occurs. The synovial sheath is rebuilt, and a smooth gliding surface develops. Fibroblasts also start to become oriented in line with the tendon's axis.
4 wk	Fibroblasts predominate in the healing area. Collagen content increases. Collagen is fully oriented with the tendon's long axis.
35 d	Collagen synthesis is completed.
42 d	Fibroblasts that have proliferated from the endotenon are the primary cells, simultaneously synthesizing collagen while contributing to collagen resorption.
2 mo	Collagen is mature and realigned along the tendon's axis.
112 d	Fibroblasts have reverted to tenocytes, type III collagen has been replaced by type I, and maturation is complete.
40-50 wk	Strength is 85%-95% normal.

Also by three weeks, the synovial sheath has been reconstituted. This is important so the tendon has a smooth gliding surface within which to move. When type III collagen has been replaced with type I collagen and the fibroblasts revert to their original status as **tenocytes**, the remodeling phase is finished. This occurs by day 112 (Gelberman, Banes, and Goldberg 1988).

When a tendon is surgically repaired, the tendon and the surrounding soft tissue, including blood vessels, fascia, and skin, all become one wound. The area is filled with a sticky gel. This gel is viscous and has the potential to become a thick, dense scar. If formed, the scar will limit the gliding of the tendon and thereby impede function of the muscle, ultimately limiting the success of rehabilitation (Peacock 1965). For normal function to return, the scar tissue must not bind together the normally separate structures at the site but instead allow the tendon to glide within its sheath, the skin to move freely from subcutaneous structures, and the blood vessels and nerves to have normal mobility so that all structures can function normally. One major factor that determines the success of this separation of elements is how long immobilization is maintained and when motion is initiated. The effects of immobilization are discussed in further detail in chapter 5.

Muscles

Although muscle tissue may heal like the other tissues we have discussed, following the same three phases to ultimately produce scar tissue, muscle has unique structures within it that permit it to also regenerate. These structures are called **satellite cells**. These cells fuse with adjacent myofibers to repair and regenerate muscle tissue. It is believed that some destruction of muscle tissue occurs daily in routine activities. This destruction also occurs when an uninjured individual exercises. The satellite cells play a role in the restoration and replacement of muscle cells routinely damaged during activity (Caplan et al. 1988). If an injury is sufficiently small, revascularized, reinnervated, and involves a muscle type that can regenerate, satellite cells replace injured muscle tissue with new muscle tissue. Table 2.6 summarizes the muscle's healing time line.

Table 2.6
Muscle Healing Time Line

Time	Activity
6 h	Fragmentation of injured muscle fibers begins. Macrophages appear.
1-4 d	Fibroblasts appear.
	Ability to produce muscle tension is progressively reduced.
1 wk	Scar tissue is seen in large muscle injuries.
	Muscle is able to produce near-normal tension.
7-11 d	Tensile strength reaches near normal.
10 d	Large number of phagocytes, primarily macrophages, are seen at the injury site.
13 d	Regenerating myotubes are seen.
18 d	Cross-striated muscle fibers appear.
6 wk-6 mo	Contraction ability is 90% normal.

In the early hours of healing, injured muscle tissue appears to follow the same route of other tissue: Phagocytes, primarily macrophages, invade the site within 6 h following an injury. Macrophages are the predominant cell in the area for the next 10 days as they work to debride the area. In the proliferation phase, muscle tissue regeneration is begun as myogenic cells are activated. These evolve into myoblasts, which fuse together to form myotubes. Myotubes are seen in the injury site by day 13. Through a complex progression of events, these myotubes become muscle fibers and are apparent in the area by day 18. Final muscle regeneration is completed with the development of the neural aspect of the neuromuscular structure. When the process is complete, satellite cell levels return to normal and resume their daily function of less-intensive, ongoing muscle tissue replacement.

Larger muscle injuries are unable to repair by regeneration and must resort to scar tissue as the means of healing. When the mass of damaged muscle is larger than 3 g (0.1 oz), the muscle heals via the scarring process and goes through the normal sequence of healing.

Cartilage

There are different types of cartilage. Hyaline cartilage dissipates loads in joints. Commonly referred to as articular cartilage, it lines the surfaces of the diarthrodial joints. Fibrocartilage transfers loads between the tendons and ligaments and the bone. Examples of fibrocartilage are found in the intervertebral disks and the temporomandibular joint. Elastic cartilage provides a flexible support to external structures and is similar to hyaline cartilage.

As a rule, cartilage is composed primarily of type II collagen. When tissue healing occurs, type I collagen is the primary resulting collagen, so the ultimate structure changes if scar tissue is produced. Cartilage does have some regenerative capability. The difficulty in cartilage healing is that cartilage is regenerated at a slower rate than scar tissue is deposited. Fibrocartilage seems to have a better capacity to regenerate than articular cartilage (Silver and Glasgold 1995).

Whether cartilage regeneration or scar tissue occurs depends on three variables: the depth of the defect, the maturity of the cartilage, and the location of the defect (Silver and Glasgold 1995). Small, full-thickness defects are repaired by regeneration of fibrocartilage, but partial-thickness defects are repaired with scar tissue. For this reason, a surgeon may opt to place burr holes in an arthritic joint to stimulate the production of fibrocartilaginous tissue to repair the defect and provide some joint protection.

The healing course of articular cartilage once again follows a sequence of events initiated with macrophages and fibrin-plug formation. Fibroblasts appear in the area to perform their rebuilding tasks. As the site advances into the remodeling phase, collagen becomes the prevalent structure. See Table 2.7 for a general outline of the sequence of events in cartilage healing.

For regeneration of cartilage to occur, the following conditions must be present (Buckwalter et al. 1988):

- Cells that will proliferate and differentiate into chondrocytes must be located in or migrate to the wound site.
- A mechanical stimulus that enhances articular cartilage formation must be present.
- Protection from excessive loads must be sufficient to allow cartilage repair without causing damage.
- A normal joint conformation must be maintained or restored.

A procedure to replace articular cartilage with homogeneous cartilage was reported by Brittberg et al. (1994) from the University of Gloteborg, Sweden. Some hyaline cartilage is first removed from the patient's unaffected joint area then grown in a lab to increase the quantity before finally being re-implanted in the cartilage defect site. This is known as the Swedish procedure. The procedure is currently being used in isolated situations and has not yet obtained approval by the Food and Drug Administration (FDA) for standard use in the United States.

Even more recent attempts have been made at the Stone Foundation for Sports Medicine and Arthritis Research in San Francisco (http://www.stonefoundation.com/frame.htm) using homogeneous grafts to transplant articular cartilage into arthritic joints without culturing the hyaline cartilage in a laboratory. This procedure is still at the experimental stage, but results have been promising.

Bone

As with other tissues, bone tissue has an inflammation phase that lasts three to four days (Heppenstall 1980), during which time fibroblasts and macrophages invade the area. The necrotic ends of the fractured bone and metabolic wastes are debrided by osteoclasts to clear the way and set the stage for the next phase.

During this next phase the bone demonstrates its ability to regenerate. Osteoblasts, bone-generating cells, invade the area via the periosteum. As these cells go to work, a callus is formed at the site of each bone fragment end. This soft callus, whose formation takes three to four weeks, is a fibrous matrix of collagen that eventually becomes bone. The callus has an internal component and an external component. The external callus immobilizes the

Table 2.7
Articular Cartilage Healing Time Line

Time	Activity
48 h	Fibrin clot is formed to fill the defect.
5 d	Fibroblasts are in the area and combine with collagen fibers to replace the clot.
2 wk	Fibroblasts differentiate, and islands of chondrocytes appear.
1 mo	Fibroblasts have been completely differentiated.
2 mo	Satisfactory repair has occurred, with the defect resembling cartilage in appearance. The majority of collagen present, however, is type I.
6 mo	A combination of type I and type II calcified cartilage has a normal appearance.

fragment ends, eventually bridges the two fragments, and allows stress to be applied to the bone without harming the fracture site before it is completely healed. By the third week, the bony ends have become united. It takes approximately 40 days from the time of injury for the fracture site to become mechanically stable. Table 2.8 demonstrates the healing time line of bone.

As the osteoblasts move along the stump ends and farther away from the blood supply, they convert to chondrocytes, which produce a layer of cartilage. The chondrocytes are in turn covered by osteogenic cells, which are also covered by a fibrous layer. This process occurs simultaneously on the external and internal layers in the bone's marrow cavity. The soft callus matures into a hard callus as the fibrous matrix converts into spongy bone. In a not fully understood process, the spongy bone converts to normal compact bone over time. In the long bones of adults, this routinely takes three to four months (Heppenstall 1980, pp. 42–44).

During the remodeling phase, the callus size is reduced, the medullary canal is reestablished, the conversion to bone tissue is finalized, and normal oxygen and electrical levels are restored (Lane and Werntz 1987, p. 55).

TENSILE STRENGTH DURING HEALING

▶ Tensile strength takes a year or more to reach near-normal levels after an injury and seldom returns to its preinjury level, but the strength of surrounding tissues may permit a return to sport participation or normal activity sooner than that.

Tensile strength is the maximal amount of stress or force that a structure is able to withstand before tissue failure occurs. In other words, it is the amount of outside force that can be applied to a muscle, tendon, ligament, or bone before it tears or breaks. Healthy tissue is able to withstand high amounts of tensile force. Once injured, however, tissue's tensile strength seldom returns to 100% of its prior level.

This is about the only fact on which researchers of tensile strength agree. Disagreements arise because of variations in research techniques, the animals and specific structures investigated, the degrees of the injuries studied, and the results of in vitro versus in vivo studies all vary. It is difficult to extrapolate findings of research with animals to humans, and it is even more difficult to obtain humans who are willing to be injured to study the in vivo effects of injury on tensile strength. Studies investigating tensile strength are limited because the tensile strength of a structure can be affected by surrounding tissues that contribute strength through their own framework, function, configuration, or attachments in the area.

The contributing strength of surrounding tissues may explain why athletes often return to full competition without becoming reinjured six months after reconstructive surgery, even

Table 2.8
Bone Healing Time Line

Time	Activity
Immediately	PMNs, plasma, and lympocytes occur.
First few hours	Fibroblasts invade the area.
3-4 d	Hematoma forms. Fractured edges become necrotic. Mast cells occur at the site.
	Macrophages remove debris. Osteoclasts mobilize in the area.
Up to 4 wk	Osteoblasts ~~Osteoclasts~~ proliferate to form soft callus. Cartilage cells are seen.
3-4 wk	Hard callus develops. Osteoclasts continue to remove dead bone. Endosteal blood supply continues to develop.
4-6 wk	External blood supply dominates.
6-10 wk	Medullary circulation is re-established.
3-4 mo	Fracture is healed, but remodeling continues.
12 wk	Near-normal strength is attained.

though the tissue has not yet regained its full tensile strength. There are many unanswered questions about the tensile strength of healing and healed tissue; nevertheless, clinicians must be aware of current knowledge, incomplete though it may be.

During the inflammation phase, normal tensile strength declines rapidly to 50% (Gelberman et al. 1988; Gelberman et al. 1982). Depending on the tissue type involved, this decline occurs in 24 h to 48 h. In the very early stage of healing, the injured site's strength derives from the fibrin clot, which is insufficient to withstand much stress. Tensile strength is at its lowest during this time. Around day 5, tensile strength begins to increase. Without significant collagen, the injured tissue relies on other structures in the area, including the granulation tissue and ground substance, for this increase in strength.

As collagen becomes more plentiful and cross-links develop, the area's tensile strength becomes greater. Collagen conversion from type III to type I and the increased number of cross-links are the core reasons for tensile strength development.

Studies have demonstrated that time for tensile strength development in muscle varies, depending on the animal investigated. Rat studies show that by six weeks after injury, 90% of normal tensile strength is achieved, and in the cat it takes six months (Caplan et al. 1988). Bone strength is returned to 83% of normal 12 weeks after injury (Grundnes and Reikeras 1992). Ligaments and tendons vary in the time it takes to achieve near-normal strength, depending on the specific structure. These tissues approach near-normal levels anywhere from 17 to 50 weeks after injury (Nordin and Frankel 1980).

Researchers agree that once an injury occurs, the structure involved never regains full tensile strength. Tensile strength initially increases rapidly after an injury, then slows and even regresses as type III collagen degrades and is replaced with type I collagen. Depending on the structure, it may take a year or more for an injured part to regain maximal tensile strength.

FACTORS THAT AFFECT HEALING

▶ Factors that affect healing include the treatment modality, drugs, surgical repair, patient's age, systemic diseases suffered by the patient, injury size, infection, nutrition, spasm, and swelling.

A number of outside influences can profoundly or subtly affect the healing process. Some of these factors can be applied by clinicians to assist or stimulate the healing process. Others can be controlled by the patient, parents, or physician. Still others, such as age and systemic diseases, cannot be controlled.

Figure 2.4 outlines the injury and healing process and the difference an effective rehabilitation program can have on tissue healing and its outcome. It is important for a clinician to know appropriate techniques that positively influence the healing process.

Treatment Modalities

Some of the treatment modalities most frequently used to enhance healing include electrical stimulation, and thermal modalities such as ice, superficial heat, and deep heat.

There is an excellent profile of modalities and their effects on tissue healing in Craig Denegar and colleagues' (2005) Athletic Training Education Series text, *Therapeutic Modalities for Musculoskeletal Injuries, Second Edition*. Refer to his text for specific information on how modalities can affect the signs of inflammation.

Ice is used during rehabilitation to reduce inflammation caused by therapeutic exercise. Occasionally after therapeutic exercise such as vigorous stretching or strengthening, signs of new inflammation, such as increased edema, may occur. Although ice will not affect existing edema, it can reduce new edema that results from overstretching or over-strengthening exercises. Remember that tissue irritation should be avoided; however, there may be occasions when it is unavoidable. At such times, ice should be used preemptively to quell new pain and edema.

Electrical stimulation during the first week after injury has been shown to enhance protein synthesis to help promote healing. It also increases the tensile strength of tendons (Enwemeka 1989). Because tendon and ligament structures are similar, it may also have the same effects when applied to ligaments.

Electrical stimulation can also be applied to muscles to relax muscle spasm. When facilitating muscle contraction, electrical stimulation may also assist in relieving local edema by

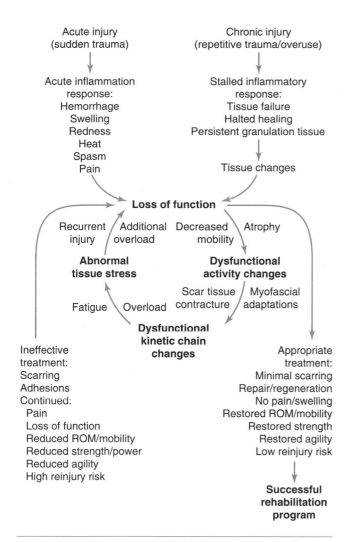

Figure 2.4   Effects of treatment on healing.
Adapted by permission from W.B. Leadbetter 1994.

pumping fluid into the lymph system, which reduces pain. With less pain, the patient may exercise more willingly.

Muscle atrophy following injury or prolonged inactivity can be retarded by electrical stimulation. After prolonged inactivity, electrical stimulation is often used to facilitate muscle contraction and encourage reactivation and recruitment of dormant fibers. During short-term denervation, it may be used to facilitate muscle contraction until nerve function is restored.

After the inflammatory phase, heat can be advantageous when applied prior to exercise. It can increase circulation to encourage healing and better exchange nutrients and waste products, relax muscles to allow better exercise execution with less pain, and reduce tissue viscosity to make an area more pliable for stretching.

Ultrasound has the benefit of producing thermal as well as mechanical effects. A contraindication to continuous ultrasound is in the acute inflammatory phase, when heat is deleterious. At that time, pulsed ultrasound is indicated. It is believed that ultrasound promotes collagen, neovascular, and myofibroblast production. As a source of deep heat, it may be a useful prestretch application for tendon and capsular adhesions that lie deeper than superficial heat can reach effectively.

It is important for the rehabilitation clinician to know the desired results and choose a modality that best facilitates those results. As the patient progresses in the rehabilitation program, fewer modalities are required because the injury is more closely approaching normal function and metabolism. For example, as the patient enters the final stages of therapeutic exercise, ice is not needed following the therapeutic exercise program. If the patient continues to have swelling or pain that requires ice application following a therapeutic exercise routine, the cause for these symptoms should be examined because these symptoms should not occur late in rehabilitation.

Drugs

The injured individual often consults with a rehabilitation clinician for information about the drugs that have been prescribed after an injury. Therefore, the rehabilitation clinician should have a basic understanding of medications, be aware of his or her own limited knowledge, and readily refer the patient to either the physician or the pharmacist for information beyond the scope of his or her knowledge.

Rehabilitation clinicians should remember certain general rules of thumb about medication. All drugs, even vitamins, have the potential to produce undesirable side effects. Any drug should be used with caution and taken according to recommendations of the physician, pharmacist, or manufacturer of over-the-counter (OTC) medications. If undesirable side effects occur, the physician should be contacted for instructions to either discontinue the medication or alter its administration. All drugs have a duration of action, the length of time that the amount of drug in the blood is above the level needed to obtain a minimal therapeutic effect. This length of time is determined by the half-life of the drug. The half-life is the amount of time it takes for the level of the drug in the bloodstream to diminish by half. The frequency with which the drug is administered is based on the half-life. The shorter the half-life, the more frequently the drug must be administered to obtain a minimal therapeutic effect. The example given in Houglum (1998) demonstrates this concept: Naproxen, with a half-life of about 14 h, is administered twice a day, whereas ibuprofen, with a half-life of around 2 h, is administered three to four times a day.

A goal of drug administration is to achieve a steady state. A **steady state** occurs when the average level of drug remains constant in the blood, that is, when the amount absorbed into the blood equals the amount removed through metabolism or excretion. After the first few administrations of the drug, the amount of drug in the bloodstream increases until this steady state is achieved. As a rule of thumb, a steady state is achieved after the dosing of the drug has continued for a time equal to 4-5 half-lives. For example, using 5 half-lives to calculate the time needed to reach steady-state, if a drug has a half-life of 12 h and is given twice a day, a steady state is achieved by the middle of the third day (5 × 12 h). If a drug has a half-life of 2 h and is administered every 6 h, a steady state occurs following the third dose (5 × 2 h), because the first dose is at time 0, the second is at 6 h, the third at 12 h, and so on. The difference between 4 and 5 half-lives is nominal: After 4 half-lives, a steady-state of 94% is reached, and is increased to 97% after 5 half-lives (Houglum et al 2005). A patient's compliance in taking medication is important for achieving a steady state and the desired results. If a patient fails to take prescribed medication, the intended results may not be achieved. By the same token, taking more than the prescribed dosage may not produce better results faster. In fact, it can be deleterious. "More is better" does not apply to drug dosages. Taking higher or more frequent doses of a drug causes higher concentrations and may cause toxic side effects. Taking two different anti-inflammatory drugs, whether they are prescription or OTC medications, should also be avoided because it is equivalent to increasing dosage and can be dangerous. These important precautions should be pointed out to the patient when taking medications.

Most drugs taken by mouth are absorbed in the small intestine. If medication is taken with liquid, a full glass of liquid is advisable, not just a swallow. The liquid helps dissolve the medication and also increases the speed with which the drug moves from the stomach to the small intestine. If a drug is to be taken with food, it is absorbed at a slower rate, but the food may reduce otherwise irritating effects on the stomach.

Other factors that alter drug absorption include exercise immediately following ingestion, since blood normally allotted to the gastrointestinal tract is shunted to working muscles. With delayed movement of medication from the stomach to the small intestine, irritation of the stomach lining may increase (Houglum 1998). For this reason, it may not be a good idea to take an anti-inflammatory medication immediately before exercise, especially when the stomach is empty.

NSAIDs

Among the most commonly prescribed drugs in medicine today are anti-inflammatory drugs (Leadbetter 1990). The most frequently used of these are the non-steroidal anti-inflammatory drugs (NSAIDs). Although research does not demonstrate a significant advantage of NSAIDs for injuries, there is enough evidence to warrant their use. The NSAIDs are used to reduce pain and promote healing by minimizing inflammation in both acute and chronic injuries. The NSAIDs reduce inflammation by inhibiting the enzymes cyclooxygenase-1 (COX-1) and cyclooxygenase-2 (COX-2). The primary reason for NSAID use in musculoskeletal injury therapy is to reduce pain by inhibiting prostaglandin (PG) production. PGs stimulate local nociceptors (pain-receptive nerve endings) and enhance edema formation by increasing vascular permeability. By limiting PG production, NSAIDs can encourage healing progression from the inflammation phase to the proliferation phase. By reducing edema and pain, range of motion and other therapeutic exercises can begin sooner to promote recovery.

Several prescription and OTC NSAIDs are now available on the market. Refer to table 2.9 for a list of commonly used NSAIDs. Individuals respond differently to each of these drugs. Generally, the amount of NSAID in the OTC dosage is half the equivalent prescription medication. One person may find better results from aspirin, whereas another may find aspirin ineffective but have great relief from ibuprofen. Another person may find that naproxen upsets the stomach but have no problem with tolmetin. Physicians commonly try a different NSAID if a patient does not respond appropriately to the first. Because each person responds differently, trial and error is often used to discover the medication that is most effective in achieving desired therapy goals.

Steroid medication is also used to control inflammation, but its use is currently limited because of its severe side effects. It is usually prescribed in large doses for a short amount of time. Administration is closely monitored by the prescribing physician because of the possible side effects.

Because NSAIDs inhibit the production of PGs through alteration of arachidonic acid metabolism, other physiological functions are also affected. Besides affecting the inflammation phase of local injuries, PGs play an important role in protecting the stomach lining.

Table 2.9
NSAIDs

Generic name	Brand name	Doses/d	Maximum daily adult dose (mg)[1]
Nonselective COX inhibitors:			
Aspirin[2]	many	4	6000
Fenoprofen	Nalfon	3-4	3200
Flurbiprofen	Ansaid	2-3	300
Ibuprofen[2]	Advil	3-4	3200
Indomethacin	Indocin	2-3	200
Ketoprofen[2]	Actron	3-4	300
Naproxen Na[2]	Aleve	2	1375
Piroxicam	Feldene	1	20
Sulindac	Clinoril	2	400
Tolmetin Na	Tolectin	3-4	2000
Diclofenac	Voltaren	2-4	150
Oxaprozin	Daypro	1	1800
Selective COX-2 inhibitors:			
Celecoxib	Celebrex	1-2	400
Valdecoxib	Bextra	1-2	40
Slightly-Selective COX-2 inhibitors			
Etokolac	Lodine	2-3	1200
Meloxicam	Mobic	1	7.5
Nabumetone	Relafen	1-2	2000

[1]Typical daily dose may be considerably less.

[2]Available without prescription.

Adapted from J. Houglum 1998.

Therefore, one of the most common side effects of NSAIDs is stomach upset. For this reason, people with a history of ulcers or allergy to aspirin should not use NSAIDs. Stomach upset, nausea, and vomiting are possible side effects and may be reason for the patient to discontinue NSAID use. Generally, the tendency for stomach upset and ulcers increases the longer a person uses NSAIDs.

NSAIDs may also be harmful to kidney and cardiac functions. Arachidonic acid plays an important role in renal physiology, so people with renal disease may not be able to use NSAIDs. Because of the heart's relationship to renal function, people with congestive heart failure should avoid NSAIDs.

Like most drugs, NSAIDs should be avoided by women who are pregnant or nursing infants since NSAIDs may be harmful to the fetus or infant.

A new family of NSAIDs was approved by the FDA in the late 1990s. These drugs primarily inhibit COX-2, by their influence on arachidonic acid metabolism. The more traditional NSAIDs are nonselective and affect both COX-1 and COX-2 to varying degrees. COX-1 enzyme is involved in many homeostatic processes in the body such as renal function, bronchial tone, platelet aggregation, temperature regulation, gastric mucosa protection, and others (Urban 2000). On the other hand, function of the COX-2 occurs primarily in the inflammation process. While the nonspecific NSAIDs inhibit both COX-1 and COX-2, the selective COX-2 inhibitors isolate their activity to the inflammation-producing activity of COX-2, so these newer NSAIDs reduce inflammation with less impact on gastric and kidney cells and other normal essential functions dependent upon COX-1.

As a rule, disregarding side effects, a drug should be continued as long as desired results are obtained. Researchers disagree about the length of time an NSAID should be administered. Generally, NSAIDs should be administered during the first two phases of healing. There is some evidence that continued use of these drugs into the third phase may slow healing (Almekinders and Gilbert 1986). It seems obvious that the most effective time to use anti-inflammatory medication is during the inflammation phase, when production of PGs is the greatest. The use of NSAIDs during the first week following injury, therefore, may be most crucial. If an individual continues to respond to the medication beyond that time, however, it may be useful to continue it into the proliferation phase. This decision, of course, is made by the physician.

Drug Interactions

Any drug can interact with other drugs also being taken to either enhance or reduce their effectiveness. This is known as drug interaction. For example, NSAIDs increase blood-clotting time by affecting the role of arachidonic acid in platelet aggregation and therefore magnify the results of drugs used in anticoagulant therapy. NSAIDs may also decrease the effectiveness of other drugs such as diuretics (medication to increase urine excretion, usually to relieve systemic swelling), beta blockers (medication to slow heart rate), angiotensin-converting enzyme inhibitors (medication to lower blood pressure), and oral hypoglycemic agents (medication taken orally to control non-insulin-dependent diabetes). Antacids delay the rate at which an NSAID is absorbed.

Other Drugs

Some medications may delay the healing process. Antibiotics, antineoplastic drugs, heparin, nicotine, and corticosteroids can all delay healing.

Other Modifying Factors

A number of other factors affect healing. Some of the factors over which the rehabilitation clinician has no control include quality of surgical repair, patient's age, systemic diseases from which the patient suffers, and wound size. Other factors such as infection, spasm, and swelling, can be reduced by appropriate and timely treatment. Nutrition can be influenced through instruction and advice to the patient.

Surgical Repair

The physician's surgical and sterile techniques have a direct effect on the healing of injuries that are surgically repaired. Infection complicates and delays the healing process. The quality of the surgeon's repair technique and follow-up care directly influences when rehabilitation can be started. If a surgeon's technique results in increased rather than decreased postoperative edema, tissue repair is delayed. If a surgeon immobilizes an injury for three months rather than three weeks, rehabilitation will be slower.

Age

Age can be a factor that alters healing. A good blood supply is crucial for any injury to heal properly. A poor blood supply delays or prevents an injury from healing properly. Blood supply is often impaired with age. Diseases associated with age also can affect healing.

Disease

Certain systemic diseases can impede healing. If a patient has diabetes, HIV, arthritis, endocrine disease, connective tissue disease, carcinoma, or other systemic diseases, extra care should be taken with healing wounds. Additionally, conditions not often seen in athletes that can delay healing include renal, hepatic, cardiovascular, and autoimmune diseases. If a patient has any of these conditions, the rehabilitation clinician is wise to be especially cautious.

Wound Size

Generally, the greater the injury, the more time necessary for healing to occur. If a patient suffers a first-degree ankle sprain, he or she may be able to participate in practice and activity the next day. However, if a patient has a second-degree ankle sprain, he or she may be unable to return to practice or normal activity for one week.

The larger the destruction of tissue and separation of tissue ends, the longer it will take for the body to debride the area and connect the stump ends. Similarly, the greater the injury, the greater the scar tissue. Scar tissue can impede rehabilitation, depending on where the scar tissue is and how long the injured site is immobilized before exercises begin.

Infection

Infection is a possibility any time an open wound occurs, whether it is an abrasion, a surgical wound, or a needle stick from an injection or aspiration. Precautions should always be taken to prevent infection, regardless of the source or size of the wound. Infection always delays healing. When an infection occurs, the wound site will have more scar tissue than it would otherwise have had.

Nutrition

Nutrition plays an important part in healing. The rehabilitation clinician should encourage the patient to have good nutrition through well-balanced meals to enhance healing. Diets lacking in protein, vitamins (especially A and C), or minerals (especially the trace minerals zinc and copper) make healing more difficult.

Muscle Spasm

Spasm is a reflex that occurs with injury as the body attempts to minimize the injury by immobilizing the area. Pain and muscle inhibition combine to diminish function. Spasms result in ischemia by restricting blood flow. Applying immediate first aid to the area is important in reducing spasm and ultimately improving the rate of tissue healing and the function of the injured part.

Swelling

The amount of swelling for similar injuries varies from one person to another. As a rule, however, the more severe the injury, the greater the swelling for all individuals. Swelling is caused by fluid in the interstitial spaces and can include blood, watery fluid from damaged cells, and plasma fluids. The body interprets extracellular blood as a foreign substance and works to rid the area of it. Edema also puts pressure on sensitive nerve endings, causes reflex muscular inhibition, and negatively affects nutrient exchange at the site of injury. These factors ultimately increase pain, reduce function, and slow healing. The greater the amount of accumulated extravascular blood and fluid, the greater the symptoms of inflammation and the longer it will take the body to progress from inflammation to proliferation. It therefore is crucial for the clinician to apply immediate treatment to minimize the edema and promote healing. Minimizing edema also reduces inflammation, pain, and loss of function.

THE ROLE OF THERAPEUTIC EXERCISE IN HEALING

▶ Application of therapeutic exercise components must be carefully coordinated with the phases of healing. Respecting tissue healing must always be a tantamount consideration when planning a successful rehabilitation program.

Now that you understand the healing process, it is time to see how this knowledge can help you design therapeutic exercise programs for injured individuals. Your knowledge of the events and timing of the healing cycle should help you know what to do and when to do it to promote the patient's safe and timely return to competition or normal activity.

The clinician can influence healing positively or negatively, depending on the treatment and when it is applied. Knowledge plays a vital part in the delivery of treatment. Knowing how to apply a treatment is the easy part. Knowing when to apply it and the consequences or benefits of applying it is more difficult.

Although immediate treatment after an injury is considered first aid, it is really the first step in rehabilitation. Sue Hillman's (2005) *Introduction to Athletic Training, Second Edition*, provides an excellent description of first-aid procedures. Therefore, they are not addressed here; refer to her text for a review.

Rehabilitation involves two aspects of treatment beyond on-site evaluation and immediate care. Therapeutic modalities are often first applied to promote healing, reduce spasm and pain, and allow the next phase of rehabilitation—therapeutic exercise—to begin. Therapeutic exercise allows the patient to resume full sport participation or normal activity. Various aspects of therapeutic exercise are discussed in detail throughout this text. This section covers only general principles. It is important to realize that rehabilitation involves the use of both modalities and therapeutic exercise. Each component serves a very different purpose and together they are used to achieve a common goal, the full recovery of the patient.

Timing of Treatment

Once the injury is stabilized, efforts to control the edema and pain are important in the early treatment phase. Even at this time, efforts can be made through therapeutic exercise to encourage the healing process. Care must be taken, however, not to disturb the newly formed, tenuous fibrin plug, which provides the injured site's primary stability and strength. Recall that in the first three days after injury, there is a lot of physiological activity at the injury site. Among other activities, macrophages are attempting to clear the site of debris so that the fibroblasts can start their task of rebuilding. Undue stress to the injury at this time reinjures the site, disrupts the fibrin clot, and causes additional edema.

In severe injuries, the rehabilitation clinician must be cautious about the amount of stress applied to the area, especially in the early healing phases. During these phases even patients with surgical repairs can begin therapeutic exercise early. Even though the injury is unable to tolerate high stresses, the patient can work toward one of the goals of rehabilitation (discussed in chapter 1): maintaining the conditioning status of uninjured parts and the cardiovascular system. For example, if a patient has had surgery on the right knee, he or she can maintain cardiovascular conditioning by performing activities such as one-legged cycling or upper-body cardiovascular activities. Upper-body weightlifting and left lower extremity resistance exercises can also be a part of the program at this time. Some evidence indicates that exercising the contralateral limb provides some gains in strength in the involved extremity (Steadman, Forster, and Silferskiold 1989).

By the end of the first week, the injured site is already entering the remodeling phase. Type I collagen is being produced, and the area becomes stronger and able to withstand more stress than in the first few days. The site of injury is still very weak compared to normal tissue, but it is able to tolerate some controlled stress. At this time, depending on the injury and the tissue involved, motion activities and in some cases, early strengthening activities are used. There are some exceptions to this general rule.

Tendon repair is one exception. Some physicians permit range of motion exercises but no strengthening exercises until the third week. Others prefer to wait six weeks or longer to begin strengthening. Some physicians allow strengthening exercises after one week because collagen fibers are being synthesized rapidly and reach their maximum levels by day 10. They feel that the collagen is strong enough at this time to start mild resistive exercises, often in the form of easy isometrics. Other physicians prefer to wait three weeks because it is then that the synovial sheath has been rebuilt to provide a smooth gliding surface for the tendon. Physicians who wait six weeks presumably do so because by then the new collagen is fairly mature and risk of rupture is significantly less. The risk of waiting too long to initiate activity following surgery is that the tendons will become bound down by scar tissue formation following surgical disruption of skin, fascia, surrounding soft tissue, and the tendon itself. It is important to know the physician's preferred protocol regarding initiation of therapeutic exercise.

As mentioned in chapter 1, flexibility must be achieved before the other physical parameters. After reading this chapter, you should appreciate the reasons for this sequence. By the end of the first week of healing, collagen is transforming from weak type III to stronger, permanent type I. The cross-links are increasing, and the bonds between the collagen are becoming stronger. As a general rule, the most effective gains in range of motion are made during the first three to six weeks after injury. Changes in motion can be made relatively easily during the first two months following surgery or severe injury. After that time the collagen becomes more mature and resistant to change. This is the reason why an ankle that has been immobilized for three months is much more difficult to restore to its former range of motion than one that has been immobilized for three weeks.

Different techniques for achieving flexibility are used at different times in the rehabilitation process. Specific flexibility techniques depend on how mature the scar tissue is. These techniques are described and differentiated in chapter 5.

Once a therapeutic exercise program has begun and flexibility activities have been initiated, strength activities should begin when it is safe to do so. Depending on the severity of the injury and the status of the patient, early strength exercises may include only isometrics. Progression of strengthening exercises is discussed in more detail in chapter 7. The rehabilitation clinician must be cognizant of the stresses applied by strengthening activities. Care must always be taken to stress the tissues enough to provide the desired results without overstressing them to cause damage. The most dangerous time for strength activities is during the inflammation phase, when there is little tensile strength in the injured area except the fibrin clot securing the injury site. Care must also be taken during the remodeling phase, when collagen is converted from type III to type I, especially following surgical repair, when tendons and ligaments are particularly vulnerable.

The therapeutic exercise program should progress as described in chapter 1. Once flexibility is achieved, emphasis is placed on progressive strength and muscular endurance activities. These exercises become more intense as the injured area increases in tensile strength through healing and the muscles, tendons, ligaments, and bones themselves gain strength from the exercises.

As the injured area's supporting structures, especially the muscles that provide dynamic control, increase their strength, exercises progress to improve the next parameter, proprioception. These activities emphasize balance, agility, speed, and coordination. The exercises become more advanced until the patient can transit into functional activities that replicate the motions and stresses of normal sport performance and activity.

The timing of the injured part's healing should always be considered in determining when the patient should progress in the program. Stresses applied to the injured part must be assessed and correlated with tissue's healing time line.

Overuse Injuries

Rehabilitation programs for overuse injuries involve somewhat different strategies from those for acute injuries because of their different causes. These differences are discussed in more detail in chapter 15. A rehabilitation program must always be designed with the healing of injured tissue in mind.

Often, an overuse injury is caused by continual or cumulative irritation to an area. The aggravating factor must first be resolved before a successful treatment program can be instituted. Once the cause has been determined, healing can begin, although it is often slower than the healing of acute injuries.

For any injury, two considerations determine the appropriate course of therapeutic exercise. The first is the usual healing sequence and timing. Knowing when the tissue is most vulnerable and how long it takes for various tissues to go through their normal healing process determines what stresses can be applied safely.

The second consideration is the individual's unique response to injury and treatment. To evaluate each person's response, examine the area for negative and positive responses to treatment. Increased edema, increased pain, and diminished function are signs that the exercise was too severe for the injury to tolerate. Asking the patient for his or her response to exercise is helpful. "Did your knee have more swelling last night?" "Was there more pain in your shoulder after the treatment yesterday?" "Was it easier or more difficult to walk on one crutch after the last treatment?" If you determine that an exercise produced undesirable effects, the appropriate action is to exclude or modify that exercise until the injured area further improves. If no deleterious effects occur, the current course of treatment is appropriate.

SUMMARY

1. Explain the differences between primary and secondary healing.

   Primary healing produces a minimal scar and occurs when the damaged edges of a wound are close to each other, whereas secondary healing produces a greater scar because the wound must heal by filling in tissue from the bottom and sides of the wound.

2. Identify the healing phases.

   The body follows a very complex and not entirely understood process of healing, going through the three phases of healing: inflammation, proliferation, and remodeling.

3. Describe the primary processes of each healing phase.

   During inflammation, neutrophil migration begins the process, fibrin-plug production prevents fluid and blood from escaping, monocyte migration rids the area of debris. Proliferation occurs when angiogenesis restores blood flow, and type III collagen is produced and fibroblasts, myofibroblasts, and collagen synthesis are at their peak. During remodeling, healing slows, wound contraction is well under way, and type III collagen is converted to type I collagen.

4. Discuss the causes for the signs of inflammation.

   Redness, localized warmth, swelling, pain, and dysfunction are all signs of inflammation. Redness occurs because of increased circulation and released chemicals, localized warmth and swelling are caused by interstitial fluid leakage and increased metabolic activity in the area, pain is caused by pressure on nerve endings from edema and damage to nerves in the area. Dysfunction occurs because of the physical restrictions of swelling, damage to structures, and the muscular inhibition from the pain.

5. Explain the role of growth factors in healing.

   Growth factors are not well understood, but present knowledge indicates that they play an important role in tissue healing. They assist in causing cell proliferation and chemotactic activity that are vital to healing.

6. Discuss the differences between acute and chronic inflammation.

   Acute inflammation occurs through a systematic progression of chemical and cellular activity. Chronic inflammation occurs when the site is unable to proceed from the inflammatory phase to the proliferation phase because granulocytes are unable to fully debride the area so that mononuclear cells persist.

7. Discuss healing characteristics of specific tissue.

   Ligaments, tendons, muscle, bone, and cartilage all follow the general healing process, but their healing also has aspects unique to their own cellular makeup. For example, muscle has myogenic cells that are able to regenerate muscle tissue, bone has osteoblasts, and tendons have tenocytes.

8. Identify the relevance of tensile strength.

   Tensile strength enables a structure to withstand stresses. Once an area is damaged, the tensile strength is not restored to 100% normal. In spite of this, a patient is able to safely return to participation if the injury has properly healed and a proper rehabilitation program has been followed.

9. Discuss factors that can modify the healing process.

   Healing of any tissue is influenced by a number of factors. Factors that can be influenced include the use of medications (especially anti-inflammatory drugs), the use of various treatment modalities, the application of first aid, edema and pain, infection, and nutrition. Other factors over which the rehabilitation clinician has no control include the physician's surgical technique and the patient's age and general health.

10. Explain the role NSAIDs play in inflammation.

    NSAIDs reduce the effects of inflammation by altering chemical production or the impact of specific chemicals on the healing process. If administered correctly, they can positively reduce the inflammation phase to promote healing.

11. Discuss the timing of treatment with the various stages of healing.

    Therapeutic exercise must be administered appropriately without causing harm to the healing tissues if the rehabilitation program is to be successful. It is important to use exercises carefully and watch for adverse effects from the exercises.

CRITICAL THINKING QUESTIONS

1. If you were Daniel in the opening scenario, how would you approach Becki to discuss whether or not she has anorexia? How could anorexia affect Becki's healing process? What could you do to counteract her anorexia? What precautions should you take to "do no harm"?

2. If a patient presented to you with Achilles tendinitis that began two weeks ago, at what stage would you estimate the tendinitis to be? What would be your criteria for determining whether it is acute or chronic?

3. A patient who undergoes an outpatient surgical repair of the elbow comes to you three days after the surgery to begin rehabilitation. Where in the healing process do you estimate this patient to be, and what healing activities are occurring? What would you do for treatment in the first three days of your treatment program? What would you do for treatment in the first three weeks of your treatment program? What factors would you consider to determine when to change the treatment program?

4. A patient with a second-degree ankle sprain that occurred four days ago comes to you for rehabilitation. If the patient was 50 years old; had diabetes, severe swelling, and cramps in the calf muscles; was on Coumadin and an oral hypoglycemic medication; and had been taking oral anti-inflammatories for the past three days, what would your treatment program include? How would your treatment be different if the patient was 22 years old; had severe swelling and cramps in the calf muscles; and had been taking oral anti-inflammatories for the past three days?

LAB ACTIVITIES

1. Identify three reliable Web sites to which you can refer for additional information on tissue healing, the stages of healing, or specific tissue healing.

2. List the types of rehabilitation techniques you would be able to use within each phase of healing.

3. Identify three medications kept either in the clinic or your own home. List what influence, if any, they may have on healing.

4. Investigate the influences growth hormones have on healing. Where are they produced in the body, how are they attracted to an injury site, and during what stage of healing would you expect them to be most evident? Why?

REFERENCES

Almekinders, L.C., and J.A. Gilbert. 1986. Healing of experimental muscle strains and the effects of non-steroidal antiinflammatory medication. *American Journal of Sports Medicine* 14:303–308.

Andriacchi, T.P., Sabiston, K., DeHaven, K., Dahners, L., Woo, S., Frank, C., Oakes, B., Brand, R., and J. Lewis. 1988. Ligament: Injury and repair. In *Injury and repair of the musculoskeletal soft tissues*, ed. S.L.-Y. Woo and J.A. Buckwalter. Park Ridge, IL: American Academy of Orthopaedic Surgeons.

Betz, P., Norlich, A., Wilske, J., Tubel, J., Penning, R., and W. Eisenmenger. 1992. Time-dependent appearance of myofibroblasts in granulation tissue of human skin wounds. *International Journal of Legal Medicine* 150:99–103.

Brittberg, M., Lindahl, A., Nilsson, A., Ohlsson, C., Isaksson, O. , and L. Peterson. 1994. Treatment of deep cartilage defects in the knee with autologous chondrocyte transplantation. *New England Journal of Medicine* 331:889–895.

Buckwalter, J.A., Rosenberg, L., Coutts, R., Hunziker, E., Reddi, A.H., and V. Mow. 1988. Articular cartilage: Injury and repair. In *Injury and repair of the musculoskeletal soft tissues*, ed. S.L.-Y. Woo and J.A. Buckwalter. Park Ridge, IL: American Academy of Orthopaedic Surgeons.

Caplan, A.B., Carlson, J., Faulkner, J., Fischman, D., and W. Garrett, Jr. 1988. Skeletal muscle. In *Injury and repair of the musculoskeletal soft tissues*, ed. S.L.-Y. Woo and J.A. Buckwalter. Park Ridge, IL: American Academy of Orthopaedic Surgeons.

Christie, A.L. 1991. The tissue injury cycle and new advances toward its management in open wounds. *Athletic Training* 26:274–277.

Connolly, J.F. 1988. *Fracture complications, recognition, prevention, and management.* Chicago: Year Book Medical.

Denegar, C., E. Saliba, and S. Saliba. 2005, 2nd ed. *Therapeutic modalities for musculoskeletal injuries.* Champaign, IL: Human Kinetics.

DiPietro, L.A. 1995. Wound healing: The role of the macrophage and other immune cells. *Shock* 4: 233–240.

Enwemeka, C.S. 1989. Inflammation, cellularity, and fibrillogenesis in regenerating tendon: Implications for tendon rehabilitation. *Physical Therapy* 69:816–825.

Gelberman, R., An, K.-A., Banes, A. , and V. Goldberg. 1988. Tendon. In *Injury and repair of the musculoskeletal soft tissues*, ed. S.L.-Y. Woo and J.A. Buckwalter. Park Ridge, IL: American Academy of Orthopaedic Surgeons.

Gelberman, R.H., Woo, S.L.-Y., Lothringer, K. Akeson, W.H., and D. Amiel. 1982. Effects of early intermittent passive mobilization on healing canine flexor tendons. *Journal of Hand Surgery* 7: 170–175.

Grundnes, O., and O. Reikeras. 1992. Blood flow and mechanical properties of healing bone. *Acta Orthopaedica Scandinavica* 63:487–491.

Heppenstall, R.B. 1980. Fracture healing. In *Fracture treatment and healing*, ed. R.B. Heppenstall. Philadelphia: Saunders.

Hillman, S. 2005. *Introduction to athletic training*, 2nd ed. Champaign, IL: Human Kinetics.

Hom, D.B. 1995. Growth factors in wound healing. *Otolaryngologic Clinics of North America* 28: 933–953.

Houglum, J.E. 1998. Pharmacologic considerations in the treatment of injured athletes with nonsteroidal anti-inflammatory drugs. *Journal of Athletic Training* 33:259–263.

Houglum, J.E., Harrelson, G.L., and D. Leaver-Dunn. 2005. *Principles of pharmacology for athletic trainers*. Thorofare, NJ: Slack, Inc.

Houglum, P.A. 1992. Soft tissue healing and its impact on rehabilitation. *Journal of Sport Rehabilitation* 1:19–39.

Kibler, W.B. 1990. Concepts in exercise rehabilitation of athletic injury. In *Sports-induced inflammation*, ed. W.B. Leadbetter, J.A. Buckwalter, and S.L. Gordon. Park Ridge, IL: American Academy of Orthopaedic Surgeons.

Kirsner, R.S., and W.H. Eaglstein. 1993. The wound healing process. *Dermatological Clinics* 11: 629–638.

Koopman, C.F. 1995. Cutaneous wound healing: An overview. *Otolaryngologic Clinics of North America* 28:835–845.

Lane, J.M., and J.R. Werntz. 1987. Biology of fracture healing. In *Fracture healing*, ed. J.M. Lane. New York: Churchill Livingstone.

Leadbetter, W.B. 1994. Soft tissue athletic injury. In *Sports injuries: Mechanisms, prevention, treatment*, ed. F.H. Fu and D.A. Stone. Baltimore: Williams & Wilkins.

Martinez-Hernandez, A., and P.S. Amenta. 1990. Basic concepts in wound healing. In *Sports-induced inflammation*, ed. W.B. Leadbetter, J.A. Buckwalter, and S.L. Gordon. Park Ridge, IL: American Academy of Orthopaedic Surgeons.

Nordin, M., and V.H. Frankel. 1980. Biomechanics of collagenous tissues. In *Basic biomechanics of the skeletal system*, ed. V.H. Frankel and N. Nordin. Philadelphia: Lea & Febiger.

Peacock, E.E. 1965. Physiology of tendon repair. *American Journal of Surgery* 109:283.

Peacock, E.E. 1984. *Wound repair*. 3rd ed. Philadelphia: Saunders.

Salter, R.B., Simmons, D.F., Malcom, B.W., Rumble, E.J., Macmichael, D., and N.D. Clements. 1980. The biological effect of continuous passive motion on the healing of full-thickness defects in articular cartilage. *Journal of Bone and Joint Surgery* 62A:1232–1251.

Silver, F.H. and A.I. Glasgold. 1995. Cartilage wound healing. *Otolaryngologic Clinics of North America* 28:847–864.

Steadman, J.R., Forster, R.S., and J.P. Silferskiold. 1989. Rehabilitation of the knee. *Clinics in Sports Medicine* 8:605–627.

Urban, M.K. 2000. COX-2 Specific inhibitors offer improved advantages over traditional NSAIDs. *Orthopedics* 23:761s-764s.

Concepts in Physics

Objectives

After completing this chapter, you should be able to do the following:

1. Define force and give an example of an internal and an external force.
2. Explain the relevance to therapeutic exercise of Newton's first, second, and third laws of motion.
3. Explain how center of gravity changes with movement.
4. Discuss how a change in base of support can change a person's stability.
5. Explain the relationship between line of gravity and base of support.
6. Explain two ways of increasing stability.
7. Identify the difference between stabilization and fixation.
8. Explain how torque can be altered in the body.
9. Identify how varying position changes a muscle's mechanical advantage.
10. Discuss the difference between mechanical and physiological advantage of a muscle.
11. Explain the importance of positioning in exercising two-joint muscles.
12. Distinguish between velocity and acceleration.
13. Discuss the relevance of elasticity, stress-strain, creep, and friction to therapeutic exercise.

Joel Edgars is working to rehabilitate Reeda Skaalie, a swimmer with a shoulder injury. The facility where Joel works has an adjustable pulley system, and he wants to use it for the series of scapular strengthening exercises he has planned for today's program with Reeda. He wants to exercise the lower trapezius, middle trapezius, rhomboids, and serratus anterior on the pulleys. Joel realizes that the muscle's physiological length, lever-arm length, and angle of pull all influence the amount of work that is done by the muscles and understands that stabilization must be a consideration, but he is at a loss as to where the pulleys should be placed to obtain the best results. Reeda is scheduled to begin the program in 30 min, so Joel must quickly figure out the pulley placement for the exercises he has in mind for today's program.

■ You had better live your best and act your best and think your best today; for today is the sure preparation for tomorrow and all the other tomorrows that follow.

Harriet Martineau, 1802-1876, Author

As Ms Martineau's words suggest, this chapter will prepare you by providing a foundation for future knowledge and understanding of therapeutic exercise technique applications. Knowing why we do what we do in therapeutic exercise is vital. Only with an understanding of theory and precepts can we adjust exercises to each injured individual's needs and develop soundly structured, knowledge-based therapeutic exercise programs. It is easy to know the hows, but knowing the whys is the difference between being a technician and a professional. A professional knows what is important and why. The concepts presented in this chapter provide the whys of therapeutic exercise so that the hows become logical and simple.

The physics concepts in this chapter are not new; they have successfully endured the test of centuries. Many of the ideas that Sir Isaac Newton and other engineers and philosophers introduced during the 1600s have profound impact on the delivery of therapeutic exercise in musculoskeletal rehabilitation today. These concepts are another vital part of the foundation of knowledge that you will need to guide a patient through a therapeutic exercise program. Without this knowledge it is difficult to apply forces correctly for stretching and strengthening, use your own body efficiently and effectively, or develop a successful therapeutic exercise program.

As you read through this chapter, you should develop an appreciation of basic physics principles that will affect the application of your clinical skills daily. These principles are not complicated, but they are vital for rehabilitation clinicians. First, concepts are presented; then examples of direct applications to daily tasks in therapeutic exercise are provided.

FORCE

▶ A force causes movement and has direction and magnitude. Gravity is a pervasive external force that affects every movement.

A **force** is something that causes movement and has direction and magnitude. A mass is moved in a specific direction when a specific amount of force is applied. In the human body, the force can be either internal or external and usually produces either a push or a pull. Internal forces, of course, are generated by the muscles. External forces can be applied by a wide variety of sources, the most basic being gravity.

Gravity is probably the most basic external force; we all deal with gravity continuously. Whether you realize it or not, it affects your every move. For example, if there were no gravity, activity as we know it would be drastically different. Although Sir Isaac Newton didn't formulate his law of gravity until the late 1600s, gravity has been around since before the beginning of earth.

Sir Isaac Newton's law of gravity states that every object attracts every other object with a force proportional to the product of their masses and inversely proportional to the square of the distance between them. Because the earth is so massive compared with the objects on its surface, gravity is commonly thought of as the force of attraction that the earth exerts on an object. Gravity is counterbalanced by the supporting surface on which a person is standing, sitting, or lying. In other words, without surfaces such as a floor, bed, or chair to balance our weight on, we would simply fall. This concept leads us to Newton's third law of motion, which will be discussed later.

NEWTON'S LAWS OF MOTION

▶ Newton's first and second laws of motion describe inertia, momentum, and acceleration. These laws explain that the faster an object already moves, the less force is needed to move it in the same direction. His third law, action-reaction, states that for every action there is an equal and opposite reaction.

The mathematician Sir Isaac Newton (1642–1727) formulated laws of motion and gravity that are used to explain movement. The three laws of motion discussed here are inertia, acceleration and momentum, and action-reaction.

Inertia

Newton's first law of motion deals with inertia: A body remains at a state of rest or remains in uniform motion until an outside force acts on it. This is one reason why it is difficult for a weak muscle to initiate the lifting of a limb, but once movement begins, it becomes easier for the muscle to continue the movement. The muscle must have enough strength not only to lift the weight of the limb but also to overcome inertia. For example, if you give assistance in the beginning of a weightlifting exercise, such as a straight-leg raise, the patient may be able to continue the exercise on his or her own once the motion has begun, provided there is enough strength to lift the limb.

Acceleration and Momentum

Newton's second law of motion deals with acceleration and momentum. It states that the acceleration of an object is directly proportional to the force causing motion and inversely proportional to the mass of the object being moved. Momentum is the amount of motion a moving object has. The formulas used to calculate acceleration and momentum make it easy to understand:

$$\text{Momentum} = \text{mass} \times \text{velocity}$$
$$\text{Mass} = \text{weight} \div \text{acceleration due to gravity}$$
$$\text{Linear velocity} = \text{distance} \div \text{time}$$

Newton's second law of motion is important in therapeutic exercise because it explains why a slow, controlled motion of an extremity requires more strength than a quickly executed movement. If strength gain is the goal, it is better to have the patient move the extremity through the motion in a slow, controlled manner.

Action-Reaction

The force of gravity is commonly referred to as weight. If this force is counterbalanced, a body does not fall to the earth. This demonstrates Newton's third law of motion: An object reacts to a force with a force of equal magnitude in the opposite direction. Stated another way, for every action there is an equal and opposite reaction. Here are a couple of everyday applications of this law: If you hold a book in your hand, your muscle force counteracts the force of gravity and prevents the book from going to the ground. Another example is a patient's lying on a treatment table: The force of gravity on the patient is counterbalanced by the upward force of the treatment table.

Newton's Three Laws of Motion

Here is a summary of Newton's first three laws:

1. **Newton's first law of motion: inertia.** A body remains at a state of rest or remains in uniform motion until a force acts on it.

2. **Newton's second law of motion: acceleration and momentum.** The acceleration of an object is directly proportional to the force causing motion and inversely proportional to the mass of the object being moved.

3. **Newton's third law of motion: action-reaction.** For every action there is an equal and opposite reaction.

Let's consider the next step, what happens when a force that is stronger than gravity causes a body to move in the direction of that force. For example, a basketball being shot is propelled by a force strong enough to move the basketball up and toward the basket. The force must not only be applied with enough intensity to get the ball to the basket, but the force must be applied in the correct direction or angle to reach the target accurately. As another example, a volleyball player jumping to block at the net must produce enough force to overcome the force of gravity; the more force applied, the higher the volleyball player jumps. To perform a straight-leg raise, a patient must exert enough muscle force at the hip to counteract gravity's pull on the lower extremity.

CENTER OF GRAVITY

▶ *Center of gravity refers to the point in the body or object around which its weight is balanced. Knowing the center of gravity of a body of an object can lead to understanding how to increase its stability.*

Every object has a **center of gravity**. It is the point in the body or an object around which its weight is balanced. If we look at a symmetrical, rigid pole, the center of gravity is easy to find; it is the point toward the middle at which the pole balances when suspended. Every body part and the entire human body itself have their own center of gravity, as noted in table 3.1. Knowing the center of gravity's location is important for knowing where to apply force and how much force to apply to move or maintain a position.

The center of gravity is harder to find in the human body because of the body's irregular shape. In the anatomic position, the body's center of gravity is generally considered to be at about the level of the S2 vertebra. It is slightly higher in men than in women and varies with individual variations in shape. It also is different in children, because their weight distribution is different from that of adults.

As the body or part of the body moves, the center of gravity changes, as seen in figure 3.1. When a sprinter is in the starter blocks, the center of gravity is much lower than when running. When a rhythmic gymnast reaches out to catch a baton, her center of gravity changes as the arm extends forward and the baton's weight is added to her body weight.

The center of gravity also changes when weight is added to the body. For example, if a track and field athlete picks up a 15.9-kg (35 lb) hammer in his left hand, his center of gravity shifts to that side. If a 91-kg (200 lb) weightlifter jerks a 68-kg (150 lb) barbell overhead, his center of gravity becomes significantly higher than vertebra S2; this is why some weightlifters have a difficult time stabilizing themselves in this maneuver.

The lower the center of gravity, the more stable the object. We see this concept commonly in athletics. For example, a football lineman protects himself from being pushed by an opponent by lowering his center of gravity.

Table 3.1
Parts of the Human Body and Their Centers of Gravity

Segmental weights and percentage of total body weight for a 68-kg (150-lb) man				
Body part(s)	kg	lb	%	Location of center of gravity
Entire body (anterior to second sacral vertebra)				
Head	4.7	10.3	6.9	In sphenoid sinus, 4 mm beyond anterior inferior margin of sella (on lateral surface, over temporal fossa, on or near nasioiniac)
Head and neck	5.4	11.8	7.9	On inferior surface of basioccipital bone or within bone 23 ± 5 mm from crest of dorsum sellae (on lateral surface, 10 mm anterior to supratragic notch above head of mandible)
Head, neck, and trunk	40.1	88.5	59.0	Anterior to 11th thoracic vertebra
Upper Limb (just above elbow joint)				
Arm	1.9	4.1	2.7	In medial head of triceps, adjacent to radial groove; 5 mm proximal to distal end of deltoid insertion
Forearm	1.1	2.4	1.6	11 mm proximal to most distal part of pronator teres insertion; 9 mm anterior to interosseus membrane
Hand	0.4	0.9	0.6	(In rest position) On axis of metacarpal III, usually 2 mm deep to volar skin surface; 2 mm proximal to proximal transverse palmar skin crease, in angle between proximal transverse and radial longitudinal creases
Lower limb (just above knee joint)				
Thigh	6.6	14.5	9.7	In adductor brevis muscle; 13 mm medial to linea aspera, deep to adductor canal, 29 mm below apex of femoral triangle and 18 mm proximal to most distal fibers of adductor brevis
Leg	3.1	6.8	4.5	35 mm below popliteus, at posterior part of posterior tibialis; 16 mm above proximal end of Achilles tendon, 8 mm posterior to interosseus membrane
Foot	1	2.1	1.4	In plantar ligaments, or just superficial in adjacent deep foot muscles; below proximal halves of second and third cuneiform bones; on a line between ankle joint center and ball of foot in plane of metatarsal II
Lower limb	10.6	23.4	15.6	
Leg and foot	4.1	9.0	6.0	

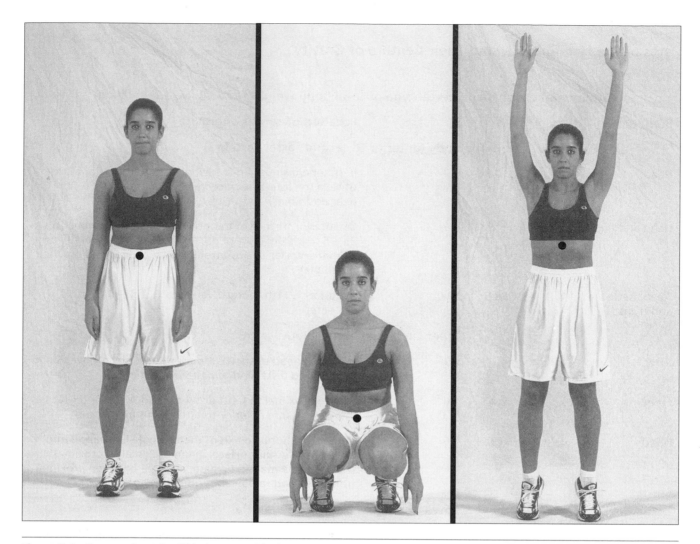

Figure 3.1   Center of gravity (●) changes with changes in body position.

STABILITY AND FIXATION

▶ Stability is a state in which a person or object is not easily thrown off balance. Fixation is a state of stabilization in which motion is restricted or prevented.

A number of factors determine a person's or object's **stability**. They all relate, however, to the relationship between the line of gravity and the base of support.

The **line of gravity** is an imaginary line that runs through the center of gravity toward the center of the earth. This line is used as a point of reference when discussing posture and is investigated in chapter 11. The line of gravity is also used to determine stability of an object. An object is most stable when the line of gravity falls within the object's base of support, as demonstrated in figure 3.2.

The **base of support**, simply referred to as the base, is the two-dimensional area between and including an object's points of contact with the supporting surface. As the example in figure 3.3 demonstrates, when you stand with your feet 15 cm (6 in.) apart, your base of support is the area of the surface that your feet contact and the area between your feet. If you spread your feet 46 cm (18 in.) apart, your base becomes larger.

Stability

An object is stable when the line of gravity falls within the base of support. A person is stable when standing upright with the line of gravity within the base of support, but if the line of gravity falls outside of that base, it is difficult to maintain balance. For the hammer thrower

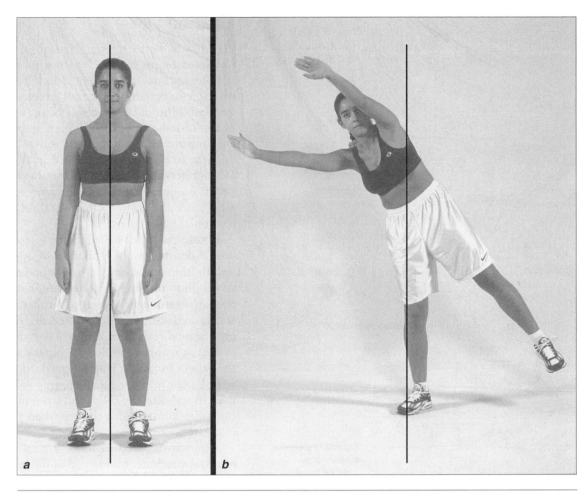

Figure 3.2   Line of gravity must fall within the base of support for the object to be stable. The larger the base of support is, the more stable the object is. According to the description above, is this patient more stable in *(a)* or *(b)*?

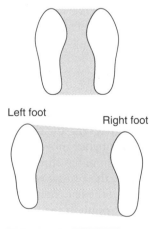

Left foot

Right foot

Figure 3.3   Base of support.

of the earlier example to maintain his balance while holding the hammer with his left hand, his center of gravity must remain inside his base of support. So what does he do to keep himself upright? He leans to the right to shift the center of gravity over his feet. The size and shape of the base of support also determines stability. The larger the base of support, the more stable the object. If you stand with your feet together, it is relatively easy for someone to push you over. If you spread your feet to give yourself a larger base of support, it is easier for you to maintain your stability and harder for someone to push you over.

The shape of the base can give additional support against external forces. A football lineman has more success in resisting an opponent's force if his feet are spread apart and in line with the direction of the oncoming player. In this position he is more likely to keep his center of gravity within his base of support and maintain stability. Most of us make these unconscious adjustments when we ride the bus or train while standing; we position our feet depending on our relation to the forward motion of the vehicle, either standing with feet side by side if we are standing sideways or positioning them in a tandem stance (one farther forward than the other) if we are facing forward, as shown in figure 3.4. In therapeutic exercise the shape and position of your base of support determines the ease with which you can provide manual resistance to a patient. For example, it is easier for you to provide manual resistance to a biceps curl while facing a seated patient if you position your feet in a forward-backward stance rather than a side-by-side stance.

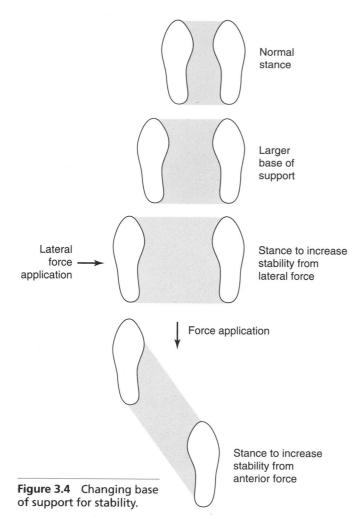

Normal stance

Larger base of support

Lateral force application →

Stance to increase stability from lateral force

↓ Force application

Stance to increase stability from anterior force

Figure 3.4 Changing base of support for stability.

Fixation

Fixation is a state of stabilization in which motion is restricted or prevented. Fixation provides a degree of stability optimal for efficient muscle function and is also desirable in certain therapeutic exercise situations. Fixation can be produced by either active muscle contraction or application of an external force. In performing an arm curl, fixation of the upper arm allows movement of the forearm to produce the desired goal of elbow flexion. When referring to the act of fixating a body segment to produce a desired motion, stabilization is the term often used, since the desired effect—stability—is the result of fixation of a body part.

Fixation is often needed in therapeutic exercise to produce a desired result. If fixation of a body segment and stabilization of the body are not applied during exercise, substitution of unwanted muscles or muscle groups can result in exercising a muscle other than the one intended, and desired results are diminished. For example, when you give manual resistance to hip abductors for a side-lying patient, it is important that the hip is stabilized to prevent the patient from using hip flexors during the exercise. On an isokinetic machine the thigh strap is the external fixator used to stabilize the thigh and prevent the patient from using hip flexors to lift the leg when the knee is moved into extension.

A muscle can produce motion from either its proximal or distal attachment. One end of the muscle must be fixated to achieve a desired motion. For example, the upper trapezius can move its proximal end to produce cervical extension and rotation or its distal end to cause scapular and clavicular elevation. To provide the greatest cervical motion, the scapula must be stabilized, and to provide the best scapular elevation, the neck must be stabilized. This stabilization is usually performed by other muscles.

Using a muscle as a stabilizer to fixate a body segment can be one way of strengthening it, especially in the early stages of a therapeutic exercise program. For example, if injured abdominal muscles are too weak or painful to perform an abdominal curl, they may tolerate a straight-leg raise; the abdominals work to fixate the trunk during this activity but do not work as hard as they would in a trunk curl.

BODY LEVERS

▶ A lever is a simple machine consisting of a rigid bar that rotates about a fulcrum. Levers are classified as first class, second class, or third class, depending on the relative positions of the fulcrum and the points where resistance and force are applied. Levers in the body can affect the force, speed, or distance of a movement.

A lever is a simple machine that contains a rigid bar and a fulcrum, or point of movement. The body moves because of its levers. It is important to know about the types of levers since levers are used continually in therapeutic exercise to produce resistance or to enhance movement.

There are three classes of levers. Each lever, regardless of its classification, has three primary components (shown in figure 3.5): the force arm (and force point), the resistance arm (and resistance point), and the fulcrum. The fulcrum is the point at which the bar rotates. In the body, the fulcrum is the joint and the bar is the bones. The resistance point in the body's lever system is the center of gravity of the body segment being moved. If an external object such as a weight is attached to the segment, the center of gravity for that segment, and thus the resistance point, changes. For example, the center of gravity for an average forearm and hand is approximately 3/7 the distance from the elbow to the fingertips. If the patient grasps a weight in the hand, the center of gravity resistance point moves more distally; the heavier

Figure 3.5   Basic lever system.

the weight, the more distally the resistance point's center of gravity moves. The resistance arm is the distance from the fulcrum to the resistance point. The force point is the point at which the force moving the lever is applied, and the force arm is the shortest distance from that point to the fulcrum. The generic term for resistance arm and force arm is *lever arm*. Since joint movement is rotational, the level arm is technically referred to as the moment arm; clinicians often interchange these two terms. Two lever arms and a fulcrum comprise a lever system. The relationship among the positions of these components determines the class of lever that is being used.

First-Class Lever

A **first-class lever** is one in which the fulcrum is located between the resistance and the force. A simple example is the seesaw. In the body an example of a first-class lever is the triceps, shown in figure 3.6: Its point of force is at its insertion on the olecranon, proximal to the joint, and the resistance force is at the center of gravity of the forearm, down the forearm 3/7 of the distance between the elbow and the fingertips. If two equal forces act against each other, the advantage will lie with the force having the longer lever arm.

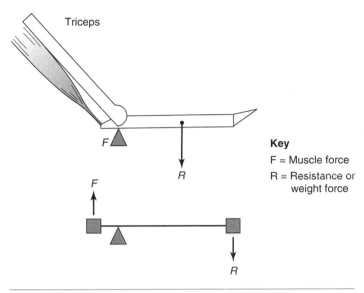

Key
F = Muscle force
R = Resistance or weight force

Figure 3.6   First-class lever.

Second-Class Lever

In a **second-class lever** the resistance point is between the fulcrum and the force. This class of lever always has a longer force arm than resistance arm. It is efficient in production of force, because the amount of force needed to move a resistance is always less than the resisting force. A typical example is the wheelbarrow. In the human body the brachioradialis, seen in figure 3.7, is an example of a second-class lever because it inserts on the forearm distal to the forearm's center of gravity.

Figure 3.7   Second-class lever.

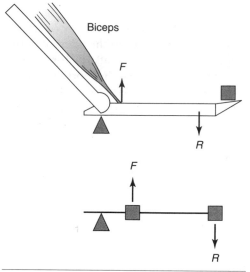

Third-Class Lever

A **third-class lever** has the force between the fulcrum and the resistance. This is an inefficient lever since the force arm is always shorter than the resistance arm, so more force is always required to move the resistance. Many of the levers of the body fall into this class. The elbow can once again be used as an example of this class of lever: As seen in figure 3.8, the biceps tendon inserts on the forearm between the elbow joint and the center of gravity of the forearm.

Figure 3.8 Third-class lever.

Effects of Levers

These classes of levers determine the body's mechanical response. They can increase or decrease the forces produced, the speed of movement of a body part, and the range of motion of the joint. If one or more of these factors increases, the remaining factors decrease. Conversely, if one or more decreases, the others increase. Figure 3.9 shows two people of equal weight at opposite ends of a seesaw. If person A is 6 ft from the fulcrum and person B is 8 ft from the fulcrum, person B can exert more torque (discussed later in this chapter) than person A, and person A moves more slowly and over a shorter distance than person B.

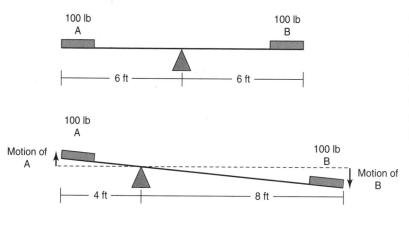

Figure 3.9 First-class lever.

Levers are classified according to the relative position of the fulcrum, force point, and resistance point. Sometimes when an outside resistance—such as a weight in a hand—is added, the class of lever changes. Recall that the brachioradialis is normally a second-class lever. If a heavy enough weight is placed in the hand, however, as seen in figure 3.10, the center of gravity (resistance point) moves more distally and can change the brachioradialis from a second-class to a third-class lever.

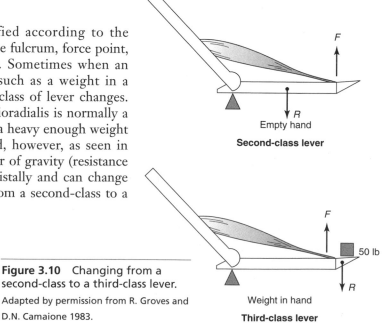

Figure 3.10 Changing from a second-class to a third-class lever.

Adapted by permission from R. Groves and D.N. Camaione 1983.

LEVERS AND FORCE

▶ The ability of a force to cause a rotational movement, or torque, is affected by the angle at which the force acts on a body part.

Linear motion is movement in a straight line, whereas angular motion is rotational movement through an arc. All joints in the body produce angular motion, but movement of the entire body through space is often linear. In other words, the rotational movement of the hips, knees, and ankles causes the body to move forward linearly, a motion known as walking.

Torque

The ability of a force to cause a rotational movement is referred to as torque. Torque is the product of the force and length of the force arm. Torque is commonly expressed in units such as Newton-meters (N · m), foot-pounds (ft · lb), or inch-pounds (in. · lb). When torque is produced, the force arm is referred to as a moment arm, but as mentioned, clinicians commonly interchange the two terms.

An increase in the length of the moment arm increases the torque produced by a force. For example, if you apply manual resistance at the thigh to a straight-leg raise, your torque is less (or you have to produce more force for the same torque) than if you positioned your hand at the ankle. With your hand at the ankle, your effort is less for the same torque production because your lever arm is longer. Conversely, if a patient has a difficult time performing a straight-leg raise against gravity, bending the knee to shorten the leg's resistance arm length may permit the patient to lift the leg without assistance.

Torque can also be altered by changing the force. Placing a 4.5 kg (10 lb) weight on an ankle produces twice as much torque as a 2.25 kg (5 lb) weight on a knee-extension exercise.

As a joint goes through its range of motion, a muscle's torque changes. This is related in part to the change in the muscle's line of pull and the angle of pull causing the moment arm length to change.

Line of Pull

Key

A = Direction of biceps force
B = Angle of pull
C = Moment arm

The line of pull of the muscle is the long axis of the muscle. The angle of pull is between the long axis of the bone (lever arm) and the line of pull of the muscle. The angle of pull and moment arm of the muscle change as the joint goes through its range of motion. As demonstrated in figure 3.11, the maximal amount of torque is produced when the angle of pull of the muscle is 90° and the moment arm is at its greatest length. In this position all the muscle's force is directed to produce rotation only. As the muscle's angle of pull increases or decreases from 90°, the part of the force that contributes to rotational motion (rotatory force) decreases, and the part that does not contribute to rotation (nonrotatory force) increases, so the ability to produce rotational motion—or torque—diminishes. How much rotatory force (vector) and how much nonrotatory force (vector) exists depends on the angle of pull and the moment arm. The nonrotatory force will tend to either stabilize the joint by providing compression or destabilize the joint by providing a distracting force, depending on the angle of pull. The farther the angle of pull is from 90°, the more force is used to stabilize or destabilize the joint and the less force is used to rotate the joint. For example, the biceps, seen in figure 3.12, has a nonrotatory force component that is pulling the ulna into the elbow and provides stability to the joint. It also has a rotatory component causing the forearm to move through its arc of motion. In

Figure 3.11 The angle of pull changes as range of motion changes. The most rotary force occurs when the muscle's angle of pull is 90°.

Adapted by permission from R. Groves and D.N. Camaione 1983.

Key

A = Line of muscle pull

B = Rotatory component of force moving the point
    through its arc of motion

C = Nonrotatory component of force pulling
    the ulna into the elbow (compression force)

D = Resistance point (center of mass of forearm)

E = Angle of pull

Figure 3.12   Rotatory and nonrotatory components of force.

Adapted by permission from R. Groves and D.N. Camaione 1983.

Figure 3.13   With this pulley arrangement, the greatest resistance is produced at 90° knee flexion.

therapeutic exercise, the mechanics of each joint and the angle of pull of the muscles surrounding the joint should be appreciated. A recently dislocated shoulder, for example, should not be placed in positions that encourage surrounding muscle to destabilize it. For this reason, early rehabilitation of this condition warrants avoiding overhead or full-external-rotation positions.

Angle of Pull

Angle of pull of a muscle is an important concept in therapeutic exercise. If you want to produce the maximal torque from a muscle, the joint must be positioned so that the muscle being worked has a 90° angle of pull on the extremity.

This concept also works for external forces applied to the body. With pulleys, the maximal resistance occurs when the angle of pull of the pulley's rope is 90° to the extremity being resisted, as shown in figure 3.13. With free weights, the maximal resistance occurs when the pull of the weight is perpendicular to the ground regardless of the extremity's position. For example, when a supine patient performs elbow flexion with a weight, the greatest resistance is at the start of the motion when the patient's elbow moves from full extension to flexion, as seen in figure 3.14. If the patient is standing or sitting, however, the maximal resistance from the weight is when the elbow is at 90°.

PHYSIOLOGICAL MUSCLE ADVANTAGES

▶ A muscle's ability to shorten is its physiological advantage. A two-joint muscle will have a better physiological advantage when it is placed on stretch at one joint while it is moving the other.

What we have been discussing thus far is the mechanical advantage of muscles, which relates to the angle of pull and moment arm of the muscles and the amount of resistance a muscle must overcome to produce motion. Physiological advantage is a muscle's ability to shorten. This is an important functional concept in therapeutic exercise. A muscle has the most physiological advantage when it is at its resting length. The resting length of a muscle is the length to which a muscle can be lengthened in a relaxed condition without producing tension or any additional stretch. For example, the greatest physiological advantage of the brachialis is with the elbow in full extension, and the greatest physiological advantage for the soleus is with the ankle in dorsiflexion.

As a muscle shortens, its physiological advantage becomes progressively less until it is unable to produce a force, as illustrated in figure 3.15. A muscle is able to shorten to about 66% of its resting length (Smith, Weiss & Lehmkuhl 1996). At that point, all the muscle's energy is used to shorten it, so no external force can be exerted.

Multijoint Muscles

If a multijoint muscle is shortened as far as possible, it will ultimately impact the position of all the joints it crosses. For example, if the hamstrings were maximally shortened, it would produce extension of the hip and flexion of the knee. However, since the muscle has used up its shortening ability, it cannot be effective in holding an isometric at its ends of motion. This condition is called *active insufficiency*. Likewise, if a multijoint muscle is elongated over both

Figure 3.14 Changes in position causes changes in resistance arm. Resistance is greatest at 0° when supine and 90° when standing.

Key

A = Combination of stretch of connective tissue and muscle elasticity
B = Active tension of muscle fiber as it is stretched
C = Passive stretch of connective tissue

Figure 3.15 Physiological advantage of muscles.

joints, there is an insufficient amount of myofilament overlap within the muscle and the muscle is unable to produce a strong contraction. This condition is called *passive insufficiency*.

Because of active and passive insufficiency, when a two-joint or multijoint muscle is worked, it should be elongated at the stabilized, unaffected joint so it can work optimally at the injured joint. For example, if you want to maximize efforts of the hamstrings during a knee exercise, the best position for the patient is sitting. If the patient is prone, the hamstrings are already shortened at the hip and will be unable to fully contract at the knee. When you want to produce as much force from a two-joint muscle as possible, the muscle should be placed on stretch at the stabilized joint as it moves the other joint. This permits all its available physiological length to be used at the desired site. When working with the finger flexors and other multijoint muscles, care must be taken to stabilize the multiple joints they cross when attempting to isolate their activity.

Summation of Forces

Summation of forces is especially important during the functional phase of a therapeutic exercise program. The **summation of forces** is a sequence of movements timed so that each movement contributes to the next movement to produce a desired outcome. For the summation of forces to be successful, the forces from each part must be correctly timed, and each successive joint from which the activity occurs must be stabilized. This is more easily understood with an example: A baseball pitcher goes through a series of sequential movements starting with the hips, progressing to the trunk, then the shoulder, the elbow, and finally the wrist and hand. Acceleration of the ball is produced by a series of rotations and extensions in each of the joints. If a ball is tossed with movement only from the wrist, it does not go as far as when it is thrown correctly using a summation of forces from all body segments. Even using only the upper extremity and not the hips and trunk produces a far less effective throw than a full summation of forces. The forces applied by the muscles in each of the joints must be precisely timed to build on the previous forces. If correct timing does not occur, the pitcher ends up using forces primarily from the arm, not the hip and trunk, and risks injury to the shoulder or elbow.

For summation of forces to occur, each joint must be stabilized in correct sequence. If this does not occur, the transfer of forces generated fails. Once a joint's desired motion is produced and the muscle's forces have been transmitted, the joint must be stabilized by a static contraction of the muscles for summation to occur. If the pitcher does not have good hip strength for stabilizing the hip and back during pitching, the pitch will be weak and demand higher forces from the upper extremity to compensate for the hip's weakness. This example not only demonstrates summation of forces but also points out the importance of two concepts in therapeutic exercise: (1) maintaining normal parameters in uninjured parts and (2) achieving normal parameters of factors, including strength, before functional activities can be resumed.

OTHER CONCEPTS IN PHYSICS

▶ Other concepts that relate to movement and the way the body responds to force include strength, work, power, energy, velocity, acceleration, elasticity, stress, strain, creep, structural fatigue, and friction.

Many physics terms have been used in this chapter. To improve your understanding and because these terms are used in later chapters, terms that are commonly used in therapeutic exercise and rehabilitation programs are defined here.

Strength

Strength is a muscle's relative ability to resist or produce a force. The greater the strength, the greater the ability to produce a force. The muscle's angle of pull, the angle of the resisting force, the muscle's length, and the speed of contraction and movement are factors that determine a muscle's strength.

The measure of a muscle's strength varies, depending on these factors and also on the method of measurement used. Using free weights to determine strength assesses the strength of the muscle at its weakest point in the range of motion. For example, if a patient is able to perform a forearm curl with a maximum weight of 14 kg (30 lb), this is the weight that the forearm flexors are able to lift at their weakest point. Although the weight of the dumbbell does not change as the forearm goes through its range of motion, the muscles' strength changes with the changing angles of pull and lever-arm lengths of the muscles force arm and dumbbell's resistance arm, and the changing physiological length of the muscles.

An isometric contraction can be used to evaluate the muscle's strength only at the specific joint position tested. The quantity of strength produced in an isometric contraction changes as the joint is positioned differently in its range of motion because of the changes in the muscle's lever-arm length, angle of pull, and physiological length. A more complete discussion of strength can be found in chapter 7.

Work

Work is the product of the amount of force (F) and the distance (d) through which the force is applied:

$$W = F \cdot d$$

Work is measured in foot-pounds (ft · lb) in the English system and joules (1 J = 1 N · m) in the metric system. If you lift a 20 lb (89 N) weight from the floor to a shelf 6 ft (1.8 m) above the floor, you would do 120 ft · lb (about 160 J) of work (6 ft · 20 lb, or 89 N · 1.8 m). When a weightlifter lifts a 250 lb (1112.5 N) barbell overhead to a height of 6.5 ft (2 m), he produces 1625 ft · lb (2225 J) of work.

Power

Power is the work per unit of time, or how fast the work is produced:

$$P = Fd/t$$

Work is done regardless of how much time it takes to perform the work. Power is a measure of the work done in a specific amount of time. In the English system it is measured in foot · pounds per second or in horsepower (1 horsepower = 550 ft · lb/s). In the metric system it is measured in joules per second or Newton-meters per second. Power is sometimes inaccurately interchanged with force.

In sports the most frequently used tests for power include the standing vertical jump and the softball throw. These activities require a sudden contraction of muscles to move the body or object in a short amount of time, thus generating a large force and great power.

Power requires strength to produce the force necessary to perform an activity with neuromuscular control to contract the muscles rapidly. Proprioception and functional aspects of therapeutic exercise programs should include power activities for patients involved in rapid activities. Keep in mind when working with athletes that power training is sport specific and requires you to understand the requirements of the patient's activity demands.

Energy

Energy is the capacity to do work. There are different types of energy. The law of conservation of energy states that energy can neither be created nor destroyed. Energy can, however, be converted from one form to another. For example, when a volleyball player serves the ball, some of the mechanical energy is converted to sound energy, but no energy is lost.

In therapeutic exercise and rehabilitation the two energy classifications that we are interested in are potential energy and kinetic energy. Potential energy and kinetic energy are often converted from one to the other. Potential energy is the capacity to do work that is stored in a body. Kinetic energy is the energy a body has because of its motion. When a moving body stops, the kinetic energy is all converted to potential energy. It is important to absorb this energy in a way that prevents injury. For example, when a gymnast dismounts from the high bar, he bends his knees to absorb the kinetic energy. When a patient performs plyometrics in the final stages of the therapeutic exercise program, the patient should move to safely absorb the kinetic energy produced by the movements in the exercise.

Velocity

Velocity is the rate of change of position. It is expressed in miles per hour (mph), feet per second (ft/s), or meters per second (m/s). *Velocity* is often interchanged with *speed*, which is not entirely accurate, but in most instances the difference is inconsequential. We use velocity to assess how well a sprinter runs the 100 m or how quickly a basketball player can get to the other end of the court on a fast break. Part of the functional examination before allowing a patient to return to activity may include an evaluation of the patient's velocity in functional activities.

Acceleration

Acceleration is the rate at which velocity changes. It is expressed in feet per second per second (ft/s²) or meters per second per second (m/s²). A sprinter coming out of the blocks at the start of a race accelerates, increasing velocity as she continues. In the final stages of a therapeutic exercise program, it is important for you to work on acceleration activities with patients for which acceleration is a factor. The therapeutic exercise program for an injured sprinter needs to include explosive strength development in the starting positions of hip flexion and knee flexion if the sprinter is to have the acceleration necessary to get out of the starting blocks.

Negative acceleration is called deceleration, the process of an object's slowing down rather than speeding up. After a baseball is pitched, the pitcher's arm goes from sudden acceleration to deceleration until the arm stops moving. It is the follow-through on an activity that provides as smooth a transition as possible from acceleration to deceleration. Poor follow-through increases the risk of injury because of the more rapid change from acceleration to deceleration. This is an important concept to recall in the final stages of the therapeutic exercise program, when activity-specific exercises are part of the program.

Gravity provides a constant acceleration of 9.8 m/s² (32 ft/s²). In other words, every second that an object falls it moves 9.8 m/s (32 ft/s) faster than it did during the previous second. If you drop a golf ball from a sufficient height, after the first second it falls at a velocity of 9.8 m/s (32 ft/s). After the next second it falls at a velocity of 19.6 m/s (64 ft/s), and after the third second it has a velocity of 29.4 m/s (96 ft/s). As Galileo discovered during the late 1500s when he dropped objects from the Tower of Pisa, this rate of acceleration occurs regardless of the object's weight if the effect of air resistance is disregarded. If you drop a ping-pong ball from the same height as the golf ball at the same time, its acceleration will be the same as the golf ball and they will hit the floor at the same time.

Conversely, a diver who jumps off a 3-m board will not hit the water at as great a speed as one who jumps off a 10-m board. Their acceleration is the same, but the diver from the 3-m board has a shorter distance to go before hitting the water; therefore, the time during which he accelerates is shorter, so his velocity by the time he hits the water is less than that of the 10-m diver.

Elasticity

Elasticity is the ability of an object to resume its former shape after a deforming or distorting force is applied. A muscle has elasticity because it can be stretched but returns to its normal length when the deforming force is discontinued. Rubber tubing or bands used in therapeutic exercise have a lot of elasticity. Steel has elasticity but less than asphalt. Ligaments have more elasticity than bone but less than muscles.

Stress and Strain

Stress is a force that changes the form or shape of a body. Strain is the amount of change in the size or shape of the object caused by the stress. Hooke's Law, developed during the 1600s by the physicist and mathematician Robert Hooke, deals with the relationship of stress and strain to elasticity: The strain is proportional to the stress producing it (so long as the strain is not too great—once the elastic limit is exceeded, permanent deformation occurs).

This concept is demonstrated in figure 3.16. The *OA* curve segment represents the elastic range. If a load is released in this range of the stress-strain curve, the object returns to its normal length. *A* is called the elastic limit,

Key

A = Elastic limit
Y = Yield point
OA = Elastic range
M = Maximum strength
AM = Plastic range
F = Failure point

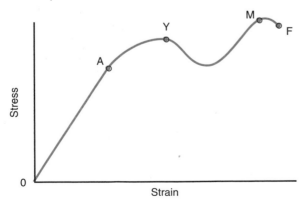

Figure 3.16 Stress-strain curve.

beyond which Hooke's law is no longer valid. Beyond the elastic range is the plastic range *AM*. When a load stresses an object into this range, a permanent change in the object's size or shape occurs. Any load that continues beyond the plastic range ultimately causes a failure of the object, *F*.

The size of these ranges varies from material to material and from structure to structure. In rehabilitation, it is important to realize the differences in the stress-strain curves of structures such as bone, muscle, tendons, cartilage, and ligaments. This knowledge is important in prevention and treatment of injuries. Some ligaments contain more elastic fibers than others, so they can withstand more stress, whereas others have fewer elastic fibers and provide more stability to a joint. Recently formed scar tissue has more elasticity than more mature scar tissue. Knowing the maturity of scar tissue determines the amount of stress and the amount of time the stress should be applied to affect a change in the scar tissue's length.

Creep

Creep occurs when a low-level stress, usually in the elastic range of the tissue, is applied over a long enough period to cause deformation of the tissue. Increasing the temperature of the tissue increases the rate of creep. For this reason, applying heat to an area before stretching may make the stretch more effective. This concept also explains why longer stretches produce better results. It also demonstrates why poor posture over time causes changes in muscles, joints, and connective tissue; sitting with your head forward for a prolonged time as you read this book will cause the ligaments and muscles of your posterior neck and upper back to lengthen, making it ultimately more difficult to resume a proper posture. Over time and with repetition of any abnormal position, permanent changes in tissue length result.

Structural Fatigue

All tissues and objects are subject to structural fatigue. Structural fatigue is the point at which a tissue or object can no longer withstand a stress, and breaks. This can occur in a sudden movement, as when a ligament is suddenly torn, or it can occur over time with an accumulation of stress. The point at which tissue failure results from long term stress is sometimes referred to as the endurance limit or fatigue failure. Breakdown of bone from cumulative trauma is called a stress fracture. Injuries caused by repeated stress, such as carpal tunnel syndrome, are called repetitive stress syndromes or overuse syndromes. Treatment of cumulative trauma injuries is different from that of acute trauma injuries and is discussed more thoroughly in chapter 15.

Friction

Friction is the relative resistance between two surfaces. It can be advantageous or deleterious, depending on the circumstances. A patient who is very weak may have difficulty abducting the thigh in supine because friction of the leg against the treatment table adds resistance. If the surface is made smoother by applying a friction-reducing agent such as talcum powder, the activity is easier.

Standing with a wide base of support, with the feet wider than the hips, stabilizes the body but requires friction. If a person takes that same stance on ice, he or she will fall because ice provides less friction than many other surfaces.

Sometimes we want to increase friction to obtain more traction and apply more force. Cleats on football shoes or tread on basketball shoes are good examples of this. When decreasing friction is desirable, such as on the uneven parallel bars in gymnastics, substances such as chalk are used to reduce friction and minimize the risk of blisters.

In therapeutic exercise, friction may not be desirable in pulley exercises because it wears out the system more quickly and makes exercises more difficult. On the other hand, it may be advantageous to have more friction to increase resistance in other exercises. For example, a patient sitting on a rolling stool and propelling it with one foot is exercising the hamstrings, as in figure 3.17a. If a patient can propel the stool without much difficulty, a weight that is attached and dragged behind the stool increases friction and provides more resistance to movement (figure 3.17b).

Figure 3.17   Use of friction in therapeutic exercise.

SUMMARY

1. Define force and give an example of an internal and an external force.

   Force is energy that causes movement and has direction and magnitude. Internal forces are generated by muscles. An example of an external force is gravity.

2. Explain the relevance to therapeutic exercise of Newton's first, second, and third laws of motion.

   Newton's first law of motion deals with inertia, the second law of motion deals with acceleration and momentum, and the third law of motion concerns action and reaction. All these laws govern how the body moves and reacts to forces that are applied to it.

3. Explain how center of gravity changes with movement.

   The body's center of gravity becomes higher if the arms are raised overhead and lower if the body crouches. If a weight is carried at the side, the center of gravity shifts to the side with the weight; to maintain balance and keep the center of gravity over the feet, the body must lean away from the weight.

4. Discuss how a change in base of support can change a person's stability.

   The narrower the base of support, the less stable is the object; the wider the base of support, the more stable it is.

5. Explain the relationship between line of gravity and base of support.

   An object is stable when the line of gravity is within its base of support.

6. Explain two ways of increasing stability.

   A person can increase stability by aligning the feet in the direction of the applied force or lowering the center of gravity while keeping it within the base of support.

7. Identify the difference between stability and fixation.

   Stability is a state in which a person or object is not easily thrown off balance. Fixation is a state of stability where motion is being restricted or prevented. When referring to the act of fixating a body segment to produce a desired motion, stabilization is the term often used, since the desired effect, stabilization, is the result of fixation.

8. Explain how torque can be altered in the body.

   Torque produced by the body can be altered most easily by changing the force-arm length, the amount of force applied, or the angle of pull.

9. Identify how varying positions change a muscle's mechanical advantage.

   As a joint moves through its range of motion, the angle of pull of a muscle changes, altering the length of the muscle's lever arm, which changes its mechanical advantage.

10. Discuss the difference between mechanical and physiological advantage of a muscle.

    A muscle's mechanical advantage has to do with its line and angle of pull and the forces it must produce to overcome a resistance, while the physiological advantage is the muscle's ability to shorten.

11. Explain the importance of positioning in exercising two-joint muscles.

    The ability of a two-joint muscle to produce force is affected by its relative length at both joints. A muscle is able to shorten to no less than about 66% its resting length, so its position at one joint affects its ability to produce force at the other joint.

12. Distinguish between velocity and acceleration.

    Velocity is the rate of change of position, whereas acceleration is the rate at which velocity changes.

13. Discuss the relevance of elasticity, stress and strain, creep, and friction to therapeutic exercise.

    Elasticity, stress and strain, and creep are all qualities that affect a tissue's ability to change its length or shape. These factors influence the type of stretch that is applied to a structure and the effectiveness of that stretch. Friction can be advantageous or detrimental, depending on the exercise and its goal.

CRITICAL THINKING QUESTIONS

1. Explain how Newton's first three laws of motion and gravity affect therapeutic exercise programs. In other words, how do inertia, acceleration, action-reaction, and gravity determine how you have a patient perform an exercise?

2. Using the concepts about base of support discussed in this chapter, describe how you can improve your base of support while giving manual resistance to hip flexion and extension on a patient who is supine. Use a partner and try the changes in your base of support to demonstrate how those changes give you an advantage or disadvantage in the manual-resistance exercise.

3. Explain how the different classes of levers apply to therapeutic exercise. Give an example of each class of lever with a different therapeutic exercise, and explain how the class of lever can change with a change in the exercise position or resistance application.

4. Describe how an elbow-flexion exercise changes when the technique or equipment used is manual resistance, rubber banding, pulley, dumbbell, weight machine, and hydraulic machine. Does the type of resistance change? What about the kind of muscle activity? What advantage of each exercise makes it different from the others?

5. In what position would you put a patient to provide maximal muscle shortening during an exercise for the hamstring? In what position should the patient be to maximize hamstring activity at the knee? at the hip?

6. Throw a ball as far as you can while standing on one foot and then with both feet on the ground. In which position are you able to throw the ball farther? What mechanical concepts come into play here?

LAB ACTIVITIES

1. State the primary planes in which the following motions occur (assume the anatomical position unless otherwise noted):

   Stair climbing

   Wrist ulnar deviation

   Turning a door knob (using the forearm with the elbow flexed to 90°)

   Using a screwdriver with the elbow extended and the arm at the side

   Cervical rotation

   Jumping jacks

   Lumbar spine sidebending

2. The following exercises are to be performed in the sitting position with the elbow straight:

   Perform shoulder flexion to 90° with a 5 lb. weight held in the hand

   Perform shoulder flexion to 90° with a 5 lb. cuff weight placed above the elbow

   Which motion is easier to perform? Why?

3. With one person lying supine on a table as the patient and the other person standing beside the table as the rehabilitation clinician, have the patient lift the leg in a straight-leg raise and return to the start position. Now have the rehabilitation clinician apply resistance to the leg with a hand on the mid thigh as the patient lifts the leg as hard as possible and returns to the start position. Next, the rehabilitation clinician applies resistance force at the knee, and in the final repetition, the rehabilitation clinician applies force at the ankle. On each repetition, the patient should push against the rehabilitation clinician as hard as possible.

   Answer the following questions:

   a. Which repetition was the most difficult for the patient? For the rehabilitation clinician?

   b. Why?

   c. Of what value is this information to you in performing a resistance exercise with a patient? In performing a manual muscle test?

4. Hold a 5 lb. weight in your hand with your elbow bent and next to your side. Now hold it out so your shoulder is in front of you at 90° and your elbow is flexed to 90°. Now straighten your elbow so the arm is fully extended in front of you.

   Answer the following questions:

   a. Calculate the torque of the 5 lb. weight for each position.

   b. How much torque do your muscles produce to hold the weight in each position?

   c. Of what value is this information to you in setting up a patient on resistance exercises?

   d. Have your partner perform a push-up in an easy, moderate, and then difficult position. What are the three positions? What is the principle upon which the difficulty increased with the exercise progression?

5. Position your partner to achieve passive insufficiency of the finger flexors. What joints do the long finger flexor tendons cross; into what position did you position each joint?

6. Position your lab partner to place the quadriceps in a passively insufficient position. Now resist the quadriceps in knee extension. What was the outcome? Why?

7. Have your partner create active insufficiency of the quadriceps. Now resist the quadriceps in knee extension. What was the outcome? Why?

8. What to the results of questions 7 and 8 demonstrate to you in terms of importance in exercises?

SUGGESTED READING

Cornwall, M.W. 1984. Biomechanics of noncontractile tissue. *Physical Therapy* 64:1869–1873.

Dumbelton, J.H., and J. Black. 1975. *An introduction to orthopedic materials.* Springfield, IL: Charles C Thomas.

Frankel, V.H., and M. Nordin. 1980. *Basic biomechanics of the skeletal system.* Philadelphia: Lea & Febiger.

Frost, H.M. 1973. *Orthopedic biomechanics.* Springfield, IL: Charles C Thomas.

Gardiner, M.D. 1981. *The principles of exercise therapy.* London: Bell.

Groves, R., and D.N. Camaione. 1983. *Concepts in kinesiology.* Philadelphia: Saunders.

Luttgens, K., and N. Hamilton. 1998. *Kinesiology: Scientific basis of human motion.* 9th ed. Boston: McGraw-Hill.

Rasch, P.J., ed. 1989. *Kinesiology and applied anatomy.* Philadelphia: Lea & Febiger.

Smith, L.K., Weiss, E.L., and L.D. Lehmkuhl. 1996. *Brunnstrom's clinical kinesiology.* Philadelphia: Davis.

Strauss, R.H., ed. 1979. *Sports medicine and physiology.* Philadelphia: Saunders.

Wilmore, J.H., and D.L. Costill. 2004. *Physiology of sport and exercise* 3rd ed. Champaign, IL: Human Kinetics.

Examination and Assessment

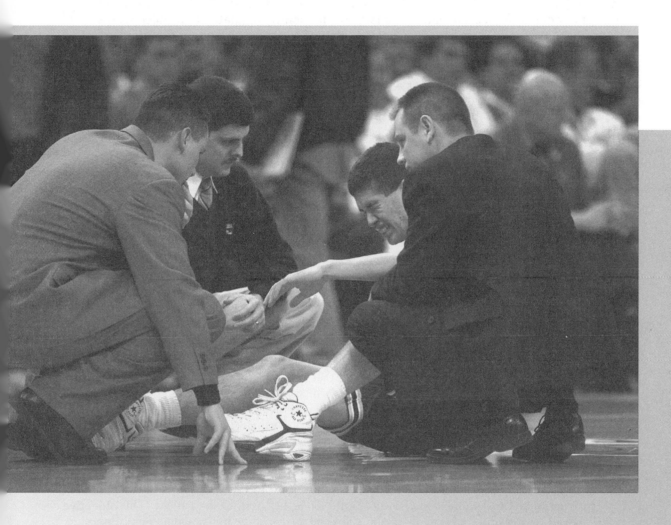

Objectives

After completing this chapter, you should be able to do the following:

1. Identify the primary factors of subjective examination.

2. Outline an objective examination procedure that includes all primary factors.

3. Explain the different types of end-feel and distinguish between normal and pathological end-feels.

4. Explain how a treatment plan is designed and upon what factors it is based.

5. Define the SOAP note and explain its significance to rehabilitation.

6. Identify two other records used in rehabilitation and demonstrate their importance.

Catherine An instructs incoming athletic training students on rehabilitation examination procedures. She has found in the past that the students' primary point of confusion is identifying the difference between examination of an acute injury for first aid and examination of an injury for rehabilitation. Instruction with her new class begins today. Her first goal is to identify the differences between an acute-injury examination and a rehabilitation examination. Catherine will then introduce the procedures for a rehabilitation examination, explain how to identify the patient's problems, how to base goals on those problems, and how to develop a plan of treatment based on the problems and goals.

Although many of the students have been exposed to record keeping for initial injuries in the athletic training clinic, few of them know the record-keeping procedures for rehabilitation. Some of them have seen SOAP notes during their observations in their freshman year, but not many of them understand what they are and how they function. In addition to SOAP notes, Catherine will introduce students to the other records used in rehabilitation. Many new students are overwhelmed with their first sight of what seems like a mountain of paperwork, but Catherine knows from experience that the paperwork becomes routine and is not the insurmountable task students initially think it to be.

■ Oh . . . I listen a lot and talk less. You can't learn anything when you're talking.

Bing Crosby, entertainer, 1903-1977

Examination and assessment of an injury serve as the foundation for a treatment program. For the rehabilitation clinician to design the most appropriate therapeutic exercise program, the patient must first be examined. Without an examination to know where deficiencies lie, the extent of the injury, and other factors that may affect a therapeutic exercise program, the rehabilitation clinician has no basis on which to decide what should or should not be incorporated in the rehabilitation program. The terms *evaluation* and *examination* are often interchanged. This text uses **examination** to indicate the means by which a rehabilitation clinician seeks information on the severity, irritability, nature, and stage of a patient's injury. The examination is composed of subjective and objective elements. The **subjective examination** is the history of the injury and the patient's experience of pain and other symptoms. It is obtained from the patient and serves to guide the objective portion of the examination. Like Bing Crosby, the clinician can learn a lot by listening to the patient. The **objective examination** discovers the observable signs and effects of the injury and involves observing, testing, and palpating the injury. The results of the subjective and objective examinations allow the rehabilitation clinician to assess the patient's injury and determine the most appropriate treatment for achieving whatever goals are established for the patient. An **assessment** is a conclusion based on the gathering of information. At the time of an initial examination, assessment is used to design a therapeutic exercise program. Once the program has been instituted, the results of the treatment are evaluated to assess the treatment's effectiveness. Finally, before the patient returns to full sport participation or normal activity, the patient is examined and assessed for readiness and ability to perform and withstand the stresses of the sport or activity. In short, an examination must precede an assessment, and both are required not only at the commencement and conclusion of a rehabilitation program, but frequently throughout the program as well.

This chapter is divided into three parts. The first part deals with subjective and objective aspects of an examination, the second part discusses assessments that are based on the examination, and the third part introduces records of these examinations assessments that should be kept throughout the rehabilitation process. This chapter concludes the presentation of the basic concepts needed to understand the whys of therapeutic exercise.

EXAMINATION: MAKING A PROFILE

▶ Information from the patient regarding the history of the injury and subjective symptoms is gathered during the subjective examination. The objective examination involves inspecting, palpating, and testing to determine the extent and severity of the injury.

The first part of performing an initial examination to determine the extent and involvement of the injury, the patient's deficiencies, and a course of treatment is to create a profile of the injury. This is accomplished by performing a subjective and an objective examination.

It is important to take an accurate and complete history before the objective examination. As Bing Crosby indicated in the opening quotation of this chapter, listening is fundamental to learning, and obtaining a history includes listening to the patient's reports of the injury. A history is only as good as the questions asked. If you expect a thorough history from the patient, you must ask questions that will reveal all that is necessary to obtain a complete picture.

Once the subjective examination is completed, an objective examination follows. This includes observations of abnormalities, palpation, and measurements of deficiencies in range of motion, strength, proprioception, and other parameters, which provide you with a clear picture of problems. A treatment program cannot be planned and delivered until you identify and assess the problems and deficiencies that the injury has caused. Problems are identified by thorough and accurate subjective and objective examinations.

Subjective Examination

The subjective examination is essentially the history of the injury and patient's report of pain and other symptoms. The subjective examination can assist in determining the extent of the injury, how aggressively the objective examination can be performed, and what to include in the objective examination. The specific questions to ask during the history vary, depending on a variety of factors such as the area injured and the severity and nature of the injury.

To obtain a thorough and accurate history, it is best to ask questions that do not lead the patient to an anticipated answer. For example, rather than ask, "Is it painful to walk?" a better question is, "What activities cause you more pain?"

The questions should be simple and straightforward. They should be presented in a logical and systematic sequence. It is best for each rehabilitation clinician to develop his or her own method or system of sequential questions that is consistent and easy to remember. This is not to say that the questions should be rigid and unchanging. Because each patient's history is different, the line of questioning will be different in each situation. The idea is to make history-taking procedures a habit that results in a consistent overall profile. When you first start out, you may need to write down questions to establish a routine for yourself, but listening to patients' responses and taking a logical and thorough history will become more automatic with experience.

History of the Injury

Allow the patient to explain in his or her own words how the injury occurred. The goal is to get an idea of the mechanism of injury, tissues involved, and extent of involvement. The patient should tell when the injury occurred, whether it occurred suddenly or gradually, immediate and later signs (e.g., immediate swelling or swelling only 24 h later), and what treatment has been provided. The patient should also say whether he or she was able to continue sport participation or activity, if the injured part remained functional (e.g., was the patient able to walk?), and what, if anything, has changed between the time of the injury and the time of your examination. Information of this type can help you determine the severity of the injury and the tissue type involved. Knowing whether ice or heat has been applied may change your impression of the injury. The involved area may be very swollen because no treatment was given, heat was applied, or the patient swells easily. If the patient has taken medication, it may mask pain or change the results of the tests you perform.

Medical History

Getting a medical history of previous injury is important. If a prior injury has occurred, it is valuable to know previous treatments. Did the patient seek medical care? Did the patient receive treatment, and if so, what specific treatment was given, how long was it provided, and what was the outcome? How many subsequent injury episodes has the patient experienced? Is the pain the same this time as it was in the past?

Recurring episodes may affect your assessment of the current problem and the treatment program you establish. For example, recurring ankle sprains can result in additional scar tissue in or around the joint, restricted soft-tissue mobility, reduced strength and proprioceptive abilities, or increased laxity and instability of the joint. Repeated muscle strains may cause tendinitis. Recurring knee meniscus lesions may lead to chronic synovitis. Over the long term, repetitive injuries to a joint may result in arthritis.

In the case of prior injuries, a report of the previous treatments provided is necessary to get a picture of prior injury management. Good management may have minimized previous injuries and left the patient with a good impression of rehabilitation, but poor management may prejudice the patient into having little confidence in rehabilitation outcomes and may also complicate the current picture. For example, if a patient presents with a knee injury and a history of prior similar injuries that were not treated, the current injury may have been caused by a weakness of the muscles and other knee structures that may prolong the current treatment. You will need to deal with effects of both the current and prior injury.

Special Questions

Special questions, such as whether the patient is taking any medications and the general health of the patient, can reveal factors that influence your understanding of the injury and your treatment plan. Does the patient have any systemic diseases that may affect treatment, such as diabetes, asthma, HIV? Has there been any unexpected weight loss lately? This may be a sign of unsuspected cancer and should be referred to the physician. Is the patient taking steroids? This can interfere with the healing process. Questions regarding difficulty with bowel or bladder control are important to ask with back injuries since a positive answer may indicate an injury to the cauda equina, which needs immediate medical attention. Knowing what tests have been performed, such as X-rays or MRI, can help you focus your examination on related tests.

Additional Information

Additional information is also useful in completing an accurate profile of the injury and the patient's expectations of the treatment program. The patient's normal level of activity and the activities to which the patient wishes to return after rehabilitation give you an idea of the patient's expectations and the physical requirements for meeting those expectations. For example, if a runner presents with a knee injury that has been getting worse over time, what does he want to be able to resume doing once the treatment is over? How far, fast, and frequently was he running before the injury? Over what kinds of terrain was he running? What kind of shoes does he use? Has he had any changes in his workouts, terrain, or other activities? Questions like these help you create an accurate profile of the patient and determine the cause of injury.

Other general questions include the patient's sport and position in that sport, if the patient is an athlete. The answers give you an idea of the amounts and kinds of stresses that may have caused the injury and the stress level that the patient's body must withstand in order to return to the sport.

When working in a high school or college athletic program, the clinician often knows the age of the patient. In a clinic, however, the ages of patients can vary greatly. The patient's age is important in identifying certain injuries and also in deciding what treatment to apply. For example, osteoarthritis is a common problem among individuals over the age of 40. Ultrasound is not a treatment choice for a 13-year-old patient with a knee injury because of the open epiphyseal plates in the knee at that age.

Does the patient hear **crepitus** (clicking or snapping) from the injured part? These are what I call the "Rice Krispies" sounds: the snap, crackle, and pop of injury. Crepitus in a joint can sound either light or coarse, depending on whether the roughening of cartilage surfaces is slight or significant. A fine crepitus sometimes can be palpated in a joint with synovial thickening, as in synovitis. Crepitus can also be felt or heard in tendinitis because of the increased thickening and friction between the tendon and its sheath. A creaking sound is heard in joints that are in the later stages of joint-surface degeneration. A clicking or popping sound can be heard with meniscal displacement in either the temporomandibular joint or the knee joint; if the clicking is painful, the meniscus may be torn. Non-painful clicks heard in joints, especially hypermobile joints, may be a normal vacuum click and of no consequence. Non-painful but sometimes loud snapping sounds are frequently the inconsequential result of a ligament or a tendon slipping over a bony prominence when a joint moves. A clunking sound is produced by a joint that is unstable and subluxes as it moves through a particular part of its motion. Repeated subluxation making this sound can eventually cause degeneration of the joint.

Pain Profile

A profile of the patient's pain assists in determining the nature and severity of the injury and what to include in your objective examination and initial treatment plan. Several questions should be asked to obtain this profile:

- *Where is the pain?* Can it be located with one finger, or is it over a larger area? Does it stay localized, or does it go to other areas? Is the pain deep or superficial? Is it in a joint or in the surrounding area? A small, pinpoint area of pain is probably a localized, minor injury or a chronic injury. A larger, more diffuse or deep area of pain probably indicates a larger or more serious injury or an acute injury.

  Pain that radiates into other areas may be referred pain caused by pressure on a nerve or myofascial referral from stimulation of trigger points. This pain and its cause need to be identified and further examined during your objective evaluation.

- *Did the pain come on suddenly or gradually?* This question helps determine the cause of injury. A sudden pain is most often seen in sport injuries and occurs with a sudden overstress of tissue, as occurs with a muscle strain or a ligamentous sprain. Gradual onset of pain occurs more often with tendinitis and other inflammations. With gradual pain, patients commonly do not seek medical assistance until the pain interferes with sport or work performance or less stressful daily activities.

  If the pain occurred gradually, how long has the patient had the pain? This determines whether the problem is acute or chronic. Acute pain is treated differently from chronic pain.

- *Is the pain constant or intermittent?* Most pain is intermittent or varies in intensity with either activity or time of day. The cause of pain that is constant and unchanging must be suspected as something other than musculoskeletal injury. Pain that is initially constant becomes intermittent with appropriate treatment.

- *How intense is the pain?* Have the patient rate the pain on a scale of 0 to 10, where 0 is no pain and 10 is "take me to the hospital, I'm dying" pain. Pain is very subjective and varies greatly from one person to another. Trying to quantify pain by assigning a number to it does not make it an objective measure but does allow relative comparisons. The patient's pain rating gives you an idea of the patient's pain tolerance and can be used later to determine changes in the patient's pain. If a patient rates pain initially as 8 and three days later as 4, your treatment program is achieving its desired goal. This numerical system gives both you and the patient a method of gauging changes. It would be improper and useless to compare one patient's pain to another's, but there is some value in reassessing the patient's pain ratings as the treatment program progresses.

- *How does the patient describe the pain? What kind of pain is it?* There is a variety of descriptors that can be used to identify pain, such as sharp, dull, aching, burning, and tingling. Musculoskeletal pain is usually deep, dull, or an ache. The pain of more acute or severe muscle injuries can be described as sharp, stabbing, or throbbing.

- *What are aggravating and easing factors? What does the patient do that causes or intensifies the pain? What relieves or reduces it?* In general, musculoskeletal pain occurs with movement and is relieved with rest. Pain from inflammation may not be relieved with rest. Prolonged positioning, such as poor sitting posture, can irritate soft tissues by applying prolonged or abnormal low-level stress to them.

• *Does the pain vary with time of day? How does the area feel in the morning? As the day progresses? By evening?* Stiffness in the morning can be related to inflammation. If the pain increases as the day progresses, it may be that the injured area lacks sufficient strength and endurance to carry on activities and becomes fatigued. Spasm and pain may intensify as the day progresses, especially in acute injuries.

• *Does the pain awaken the patient at night?* Musculoskeletal pain can worsen at night enough to disturb the patient's sleep. Inflammation and bone pain can also cause sleep disturbances. Inflammation pain that causes sleep disturbances indicates a bigger problem than pain that does not disturb sleep. If pain disturbs sleep, ask the patient how many times this occurs in a night and how long it takes to return to sleep. The answers to these questions give you an idea of the irritability of the injury. The more frequent the disturbances and the longer it takes the patient to return to sleep, the more irritated the injury.

The intensity of the pain, the kinds of activities that aggravate it, how long a patient can perform an activity before the pain increases, and how long it takes to reduce the pain once it has increased also indicate the **irritability** of the injury. The more irritable an injury is, the greater the pain, the more easily pain is increased with even low-level activity, and the longer it takes to ease. Corrigan and Maitland (1989) define an injury as being irritable when only a moderate amount of activity increases the pain and pain lasts for an hour. When an injury is not irritable, the patient feels only a momentary pain after stress.

Objective Examination

Once you have completed your subjective examination by taking the history of the injury, determining the patient's activity level and performance expectations, and profiling the pain and injury, it is time to perform your objective examination. Your goal is to determine exactly the structure or structures involved and the extent of the injury's effects so that you can determine your course of treatment.

Before you begin your physical examination, you already have a lot of information about the injury. This information guides your objective examination. From your subjective examination you have an idea of the nature of the problem, the severity and irritability of the injury, how aggressive or cautious you should be in performing your objective examination, which special tests to use, and which contraindications to consider. Although you may expect certain findings from your objective examination, it is important to keep an open mind and look at all possibilities for the injury and the tissues involved. Do not assume that you know what the diagnosis is until you have a total picture based on the accumulated information from both the subjective and objective segments. Narrowing your scope of vision may lead you to an inaccurate conclusion and to create an inappropriate rehabilitation program.

If an injury is irritable, your objective examination should be brief, relatively gentle, and less stressful to the injury. On the other hand, if an injury is not irritable, your examination can be more aggressive. A second degree sprain that occurred two days ago, that now exhibits a lot of swelling, causes persistent pain that increases with any active or passive range of movement, and causes pain with weight bearing is considered irritable and requires a gentle, brief examination to determine initial treatment. At a later stage when the injury is less irritable, a more aggressive and complete examination can be performed. Right now, however, your evaluation goal is to determine what treatment will best relieve current symptoms so that the patient can begin an effective rehabilitation process.

If a patient is able to walk without pain and has minimal edema, your objective evaluation can be more aggressive to determine the extent of the injury, the tissues involved, and the treatment approach that will most effectively return this patient to participation or normal activity.

A **comparable sign** is an active or passive movement that reproduces the patient's pain symptom, (Maitland 1991). Although it is not always easy to achieve a comparable sign in an objective examination, the rehabilitation clinician usually attempts to produce one.

Observation and Visual Inspection

Your visual inspection starts the moment you see the patient enter your facility. How is the patient walking? What is the posture and gait? General observations give you information about the severity of the injury and the items to inspect in your examination. For example, if the patient complains of medial knee pain and has excessively pronated feet, part of the problem may result from the feet and not the knee. If a patient has hip pain and genu valgus, weakness or structural anomalies at the knee may be contributing to hip pain.

Other general observations include noting whether the patient requires any assistive devices, such as a brace or crutches. Is the patient reluctant to move the injured part? Noting any abnormal movements, posture, or behavior helps you complete your picture of the injury. For example, if a patient enters your facility walking with crutches, you already know that gait training will eventually be a part of your treatment program. If you see a patient limping into the room, you should examine the entire lower extremity for weakness, because limping can cause weakness of improperly used muscles very quickly.

Your visual inspection of the injured area includes noting any abnormalities in the extremity that need more discriminate examination. Is there edema present, and if so, how much? Is there any discoloration, rash, wound, deformity, or atrophy present? If there is discoloration, does it appear distal to the injury, indicating that the patient probably did not elevate and correctly treat the injury when it occurred, or is the discoloration around the injury or proximal to it? Is there a scar, and if so, is it healed, does it look infected or excessive, and how recent does it appear to be?

Range of Motion

Range of motion of any joint can be normal, excessive (hypermobile), or less than normal (hypomobile). Normal ranges of motion for specific joints and how to measure them are discussed in chapter 5. Examination of the quality and quantity of available joint mobility investigates the capsule and ligamentous stability of the joint.

Active Range of Motion

Active range of motion (AROM) is the amount of movement produced by an individual without assistance (figure 4.1). Active range of motion depends on the amount of pain caused

Figure 4.1 Active range of motion.

by active movement of the part, the willingness of the patient to move it, the strength of the muscles moving the joint, and the available range of motion of the joint. Pain may not be the only reason a patient is reluctant to move a part through its range of motion. For example, the patient may be apprehensive of reinjury. When evaluating active range of motion, the rehabilitation clinician must consider the patient's position and be aware of gravity's effect on movement. For example, in a test of shoulder-flexion range of motion, a sitting patient has to overcome the greatest resistance to gravity at midrange, but in a supine position gravity's effect is greatest in the initial stages of movement. If a patient is unable to raise her arm overhead when sitting, the rehabilitation clinician should have the patient lie supine to see whether additional active motion is possible when gravity has less impact on shoulder-flexor strength in that position.

Restricted joint motion may have a number of causes. Swelling, tightening of the joint capsule and ligaments, loss of flexibility in muscles, and a mechanical blockage, such as a loose body or osteophyte, can by themselves or in combination prevent a patient from achieving full range of motion. As your examination proceeds, the cause should be revealed.

It is also important to observe the quality of movement. Is the movement full and fluid, or is it irregular, hesitant, or jerking? Does it occur through substitution of other muscles? If active motion causes pain, where in the motion does it occur? Does the pain occur midrange through an arc of motion? This often indicates an irritated structure, such as the shoulder's supraspinatus tendon or a disk protrusion in the spine.

Information regarding the patient's ability to move helps you to determine what to include in your rehabilitation program, such as pain-relief measures, joint motion and strength exercises, and coordination and functional activities.

Passive Range of Motion

Passive range of motion is the amount of movement produced without any active participation by the patient (figure 4.2). Passive joint motion can be divided into two categories:

Figure 4.2 Passive range of motion.

physiological and accessory. **Physiological joint motion** is movement that can also be performed actively by the individual. Physiological motion is also called cardinal motion. **Accessory joint motion** is motion that cannot be performed actively but is necessary for full active motion to occur.

Passive physiological range of motion is the motion a joint attains when you move it while the patient remains relaxed. It is usually greater than the active range of motion in both injured and uninjured joints. As you move the joint through its motion, the patient should tell you when and where pain occurs in the motion. You should observe the patient's facial expressions, which also may indicate pain. The joint should be moved as far into the pain and through the range of motion as the patient can tolerate.

Once again, note the quantity and quality of the motion, whether passive motion causes pain, and if so, where in the motion the pain occurs. Pain that occurs with passive movement may be the result of stretching either inert structures, such as ligaments and capsules, or active structures, such as muscles. As you move the part through its motion, it is also important to note the end-feel of the movement.

If a joint's movement is normal and painless, **overpressure** is applied to truly assess full, painless motion. The pressure should be moderate and achieve slightly more motion as the joint is brought to its end range, but the motion should remain painless. To truly consider a joint as normal, firm overpressure must produce a painless and full range of motion (Maitland 1991).

End-Feel of Movement

The **end-feel** of a joint's movement is the nature of resistance that is felt at the end of a range of movement. The end-feel can be normal or pathological, depending on the particular joint and the extent of its range of motion compared to what's expected. Kessler and Hertling (1983) list normal and pathological end-feels for a variety of tissues. End-feels that can be either normal or pathological include capsular, bony, soft-tissue approximation, and muscular. Some end-feels are pathological because they occur only when there is tissue injury. These include muscle spasm end-feel, boggy end-feel, springy end-feel, and empty end-feel.

A capsular end-feel is a firm, leathery sensation when bringing a joint to the end of its motion. It is firm but not hard. If you move a normal, uninjured shoulder into full lateral rotation you will feel a firm, leathery end-feel. A capsular end-feel can also be felt in a pathological joint, such as a knee that has no edema or inflammation but does have limited mobility.

A common example of a normal bony end-feel is that of the elbow in full extension with the olecranon process moving against the olecranon fossa. It is a sudden-stop end-feel. In pathological states, the sensation is the same, but it occurs because of an abnormal condition, such as a bony growth or fracture malunion, and the total motion is less than normal.

Soft tissue approximation end-feels occur when two muscle bellies meet to prevent further movement. A normal example is the anterior upper arm and forearm meeting in elbow flexion. The sensation is soft at the end of the movement.

A muscular end-feel is softer, less abrupt, and more rubbery than a capsular end-feel. It has a spring to it, much like what is felt when performing a straight-leg raise that is restricted by the hamstring muscles. The muscular end-feel is different from a muscle spasm end-feel in that the muscle spasm end-feel is more abrupt and usually causes pain. A rebound of the muscle as it reflexes into a contraction in response to the stretch is felt only in pathological conditions.

A boggy, soft, mushy end-feel is usually observed with joint effusion, when fluid within the joint prevents full motion. While the sensation of movement is boggy, the fluid's pressure blocks normal motion. It is common for this sensation to follow capsular joint movements, but this sensation occurs before the capsular end-feel is achieved.

A springy end-feel occurs from the mechanical block of a loose body and indicates an internal derangement. It is most commonly seen in the knee, where loose bodies of cartilage or meniscal flaps can stop normal joint movement.

An empty end-feel is not common. There is no resistance to joint movement because the ligamentous and capsular restrictions are gone, and there is too much pain with muscular restriction for the patient to voluntarily stop the movement. In the absence of any ligamentous injury, acute bursitis or a neoplasm should be suspected with an empty end-feel.

Accessory Joint Mobility

The other portion of passive motion, accessory joint motion, must also be evaluated to determine overall joint mobility. Accessory joint motion is motion that cannot be produced actively by the patient but is necessary for full, normal motion of a joint. Accessory joint motion is evaluated by joint mobilization techniques. A good example of accessory joint motion is longitudinal rotation of the finger on the metacarpophalangeal joint (figure 4.3). It is not a motion that the patient can produce by any muscle activity, but you can rotate the phalanx easily by grasping the finger and rotating the proximal phalanx on its metacarpal. This accessory rotation must be present for full, active finger flexion-extension to occur. Specific joint mobilization techniques for treatment are the same as those used in examination and are discussed in chapter 6.

Figure 4.3 Accessory joint mobility.

A joint can be normal in its mobility, hypermobile (excessive mobility), or hypomobile (restricted mobility). Joints that are hypomobile may be so because of muscle spasm protecting the area or because of restriction of ligamentous and capsular structures. Adhesions within the capsule can occur following injury, surgery, or immobilization. If you determine that a joint lacks full capsular mobility, part of your treatment plan should include joint mobilization techniques.

In examination of physiological and accessory joint mobility, you are looking for signs of stiffness in the joint, amplitude of available mobility, quality of motion, end-feel, and motion that is pain free. The best examination of the quality and quantity of stiffness and amplitude of motion is made by comparing the joint with its counterpart. Hypermobility of a joint can be considered normal for the individual if it is bilateral. Accessory joint motions should be pain free throughout a normal range of movement.

Resistive Range of Motion: Muscle Strength

Examining muscles surrounding the injured area involves investigation of their strength and endurance in addition to their motion. There are a number of procedures that can examine muscular strength and endurance. The most common technique is isometric strength testing (figure 4.4). Other techniques can be used and are discussed in chapter 7.

Isometric testing for a quick determination of muscular strength is usually performed in a midrange or end-range joint position to measure gross muscle-group strength. This method of strength examination is called a **manual muscle test** and is discussed in detail in chapter 7 along with other methods of strength examination. Table 4.1 lists the muscle strength grades used in a manual muscle test. A more extensive table is seen in chapter 7.

Special Tests

Special tests are used in the examination to determine the aggressiveness of the treatment program and at what point the patient should begin the program. For example, if a patient

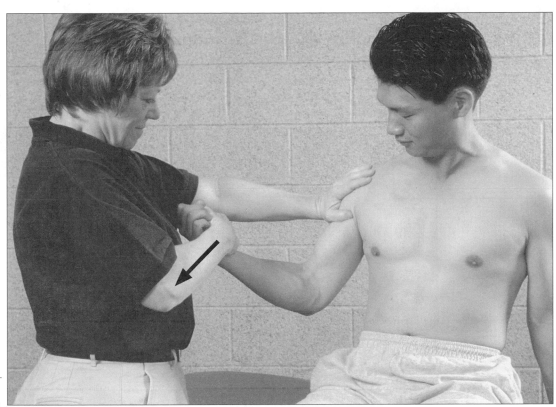

Figure 4.4 Muscular strength testing.

Table 4.1
Muscle Strength Grades

Numerical grade	Qualitative grade	Definition
5	Normal (N)	Able to resist maximum force throughout a full range of motion in a gravity-dependent position
4	Good (G)	Able to resist some force throughout a full range of motion in a gravity-dependent position
3	Fair (F)	Able to move the segment through a full range of motion against gravity but without resistance
2	Poor (P)	Able to move the segment through a full range of motion but not against gravity
1	Trace (T)	Palpation reveals a contraction of the muscle but no limb motion occurs
0	Zero (0)	No perceptible contraction is present

has an ankle sprain with a positive anterior drawer test, you should avoid aggressive dynamic proprioception examination in weight bearing until the patient's ankle has increased strength sufficiently to keep the ankle stabilized during those activities. If, on the other hand, a patient has a mild sprain and a negative anterior drawer sign, you can include those examination activities in the initial examination.

Neurological Tests

If your examination demonstrates neurological changes, neurological testing is warranted. These special tests include examination of sensory, motor, and reflex parameters (figure 4.5).

Special tests are outlined in detail in Shultz, Houglum, and Perrin's (2005) book in the Athletic Training Education Series, *Examination of Musculoskeletal Injuries.*

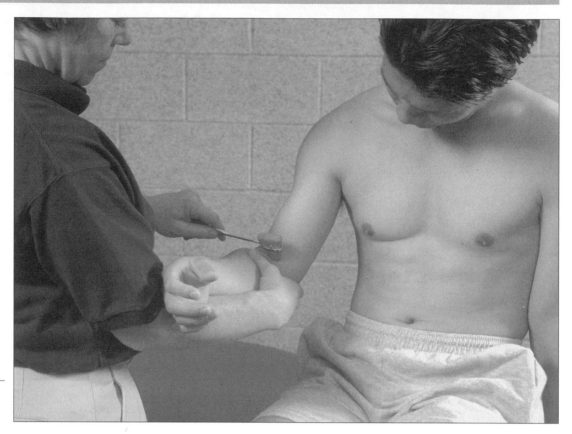

Figure 4.5 Reflex test for neurological examination.

Many professionals, including Corrigan and Maitland (1989), advocate using neurological testing for any signs or symptoms distal to the acromion in the upper extremity and distal to the gluteal fold in the lower extremity. This rule of thumb is especially warranted if you did not witness the injury incident and the patient is unsure of the nature of the injury. If neurological deficiencies are noted, impingement on the nerve root is possible and should be addressed in the treatment program.

Palpation

Palpation of the site is performed after the other tests are completed because palpation can irritate the tissues and lead to cause inaccurate conclusions. This sequence in a rehabilitation examination is different from that in an examination at the time of injury. One of the primary reasons for this is that it is not always clear during a rehabilitation examination what structures are involved until the examination is nearly complete, but if you have seen the injury occur, there is usually less question of what structures are involved. If palpation is performed early in a rehabilitation examination, before a good profile of the injury is obtained, the rehabilitation clinician may end up palpating a structure that is not actually injured, reducing the patient's confidence and wasting time.

Several structures are examined through palpation. Skin and subcutaneous tissue are examined by light touch for temperature, tone, and edema. Light movement of the skin and subcutaneous tissue against underlying structures shows any excessive rigidity or adhesions of tissue, as commonly seen following prolonged immobilization or excessive edema with immobilization. If movement between the subcutaneous tissue and underlying structures is impaired, a loss of motion is present. Deficiencies of these type warrant soft-tissue mobilization techniques as part of the treatment plan.

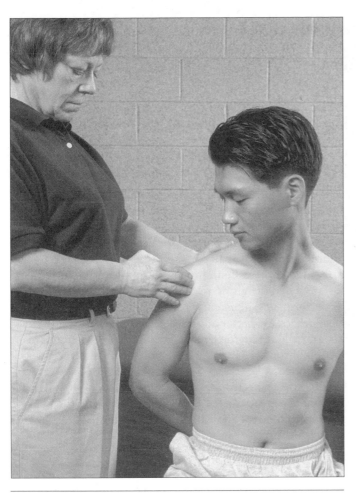

Figure 4.6 Palpation.

Palpation of fascia, muscles, ligaments, and tendons for tenderness, trigger points, and texture is important in examining causes of pain, motion restriction, and irritability (figure 4.6). Examination of these structures starts with light palpation of superficial structures; if the area's irritability permits, palpation pressure then increases to palpate deeper structures. Palpation of deeper structures requires a sensitive touch, not heavy pressure. For example, in palpating the midback area, light palpation is first performed to examine skin and subcutaneous mobility. Then slightly deeper palpation allows examination of the rhomboids and trapezius. Even deeper palpation is required to examine the paraspinal muscles. The deepest palpation in this region allows examination of the costovertebral joints. If palpation is too vigorous, accurate examination of tender structures is not possible. Palpate only as deeply as necessary to obtain the information you seek.

Areas of tenderness are detected by palpation. Areas of spasm, crepitus, nodules, and scar tissue can also be palpated. Palpation reveals specific sites of tenderness and the tissue type involved. Palpation is also used to examine consistency, mobility, and abnormalities of underlying tissue. Gaps, rigidity, loss of normal mobility, woodiness, nodules, and other textures and tissue quality are recorded and used later to form the assessment.

Functional Testing

Functional tests are not always performed at the time of the initial rehabilitation examination. When they are performed can vary. Sometimes they may be used after palpation and after other factors have been examined, and sometimes they may be incorporated before palpation to assist you in further identifying deficiencies. The irritability and severity of the injury dictate if and when these tests are appropriate. These tests determine whether specific activities produce pain, the injured part's ability to perform an activity, and the quality of movement during the activity. Agility, coordination, and proprioception play key roles in a patient's ability to perform functional tasks. Simple functional tests include having the patient perform a squat while you look for smoothness of movement, full motion, and an ability to keep the feet flat on the floor.

Standing on one foot (figure 4.7), standing on toes, walking on toes, walking on heels, jumping, running, and cutting are other functional tests used to determine functional ability and quality. More advanced functional testing can include sport-specific or activity-specific skills.

Examination Results

Once you have accumulated all the information from the subjective and objective portions of your examination, you are ready to make a well-informed assessment and determine the diagnosis and problems that should be addressed in the treatment plan. The treatment program is designed to resolve these issues and achieve the goals that you and the patient set.

▶ Assessment involves identifying problems based on information from the evaluation, setting goals to address those problems, and planning the treatment program for achieving those goals.

ASSESSMENT: PLANNING FOR ACTION

Once the subjective and objective examinations are complete, you interpret the information you have accumulated from the subjective and objective parts. This is where you express your opinions as a health care professional regarding the patient's problems, potential, and progress (Borcherding 2000). Your judgment as to the patient's response to treatment, expected outcomes, functional limitations, and ability to perform is also included in this section.

Figure 4.7   Functional testing.

Problems to Overcome

The rehabilitation clinician identifies the diagnosis and problems that the injured individual must overcome in order to return to full competition. Several simultaneous problems may need to be addressed, including subjective findings of pain and swelling or objective findings of reduced joint mobility or strength. Inability to perform can be an additional problem.

Progress and Potential

The assessment section is where the clinician expresses his or her opinion of the patient's progress, response to treatment, and potential for success in rehab. Is the progress as expected, are the complaints of the patient reasonable or exaggerated from objective findings, is the patient working hard in his or her rehab program? Does the patient show enthusiasm or is the patient difficult to motivate? Is the patient's poor trunk stability contributing to poor agility? Any observations of the patient's performance, deficiencies, issues needing to be addressed, concerns, changes for the better or worse, or other points the clinician feels should be noted are recorded here. The assessment section is really the only portion of the SOAP note where you are able to record your professional judgments.

After the subjective, objective, and assessment portions of the examination or treatment are provided, the plan is next. Within the plan are included goals for treatment and what the clinician intends to do with the patient during the next session.

Goals for Treatment

This process includes creating a list of problems and a list of goals. The goals address the problems, and the problems are based on the findings of the examination.

Once the problems are identified, the treatment program and its goals can be outlined. The general goals most often are to remove or reduce the problems and return the patient to full competition. Specific goals may include relief of pain and swelling and restoring normal levels of joint mobility and strength. For every problem listed, there should be a goal to address and resolve it. A goal should not be listed if a problem has not been identified. For example, a goal to relieve spasm should not be listed if spasm is not present. There is a direct relationship between the problems identified by an evaluation and the goals that are sought through the treatment program.

Both short-term and long-term goals should be set with specific objective aims regarding the activity to be accomplished (i.e., walk 2 flights of stairs), any conditions under which it may be achieved (i.e., without assistive devices) and the time frame within which it should be accomplished (i.e., in one week), as discussed in chapter 1. The goals should be objective and measurable. The time it will take to achieve short-term and long-term goals should be estimated. A common duration for a short-term goal is two weeks. You should estimate how far you expect the patient to progress in the next two weeks of your therapeutic exercise program and base your short-term goals on those estimates. The long-term goals are the final goals that the patient will achieve.

Some long-term goals are achieved sooner than others during the course of the treatment program. For example, full flexibility is achieved before full agility and coordination. A short-term goal for week 6 of a rehabilitation program following ACL reconstruction surgery might be 100% range of motion of the knee, 50% normal quadriceps strength, and 30% normal agility. Once full range of motion is achieved, the maintenance of full motion becomes a goal.

Plan For Treatment

After the goals have been outlined, a plan of action to achieve those goals can be designed. The **plan of treatment program** includes the frequency and duration of the treatment and the components included. The plan in a treatment note may change depending on the patient's response to the previous treatment. For example, the clinician may have recorded in the plan of the last treatment: "P: Begin jogging activities next treatment", but if the patient reports that the injury has been more painful since the last treatment, the clinician may choose to defer jogging activities and attend to the issue causing the increased pain first.

Various factors are involved in the treatment program, depending on the problems and goals that have been identified. For example, if goals include relieving swelling and pain and increasing range of motion and strength, modalities to reduce swelling and pain are included. Active range of motion may also be used to relieve these problems. Joint mobilization, range-of-motion exercises, massage, and home exercises may all be used to increase range of motion. Resistive exercises to increase strength may start with isometrics or more aggressive exercises, depending on the patient's ability and restrictions. Just as goals are designed to fit the problems, the plan is designed to achieve those goals.

A good therapeutic exercise program changes as the patient's problems decline and his or her status improves. As short term goals are achieved, new short term goals are set. To meet those goals, new treatment techniques must be planned. For example, if the patient achieves a short term goal of balancing in a stork stand for 30 s, a new goal should be established to further challenge the patient to achieve normal balance and progress to agility tasks.

The final short-term goals are actually the long-term goals. The patient progresses in the treatment plan until only the long-term goals are left. Once these are achieved through the treatment plan, the final treatment goal of returning the rehabilitated individual to full participation.

Continual Examination and Assessment

Examination and assessment take place before treatment, after treatment, and periodically throughout treatment to determine whether a specific technique is achieving its goals. For example, an examination before applying modalities determine the extent of muscle spasm present. An examination at the conclusion of the modality treatment assesses the success and efficacy of the modality. Similarly, an examination before applying a joint mobilization technique determines the quantity and area of joint restriction. An examination during the treatment determines whether joint mobility is improving as the mobilization technique is applied. An examination following the joint mobilization technique determines its effectiveness: Did your treatment achieve the improvements in pain reduction, range of motion, and joint mobility that you expected? How much motion has been gained?

The only way to assess whether the treatment is producing the desired effects is to continually examine and reexamine. Examination and assessment are also performed after exercise. Sometimes the exercise effects are determined immediately: Was the patient able to perform the exercise correctly? Could the patient have tolerated a higher resistance or more repetitions? Did the patient favor the injured extremity during the exercise? At other times the effectiveness and appropriateness of exercise are determined at the next treatment session: Did the patient suffer any unwanted side effects, such as more pain or edema after the exercise? Was there any muscle soreness without pain and edema? Your pretreatment findings determine your treatment for the day and also indicate whether you are providing the patient with an appropriate exercise program and what changes should be made in the exercises to achieve your goals.

The patient's response to the treatment must be assessed so that the program can be changed appropriately when necessary. Without ongoing examination and assessment, the rehabilitation clinician is unable to determine when to advance a patient, what techniques to use, how much force to apply in treatment techniques, and whether a treatment is beneficial or harmful to the patient. The process is also necessary for designing and following an appropriate treatment plan. An examination and assessment are made before, during, and after each treatment and from one treatment session to the next.

Functional Examination

As the therapeutic exercise program advances, more and more functional activities are incorporated. Functional activities are covered in detail in chapter 10. As the patient nears the end of the therapeutic exercise program and is preparing to return to sport participation or normal activity, it is important for the rehabilitation clinician to examine the patient's abilities and readiness to return to full participation. This is accomplished through functional testing. Specific functional activities vary from activity to activity, from sport to sport, and from one position to another within a sport. For example, a soccer offensive wing and a soccer goalie perform different activities. A gymnast has different functional requirements and should be examined differently from a basketball player. A warehouse worker has different physical demands than an editor. It is your responsibility to appreciate these differences, know functional examination tools that appropriately test the necessary skills of different sports, positions, and occupations, and accurately assess the patient's readiness to return to full participation.

KEEPING REHABILITATION RECORDS

▶ Record keeping is essential for judging the treatment's effectiveness, for communicating with other care givers, as a reference in the event of reinjury, and as a legal document.

Record keeping sometimes can seem overwhelming to medical professionals, but it is a crucial part of the treatment process. It reports the patient's initial levels of ability and performance, the effects of treatments, and the final outcomes of a rehabilitation program. It is important to keep accurate records because they can be referred to later to determine progress, they can be used by other rehabilitation clinicians to provide consistent treatment, and they are legal documents. Because medical records are legal documents, all records that are not typed must be recorded clearly and legibly in pen, not pencil. Recorded items should not be erased, blacked out, or covered with correction fluid; an error should be noted with one line drawn through it and your initials next to it, indicating that you have altered the record. You should always sign or initial and date the record after completing notes.

Recording the Examination

Many different formats can be used to record the examination. Most directors of athletic training clinics and other health care facilities develop their own forms for use in the facility. Preprinted forms are easy to use and provide consistency and thoroughness in examinations. Forms can offer a detailed list or a general outline, but they should include all the necessary information discussed in this chapter. A human figure on the form is also convenient so that the specific area of injury can be easily marked. Figures 4.8a and 4.9 are examples of detailed and general examination forms respectively. Figure 4.8b is a sample of a completed examination form.

The record should include information from the patient's subjective examination, including the injury site and onset; history and previous treatment of prior injuries; pain profile; additional medical problems; special questions; patient's activities, such as occupation or school demands; and if the patient is an athlete, the patient's sport and position. Any tests that have been ordered and their results should be included as well.

REHABILITATION EXAMINATION

Name _____   Date _____

Medical Diagnosis _____   DOI _____

Age_____ Occupation/Sport _____M.D. _____

Activity level_____

Current history:

Previous history:

Pain:

    Area:

    Description:

    Intensity: (0= no pain; 10 = "take me to the hospital, I'm dying")

    Aggravating factors:

    Easing factors:

    24-hour profile: AM:

             As day progresses:

                Evening:

                Night:

Special questions:

    GH: WL: X-rays: CE:

                                Steroids: Meds:

Patient's goals:

(continued)

Figure 4.8a Detailed examination form.

OBJECTIVE EXAMINATION

Observation/Inspection:

Range of motion/Flexibility:

```
          FB
           |
    L ——————+—————— R
           |
          BB
```

Strength/Endurance: Special tests:

Tension signs: Neurological signs:

Accessory movements:

Palpation:

Problems:

Goals:

Recommendations/Plan:

Initial treatment:

_____

Rehabilitation clinician

Figure 4.8a *(continued)*

REHABILITATION EXAMINATION

Name __Samuel Jole_____ Date __5-16-06__

Diagnosis __ACL reconstruction, left knee_____ DOI __4-01-06__

Age __20__ Occupation/Sport __student/ basketball team__ M.D. __E. Jesness__

Activity level __varsity BB until injured in game; currently going to class__

Current history: Injured Ⓛ ACL landing from a lay-up during game at home. Seen immediately by team MD; referred to Dr. Jesness for ortho consult. OP Sx: 4-16-06 for reconstruction with ipsilateral quad tendon. Immed post-op, WB to tol with 2 crutches, but now WB with 1 crutch. Brace set at 0°-90°; to ↑ today to 110°.

Previous history: No prior knee injury. Ankle sprain x6 yrs with good post-injury rehab; no problems since.

Pain:

Area: Ⓛ Ant knee around patellar tendon surgical site.

Description: Normal post-op pain.

Intensity: (0= no pain; 10 = "take me to the hospital, I'm dying")   2-4/10

Aggravating factors: Prolonged standing and walking.

Easing factors: Getting off the leg.

24-hour profile: AM: Stiff.

As day progresses: Loosens up and feels good by mid-day

Evening: Tired with some soreness, especially if swelling from doing too much is there.

Night: No sleep disturbance any more. Had trouble sleeping first few days post-op. Still sleeping with brace but no problems; he's gotten used to it.

Special questions:

GH: Neg   WL: None   X-rays: MRI: +RACL   CE: NA

Steroids: None   Meds: Pain meds given but none taken, denies other meds.

Patient's goals: Return to BB ASAP

(continued)

Figure 4.8b Detailed completed examination form.

OBJECTIVE EXAMINATION

Observation/Inspection: Amb well c̄ 1 crutch, brace. Removes brace easily. Mod edema around knee, slightly warm. Well-healed surgical scars over P. tendon and arthroscopic window sites. Ecchymosis in distal knee and proximal leg. Edema 4 cm above joint line: L is 2 cm larger than R. Midbelly of calf is 1 cm smaller on L, and mid-thigh is 5 cm smaller on L. Unable to stand on L LE s̄ assist.

Range of motion/Flexibility:

Strength/Endurance:
L hip: grossly 4/5; L ankle: grossly 4/5
L knee flex = 4-/5; ext = 2+/5
R LE = WNL throughout
Unable to perform a complete quad set.

Special tests: Deferred

Tension Signs: Deferred

Neurological signs: N/T

Accessory movements: L Patella: 50% restricted in all planes
L tibiofemoral joint: deferred for now

Palpation: Warmth around knee, as expected. Some tenderness over surgical sites. Swelling is boggy but no thickness palpated. Light spasm in gastroc-soleus, hamstrings.

Problems: Weakness and reduced endurance in L LE; Reduced motion in L knee; reduced mobility of L patella; reduced balance; mod edema around L knee; mild pain; abnormal gait; reduced level of activity.

Goals: Pt. to have: No pain, spasm in 1 week; No significant edema in 10 days; full AROM in 3 weeks; normal strength in 10-15 weeks; normal proprioception and balance in 4 weeks; normal ambulation s̄ assistive devices in 2 weeks. Good agility in 4-5 months. Return to full optimal function c̄ BB team in 6 months.

Recommendations/Plan: Per ACL protocol: relieve pain, spasm, edema within next 2 weeks. Patellar mobs for mobility; grade II tibiofemoral mobs for pain relief. Instructions in gait training with progression to ambulation without crutch. Progress as tol.

Initial treatment:

O: Following examination:
Pulsed interferential current to R knee x 15 m for edema, spasm relief.
Patellar mob for inf, sup, med, & lat: each II 1 x 30 s, III 2 x 45 s.
AROM with wall slides to tol x 5 m.
Assisted SLR, 2 x 5, then indep SLR 3 x 5.
Standing wt transfer L-R with verbal cueing for proper hip motion.
M.R. to L hip ab, ad, flex, ext; knee flex—all to fatigue x1 set.
HEP: instructed in quad sets; to perform 10 q 2 hr.
Ice after ex. L knee AROM after rx: 15-95° and edema ↓ by 1 cm.
A: Pt tired easily with strength ex; low endurance. Required some assistance with quad set, but was able to perform it well by end of rx. Pt appeared less apprehensive to move the R LE after rx.
Spasm seems nearly resolved after rx.
P: Cont with modalities to ↓ pain, edema, spasm; add SAQ, IV patellar mobs next rx; if knee flex is 110°, start on stationary bike.

Susan Moline
_____
Rehabilitation clinician

Figure 4.8b *(continued)*

Name:

Subjective/History:

Objective/Findings:

Assessment/Problems:

Plan/Goals:

Date _____

_____
Rehabilitation clinician

Figure 4.9 General examination form.

The objective portion of the form should include observations and inspections; examination findings on range of motion, strength, joint mobility, soft-tissue mobility, and neurological signs; palpation findings; and special test results.

A list of problems and a list of goals are a routine part of the examination form. The final portion of the examination form is the presentation of the treatment plan. A copy of the examination is frequently forwarded to the physician as a professional courtesy. It also completes the physician's records and helps the rehabilitation clinician and the physician to communicate and coordinate their treatment plans and goals.

Recording the Treatment

Recording your treatment sessions is as important as recording your examination (figure 4.10). A common method of record keeping is the SOAP (subjective, objective, assessment, and plan) note, which is thoroughly described in Borcherding (2000). SOAP notes are the most commonly used system of problem-oriented record keeping in the medical profession. SOAP notes are clear, concise, and easily understood, and they provide a plan of action for medical care and treatment.

Additional information on SOAP notes appears in *Management Strategies in Athletic Training*, third edition (Ray 2005).

S: Subjective

Subjective notes are what the patient says. Direct quotations should be used. A common mistake is to put the clinician's impressions or assessments in this category. For example, a statement such as "The patient seems depressed" is incorrect. A more correct statement would be, "The patient states that he is having trouble sleeping, has lost his appetite, and doesn't feel like working on his rehabilitation program."

O: Objective

Objective notes record what is done in the treatment session. They also include any objective measurements or examination and test results, for example, "ROM L knee = 115°. Leg press, L with 90 lb, 3 × 15. Heel raises on L only, 3 × 20, no wt. Ice L knee 3 × 15 min." Many organizations use an exercise record sheet as part of their objective reporting. Figure 4.11a is a sample of an exercise record sheet, and 4.11b is an example of how an exercise record sheet could be filled out for a few treatment sessions. This is particularly useful in rehabilitation, where many exercises are included from one treatment session to the next. It saves time by reducing paperwork and needless repetition, yet still provides an accurate record of treatment.

A: Assessment

The assessment is your interpretation of the problems being addressed and how the patient and the injury responded to the treatment. Here is an example: "Patient continues to walk with an antalgic gait secondary to pain in the medial knee joint. His range of motion and strength are improving but remain deficient. He seems to be depressed about the injury but is willing to perform all activities in the treatment session."

P: Plan

This is the treatment plan. What will you do with the patient at the next treatment session? Continuing with the patient in the previous examples, the plan may be written like this: "Add beginning agility activities of stork standing and balance board next treatment. If pain persists, use electrical stimulation to reduce pain. Continue strengthening program progression as tolerated, add weight to heel raise, and increase repetitions on leg press. Patient to see ortho next Monday."

TREATMENT NOTES

Patient _____ Diagnosis _____

Date: _____

S: _____

O: _____

_____

_____

A: _____

_____

P: _____

_____

_____
Rehabilitation clinician

- -

Date: _____

S: _____

O: _____

_____

_____

A: _____

_____

P: _____

_____

_____
Rehabilitation clinician

- -

Date: _____

S: _____

O: _____

_____

_____

A: _____

_____

P: _____

_____

_____
Rehabilitation clinician

Figure 4.10 Rehabilitation treatment form.

EXERCISES

Name _____   DX _____

M.D. _____   Precautions _____

DATE

EXERCISE												

Figure 4.11a Exercise record sheet.

EXERCISES

Name: Samuel Jole DX: L Bicipetal Rupture

M.D.: E. Jesness Precautions DOI: 4-16-06

EXERCISE	DATE 5/20 Reps/Wt	5/22 Reps/Wt	5/24 Reps/Wt	5/27 Reps/Wt	5/29 Reps/Wt	6/1 Reps/Wt	6/3 Reps/Wt	Reps/Wt	Reps/Wt	Reps/Wt	Reps/Wt	Reps/Wt
Biceps curl	2×15 / 15#	2×20 / 15#	2×12 / 20#	15,12 / 20#	2×15 / 20#	20,15 / 20#	2×20 / 20#					
French curl	2×10 / 8#	2×12 / 8#	15,12 / 8#	2×15 / 8#	20,15 / 8#	20,17 / 8#						
Wall pushup			2×20 / 0	3×15 / 0	3×15 / 0×	2×20 15 / 0	3×20					
Military press-up			15,12 / 15#	2×15 / 15#	2×15 / 15#	20,18 / 15#						
Supination						2×12 / 4#	17,15 / 4#					
Pronation						2×12 / 8#	18,16 / 8#					

Figure 4.11b Partially completed exercise record sheet.

Additional Records

Additional records help to form a complete synopsis of treatment and progression for a patient. They provide a well-rounded perspective of progress, a summary of overall results, and a reference in the event of future injury.

Progress Note

When the patient is seen for follow-up visits by the physician, a brief progress report in a SOAP format is often sent with the patient, and a copy is kept in your records as well. An example of a progress note is seen in figure 4.12a and a completed progress note is seen in figure 4.12b. The progress note provides the physician with a written record of the rehabilitation program and the patient's progress. It also allows communication between the rehabilitation clinician and the physician and helps to ensure that both are on common ground in the patient's care.

Additionally, the progress note provides you with a regular summary of the changes in the patient's condition. Objective and subjective changes that occur over time are sometimes difficult to assess when working with a patient regularly but are easily seen with a glance at your progress notes. You can judge more easily whether the patient is progressing appropriately.

Discharge Summary

When the patient has achieved the long-term goals that were established at the outset of the rehabilitation program, a brief discharge summary is completed, one copy is sent to the physician, and another is kept in your files (figure 4.13). A discharge summary is important because it indicates the completion of the patient's rehabilitation program. It states the patient's condition at the time of discharge and summarizes the program and its duration. If the patient suffers another injury to the same area, the discharge summary also provides a quick reference to the patient's response to treatments, willingness to work in a therapeutic exercise program, and any deficiencies that may have resulted from the previous injury.

Outcomes

Assessment of outcomes is important in health care records. It can assist the clinician in providing useful information on patient perceptions of treatment quality and effectiveness. Outcomes can also be valuable when clinicians bill for their services; third party providers often require evidence of outcomes for reimbursement. More detailed outcomes information is presented in chapter 1.

Diploma

An optional bit of paperwork that usually is a pleasure instead of drudgery is a rehabilitation diploma (figure 4.14). A diploma printed on special paper for a patient who successfully completes a rehabilitation program is often well earned and coveted. It provides a bit of motivation for patients. Patients with whom I have worked have cherished and even framed their rehabilitation diplomas. Successful completion of a rehabilitation program involves dedication, hard work, and diligence, so a diploma is a well-deserved reward.

REHABILITATION PROGRESS REPORT

NAME _____ DATE _____

DIAGNOSIS _____

NUMBER OF TREATMENTS _____

==

SUBJECTIVE:

OBJECTIVE:

ASSESSMENT:

RECOMMENDATIONS/PLAN:

_____
Rehabilitation clinician

Figure 4.12a   Rehabilitation progress report.

REHABILITATION PROGRESS REPORT

NAME <u>Samuel Jole</u>   DATE <u>2-15-06</u>

DIAGNOSIS <u>L ACL reconstruction (2-01-06)</u>

NUMBER OF TREATMENTS <u>8 Daily treatments</u>

==

SUBJECTIVE: Patient reports that he feels the treatments are helping him. He states he is now able to sleep the entire night without waking with pain.

OBJECTIVE: Patient was started on treatments at 3 days post-op on 2-4-06. Initial treatments were provided to decrease post-op pain, edema, and muscle spasm in the quadriceps. At 10 days post-op active and active assistive ROM was started and is provided on a daily basis.
AROM of L knee: 20° to 110°
Strength of LLE: Knee flexion = 4/5; knee extension = 3+/5; hip abduction, extension, and adduction = 4/5; hip flexion = 4–/5; ankle dorsiflexion and plantar flexion = 4+/5.
Gait: Pt is ambulating with the knee brace set at 15° to 120° as per MD orders. He is able to ambulate without the crutches for community distances.
Swelling: Girth at 4 cm proximal knee = 1 cm more on L, down from 3 cm at time of first treatment.
Pain: Decreased from 6/10 to 3/10 since initial treatment.

ASSESSMENT: Pt is making gains with improvement in pain and edema levels. ROM is lacking more than is expected at this time, but patient appears reluctant to move the knee outside the brace without supervision.

RECOMMENDATIONS/PLAN:

Continue with ROM activities to gain full passive extension and flexion to 130° within 2 weeks. Encourage pt to perform home exercise program for ROM gains. Isometric exercises for knee muscles, manual resistance to the hip, and body weight resistance exercises to the plantar flexors will be initiated tomorrow (2/16) as per ACL protocol.

Susan Moline
_____
Rehabilitation clinician

Figure 4.12b   Completed rehabilitation progress report.

REHABILITATION DISCHARGE SUMMARY

NAME _____ DATE _____

DIAGNOSIS _____

NUMBER OF TREATMENTS _____

INITIAL TREATMENT DATE _____ FINAL TREATMENT DATE _____

==

DISCHARGE STATUS:

    PAIN/SWELLING: _____

    ROM: _____

_____

    STRENGTH: _____

_____

    FUNCTION: _____

_____

    RECOMMENDED HOME PROGRAM: _____

_____

    GOALS ACHIEVED: _____ YES _____ NO

    REASONS FOR DISCHARGE: _____

_____

_____
Rehabilitation clinician

Figure 4.13 Rehabilitation discharge summary.

Diploma

This is to certify that

_____

Has satisfactorily completed and endured the rigors of rehabilitation and the trauma

of treatment prescribed for graduation from this facility, and is awarded this diploma

for rehabilitation of _____

_____
REHABILITATION CLINICIAN

_____
DATE

Sports Medicine

Seal of Approval

State University of Science and Technology

Figure 4.14 Rehabilitation diploma.

SUMMARY

1. Identify the primary factors of subjective examination.

   The subjective portion of the examination should include a history of the injury, pain profile, medical history, special questions, and additional questions about factors that may affect the injury.

2. Outline an objective examination procedure that includes all primary factors.

   The objective portion of the examination includes observation and visual inspection, examining active and passive physiological and accessory range of motion, strength tests, special tests, palpation, and functional tests if appropriate.

3. Explain the different types of end-feel and distinguish between normal and pathological end-feels.

   Typical normal end-feels include capsular, bony, soft tissue, and muscular, although these can also be abnormal, depending on the tissue involved. Other abnormal end-feels are springy, boggy, and empty.

4. Explain how a treatment plan is designed and upon what factors it is based.

   A treatment plan is developed after an assessment is made of the results of the examination. A list of problems based on the findings dictates a list of treatments to relieve those problems.

5. Define the SOAP note and explain its significance to rehabilitation.

   A SOAP note is a common method of record keeping. It includes subjective reports from the patient, objective treatment provided, assessment of the results of and tolerance to the treatment, and plan of treatment for the next session. It provides a record of progress and allows consistency of treatment.

6. Identify two other records used in rehabilitation and demonstrate their importance.

   A progress note to the physician, written when the patient returns to the physician for follow-up visits, and a discharge summary when the patient returns to sport participation are common rehabilitation records.

CRITICAL THINKING QUESTIONS

1. Describe the difference between an examination that occurs at the time of an injury and one that occurs before a rehabilitation program is started. Why are these differences important? What information may be different from one evaluation to the other?

2. Since pain is often the dominant complaint, an accurate pain profile provides you with a better idea of its source and how to proceed in your treatment program. Can you identify the most common types of pain and what they classically indicate? How does duration or intensity of pain influence the treatment you provide?

3. Your objective examination is based on the results of the subjective examination. How would your objective examination of a patient who reports severe pain most of the time compare with an examination of a patient who has minimal pain most of the time with occasional severe pain? If the patient's pain prevents you from performing all the tests you would like, what does your objective examination include, and what do you do for treatment?

4. Is it possible to have a goal without a problem? Is it possible to have a problem without a goal? How are these two factors related? If the goals change, does that mean the problem has changed?

5. You have been newly hired at a university that has not kept medical records beyond the initial injury incident report and daily athletic training clinic visitation record. How would you change the system to make it more compliant with record-keeping standards for medical facilities? What forms would you develop to make the process as simple as possible? What minimum record-keeping requirements would you put into place? What are the justifications for these changes?

LAB ACTIVITIES

1. Indicate which of the following statements are S statements, which are O statements, which are A statements, and which are P statements:

   a. Pt c/o L wrist pain.

   b. Pt will demonstrate a normal gait pattern 95% of the time within 3 wk.

   c. Flexion in lying reproduces pt's worst R LE pain.

   d. Pulsed US @ 1.5-2.0 W/cm^2 to R upper trap for 5 min.

   e. States onset of pain was in July 2002.

   f. AROM: WNL bilat LEs.

g. ↑ AROM R shoulder to WNL within 2 mo.

h. Will inquire if pt can be referred to orthopedist.

i. Pt was too groggy following pain medication and could not follow instructions well.

2. Write the two-week goals for each of the following scenarios:

Scenario A:

Dx: Fx R tibial plateau. Long leg cast applied 8/30/03

O: Amb: Not attempted; MD wants pt to begin with crutches, NWB R LE

A: Pt. has difficulty with standing; this may be a slow process based on pt's initial reaction to treatment.

P: Long-term goal: Indep amb c̄ crutches for unlimited distances on level surfaces & stairs within 1 mo.

Short-term goal: _____

You estimate that the pt will be able to ambulate 100 ft × 2 on level surfaces and require minimal assistance on stairs in 1 wk.

Scenario B:

Dx: Neck strain

S: c/o neck pain of an intensity of 9/10 with any movement of the neck.

O: AROM: 0-5° cervical rotation L & R

A: May have neck pain for a few weeks.

P: Long-term goal: ↑ neck AROM to WNL & pain free within 1 mo.

Short-term goal: _____

You judge that the patient will be able to move her head to ~10° of rotation to either side in 2 days.

3. Read the following report and convert it into a SOAP note:

When I saw the patient this morning he reported that he didn't sleep well after his last treatment session. He reported that the pain in his right shoulder was more intense than it usually was after the treatment, going from a 3 to a 6 on the 10-point scale, and thinks that it might be because of the new strength exercise that was added last time. Since he was more sore today I decided not to continue with the overhead lat pulldown exercise with 60 pounds we started last time and keep his shoulder exercises no higher elevation than 90°. I started out with ultrasound to the supraspinatus tendon at 1.5 w/cm² for 5 minutes. The ultrasound was followed by some joint mobilization, grade II for distraction, then grade III for anterior-posterior glides and inferior glides for about 5 minutes, and then I finished with more grade II distractions. After the mobilization he did his stretching exercises. The stretching exercises included stretches for 30 seconds each to his shoulder lateral rotators, flexors, abductors, and horizontal abductors. The strengthening exercises I had him do today included wall push-ups for 2 sets of 20, shoulder medial rotation in sidelying on his right side with 7 pounds for 3 sets of 15, shoulder lateral rotation in sidelying on his left side with 5 pounds for 3 sets of 15, shoulder abduction with him in standing using 5 pounds and going to only 45° for 3 sets of 20. I finished his treatment today with ice to the shoulder for 15 minutes. I instructed him to do only his usual range of motion exercises for flexion, abduction, lateral rotation, and horizontal adduction for his home program until the pain subsides to where it was before the last treatment. I also told him to put ice on the shoulder at home if the pain increases again. He said he felt better after today's treatment and thought he would sleep better tonight. Next time I'll see how he feels before we start his program. If he is better I will try the lat pulldown exercise again but with less weight. If he still has more pain, I think I should probably refer him to the doctor.

4. For two weeks you have been treating a soccer player with an old hamstring strain that has not resolved. He has been on your program for two weeks, and you want to examine how his progress has been with the treatments you have performed.

   a. What tests will you perform?

   b. How will you know if your treatment program has been effective?

   c. What soccer activities will you have him perform as part of his functional activities?

5. Three days ago a gymnast suffered a grade II ankle sprain. You are going to start her on rehabilitation today.

   a. What will you examine before you begin her program?

   b. What will be the determining factors in what to include in your program today?

   c. How will you know if you have provided an appropriate program for her?

6. An athlete comes to you, reporting that she has pain in her knee but she doesn't remember injuring it recently. What questions would you ask her? What is your reason for asking each question?

7. With your lab partner lying on the treatment table, go to the end range of the following motions and describe what you feel for each end-range position:

   a. Elbow extension

   b. Elbow flexion

   c. Knee extension

   d. Knee flexion

   e. Subtalar inversion

   f. Shoulder flexion

   g. #2 MCP extension

REFERENCES

Borcherding, S. 2000. *Documentation manual for writing SOAP notes in occupational therapy.* Thorofar, NJ:Slack.

Corrigan, B., and G.D. Maitland. 1989. *Practical orthopedic medicine.* London: Butterworth.

Kessler, R.M., and D. Hertling. 1983. *Management of common musculoskeletal disorders.* Philadelphia: Harper & Row.

Maitland, G.D. 1991. *Peripheral manipulation.* London: Butterworth-Heinemann.

Ray, R. 2005. *Management strategies in athletic training.* 3rd ed. Champaign, IL: Human Kinetics.

Shultz, S.A., Houglum, P.A., and D.H. Perrin. 2005. *Examination of musculoskeletal injuries.* 3rd ed. Champaign, IL: Human Kinetics.

II

Therapeutic Exercise Parameters and Techniques

Once the 'what' is decided, the 'how' always follows. We must not make the 'how' an excuse for not facing and accepting the 'what.'

Pearl Buck, novelist, 1892-1973

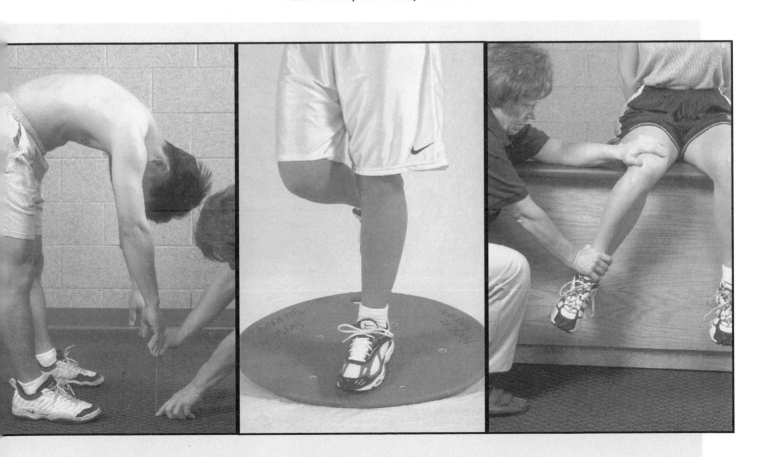

The next six chapters delve into specific techniques for restoring range of motion and flexibility, muscular strength and endurance, coordination and agility, soft-tissue and joint mobility, and functional and sport-specific activities.

Recall from part I that the parameters of normal function are emphasized in a logical sequence, each one building on the previous ones, throughout the therapeutic exercise program. This part follows that sequence in the presentation of topics. In chapter 5, range of motion and flexibility are discussed. What normal joint motion is and how to achieve it are presented. Chapter 6 extends the material of chapter 5 in that it deals with soft-tissue and joint pathology that may interfere with normal motion. The various techniques commonly used to resolve problems in these areas are discussed.

Progressing along the rehabilitation sequence, strength and muscular endurance are discussed in chapter 7. The various types of strengthening techniques, equipment used, program progressions, and precautions are also introduced.

Proprioception—including balance, agility, and coordination—is discussed in chapter 8. Progression from a static to a dynamic program is also included.

Chapter 9 presents information on plyometrics—activities that require flexibility, strength, endurance, and proprioception. Plyometrics are often incorporated into a rehabilitation program before functional exercises.

Chapter 10 presents functional exercises and their concepts. Functional and sport-specific exercises are the final progression of a total therapeutic exercise program.

The words of Pearl Buck apply directly to your education in rehabilitation. As you read through the chapters of this part, the relevance of the information presented in part I will become clear. By the time you complete part II, you will have the knowledge of the 'what' needed for parts III and IV, where general and specific programs for injuries are presented. Parts I and II are your gateway to understanding and appreciating the 'how' of practical program applications and concepts in parts III and IV. By the time you have completed this book, you will be able to use your mind to apply what you have learned in developing your own rehabilitation programs.

Range of Motion and Flexibility

Objectives

After completing this chapter, you should be able to do the following:

1. Define the differences between range of motion and flexibility.

2. Explain the differences in structure of loose connective tissue and dense connective tissue.

3. List the deleterious effects of prolonged immobilization.

4. Discuss the mechanical properties of plasticity, elasticity, and viscosity of connective tissue.

5. Explain the physiological properties of creep and stress-strain and how they affect stretching techniques.

6. Discuss the neuromuscular influences of the muscle spindle and GTO on stretching muscle.

7. Explain the procedure for measuring range of motion with a goniometer.

8. Discuss the active and passive methods for stretching.

9. Identify two mechanical assistive devices used to increase range of motion.

10. List contraindications, indications, and precautions of stretching.

11. Discuss the progression of a stretching exercise program.

As a senior athletic training student, Anthony Johns is on his first sports medicine clinical rotation. His first patient today is a new shoulder patient. Anthony knows from his past experience that he will measure the shoulder, elbow, and wrist ranges of motion in all their planes of movement. He also knows that the patient had a rotator cuff repair, but he does not know when the surgery was performed, what specific repair was used, or the physician's post-operative restrictions on shoulder motion. He anticipates, though, that there may be some limitations and precautions that must be respected. Although there should be no limitations on elbow and wrist motions, if the shoulder has been immobilized in a sling, there may be some loss of motion in the elbow that must be evaluated and addressed.

■ **Education is not the filling of a pail, but the lighting of a fire.**

William Butler Yeats, 1865-1939, Irish poet, dramatist, and Nobel laureate

By now you realize that a rapid restoration of range of motion and flexibility is important in a therapeutic exercise program. The aim of this chapter is to light the fire of knowledge in you, as William Butler Yeats suggests, by showing you ideas and techniques for flexibility. This chapter introduces the deleterious effects of prolonged immobilization, defines the differences between range of motion and flexibility, discusses the various methods and progressions for achieving full motion, identifies normal levels of motion throughout the body, and investigates the equipment that is used to evaluate motion.

At the conclusion of this chapter, the consequences of establishing or not establishing normal motion and of delaying the process should become clear. You will also know the techniques and skills needed for successfully restoring range of motion, and you will acquire an awareness of the precautions that should be taken and the progression that should be used.

DEFINING FLEXIBILITY AND RANGE OF MOTION

▶ Flexibility is a musculotendinous unit's ability to elongate, whereas range of motion is a joint's mobility, which is affected by many tissues in and around the joint.

Range of motion and flexibility are closely related. Although the terms are often used interchangeably, their definitions are different.

Flexibility refers to the musculotendinous unit's ability to elongate with application of a stretching force. The amount of flexibility of an area is generally thought of as its stiffness, suppleness, or pliability. Prolonged loss of flexibility can cause reduced range of motion.

Range of motion is the amount of mobility of a joint and is determined by the soft-tissue and bony structures in the area. The status of soft tissues—including muscles, tendons, ligaments, capsule, skin, subcutaneous tissues, nerves, and blood vessels—all affect the range of motion of a joint. If a patient has impaired flexibility, range of motion is also limited.

Clinically, range-of-motion measurements are used to quantify both range of motion and flexibility. Although there is a technical distinction between the two, clinical interpretations make differences less clear. For this reason, range of motion and flexibility are used interchangeably in this text.

CONNECTIVE-TISSUE COMPOSITION

Mobility of the musculoskeletal system is determined by the composition of connective tissue and the orientation of the various soft-tissue structures. Connective tissue of soft-tissue structures is composed of collagen, elastin, reticulin, and ground substance. The quantities

▶ Connective tissue supports the body and provides it with its framework. It is composed of many different kinds of cells and fibrous and ground substances that form in various combinations, depending on the specific connective tissue type. These connective tissues vary in the types, orientation, and linking of their fibers, which affect their ability to withstand stress.

of these substances vary according to the specific structure and determine the characteristics of the structure. For example, there is more collagen in ligament and more elastin in skin.

Collagen provides tissue with strength and stiffness. Recall from chapter 2 that the collagen fibers bind themselves together, and the more binding between the fibers, the greater the tensile strength and stability of the structure. Collagen fibers are five times as strong as elastin fibers.

Elastin fibers provide the structure with extensibility. They are able to withstand elongation stress and return to normal length. Tissues that have more elastin have more flexibility.

Reticulin fibers are essentially type III collagen fibers. They are weaker than type I and are considered temporary. They are particularly important during repair following injury.

Ground substance is a structureless organic gel that serves to reduce friction between the fibers, maintains spacing between the fibers to prevent excessive cross-linking, and transports nutrients to the fibers.

Connective-tissue composition varies according to structural differences and the amount of motion required. The fiber arrangement of **areolar (loose) connective tissue** is unorganized and loose with relatively long distances between the cross-links. Loose connective tissue's open network is composed primarily of thin collagen and elastic fibers that are interlaced in several different directions. This arrangement provides the structure with tensile strength as well as pliability. Skin is an example of areolar connective tissue.

Tendons are an example of a structure containing more highly organized connective tissue with parallel collagen fibers and more cross-links. This arrangement allows **dense connective tissues** to resist high-tensile loads and still provide some flexibility. Ligaments are similar to tendons in their structure except that their fiber arrangement is not as regular. Their collagen fibers are primarily parallel, but there are also spiral and oblique arrangements.

Between the structural extremes in the arrangement, orientation, and quantity of fibers and cross-links in skin and tendons are structures such as ligaments, capsules, and fascia. Even within these categories fiber arrangements vary. For example, ligaments that must resist higher forces have more organized fiber arrangements with greater quantities of cross-links.

Areolar connective tissue is present between the tissues in areas where motion occurs, such as joint capsular fascia, intermuscular layers, and subcutaneous tissue. Areolar connective tissue permits movement in all directions.

EFFECTS OF IMMOBILIZATION ON CONNECTIVE TISSUE

▶ Immobilization causes changes that result in loss of motion in all tissues. Increased collagen cross-links, loss of ground substance, and fibrosis all impair the flexibility of connective tissue.

Connective tissue is continually replaced and reorganized as a part of normal body function. As a part of the reorganization process, connective tissue normally tends to shorten (Kottke, Pauley, and Ptak 1966). To combat this tendency, normal motion is maintained through daily activity. If motion is restricted, either voluntarily or passively, rapid changes in the structure and function of connective tissue can be seen. Immobilization following injury is sometimes necessary to protect the area and permit the healing process to occur unimpeded. Immobilization, however, can also be detrimental. Depending on how long an area is immobilized, the changes in connective tissue can be either permanent or reversible. Although it does not take long for changes to occur, the longer the period of immobilization, the more difficult the restoration to normal becomes.

To understand the problems that must be addressed to restore normal range of motion and other lost parameters of an affected area, you must first be aware of the changes that occur with immobilization. Immobilization affects all tissue, from bone to soft tissue, including tendon, ligament, capsule, muscle, skin, and subcutaneous structures.

General Changes in Soft Tissue

Soft-tissue changes are seen following even one week of immobilization and are increased by edema, trauma, and impaired circulation (Kottke & Lehmann 1990). Immobilization

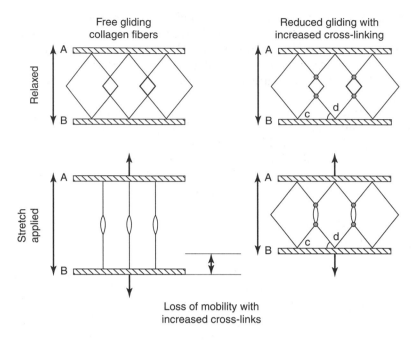

Figure 5.1 Collagen cross-links reduce mobility.

Adapted by permission from Woo et al. 1975.

causes a loss of ground substance, which in turn results in less separation and more cross-link formations between collagen fibers. The fiber meshwork contracts so that the tissue becomes dense, hard, and less supple. If a normal joint is immobilized for four weeks, the dense connective tissue that forms prevents normal motion.

In the presence of injury, the newly formed fibrin and collagen fibers are laid down in a haphazard way when the area is immobilized. The increase in newly formed cross-links impairs motion. Although cross-links are necessary for collagen strength, excessive cross-link formation can restrict normal movement of collagen tissue (figure 5.1). After two weeks of immobilization, an injured joint has reduced motion because of these connective tissue changes. Remember also that as scar tissue forms, the natural process of wound contraction augments the injured area's motion loss.

When edema is combined with immobilization, fibrosis increases, probably as a result of more tissue fluid protein and metabolites in the area along with deficient local metabolism. The end result is less tissue mobility. Fibrosis further increases when circulation is impaired, either because of age or local conditions. Edema acts like a glue to bind down tissue structures, especially if its presence is prolonged.

Even when an area is immobilized, connective tissue continues its process of remodeling and reorganizing. Without movement, as collagen is laid down, it forms a dense, hard meshwork of sheets or bands with a loss of normal suppleness. Collagen fibers then form between the connective tissue's reticular fibers and also from one structure to another, "gluing down" the area. The result is restricted motion where normal areolar connective tissue would have permitted one tissue type to freely flow over another. Muscle tissue becomes restricted by fascia, tendons lose their ability to move against subcutaneous tissue, and ligaments adhere to capsules.

Immobilization produces structural weakness as well as a loss of tissue mobility. Weakness occurs because of a decrease in collagen mass. This is believed to occur because of the reduction in applied load or stress when a part is immobilized. Klein et al. (1989) demonstrated that if motion is allowed in a non-weight-bearing extremity, the integrity of the ligaments is not lost. Immobilized, non-weight-bearing limbs also lose bone density. When possible, therefore, activity should be instituted for non-weight-bearing extremities until weight bearing and a full therapeutic exercise program are allowed.

Effects on Muscle Tissue

Changes in muscle tissue following immobilization include reductions in muscle fiber size, number of myofibrils in the muscle, and oxidative capacity. As these changes occur, there is an increase in the fibrous and fatty tissue in the muscle and a reduction in the intramuscular capillary density. These changes, which cause the muscle to become smaller and weaker, can be seen after two weeks of immobilization. The longer a muscle is immobilized, the greater the number of muscle fibers that degenerate and the greater the quantity of fibrous and fatty tissue. As the muscle becomes weaker, loses its motion, and is kept immobilized, the normal neural feedback system of movement is lost. The combination of these factors along with changes in the ligaments impairs proprioception (Montgomery and Steadman 1985).

Histological changes in immobilized muscle include decreased levels of adenosine triphosphate (ATP), adenosine diphosphate (ADP), creatine phosphate (CP), creatine, and glycogen. When the immobilized muscle works, more than the normal level of lactic acid is produced. These changes, along with a reduction in mitochondrial production and size, cause a reduction in the oxidative capacity of the muscle, which causes the muscle to fatigue more quickly and easily. Several clinical observations can be made of immobilized muscle. The most obvious change is that the muscle is smaller in size. It is also unable to produce as strong a contraction and cannot sustain activity for as long a time as before immobilization. Additionally, the muscle is slower to respond to a stimulus when it contracts.

Many of these changes occur within the first few days of immobilization. A decrease in muscle size (atrophy) and mitochondrial production are seen within the first five to seven days of immobilization. The rate of atrophy, however, varies from one muscle to another. For example, when the thigh is immobilized, the quadriceps becomes weaker and smaller at a faster rate than the hamstrings.

Effects on Articular Cartilage

Articular cartilage also suffers changes from immobilization. These changes depend on the position of immobilization, the duration of immobilization, and whether the joint bears weight or not during the immobilization. Generally, the mechanical properties decay: The cartilage becomes thinner, the proteoglycan concentration decreases, and the matrix organization is reduced (Buckwalter 1996). In joints where articular surfaces are not in contact with each other, the articular cartilage of those surfaces changes. In addition, necrosis of articular cartilage has been seen when constant pressure between the joint surfaces is maintained during immobilization. Immobilization also increases the amount of fibrofatty tissue that ultimately becomes scar tissue within the joint.

Buckwalter (1996) indicated that with continued immobilization, joints suffer irreparable damage. These changes include contracture of the joint because dense, fibrous tissue forms around the joint and in muscles that cross the joint; reduction of the articular cartilage lining of the joint surfaces; and replacement of the normal joint cavity by fibrofatty tissue. How long before the process becomes irreversible has not yet been definitively established in humans. In rats it occurs after 60 days of immobilization (Evans et al. 1960). In rabbits irreversible changes were seen after immobilization for six weeks (Finsterbush and Friedman 1975). Studies performed on animals also demonstrate that the longer an extremity is immobilized, the longer it takes to establish preimmobilization parameters. It is presumed that, at least in this regard, human tissue is no different.

Effects on Periarticular Connective Tissue

Periarticular connective tissue is soft tissue surrounding the joint, such as ligaments, the joint capsule, fascia, tendons, and synovial membranes. As with muscle and articular cartilage, all these structures are adversely affected by immobilization. The connective tissue becomes thick and fibrotic. Normally, the ground substance, a viscous gel that contains GAGs and water, serves to separate the collagen fibers, lubricate the area, and keep the fibers gliding freely. During immobilization the GAG and water content of the ground substance is reduced, causing a diminution of extracellular matrix. The combination of changes in ground substance, increased collagen cross-links, and continued normal collagen processing diminishes tissue mobility. The clinical impact of these changes is a loss of motion of the affected joint.

With all these dramatic changes from immobilization, it makes sense to minimize the duration of immobilization. Immobilization is important and necessary after some injuries and surgeries, and some require longer immobilization than others. It is in the best interest of the patient, however, to base the time of immobilization on the time course of injury and healing that was discussed in chapter 2.

Recall that collagen formation is well under way after seven days. The injury has gone from inflammation to proliferation and is entering the start of the remodeling phase. By day 21 the remodeling phase is in full swing, and the permanent structure is emerging. Although there are exceptions, gentle range-of-motion activities may be started by day 7 and certainly should be instituted by the third week following injury or surgery. From a biological standpoint, the initiation of range-of-motion activities depends on the severity of the injury, the tissue and body part involved, and the surgical repair technique used. From a practical standpoint, it is also determined by the patient's ability and status, the philosophy of the physician, the physician's confidence in his or her own surgical repair, and the abilities of the rehabilitation clinician.

EFFECTS OF REMOBILIZATION ON CONNECTIVE TISSUE

▶ Remobilization enhances recovery. It prevents abnormal collagen cross-link formation and increases fluid content in the extracellular matrix of connective tissue.

Recent awareness of the deleterious effects of immobilization has changed how acute and surgically repaired injuries are treated. It is now more rare to cast a knee after surgery than it was in the early 1980s. It is also uncommon to see injuries other than bone fractures immobilized for more than a few weeks.

Just as there are many disadvantages to prolonged immobilization, there are many advantages to early remobilization.

Effects on Muscle fibers

Muscle fibers generally recover from immobilization. Initially, the recovery is rapid, but as it continues, the rate of change slows until full recovery is achieved. Injured muscle responds best to a short period of immobilization followed by active motion. Movement causes a more rapid absorption of hematoma, an increase in tensile strength, and improved myofiber regeneration and arrangement for an effective overall recovery. Adhesions of muscle to fascia with immobilization can reduce the muscle's flexibility and affect joint range of motion. Techniques for treating these restrictions are discussed in chapter 6.

Effects on Articular Cartilage

Less articular cartilage degeneration occurs if both joint motion and weight bearing are allowed, even on a limited basis. Controlled weight bearing or loading of articular cartilage may even encourage repair of damaged cartilage. Overall, research findings consistently indicate that a joint, after injury, responds best to a rehabilitation program that provides controlled loading and movement, which stimulate proteoglycan and chondrocyte production.

Effects on Periarticular Connective Tissue

Remobilization of periarticular connective tissue prevents abnormal cross-link formation and helps to maintain the fluid content of the extracellular matrix so that proper fiber distance can be maintained (Donatelli and Owens-Burkhart 1981). Fatty tissue buildup around the joint limits mobility and must be broken by techniques such as stretching and joint mobilization. Stretching techniques are discussed later in this chapter, and joint mobilization is introduced in chapter 6.

MECHANICAL PROPERTIES AND TISSUE BEHAVIOR IN RANGE OF MOTION

▶ A tissue's mechanical properties, such as plasticity, elasticity, and viscoelasticity, affect its response to force and thus to stretching.

Even when an extremity is not immobilized, injury or surgery causes scar-tissue formation, which can lead to adhesions of connective tissue and increased fibrosis. In most cases, whether in healthy or injured individuals, restricted range of motion is the result of limited connective-tissue extensibility. Connective tissue is contained in joint capsules, ligaments, tendons, and fascia. Although muscles are not composed primarily of connective tissue as these other structures, they are surrounded by an extensive fascial network that affects their flexibility and response to stretch. The flexibility of all tissues that rehabilitation clinicians deal with in the treatment of injuries is influenced by connective tissue.

To determine the most effective ways to increase the range of motion of injured parts, it is important to review the physiology of connective tissue. Stretching exercises can affect the noncontractile element of all connective tissue. Because collagen gives a structure its tensile strength, resilience, and form, it is also the primary component that restricts range of motion and therefore should be the primary target of stretching exercises.

Remember that body parts are three-dimensional and respond to forces in three dimensions. When stress is applied, a structure's response depends on the direction, duration, and magnitude of the force and the specific fibers involved.

Mechanical Properties of Connective Tissue

To effectively apply stretching forces to collagen, you must first understand its mechanical properties. Collagen is elastic, viscoelastic, and plastic. Connective tissue possesses all these qualities simultaneously (figure 5.2). When connective tissue is stretched, all three qualities may be affected. If we separate the properties and look at them individually, it might be easier to understand how collagen functions and what we can do to influence it. Plasticity allows the connective tissue's length to change, while elasticity allows some restoration of normal length. The effectiveness of the stretch depends on the amount of collagen and elastin in the gross structure. The effectiveness of the stretch also depends on the amount of force applied, the duration of the stretch, and the temperature of the tissue. The physical properties of collagen also influence the effectiveness of a stretch.

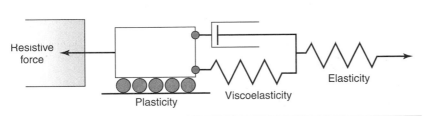

Figure 5.2   Connective tissue stretch model. Connective tissue possesses qualities of plasticity, viscoelasticity, and elasticity.
Reprinted from Viidik 1973.

Figure 5.3   Elasticity.
Reprinted from Viidik 1973.

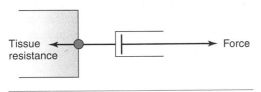

Figure 5.4 Viscosity.
Reprinted from Viidik 1973.

Figure 5.5   Viscoelasticity.
Reprinted from Viidik 1973.

Elasticity

Elasticity is the ability to return to normal length after an elongation force or load has been applied. This restoration of length occurs because of its stored potential energy. Elastic material is commonly symbolized by a spring in engineering models (figure 5.3). Elasticity is observed when you give a rubber band a brief pull; when you release the force, the rubber band returns to its normal length.

Viscoelasticity

Viscoelasticity is demonstrated by substances that have both elastic and viscous properties. **Viscosity** is the resistance to an outside force that causes a fluidlike, permanent deformation. No potential energy is stored in a viscous object, so there is no energy to permit its return to normal length; the energy is released as heat before it can be stored. Viscosity is represented by a hydraulic cylinder, as in figure 5.4. Elasticity provides some recovery to a former condition. **Viscoelasticity**, then, is the ability of a structure to resist change of shape when an outside force is applied but an inability to completely return to its former state after changing shape. Viscoelasticity is commonly represented as a combination of a spring and a hydraulic cylinder (figure 5.5).

Plasticity

Figure 5.6 Coulomb friction model.

Reprinted from Viidik 1973.

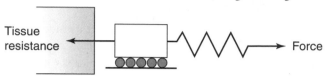

Figure 5.7 St. Venant body.

Reprinted from Viidik 1973.

Plasticity

Plasticity is the ability of a substance to undergo a permanent change in size or shape after a deforming force is applied. An example of plasticity is pulling a ball of putty; the putty changes in length and does not return to its former condition when you release your force. Plasticity is commonly represented by the Coulomb model of dry friction, as seen in figure 5.6. In the Coulomb model, if the force applied to a structure is greater than the friction, movement occurs; if the applied force is less than the friction force, no movement will take place. So it is with plasticity of collagen: Change in length occurs when the applied force is greater than the force holding collagen fibers attached to one another. The St. Venant body (figure 5.7), however, is a more practical representation of biological tissue, which has both plastic and elastic components. In this model, when a load is applied to the structure, it responds elastically until the friction force is exceeded. At that point a plastic deformation occurs. When the load is released, there is some change in the structure's length because of the plastic deformation, but there is some return toward normal length as well because of the elastic component of the tissue.

Physical Properties of Connective Tissue

The physical behaviors of connective tissue include force relaxation and creep. They are both time-dependent responses that rely on the duration of the outside force and the rate at which it is applied. **Force deformation** is the amount of force that is applied to maintain a change of length or other deformation of tissue. It results in a relaxation of the tissue. If the force is applied too quickly and viscoelastic and plastic changes occur that are faster or greater than the tissue can tolerate, an injury can result (figure 5.2).

Creep

Creep is the elongation of tissue when a load, usually a low-level load in the plastic range, is applied over an extended period of time. The result is a permanent change in the tissue's length. Creep is time dependent, so a load that is applied for a longer time is more effective in causing a change in tissue length than a load that is applied and released quickly. Increasing the tissue's temperature increases the rate of creep. In functional terms, applying heat to a muscle before stretching it permits a better stretch.

If a load is applied in the elastic range, the structure gradually returns to normal length once the load is released. This does not cause a permanent change in tissue length.

A structure's length can also be affected by structural fatigue. Fatigue of a structure occurs when it is loaded repetitively below the failure point until the cumulative stress results in failure. The greater the load, the fewer the repetitions necessary for failure to occur. The point at which structural fatigue causes tissue failure is referred to as **fatigue failure** or **endurance limit**. When structural fatigue occurs in bones it is called a stress fracture; when it occurs in tendons, as an overuse injury, it is called tendinitis.

Stress-Strain

As was discussed in chapter 3, the load required to change the length of connective tissue is directly related to the tissue's strength, and the tissue's strength is directly related to its ability to resist a load. This relationship is defined by **Hooke's law**, which states that the strain (deformation) of an object is directly related to the object's ability to resist the stress (load), and is illustrated by the stress-strain curve. **Stress** is a force that changes the form or shape of a body. Connective tissue is subject to three types of stress: tension stress (stretching force), compression stress (from muscle contractions and weight bearing on joints), and shear force (force applied parallel to the cross section of the tissue).

Strain is the amount of deformation that occurs when a stress is applied. Each tissue has a stress-strain curve that represents its own specific ability to resist deforming forces. Although

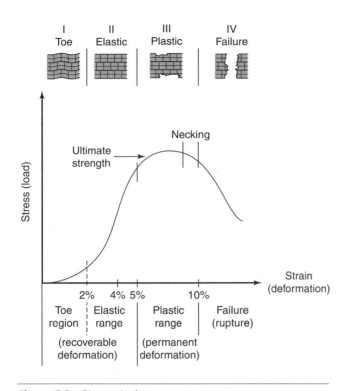

Figure 5.8 Stress-strain curve.
Reprinted by permission from D.L. Butler et al. 1978.

different tissues' stress-strain curves may differ in timing and magnitude, they share the same general characteristics. The specific reactions of a tissue to a load that are illustrated by this curve can be seen in figure 5.8.

The initial portion of the stress-strain curve is referred to as the toe region. In connective tissue the collagen fibers have a wavy crimp arrangement at rest. The toe region accounts for 1.5% to 4% of the total collagen fiber lengthening that is possible (Butler et al. 1978). As a force is applied, the fibers are stretched into the elastic range. As the slack in the collagen is taken up, it loses its wavy appearance. At a macroscopic level, no resistance is felt until the tissue is brought to the end of the elastic limit. In the elastic range a collagen fiber elongates to 2% to 5% of its total possible elongation (Butler et al. 1978). The tissue's full normal range of motion is in the elastic range. If the force is released in this range, the tissue will return to its prestretch length.

At the yield strength point, the stress loads the tissue beyond its elastic range and into its plastic range. Tissue loaded into this range undergoes permanent elongation. This is the result of the failure of a few of the collagen fibers to withstand the stress and a disruption of the cross-links. Collagen fiber can fail through a number of mechanisms, including a failure of the force-relaxation response when a load is applied too quickly for the collagen's viscoelastic and plastic adaptations to occur. Fibers also tear if the creep response causes too much deformation too quickly. This deformation can occur either in one episode or from accumulated stress from a number of lesser loads. This failure of isolated collagen fibers occurs unpredictably and results in an increase in range of motion.

Two factors within the plastic range should be respected. **Ultimate strength** is the greatest load that a tissue can tolerate. After this point the fiber length changes without application of any additional load. The point of ultimate strength is not always achieved. There may be a necking region prior to failure of the tissue, where the tissue's strength noticeably decreases so that less stress is needed to cause a change in the tissue's length. When this occurs, failure of the tissue is often imminent if the stress application continues.

Fatigue failure is the point at which the tissue is unable to tolerate continued stress and then ruptures. In collagen this occurs when the fiber is stretched to 6% to 10% beyond its resting length (Butler et al. 1978).

The general shape of the stress-strain curve is seen in figure 5.8, but the specific shape of the curve varies from one structure to another. Some additional factors influence the failure point of the whole structure rather than just the connective tissue. Tissue width is one of these factors. A structure's larger cross-sectional size indicates more fibers, so more stress is required to produce failure of the structure. The tissue's slack length is another factor. Longer tissues can withstand greater forces because they have more slack. For example, if two pieces of rope have the same number of fibers but one is twice as long as the other, the longer rope can tolerate greater deformation before breaking. The microstructure of the tissue and the orientation of the structure to the forces applied also influence the ability of the ligament or tendon to withstand deforming loads.

Given these physical and mechanical properties of connective tissue, some methods of stretching can be more effective than others for increasing range of motion. Using the principle of creep, a low load applied over a period of time can effectively remodel collagen bonds to increase range of motion. Stretches that take advantage of creep are more effective in remodeling collagen and maintaining range of motion increases than other stretching methods. This type of stretching is commonly referred to as prolonged stretching and is discussed later in this chapter.

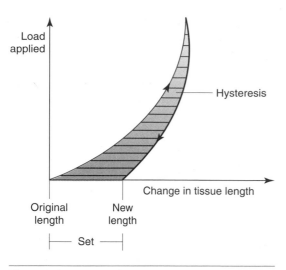

Figure 5.9 Hysteresis.

Adapted by permission from Bogduk and Twomey 1987.

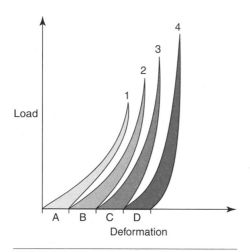

Figure 5.10 Deformation with hysteresis in repetitive stretching.

Reprinted from Viidik 1973.

▶ Muscle spindles and Golgi tendon organs are sensitive to tension in the muscle and its tendons, respectively, and protect these structures from abrupt changes in tension.

Hysteresis

Repetitive stretching with submaximal loads can also be effective in increasing range of motion. Energy in the form of heat is released when stress is applied to tissue. As the tissue is heated with repetitive stretches, the tissue is more easily stretched. When tissue is unable to keep pace with the forces, with each successive load application, it elongates more. This response is called **hysteresis**. When a load is released, the tissue returns to its normal length at a different rate from that of stretching it. When a new length is achieved with this process, the change in length is referred to as the *set*, as seen in figure 5.9.

As the tissue changes length and is heated with the stretch, higher-level loads are tolerated in later repetitions. In other words, the tissue's failure load increases, so a greater force can be applied to produce a greater tissue deformation, as seen in figure 5.10. An example of this is when a **proprioceptive neuromuscular facilitation (PNF)** stretch is applied, released, and then reapplied to a patient's hamstrings; in the second stretch, the patient's hamstring is stretched farther and the patient can tolerate a slightly greater stretch force.

NEUROMUSCULAR INFLUENCES ON RANGE OF MOTION

In addition to the physical and mechanical properties of connective tissue, neurological factors influence the effectiveness of stretching techniques in increasing range of motion of a structure. Neurological components that affect a muscle's ability to respond to a stretching force include the muscle spindle and the Golgi tendon organ (GTO). The muscle spindle is much more complex than the GTO.

Muscle Spindle

There is a variation in the ratio of muscle spindles to muscle fibers in each muscle. Generally, the more precise the movement required of a muscle, the lower the ratio of muscle fibers to muscle spindles. A typical muscle fiber is often referred to as an **extrafusal fiber**. Muscle spindles vary in length and diameter, but all lie between and parallel to the extrafusal muscle fibers. The muscle fibers contained by the muscle spindle are called **intrafusal fibers.**

Entering the intrafusal muscle fiber are three efferent nerve fibers: alpha, beta, and gamma nerves, as noted in figure 5.11. Exiting the intrafusal fibers are the Ia, Ib, and II afferent, or sensory, fibers. The muscle spindle is composed of these nerve fibers, the intrafusal muscle fibers, and the sac that surrounds these structures. There are two types of intrafusal fibers, and each has a different function within muscle spindles. One type, the **nuclear bag fiber,** has an enlarged center region with two or three nuclei stacked beside each other. The shorter, thinner fibers are called **nuclear chain fibers,** and their nuclei are arranged in single file in the center region. Although both are sensitive to stretch, the nuclear bag fiber has more elasticity and is therefore sensitive to the velocity of the stretch.

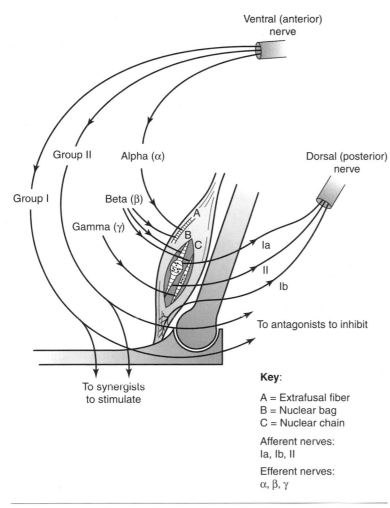

Ventral (anterior) nerve

Group II   Alpha (α)

Dorsal (posterior) nerve

Group I   Beta (β)

Gamma (γ)

A

B

C

Ia

II

Ib

To antagonists to inhibit

To synergists to stimulate

Key:

A = Extrafusal fiber
B = Nuclear bag
C = Nuclear chain

Afferent nerves:
Ia, Ib, II

Efferent nerves:
α, β, γ

Figure 5.11   Muscle spindle and Golgi tendon organ.

Adapted from Brown 1980.

An afferent Ia nerve fiber wraps around the center region of the intrafusal fibers. This nerve ending is sometimes called a *primary ending* or an *annulospiral ending*. The secondary or II afferent nerve endings are at the ends of the intrafusal muscle fibers, primarily on nuclear chain, and are sometimes called *flower-spray endings* because of their appearance. Because of the structure of Ia nerve fibers, they respond much more quickly to stimulation than the II nerves. The Ia nerve fibers are sensitive to a quick stretch, and both Ia and II nerve fibers respond to a static stretch (Eldred 1967).

Because the intrafusal fiber is attached to the connective tissue surrounding extrafusal muscle fibers, the intrafusal muscle fiber is sensitive to changes in the muscle's length. Both the afferent nerve fibers in the muscle spindle transmit signals to the spinal cord regarding changes in the muscle's length and the velocity and duration of a stretch. An efferent response is sent to both the intrafusal and extrafusal muscle fibers to permit the muscle to react to the stimulation. Gamma efferent fibers transmit to the intrafusal muscle fibers, and alpha efferent fibers transmit to the extrafusal muscle fibers to cause a muscle contraction. Once the muscle contracts and shortens, stress and stimulation of the muscle spindles cease.

In addition to stimulating the muscle in which they lie, group I nerve fibers of a muscle send a branch to synergistic muscles and antagonistic muscles. The result is simultaneous stimulation of synergistic muscles and inhibition of antagonistic muscles. Group II nerve fibers also transmit to the synergistic and antagonistic muscles, but they use another neuron link to complete the transmission. The impact of stimulating synergistic muscles will become more apparent in chapter 7 during the discussion of proprioceptive neuromuscular facilitation (PNF).

Golgi Tendon Organs

Like the muscle spindle, the **Golgi tendon organ (GTO)** also functions as a protective mechanism. GTOs are not as sensitive to stretch as muscle spindles are, but they are very sensitive to contraction and tension that occur in a muscle.

GTOs, located at the distal and proximal muscle-tendon junctions, are long, delicate, tubular capsules that contain a cluster of Ib nerve fibers. These nerve fibers originate on the tendon's fascicles. The protection performed by the GTO is known as **autogenic inhibition**. When the GTO is stimulated, its activity causes simultaneous inhibition of the alpha motor neuron of its own muscle and internuncial activation (between afferent and efferent neurons) of the antagonistic muscle.

The result of the combined reactions of the muscle spindle and the GTO is seen in functional activities. If a muscle is stretched quickly, the muscle spindle produces a **monosynaptic response**, which is a rapid reflex motor response resulting from a direct neural connection between a sensory (afferent) and motor (efferent) nerve without an intermediary neuron.

A monosynaptic response is the most rapid response because an intermediary nerve is not involved. If a stretching force is applied too quickly, the muscle being stretched reflexively responds secondarily to stimulation of the muscle spindle. This is a potential problem with ballistic stretching that is discussed later in this chapter. On the other hand, if a stretch is applied slowly, the GTO inhibits muscular contraction. This may actually provide better relaxation of the muscle to improve the effectiveness of the stretch.

DETERMINING NORMAL RANGE OF MOTION

▶ Normal range of motion is different for each joint, each patient, and each sport and position.

Before you can determine whether a joint has deficient range of motion, you must first know the normal range of motion. Only then can you decide whether stretching exercises should be included in the therapeutic exercise program. Table 5.1 demonstrates that there is some dispute among authors as to what is considered normal, though all are within close range of one another. Differences are probably due to the populations each author measured to achieve the data. Age and sex of the subjects and the positions in which measurements are taken all affect measurement results. Regardless of whose data are used, they can provide rehabilitation clinicians with a guideline for expectations of normal range of motion.

Each patient's normal range of motion is actually determined by comparison with the contralateral part. It is also based on the demands of the individual's activities. For example, normal range of motion for shoulder external rotation is different for a baseball pitcher and for a football lineman.

It is important for you to become familiar with normal ranges of motion. Without this knowledge, it is impossible to determine when a problem exists. If problem areas are not identified, proper therapeutic exercise programs cannot be designed, and the rehabilitation program cannot be successful.

MEASURING RANGE OF MOTION

▶ Range of motion is typically measured with a goniometer. Good technique is essential for measuring accurately and consistently.

Now that you have been introduced to the physiological constructs that determine range of motion and to the normal values of range of motion, you are ready to learn how to measure range of motion.

Equipment

Range of motion is usually measured with an instrument known as a **goniometer**. It is essentially a protractor with a stationary arm and a movable arm, as shown in figure 5.12. It can measure up to either 180° or 360°. Many varieties of goniometers have been designed to measure different joints. Other devices have been designed either to measure specific body segments or to make measurement easier. For example, the Leighton flexometer has a weighted, 360° dial with an enclosed needle; it is attached with a strap to the body part that is being measured. An inclinometer is a device similar to a flexometer and is used to measure degrees of rotation on a 360° dial; it is commonly used for the cervical spine. An elgon, or electrogoniometer, was developed by Karpovich et al. (1959) and uses a potentiometer rather than a protractor. It is used to measure primarily dynamic motion, as it is less accurate with static motion. The number of joints that it can be used to measure is also limited. Another electrogoniometer, the Penny and Giles, is shown in figure 5.13.

Figure 5.12 Goniometers come in different sizes to measure various body segments. They are most often 360° or 180°.

Table 5.1

Examples of Normal Ranges of Motion in Upper and Lower Extremities According to Various Authors

Joint Motion	Hoppenfeld (1976)	Daniels & Worthingham (1972)	A.A.O.S. (1965)	Kendall & McCreary (1983)	Kapandji (1980)	Esch &Lepley (1974)	Gerhardt & Russe (1975)
Shoulder							
Flexion	180	—	180	180	180	170	170
Extension	45	50	60	45	50	60	50
Abduction	180	—	180	180	180	170	170
Lateral rotation	45	90	90	90	80	90	90
Medial rotation	55	90	70	70	95	80	80
Horizontal abduction	—	—	—	—	—	—	30
Horizontal adduction	—	—	135	—	—	—	135
Elbow							
Flexion	135+	145-160	150	145	145-160	150	150
Forearm							
Supination	90	90	80	90	80	90	90
Pronation	90	90	80	90	85	90	80
Wrist							
Extension	70	70	70	70	85	70	50
Flexion	80	90	80	80	85	90	60
Radial Deviation	20	—	20	20	15	20	20
Ulnar Deviation	30	—	30	35	45	30	30
Thumb, carpometacarpal							
Abduction	70	50	70	80	50	—	—
Flexion	—	—	15	45	—	—	—
Extension	—	—	20	0	—	—	—
Opposition	**Tip of thumb to tip of 5th finger**						
Thumb, metacarpophalangeal							
Flexion	50	70	50	60	80	—	—
Thumb, interphalangeal							
Flexion	90	90	80	80	80	—	—
Digits 2-5, metacarpophalangeal							
Flexion	90	90	90	90	—	—	—

(continued)

Table 5.1
(continued)

Joint Motion	Hoppenfeld (1976)	Daniels & Worthingham (1972)	A.A.O.S. (1965)	Kendall & McCreary (1983)	Kapandji (1980)	Esch &Lepley (1974)	Gerhardt & Russe (1975)
Extension	45	30	45	—	—	—	—
Digits 2-5, proximal interphalangeal							
Flexion	100	120	—	—	—	—	—
Digits 2-5, distal interphalangeal							
Flexion	90	80	—	—	—	—	—
Subtalar joint							
Inversion	—	—	35	35	52	30	40
Eversion	—	—	20	20	30	15	20
Ankle							
Dorsiflexion	20	—	20	20	20-30	10	20
Plantar flexion	50	45	50	45	50	65	45
Knee							
Flexion	135	140-160	135	140	135	135	130
Hip							
Flexion	120	115-125	120	125	120	130	125
Extension	30	15	30	10	30	45	15
Abduction	45-50	45	45	45	45	45	45
Adduction	20-30	—	30	10	30	15	15
Medial rotation	35	45	45	45	45	33	45
Lateral rotation	45	45	45	45	60	36	45

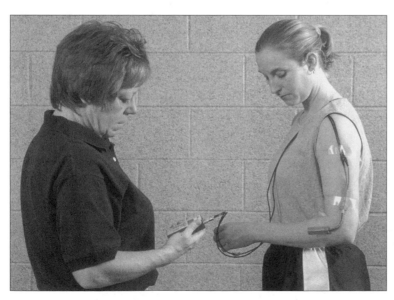

Figure 5.13 Penny and Giles electrogoniometer.

Trunk motion is difficult to measure with a standard goniometer. Using the Moll and Wright (1971) method (figure 5.14), marks are made at the top and bottom of the lumbar spine. A metal tape measure is used to measure the difference in distance between the two marks in flexion, extension, and normal standing. This measure is relative to the individual being tested and cannot be used to determine an individual's deviation from normal, because standards have not been established and would probably be difficult to determine.

Figure 5.14   Moll and Wright spinal ROM method.

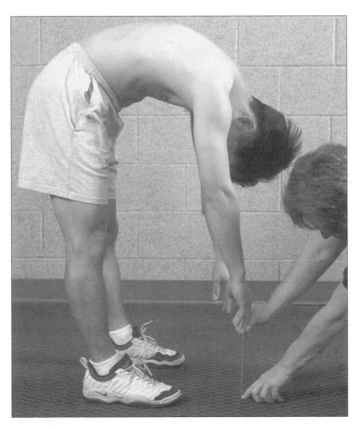

One of the most common methods for measuring trunk flexion is the fingertip-to-floor method, demonstrated in figure 5.15. The person stands with trunk flexed, and the distance between the fingertips and the floor is measured. Side bending (figure 5.16) also produces a relative measurement, recorded as the distance from the fingertips to either the fibular head or the floor. Although this method may not be as accurate as others and does not isolate the structure being assessed (i.e., the lumbar spine), it can be reproduced in the same individual so that changes can be evaluated.

Application

To measure accurately with a goniometer, the most common tool for evaluating range of motion, placement of the protractor and arms is important. The arms of the goniometer are placed along the length of the two limbs forming the joint. If placed correctly, the pivot point of the protractor should be lined up over the axis of motion of the joint. For correct alignment, the limbs being measured should be exposed. With

Figure 5.15   Measuring trunk flexion.

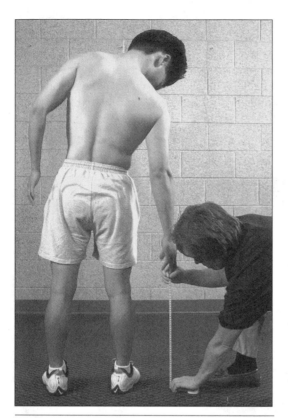

Figure 5.16 Measuring lateral trunk flexion.

some exceptions, the goniometer is placed along the central lateral aspect of the limb. Figure 5.17 demonstrates measuring techniques for some joints.

Range of motion is measured in either a 180° or 360° system using either a 180° or 360° goniometer. In the 360° system, 0° is overhead and 180° is at the feet. In the 180° system, 0° is at the start of the range in the anatomical position and 180° is at the end. Either system is valid and can be used to measure range of motion. The most common system used for musculoskeletal injuries is the 180° system. There is some variation in both systems for measurements of inversion, eversion, supination, pronation, and lateral flexion.

Accuracy

A rehabilitation clinician's ability to accurately measure range of motion depends on his or her training, experience, and attention to detail. Even an experienced clinician with good equipment can expect accuracy only within 3° to 5° of true values. It is, therefore, vital to be as consistent as possible. Careful attention to the placement of the goniometer arms and making sure that the axis of the goniometer coincides with the joint's axis of rotation are very important to assure accurate measurements. Check the goniometer placement, adjust the patient's position if necessary to achieve correct body segment alignment, and then check again before recording your final measurement to help ensure accuracy. Consistent measurements depend on your attention to these details. If your technique is good, your measurements should be reliable. If your technique varies, your results will be inconsistent and of no use to you, the patient, or anyone else. If your technique is accurate, other clinicians (assuming their technique is also good) should obtain measurements that are the same or within 5° of yours.

Interpretation of range-of-motion measurements can be clouded by a variety of conditions. The position in which the patient is placed, whether active or passive motion is measured, pain occurring with motion, spasm, voluntary resistance to movement, wounds, and the patient's willingness to move the part can all affect measurements. You should note such conditions in your record.

Recording Range Of Motion

Range of motion records are indicated first of all by the joint and motion measured, and then by the type of motion measured: active range of motion (AROM) or passive range of motion (PROM). Degrees are most often recorded based on a 180° scale, so if a 360° is used, it should be indicated as such. 0° is usually the position of neutral as in pronation-supination and plantar flexion-dorsiflexion or in full extension such as knee and elbow extension. If a patient is unable to achieve full extension (0°), the point at which the patient is able to move is recorded along with the end point of motion in the opposite direction. For example, if a patient was lacking 15° from full extension and was able to flex the knee to 100°, the record would show: knee extension-flexion = 15° to 100°. Sometimes a clinician will record the amount of degrees lacking from extension as a minus (–) number, such as –15°. This can be misleading, however, in that it may also be interpreted as 15° of hyperextension.

Right lateral bend | Neutral | Left lateral bend

Figure 5.17 Goniometer placement for measuring *(a)* shoulder flexion, *(b)* elbow flexion, *(c)* hip medial rotation, *(d)* knee flexion, *(e)* ankle plantar flexion, and *(f)* cervical lateral flexion. The center of the goniometer is placed over the joint's center (axis of motion). Alignment of the goniometer's stationary and movable arms and fulcrum must be accurate for reliable measurements.

TERMINOLOGY IN GONIOMETRY

▶ Standard terminology and frames of reference to describe bodily movements and range of motion make your records usable by others.

To ensure accurate interpretation of your results by those to whom your report is sent or by those who refer to your notes, you and your readers should use common terminology. Table 5.2 gives common terms used in goniometry.

Body motion can be divided into three planes: sagittal, frontal or coronal, and horizontal or transverse. Their frame of reference is the anatomical position, which is the body standing erect with the hips and knees in extension, the feet facing forward, the elbows and wrists in extension, the hands at the sides, and the palms facing forward.

Table 5.2
Goniometric Terms

Term	Definition
sagittal plane	The anterior-posterior vertical plane through which the longitudinal axis passes and that divides the body into right and left halves.
frontal (coronal) plane	Any vertical plane that divides the body into front and back parts.
transverse (horizontal) plane	A plane that divides a section of the body into upper and lower parts. It is parallel to the horizon.
flexion	Bending a joint so that the two body segments approach each other and decrease the joint angle.
extension	Straightening a joint so that the two body segments move apart and increase the joint angle.
abduction	Lateral movement of a limb or segment away from the midline of the body or part.
adduction	Lateral movement of a limb or segment toward the midline of the body or part.
medial rotation	Rotation of a joint around its axis in a transverse plane toward the middle of the body. Also called *medial rotation*.
lateral rotation	Rotation of a joint around its axis in a transverse plane away from the midline of the body. Also called *lateral rotation*.
supination	Movement of the palm forward or upward into the anatomical position. Also, the multiplanar rotation of the subtalar and transverse talar joints that includes plantar flexion, adduction, and inversion.
pronation	Movement of the palm backward or downward so that the palm faces in a posterior direction, opposite the anatomical position. Also, a multiplanar rotation of the subtalar and transverse talar joints that is the combination of dorsiflexion, abduction, and eversion.
inversion	Inward turning motion of the foot that causes the bottom of the foot to face medially.
eversion	Outward turning motion of the foot that causes the bottom of the foot to face laterally.
dorsiflexion	A flexion of the ankle that causes the dorsum (top) of the foot to move toward the lower leg so that the angle of the ankle decreases.
plantar flexion	An extension of the ankle that causes the dorsum (top) of the foot to move away from the lower leg so that the angle of the ankle increases.
radial deviation	A movement of the wrist toward the thumb side of the forearm. Also called *radial flexion*.
ulnar deviation	A movement of the wrist toward the little-finger side of the forearm. Also called *ulnar flexion*.
opposition	A diagonal movement of the thumb across the palm of the hand to permit it to make contact with one of the other four fingers.
depression	A downward movement of the scapula.
elevation	An upward movement of the scapula.
protraction	A forward movement of the scapula. Also called *scapular abduction*.
retraction	A backward movement of the scapula. Also called *scapular adduction*.
upward rotation	A movement of the scapula that causes the glenoid to face forward and upward. The inferior angle of the scapula moves laterally away from the spine, and the scapula slides forward.
downward rotation	A movement of the scapula that causes the glenoid to face downward and backward. The inferior angle of the scapula moves medially, and the scapula slides backward.
horizontal flexion	A motion of the upper extremity in a transverse plane toward the midline of the body. Also called *horizontal adduction*.
horizontal extension	A motion of the upper extremity in a transverse plane away from the midline of the body. Also called *horizontal abduction*.

Motions of flexion and extension occur in the sagittal plane. Motions in the frontal plane include abduction and adduction at the shoulders and hips. Transverse plane movement includes hip and shoulder rotation, pronation, and supination in the anatomical position. Although discussions of range of motion refer to these planes, functional activities usually involve oblique planes of motion that include all three conventional planes.

STRETCHING TECHNIQUES

▶ Stretching can be active, passive, or a combination of the two. Knowing the indications, contraindications, and proper precautions for stretching is necessary to safely and effectively use any stretching technique.

When an individual has an injury that results in deficient range of motion, several techniques can be applied to restore range of motion, depending on your preference and skill, the type of tissue restriction involved, the extent of the injury, and the duration of the loss of motion. Continuous passive motion machines and other mechanical devices are discussed later in this chapter. Joint mobilization and various techniques of soft-tissue mobilization are investigated in chapter 6.

Probably one of the most common methods of increasing range of motion is stretching exercises. Many researchers have investigated various methods and techniques in search of the best and most effective way to gain range of motion. Unfortunately, the answer remains elusive. One of the problems is that many of the research studies investigating stretching methods have been performed with normal, uninjured subjects or with animals. Some of the investigations are not sound, objective, or reproducible. Studies, as yet, have failed to provide answers regarding the best method of stretching for patients. Needless to say, we must rely on our knowledge of injury, healing, and the physiology of connective tissue more than on specific investigations to determine the best way to stretch an injured area.

Regardless of the type of stretch used, the application of heat before the stretch produces a better stretch. Heat can be applied either passively or actively. An example of a passive heat application is the application of a hot pack before stretching. A better method is active heat application, in which the patient performs a warm-up activity, such as exercising on a stationary bike, stair climber, or upper-body ergometer, before stretching. A hot pack provides superficial heat, but an active exercise increases the deeper tissues' temperature more effectively and more safely than a passive modality (Saal 1987).

Active Stretching

Stretching exercises can be divided into active stretching, passive stretching, and a combination of the two. Active stretching includes flexibility exercises that are performed by the patient without outside assistance from either another person or a machine (figure 5.18). Depending on the duration and repetitions of the active stretch, it affects the elastic range of connective tissue and may have some effect on the plastic range. Studies on the effects of stretching on injured patients have yet to be identified (Shrier and Gossal 2000). However, based on the results of four studies on normal subjects (Garrett 1990; Bandy et al. 1997; McNair and Stanley 1996; Taylor et al. 1990) and my clinical observations of patients, I feel the best application of active stretching is a 15 to 30 s hold for four to five repetitions of an exercise. For patients who have significant loss of motion, repeated stretch sessions throughout the day may be beneficial; although there have not been any studies demonstrating that repeated sessions are beneficial, reason indicates the possibility that they may be, especially during scar-tissue formation and contraction. If the individual is participating in sport activities, the stretches should also be performed after the activity.

Because of the phenomenon of antagonist inhibition, if the individual contracts the opposing muscle, relaxation of the muscle being stretched increases. This results in a more effective stretch. For example, a better stretch occurs when the patient actively contracts the quadriceps as the hamstrings are being stretched. It is believed that a strong relationship

Figure 5.18 Active stretch.

between muscles and their antagonists affect muscle flexibility. It is believed that an agonist muscle is shortened when its antagonist is weaker, preventing a balance between the two and resulting in a loss of range of motion (Sahrmann 2002). If the antagonist is facilitated, the agonist becomes inhibited, which allows a restoration of normal flexibility. You can perform this quick experiment on yourself to see the impact of agonist inhibition on increasing muscle flexibility. Do not perform this activity if you have a lumbar disk injury. In a standing position, first evaluate your hamstring flexibility by attempting to touch your toes, keeping your knees straight. Return to an upright position. Now bend over at the waist to touch your toes but with your knees bent to prevent a stretch of the hamstrings. Keeping your hands on your toes, straighten your knees by tightening the quadriceps. Repeat this activity three or four times. Now return to a full standing position, and reevaluate your hamstring flexibility by attempting to touch your toes, keeping your knees straight. You should be able to reach farther than on your initial attempt. This improvement occurs because the contraction of the quadriceps causes a reciprocal inhibition of the hamstrings, so the hamstrings are able to relax and allow elongation to occur.

The effects of this reciprocal inhibition demonstrate the need to accompany any stretching technique with strengthening exercises to maintain newly acquired muscle length. Strengthening exercises also assist in restoring balance between agonist and antagonist muscle groups. This topic is discussed in later chapters.

Passive Stretching

Passive stretching includes a variety of methods, including short-term and long-term stretches. Passive stretching involves the use of equipment or another person, and the patient does not assist in the stretch activity (figure 5.19). A typical example of a short-term passive stretch is when the clinician moves the patient's injured part through its range of motion and applies a stretch at the end of the motion. Madding et al. (1987) found that a 15 s stretch is just as effective as a 2 min stretch in healthy individuals, so in the interest of time, they recommended that individuals use a 15 s stretch. Although a short-term, passive stretch affects primarily the elastic range of connective tissue, it may be more effective in producing changes in the plastic range than an active stretch, because a passive stretch may be applied longer or with a slightly greater force than the patient can apply unassisted.

When applying a stretch, the part should be moved to the end of its free motion. The proximal segment of the joint being stretched should be stabilized to prevent its movement while a firm pressure is applied to the distal segment. A steady pressure is applied until the slack of soft tissue is taken up and the joint is tight. The joint is then moved slightly beyond this point. The patient should feel a stretch or tension, but not pain. If a two-joint muscle is being stretched, first one joint is positioned in the muscle's lengthened position, then the second joint, until maximum muscle length is achieved. The stretch is repeated four to six times.

The most effective stretches involve the steady application of force over a period of time. This prolonged passive stretch causes a better plastic deformation of connective tissue, primarily because of the length of time it is applied. Although research has yet to define how long a prolonged stretch should be applied, Kottke, Pauley, and Ptak (1966) suggested 20 min in clinical application. Although prolonged stretching is the most effective of all stretching techniques, it seems to be the least investigated (Light et al. 1984). A prolonged stretch is applied with

Figure 5.19 The patient does not assist in passive stretch. The stretch here is provided by gravity and further assisted with weights on the leg.

a reduced load. Two articles by Warren, Lehmann, and Koblanski (1971, 1976) reported that the amount of time required for a prolonged stretch to change connective tissue length is inversely proportional to the amount of force used. As with short-term stretches, research is lacking on prolonged-stretching effectiveness on scar tissue. One study investigated normal subjects with a prolonged stretch of 3 min but used full body weight as the force; they found significant linear increases in motion because of the great amount of force applied over a 3 min period (Pratt & Bohannon 2003). Most of the time, however, prolonged stretches applied to healing tissue is not that intense, so to influence changes in the scar tissue's plastic range, stretch time is increased. A prolonged stretch is effective in increasing motion because of its impact on the stress-strain curves of tissue and the creep phenomenon, discussed earlier in this chapter.

When using prolonged stretches, the part being stretched should be stabilized to permit the load to stretch the correct tissue. This stabilization can be provided either by the weight of the body or part or by a mechanical device such as a weight or strap. The stretch is applied slowly and steadily to the point of tightness. The segment is then secured in this position and held for the desired amount of time. If a two-joint muscle is stretched, the secondary joint should be placed in a position that elongates the muscle. For example, if the knee is stretched in extension, the patient should sit to elongate the hamstrings at the proximal end where it crosses the hip joint. The patient commonly does not feel much, if anything, when the stretch is first applied. Within 5 to 10 min, however, the patient will feel the stretch's effect. The minimal prolonged stretch duration is usually about 15 to 20 min; if the patient cannot tolerate the stress, the force should be reduced to allow the patient to stretch for the desired time.

The part placed in a prolonged stretch can feel very stiff once the stretch load is removed. The patient should be cautioned about this prior to releasing the stretch. Gentle, active range-of-motion activities help to relieve the stiffness. The stretch should be released slowly. As the stretch is released, the patient should be advised to simultaneously contract the stretched muscle to reduce the discomfort and stiffness.

Proprioceptive Neuromuscular Facilitation

The combination of active and passive stretching is often referred to as neuromuscular facilitation or proprioceptive neuromuscular facilitation (PNF). Although PNF can be used as a strengthening technique, it also is useful for gaining range of motion. A more extensive discussion of PNF principles is presented in chapter 7. Of the various PNF techniques used to increase motion, the most frequently used are the hold-relax, contract-relax, and slow reversal-hold-relax techniques (figure 5.20).

There are two technique patterns used in PNF: agonistic and antagonistic. The *agonistic muscle pattern* occurs when the muscle is contracting toward its shortened state. The *antagonistic muscle pattern* is diagonally opposite to the agonistic pattern and occurs when the muscle is approaching its lengthened state.

In each of the descriptions that follow, it may be easiest to visualize an example. Think of a hamstring muscle that is tight and you are trying to improve its flexibility. In this example, the hamstrings group is the antagonist and the quadriceps group is the agonist.

The *hold-relax* technique is a maximal isometric contraction of the antagonist (hamstrings) in all three planes of movement at the end range of the agonist (quadriceps) range that is followed by a relaxation of the hamstrings. The agonist is then used actively without resistance to increase motion of the antagonist (hamstrings). Rotation must be a component motion of the movement pattern.

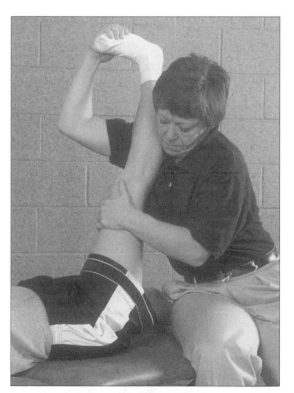

Figure 5.20   PNF stretch.

This technique is used to relax muscle spasm. For example, if a biceps is in spasm and limits elbow extension, the elbow is moved into as much extension as possible, and the biceps is tightened progressively until a maximum effort against pronation resistance is produced by the biceps for 5 to 10 s. The patient is then instructed to relax the biceps and actively extend the elbow without resistance. This process is repeated four to five times or until the desired results are achieved. The isometric contraction of the muscle facilitates a better relaxation of that muscle.

The *contract-relax* technique is used with patients who have limited range of motion. With the patient's restricted joint placed at the end-range in the agonistic (quadriceps) pattern, the clinician provides isotonic resistance against the antagonist muscles (hamstrings) to allow diagonal and rotational motion to the end range. When the patient relaxes the muscle, the clinician moves the part passively into the agonistic muscle pattern to stretch the antagonist (hamstrings). The process is repeated several times.

The *slow reversal-hold-relax* technique uses concentric contraction of the agonist (quadriceps) into the range-limited motion of the hamstrings followed by an isometric contraction of the antagonist (hamstrings). This is followed by relaxation of the antagonist (hamstrings), then concentric movement by the agonist (quadriceps). The clinician provides maximal isometric resistance against the rotational component of the movement. All the PNF stretches are useful when the primary resisting factor is a shortening of the antagonist caused by muscle spasm or loss of motion. Table 5.3 summarizes the three PNF techniques for improving flexibility.

Various investigations have compared the different types of short-term passive, active, and combination stretching procedures. Many investigators conclude that PNF stretches are more effective than other active or short-term passive stretches (Sady et al 1982; Prentice 1983). Others conclude that PNF techniques are either no different or less advantageous over other stretching techniques (Sullivan et al 1992; Church et al 2001). The body parts stretched, duration of stretches, frequency, and duration of studies vary widely among the investigations. With so many variables, it is not surprising that little or no consensus has been reached on specific methods, duration, and frequency of these stretching techniques.

Ballistic Stretching

Ballistic stretching is the use of quick, bouncing movement through alternating contraction and relaxation of a muscle to stretch its antagonist. This type of stretch is not used much in rehabilitation because of the damage it can cause to already injured tissue. The physiological characteristics of connective tissue and muscle discussed previously in this chapter provide an understanding of the dangers of ballistic stretching in therapeutic exercise:

- Ballistic stretching stimulates both the muscle spindles and GTOs. These structures normally oppose stretch reactions to protect the muscle from injury, but with uncoordinated firing, their protective mechanisms are ineffective.

Table 5.3

PNF Techniques to Gain Flexibility

Technique	Muscle activity
Hold-relax	Muscle is brought to end-motion, isometric of tight muscle, relax, stretch via contraction of opposing muscle.
Contract-relax	Muscle is brought to end-motion, isotonic contraction of tight muscle, relax, passive movement to end-range.
Slow reversal-hold-relax	Opposing muscle contracts to bring tight muscle to end-range, isometric contraction of tight muscle, relax, stretch via contraction of opposing muscle.

- Control of the stretch is limited by the velocity of the force applied in the stretch. Plastic deformation is related to the magnitude and duration of the force. A greater force over a shorter period of time is likely to cause failure of the structure, risking injury to the connective tissue. Injury will result in more scar tissue formation that ultimately decreases flexibility.

Ballistic stretching is used most often by normal, healthy people in sport activities and serves well to increase dynamic flexibility. In unhealthy tissue, however, the risk of causing further injury is too great for ballistic stretching to be considered a viable technique in rehabilitation.

Assistive Devices

In addition to equipment such as weights, pulleys, and straps for providing prolonged stretch to areas of limited motion, many devices are commonly used to assist in regaining range of motion.

Continuous Passive Motion Machines

A continuous passive motion (CPM) machine is sometimes used following surgery to restore range of motion. Although now used less frequently, a CPM can help counteract the deleterious effects of immobilization and reduce pain and edema after surgery. Because range of motion is more quickly restored with the use of a CPM, the patient is able to begin active exercises sooner to ultimately shorten the recovery and rehabilitation time following surgery. CPMs are designed for a variety of joints, including the knee, ankle, elbow, wrist, and shoulder. An example of a knee CPM is seen in figure 5.21.

Splints

Splints also assist in prolonged stretching of restricted joints. After injury the collagen and connective tissue that produce scarring become progressively more difficult to

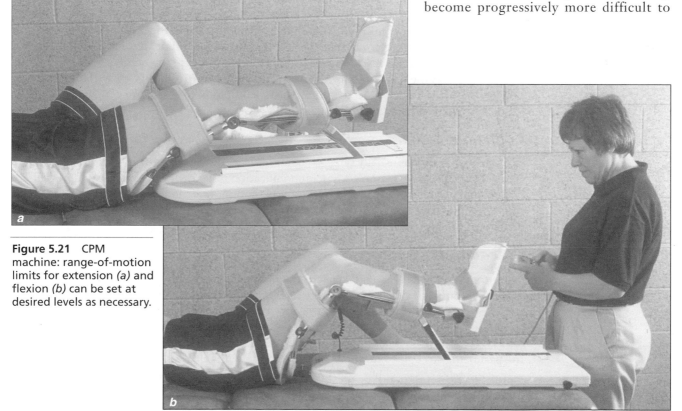

Figure 5.21 CPM machine: range-of-motion limits for extension *(a)* and flexion *(b)* can be set at desired levels as necessary.

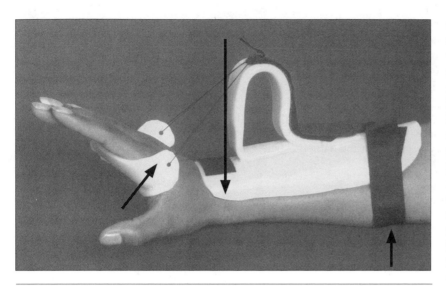

Figure 5.22 Splint to increase range of motion. Notice the 3-point system used to provide the stretch force.

stretch as the cross-links become more numerous and the collagen more mature with time. Prolonged stretching for more than 20 min is often needed with very mature or restricted scar tissue. In such instances, various splints that apply a low-level, continual stretch force are often most beneficial. They commonly use a three-point lever-and-spring system to provide a low-level, continual load (figure 5.22). These devices are used to stretch connective tissue surrounding joints and not to change muscle length. The magnitude of the load and the angle at which it is applied can be adjusted to meet the individual patient's needs. A splint can be worn for several hours at a time to cause effective plastic deformation of connective tissue.

Indications, Contraindications, and Precautions

Before applying a stretch to increase range of motion, you must first know when stretching is indicated, when you should not use stretching, and precautions for its use.

Indications

As part of a patient evaluation performed in rehabilitation, the clinician determines deficiencies in range of motion, the structures causing the loss of motion, and the status of the tissue. Is the loss a result of recent scar tissue formation, adherent and mature scar tissue, spasm, edema, postural deformities, or weakness of opposing muscles? If ligaments, capsules, muscles, fascia, skin, or other soft tissue is shortened because of scar tissue or adhesions, stretching exercises are indicated. Stretching is also indicated in the presence of contractures and structural deformities from injury or posture changes over time. If weak muscles are overpowered by opposing tight structures, flexibility of the restricted structures must accompany strengthening of the weak muscles for the treatment program to be effective. If muscle spasm or edema contributes to reduced motion, the rehabilitation program must include modalities and activities to address these problems.

Contraindications

Although stretching is usually safe, it is contraindicated when certain conditions are present. These include recent fractures when immobilization is necessary for healing and movement is detrimental to it, a bony block that restricts motion, infection in a joint, acute inflammation in a joint, extreme and sharp pain with motion, and when tightness of soft tissue actually contributes to an area's stability.

Precautions

Precautions should be taken to ensure the most effective application of the stretch and to prevent harm from the stretch. Before applying any treatment, you should always explain to the patient what you will do and the sensations and outcome to expect. A patient who is apprehensive and unable to relax will not receive an effective stretch treatment.

The force applied in a stretch should cause sensations of tension, perhaps unpleasant, in the part being stretched but not residual pain following release of the stretch. This is true for active and passive stretching. It is important that the patient understands that during active stretches the sensation of a stretch is necessary, but it should be without pain. Residual pain beyond a brief transitory tenderness, especially accompanied with new edema within a 24-hour period post-treatment, is an indication that the stretch has been too aggressive. The stretch should be less forceful to cause proper plastic changes without unwanted damage.

Vigorous stretching of areas that have been immobilized for a period of time should be used with extreme caution and even avoided in the early stretching stages. Recall that immobilization reduces the tensile strength of many connective tissue structures, including tendons and ligaments, so caution should be used when stretching these structures.

Stabilization of the area is necessary to properly apply the stretch force and to stretch the correct structures. During both active and passive stretches, the part should be positioned so that the force affects only the targeted structures. For example, if a patient is stretching the left hamstrings in a standing position with the left foot on a chair or bench, the foot should be facing the ceiling, not rotated so that the adductors, not the hamstrings, are stretched. When stretching a muscle that traverses two or more joints, the other joints must be positioned so that the muscle is elongated throughout its entire length. For example, to stretch the quadriceps, place the hip in extension with the knee in flexion to fully elongate the rectus femoris portion of the quadriceps.

In active and passive stretches, the muscle being stretched should be relaxed for optimal results. If a muscle tenses, it will resist the stretch and make it ineffective. For this reason, careful positioning and analysis of positions is important. For example, standing bent over from the waist to touch the floor with the fingertips is an ineffective position for stretching the hamstrings, since the hamstrings must work isometrically to hold the position and cannot relax. By the same token, if a passive stretch is too forceful and causes a reflex or voluntary muscle contraction, the stretch will be both ineffective and painful to the patient.

Once full range of motion is achieved following an injury, maintenance flexibility exercises need to be continued. With the continued contraction of connective tissue as scar tissue matures, loss of motion also tends to continue. This is why a patient can achieve full range of motion in one session of therapeutic exercise and return for treatment the next day with less than full range of motion. Until the healing process is complete, special attention must be paid to maintaining full range of motion even after it is achieved.

The release of the stretch force is as important as its application. Both should be done slowly. A quick application or release of a stretch, especially release of a prolonged stretch, can be very uncomfortable. Begin applying the stretch slowly, and do not apply more force until you know the patient can tolerate it.

Some pain and stiffness are normal after release of a stretch, especially a prolonged stretch. As mentioned earlier, these symptoms can be relieved by contracting the agonist as the stretch is released and following the stretch with gentle, active range of motion exercises.

If a stretch is painful, gentle traction applied to the joint during the stretch may relieve the pain. If this is not successful in relieving the pain, reduce the stretch load. A stretch should not be painful.

A stretch force affects all soft tissue in the area where the force is applied. Knowing exactly which tissues are affected has thus far eluded researchers. The structures affected may include the joint capsule, ligaments, surrounding tendons, muscles, fascia, nerves, skin, and subcutaneous tissue.

EXERCISE PROGRESSION

▶ The choice of stretching technique depends on the tissues involved, the stage of healing, the patient's motivation, the time and facilities available, and other factors of the injury.

Common questions regarding therapeutic flexibility exercises are when to use them and which stretching exercises to use. The information presented in this chapter and in chapter 2 provides the answers. If motion is permitted immediately following injury, active range of motion may be all that is necessary to regain motion. Active motion is the first choice because it does not require outside assistance, so the patient can perform it frequently and independently throughout the day when it is convenient. Frequent flexibility exercise sessions throughout the day can be an effective way to increase flexibility.

Following major surgery, the physician may order the use of a CPM machine for involved areas that require close monitoring. A CPM machine does not harm the surgical site, yet provides immediate postoperative motion, reduced pain, and less edema than limited post-operative motion. The use of CPM machines is not as prevalent today as it was when they were first introduced; surgeons have discovered that active motion within safe bounds can also produce similar beneficial results.

Other techniques may be needed after immobilization. To some extent, the method of stretching depends on the length of immobilization, the tissues affected by the immobilization, the patient's motivation, and the rehabilitation clinician's facilities and availability. Recall that collagen appears in a wound within three to five days following an injury. By the seventh day, collagen abounds, and the forming scar tissue begins to contract. This contraction continues into the final phase of healing and requires stretching exercises to maintain range of motion even after full motion has been achieved.

If scar tissue is relatively new and still pliable, active and short-term passive stretches are effective to increase motion. PNF stretching techniques can also be utilized with success. When scar tissue is more mature and well into the remodeling phase, however, prolonged-stretching techniques should be the main part of the stretching program. Short-term and active stretches accompanying the prolonged stretches help to reinforce the effects.

In particularly difficult situations where scar tissue is more than three to four months old and range of motion is still deficient, prolonged-stretch machines can be used to achieve maximal range of motion. The degree of plastic deformation of connective tissue required at this point to effect change in range of motion requires a very prolonged stretch.

SPECIAL CONSIDERATIONS

▶ The anatomy of the specific structure to be stretched determines the most appropriate stretch application.

As with application of any therapeutic exercise technique, application of stretching techniques requires common sense and consideration of the specific structure to be stretched.

Trunk

The most important consideration in stretching the trunk is to avoid any stretch that causes pain or a change in sensation down either leg.

Upper Extremity

When stretching the shoulder, the scapula must be stabilized. If it is not, the stretching force is distributed into the scapular muscles, and gains in motion may not be actual gains in the intended area.

When stretching the elbow, remember that several muscles acting at the elbow also cross the shoulder, so the shoulder should be positioned and stabilized before stretching the elbow. Because the elbow flexors and extensors work in both supination and pronation, stretches for those muscles should be performed in both positions. One possible side effect of vigorous elbow stretching is myositis ossificans, especially in youth. For this reason, elbow stretches should be performed with caution. Active stretches and reciprocal inhibition techniques may help to prevent this problem.

When stretching the wrist, the distal force should be applied over the metacarpals, not the fingers. The patient's fingers should remain relaxed during the stretch, since the extrinsic finger flexors and extensors cross the wrist and can affect the stretch if they are not relaxed.

Lower Extremity

The ankle and foot contain many joints and soft-tissue structures. When stretching these areas, the location where the joint's tendons cross and the appropriate force application must be considered to produce the desired results.

The position of the hip affects stretching the knee. Since both the knee flexors and extensors cross the hip joint, the effectiveness of the stretch is determined by the position in which the hip is placed during the stretch.

When stretching the hip, the pelvis must be stabilized. If the pelvis is not stabilized, as with the scapula during shoulder stretching, movement occurs in this segment, and an increase in hip range of motion is sacrificed to the pelvis.

Caution must be used when stretching hip rotators with the knee in flexion and the force applied at the lower leg. This position offers the rehabilitation clinician a tremendous lever arm advantage and reduces the force required to cause hip joint subluxation, especially in patients who have undergone prolonged immobilization, recent fracture, or recent dislocation.

SUMMARY

1. Define the differences between range of motion and flexibility.

   Range of motion is the amount of mobility of a joint, and flexibility is the musculo-tendinous unit's ability to elongate with application of a stretching force. Both are closely related and are often used interchangeably.

2. Explain the differences in structure of loose connective tissue and dense connective tissue.

   The primary tissue that determines range of motion is connective tissue. The fiber arrangement of loose connective tissue, such as skin, is unorganized and loose with relatively long distances between the cross-links. Dense connective tissue, such as tendons and ligaments, is highly organized with parallel collagen fibers and more cross-links.

3. List the deleterious effects of prolonged immobilization.

   Each tissue type is affected by immobilization differently, but some general changes are seen in all tissues. These include a loss of ground substance, which in turn results in less separation and more cross-links between collagen fibers. The fiber meshwork contracts, so the tissue becomes dense, hard, and less supple. The more severe effects occur with more prolonged immobilization. If a normal joint is immobilized for four weeks, the dense connective tissue that forms prevents normal motion.

4. Discuss the mechanical properties of plasticity, elasticity, and viscosity of connective tissue.

   Connective tissue's plastic quality allows its length to change, while its elasticity allows some return toward normal length. Viscoelasticity is a combination of elastic and viscous properties that allows either a change in length or a return to former length after stretching, depending on the speed, duration, and magnitude of the stretch force applied.

5. Explain the physiological properties of creep and stress-strain and how they affect stretching techniques.

   Creep permits a gradual change in tissue length with the prolonged application of a stretch force, and the stress-strain curve describes a tissue's ability to withstand stresses and the strains they produce. If a stretch force is applied beyond a tissue's stress-strain limits, deformation occurs.

6. Discuss the neuromuscular influences of the muscle spindle and GTO on stretching muscle.

   The muscle spindle and GTO are neuromuscular protective mechanisms that attempt to reduce the stress-strain forces on the musculotendinous unit.

7. Explain the procedure for measuring range of motion with a goniometer.

   To measure a joint's range of motion, the goniometer's stationary arm is placed along one segment, and the movable arm is aligned along the segment on the other side of the joint. The protractor portion of the goniometer is placed over the joint's axis of rotation.

8. Discuss the active and passive methods for stretching.

    Active stretching uses the antagonistic muscles to provide the stretch force to the agonist. In passive stretching, outside assistive devices or another person provide the force to gain additional range of motion.

9. Identify two mechanical assistive devices used to increase range of motion.

    CPMs and splints are commonly used as external devices to gain additional motion. CPMs are sometimes used after surgery to counteract the deleterious effects of immobilization. Splints can be used to apply prolonged stretch to joints restricted by mature or very restricted scar tissue.

10. List contraindications, indications, and precautions of stretching.

    Indications for stretching include a shortening of ligaments, capsules, muscles, fascia, skin, and other soft tissue by scar tissue or adhesions. Some precautions include explaining to the patient the technique and expected sensations before application, applying and releasing the force slowly and steadily, and avoiding pain. Contraindications include recent fractures, inflammations, infections, and extreme pain.

11. Discuss the progression of a stretching exercise program.

    The type of flexibility exercise applied depends on a number of considerations, including the age of the scar tissue, the stage of healing, available equipment, the patient's motivation and pain tolerance, and the tissue involved. If the scar is in the early remodeling phase of repair, active exercises may be sufficient. If the scar tissue is more mature, a more prolonged stretch that affects the plastic range of the tissue is probably indicated.

CRITICAL THINKING QUESTIONS

1. How would you stretch the quadriceps muscle if you did not want to fully lengthen the rectus femoris? In what bodily position is the rectus femoris included in the quadriceps stretch? Try these two positions with a partner. Does the knee motion change in the different positions? If so, what does that tell you?

2. Over the course of a week, stretch a partner's hamstrings using a different technique each day: a passive technique with a 15 to 30 s hold, a contract-relax-stretch PNF maneuver, a ballistic stretch, and a prolonged stretch for 15 to 20 min. Measure the hamstring length immediately after the stretch is released. Which technique gives you the greatest change in hamstring length? Measure the hamstrings 24 h after each stretch and notice the change. Why does this occur? Do any of the physical properties of creep, stress-strain, or hysteresis influence the changes?

3. If you are measuring a patient's shoulder range of motion, in what position should he or she be for the most accurate measurements? Why? What position would be least accurate when measuring a weak shoulder? Why?

4. Explain why active range of motion is not usually as great as passive range of motion. Can you think of exceptions to this generalization and explain why they occur?

5. If a patient had a condition in which the GTOs did not respond to stimuli, what would be the result? Could this be harmful during normal activity?

6. If you did not have a goniometer small enough to measure finger joint range of motion, what could you use to record flexibility in each finger joint? How can you measure trunk motion without a goniometer?

7. What is the most effective stretch for a patient who has a tight Achilles tendon? Why would you select that stretch?

LAB ACTIVITIES

1. Measure active and passive range of motion with a goniometer on the following motions. Watch for substitutions as you measure to be sure the patient is going through the range of motion correctly.

   a. Ankle dorsiflexion

   b. Knee extension

   c. Hip abduction

   d. Shoulder flexion

   e. Elbow flexion

   f. Wrist lateral flexion

   g. #1 MCP abduction

2. Measure active and passive range of motion of knee flexion with the patient in seated and prone positions. Why do the measurements change with position changes?

3. What is normal motion for the following movements?

   a. Shoulder abduction

   b. Elbow flexion

   c. Wrist extension

   d. Supination

   e. PIP flexion

   f. Hip lateral rotation

   g. Knee flexion

   g. Ankle inversion

4. Measure hip abduction with the patient lying supine and the foot facing the ceiling so there is no lateral rotation. Now have the patient laterally rotate the leg, and then abduct it. Which position provides the greatest motion? Which measure should you record as the patient's motion? Why? How does the information received from this exercise relate to other joint measurements?

REFERENCES

American Academy of Orthopaedic Surgeons. 1965. *Joint motion: Method of measuring and recording.* New York: Churchill Livingstone.

Bandy, W.D., Irion, J.M., and M. Briggler. 1997. The effect of time and frequency on flexibility of the hamstring muscles. *Physical Therapy.* 77:1090–1096.

Buckwalter, J.A. 1996. Effects of early motion on healing of musculoskeletal tissues. *Hand Clinics* 12: 13–24.

Butler, D.L., Grood, E.S., Noyes, F.R., and R.F. Zernicke. 1978. Biomechanics of ligaments and tendons. *Exercise and Sport Sciences Reviews* 6:125–281.

Church, J.B., Wiggins, M.S., Moode, F.M., and R. Crist. 2001. Effect of warm-up and flexibility treatments on vertical jump performance. *Journal of Strength & Conditioning Research.* 15:332-336.

Donatelli, R., and A. Owens-Burkhart. 1981. Effects of immobilization on the extensibility of periarticular connective tissue. *Journal of Orthopaedic and Sports Physical Therapy* 9:67–72.

Eldred, E. 1967. Peripheral receptors: Their excitation and relation to reflex patterns. *American Journal of Physical Medicine* 46:69–87.

Esch, D., and M. Lepley. 1974. *Evaluation of joint motion: Methods of measurement and recording.* Minneapolis: University of Minnesota Press.

Evans, E.B., Eggers, G.W.N., Butler, J.K., and J. Blumel. 1960. Experimental immobilization and remobilization of rat knee joints. *Journal of Bone and Joint Surgery* 42A:737–758.

Finsterbush, A., and B. Friedman. 1975. Reversibility of joint changes produced by immobilization in rabbits. *Clinical Orthopaedics & Related Research* 111:290–298.

Garrett, W.E., Jr. 1990. Muscle strain injuries: Clinical and basic aspects. *Medicine and Science in Sports and Exercise* 22:436–443.

Gerhardt, J.J., and O.A. Russe. 1975. *International SFTR method of measuring and recording joint motion.* Bern: Huber.

Hoppenfeld, S. 1976. *Physical examination of the spine and extremities.* New York: Appleton-Century-Crofts.

Kapandji, I.A. 1986. *The physiology of the joints. Vol. 2. Lower limb.* 5th ed. New York: Churchill Livingstone.

Karpovich, P.V., Herden, E.L., Jr., Asa, M.M., and G.P. Karpovich. 1959. Electrogoniometer: A new device for study of joints in action. *Federation Proceedings* 18:79.

Kendall, F.P., McCreary, E.K., and P.G. Provance. 1993. *Muscles: Testing and function.* 4th ed. Baltimore: Williams & Wilkins.

Klein, L., Heiple, K.G., Torzilli, P.A., Goldberg, V.M., and A.H. Burstein. 1989. Prevention of ligament and meniscus atrophy by active joint motion in a non-weight-bearing model. *Journal of Orthopaedic Research* 7:80–85.

Kottke, F.J., Pauley, D.L., and R.A. Ptak. 1966. The rationale for prolonged stretching for correction of shortening of connective tissue. *Archives of Physical Medicine and Rehabilitation* 47:345–352.

Kottke, F.J. and J.F. Lehmann. 1990. *Krusen's handbook of physical medicine and rehabilitation.* 4th ed. Philadelphia: Saunders.

Light, K.E., Nuzik, S., Personius, W., and A. Barstrom. 1984. Low-load prolonged stretch vs. high-load brief stretch in treating knee contractures. *Physical Therapy* 64:330–333.

Madding, S.W., Wong, J.G., Hallum, A., and J.M. Medeiros. 1987. The effect of duration of passive stretch on hip abduction range of motion. *Journal of Orthopaedic & Sports Physical Therapy* 8: 409–416.

McNair, P.J., and S.N. Stanley. 1996. Effect of passive stretching and jogging on the series elastic muscle stiffness and range of motion of the ankle joint. *British Journal of Sports Medicine* 30:313–317.

Moll, J., and V. Wright. 1971. Normal range of spinal mobility: A clinical study. *Annals of the Rheumatic Diseases* 30:381–386.

Montgomery, J.B., and J.R. Steadman. 1985. Rehabilitation of the injured knee. *Clinics in Sports Medicine* 4:333–343.

Pratt, K. and R. Bohannon. 2003. Effects of a 3-minutes standing stretch on ankle-dorsiflexion range of motion. *Journal of sport rehabilitation.* 12:162-173.

Prentice, W.E. 1983. A comparison of static stretching and PNF stretching for improving hip joint flexibility. *Athletic Training.* 18:56-59.

Saal, J.S. 1987. Flexibility training. In *Rehabilitation of sport injuries,* ed. J.A. Saal. Philadelphia: Hanley & Belfus.

Sady, S.P., Wortman, M., and D. Blanke. 1982. Flexibility training: ballistic, static or proprioceptive neuromuscular facilitation. *Archives of Physical Medicine & Rehabilitation.* 63:261-263.

Sahrmann, S. 2002. *Diagnosis and treatment of movement impairment syndromes.* St. Louis: Mosby.

Shellock, F.G., and W.E. Prentice. 1985. Warming-up and stretching for improved physical performance and prevention of sports-related injuries. *Sports Medicine* 2:267–278.

Shrier, I. and K. Gossal. 2000. Myths and truths of stretching. Individualized recommendations for healthy muscles. *Physician and Sportsmedicine.* 28: 57-63.

Sullivan, M.K., DeJulia, J.J., and T.W. Worrell. 1992. Effect of pelvic position and stretching method on hamstring muscle flexibility. *Medicine & Science in Sport & Exercise.* 24:1383-1389.

Taylor, D.C., Dalton, J.D., Jr., Seaber, A.V., and W.E. Garrett, Jr. 1990. Viscoelastic properties of muscle-tendon units: The biomechanical effects of stretching. *American Journal of Sports Medicine* 18:300–309.

Warren, C.G., Lehmann, J.K., and J.N. Koblanski. 1971. Elongation of rat tail tendon: Effect of load and temperature. *Archives of Physical Medicine and Rehabilitation* 52:465–474.

Warren, C.G., Lehmann, J.K., and J.N. Koblanski. 1976. Heat and stretch procedures: An evaluation using rat tail tendon. *Archives of Physical Medicine and Rehabilitation* 57:122–126.

CHAPTER 6

Manual Therapy Techniques

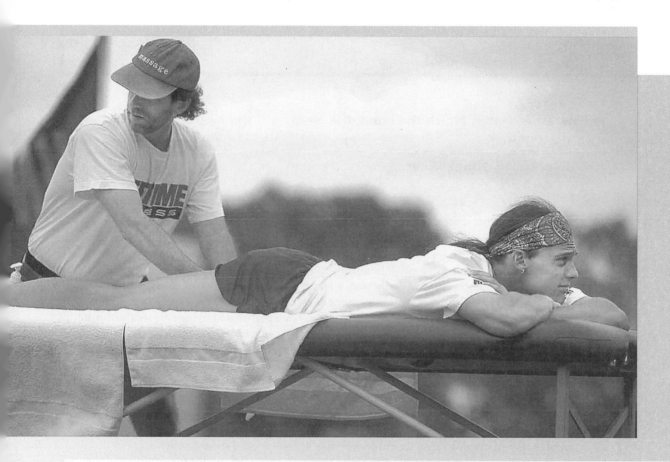

Objectives

After completing this chapter, you should be able to do the following:

1. Discuss the three techniques of massage and their indications, precautions, and contraindications.

2. Explain the progression of myofascial restriction after an injury.

3. Discuss the techniques for myofascial release.

4. Explain the theory of the mechanism of myofascial trigger points.

5. Discuss the ice-and-stretch trigger point release theory.

6. Explain the concave-convex and convex-concave rules.

7. Define joint mobilization grades of movement.

8. Discuss the direction of glide and traction in relation to the treatment plane.

9. Explain the double-crush syndrome.

10. Discuss the dangers of neural mobilization.

11. Describe one neural self-mobilization technique for the upper extremity and one for the lower extremity.

Michael Turner, certified athletic trainer for a Division III college, had never seen scar tissue adhesions like the ones he encountered in his most recent rehabilitation case. Over 6 months ago, one of the softball players, Emilie, had suffered a severe cleat laceration along her entire forearm when an opposing player sliding into second base ran the bottom of her shoe into Emilie's forearm. The forearm required over 30 stitches. Although Emilie hadn't suffered any immediate loss of motion from the scar, she was now losing some elbow and wrist motion because the scar tissue was pulling on both joints. When Michael palpated the forearm, he could feel a lot of hard, unyielding scar tissue adhesions below the skin. He knew he had to soften the scar tissue and mobilize the tissue below the skin if Emilie was to have normal elbow and wrist motion. He also knew he would have to show Emilie some soft-tissue techniques that she could perform on her own throughout the day to reinforce his efforts in the athletic training clinic.

■ **Fine art is that in which the hand, the head, and the heart of man go together.**

John Ruskin, British Writer

Manual therapy is the use of hands-on techniques to evaluate, treat, and improve the status of neuromusculoskeletal conditions. A variety of structures, including joints and soft tissue, are affected by procedures that come under the category of manual therapy. The various procedures in this category are defined according to the tissues and structures they influence. This chapter discusses some of the more commonly used manual therapy procedures and techniques. Manual therapy techniques are considered by many medical professionals to be subjective because little quantitative research has been performed to investigate the efficacy of such treatment techniques. It is difficult to create an objective research design of these treatments because the specific application, direction, duration, and amplitude of a force can vary from one health care provider to another. With these variations come a variety of outcomes, so a truly objective assessment of treatment effectiveness is difficult, if not impossible. Most of the benefits recorded are considered anecdotal because of their subjective, rather than objective, basis. Manual therapy techniques, however, deserve attention and application because of these overwhelming clinical reports of successful outcomes. Certain common principles apply to all manual therapy techniques if they are to be used successfully.

It is important for you to keep in mind these common principles for applying all manual therapy techniques:

- The patient should be in a comfortable position.
- You should be in a comfortable position.
- You should always use good body mechanics.
- Feedback from the patient throughout the treatment is necessary for proper application of the technique and appropriate pressure.
- Your fingernails should be clean and trimmed. As a general rule, the nail should not extend beyond the fingertip pad.
- You should explain to the patient before applying the technique what will be done and what sensations to expect. The patient should be warned whether any discomfort may be felt and should tell you whether less pressure or discomfort is desired during the treatment.
- The patient's condition must be assessed before, during, and at the conclusion of the treatment.

- The appropriate manual therapy technique must be correctly applied for a successful result.
- Precautions and contraindications must always be respected.
- If you are unsure, do not perform the technique.

CRITICAL ANALYSIS

▶ Evaluation and assessment are important for selecting appropriate manual therapy techniques.

The foundation of any manual therapy technique is your ability to critically think and to analyze the patient's condition to determine the best and most appropriate course of action. This practice involves understanding the injury and healing process, identifying the structures and problems involved, analyzing the situation and all its parameters to decide on a plan of action, and critically appraising the results of the treatment plan to determine its effectiveness or the need to change it. Critical analysis and examination with continual reassessment are key to effective manual therapy application and outcomes.

There is no cookbook method for applying manual therapy. You must be able to use your skills of observation, palpation, analysis, and technique application. As with other aspects of rehabilitation, analysis and deductive reasoning are skills vital to a successful outcome of manual techniques. The rehabilitation clinician is a detective in search of answers to problems. Detective skills in the assessment of clinical findings and deduction of logical expectations must be continually used throughout the manual therapy process.

Depending on the specific injury and resulting impairments, you may choose to use more than one manual therapy technique. Evaluation and deductive reasoning allow you to select treatment techniques that can best reduce the impairment and improve the functional ability of the injured athlete.

Whatever techniques you choose, your selection should be based on individual findings, not on rote or cookbook decisions. Always approach an injury with an open mind and maintain flexibility in your treatment options. Each patient must be individually and objectively assessed to determine the best course of treatment. Two patients may have shoulder pain and loss of motion, but the causes and courses of treatment may be very different for each of them. A successful treatment program depends on your evaluation skills as much as on your treatment skills.

MASSAGE

▶ Effleurage, petrissage, and friction massage are techniques that can relax muscles, improve blood and lymph flow to reduce edema, reduce pain, and improve soft-tissue movement.

Many types of massage are used in a number of applications to achieve a variety of goals. A sports massage is frequently used either before or after competition in what is known in non-medical circles as a rubdown. Even though massage is used in non-medical situations, it still produces a physiological effect. The use of massage for non-pathological conditions, however, is not discussed in this text. The range of techniques most commonly used in the injury treatment is briefly described in this section.

Definition of Massage

Massage is the systematic and scientific manipulation of soft tissue for remedial or restorative purposes. Massage affects various systems of the body through its influence on reflex and mechanical processes to produce desired results.

Effects of Massage

Massage produces reflex physiological and mechanical effects in the area treated. Repetitive pressure stimulation without irritation to the skin causes transmission from peripheral receptors to the spinal cord and brain, which results in relaxation of muscles and dilation of blood vessels. Mechanical effects improve blood and lymph flow, promote mobilization of fluid, and stretch and break down adhesions to ultimately assist in reducing edema and improving tissue mobility. The overall end result is relaxation of muscles, dilation of local capillaries, increase in lymph flow to reduce edema, reduction of pain, and improvement in soft-tissue movement. The specific effects vary, depending on the type of massage given.

Types of Massage

Although there are many different massage techniques, three primary techniques are used in treating injuries to achieve the effects mentioned earlier. The French terms for many of these techniques were first introduced by Peter Ling of Sweden, who traveled widely in Europe (Beard and Wood 1969).

Figure 6.1 Effleurage: Stroking motion begins distally and moves proximally toward the heart. Elevating the segment during treatment further assists in edema reductions.

Effleurage

Effleurage, or stroking, is a massage that is performed by running the hand lightly over the skin's surface. The direction of the stroke moves distally to proximally (figure 6.1). Effleurage is used to assist in venous and lymphatic flow to decrease edema and aid in muscle relaxation. If the technique is used primarily to treat edema, it should be performed with the part in a position so that gravity can assist the flow. The pressure should be applied firmly and deeply but not heavily. The direction should be toward the heart.

Figure 6.2 Petrissage: skin and underlying tissue are kneaded and lifted to improve tissue mobility, relax muscle, and promote circulation.

Petrissage

Compression and kneading fall under the category of petrissage. In this technique the soft tissue is grasped and manipulated intermittently so that there is movement between the skin's under-lying structure and the muscle (figure 6.2). Although the stroking movement is constant, the pressure is intermittent. The tissue is grasped and released with varying degrees of pressure so that the action's mechanical effects reduce edema.

This technique is often preceded and followed by a stroking technique for relaxation. Petrissage is used to promote circulation, relax muscle, mechanically assist fluid exchange, and improve mobility of muscle tissue.

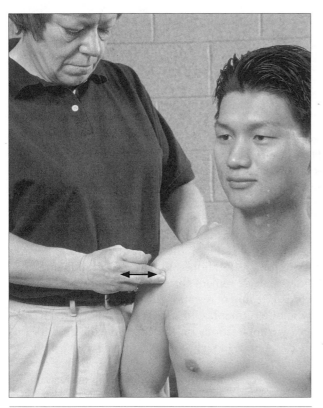

Figure 6.3 Friction massage across the biceps tendon will loosen adhesions and stimulate circulation.

Friction

Friction is a deep-pressure movement of superficial soft tissue against underlying structures (figure 6.3). Sometimes the underlying structure is bone or another hard surface, and sometimes it is soft tissue, such as muscle or fascia. The intent is to loosen scar tissue and adhesions of deeper parts, such as tendons, ligaments, and joint capsules, to improve movement and gliding of these structures. Friction also helps to stimulate circulation of the local area. It usually is applied through firm pressure by either the thumb or finger pads in a crisscross or circular motion.

Indications

The indications for massage are related to its effects. Relief of pain, muscle relaxation, reduction of swelling, and mobilization of adherent scar tissue are all appropriate indications for the use of massage. The specific technique selection is based on the evaluation findings. Recent edema secondary to trauma is an indication for effleurage and petrissage massage techniques. Friction massage is indicated when scar tissue restriction of superficial tissue can be palpated and in inflammatory conditions where adhesions play a role in continued symptoms, such as tendinitis and bursitis.

Contraindications

Massage is contraindicated when the technique may aggravate the condition or cause additional harm to the patient. Contraindications include the presence of infection, malignancies, skin diseases, blood clots, and any irritations or lesions that may spread with direct contact.

Precautions

When you apply massage to the patient, both the patient's skin and your hands should be clean. Your hands should be warm and your nails should be trimmed so as not to cause a laceration or abrasion. Rings, watches, and wrist jewelry should be removed for the same reason. A lubricant is used to reduce friction when using effleurage. Less lubricant is used with petrissage, and still less is used with friction massage. Too much lubricant with friction massage does not allow the presence of enough friction to be effective, and too much lubricant with petrissage makes it difficult to lift or grasp the tissue.

Application

Before beginning the massage, position the patient comfortably with the part to be massaged properly exposed. If the massage is to reduce edema, elevate the part to enhance lymphatic flow. Explain the procedure to the patient and instruct the patient to inform you if he or she feels pain with the massage.

When using effleurage or petrissage, the pressure of the massage strokes should be toward the heart, and the hands should not lose contact with the skin. On the return stroke, continue lightly touching the part. Keep your hand in good contact with the part and your fingers together, not spread apart. The rhythm of the stroke should be even and slow to promote relaxation. Maintain a comfortable position during the treatment and use proper body mechanics.

When using friction massage, it is important to warn the patient that some discomfort may be felt but that it will not be lasting. The thumb or finger pads are used on a small, localized surface in a cross pattern. A firm, consistent pressure and rhythm are also important. A small area at a time is massaged until the discomfort of the massage subsides and you can palpate an increase in tissue mobility. The massage is applied in a "cross" pattern perpendicular to the tissue's fiber arrangement.

MYOFASCIAL RELEASE

▶ Myofascial release involves manual contact to evaluate and treat soft-tissue restriction and pain, relieve symptoms, and improve motion and function. It is commonly used to treat the restricted fascia associated with the skin, subcutaneous tissues, and other superficial structures.

Myofascial release is a close relative to massage. They both involve manual contact with the patient, and they both use the sense of touch to evaluate the problem and the effectiveness of the treatment. They also both include the use of pressure and tissue stretch to produce results.

There are many different techniques of myofascial release, but they all are essentially variations of the same principle: The use of manual contact for evaluation and treatment of soft-tissue restriction and pain with the eventual goal of the relief of those symptoms to improve motion and function. There are different names for these techniques: myofascial release, myofascial stretching, strain-counterstrain, Rolfing, soft-tissue mobilization. Because of the individual variations in application, forces, duration, and precise technique, reliable research results on the efficacy of myofascial release remain elusive. Clinical observations and anecdotal reports of those who have recorded treatment results is currently the best barometer by which to judge the results of this type of treatment. Ultimately, treatment effectiveness must be assessed by the results of your own applications on the patients you treat. In this section, some of the more commonly used myofascial techniques are introduced briefly.

Before describing the various myofascial release techniques, their theoretical basis is discussed. The different myofascial release systems cannot be appreciated without understanding their basis.

Fascia

Fascia is a continuous structure that surrounds and integrates tissues and structures throughout the body. Fascia varies in density and thickness and is interconnected with the structures it surrounds. It can affect the relationship among the structures it encompasses (their physical orientation to each other, their chemical relationship, or their physiological relationship, e.g., what tissues are served by which blood vessels or nerves). Fascia is vital for tissue form, lubrication, nutrition, stability, integrity, function, and support.

Throughout the body, fascia is divided into three layers. The superficial layer is attached to the undersurface of the skin. Within this superficial layer lie capillaries, lymph vessels, nerves, and fat. Because this layer is a loosely knit structure made of fibroelastic and areolar connective tissue, it permits the skin to move in many directions over the underlying structures. It is also a place where edema accumulates following injury.

Deep fascia is dense connective tissue that surrounds and separates deeper structures, such as muscle, tendon, joints, ligaments, and bone. Because of its stiffer, firmer structure, deep fascia is less able to accommodate edema, which can cause problems, such as compartment syndromes in the lower leg.

The final layer is subserous fascia, which surrounds internal organs. Its loose areolar connective tissue contains channels where fluid assists in providing the organs with lubrication. Myofascial release techniques are not used to treat fascia surrounding visceral organs.

Fascia contains collagen, elastin, cellular components, and ground substance. The elastin within fascia allows the structure to return to its original shape when applied stresses are released. Fascia also responds with plastic deformation when prolonged forces are applied. Creep and hysteresis, discussed in chapters 3 and 5, are properties of fascia and are used in myofascial release techniques.

Although fascia has high tensile strength and is able to tolerate multidirectional compressive, stretch, and sheer forces, an injury can profoundly affect fascia. The fascia's normal biomechanics can be altered to cause either a temporary or permanent deformation, depending on the load, duration, and type of stress applied to the fascia. Injury to fascia causes a change in the biochemical structure of the ground substance, and the scar tissue that forms after injury can interfere with normal fascia functions. The fascia's reduced ability to provide skin, subcutaneous, muscle, and other tissue with normal motion, support, lubrication, and other functions can cause extended disability and prolonged symptoms following injury and repair if not treated properly.

Myofascia maintains an intimate relationship with the muscle it covers and surrounds. The two provide the combined contractile and noncontractile properties of muscle. Myofascia assists in increasing muscle strength during eccentric contractions. It helps provide structure and form to the muscle, lubrication between muscle fibers and muscles, and nutrition for the muscles. It also bears the blood and lymph vessels and nerves for the muscles. In short, myofascia provides vital support to permit normal muscle function.

Nonacute Biomechanical Forces

When injury or unbalanced biomechanical forces are applied to myofascia, its ability to support normal muscle function is impaired. This can lead to pain, loss of motion, and less than optimal function performance. Dysfunction causes additional changes in the myofascia.

In pathology that occurs over time—for example, the swimmer who has developed poor posture—muscle imbalances are often the cause. As noted in figure 6.4, the process may start with a minor trauma or injury. It causes a change in the muscle, perhaps as a part of its withdrawal reflex to the injury. This muscle change eventually causes an imbalance of muscle strength between an agonist group and its antagonist group. Muscle imbalances lead to changes in neuromuscular response and coordination, which lead to further imbalances, until the structure reaches a point where the imbalance and resulting increased tissue stress cause symptoms that impair performance and require treatment.

The patient can inadvertently start this cycle through the activities he or she performs. If the swimmer with poor posture concentrates on pectoralis strengthening without also working on antagonist strength, or uses only strokes that emphasize anterior and not posterior muscles, eventually a muscle imbalance will occur. Awareness of muscle imbalance is important in treating patients with loss of motion. Muscle imbalances are discussed more thoroughly in chapter 7.

It is also important to realize that exercise is a vital collaborative adjunct of myofascial release treatments in a successful rehabilitation program. Myofascial techniques release restricted areas, but exercises for flexibility and strength reset neurological programming. Together they cause permanent positive changes in the affected tissues.

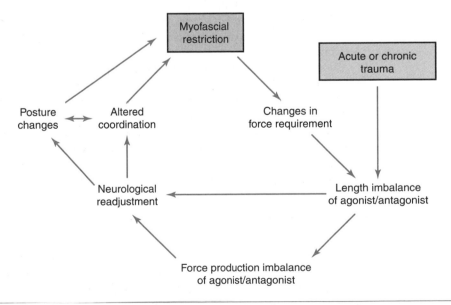

Figure 6.4 Pathology of myofascial restriction: Myofascial restriction can occur within a short time from acute injury and scar-tissue formation or gradually from minor but progressive alterations from repeated low-level trauma.

Acute Biomechanical Forces

Previous chapters have already addressed the biomechanical causes of fascial restriction following acute injury. Scar tissue is less extensible and creates a localized connective tissue meshwork that extends tentacles outward, much like a shattered plate glass window, to adjacent locations and can limit normal tissue mobility. Recall from the discussion of immobilization in chapter 5 that the scar tissue matrix can restrict neurovascular and lymph vessels and reduce local metabolism. With reduced metabolism a fluid imbalance further adds to the area's reduced mobility and continued inflammation. Less motion causes a loss of GAGs and promotes increased cross-link formations. Mobility between fibers becomes restricted through this process.

In addition to the scarring that occurs with acute injury, spasm also can influence the myofascial system by producing prolonged tightness in one area that causes another area to compensate with prolonged looseness, initiating a cycle of imbalance and myofascial pathology. It is important to evaluate for fascial restrictions in both acute and nonacute injuries.

Terminology

The term *myofascial release* is common and is frequently used in the techniques described here, but it is actually a misnomer. Myofascial release implies the treatment to myofascia. Although myofascia can certainly be the target of treatment, it is not always the targeted tissue nor the only tissue treated. For example, to relieve fascia contractures and restriction of skin and subcutaneous tissue mobility following edema and immobilization, myofascial release techniques actually commonly treat the fascia associated with skin, subcutaneous tissue, and other superficial structures that have limited mobility, not the muscle's fascia.

Even when the target tissue is myofascia, other structures may also be affected by treatment because of secondary restriction in the area. With subcutaneous restriction following edema and immobilization, for example, myofascial structures may be restricted and require myofascial release treatment, but the areas restricted subcutaneous and skin structures are also treated when the myofascia is treated.

Palpation

Palpation is fundamental in myofascial release. Not only is it required for an examination of the area, but continual palpation is performed during the treatment. The soft tissue's extensibility, movement, end-feel, and response to treatment are continually palpated during and after the treatment. Adjustments are made as the area is palpated and examined during the treatment.

Normal tissue has no tenderness when palpated. Normal tissue also has a springy end-feel that can be palpated when pressure to the tissue is released. This springy end-feel is present in normal tissue regardless of the tissue's excursion. Tissue mobility varies according to the body part and tissue type, but the springiness of the end-feel is consistent. In myofascial techniques, palpation also includes feeling the release in the tissues during the treatment. This release is the treatment goal and is necessary for restoring tissue mobility and balance. The release that is palpated has been described as the tissue giving way, letting go, relaxing, or melting as ice with a hot knife going through it.

Superficial to Deep Structures

When examining and treating with myofascial release techniques, you should move from superficial structures to deeper structures to avoid a mistake in identifying the structure or tissues that are restricted. Techniques should be applied with the least amount of force that is appropriate for achieving the established goals. More force is often indicated when scar tissue adhesions and reduced mobility are present, but the additional force is applied only after examining and assessing the area and determining the patient's tolerance.

Autonomic Effects

Neuroreflex changes can sometimes result from the use of myofascial techniques. Myofascial restriction can cause autonomic changes, so it is not surprising that when restriction is released, the autonomic system can be affected. If pain and myofascial restriction cause changes in skin color, moisture, temperature, and sensation, then their release will also cause changes in those signs and symptoms.

Afferent sensations are transmitted to the dorsal horn of the spinal cord. The dorsal horn is a processing center that receives and redirects information. It can send an impulse directly out the spinal cord as a reflex efferent response, or it can send the information to the subcortical or cortical level of the brain, where it is interpreted and a response is formulated and returned down the spinal cord to the appropriate locale.

The patient may experience an autonomic response when the myofascial treatment is particularly effective. The patient's sympathetic system is stimulated, and the patient demonstrates symptoms such as increased pulse rate, sweating, and blood pressure changes. Less intense responses include sensations of burning, tingling, stinging, or heat in the area being treated (Sutton and Bartel 1994). Although these sympathetic responses are unusual, you should be aware that they may occur and be prepared to respond appropriately.

Treatment Techniques

Because there are many different ways to apply myofascial techniques, only general application techniques regarding time, frequency, pressure, and palpation are introduced here. This is by no means an exhaustive list of myofascial techniques. It is, however, a list of the more commonly used techniques.

General Guidelines

In the beginning, it may be necessary to restrict the treatment time to 3 to 5 min and increase it as the patient's tolerance and the response of the area indicate. Daily treatment can be beneficial. If bruising occurs, the technique is too aggressive. Because bruising causes additional scarring and adhesions, it should be avoided. Bruising is not a desirable reaction, but a short-term redness of the skin in the area should be expected.

There are many different ways to apply myofascial release techniques (Manheim 1994). Palpation and relaxation by the rehabilitation clinician are basic to applying myofascial techniques. If you are relaxed you will have more sensitivity in your hands and fingertips to palpate the area being treated. An exercise to illustrate this idea is to take a dime in your fingertips, close your eyes, tense your arm from the shoulder to the fingers, and try to feel the nose on the portrait. Then relax your entire arm and try to feel the nose. It should be easier to locate the nose when your arm and hand are relaxed. To ensure both the patient's and your relaxation, you should both be in comfortable positions.

In one of the most frequently used techniques, both hands move longitudinally in opposite directions while stretching the tissue (figure 6.5). In another variation, only one hand applies the treatment while the other hand stabilizes or supports

Figure 6.5   In longitudinal myofascial release, fascial tissue between the hands is stretched.

the tissue. The treatment hand applies pressure through the finger pads, thumb, knuckles, or heel of the hand (figure 6.6). The pressure can also be applied by the forearm or elbow, depending on the size and location of the area being treated. The stabilizing hand anchors the tissue so that the pressure can be applied in the direction of the restriction. The tissue's slack is taken up, and a steady pressure into the restriction is continued until the area releases or for about 90 s.

The amount of pressure applied is determined by the tissue involved and the sensitivity of the area, but it is generally a low-load, sustained pressure.

Figure 6.6 Alternative myofascial release applications using (a) finger pad, (b) knuckle, or (c) elbow.

Figure 6.7   J-stroke.

J-Stroke

A J-stroke is a common technique that is used on limited areas of tightness and on longitudinal scars. The technique is used in these situations because of its multidirectional stretch. As shown in figure 6.7, the treatment hand draws short Js across the restricted area.

Oscillation

When muscle spasm is present, an oscillating pressure technique can be used. This technique involves a rhythmic, back-and-forth application of a low-load pressure while maintaining constant contact.

It is designed to relax the muscle by reducing the spasm and relieving the patient's guarding of the area. It can be applied with finger pads for small areas, as shown in figure 6.8, or with the palms for larger areas.

Wringing

In areas of generalized or multidirectional restriction, a technique referred to as *wringing* can be effective. In this technique both hands are used for treatment. The hands are placed on the area in similar positions. They are then rotated on the extremity in opposite directions to twist or wring the tissue, as in figure 6.9. This same technique can be used on smaller areas using the two thumbs in the same manner.

Figure 6.8   Oscillation.

Figure 6.9   Wringing: a generalized, multidirectional release technique.

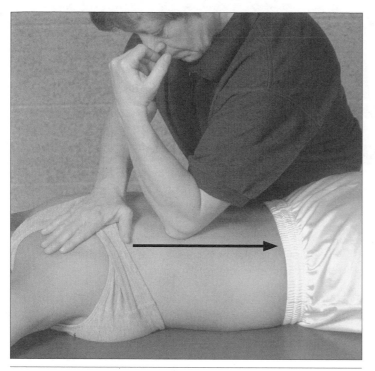

Figure 6.10 Stripping: a deep tissue release using one hand to stabilize and the elbow to treat.

Stripping

The stripping technique is used as a deep-tissue release. It is similar to the general technique described earlier, but it is applied to deeper tissue. Knuckles and elbow are frequently used in this technique (figure 6.10) but, the finger pads can also be effective over small areas. The pressure is slow, consistent, and deep. It is uncomfortable for the patient, but if it can be tolerated, it is effective in breaking up deep adhesions.

Arm Pull and Leg Pull

The arm pull and leg pull are gross techniques applied to generalized tightness in the upper and lower extremities, respectively. These techniques involve the application of longitudinal traction to the arm or leg from the hand or foot with the patient lying supine (figure 6.11). As the traction is applied, the extremity is slowly moved into abduction and rotation. When tissue resistance is felt, the motion is stopped, and the position is maintained until you feel the extremity release. Once the area releases, the extremity is moved through its arc of motion into the new area of restriction, and the sequence is repeated until an end position is reached.

Figure 6.11 Arm pull: a generalized technique in which traction is applied to the arm while moving it into abduction and rotation to the point of resistance. Movement through an arc of motion continues following the resistance after the extremity releases.

Precautions

As with any treatment, you should take precautions with this application. Myofascial release should be used cautiously on new scars. The new tissue is fragile because of its reduced tensile strength. It also may have increased sensitivity and limited tolerance to pressure.

Care should also be used with patients with reflex sympathetic dystrophy (RSD). RSD is exacerbated with pain, so treatments should avoid pain.

Bruising should also be avoided. This is especially true when the purpose of the treatment is to improve scar tissue mobility, because bruising produces more scar tissue.

The patient should be warned that sensations of pain, tingling, burning, and warmth are normal with this technique. The patient should also be instructed to inform you if any additional sensations are felt.

Contraindications

Contraindications for the use of myofascial techniques include malignancy, hypermobile joints, recent fractures, hemorrhages, sutures, osteoporosis, local infections, and acute inflammations (Sutton and Bartel 1994). As always, contraindications should be respected, and treatment in the presence of these conditions should be avoided.

MYOFASCIAL TRIGGER POINTS

▶ A myofascial trigger point is an area of tenderness in a muscle or its fascia that can cause referred pain and is palpated as a taut band with a nodule. Ice stroking, ischemic compression, stripping, and PNF are techniques often used to treat trigger points.

Two of the most recognized names in the study of myofascial trigger points are Janet Travell and David Simons. They devoted their professional lives to understanding and treating trigger points and are world-recognized leaders on the topic. Most of the information presented here is the result of their findings. For additional information on trigger points, see Travell (1976), Simons (1981), and Travell and Simons (1983, 1992).

Myriad terms are often used interchangeably with myofascial trigger point. Some of the more commonly used terms include myalgia, fibrositis, muscular rheumatism, fibroplastic syndrome, myositis, and myofascitis.

Definition of Trigger Point

Travell and Simons (1983) define a trigger point as a "focus of hyperirritability in a tissue that, when compressed, is locally tender and, if sufficiently hypersensitive, gives rise to referred pain and tenderness, and sometimes to referred autonomic phenomena and distortion of proprioception." Trigger points can be located in cutaneous, fascial, myofascial, ligamentous, and periosteal tissue. The discussion here is limited to myofascial trigger points.

A myofascial trigger point involves a taut band of muscle tissue and its surrounding fascia, hence the name. A central focal point of local tenderness can be palpated as a nodule within the taut band. Compression of this point often refers pain to other areas or causes an autonomic response.

Travell and Simons (1983, 1992) identify two types of trigger points: active and latent. An active trigger point is one that is always tender and can produce referred pain whether the muscle is active or inactive. The muscle can also display weakness and reduced motion. When an active trigger point is palpated with a rolling pressure crosswise against the muscle fibers, the muscle fibers are stimulated to produce a localized twitch response. This palpation technique is called a snapping palpation and is performed using firm, constant pressure and moving the fingertips across the muscle fibers as if plucking a guitar string. The local twitch response is an involuntary contraction of the muscle fibers in response to the snapping palpation (Travell and Simons 1983). Sometimes this response is incorrectly called a *jump sign*. A jump sign is also a reflex response but is a reaction of wincing or withdrawal.

A latent trigger point is painful only when it is palpated. Normal muscles do not have areas of tenderness, sites that elicit a local twitch response, or palpably taut bands.

Trigger Point Characteristics

Trigger point tenderness is often described as a dull ache and can be merely uncomfortable or very intense. Pressure on the trigger point can elicit a referred pain pattern that is unique for each muscle. The more irritable the trigger point, the more severe and extensive is the referral pattern. For detailed trigger point referral patterns, refer to the two texts that Simons and Travell have written on this topic (1983, 1992). The earlier publication deals with referral patterns of the upper extremities, and the more recent text addresses lower-extremity referral patterns.

The referral patterns do not follow neurological referral patterns; this is an important distinction. The sensation of trigger point referral pain is also different from neurologically referred pain. Trigger point pain is often described as a deep ache. Occasionally, a trigger point pain is described as a sharp or stabbing pain, and rarely is it described as burning. Referred sensation from peripheral nerve entrapment or nerve root irritation, however, is evidenced by prickling, tingling, or numbness.

Myofascial trigger point pain becomes amplified by muscle activity (especially strenuous activity), passive stretch of the muscle, direct pressure of the trigger point, prolonged stationary periods followed by moving (such as getting up in the morning or standing after prolonged sitting), repeated or sustained muscle activity, and cold. On the other hand, myofascial trigger points are relieved with short periods of rest; heat accompanied by slow and sustained stretches; short-term, low-level activity; and specific treatment techniques that are discussed later in this chapter.

Trigger Point Causes

Trigger points can be activated by various factors, including injury, overload, fatigue, and chilling. Acute conditions that can activate trigger points include fractures, sprains, dislocations, muscle impact injuries, and the stress of excessive or unusual exercise that the body is unable to tolerate. Overload of the muscles from a prolonged stationary posture, prolonged muscle immobilization in a shortened position, and nerve compressions are the most common causes of gradual trigger point onset. The exact mechanism of trigger point production; however, is only theoretical at this time. Travell and Simons (1983) have proposed a theory that involves the contractile activity of a muscle: During contraction of a normal muscle fiber, calcium that is stored in the fiber's sarcoplasmic reticulum is rapidly released when the contraction begins and then reabsorbed in the presence of ATP when the contraction terminates. This process is triggered by a brief nerve impulse called an action potential. A contraction is the result of the shortening of the sarcomere when its cross-bridges pull the actin and myosin filaments over each other (figure 6.12). If an injured muscle fiber's sarcoplasmic reticulum is damaged, its calcium stimulates the sarcomere to produce a sustained contraction as long as ATP is present to provide the energy for the activity. This runaway metabolic activity no longer needs an action potential to continue the sustained contraction; it can continue on its own as long as the calcium and ATP are present together. Once the calcium becomes depleted, the trigger point may continue to exist, but the mechanism for its persistent presence remains theoretical as yet. Travell and Simons (1983) propose that with a near- exhaustion of local ATP levels, localized muscle contractions that do not require action potentials may take over. Without any ATP, the sarcomere's filaments cannot release from each other and remain fixed in their contracted position.

Vasoconstriction of the area occurs probably either because of a localized reflex response or stimulation of the central nervous system and autonomic system through the trigger point. This simultaneously reduces local circulation and increases metabolic needs. The release of nerve-sensitizing and ischemia-causing substances such as histamine, serotonin, kinins, and prostaglandins (mentioned in chapter 2) may be the cause of continued, localized, runaway metabolic activity. Travell and Simons (1983, 1992) propose that these substances, which are released following an injury, increase the metabolic demands and sensitize afferent nerve endings to make them hyperirritable to mediate referred pain, autonomic and motor neutron responses, and cause trigger points.

Figure 6.12 Normal skeletal muscle structure and a sarcomere in shortened and lengthened conditions.

Trigger Point Examination

As part of the total treatment plan, the causes of the patient's pain must be accurately assessed to rule out trigger points as a possible factor. Observation and examination of the patient's posture, range of motion, weakness patterns, pain areas, and history are all required to determine the patient's injury and rehabilitation needs. It is sometimes easier to identify patterns if the areas of pain are indicated on a figure drawing like the one in figure 6.13.

A compression test over the muscle can detect taut bands, nodules, and local and referred pain. A local twitch response confirms the presence of a trigger point. A taut band is palpated by stretching the muscle until the taut fibers are pulled to the point of discomfort without pain while the overall muscle remains slack. The taut band feels like a cord within the muscle. Begin at the distal attachment and palpate with either the pad of the thumb or two or three fingers along the taut band toward the fibers' proximal attachment to locate the trigger point within the band. It is an area of increased tenderness and feels like a hard ball within the taut band.

A local twitch response can be elicited along the taut band by performing a snapping palpation of the band. A snapping palpation is done by placing the muscle in a relaxed, neutral position and strumming the fibers with pressure perpendicular to the fiber alignment, much like strumming a guitar. In a positive response the taut band twitches. The more closely the pressure is applied to the trigger point of the taut band, the more vigorous is the response. This technique works most effectively on superficial muscles.

Trigger Point Treatment

Travell and Simons (1983, 1992) and Cyriax (1977) advocate the use of trigger point injection as an effective method of treatment, but this treatment is neither appropriate nor legal for rehabilitation clinicians. When an active trigger point does not respond to the treatment techniques presented here, it may be useful to refer the patient to a physician who can inject the site.

Three primary methods of myofascial trigger point treatments are discussed briefly here. For additional information, refer to the Travell and Simons texts (1983, 1992), the source of the techniques described next.

Ice-and-Stretch

Fluorimethane as a cold spray was formerly used as a common treatment for myofascial trigger points. Now that we are more aware of the harm that chlorofluorocarbons cause to the

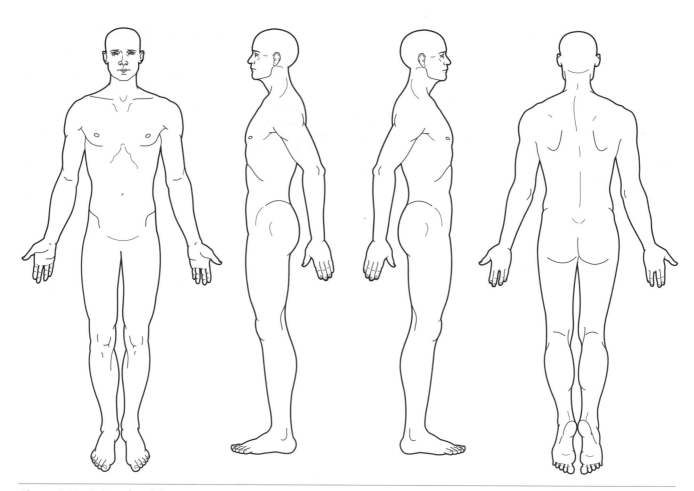

Figure 6.13 Pain-referral figure.

atmosphere, Fluorimethane is not used as often; those who are environmentally concerned have replaced cold spray with ice stroking using an icicle. An "icicle" is made by placing a tongue depressor in a cup of water and freezing the water. Before applying the icicle to the skin, the paper or styrofoam cup is torn back and covered with thin plastic wrap to avoid getting any cold water on the patient's skin; keeping the skin dry throughout the treatment maintains the contrast between the warm skin and the cold ice. Since ice rather than Fluorimethane spray is safer for the environment and less costly, the cold-and-stretch technique will be referred to throughout this text as "ice-and-stretch".

Before application, the patient should be instructed to relax. Applying just enough pressure on the trigger point area to produce the referred pain may help the patient understand why your treatment is not being applied directly to the area of pain. The patient is placed in a comfortable position with the skin exposed and the body part supported to permit full relaxation. Before treatment the part is moved through its range of motion so you and the patient can judge changes made by the treatment. With the muscle anchored at one end, the ice or cold spray is applied in a sweeping motion in parallel strokes in only one direction over the length of the muscle and then over the referred pain pattern. As the ice is applied in a rhythmic, unhurried fashion, a slow, continual, passive stretch is applied progressively to the muscle. Any one area of the skin should receive only two to three strokes of ice before rewarming to achieve optimal results of the ice-and-stretch technique (figure 6.14). The rate at which the ice is moved over the skin is approximately 4 in/s (10 cm/s). The stretch force should be light enough that it does not elicit a stretch reflex from the muscle but strong enough to be effective. As a muscle releases, you must be able to detect the relaxation and place the muscle in a new stretch position that takes up the slack and provides the same level of tension on the muscle. The application and release of the stretch force should be done

Figure 6.14 In the ice-and-stretch technique, ice strokes are applied in sweeps that include the muscle, its trigger points, and its referred pain areas. The ice is applied in a rhythmic fashion while a gentle stretch is applied to the muscle.

smoothly and gradually, not quickly. A hot pack can be immediately applied to further relax the muscle. The patient can also assist the stretch by contracting the antagonist, but you must monitor the contraction so as to prevent a co-contraction of the agonist and antagonist. The ice-and-stretch technique can be repeated for several cycles after the skin has been rewarmed, depending on the results of treatment, the patient's response, and desired goals.

Theory of Effectiveness

It is believed that this technique is effective because of two mechanisms, although they have not been confirmed through research. The gate theory of pain presented by Melzak (1973) and the modified gate control theory advanced by Castel (1979) postulate that sudden cold and touch sensations inhibit the pain cycle by blocking transmission of pain signals. Active trigger points activate the pain-spasm response. Ice stroking inhibits the pain-spasm cycle and allows the muscle to respond to the stretch (figure 6.15).

The second factor is mechanical: If a muscle is stretched, its sarcomere elongates and releases the actin and myosin elements enough to end the sustained muscle fiber contraction.

Ischemic Compression

Another myofascial trigger point release is ischemic compression. In this technique, pressure is applied slowly and progressively over the trigger point

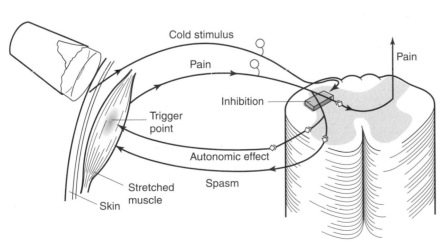

Figure 6.15 Effect of trigger point release on neural pathways: The sudden cold and touch afferent stimulation facilitates a presynaptic inhibition to "close the gate" to pain transmission.

Adapted by permission from D.G. Simons, J.G. Travell, and L.S. Simons 1999.

as the tension in the trigger point and its taut band subsides. Pressure is maintained until the tenderness is gone or the tension is released. This is followed by stretching the muscle. Before application, the patient should be informed that some discomfort may occur.

Stripping

A third technique is stripping massage, a deep-stroking massage applied with minimal lubrication on the fingertips. A firm pressure is used along the length of the taut band. The pressure increases progressively with each successive pass along the muscle. A milking movement from the distal to proximal end of the muscle goes over the trigger point at the rate of about 1 in. (2.5 cm) every 3 s. As the effects of the technique become apparent, the taut band relaxes, the trigger point nodule softens, and the area ceases to be tender and no longer refers pain.

The ischemia produced by the pressure of the ischemic compression or stripping massage techniques is believed to cause a reflexive hyperemia that returns the site to a normal condition (Travell and Simons 1983).

Proprioceptive Neuromuscular Facilitation and Other Techniques

The PNF techniques of contract-relax and reciprocal inhibition, which were introduced in chapter 5 and are discussed further in chapter 7, are also effective in relaxing myofascial trigger points. In addition, various other techniques are used in the treatment of myofascial trigger points. Modalities such as hot packs, ultrasound, and electrical stimulation are also frequently used as adjuncts to enhance the effectiveness of treatments.

Precautions

Before application, an accurate history should be taken and the patient's condition assessed to determine whether trigger point therapy will be effective. Trigger point therapy is not as effective on scar tissue adhesions as on myofascial restrictions.

The patient should relax for optimal treatment results. The stretch applied should be passive without any contraction of the agonist. If the patient is able to isolate the antagonist and if you can monitor the patient's response, contraction of the antagonist may improve treatment results, as long as the stretched muscle remains relaxed. Cold is not as effective if it is applied too quickly or repetitively over the same area. The stretch should be applied slowly and should not cause painful spasm or prevent the patient from relaxing, but it should be sufficient to produce the desired results.

The cause of the myofascial trigger point must be corrected for the treatment to be successful, particularly if the cause is poor posture or chronic stress of the muscle. The cause can be corrected with flexibility and strengthening exercises and patient education and instruction.

Prolonged direct pressure over nerves and blood vessels should be avoided. The pressure should be discontinued if the patient complains of tingling or numbness.

MUSCLE ENERGY

▶ Muscle energy techniques are used to treat joint malalignments. These techniques involve the precise and controlled voluntary contraction of a muscle against a counterforce provided by the rehabilitation clinician, followed by a passive stretch.

Like many manual therapy techniques, muscle energy techniques have their origin in osteopathic medicine. Fred Mitchell, DO, originally developed muscle energy techniques which others have since modified.

Definition of Muscle Energy

According to Greenman (1996), muscle energy is a manual technique that involves the voluntary contraction of a muscle in a precisely controlled direction, at varying levels of intensity, against a distinct counterforce applied by the rehabilitation clinician. Essentially, muscle energy is the use of muscle contraction to correct a joint's malalignment.

Muscle Energy Theory

Muscle energy theory is based on the premise that joint malalignments occur when the body becomes unbalanced. Malalignment may be the result of a muscle spasm, a weakened muscle overpowered by a stronger muscle, or restricted mobility. The muscle contraction used to correct a malalignment may be **isometric, concentric,** or **eccentric.** The patient controls the magnitude of contraction, and the clinician positions the patient and provides the resistance to change the treated joint's alignment.

In malalignments, movement is restricted by what Mitchell identifies as a barrier. A **barrier** is not the end of the existing range of motion, but a resistance that is felt when a part is moved through its passive range of motion. For example, you can passively move the leg of a patient with a tight hamstring in a straight leg raise. Although the hip may be able to go through its full motion, you will feel a resistance because of tightness in the hamstring at some point before the end of its motion. Where in the motion this resistance is felt depends on how tight the hamstring is.

Isometric muscle contraction is most commonly used when treating the spine with muscle energy techniques, whereas isotonic contraction is more frequently used when treating the extremities. Briefly reviewing muscle physiology principles can help you understand how muscle energy techniques work. When the patient contracts a muscle against an external resistance, the contracting muscle causes the neurological response of reciprocal innervation. In other words, the contracting muscle causes relaxation of the antagonist and contraction of synergists through responses of Golgi tendon organs and muscle spindles via spinal cord and cortical reflexes. After the isometric contraction, the antagonist relaxes enough to permit a stretch. Its relaxation also impedes its inhibition of the contracting muscle to permit a more normal force-counterforce balance between the agonist and antagonist. Repeated contractions combined with passive stretches then provide additional motion gains and improved muscle balance.

It is believed that these muscle contractions and changes in muscle length affect the surrounding fascia and connective tissue. Since the technique is an active one, requiring the active participation of the patient, muscle physiology is affected and can result in postexercise soreness secondary to metabolic waste buildup and a change in the fascial length. You should warn the patient that muscle soreness may occur and avoid overpowering the patient or overdoing the activity. Because the forces used are relatively low and the techniques involve an active motion and a passive stretch, the only contraindications to muscle energy techniques are recent or nonunion fractures.

Components of Muscle Energy Technique

The components necessary for muscle energy techniques are an accurate determination of the cause and best treatment of the malalignment, a specific joint position, a precise active muscle contraction performed by the patient, an appropriate counterforce produced by the rehabilitation clinician, and an applied stretch force that results in increased motion without pain.

Before you can determine the appropriate muscle energy technique to apply, you must determine through an examination the presence of a malalignment and the cause of the malalignment.

Once you determine that muscle energy would assist in correcting the deficiency, you must determine the most effective position for the muscle energy technique. The patient's injured part is then positioned at the end of the barrier, and the patient is instructed on the type of muscle contraction desired. While the patient actively contracts the muscle, you apply the appropriate resistive force with the correct direction, duration, and magnitude.

Isometric contractions are used for muscle energy techniques on the spine, and isotonic contractions are used for muscle energy techniques on the extremities. If the contraction is isometric, you should provide only about 2 ounces of force. The isometric contraction is not strong but should be sustained and light. It should be sustained for 5 to 10 s, and the length of the muscle should not change.

Figure 6.16 Muscle energy release to gain knee extension: With the lower leg in lateral rotation and the foot in dorsiflexion, the patient rotates the lower leg medially while you provide a smooth resistance throughout the full movement. Once the patient relaxes the muscles, the lower leg is laterally rotated to its new barrier.

If an isotonic contraction is used, enough counterforce should be provided to allow motion at an even, controlled speed. The muscle contraction should be forceful and through the muscle's full range of motion.

For either an isometric or an isotonic contraction, it is important for you to permit full relaxation of the muscle after the contraction before stretching the joint to a new barrier position. This allows the muscle to enter its refractory period (time of relaxation) following its contraction and achieve optimal stretch results. The technique is repeated three to five times for the best results. The greatest changes are seen after three repetitions; clinical observations indicate that more than five repetitions produce little additional benefit.

Application

A couple of examples can demonstrate the application of muscle energy techniques. In the first example, an isotonic contraction is illustrated. Let us look at a basketball player who has undergone rehabilitation after an ACL reconstruction. After many varied attempts to attain full motion, she still lacks full extension. You must investigate possible alternative methods for relieving the problem:

1. *Assessment of the problem.* You have determined that the lack of extesion is the result of restricted lateral rotation of the tibia on the femur.

2. *Specific joint position.* The patient sits with the lower legs hanging over the table. You position the ankle in dorsiflexion and the lower leg in lateral rotation to their barrier (figure 6.16).

3. *Precise active contraction by the patient.* The patient contracts the thigh muscles to move the lower leg into medial rotation through the full range of motion.

4. *Appropriate counterforce.* While the patient contracts the muscles and moves the joint, you offer resistance that permits a smooth, controlled movement into medial rotation for 5 s. Guide the lower leg through the correct plane of motion while offering resistance.

5. *Stretch force.* Instruct the patient to relax while holding the lower leg at its end position, wait to feel the muscles fully relax, then apply a stretch into lateral rotation to a new joint position where the new barrier is felt. This technique is repeated three to five times. Reexamine for range-of-motion changes after final repetition.

In the next example, isometric contractions are used in a muscle energy technique applied to a soccer player who collided with another player and suffered a direct blow to the right anterior ilium. The contusion is resolved, but she continues to complain of groin pain that goes down her leg. The physician has ruled out a disk injury and reports to you that the problem may be coming from his pelvis. You are given the challenge of evaluation and treatment of the patient's injury:

1. *Assessment of the problem.* Your examination reveals that there is an inflare of the right ilium. Other tests for lumbar dysfunction have ruled out injury to the low back. You determine that muscle energy techniques would be an appropriate treatment.

2. *Specific joint position.* With the patient lying supine, the right leg is placed in a figure-4 position with the right knee flexed, the hip abducted and flexed, and rotated so the outside of the ankle is placed on the distal left thigh to the barrier point. Stabilize the patient's pelvis by placing your left hand on the left anterior superior iliac spine and the right hand on the patient's medial right knee. Then apply enough pressure on the knee to move the right hip to its end position of lateral rotation.

3. *Precise active contraction by the patient.* Ask the patient to contract isometrically in an attempt to move the leg into medial rotation, pulling the knee toward the left shoulder as you provide resistance to prevent the motion from occurring. The isometric contraction is held for 5 to 10 s.

4. *Appropriate counterforce.* The amount of resistance applied by the patient is not great: less than a pound of resistance. Since the contraction is isometric, you must instruct the patient to match your force and not to overpower the resistance you provide (figure 6.17).

5. *Stretch force.* As in the previous example, instruct the patient to relax while you support the extremity at its end position, wait to feel the muscles fully relax, then apply a stretch into lateral rotation and abduction by pushing the right knee toward the table to the new barrier. The process is repeated three to five times. After the final repetition, passively return the leg into hip and knee extension. Reexamine for alignment and pain.

The majority of muscle energy techniques must be accompanied by exercise to effectively treat the problem. You must understand the mechanics of the change that occurs with muscle energy treatment in order to correctly use accompanying active stretches. As an example, you could instruct the soccer player with the iliac inflare to perform a stretch similar to the position used in the treatment. It is also necessary for the patient to progress to strengthening exercises that support the stretching exercises, such as hip lateral rotation or hip adductor strengthening exercises.

JOINT MOBILIZATION

▶ Joint mobilization involves passive movement of a joint to relieve pain or restore mobility. Proper application requires knowledge of joint mechanics, normal range of motion, and proper technique.

Joint mobilization is one of the most commonly used manual therapy techniques in the treatment of restricted joint motion. Manipulation and mobilization are not new concepts. Hippocrates (460–355 b.c.) used these techniques in his medical practice and recorded various methods of manipulating bones and joints.

Through the years a variety of approaches to manipulation and mobilization have been developed. More recent schools of thought have been influenced by the teachings of manual clinicians such as Geoffrey Maitland, Freddy Kaltenborn, James Cyriax, James Mennell, and Stanley Paris. Table 6.1 identifies the main distinctions of each of these manual therapists' approaches.

Figure 6.17
Muscle energy release to correct ilium inflare.

Table 6.1
Manual Therapy Schools of Thought

Sources	Key distinction
James Cyriax	Uses selective tension techniques to identify faulty structures in the examination. Emphasizes the need for soft-tissue massage and frequently uses injection of muscle trigger points. Believes the disk is the primary source of low-back pain and uses nonspecific spinal techniques designed to move the disk to relieve nerve root pressure.
Freddy Kaltenborn	Arthrokinematics. The techniques incorporate the influence of muscle function and soft-tissue changes in the manifestation of the patient's loss of function. The techniques are eclectic and very specific.
Geoffrey Maitland	Uses primarily passive accessory movements to restore function after an extensive assessment based on information from the patient's subjective examination (history) and the evaluator's objective assessment. The movements are oscillations, the techniques are specific, and the goal is to relieve what he terms "reproducible signs."
James Mennell	Feels that "joint play" is key to normal joint function. Emphasizes the importance of the small accessory movements as necessary for full joint motion to occur. Techniques are more specific for the extremities than for the spine.
Stanley Paris	Incorporates both chiropractic and osteopathic orientations in his eclectic approach to normalization of arthrokinematics, especially joint play and component motions. As a general rule, the patient's pain is not used to guide treatment.

Definition of Joint Mobilization

Joint mobilization is on a continuum with manipulation. They both involve passive movement of a joint, but mobilization is under the patient's control in that voluntary contraction of a muscle will stop the movement. Manipulation is at such a speed that the patient is unable to stop the motion. Mobilization is frequently performed by rehabilitation clinicians, but manipulation is not. Manipulation is most commonly performed in chiropractic applications, and is beyond the scope of this book.

Joint Motion

There are two types of joint motion: physiological and accessory. Physiological joint motion is movement that the patient can do voluntarily, such as flexion and abduction. Accessory motion is necessary for normal joint motion but cannot be voluntarily performed or controlled.

There are two types of accessory motion: joint play and component motion. Both component motion and joint play are necessary for full motion. Component motions are not capsular, but they accompany physiological motion. The rotation of the clavicle during shoulder flexion is an example of a component motion. Joint play occurs within the joint and is determined by the joint capsule's laxity. If you grasp and twist a finger, you can feel the joint play of the metacarpophalangeal joint.

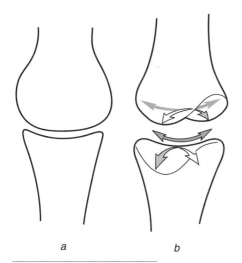

Figure 6.18 Joint surfaces of *(a)* ovoid and *(b)* sellar joints.

Arthrokinematics

Arthrokinematics refers to the motions between the bones that form a joint. There are five types of motion that occur within a joint: roll, slide, spin, compression, and distraction. These motions permit greater motion of a joint and can occur only with appropriate joint play. This concept is vital to understanding how joint mobilization works and how it can be applied.

Most joint surfaces are concave, convex, or both. Joints that have one concave and one convex surface are called *ovoid* (figure 6.18a). Joints that have a surface that is concave in one direction and convex in another with the opposing surface convex and concave in complementary directions are called *sellar* or *saddle joints* because of their similarity to a saddle (figure 6.18b). The shape of the joint determines its arthrokinematic motions.

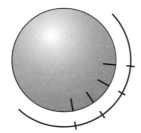

Figure 6.19 Roll: different points on one surface come in contact with different points on the second surface.

Roll

Roll occurs on incongruent surfaces when a new point of one surface meets a new point of the opposing surface (figure 6.19). Rolling occurs in combination with sliding or spinning in a normal joint. Roll occurs in the direction of bone movement.

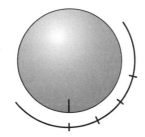

Figure 6.20 Slide: one point on a surface comes in contact with different points on a second surface.

Slide

Slide occurs on congruent surfaces when one point of one surface contacts new points on the opposing surface (figure 6.20). Like rolling, sliding does not usually occur by itself in normal joints. When a passive mobilization technique is applied to produce a slide in a joint, the technique is referred to as a glide. The more congruent a joint is, the better it responds to gliding mobilization techniques to gain mobility.

Figure 6.21 Spin: a segment rotates about a stationary mechanical axis.

Spin

Spin occurs when one bone rotates around a stationary axis (figure 6.21). Like rolling and sliding, spin does not occur by itself during normal joint motion.

Figure 6.22 Compression

Figure 6.23 Distraction.

Compression

Compression is a decrease in the space between two joint surfaces (figure 6.22). Compression adds stability to a joint and is a normal reaction of a joint to muscle contraction. Some compression occurs during a roll on the side in the direction of the motion.

Distraction

Distraction of a joint occurs when the two surfaces are pulled apart (figure 6.23). A gentle distraction can relieve pain in a tender joint. Distraction is often used in combination with joint accessory mobilization techniques to further stretch the capsule.

Concave and Convex Rules

Knowing which type of joint is being treated and keeping in mind the concave and convex rules (figure 6.24) is basic to the application of correct mobilization techniques. In these rules, one joint surface is mobile, and the other is stable. The concave-convex rule states that concave joint surfaces slide in the same direction as the bone movement (figure 6.24). The convex-concave rule states that convex joint surfaces slide in the opposite direction of the bone movement. For example, if the thigh is stabilized to prevent the femur from moving at the knee, the tibia's concave joint surface slides posteriorly when the tibia moves posteriorly from extension to flexion. In contrast, if the glenoid is stabilized at the shoulder, the humerus's convex shoulder joint surface slides inferiorly as the arm is moved superiorly into abduction. In other words, if you want to increase knee flexion, your mobilization force on the tibia is in an anterior-to-posterior (AP) direction. If you want to increase knee extension, you apply a posterior-to-anterior (PA) mobilization force. On the other hand, when mobilizing the shoulder, if you want to increase shoulder flexion, you would apply an AP force.

Capsular Patterns of Motion

As discussed in chapter 5, all joints have expected, or normal, ranges of motion, and various causes can prevent normal motion. When loss of motion is caused by tightness within the joint capsule, specific characteristic changes are seen in the pattern of motion loss and are referred to as a capsular pattern. Table 6.2 indicates the capsular pattern for most joints. When you examine a joint's range of motion, knowing both the joint's normal degree of motion and the typical pattern of capsular restriction is necessary. When a capsular pattern is present, full joint motion will not be attained until the capsular tightness is addressed. A capsular pattern indicates that at least some of the loss of motion is due to tightness within the capsule and that joint mobilization should be included in the treatment program. A noncapsular pattern indicates that structures other than the capsule are preventing normal motion and that joint mobilization will not significantly contribute to range-of-motion gains.

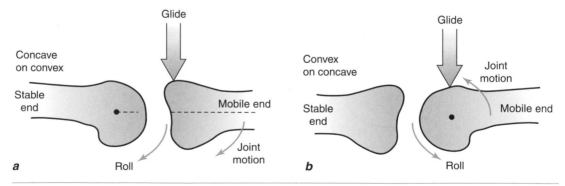

Figure 6.24 Rules for concave and convex joint surfaces. *(a)* Concave-convex rule: Joint mobilization glide force is applied in same direction of bone motion. *(b)* Convex-concave rule: Joint mobilization glide force is applied in the opposite direction of bone motion.

Table 6.2
Capsular Patterns

Joints	Capsular pattern
Glenohumeral	Lateral rotation is more limited than abduction. Abduction is more limited than flexion. Flexion is more limited than medial rotation.
Elbow	Flexion is more limited than extension. Supination and pronation are equally limited.
Wrist	Flexion and extension are equally limited. Pronation and supination are mildly limited at the distal radioulnar joint.
Finger	Abduction is more limited than adduction of the thumb CMC. Flexion is more limited than extension of the MCPs and IPs.
Hip	Medial rotation, abduction, and flexion are more limited than extension. Generally, no limitation of lateral rotation.
Knee	Flexion is more limited than extension.
Ankle Talocrural Subtalar	Plantar flexion is more limited than dorsiflexion. Inversion is more limited than eversion.
Foot and toes 1st MTP 2nd-5th MTP IP joint	Extension is more limited than flexion. Variable. Extension is more limited than flexion.
Lumbar spine	If a left facet is limited: Forward bending (FB) produces a deviation to the left. Side bending right (SBR) is limited. Side bending left (SBL) is unrestricted. Rotation left (RL) is limited. Rotation right (RR) is unrestricted.
Cervical spine	If a left facet is limited: FB produces some deviation to the left. SBR is unrestricted. SBL is comparatively unrestricted. RL is comparatively unrestricted. RR is most limited.

CMC = carpometacarpal; MCP = metacarpophalangeal; IP = interphalangeal; MTP = metatarsophalangeal.

Effects of Joint Mobilization

As with many manual therapy techniques, the exact effects of joint mobilization are unknown, and many reported benefits are anecdotal with little objective evidence to identify their effects. Nonetheless, many clinicians report consistent, positive results from their treatments, so it is assumed within the allied health and medical world that some biochemical, biophysiological, or biomechanical benefits are produced by the techniques.

Neurophysiological Effects

Hertling and Kessler (1990) report that joint mobilization stimulates the joint's mechano-receptors to decrease pain. Small-amplitude joint mobilization oscillations stimulate the mechanoreceptors that inhibit the transmission of nociceptive stimulation from the spinal cord and brain stem. Small-amplitude and mild joint mobilization oscillations also affect muscle spasm and muscle guarding. Inhibition of nociceptive stimulation results in relaxation.

Nutritional Effects

Distraction or small gliding movements can cause synovial fluid to move within the joint. The avascular articular cartilage within a joint depends on synovial fluid movement for its nutritional needs and nutrient-waste exchange. In edematous and painful joints, these movements can improve nutrient exchange to prevent deleterious effects of joint swelling and immobilization.

Mechanical Effects

More aggressive mobilization techniques can improve the mobility of hypomobile joints. Immobilized joints that have lost their normal range of motion develop collagenous adhesions and thickened connective tissue. Mobilization techniques that stretch collagen structures into their plastic range of deformation increase the tissue's mobility and improve the joint's motion. Mobilization not only stretches capsular tissues but also effectively loosens or breaks down adhesions to improve mobility (Kaltenborn 2002).

Cracking Noise

Occasionally, a mobilization or joint movement produces a cracking sound. When tension is produced in a synovial joint, increased pressure within the joint causes a vaporization of gas within the synovial fluid. When the gas is liberated as the gas bubble forms then collapses, the joint space expands. The collapse of the gas bubble causes the noise (Corrigan and Maitland 1989). Initial reports indicated that the gas formed was nitrogen, but it is now believed to be carbon dioxide.

Following this cracking, joint mobility often increases. This is believed to occur because of the expansion of the joint capsule from the increased pressure and the reflex relaxation of surrounding muscles through stimulation of inhibitory mechanoreceptors (Paris and Patla 1988). This increased joint mobility can be advantageous or disadvantageous. It is advantageous for hypomobile joints. For hypermobile joints, a reduction of muscle tone along with an increase in joint laxity can lead to increased joint stress and pain; the muscles reflexively tighten and cause additional discomfort. Although "cracking" one's back or neck may offer temporary relief, Paris and Patla (1988) believe that such joint cracking may increase the risk of disk injury. When cracking occurs repeatedly in the spine, the joints become unstable. Conversely, when it occurs repeatedly in the extremities, as when cracking the knuckles, the joint capsule eventually becomes thickened and increases the joint's stiffness.

Application of Joint Mobilization

Before you apply joint mobilization, you must identify the forces and excursions that can and should occur as well as what is considered "normal" for a joint and the individual. These issues are discussed in the following sections.

Grades of Movement

Movements used in joint mobilization are divided into four grades, indicated I, II, III, and IV. Manipulation uses grade V. The grading is based on the amplitude of the movement and where within the available range of motion the force is applied. Grades I and IV are small-amplitude movements performed at the beginning and end of the range, respectively. Grades II and III are large-amplitude movements. Grade II movement does not reach the limits of the range, whereas grade III movement is performed up to the limit of the available range. These grades overlap somewhat, as seen in figure 6.25. Grade V is the manipulation grade and is usually small in amplitude and beyond the end range of a restricted joint.

The amount of motion within each grade is relative to the specific joint and to the available motion within that joint. For example, a normal glenohumeral joint has larger grade I, II, III, and IV movements than a severely restricted glenohumeral joint and certainly larger movement than a metacarpophalangeal joint.

Grades I and II are generally used to relieve pain in joints. Oscillations in these grades stimulate joint mechanoreceptors to inhibit nociceptive feedback into the joints. These grades often are also used before and after treatment with grades III and IV, beforehand to relax the joint and afterward to relieve discomfort that the more aggressive grades may have caused.

Grades III and IV are used to gain motion within the joint. These grades stretch the capsule and connective-tissue structures that limit joint mobility. They can be uncomfortable but are not necessarily so.

Oscillatory motions are most often used with the various grades of movement. Sustained joint-play motions can also be used. The sustained techniques involve only three grades: I, II, and III. Their grade definitions are slightly different from those of oscillatory motions: Grade II goes to the end point of resistance, and grade III is essentially a stretch of the joint, going toward a normal joint's limit (figure 6.26). The techniques discussed here use the oscillatory motions, since they are the most common.

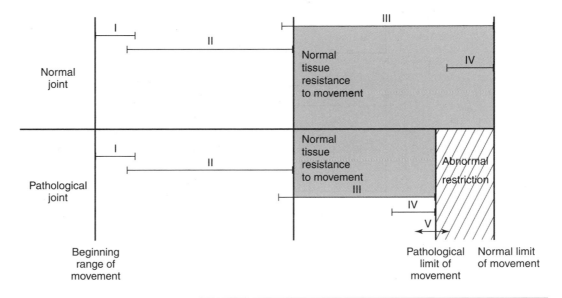

Figure 6.25 Grades of movement in a normal and a restricted joint: Grades I and II do not reach the limits of movement. Grades III and IV do reach the limits of movement. Grades I and IV are small amplitude, while grades II and III are large amplitude.

Adapted by permission from G. Maitland 1991.

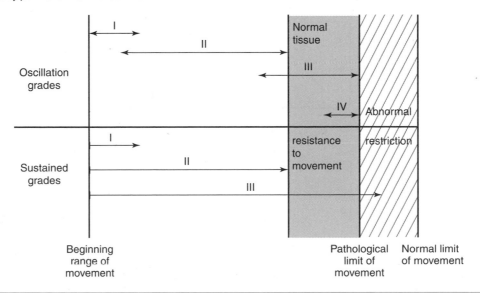

Figure 6.26 Sustained versus oscillation mobilization.

Figure 6.27 Movement diagram.

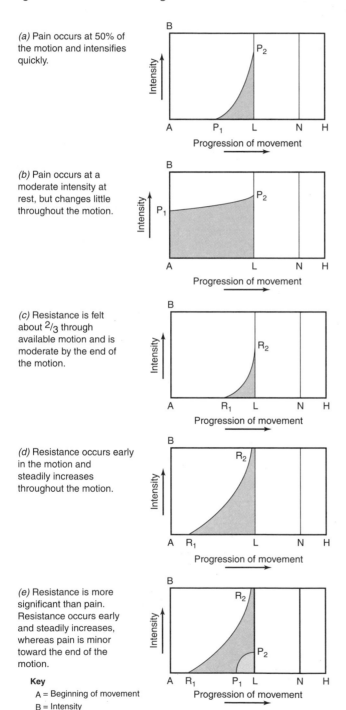

(a) Pain occurs at 50% of the motion and intensifies quickly.

(b) Pain occurs at a moderate intensity at rest, but changes little throughout the motion.

(c) Resistance is felt about 2/3 through available motion and is moderate by the end of the motion.

(d) Resistance occurs early in the motion and steadily increases throughout the motion.

(e) Resistance is more significant than pain. Resistance occurs early and steadily increases, whereas pain is minor toward the end of the motion.

Key
A = Beginning of movement
B = Intensity
H = Hypermobile range
L = Abnormal limit of ROM
N = Normal limit of ROM

Figure 6.28 Pain and resistance on movement diagrams.

Movement Diagram

A movement diagram is a visual aid that can sometimes be helpful in determining which mobilization grade to use in a treatment. Either physiological or accessory movements can be diagrammed. A movement diagram is shown in figure 6.27. AN is the normal range of motion of a joint; A is the beginning of motion, and N is the normal limit of a motion. L is the abnormal limit of motion. H indicates a joint's hypermobile range. B is the intensity of a treatment technique.

You mark on the movement diagram where the patient reports pain. P in figure 6.28 represents where within the range of motion the patient reports pain and the intensity of the pain; P_1 indicates where the pain starts, and P_2 the intensity of pain at the end of motion. R_1 indicates where you first feel resistance during a passive movement of the joint, and R_2 is the intensity of the resistance at the end of the motion. If the patient has pain at rest, the P curve begins at A and is placed at a height on the vertical scale that corresponds to the intensity of pain reported by the patient. If the pain is mild, the mark is placed low on the AB line; if pain is moderate, the mark is placed higher (figure 6.28b). If the patient reports the start of pain at 50% of possible motion, P_1 is placed at the midpoint of the AL line (figure 6.28a). If the pain occurs gradually but progressively over the length of the motion, a gradually sloping upward line is drawn, but if pain begins suddenly and quickly intensifies, a steep line is used.

To determine where R is drawn, you passively move the joint through its available range and indicate on the graph where the start of the restriction can be palpated. If the restriction begins abruptly and inhibits motion, a steep, rapidly climbing line is drawn. If restriction is more gradual, a line with a gentler slope is drawn.

Once you complete a movement diagram, you can easily assess the treatment needs and determine whether to attend to the patient's pain or joint restriction first. If the pain is not significant, you may choose to treat the restriction first, but if pain appears more intense and increases more quickly than resistance on the movement diagram, pain should be relieved before restriction is treated.

Until you understand joint mobilization techniques and grades and develop the skill to palpate and evaluate pain and resistance, it is a good idea to draw a movement diagram on paper or in your head. It will help you determine what you need to treat first and what grades of mobilization are most appropriate.

Normal Joint Mobility

Determining normal and abnormal joint mobility requires practice and familiarity with the patient. Because joint mobilization is a manual therapy, you must develop your sense of touch so that you can detect what is normal for any particular joint. This can be done only through practice on normal subjects. Once normal mobility is identified, abnormal mobility is easier to recognize. Mobility that is normal for a glenohumeral joint is not normal for a wrist joint.

Normal mobility also varies for different populations and is determined by factors such as age, disease, occupation, sport, and position in a sport. For example, a 40-year-old man will not have the same normal lumbar spine mobility as his 15-year-old son has. Even though they may both have normal vertebral mobility, what is considered normal for the father is not normal for the son. Age plays a role in determining normal joint mobility.

Athletes from different sports also demonstrate various degrees of normal joint mobility. For this reason, it is important to compare the joint being treated with the contralateral side to assist in determining normal mobility for that individual. For example, a baseball pitcher may have a hypermobile glenohumeral joint when compared with a football lineman. A ballet dancer may have a hypermobile hip compared with a shot-putter. You must consider the specific needs and demands of a sport or activity and even of a position within the sport when determining an individual's normal joint mobility.

Close-Packed and Loose-Packed Positions

The relative position of the joint surfaces must be considered prior to applying joint mobilization techniques. In a close-packed position, the joint surfaces are most congruent with each other (table 6.3). The convex surface of one bone is in complete congruence with the opposing concave surface of the other bone. The ligaments and capsule are taut, and the joint surfaces cannot be easily separated with traction. Joints are not initially mobilized in a close-packed position, but

Table 6.3
Resting and Close-Packed Joint Positions

Joints	Resting	Close packed
Fingers		
Metacarpophalangeal	20° flexion	1: Full opposition 2-5: Full flexion
Interphalangeal	20° flexion	Full extension
Wrist	0°	Full flexion
Elbow		
Humeroulnar	70° elbow flexion with 10° supination	Full extension
Humeroradial	Full elbow extension with full supination	Midflexion with midpronation
Radioulnar	70° elbow flexion with 35° supination	Full pronation or full supination
Glenohumeral	55° flexion with 20°-30° horizontal abduction	Full abduction with full lateral rotation
Hip	30° flexion, 30° abduction with slight lateral rotation	Full extension, medial rotation, and abduction
Knee		
Tibiofemoral	20°-25° flexion	Full lateral with lateral tibial rotation
Patellofemoral	Full knee extension	Knee flexion
Ankle and midfoot		
Talocrural	10° plantar flexion	Full dorsiflexion
Subtalar and midtarsal	Midrange of inversion and eversion	Full inversion
Forefoot and toes		
Metatarsophalangeal 1	20° dorsiflexion	Full dorsiflexion
Metatarsophalangeal 2-5	20° plantar flexion	
Interphalangeal	20° plantar flexion	

this position can be used to stabilize an adjacent joint before applying mobilization forces to another joint. For example, if you want to mobilize a proximal interphalangeal joint, the metacarpophalangeal joint can be positioned in full flexion, the close-packed position, to stabilize the proximal segment.

A **loose-packed position** is any position that is not close packed. The articular surfaces are not totally congruent, and some portions of the capsule are lax. Examinations and early mobilization techniques should both be performed with a joint in its maximum loose-packed position. This position is often referred to as a joint's **resting position**. See table 6.3 for a list of resting and close-packed positions for the joints. As a general rule, extremes of joint motion are close-packed positions, and midrange positions are loose-packed positions.

Rules for Application

Before applying mobilization techniques, you should understand the following rules and use them as guidelines for all joint mobilization treatments:

1. The patient should be relaxed.

2. Before application, explain to the patient the purpose of the treatment and what sensations to expect.

3. Joint physiological and accessory mobility are assessed before and after the treatment. It may be necessary to check accessory mobility at various points within the physiological range.

4. Compare the joint to be treated with the contralateral joint to determine what is normal for the patient.

5. Determine treatment goals before treatment.

6. Grades I and II are used to relieve pain. Grades III and IV are used to increase mobility.

7. Stop the treatment if it is too painful for the patient.

8. Initial mobilization is performed in a resting position.

9. One segment, usually the proximal joint segment, is stabilized, while the other is mobilized.

10. Your hands should be as close to the joint as possible.

11. The larger the surface area of contact, the more comfortable is the force application for the patient. When you use the entire hand, the fingers should be together, and as much of the finger and palm surface as possible should contact the patient's extremity.

12. Always use good body mechanics, and use gravity to assist the mobilization technique whenever possible.

13. The direction of the mobilization force is either parallel or perpendicular to the treatment plane. The treatment plane lies on the concave articulating surface, perpendicular to a line from the center of the convex articulating surface (figure 6.29). Traction is applied perpendicular to the treatment plane, and gliding is applied parallel to it. The treatment plane can change with a change in a joint's position. Carefully determine the joint's treatment plane before application.

Figure 6.29 Direction of force application. The application is either perpendicular or parallel to the treatment plane.

14. Always apply the concave-convex and convex-concave rules when determining in which direction to apply the mobilization force.

15. Emphasize one plane of motion at a time, although more than one plane may be treated in a session.

16. The patient's response determines the selection of oscillating or sustained techniques. Oscillation is used more often than sustained techniques for pain relief. Gains in range of motion can be achieved by either oscillation or sustained techniques.

17. The patient's comfort and tolerance determine the speed and duration of treatment. Oscillation techniques should be applied smoothly and regularly at the rate of two to three oscillations per second and should be repeated for 1 to 2 min for pain and 20 to 60 s for tightness. Sustained techniques are applied for only about 10 s in painful joints and repeated several times between bouts of rest. For tightness, sustained techniques are held for 10 to 30 s, depending on the patient's tolerance, and repeated three to five times.

18. Begin and end mobilization treatments for increasing range of motion with grade I or II distraction oscillations to facilitate relaxation at the start of treatment and relieve pain following treatment.

19. Progression is individually determined by the patient's response to the treatment. You must assess the patient's response to treatment in terms of pain, changes in joint mobility and range of motion, and the patient's psychological reaction to determine whether changes in the mobilization techniques are warranted. Progression can involve increasing the length of the treatment, increasing the grade if treating a hypomobile joint, or changing the joint to a less loosely packed position.

20. Mobilization techniques should be accompanied by therapeutic exercise to reinforce the gains made with the treatment. The goal of treatment is to make positive changes in pathological conditions, so therapeutic exercises, such as flexibility or strengthening exercises, are most often indicated.

Indications

There are two main indications for the use of joint mobilization techniques. The first is joint pain. Grade I and II oscillations are used to relieve pain. The other indication is a hypomobile joint, which is determined by a capsular pattern of joint motion and less mobility than the contralateral joint.

Precautions and Contraindications

Absolute contraindications to joint mobilization include malignancy, tuberculosis, osteomyelitis, osteoporosis, fracture, ligamentous rupture, and herniated disks with nerve compression. Joint effusion is a contraindication, since the capsule is already swollen from the extra fluid in the joint. Grade I and II mobilizations may be used to relieve pain, but grade III and IV techniques should be avoided. Relative contraindications, which are determined by the rehabilitation clinician's skills and expertise, or precautions include osteoarthritis, pregnancy, flu, total joint replacement, severe scoliosis, poor general health, and a patient's inability to relax. Precautions should also be taken when treating hypermobile joints using the pain-relieving grades. If you doubt whether to use joint mobilization, err on the side of caution and refrain from its use.

▶ Neural mobilization should be used with extreme caution and only as a last resort when other treatment techniques have failed.

NEURAL MOBILIZATION

Of all the manual therapy techniques, neural mobilization is the most dangerous and must be used with care and precision. The rehabilitation clinician must not take its use lightly. Neural mobilization is discussed here so that you can be aware of its proper use and possible consequences.

Fascial Connection

Like the myofascial system, the neural system is continuous throughout the body. It too is surrounded with fascia and can be affected by direct and indirect injuries to fascia and adjacent tissues. The effects of neural injury, like those of fascial injury, can refer to distant areas. The referred pain of neural injuries is different from myofascial pain referral patterns, however.

Afferent System

Referred pain from nerve-tissue injury follows the neural pathways and is described as tingling or burning. It can also jump from one area to another or progress along a neural pathway. The type of pain the patient reports is related to the nerve fiber carrying the impulse. Peripheral afferent nerve fibers that carry painful signals are called nociceptive fibers. The stimuli that activate pain fibers include mechanical forces, chemical irritants, and hot or cold temperatures. The A-delta and C fibers respond to pain stimuli that result in a pain-reflex withdrawal. They are myelinated afferent fibers that are excited by a mild mechanical stimulus. The A-alpha afferents are high-threshold mechanoreceptors that can also respond to temperature stimuli. The A-delta fibers are stimulated in sudden injuries, such as an ankle or knee sprain. About 75% of peripheral pain receptors are C fibers and respond to both mechanical and chemical stimuli. They can also spark the release of histamine through their excitation of mast cells and action as vasodilators. An insect bite, for example, can cause this activity. C fibers are also stimulated by swelling and stiffness and cause the aching sensation that occurs with these conditions. C fibers and A-delta fibers both respond to inflammation.

Once these fibers enter the dorsal horn of the spinal cord, many connections to both inhibitory and excitatory neurons are possible. The impulse can travel up the spinal cord to the thalamus and cortex. Stimulation of the cortex registers conscious pain sensation. Stimulation of the midbrain produces an inhibitory response through the release of endogenous analgesics (pain relievers that the body produces). Normal neural tissue does not refer pain at rest or during normal movement or activity. Pathological conditions, however, can produce referral patterns both proximally and distally from the site of pathology. This pain-referral pattern is referred to by Butler (1994) as pathoneurodynamics. The source of pathoneurodynamics can be either intraneural or extraneural, coming from injury either to the nerve itself or to the surrounding tissue that interacts with the nerve. In either situation, the physiology and mechanics of the nerve can be disrupted.

Susceptible Sites

Given that the nervous system, like the fascia system, is in intimate contact with other tissues throughout the body, it makes sense that when an area suffers an injury, neural tissue may also be affected. Certain nerves are susceptible to injury because of their location or pathway. Butler (1991) has identified these five susceptible sites:

1. In soft tissue or bony tunnels. A good example of this is the median nerve as it passes through the carpal tunnel at the wrist.

2. Abrupt neural branches, particularly in areas where the nerve's ability to move within the surrounding structures is limited. For example, the common plantar digital nerve in the web space between the third and fourth toes has limited movement, is formed from an abrupt junction of the lateral and medial plantar nerves, and is a common site for Morton's neuroma.

3. In areas where the nerves are relatively fixed. The common peroneal nerve as it traverses around the fibular head is an example of a relatively fixed nerve with little mobility.

4. High-friction areas where nerves are close to unyielding interfaces. Two examples are the nerves passing through the plantar fascia in the foot and the brachial plexus passing over the first rib.

5. Tension points, such as the tibial nerve in the popliteal fossa, where abnormal stress can be placed on the nerve.

Previous Trauma

Previous trauma can predispose an area to neural symptoms later. Like all other tissue, nervous tissue is surrounded by layers of fascia that serve to support and supply nutrients to the nerves. If a nerve is injured, it undergoes the healing process discussed in chapter 2. Scar tissue can be produced by the nerve, its surrounding fascia, and the other structures involved in the injury. The result can be a binding of the nerve that can affect its neurobiomechanics and neurophysiology.

Even an injury not directly involving neural tissue can affect the nervous system. Locally damaged blood vessels and ensuing edema can cause neural changes. The nervous system is very dependent on a continuous blood flow for survival and for functioning. Although the nervous system constitutes only 2% of the body's mass, it uses 20% of the circulating blood's oxygen supply (Dommisse 1975). Because nerve tissue has no means of storing reserves, if the blood supply is interrupted, damage to the nerve tissue can result from a lack of adequate oxygen and nutrients.

Nerve tissue damage secondary to either edema or vascular insufficiency results in connective tissue fibrosis. A tethering effect on the nerve by the restriction of the scar tissue can reduce the flexibility and mobility of the neural tissue. Ultimately, symptoms of abnormal neural tension can occur in locations along the nervous system other than the site of injury. According to Butler (1991), this transpires because the mechanical alterations in one nerve location can alter tissue tension throughout the nervous system, impaired neural stimulation at one site can affect the entire neuron, mechanical changes from an injury are accompanied by vascular changes, and an abnormal nerve impulse can cause abnormal neural firing elsewhere in the nervous system.

Double-Crush Syndrome

The condition in which an injury at one site produces signs and symptoms at another site is sometimes referred to as the double-crush syndrome or phenomenon (Upton and McComas 1973). An example of this is carpal tunnel syndrome. In some cases of carpal tunnel syndrome, the cause is actually a neural lesion in the cervical spine. This should be ruled out, especially in cases of bilateral carpal tunnel syndrome. In patients who have a history of cervical injury and present with complaints of elbow or wrist pain bilaterally or unilaterally, a double-crush syndrome should be ruled out. Likewise, if a patient complains of bilateral shin splints or foot pain, you should investigate prior low-back injury and suspect a possible central lesion. Multiple-crush syndromes can be seen in patients who report more than one area of pain. For example, a patient who has a history of neck injury and reports midthoracic, elbow, and wrist pain should be evaluated for a multiple-crush phenomenon.

The term *crush* is a misnomer, since the injury is not necessarily a crush injury. The syndrome is actually caused by scarring and fibrosis, restricted blood flow, alterations in neural stimulation, or some combination of these. This pathology progressively increases pressure and friction on the nerve until symptoms of pain distal to the site of origin occur.

Symptom Profile

Although a patient may use many adjectives to describe neural pain, it is often described as a deep, burning, aching, or heavy sensation. It can occur along the nerve's pathway, jump from one area to another, and clump around joints or tension areas. It can be constant or intermittent, although a constant pain is more indicative of inflammation and compressive pathology. Sometimes the pain is worse at night, and sometimes it is worse at the end of the day.

Pain that occurs because of local neural ischemia is described as sharp or knifelike. Ischemia-related pain lessens with easy motion and worsens with overuse. Sometimes an inflammation can cause a sharp pain, but it is generally an ache at the end of the day with stiffness in the morning or after prolonged inactivity. An inflammation-based pain feels better with gentle activity and worse with rest.

A good history of injuries and evaluation of the location and patterns of pain can help detect the source of the patient's pain. The following types of pain should be examined for neural origins: pain that occurs in susceptible neural-tissue areas, such as the carpal tunnel and fibular head; symptoms that do not match the common pain patterns; and pain that follows a dermatome, or sensory-nerve distribution.

Treatment

Treatment can be either direct or indirect. Direct treatment techniques are the same as those used in examination of neural tissue. Indirect treatment techniques can be as simple as changing posture and often involve altering a soft-tissue structure, which affects the nerve. A hamstring stretch can affect the sciatic nerve, and a cervical stretch can affect the brachial plexus.

There are several different direct neural mobilization techniques. Only a few of the more common ones are discussed here. Before these techniques are discussed, however, you should understand that neural mobilization is not a common treatment and should be used only as a last resort. Any of the neural techniques can easily injure the patient, so extreme caution must always be used in deciding whether and when to apply the technique and in applying the treatment. It is impossible to overstate this point. Even the most experienced rehabilitation clinicians use neural mobilization only after all other modes of treatment have failed and only when benefit to the patient from its application is strongly indicated. It is used always with extreme caution, because it can further injure the patient. Precautions and contraindications are discussed later in this chapter. Neural mobilization techniques should be used only when the rehabilitation clinician knows the pattern of application and the expected outcome of the treatment.

Techniques

Seven neural tension tests are commonly used: one for the spine, three for the lower extremity, and three for the upper extremity. The spine test is passive neck flexion (PNF). The lower-extremity tests include straight-leg raise (SLR), slump test, and prone knee bend (PKB). The upper-limb tension tests are identified as ULTT1, 2a, 2b, and 3. The lower-extremity tests assess the sciatic and femoral nerves, while the upper-extremity tests assess the median, radial, and ulnar nerves, respectively. These test procedures are also used as treatment techniques. You must accurately apply the mobilization technique and assess for symptoms, responses, range of motion, and resistance before and after the treatment. All these techniques can be applied either proximally to distally or vice versa. The direction of application may produce varying results, depending on the location and cause of the irritation or restriction. The positions described here are described in detail by Butler (1991). His text and courses are recommended for readers who have an interest in pursuing neural mobilization techniques.

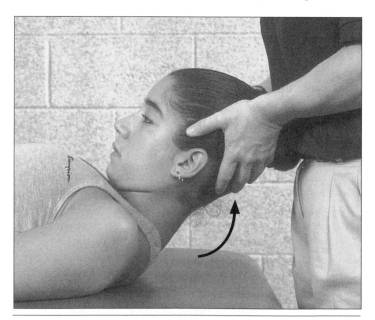

Passive Neck Flexion

PNF can be used by itself to examine spine disorders or along with the lower-limb or upper-limb tests. PNF can be performed with the patient sitting or lying supine. In the supine position, the patient lies supine without a pillow. The patient initiates the motion by lifting the head off the table (figure 6.30). The rehabilitation clinician places his or her hands under the head to support it and moves the neck into flexion while the patient remains relaxed.

Figure 6.30 In passive neck flexion the patient's head is supported as the neck is passively flexed.

Figure 6.31 Straight-leg raise: Tension is applied to the sciatic nerve. With the knee straight, additional neural stress can be applied with ankle dorsiflexion, hip adduction and internal rotation, and neck flexion.

Figure 6.32 Prone knee bend: Tension is applied to the femoral nerve with passive hip extension and knee flexion.

Straight-Leg Raise

Straight-leg raise (SLR) is sometimes referred to as Leseague's test or Lazarevic's test. The patient lies supine without a pillow, and the rehabilitation clinician places one hand on the foot and the other on the quadriceps just proximal to the patella. The leg is lifted by the hand on the Achilles, while the hand on the quadriceps keeps the knee from flexing. If enough flexibility is present, the heel may be placed on the rehabilitation clinician's shoulder (figure 6.31). Neural tension may be increased in the SLR with the addition of ankle dorsiflexion, ankle plantar flexion with inversion, hip adduction, hip medial rotation, or passive neck flexion, individually or in combination.

Prone Knee Bend

Prone knee bend (PKB) is similar to a quadriceps stretch. With the patient prone and the head turned to the side being treated, the rehabilitation clinician grasps the lower leg above the ankle and flexes the knee to move the heel toward the buttock while maintaining slight hip extension (figure 6.32). PKB is used to examine or treat anterior thigh and groin pain.

Slump Test

The slump test should not be used on patients who have an irritable disorder. With the patient sitting on a table in a slumped or sagging position and the hands behind the low back, the rehabilitation clinician applies pressure to the shoulders to bow the spine without changing the hip position. The patient then brings the chin down to the chest, and the rehabilitation clinician applies slight overpressure to the head (figure 6.33a). The patient then extends one knee and follows this motion with ankle dorsiflexion while keeping the knee extended (figure 6.33b). Neck flexion pressure is released slowly. This technique must be applied with extreme caution; it is used as a test, not a treatment, because of its forceful application. It is used to assess the response of the nervous system to treatment. If the patient reports results before the entire technique is applied, it is not necessary to go through the full procedure. This procedure is not recommended for patients with a suspected disk injury.

Upper-Limb Tension Test 1

ULTT1 is also called the brachial plexus tension test or Elvey's test. It is used to test the median nerve and to treat symptoms in the thoracic spine, neck, and arm. The patient should have full range of motion of the entire upper extremity and neck and should not have an irritable disorder. The patient lies supine; if treating the left upper extremity, you hold the patient's left hand with your right and place the patient's left upper arm along your left thigh. Place your left hand on top of the patient's shoulder and apply a stabilization force on the shoulder girdle to prevent elevation throughout the treatment (figure 6.34a). Then abduct the patient's arm to about 110° while keeping it in contact with your thigh (figure 6.34b). Laterally rotate the patient's shoulder, then supinate the forearm, and extend the wrist, thumb and fingers, and elbow, in that order. The patient then flexes the neck laterally away from the left side (figure 6.34c).

Figure 6.33 Slump test: (*a*) The shoulders are passively pushed downward to bow the spine and the chin is brought to the chest. While in this position, one knee is extended with the ankle dorsiflexed. (*b*) Maintaining the leg position, the neck pressure is slowly released.

Figure 6.34 Upper-limb tension test 1 for the median nerve.

Figure 6.35
Upper-limb tension test 2a for the median nerve.

Upper-Limb Tension Test 2a

Because shoulder girdle depression has such a significant impact on the brachial plexus, this position was developed by Butler (1991), who feels that ULTT2a is a more effective position than ULTT1. If the left arm is being treated, the patient lies on a slight diagonal on the table, with the head toward the left side and the left scapula off the table. You stand at the top of the patient's shoulder with your right thigh against the patient's shoulder. Your right hand holds the patient's elbow and the left hand crosses over to hold the wrist. Your thigh depresses the patient's shoulder girdle (figure 6.35a). Bring the patient's arm to about 10° of shoulder abduction, extend the elbow, and laterally rotate the arm. Slide your right hand down to the patient's hand and extend the patient's wrist, fingers, and thumb (figure 6.35b).

Upper-Limb Tension Test 2b

ULTT2b tests the radial nerve and is used to treat cervical, thoracic, and upper-extremity disorders, especially those involving the radial nerve. The patient and rehabilitation clinician are positioned as for ULTT2a. The hand placement, shoulder girdle position, and elbow extension are the same (figure 6.36a). You then medially rotate the patient's shoulder, pronate the forearm, and after moving your left hand to the patient's hand, flex and ulnarly deviate the patient's wrist and flex the patient's fingers and thumb (figure 6.36b).

Upper-Limb Tension Test 3

ULTT3 is used to test the ulnar nerve and to treat ulnar-nerve restrictions. The patient and rehabilitation clinician begin in the position described for ULTT1, with the patient's right shoulder girdle depressed and the patient's right arm resting on your right thigh (figure 6.37a). Externally rotate the patient's shoulder, then abduct the shoulder, flex the elbow, extend the wrist, and extend the fourth and fifth fingers (figure 6.37b). The patient can additionally flex the neck laterally away from the arm being treated.

Application

Tension tests should be performed before all neural mobilization treatments to determine the appropriate force to apply during treatment. Pretreatment and posttreatment tension tests should be used to assess the patient's symptom response and the resistance of the tissue. Symptom responses include pain, numbness, and tingling; the rehabilitation clinician must know when and where in the motion these symptoms may occur to avoid them during the treatment. Identifying where tissue resistance occurs determines the extent of application for the mobilization technique and helps the clinician evaluate the results of the treatment.

Figure 6.36 Upper-limb tension test 2b for the radial nerve.

Figure 6.37 Upper-limb tension test 3 for the ulnar nerve.

Extreme caution must be employed when using neural mobilization to treat irritable conditions that affect neurophysiology. Unless the rehabilitation clinician has taken postgraduate courses on this topic, he or she should refrain from using neural mobilization on irritable conditions.

Caution also should be taken when using neural mobilization techniques to treat nonirritable conditions. These conditions are likely to have pathomechanical causes and secondary fibrosis, connective-tissue adhesions, and restriction of normal tissue mobility. Neural mobilization techniques to treat these conditions enter into the resistance range of grade III and IV motions, but pain should still be avoided. As a rule, grade III motions produce less pain than grade IV.

Throughout the treatment the patient's symptoms must be monitored. Initial treatment should not cause or increase symptoms. A constant dull ache and sensations of pins and needles should be avoided. The patient should be relaxed throughout the treatment.

The duration, amplitude, and number of repetitions can be changed as the treatment progresses and the patient responds positively to treatment. A sequence of slow oscillations can last 20 to 30 s, followed by a reassessment of the patient's condition. A sustained movement should be released if symptoms occur and should last no longer than 10 s even without symptoms. Sustained movement and oscillations can be repeated a number of times as the treatment progresses so that the treatment lasts for several minutes. The amplitude can be increased until some symptoms are produced, although the minimal force needed to achieve a positive response is all that is necessary. Complementary techniques, including muscle energy, myofascial mobilization, cross-friction massage, and neural self-mobilization, can also be added.

Self-Mobilization

If neural mobilization techniques provide positive results, it may be beneficial for the patient to perform self-treatment techniques. Along with these techniques, the patient's program should include therapeutic exercises and corrective techniques that can resolve the problem's precipitating factors.

Self-mobilization techniques for the lower limbs are easier to apply than those for the upper limbs. One of the more difficult tasks in self-mobilization of the upper limb is maintaining scapular depression during the activity. Specific instructions on correct application and proper sequencing must be given to the patient to ensure the best results. It is important that the patient demonstrate proper execution of the technique to the rehabilitation clinician before he or she attempts the technique without supervision. Figure 6.38 demonstrates lower- and upper-limb self-mobilization tension techniques.

Precautions

Again, neural mobilization techniques should be applied only as a last resort after other treatment techniques have been unsuccessful. These techniques should be used only with extreme caution and continual feedback from the patient about the area's response to the treatment. Reproduction of painful symptoms should be avoided, especially numbness and tingling sensations. The slump test and the upper-limb tension tests are complex maneuvers that can involve many structures and therefore require consistent care and discretion. It is much easier to irritate upper-limb nerves than lower-limb nerves, because the upper-limb nerves are smaller and traverse more complicated paths around bones and through muscles than those of the lower limbs.

A worsening disorder, indicated by increased symptoms, is an indication to stop the technique. The rehabilitation clinician should always apply treatment carefully and err on the side of caution if he or she has any doubts about the treatment.

Diabetes, AIDS, and other systemic diseases can weaken the nervous system. Extra care should be taken when applying neural mobilization techniques to patients with these conditions.

Figure 6.38 Self-mobilization. *(a)* Sciatic nerve stretch: Patient lies supine with one leg flexed at the hip and hands clasped behind the thigh. In this position, the lower leg is raised into a straight-leg position. *(b)* Brachial plexus stretch (median nerve): Patient places the hand on the wall at shoulder level with the elbow straight. Maintaining the hand flat on the wall, the patient rolls away from the hand. *(c)* Combined straight-leg raise and prone knee bend stretch: Patient assumes a seated hurdler's stretch position with one leg flexed behind and the other extended in front. The patient reaches forward toward the foot. *(d)* Ulnar nerve stretch: Sidelying, the patient supports the head with the hand. The elbow is flexed and elevated above the shoulder. *(e)* Femoral nerve stretch: Standing, the patient flexes the knee and grasps the foot behind the buttock. *(f)* Radial nerve stretch: With both hands behind the back and the elbows straight, the uninvolved hands grasps the involved hand and passively moves the wrist into extension and pulls the arm across the body. *(g)* Slump: With feet positioned in neutral against a wall, the patient sits with knees extended and slumps the shoulders, moving the chin to the chest.

192

Whereas the circulatory system closely follows the nervous system throughout the body, care should be taken with individuals who have circulatory system disturbances. If a nerve is mobilized, the circulatory structure next to it is also mobilized.

Contraindications

Contraindications to neural mobilization include malignancies of the nervous system or vertebral column, acute inflammatory infections, areas of instability, and spinal cord injuries. Suspected disk lesions, cauda equina lesions (suggested by changes in bowel or bladder function or changes in perineal sensations), dizziness related to vertebral artery insufficiencies, and any central nervous system disorder, such as spina bifida or multiple sclerosis, are also contraindications. Worsening neurological signs are another important contraindication.

SUMMARY

1. Discuss the three techniques of massage and their indications, precautions, and contraindications.

   The primary massage techniques used in rehabilitation include effleurage, or stroking; petrissage, or kneading; and friction. They are used to relieve pain, relax muscles, reduce swelling, and mobilize adherent scar tissue. Massage should be avoided in the presence of infection, malignancies, skin diseases, blood clots, and any irritations or lesions that may spread with direct contact. Precautions include clean hands and body surface to be treated, explaining the procedure before application, removing jewelry that may interfere with the application, using warm hands and massage medium, and draping the body part appropriately.

2. Explain the progression of myofascial restriction after an injury.

   Myofascial restriction occurs following an injury as scar tissue is formed and adhesions occur between the newly formed tissue and adjacent structures. Immobilization following an injury can also lead to myofascial restriction and loss of tissue mobility.

3. Discuss the techniques for myofascial release.

   The primary techniques for myofascial release include J-stroke, oscillation, wringing, stripping, and arm or leg pull.

4. Explain the theory of the mechanism of myofascial trigger points.

   The theory of myofascial trigger points is that a damaged sarcoplasmic reticulum interferes with normal muscle fiber activity. The calcium of the damaged sarcoplasmic reticulum stimulates the sarcomere to produce a sustained contraction as long as ATP is present. The sustained contraction no longer needs an action potential to continue, as long as the calcium and ATP are present together. Ischemic-causing substances also make afferent nerve endings hyperirritable to mediate referred pain, autonomic response, and motor-neuron response.

5. Discuss the ice-and-stretch trigger point release theory.

   According to the gate theory of pain, the sudden, brief application of cold inhibits the pain-spasm cycle and provides muscle relaxation and pain relief, especially when accompanied by a stretch.

6. Explain the concave-convex and convex-concave rules.

   Joint mobilization techniques are based on these rules. The concave-convex rule states that concave joint surfaces slide in the same direction as the bone movement, and the convex-concave rule states that convex joint surfaces slide in the opposite direction of the bone movement.

7. Define joint mobilization grades of movement.

   Movements in joint mobilization are divided into four grades. Grade I is small-amplitude movement in the beginning range of motion, grade II is large-amplitude movement in the middle of the nonrestricted range of motion, grade III is large-amplitude movement to the restricted range of motion, and grade IV is small-amplitude movement to the restricted range of motion.

8. Discuss the direction of glide and traction in relation to the treatment plane.

   Glide movements during mobilization should be parallel to the treatment plane, and traction is perpendicular to the treatment plane.

9. Explain the double-crush syndrome.

   A double-crush syndrome occurs when an injury at one site produces signs and symptoms at another site, so although a patient reports pain at one area, the actual injury is in another area. For example, patients with neck injuries commonly report pain in the arm.

10. Discuss the dangers of neural mobilization.

    Neural mobilization is used very carefully and only as a last resort. Incorrect use can result in nerve injury.

11. Describe one neural self-mobilization technique for the upper extremity and one for the lower extremity.

    Extreme care must be taken with any neural mobilization technique. Examples of neural self-mobilization techniques include the prone knee bend for the femoral nerve, the straight-leg raise for the sciatic nerve, and sidelying on the elbow with the hand on the face for the ulnar nerve.

CRITICAL THINKING QUESTIONS

1. What problem would you suspect if, during a myofascial release treatment, a patient began to sweat and became pale? What steps would you take to relieve the symptoms? Why might this occur?

2. A patient you are treating for a shoulder injury has range-of-motion measurements of 120° flexion, 90° abduction, and 40° lateral rotation. What techniques would you use to improve range of motion? Why? If the patient's motion was 120° flexion, 125° abduction, and 70° lateral rotation, what techniques would you use to improve motion? Why?

3. A patient who had surgery on his ankle three months ago has severe joint and soft-tissue restriction of all motions. There is more loss of plantar flexion than of dorsiflexion, and the soft tissue around the ankle feels very stiff. What techniques would you use to improve motion and why? Which techniques would you emphasize the most and why?

4. If you give a patient a straight-leg-raise exercise to stretch the hamstrings and she complains of calf pain when performing it, what would you instruct the patient to do? What are the possible causes of the patient's complaints, and what precautions should you take?

5. A patient complains of shoulder-blade pain with some arm movements and has headaches. What are the possible causes of the patient's complaints? What treatments would you initiate, and why would you select those techniques? Would you give the patient any home program, and if so, what would it include?

6. If you were Michael, the certified athletic trainer in the scenario described at the beginning of this chapter, what techniques would you use to relieve the soft-tissue adhesions of Emilie's forearm? What home activities would you give her to increase soft-tissue mobility on her own?

LAB ACTIVITIES

1. Apply grades I, II, III, and IV to the tibiofemoral joint in anterior-posterior glides on your lab partner. Feel what the relative amounts of force and motion are for each grade. Now apply the same grades to your lab partner's #2 MCP joint. What are the relative amounts of force and motion for this joint? How do they compare with those of the knee joint? Where in the mobility of the joint do you feel the resistance begin?

2. Apply grades I, II, III, and IV to your lab partner's glenohumeral joint. Feel for where the resistance begins. Does it get greater as you move the humerus through the glenoid fossa or does it stay at a relatively same level of resistance throughout the mobilization? How does the amount of mobility for each of the grades compare with those you found in the knee and MCP joints?

3. Apply a posterior–anterior joint mobilization glide on the talocrural joint of each member in your class. Can you feel a difference among the different individuals? How are they different?

4. Actively and passively abduct and adduct the MCP joints in various positions of flexion and extension. Describe the difference in motion available at the joint. Which position would you classify as closed packed and which position would you classify as the resting position?

5. An athlete suffered a fracture of the midradius when he was tackled in football three weeks ago. The forearm, wrist, and elbow were in a cast for the past three weeks, but the physician wants you to begin joint mobilizations on him today. What is the purpose of the joint mobilizations? What will you be feeling for as you examine the mobility in his elbow and wrist joints? How will you determine whether or not joint mobilization is appropriate for this patient?

6. Apply myofascial release to your lab partner's back using a J-stroke. What type of injury or fascial restriction would benefit from this technique? Give an example of a condition that would not benefit from this technique but would from another myofascial technique. Why?

7 Apply an oscillation myofascial technique to your lab partner's forearm. What type of injury or fascial restriction would benefit from this technique?

8. Apply a wringing myofascial technique to your lab partner's forearm. What type of injury or fascial restriction would benefit from this technique?

9. Apply a stripping myofascial technique to your lab partner's hamstring. What type of injury or fascial restriction would benefit from this technique?

10. About midthigh on the medial aspect you are likely to find trigger points in your lab partner's hamstrings. Locate a trigger point in this area and apply a trigger point pressure technique. How much pressure should you apply? What will be your guidelines in determining the amount of pressure used? Are you able to feel the trigger point relax as you continue to hold the pressure on it? How does this type of manual therapy compare to the myofascial techniques investigated in questions 6-9 above? What kinds of problems would lend themselves to each technique?

11. A patient with rotator cuff repair has had the left arm in a sling for the past 3 weeks. He comes to you today, 3 weeks after the surgery because his physician wants him to begin rehabilitation today. How can you determine if the patient will need manual therapy? How can you determine what type of manual therapy he will need? What kinds of problems would you expect him to have at this stage? What would today's treatment include? What would you avoid doing with him today? How will you know if your techniques are beneficial? Justify each of your answers.

REFERENCES

Beard, G., and E.C. Wood. 1969. *Massage principles and techniques.* Philadelphia: Saunders.

Butler, D.S. 1991. *Mobilization of the nervous system.* New York: Churchill Livingstone.

Butler, D.S. 1994. *Mobilization of the nervous system. Level II. 1996/97 course handbook.* Marina Del Rey, CA: Neuro Orthopedic Institute.

Castel, J.C. 1979. *Pain management: Acupuncture and transcutaneous electrical nerve stimulation techniques.* Lake Bluff, IL: Pain Control Services.

Corrigan, B., and G.D. Maitland. 1989. *Practical orthopedic medicine.* Boston: Butterworth.

Cyriax, J.H. 1977. *Textbook of orthopedic medicine.* Vol. 2, *Treatment by manipulation, massage and injection.* Baltimore: Williams & Wilkins.

Dommisse, G.F. 1975. Morphological aspects of the lumbar spine and lumbosacral region. *Orthopedic Clinics of North America* 6:163–175.

Greenman, P.E. 1996. *Principles of manual medicine.* Baltimore: Williams & Wilkins.

Hertling, D., and R.M. Kessler. 1990. *Management of common musculoskeletal disorders: Physical therapy principles and methods.* 2nd ed. Philadelphia: Lippincott.

Kaltenborn, F.M. 2002. *Mobilization of the extremity joints Vol 1. The extremities.* 5th ed. Minneapolis: OTPT.

Manheim, C.J. 1994. *The myofascial release manual.* 2nd ed. Thorofare, NJ: Slack.

Melzak, R. 1973. *The puzzle of pain.* New York: Basic Books.

Paris, S.V., and C. Patla. 1988. *E1 course notes: Extremity dysfunction and manipulation.* St. Augustine, FL: Patris.

Simons, D.G. 1981. Myofascial trigger points: A need for understanding. *Archives of Physical Medicine and Rehabilitation* 62:97–99.

Sutton, G.S., and M.R. Bartel. 1994. Soft-tissue mobilization techniques for the hand therapist. *Journal of Hand Therapy* 7:185–192.

Travell, J. 1976. Myofascial trigger points: Clinical view. In *Advances in pain research and therapy,* vol. 1, ed. J.J. Bonica and D. Albe-Fessard. New York: Raven Press.

Travell, J.G., and D.G. Simons. 1983. *Myofascial pain and dysfunction: The trigger point manual.* Vol. 1. Baltimore: Williams & Wilkins.

Travell, J.G., and D.G. Simons. 1992. *Myofascial pain and dysfunction: The trigger point manual.* Vol. 2. Baltimore: Williams & Wilkins.

Upton, A.R.M., and A.J. McComas. 1973. The double crush in nerve entrapment syndromes. *Lancet* 2:359–362.

SUGGESTED READING

Åstrand, P.O., and K. Rodahl. 1977. *Textbook of work physiology.* New York: McGraw-Hill.

Breig, A. 1978. *Adverse mechanical tension in the nervous system.* Stockholm: Almqvist & Wiksell.

Grieve, G.P. 1984. *Mobilisation of the spine.* New York: Churchill Livingstone.

Kenneally, M., Rubenach, H., and R. Elvey. 1988. The upper limb tension test: The SLR of the arm. In *Physical therapy of the cervical and thoracic spine,* ed. R. Grant. New York: Churchill Livingstone.

Lee, D. 1986. Principles and practice of muscle energy and functional techniques. In *Modern manual therapy of the vertebral column,* ed. G. Grieves. New York: Churchill Livingstone.

Mackinnon, S.E. 1992. Double and multiple crush syndromes. *Hand Clinics* 8:369.

Rubin, D. 1981. Myofascial trigger point syndromes: An approach to management. *Archives of Physical Medicine and Rehabilitation* 62:107–110.

Wood, E.C., and P.D. Becker. 1981. *Beard's massage.* Philadelphia: Saunders.

Muscle Strength and Endurance

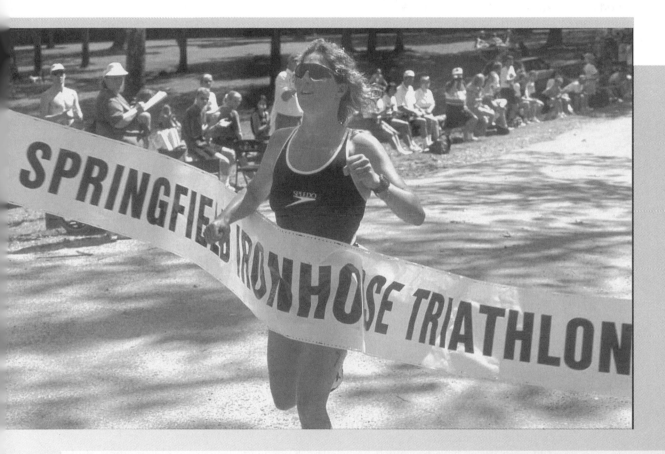

Objectives

After completing this chapter, you should be able to do the following:

1. Describe the sarcolemma and its function in muscle activity.

2. Identify the elements of a motor unit.

3. Explain how an action potential is transmitted.

4. Explain the differences between fast-twitch and slow-twitch muscle fibers.

5. Discuss the relationship between muscle strength, endurance, and power.

6. Identify the various types of dynamic activity.

7. Discuss the differences between open and closed kinetic chain activity.

8. Identify the various grades of manual muscle testing.

9. Discuss the grades of muscle activity.

10. List the PNF techniques commonly used in rehabilitaion and their purposes.

11. Identify four principles of strengthening exercises.

Now that Matthew Carlson, certified athletic trainer for the local high school, has achieved good range of motion in Kamryn's knee, he is ready to begin a more aggressive strengthening program. Early in the season, Kamryn injured her knee during gymnastics practice. She underwent rehabilitation but continued to have difficulties with the knee throughout the season. Three weeks ago she underwent an arthroscopy for a partial meniscectomy.

Matthew wants Kamryn to progress in a good rehabilitation program with effective, efficient, and appropriate strengthening exercises, but he's having difficulty deciding what equipment to use. Fortunately, the high school's booster club has been very generous to his athletic training program and has furnished his athletic training facility with a nice variety of rehabilitation equipment. He wants to do a combination of open and closed kinetic chain activities. Until now he has used manual resistance and body-weight resistance to provide strengthening activities, but at this point in Kamryn's program, more resistance would be beneficial.

■ **It's what you learn after you know it all that counts.**

John Wooden, basketball coach, 1910 –

Coach John Wooden's words are worth considering as you begin reading about a topic that you may think you already know well. Even if you possess a good deal of knowledge, you cannot assume you will know best how to apply that knowledge. As you read this chapter, you will discover that much about muscle strength is yet to be learned. This text does not come close to presenting the body of knowledge available; however, the discussion covers the importance of muscle strength, the methods of achieving it, and the ways in which rehabilitation clinicians can maximize muscle strength and endurance development in a therapeutic exercise program for injured individuals.

As you read this chapter, keep in mind that many of the concepts presented are not black and white but shades of gray. There is not necessarily a single answer for even simple questions such as *What is the best number of repetitions for increasing muscle endurance?* The "best" answer will emerge through your ability to combine the knowledge you obtain from this text with your own observation skills and common sense. This combination will enable you to determine your own best answers about what strengthening program will be most effective for a particular patient.

One can never have too much knowledge. Knowledge leads to understanding, understanding leads to appreciation, appreciation leads to respect, and respect leads to appropriate application. The greater your understanding of the "whys" and "hows," the less dangerous will be your application of the knowledge you possess.

Accordingly, then, the chapter begins with physiological and biomechanical information to help you achieve a true understanding of the rationale for techniques. The progression will provide you with additional skills so that you can design and build your own therapeutic exercise program for any patient, regardless of any obstacles or complications associated with the patient's injury profile.

MUSCLE STRUCTURE AND FUNCTION

▶ The motor units in muscle consist of the nerve, or motor neuron, and muscle fibers. Within the fibers are small contractile elements called sarcomeres, and within the sarcomere are filaments called actin and myosin. Muscle function involves various processes that occur when a motor unit is stimulated by an excitatory impulse.

Before you can learn how to affect strength and muscle endurance, you must have an understanding of muscle structure and function. Such awareness serves as a foundation for understanding how strength changes occur, why certain techniques are applied, and what procedures will provide the best results.

Structure

Previous chapters have addressed the intimate relationship between connective tissue and other tissue throughout the body. Muscle also contains layers of connective tissue. The outer connective tissue layer covering the entire muscle is the epimysium; the layer covering muscle fascicles or groups of fibers is called the perimysium; and the connective tissue layer covering each muscle fiber is the endomysium. The endomysium is continuous with the muscle fiber's membrane, the sarcolemma. This macrostructure of muscle is shown in figure 7.1.

As mentioned in previous chapters, a motor unit is composed of the nerve, or motor neuron, and the muscle fibers that it innervates (figure 7.2). The number of motor units in any muscle depends on the size and the function of that muscle. For example, in a small muscle that performs primarily finely tuned activities, such as the intrinsic muscles of the hand, the ratio of muscle fibers to neurons is small. Larger muscles used primarily for gross motor activities, such as the gastrocnemius, have a much higher ratio of muscle fibers to neurons. Table 7.1 provides some examples of average numbers of muscle fibers in motor units of various muscles.

Figure 7.1 Muscle structure.

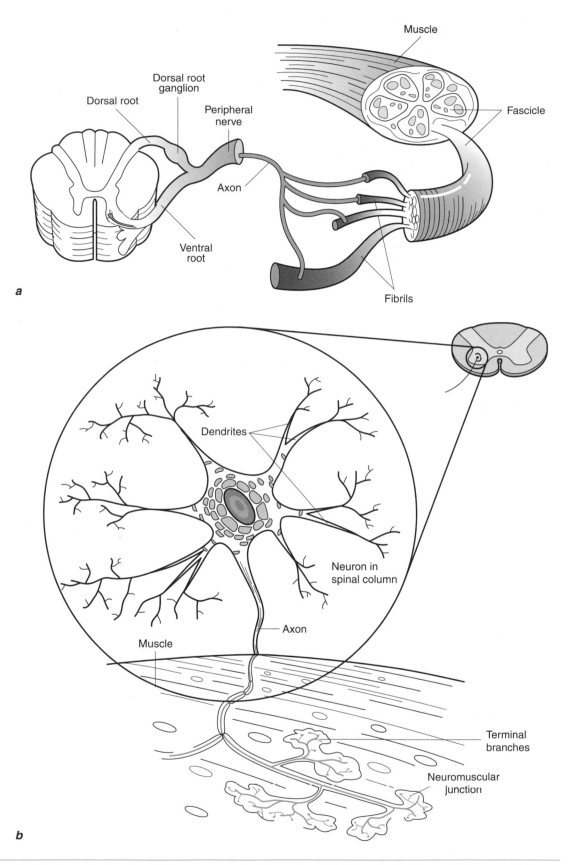

Figure 7.2 Motor unit: *(a)* schematic drawing of the components of a motor unit—the anterior horn cell, its axon and terminating branches, and the muscle fibers it innervates; *(b)* one neuron from the spinal cord with its axon extending into the muscle. The number of muscle fibers a single motor unit innervates can range from a few to several thousand (Johnson and Wiechers 1982).

Table 7.1

Average Number of Muscle Fibers in a Motor Unit in Different Skeletal Muscles

Muscles	Muscle fibers/Motor unit
Biceps brachii	750
Brachioradialis	> 410
Opponens pollicis	595
Platysma	25
Tensor tympani	8
Medial gastrocnemius	~ 1600-1900
Tibialis anterior	~ 560-660

Adapted from Enoka 1995.

a

b

Figure 7.3   Filament arrangements: *(a)* cross-sectional view; *(b)* longitudinal view. Note hexagonal arrangement of thin filaments around thick filaments; triangular arrangement of thick filaments.

The sarcomere is the smallest contractile element of a muscle fiber. The extrafusal fibers, or myofibrils, contained within the sarcomere are called actin and myosin. Myosin fibers are the thicker filaments—with diameters about 1/10,000 that of a hair strand (16 nm)—and are surrounded in a hexagonal pattern by smaller actin filaments. A three-dimensional model shows that the myosin filaments form a triangular pattern in relationship to each other—so in a sarcomere there are six actin filaments around each myosin filament and three myosin filaments around one actin filament (figure 7.3).

Within a sarcomere, the actin and myosin are arranged longitudinally from Z-disk to Z-disk, where the actin filaments are anchored on either end of the sarcomere. The myosin filaments are in the equatorial center of the sarcomere and anchored with each other at the M-bridge in the center of the H-zone (figure 7.4). The A-band contains myosin and actin filaments, whereas the I-band contains only actin filaments. Because of the myosin filaments the A-band is darker; the combination of the A-band and the I-band gives skeletal muscle its striped appearance—hence the name, striated muscle.

Function

When a motor unit is stimulated by an excitatory impulse called an action potential, the myosin cross-bridges flex and pull the actin filaments toward the center of the sarcomere. During this process the H-band becomes smaller and the Z-disks are stretched toward the sarcomere's equatorial center to produce a shortening of the sarcomere. The theory that describes this process is called the *sliding filament theory*.

When the sarcomere is lengthened, the H-zone gets larger; when it shortens, the H-zone gets smaller. During lengthening and shortening of the sarcomere, the length of the filaments does not change. Only the relative sizes of the areas of the sarcomere that do not contain myosin (I-band) or actin (H-zone) change (figure 7.5).

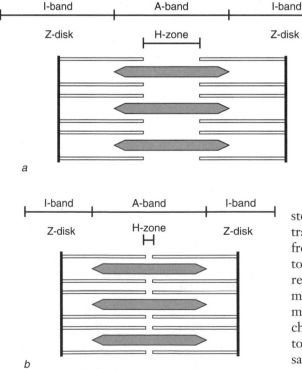

Figure 7.4 Longitudinal *(top)* and cross-sectional *(bottom)* diagrams showing the principal elements of the sarcomeric cytoskeleton *(black)* and the thick and thin filaments *(blue)* forming the contractile apparatus.

The biochemical process that causes this shortening is rather complex and occurs instantaneously. There are two tubular systems vital to the activity of the sarcomere. The **sarcoplasmic reticulum** is an internal tubule system that is arranged parallel to and surrounds the sarcomere in a fishnet mesh arrangement and that terminates near the Z-disks. The transverse tubule (T-tubule) system extends into the inner aspects of the fiber to encircle the myofibrils and also runs perpendicular to the sarcoplasmic reticulum. The T-tubules terminate near the Z-disks between two sarcoplasmic reticulum tubules in a triad arrangement (figure 7.6). The sarcoplasmic reticulum stores calcium ions that are released when an action potential is transmitted from the afferent nerve. The calcium ions are released from the sarcoplasmic reticulum and sent through the T-tubules to the Z-disks. The calcium ions then bind to the **troponin**, a regulatory protein located at regular intervals along the actin filament. This in turn causes a shift in **tropomyosin**, another protein molecule in the actin filament to which troponin is bound. This chemical process permits the head of the myosin cross-bridges to attach more readily to the actin and cause a shortening of the sarcomere (figure 7.7).

Figure 7.5 Changes in sarcomere length: *(a)* on stretch; *(b)* shortened.

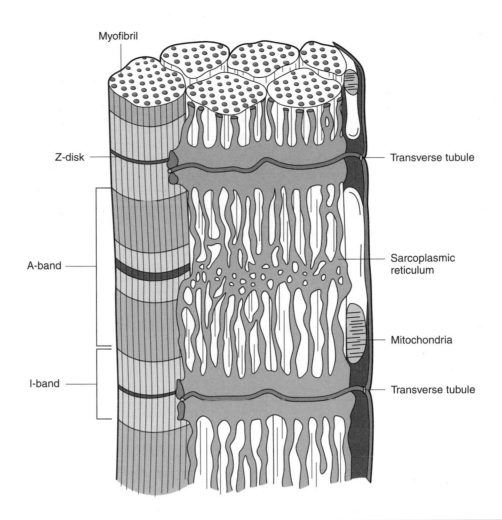

Myofibril

Z-disk

A-band

I-band

Transverse tubule

Sarcoplasmic reticulum

Mitochondria

Transverse tubule

Figure 7.6 Tubule system.

The cross-bridges contain an enzyme, myosin **ATPase,** which is a catalyst that breaks down the **adenosine triphosphate (ATP)** into **adenosine diphosphate (ADP)** and phosphate for energy production. This is the energy source for the sarcomere activity. As long as calcium ions are present and ATP hydrolysis occurs to permit the cross-bridges to re-cock, the activity can continue. As long as calcium ions are available and energy production through ATP conversion can cause the cycle of cross-bridge attachment-release-re-cocking to occur, muscle activity is sustained. On the other hand, if calcium ions are recaptured in the sarcoplasmic reticulum or ATP production and conversion is not continued, the muscle relaxes.

Because the positively charged calcium is stored in the sarcoplasmic reticulum and not the actin, during muscle inactivity the actin and myosin are not bound by cross-bridges. At rest, they are separated from each other because the negatively charged ATP is bound to the myosin filament's cross-bridges and the actin filaments are also negative. When an excitatory impulse is sent to release the calcium ions, the calcium ions bind with the ATP on the myosin filaments' cross-bridges and neutralize the ATP's negative charge. Since the myosin remains negatively charged, the actin now binds with the myosin. When the cross-bridges fold in toward the trunk of the myosin, the ATP comes into contact with the myosin's ATPase. When this enzyme breaks down the ATP, the actin and myosin break contact as the ATP becomes negatively charged once again. Through a variety of energy systems, the ADP that is released from ATP breakdown is reformed again into ATP. If an excitatory stimulus continues, this cycle is repeated.

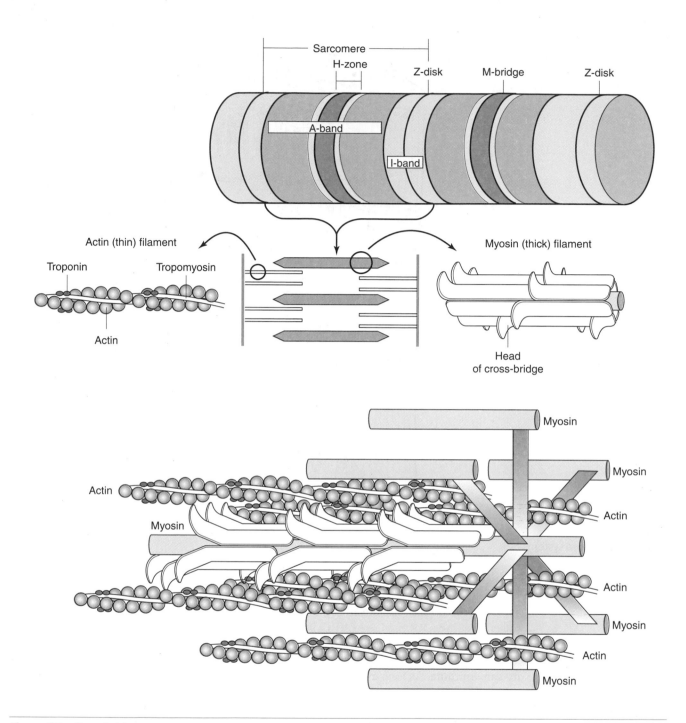

Figure 7.7 Cross-bridges.

Adapted by permission from National Strength and Conditioning Association 2000.

The sarcoplasmic reticulum also contains mitochondria. Mitochondria are the most metabolically active part of the sarcomere because they contain the substances needed for metabolism. They store the glycogen used for energy production. They also contain the enzyme that is used to metabolize lactic acid for energy to form ATP. The more mitochondria present in the sarcoplasmic reticulum, the more active the muscle.

One motor unit can innervate several muscle fibers in a muscle. These fibers are spaced throughout the muscle and are not necessarily in proximity to one another. Because the lengths of the nerve's end plates vary according to the distance between the motor point and the muscle fiber that the nerve stimulates, the impulse does not reach all of the muscle fibers at the same time. This causes an asynchronous firing of the muscle fibers. This asynchronous firing of a single motor unit produces a smooth muscle contraction.

NEUROMUSCULAR PHYSIOLOGY

▶ The physiological properties of skeletal muscle include irritability, contractility, viscosity, extensibility and elasticity, fatigue, and summation.

As mentioned in the preceding chapter, many sensory receptors provide input to the central nervous system and can influence the neuromuscular system. Figure 7.8 indicates that various sensory receptors on the skin—including the free nerve endings that perceive pain and temperature, the Meissner's corpuscles that receive light touch sensation, and the Pacinian corpuscles that perceive pressure sensation—all transmit afferent impulses to the central nervous system. These impulses can be interpreted at various levels within the central nervous system, including the spinal cord, brain stem, cerebellum, and cerebral cortex. Once received and interpreted, a response is transmitted down the spinal cord through appropriate spinal pathways to the anterior horn and along efferent nerves to the motor structures that will respond to the impulses they receive.

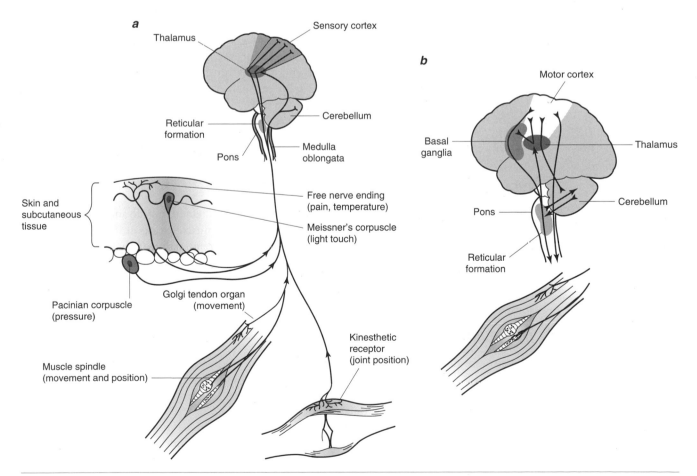

Figure 7.8 Neural pathways: *(a)* sensory; *(b)* motor.

When an impulse is strong enough to produce an action potential, the motor neuron fires and all of the muscle fibers that it supplies respond; this is in accordance with the **all-or-none principle**. Within the muscle itself, a few or many motor units can be facilitated to fire at one time. As a rule, the more motor units recruited, the stronger the muscle's response. The stimulation of an electrical impulse, an action potential, is carried along the motor neuron to the neuromuscular junction. At this junction the action potential causes the release of a chemical, acetylcholine, which in turn stimulates the sarcolemma to release its calcium ions, beginning the muscle activity just described. When this occurs once, the result is a muscle twitch.

Na⁺   Cl⁻   K⁺

K⁺   A⁻   Na⁺   Cl⁻

Figure 7.9   Resting membrane potential.

+ + + + + + + + + + +

‒ ‒ ‒ ‒ ‒ ‒ ‒ ‒ ‒ ‒

‒ ‒ ‒ ‒ ‒ ‒ ‒ ‒ ‒ ‒

+ + + + + + + + + +

Figure 7.10   Arrangement of charges on the membrane of an axon.

Resting Potential

The wall of a nerve or muscle cell membrane has a resting potential. There are positive and negative ions in the intracellular and extracellular fluids of the nerve and muscle cell membranes. The extracellular fluid contains many sodium (positive) and chloride (negative) ions. Inside the cell are many potassium (positive) ions, protein molecules (A–), and some chloride (negative) ions (figure 7.9). This distribution of ions produces a resting potential of the cell. If a microelectrode is placed on the inside and outside of a cell, it will show that an axon's intracellular fluid is 70 to 90 mV. This is represented by figure 7.10, which demonstrates the interior negative charge and exterior positive charge of the cell membrane. There is a natural tendency to attempt to attain an equilibrium of the ions. The task of keeping the balance of ion concentration in check—because the potassium tends to "want" to leak out of the cell and sodium to leak into it—is the responsibility of the sodium-potassium pump. This constant level of activity produces a net resting membrane potential average of approximately –85 mV.

When an excitation impulse occurs, a change in the electrical charge along the cell membrane occurs and produces an action potential. The membrane potential goes from negative to positive and quickly returns to negative once the impulse has passed. This process takes probably no longer than .5 ms (Clarke 1975) and is much like throwing a rock into water and producing one wave. The rock serves as the initial stimulus, and the wave is the depolarizing impulse that is sent along a nerve axon or muscle fiber, creating a brief change and then returning the water to its original calm. The process continues until the wave hits the shore, its final destination.

Physiological Properties

Skeletal muscle physiological characteristics are unique to skeletal muscle and are vital for the muscle's normal functions. It is important to know how a muscle works at its cellular level in order to fully appreciate how it responds to demands we place on it during therapeutic exercise. It is also important to know the normal responses of muscle so that when an injury occurs, you are able to recognize what alterations in therapeutic exercises will provide appropriate demands but not aggravate a muscle injury. The following sections provide a brief look at some of the physiological properties.

Irritability

The amount of stimulation required to initiate the response of a muscle fiber is determined by the irritability of the motor unit. Irritability is a physiological property of skeletal muscle. To cause a response, a minimum amount of stimulation—called threshold stimulation—is necessary. A sub-threshold stimulation level causes no muscle activity. If the stimulus is above the threshold level, the response is greater because either more motor units are affected or the duration of discharge of impulses along one motor unit is increased.

If a muscle fiber is stimulated for about 1 ms (Brown 1980), the membrane depolarizes and is unable to be immediately re-stimulated. This is called the **absolute refractory period**. In other words, a muscle fiber cannot respond to two stimuli that are less than .001 s apart. There is a **relative refractory period** when the membrane becomes partially re-polarized and can respond if the stimulus is greater than the normal threshold level.

The **refractory period** includes a latent period during which there is a momentary cessation of activity as the area is prepared to fire. The latent period not only occurs in the electrical phase of contraction, but is also seen in the energy production and mechanical results of the response as shown in figure 7.11. Once the depolarization of the membrane occurs, the energy changes are facilitated and the mechanical response of the muscle is produced.

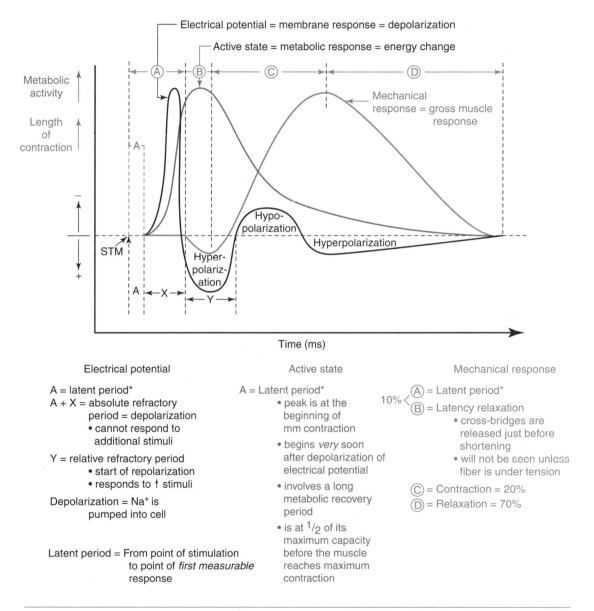

Figure 7.11   Time relationship of electrical, chemical, and mechanical responses in a simple muscle twitch.

Contractility

After depolarization, the mechanical response is the contraction. This is the second physiological property of skeletal muscle—simply the ability to contract. In a muscle fiber it is a simple twitch response. One contraction, or twitch response, occurs for each stimulus. If a muscle is to sustain a contraction, multiple succeeding stimuli must be produced. The **contraction phase** of a mechanical response follows a 10% latency period and occurs through the next 20% of the cycle. As seen in figure 7.11, the mechanical response is delayed longer than the electrical and metabolic responses because of the series elastic component of the muscle fiber.

Viscosity

Viscosity is the internal resistance that limits the rate of muscle contraction. The general rule is that the faster the rate of muscle contraction, the greater the internal resistance and the less the external force that can be exerted. At faster speeds, more force is required to lift the same weight. Water provides a good example of viscosity. If you put your arm under water, you will find that moving your hand slowly through the water is relatively easy. But if you move your hand as fast as you can, you'll notice that you need much more strength.

This is an important property to recall when you are instructing a patient in a therapeutic exercise program. For example, if you want a wrestler with an injured ankle to lift 22.5 kg (50 lb) in a slow heel-raise exercise, you should not expect him to be able to lift the same weight in a faster heel-raise exercise and perform as many repetitions as he can at the slower speed, using the same control and range of motion.

Extensibility and Elasticity

A muscle's individual fibers follow Hooke's law: Stress applied to a stretch of a body is proportional to the strain (change in length) that is produced as long as the elasticity limit of the body is not exceeded. Because of the fiber's elastic components, when a stretch is applied, there is some return to the fiber's original length; but because the fiber also contains plastic elements, there is some change in length if the force applied is of sufficient magnitude or duration. These principles are discussed in chapter 5.

As a muscle is stretched, it becomes more **extensible** because its connective tissue is heated and stretched with the activity. On the other hand, if a part is inactive, it gets stiff. The connective tissue around joints gel rather than remaining fluid, and motion becomes restricted (Kottke 1982). If an area has reached this state and is stiff, overstretching it can cause tearing of capillaries and connective tissue. This stiffness can be overcome by active exercise. Active exercise before stretching helps to increase the muscle's temperature, reduce its viscosity, and relieve the stiffness. Overall, a stretch is more effective if done after a warm-up of active exercise.

Contracture

Contracture is a failure of relaxation of a muscle. Relaxation is a normal metabolic process of a muscle following contraction. Many believe that the onset of fatigue causes both a decrease in the ability to produce an initial maximal contraction output and a decrease in the ability to reach a maximum relaxation level. One theoretical explanation is a lactic acid buildup in the muscle as demonstrated in figure 7.12. As the muscle fatigues, the resting length shortens.

Contracture is one reason for the importance of stretching after exercise. As the muscle fatigues with activity, the fibers shorten and do not resume their normal resting length. One theory is that over a period of time, the gross muscle loses flexibility if stretches are not performed to regain the normal resting length of the fibers.

Contracture is also the reason you should have the patient perform more-strenuous and more-demanding therapeutic exercises early in the day's rehabilitation session. As the patient

Figure 7.12   Contracture.

fatigues and the muscle fibers' resting length decreases, the muscle's ability to perform the activity correctly becomes limited, so the risk of injury increases. The more difficult and challenging activities should be performed early in the day's session to ensure good results.

It is important not to confuse muscle contracture with an orthopedic contracture, which is a connective-tissue shortening that causes a reduced range of motion. Nor should you confuse contracture with a **muscle spasm**, which is a prolonged reflex muscle contraction.

Fatigue

The property of fatigue is closely related to contracture. Fatigue can result either from exhaustion of a muscle with prolonged activity or from failure of the circulatory system to provide the necessary nutrients to continue muscle activity. One agent responsible for local muscle fatigue is **lactic acid.** A by-product of muscle activity, lactic acid increases after intense or prolonged muscle contraction because there is not enough oxygen available to oxidize the lactic acid. In a resting muscle, the quantity of lactic acid is 0.5 to 2.2 mmol/kg of muscle, but in a muscle that is exercised to exhaustion, the lactic acid level is 25 mmol/kg of muscle (Stone and Conley 1994). Lactic acid is measured as small amounts leak from the muscles into the blood. As activity increases the amount in the blood increases and is used as an index for calculating how vigorously the patient is working. Lactic acid buildup is associated with muscle tiredness and pain. The ability to tolerate increased levels of lactic acid varies from one person to another and is to some extent a determining factor in endurance. Endurance training does not change the levels of lactic acid buildup, but it can make the individual more tolerant of the pain produced by the lactic acid.

Lactate levels are influenced by the intensity of the activity, the exercise duration, the state of training, initial glycogen levels, and muscle fiber type (Stone and Conley 1994). The type II, fast-twitch fibers produce lactic acid at a higher rate than the type I, slow-twitch fibers. High-intensity activities such as sprints and weight lifting produce higher levels of lactic acid than low-intensity prolonged activities such as distance running and aerobic exercises. Individuals who are conditioned tolerate higher levels of lactate better than untrained individuals.

If you are working with a patient who has become severely deconditioned because of prolonged inactivity, you need to keep this factor in mind, especially in the early sessions of the therapeutic exercise program when the deconditioning may be more severe. The patient's ability to tolerate exercise intensity changes in severe deconditioning, so earlier exercise sessions require more rest periods than later sessions.

The muscle's circulation is impeded more with sustained isometric activity than with either isotonic or brief isometric activity. The sustained activity of the muscle restricts blood so that fatigue occurs more quickly than with other types of muscle activity. You need to consider this when designing a therapeutic exercise program. The section "Relationship between Muscle Strength and Muscle Endurance" deals more extensively with recovery from fatigue.

Summation

If a second twitch is produced before a muscle fiber completely relaxes, a greater force is produced. This phenomenon, known as **summation of forces,** is similar to what occurs when a moving car is hit from behind—the car will move forward with a greater force than it did before it was hit. If a series of stimuli is delivered to the muscle fiber at a rapid frequency, the muscle fiber produces a **tetany**, a sustained maximal contraction (figure 7.13). While tetany is a sustained muscular contraction, **tetanus** is an intermittent contraction that is noted by a fibrillating tremor (figure 7.13, C). An asynchronous discharge of several motor units produces a smooth mechanical contraction of a muscle.

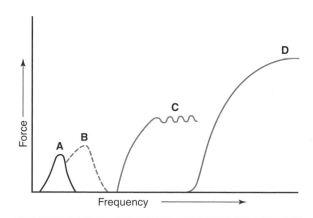

Figure 7.13 Twitch, twitch summation, tetanus, and tetany of a motor unit: A, single twitch; B, force resulting from summation of two twitches; C, tetanus; D, tetany, sometimes called a fused tetanus.

Adapted by permission from National Strength and Conditioning Association 2000.

FAST- AND SLOW-TWITCH FIBERS

▶ The fast-twitch and slow-twitch fibers of skeletal muscle differ in appearance, metabolic capabilities, and contraction characteristics.

Skeletal muscle is composed of **fast-twitch** and **slow-twitch fibers**. The ratio of these fibers varies within the individual from muscle to muscle, and from individual to individual for the same muscle. In other words, one sprinter may have more fast-twitch fibers in the quadriceps than another sprinter does, and may have more fast-twitch fibers in the quadriceps than in the hamstrings. The ratio is determined by genetics and muscle demands. Whether or not a fiber can convert from one fiber type to another is an unresolved question; but a muscle that is considered an antigravity muscle, such as the soleus, tends to have more slow-twitch fibers than a muscle that is used more for locomotion and fast or powerful movements, such as the quadriceps, which has a combination of fast- and slow-twitch fibers.

The two fiber types have different appearances, metabolic capacities, and contraction characteristics. Their names are based on their relative speed of activity. The slow-twitch fibers, sometimes referred to as type I fibers or slow oxidative fibers, are darker and take about 110 ms to reach their peak tension when stimulated (figure 7.14). The fast-twitch fibers, sometimes called type II fibers or fast oxidative fibers, are lighter in color and reach their maximum tension approximately 50 ms after being stimulated (Wilmore and Costill 2004) (figure 7.15). The slow-twitch fibers have a slower-acting myosin ATPase, and the fast-twitch fibers have a faster-acting myosin ATPase, so the ATP is converted more quickly to produce energy faster for the fast-twitch fibers than for the slow-twitch fibers. The fast-twitch fibers also have a more extensive sarcoplasmic reticulum, allowing a more efficient delivery of calcium ions to permit a quicker fiber response to stimulation. The slow-twitch fibers have a greater quantity of mitochondria, more myoglobin, and more glycogen stores, so they are better equipped for prolonged or sustained activity (table 7.2).

Figure 7.14 Fast- and slow-twitch fibers.
Reprinted by permission from Wilmore and Costill 2004.

Fast-twitch fibers are divided into three sub-classifications: type IIa, IIb, and IIc. Very little is known about type IIc. These fibers are found in very small quantities in muscles, approximately 1% to 3% on average. Type IIa and type IIb fibers are approximately equal in quantity in an average muscle (Wilmore and Costill 1999). Although the differences between these fast-twitch fibers are not yet understood, the type IIa fibers are more often recruited during muscle activity than the other type II fibers. Since type IIb fibers require a greater stimulus to fire, they are not recruited in low- or medium-intensity activities but are used in high-intensity activities such as the 100-m swim.

The slow-twitch fibers have more mitochondria than the fast-twitch fibers. Since mitochondria are the primary energy-storage facilities for the cells, they give the fibers a greater potential to produce a greater oxidative capacity. The higher mitochondria count and related increased myoglobin and blood supply account for the cells' red color.

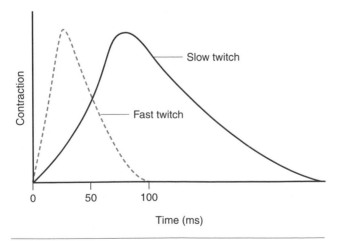

Figure 7.15 Contraction-relaxation curves for fast-twitch and slow-twitch skeletal muscle fibers.

Table 7.2

Differences Between Type I and Type II Muscle Fibers

Characteristics	Type I	Type II
Speed	Slowest	Fastest
Axon size	Smaller	Larger
Color	Red	White
Conduction velocity	Slow: 110 ms	Fast: 50 ms
Fatigue resistance	Greatest	Least
Recruitment threshold	Lower	Higher
Firing rates	Lower minimum and maximum	Higher minimum and maximum
Myosin ATPase	Slow acting	Fast acting
Mitochondria	Greater number	Smaller number
Activity	Endurance	Brief bursts

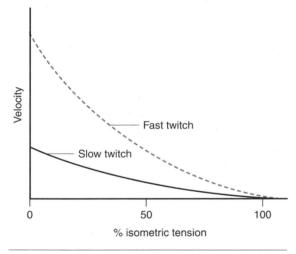

Figure 7.16 Force-velocity curves for fast-twitch and slow-twitch skeletal muscle fibers.

With a greater energy source available, the slow-twitch fibers are able to sustain activity for a longer time than the fast-twitch fibers. For this reason they are considered endurance fibers and are the fibers primarily responsible for an individual's ability to perform low-intensity endurance activities such as a marathon.

Fast-twitch fibers have fewer mitochondria and less ability to sustain activity. Their activity is anaerobic, so they fatigue quickly. However, they are capable of producing a more powerful output and are responsible for high-power, short-term activities such as a 400-m sprint (figure 7.16). A factor that allows fast-twitch fibers to produce stronger forces is the fast-twitch motor unit's higher content of muscle fibers in comparison to a slow-twitch motor unit. The greater number of responding muscle fibers causes a greater force production.

MUSCLE STRENGTH, POWER, AND ENDURANCE

▶ Muscle strength is the maximum force a muscle can exert, and power is strength over a distance for a specific time. Endurance is the ability to prolong an activity. Exercises for muscle strength and endurance lie on a continuum from low to high repetitions with high to low resistance.

Before discussing how to improve muscle function, it is necessary to identify the components involved.

Muscle Strength

Strength is the maximum force that a muscle or muscle group can exert. In healthy individuals it is usually measured in 1-RM, the one-repetition maximum. A 1 RM is the weight that a muscle or muscle group can lift for only one repetition. If an individual can perform only one repetition of a forearm curl with 20.5 kg (45 lb), that is his 1 RM, or strength, for the forearm curl. A person who can lift 22.5 kg (50 lb) for 1 RM in a forearm curl has twice the strength of someone who has a 1 RM of 11.3 kg (25 lb).

Power

Power is strength that is applied over a distance for a specific amount of time. Power is involved in most athletic events and is strength incorporated with speed. The volleyball player who can leg press 180 kg (400 lb) in half the time it takes a basketball player to lift the same weight has twice the power of the basketball player. Power is represented mathematically by this formula:

$$P = F \times D/T,$$
$$\text{where } P = \text{power},$$
$$F = \text{force},$$
$$D = \text{distance, and}$$
$$T = \text{time}$$

You may recall from chapter 3 that work is force × distance. In essence, power is work performed over time. Power increases either through performance of the same amount of work in less time or through an increase in the amount of work performed in the same amount of time.

Speed, however, depends on coordination, efficiency of movement, and timing (Stamford 1985). These elements are developed later in the therapeutic exercise program than strength because, to some extent, they depend on the patient's strength. Since power involves the element of speed, ways of improving power are discussed in chapter 9.

Muscle Endurance

Muscle endurance is the ability of a muscle or a muscle group to perform repeated contractions against a less-than-maximal load. A muscle's endurance, or ability to prolong activity, depends on the status of the energy systems available and the forces resisted. With advanced conditioning levels, circulatory and local metabolic exchanges improve. The greater the forces resisted, the more quickly fatigue occurs. If a person's 1 RM on a bench press is 136 kg (300 lb), the person will be able to lift 68 kg (150 lb) for more repetitions before fatiguing than if that individual lifts 113 kg (250 lb).

Relationship Between Muscle Strength and Muscle Endurance

Muscle strength and muscle endurance can be placed on a continuum of exercise. High-intensity, low-repetition exercises, at one end of the continuum, emphasizes primarily strength gains. Low-intensity, high-repetition exercises, at the other end of the continuum, produces primarily muscle endurance gains.

High-intensity exercises that are performed for 3 to 9 repetitions appear to best emphasize strength (Berger 1962). A high-intensity exercise is defined as one that is at least 90% of the 1 RM (Wathen 1994). Low-intensity exercises performed for 20 or more repetitions at an intensity of 70% of the 1 RM emphasize primarily muscle endurance improvement. Exercises that are moderate intensity—at 70% to 90% of the 1 RM—and are performed for 6 to 12 repetitions provide gains in both strength and muscle endurance, although not as much as when either strength or muscle endurance is emphasized individually. Most researchers have found that in order to produce strength gains, an exercise must provide resistance levels of at least 66% of the muscle's maximum. Endurance gains can be made by increasing strength through high-resistance, low-repetition exercises, but not as effectively as by increasing the repetitions of an exercise. Conversely, some strength gains can be achieved with high-repetition exercises, but not as well as with high-resistive, low-repetition exercises. As a general recommendation, if your primary emphasis is strength, perform no more than 10 repetitions; but if your goal is primarily endurance increases, repetitions from 15 to 20 are advised. The closer the exercise resistance is to the maximum resistance, the fewer repetitions performed in the exercise; the further from the maximum resistance the exercise resistance is, the more repetitions performed. The relationship between muscle strength and muscle endurance, relative to the repetitions used to make gains in each of the parameters, is seen in figure 7.17.

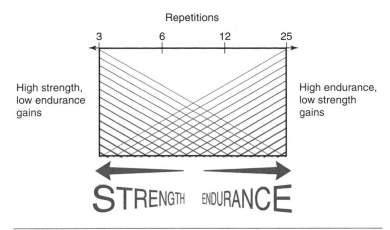

Figure 7.17 Relationship between muscle strength and endurance. Greater strength gains are achieved with lower repetitions and higher resistance, whereas greater endurance gains are achieved with higher repetitions and lower resistance.

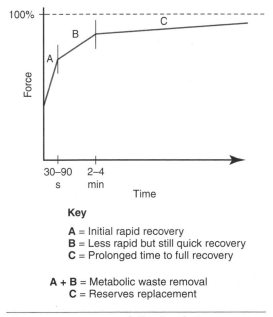

Key

A = Initial rapid recovery
B = Less rapid but still quick recovery
C = Prolonged time to full recovery

A + B = Metabolic waste removal
C = Reserves replacement

Figure 7.18 Recovery following fatigue.

The amount of work performed by a muscle during an exercise program is referred to as training volume. Training volume is based on the number of sets of each exercise, the number of repetitions completed of each set, and the amount of resistance (Feigenbaum and Pollock, 1999). Most research that has looked at training volume have used normal subjects; the response differences between healthy and injured subjects and the optimal recommendations for training volume for injured patients are yet to be determined.

Working a muscle optimally and to fatigue requires a recovery period between sets. Several studies have addressed the relationship between fatigue and recovery of muscles, both in isometric and in isotonic activities. The recovery following fatigue from isotonic exercise is slower than that from isometric exercise, but the recovery curves have similarities. As seen in figure 7.18, the recovery rate is rapid within the first 30 to 90 s. The rate of recovery then declines slightly over the next couple of minutes before making another rate change to a very gradual return to full recovery that takes place over a longer time period. The exact time of recovery depends on the study design and the type of exercise investigated, but all researchers have found a similar curve for the recovery pattern. When the activity is isokinetic, it takes approximately 4 min for a muscle to recover to 90% to 95% of its initial torque levels following an exercise bout to fatigue (Sinacore, Bander, and Delitto 1994). Recovery from isometric and isotonic exercises to fatigue occurs most rapidly in the first minute—58% and 72%, respectively. After the first minute, the recovery from isometric activity occurs at about a 35% faster rate than from isotonic activity (Clarke 1971). In all of these types of exercise recovery, there is an initial burst of recovery within 30 to 90 s. This is followed by a slightly slower but still rapid recovery. In the final phase of recovery, it takes more than 40 min for the muscle to return to pre-fatigue strength levels. On the basis of his findings, Lind (1959) extrapolated the probability that it would take more than 90 min for a muscle to fully recover.

Because of these differing recovery rates, a presumption has been that there are different recovery systems that lead to the muscle's overall recovery following exercise to fatigue (Lind 1959). The initial rapid recovery is thought to occur because of the removal of lactic acid and other buildup of metabolites that took place during the activity. The slower recovery may involve replacement of the muscle's metabolic reserves that were depleted during the activity.

These fatigue recovery findings have an impact on your therapeutic exercise program design. For example, if you are treating a hockey player with a quadriceps strain and he or she performs a leg press to fatigue, you should allow a 1/2 - to 1-min recovery before the next exercise set. If you are using an isokinetic machine to rehabilitate the quadriceps, the recovery time should be 2 to 4 min. With the use of isometric exercises, the rest between sets should be about 1 min.

Sometimes it is not possible to employ high-intensity exercises even though strength gains are needed. This situation is common, especially in early stages of therapeutic exercise when the patient's pain limits the resistance tolerated. In such cases, it helps to remember that the patient can still achieve strength gains using low-resistance, high-repetition exercises. For example, if a gymnast develops a patellar tendinitis and is unable to tolerate much weight during a leg press, he or she can use less weight and lift it for more repetitions to build the needed quadriceps strength. Later in the program as the quadriceps strength improves, the patient can use higher-resistance and lower-repetition exercises.

The number of repetitions a patient performs depends on several factors, including the patient's pain tolerance, the phase of the healing process, and the demands on the patient after return to competition. For example, a football defensive lineman's therapeutic exercise program is primarily strength based; a soccer player's program involves endurance exercises; and a basketball player—whose sport demands both strength and endurance—will have a program that emphasizes both strength and endurance exercises. If a patient begins a therapeutic exercise program one week after surgery, the resistance exercises are mild so as not to cause undue stress on newly forming tissue.

High-resistance, low-repetition exercises produce hypertrophy of the fast-twitch, type II muscle fibers. Moderate-resistance, higher-repetition exercises produce a more general increase in hypertrophy by affecting the size of both type I and type II fibers.

As a rehabilitation clinician, you must possess knowledge of injuries and sport performance requirements and must use good judgment to determine what level of resistance exercises to incorporate into the patient's therapeutic exercise program. Appreciating the patient's injury and having a sound knowledge of strengthening activities provide a good basis for making those judgments.

FORCE PRODUCTION

▶ Muscle force production is determined by the angle of the joint, the side of the muscle and its fiber arrangement, the speed of contraction, and the muscle fibers that are activated.

Some of the concepts in this section were introduced in chapter 3, but they are worth a brief review here. Putting together all the factors that determine strength output of a muscle not only helps clarify the concepts discussed in chapter 3, but also enables you to more fully appreciate the therapeutic exercises that can improve a patient's strength.

Muscle strength is determined by the angle of the joint, the length of the muscle and the sarcomere, the size and fiber arrangement of the muscle, the speed of contraction, and the number and type of muscle fibers activated. Let's look at each of these factors briefly.

Joint Angle

As you recall from chapter 3, joint movement is the result of a muscle's pull on the joint. The amount of force directed toward causing rotation of the joint (movement) and the amount of force directed at compression or distraction of the joint (stability or instability) are determined by the angle of the joint and the vector forces that are produced. Since movement around a joint is rotational, the force is called torque. Torque is determined by the amount of applied force and the length of the lever arm: $T = F \times D$ (torque = force times distance). As the joint moves through its motion, the lever arm length changes, causing a change in the muscle's torque. For example, when a patient performs a biceps curl, as the elbow moves from 90° flexion to 125° flexion, the lever arms of the resistance and the biceps shorten. Since the lever arm of the resistance (weight) undergoes a greater change than the lever arm of the biceps, the weight gets easier to lift by the time the patient has completed the full motion, as seen in figure 7.19. In terms of joint angle, the greatest force production occurs when the tendon's lever arm is at its greatest length.

Length-Tension

A muscle's strength production involves both active and passive elements. The active component is the motor unit; the passive component is the connective tissue surrounding the whole muscle, its fascicles, and its fibers. A muscle's ability to actively shorten lessens as the length of the muscle diminishes. In shortening, the muscle uses only its active component. At a muscle's shortest position, all of the cross-bridges between the fibers' actin and myosin filaments are used up. If, however, the muscle is lengthened before it shortens, its passive component, the connective tissue element, becomes taut and produces an additional resistive force because of its elasticity. The optimal length of a muscle to produce increased strength—because of the combined release of elastic energy from the passive elements and the actin-myosin cross-bridging from the active elements—is slightly beyond its resting length (figure 7.20). Stretching the muscle beyond that point further separates the actin and myosin to cause less cross-bridging, so that less force, rather than more, is produced.

When it is desirable to achieve a maximum force from a muscle, it is advantageous to produce a quick stretch of the muscle to use its elastic energy component. This factor is frequently utilized in activities such as proprioceptive neuromuscular facilitation and plyometric exercises, both of which are discussed later.

The length-tension factor requires additional consideration for multijoint muscles. The performance of a muscle that crosses more than one joint is profoundly affected by the position of both joints. For example, if you are working with a patient's injured knee and want to obtain a maximal contraction from the hamstrings, the beginning position to the hamstrings on stretch is with the hip in flexion and the knee in extension. If the exercise is performed with the patient prone, the hip is extended and the hamstring is already in a partially shortened position. In this position, it is impossible to apply a preexercise stretch to the hamstring muscle.

Although it is universally accepted that as a muscle fiber shortens, its ability to create force

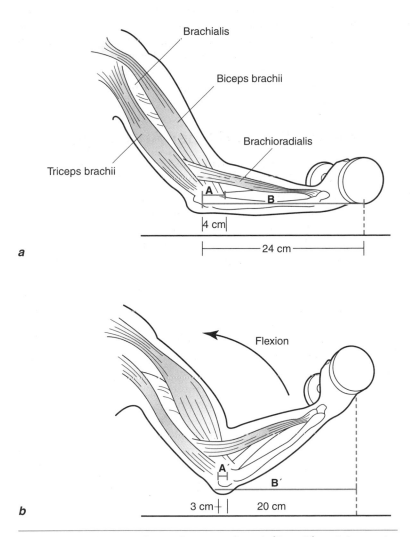

Figure 7.19 Change in biceps lever-arm length (A to A') and change in resistance lever-arm length (B to B') with different joint angles.

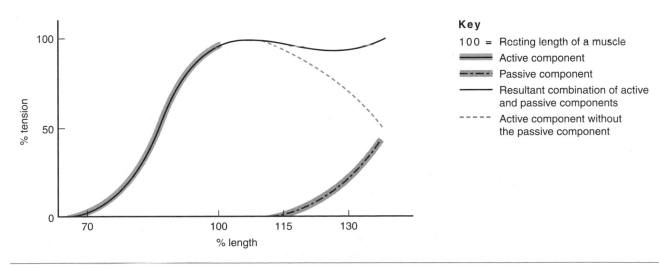

Figure 7.20 Length-tension factior: Because of the active and passive muscle-tissue elements, a muscle produces its greatest strength slightly beyond its resting length.

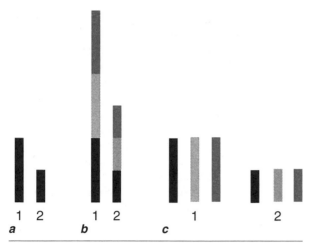

Figure 7.21 Fiber arrangement: (*a*) one fiber. (*b*) three fibers in series. (*c*) three fibers in parallel. Three fibers in series are able to shorten much farther than only one fiber, but three fibers in parallel are able to produce much more force than three fibers in series. 1 for each muscle is the resting length; 2 is the shortened length.

diminishes, how short a fiber is able to become is unanswered. Studies have looked at muscle fiber length and determined that a fiber can shorten to about 70% of its longest length (Lieber 1992). However, these studies used isometric contractions, not isotonic contractions, so the information obtained from these studies cannot be extrapolated to functional motion (Lieber 1992).

Muscle Size and Fiber Arrangement

Muscle fibers are arranged in series or in parallel with each other. Those muscles with series arrangements are longer muscles that are able to produce a greater shortening velocity. The muscles with parallel fiber arrangement have a larger cross-sectional area and are able to produce a greater force. As a simplified example, if a muscle is composed of three muscle fibers that are placed end to end and are stimulated to contract simultaneously, the muscle will shorten three times as much as a muscle with one fiber (figure 7.21). The muscle with the three fibers in a side-by-side (parallel) arrangement, however, will produce a contraction three times as powerful as a muscle with one fiber.

There is a direct correlation between a muscle's cross-sectional size and its strength. The cross section is the width of the muscle taken at an angle perpendicular to the length of the fiber. The cross section is greater when muscle fibers are arranged at angles to the axis of the muscle. Because of its featherlike appearance, this is called a pennate arrangement. The more pennates in a muscle, the greater the cross section. Those muscles with pennates tend to be force-producing muscles, not shortening-velocity muscles. Whereas the sartorius is an example of a shortening-velocity muscle, the gastrocnemius is an example of a multipennate muscle. The angle of pennation of any specific muscle varies from one person to another. Hunter (1994) believes that even if two people have the same size muscle, the angle of pennation may be a factor in the differences between their strength and speed.

Speed of Contraction

When a muscle shortens, the force produced is inversely proportional to the velocity of shortening. Billeter and Hoppeler (1992) assume that this occurs because there are fewer cross-bridges between actin and myosin filaments with a higher velocity shortening. For example, a patient who lifts 22.5 kg (50 lb) quickly finds that same weight relatively easy to lift when performing the activity more slowly.

When a muscle lengthens, the force is directly proportional to the velocity of movement. For example, when using a lengthening activity in therapeutic exercise, the patient is able to tolerate more resistance than with muscle-shortening activities. A variety of studies have addressed the relationship between force production and muscle length. One study (Horto-bagy and Katch 1990) showed that force production using a muscle-lengthening activity is 120% to 160% more than with a muscle-shortening activity. Other investigators (Wilmore and Costill 1999) believe that this figure is close to 130%.

Number and Type Of Muscle Fibers

As mentioned earlier, larger muscles are able to produce more force than smaller muscles. Fast-twitch fibers are able to produce more force than slow-twitch fibers because there are more muscle fibers in each motor unit of the fast-twitch fibers. If you are rehabilitating two patients with knee injuries and similar-sized quadriceps, the patient with more fast-twitch fibers is able to produce a stronger output of the quadriceps than the patient with fewer fast-twitch fibers in the quads. For this reason, it is fruitless to compare one patient to another and expect the two to be able to perform equally even if they are the same size and have similar injuries.

TYPES OF MUSCLE ACTIVITY

▶ Muscles perform several types of activity: Static activity occurs when there is tension but no change in the muscle's length. Dynamic activity occurs when there is a change in the muscle's length. Isotonic and isokinetic activity are particular types of dynamic activity.

Although some authors refer to the types of muscle activity as muscle contraction, it is not entirely accurate. Contraction implies a shortening of the muscle, but as you will see, a muscle does not always shorten when it acts. Therefore "muscle contraction" is referred to here as *muscle activity or movement*. There are two types of muscle activity, static and dynamic. **Static activity** is also called **isometric**. **Dynamic activity** is divided into **isotonic** and **isokinetic**. Isotonic activity is further divided into **concentric** and **eccentric** movements.

Static Activity

Static, or isometric, activity is produced when muscle tension is created without a change in the muscle's length. Static activity is used not only in therapeutic exercise but also in daily activities and sport participation. Trunk muscles act statically to provide a stable base for arm and leg movements. The shoulder acts as a stabilizer when a patient moves the elbow and hand. The advantage of isometrics is that this type of activity can strengthen a muscle without imposing undue stress on injured or surgically repaired structures. For example, in situations such as a recent fracture or a surgical repair in which movement is restricted or limited, isometrics can begin early in the therapeutic exercise program until full motion is indicated. Isometrics can also be used when the muscle is too weak to offer sufficient resistance against gravity or other outside forces. The disadvantage of isometrics is that strength gains are isolated to no more than 20° within the angle at which the isometric is performed. It is important to remember to caution the patient to avoid a **Valsalva maneuver** during isometric exercises. Valsalva occurs when the patient holds his or her breath, causing an increase in intrathoracic pressure. This can in turn impede venous return to the right atrium, leading to an increase in peripheral venous pressure (increasing blood pressure) and reducing cardiac output because of lowered cardiac volume. If you see a patient holding his or her breath during exercise, remind the patient to breathe in order to avoid the valsalva maneuver risk.

If a maximal effort is exerted in an isometric exercise, tension within the muscle progressively decreases because of fatigue. At 5 s the tension is 75% of the tension exerted at the start of the isometric activity. By 10 s, the strength drops to 50% of the original tension (figure 7.22). Because of this fatigue factor, no one has the ability to produce a sustained maximal contraction. An example of this is when you assist in carrying a stretcher with an injured person on it. As the upper extremity muscles performing the isometric activity of grasping the stretcher begin to fatigue, the muscles start to burn, and the transport team has to stop because someone will request a rest if it takes more than a short time to carry the patient.

This concept is important to remember when a patient performs isometric exercises in a therapeutic exercise program. It is unnecessary for a maximal isometric activity to be performed for more than 5 to 10 s at a time; 6 s is the recommended duration for one maximal isometric exercise (Hettinger and Müller 1953). The number of repetitions and frequency of exercise throughout the day depend on the condition of the muscle, the ability of the body part to move, and the phase of the healing process.

Strength gains are achievable if the muscle's effort is 66% to 100% of its maximum output. Efforts at 35% to 66% of maximal isometric output produce some gains in strength, but the increase is slow. Most daily activities, apart from sport activities, produce periodic tensions of 20% to 35% of maximum. This level of output maintains strength. If a muscle is immobilized and rendered inactive, there may be a range in loss of strength from 8% a week (MacDougall et al. 1980) to 5% a day (Muller 1970).

Keep in mind that it takes about one week to increase strength by 5% (MacDougall et al. 1980) to 12% (Muller 1970). These numbers may vary from one study to another because of the different protocols researchers use, but all the data make

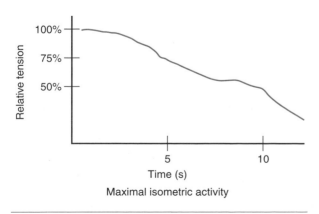

Figure 7.22 Maximal isometric force production.

a similar point: The rate of strength lost is much quicker than the rate of strength regained. In essence, it may take up to a week to recover the strength lost in one day of inactivity. This realization highlights how important it is to keep a muscle active if activity is causing no deleterious effects. If an injured part must be kept immobilized, isometric exercises can become very important in retarding atrophy and weakness.

Dynamic Activity

The term *dynamic* in relation to activity implies a change in the position of a muscle. Dynamic activity is further defined by the specific types of activity that occur.

Isotonic Activity

Isotonic activity is dynamic in that it involves a change in the muscle's length. If the muscle shortens, the activity is called *concentric*. If the muscle lengthens, the activity is called *eccentric*. Although you can isolate muscle activity to produce either concentric or eccentric motion, most sport and daily activities involve the use of both concentric and eccentric actions. For example, lifting a weight in an elbow curl is a concentric action, and lowering the weight is an eccentric action. Likewise, jumping for a basketball rebound is a concentric action that is preceded and followed by an eccentric action.

An eccentric action can produce about 30% more force than a concentric action (Wilmore and Costill 1999). For example, if an 18-kg (40-lb) weight can be lifted in a curl exercise concentrically, the same muscle can lift 23.5 kg (52 lb) eccentrically when the arm is lowered. It is believed that the muscle's noncontractile elements provide the additional forces during eccentric activity that permit increased muscle loading.

There are several other contrasts between concentric and eccentric activity. Although it takes more energy to perform a concentric action, there does not seem to be any difference in strength gains between the two types of exercise. As the speed of a concentric activity increases, the muscle's ability to produce force decreases. The opposite is true for eccentric exercises: As speed increases with eccentric exercise, the force increases initially, then eventually levels off or decreases. The differences in speed and force production of concentric and eccentric activity are demonstrated in figure 7.23.

There is also a greater likelihood of delayed-onset muscle soreness with eccentric exercise. Although the research is not conclusive, some believe that this is the result of a combination of damage occurring to muscle membranes and a secondary inflammatory reaction within the muscle (Wilmore and Costill 1999).

You can prevent this delayed-onset muscle soreness by taking a few precautionary steps when executing a therapeutic exercise program that incorporates eccentric exercise. One way is to avoid eccentric exercises early in the program when the muscles are particularly weak. Another way is start at a lower level of intensity and gradually increase the intensity as the patient is able to tolerate higher-level exercises. Delayed-onset muscle soreness (DOMS) is generally less of a problem as the patient becomes stronger and becomes accustomed to higher levels of exercise intensity. The occurrence of DOMS does not necessarily mean you should limit therapeutic exercise in subsequent sessions, but you should realize that the patient may not be able to offer as great an effort if DOMS is present. You should make a decision regarding the use of eccentric exercises in advance and determine whether risking a reduced-intensity session the next treatment day outweighs the benefits of providing eccentric exercises and risking muscle soreness. This is an individual determination that you should base on the patient's tolerance and motivation,

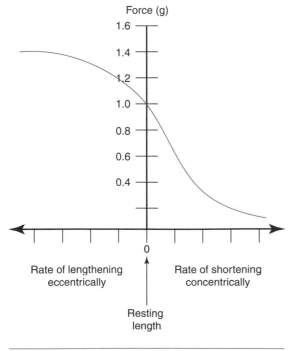

Figure 7.23   Concentric-eccentric force-length relationship.

Adapted from P.-O. Åstrand and Rodahl 1986.

the goals for therapeutic exercise, the level of healing, and the patient's current strength status.

The term *isotonic* means "having the same tension." It is, in fact, inaccurate, because the amount of tension produced by the muscle varies throughout the range of motion. The amount of tension produced depends on lever arms and the physiological principles previously discussed. The greatest amount of tension created in an isotonic activity is actually the force that the muscle or muscle group can produce at its weakest position in the motion. For example, if a patient lifts 18 kg (40 lb) in an elbow curl, that weight is the maximum the elbow flexors can exert at their weakest point. If the patient performs the exercise while standing, the weakest point occurs when gravity is at its greatest, with the elbow at 90° flexion. The elbow flexors can lift more than 18 kg at the beginning of the motion and at the end of the motion as gravity's lever arm length shortens. They can also lift more in the beginning of the motion, where the muscles are at their greatest physiological length, than they can at the end of the motion when they are at a physiological disadvantage. Because the elbow flexors can lift no more than 18 kg at 90°, the maximum weight the patient can lift through the full range of motion is 18 kg. By the same token, because the weight feels relatively lighter in the beginning and at the end of the motion, the patient is able to lift the weight at a faster speed during those parts of the motion. As the weight becomes more difficult to move around the 90° range of motion, the patient's movement slows down.

Isokinetic Activity

Isokinetic activity is a dynamic activity in that it involves motion. It differs from isotonic activity, however, in that the velocity is controlled and maintained at a specific speed of movement. Isokinetic means "having the same motion" and refers to the unchanging speed of movement that occurs during these activities. Whereas the speed of motion remains constant, the amount of resistance provided to the muscle varies as the muscle goes through its range. To return to the example of the elbow curl, if the exercise is isokinetic the patient's elbow moves through its motion at a uniform speed, but maintaining that uniform speed requires varying the amount of resistance. In that part of the motion where an isotonic exercise would be easy, the resistance in an isokinetic exercise is greater; and where the isotonic exercise would be normally more difficult, the resistance offered isokinetically is less in order to accommodate the varying strength of the muscle group as it goes through a constant motion. It is assumed in isokinetics that the patient provides a maximal output throughout the exercise. Isokinetics is sometimes called **accommodating resistance** exercise because of the change in resistance given throughout a range of motion. Today's equipment makes it possible to perform isokinetic activities isometrically, eccentrically, and concentrically. Although isokinetics was very popular during the 1970s and 1980s, closed kinetic chain activities are the current trend.

OPEN AND CLOSED KINETIC CHAIN ACTIVITY

▶ The differences between open and closed kinetic chain activities relate to whether or not the distal segment moves freely in space (open) or does not (closed).

A kinetic chain is a series of rigid arms linked by movable joints. This is a mechanical description of the body. **Open kinetic chain (OKC)** and **closed kinetic chain (CKC)** within the body are identified in terms of the distal segment of the extremity, the hand or foot. The kinetic chain is open when the distal segment moves freely in space. Kicking and throwing a ball are open kinetic chain activities. A kinetic chain is closed when the distal segment is weight bearing and the body moves over the hand or foot. Running and a handstand are closed kinetic chain activities. Generally, open kinetic chain athletic activities produce high-velocity motions such as throwing a ball or swinging the lower leg during running; closed kinetic chain activities are functional activities that place lesser shear forces on the joints, so they are generally safer to use earlier in a therapeutic exercise program.

Both OKC and CKC systems involve a relationship between one joint and the others within the chain. This is important to remember in therapeutic exercise, because if you ignore the other joints within the chain when rehabilitating an injured joint, success of the program will be elusive. Function of one joint is not exclusive: The function of one joint determines the function of the other joints within the chain. Abnormal stresses applied to an injured joint

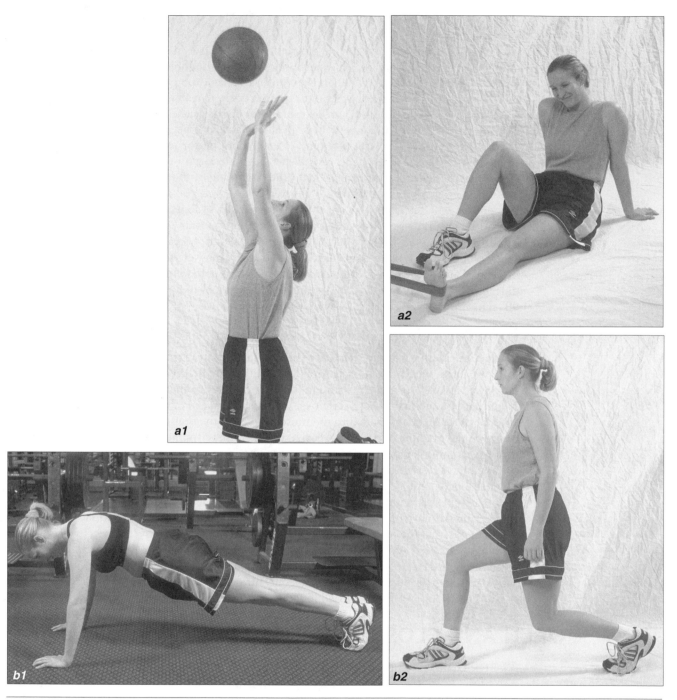

Figure 7.24 Open *(a)* and closed *(b)* kinetic chain activities for the upper *(a1, b1)* and lower *(a2, b2)* extremities.

are transmitted to and absorbed by other structures within the chain and have the potential to cause additional problems if those stresses are not tolerated by those other areas. For example, if a baseball pitcher has a weak shoulder and is unable to keep the arm elevated correctly during the pitch, he or she may develop elbow pain because of the additional stress transmitted by the abnormal force application at the shoulder.

Lower-extremity activities in sport are primarily CKC events. They can involve isometric, concentric, and eccentric activities. Closed kinetic chain exercises can be used to improve strength, power, stability, balance, coordination, and agility and are capable of generating large forces but relatively low velocities of movement. Lower extremity closed kinetic chain activities are functional in that they occur in normal activities from walking and standing to running and jumping. In a CKC, no link within the chain can move independently of the others; all are affected by movement of one segment. For this reason, the inadequacies of a weak link in the chain can be compensated for by other links within the chain, but additional stresses are generally applied to those other links. When upper or lower extremities are weight bearing, they function in a closed kinetic chain.

Open kinetic chain activities are also used in daily activities and in sport. Examples of OKC activities are kicking, throwing, and lifting lower body weights in a seated position, as in performing knee extensions. Even part of the running or walking cycle involves an OKC activity. In an OKC, any link in the chain is free to move independently of the other links. Generally, the forces generated by an OKC are small but the velocities are large. Body parts that operate in an OKC are non-weight bearing.

Open and closed kinetic chain activities are produced in both upper and lower extremities (figure 7.24). But different stresses are applied to the body by the two types of activities. The differences in stresses occur because the motion is different. In OKC activity, the proximal segment initiates the movement for the distal segment. For example, the shoulder motion initiates the movement at the hand. In CKC activity, there is compression of the joints, and stabilization occurs because of coactivation of opposing muscle groups. In a squat, the quadriceps work eccentrically while the hamstrings activate to counteract knee flexion movement. The result is stabilization of the knee through simultaneous activity of opposing muscle groups.

Continuing to look at the knee, in OKC knee flexion, only the hamstrings are working. In OKC knee extension, the quadriceps perform the motion while the hamstrings remain quiet. This exercise increases the moment force of the leg as it goes from flexion to extension. Moment force is the product of the amount of force (weight of the leg) and the perpendicular distance from the joint to the distal end of the limb (lever arm). In other words, as the leg is brought into extension, the work required to lift the lower limb increases because the moment arm of the resistive force increases. This not only requires more strength as the leg reaches terminal extension, but in an OKC the knee suffers a high shear force with an active contraction of the quadriceps as the knee goes from flexion to extension, especially during the last 30°. This shear force results from the anterior translation of the tibia as it is pulled by the quadriceps tendon. In a CKC, the shear force is counteracted by a co-contraction of the hamstring. The end result is reduced stress on the knee during terminal extension, especially the anterior cruciate ligament, and increased stability of the joint through the simultaneous contraction of the hamstrings and quadriceps in a closed kinetic chain exercise.

Although CKC exercises are more functional than open ones, in situations when the patient is non-weight bearing it may be necessary to use open kinetic chain exercises. The advantage of OKC activities in this situation is that strengthening activities need not be delayed until weight bearing is permitted. Open kinetic chain exercises also isolate muscles that are weak, so that correct emphasis can be placed on weaker muscles. One precaution in the use of CKC exercises is that because more than one muscle group is used, substitution of stronger muscles rather than correct use of weaker muscles is always a possible pattern and should be corrected when observed. A therapeutic exercise program should include a combination of open and closed kinetic chain exercises for optimal results.

EVALUATING MUSCLE STRENGTH

▶ Rehabilitation clinicians evaluate the strength of muscles with various types of machines or through manual muscle testing.

Chapter 3 addressed the idea that joint motion is produced by the muscles applying force in an arc of motion. The amount of tension a muscle produces is determined by its lever arm length and its angle of pull. In functional situations you do not need to calculate the amount of force produced, but you should have an idea of the relative strength of the muscle.

Evaluation Equipment

Strength can be objectively determined in a variety of ways. Isokinetic devices, to be considered later, can evaluate isokinetic strength; cable tensiometers can measure isometric strength; and free weights or weight machines can measure 1RM maximum isotonic strength (figure 7.25).

Figure 7.25   Strength evaluation: *(a)* isokinetic testing, *(b)* 1 RM.

Figure 7.26   Special test equipment: *(a)* Grip dynamometer measures hand-grip strength, and *(b)* pinch dynamometer measures finger-pinch strength.

Instruments that measure strength of specific areas or muscle groups are also available. For example, the grip dynamometer and the pinch dynamometer (figure 7.26) measure grip and finger pinch strength, respectively.

Manual Muscle Test

Not everyone has an isokinetic machine or cable tensiometers, however, and establishing a 1 RM for an injured extremity may not be appropriate. The 1 RM is an isotonic measure used most often with healthy individuals; 1 RM is not often used to assess strength in therapeutic exercise because it imposes too much stress on an injured part and may aggravate the injury.

The more universal, efficient, and readily available method of evaluating strength is the manual muscle test (MMT). The basis of this test is assessment of the muscle's ability to move a joint through its normal range of motion in as isolated a manner as possible. Depending on the muscle's strength, gravity is eliminated, used by itself, or used in conjunction with an outside manual force applied by the clinician. The muscle's strength is graded from 0 to 5; sometimes verbal grades, from 'no function' to 'normal', are used instead.

Manual muscle testing grew out of the need to identify and grade muscle strength in patients with polio. The MMT, based on strength relative to gravity and resistance, was developed and first used by a New York physician, Robert Lovett, in 1912. Lovett later collaborated with a physiologist, Dr. E.G. Martin, and published the tests in 1916. These first tests used the verbal scoring system. During the 1920s and into the 1950s, others further refined and redefined Lovett's MMT. In 1932 Dr. Arthur Legg in collaboration with physical therapist Janet Merrill published a book on muscle testing using the numerical scale with plus and minus designations for all except the two lowest strength grades (Hislop and Montgomery 2002). Over the years the MMT scale has evolved and been redefined as clinical trials and studies provide clearer pictures of its clinical value and limitations. The currently used grades are summarized and defined in table 7.3.

Table 7.3
Muscle Strength Gains

% Normal strength	Number grade	Letter grade	Qualitative grade	Definition
100%	5	N	Normal	Full range of motion against gravity and is able to tolerate full manual resistance to movement.
	4+	G+	Good +	Full range of motion against gravity and is able to tolerate nearly full resistance to movement.
75%	4	G	Good	Full range of motion against gravity and is able to tolerate moderate, but not full, resistance.
	4–	G–	Good–	Full range of motion against gravity and is able to tolerate some resistance .
	3+	F+	Fair +	Full range of motion against gravity and is able to tolerate minimal resistance through a partial range of motion.
50%	3	F	Fair	Full range of motion against gravity. The muscle is unable to go through its full range of motion if resistance is provided in an antigravity position. It may be able to tolerate resistance when gravity is eliminated.
	3–	F–	Fair–	Full range of motion against gravity but with difficulty.
	2+	P+	Poor +	Full range of motion with gravity eliminated. The muscle is unable to go through its full range of motion in an antigravity position. It may be able to tolerate mild resistance through a partial range when gravity is eliminated.
25%	2	P	Poor	Full range of motion with gravity eliminated. The muscle is unable tolerate resistance in a gravity-eliminated position.
	2–	P–	Poor–	Full range of motion with difficulty in a gravity-eliminated position.
	1+	T+	Trace +	Partial range of motion is possible with gravity eliminated.
10%	1	T	Trace	There is evidence of a muscle contraction but no joint motion occurs. A flicker of tension in the tendon may be seen or palpated, but the joint does not move.
0%	0	0	Zero	No evidence of contractility of the muscle. Facilitation produces no voluntary muscle response.

Since the development of these grades, it has become common practice to further define the scoring through the use of plus (+) and minus (–) signs. Just as with school grades, the +/– system in muscle grading defines the gray areas into which scores sometimes fall. For example, a deltoid that offers minimal resistance to antigravity with resistance is less than a grade 4 and more than a grade 3, so the clinician grades it as 4–. The grade is recorded as 4–/5, indicating that the strength of the muscle is 4– on a 5-point scale. If a muscle has some motion against gravity but not full range of motion, the rehabilitation clinician may give it a 3–/5 grade. If it has full motion in a gravity-eliminated position and is able to tolerate some resistance in this position but still is unable to go through a full range of motion in an antigravity position, its grade is 2+/5. The plus (+) and minus (–) system is not usually used within the average population for any grades except grades 2 and 3 (Hislop & Montgomery 2002); however, in the athletic population where there may be a significant difference between grades 4 and 5, the plus and minus system is commonly used.

When the clinician provides manual resistance to a muscle, the position most commonly used for the resistance in grade 4 and 5 muscle tests is an antigravity (against gravity) position with the muscle at the end of its range. Before a resistance is given to a muscle, the muscle actively moves the joint through its full range of motion. If that is successful, the clinician then applies manual resistance to determine the strength grade. Resistance can be applied through the full range of motion or at specific positions within the motion to determine strength. If testing positions are different from the standard positions, this should be noted on the record.

When applying a resistance force, you should exert the pressure in a direction that is opposite to the muscle's line of pull, providing stabilization if needed to permit isolated testing of the specific muscle or groups you are evaluating. Give the resistance on or near the joint distal to the joint being tested. Avoid placing your hand on the belly of the muscle being tested. Give the resistance gradually, building it up as you see that the patient is able to accept more resistance until you have determined the maximal resistance tolerated. Provide the maximum resistance possible to obtain an accurate result: If the muscle is able to tolerate more resistance than you have provided, the score may be inaccurate. Compare to the opposite side to determine what is "normal" for the patient. What is "normal" for a golfer may not be "normal" for a football lineman; what is "normal" for a recreational sprinter may not be "normal" for a competitive sprinter.

If a muscle is unable to perform a movement through its full range of motion in an antigravity position, it is placed in a gravity-eliminated test position to determine whether it has at least grade 2/5 strength. If full motion in an antigravity position is possible, resistance can be provided in this position to determine whether a 2+/5 strength is present. Figure 7.27 presents examples of strength testing of the hip, knee, ankle, shoulder, elbow, and wrist muscles.

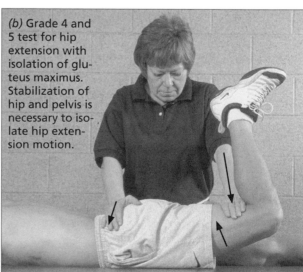

(a) Grade 4 and 5 test for hip extension with gluteus maximus and hamstrings. Note stabilization of hip to prevent pelvic rolling or hip flexion.

(b) Grade 4 and 5 test for hip extension with isolation of gluteus maximus. Stabilization of hip and pelvis is necessary to isolate hip extension motion.

Figure 7.27 Manual muscle tests.

(c) Grades 4 and 5 test for hip medial rotators: While stabilizing the thigh, resistance is applied to the leg against medial rotation movement.

(d) Grade 3 test for hip medial rotators: Patient should not lower the knee or roll the pelvis as the hip is moved through lateral rotation.

(e) Grade 4 and 5 test for hip lateral rotation: the thigh is stabilized while resistance is applied to the lower leg against hip rotation movement.

(f) Grade 3 test for hip lateral rotation: While stabilizing the pelvis, the hip is moved through a full range of external rotation.

(continued)

(h) Grade 1 test for hip lateral rotation: Hip lateral rotators are palpated as the patient performs the movement. The upper hand stabilizes the pelvis.

(g) Grade 2 test for hip lateral rotation: As the patient moves the hip through a full range of motion, the pelvis is stabilized to isolate movement.

(i) Grade 4 and 5 test for hip adduction: Resistance is applied to the thigh during movement into adduction while avoiding hip flexion or rotation substitution.

Figure 7.27 *(continued)*

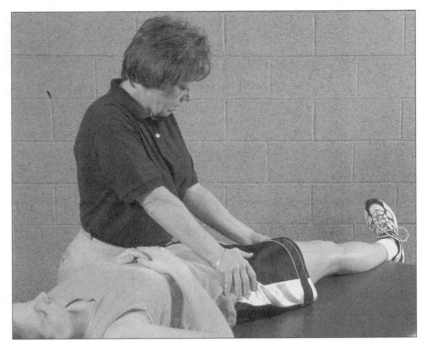

(j) Grade 1 and 2 test for hip adduction: While stabilizing the pelvis and palpating the hip adductors, movement into adduction is attempted. Watch for hip rotation or flexion substitution.

(k) Grade 4 and 5 test for knee extension: With one forearm under the thigh to elevate the thigh and protect it against the table surface, resistance is provided against knee extension motion.

(l) Grade 3 test for knee extension: While the thigh is stabilized, the knee is extended through a full range of motion without resistance.

(continued)

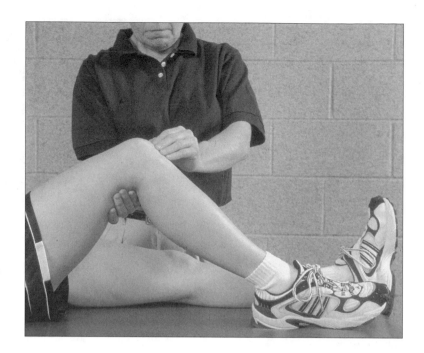

(m) Grade 1 test for knee extension: With the quadriceps on stretch in knee flexion, the quadriceps tendon is palpated as the knee is actively extended.

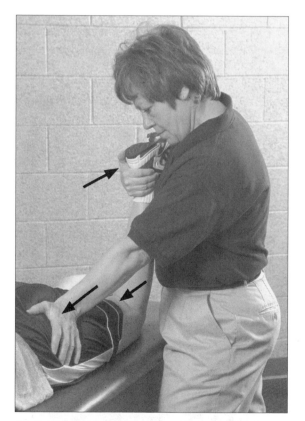

(n) Grade 4 and 5 test for knee flexion: With the hip and pelvis stabilized, resistance at the ankle is provided to knee flexion. Resistance to leg rotation can be simultaneously provided to isolate medial and lateral hamstrings.

(o) Grade 4 and 5 test for shoulder lateral rotators: While stabilizing the arm, downward resistance is applied at the forearm.

Figure 7.27 *(continued)*

(p) Grade 4 and 5 test for lower trapezius.

(q) Grade 3 test for lower trapezius.

(r) Grade 3 test for tibialis anterior: While the hip is stabilized, the foot is moved into dorsiflexion and inversion through a full range of motion. The test may be performed in sitting or standing.

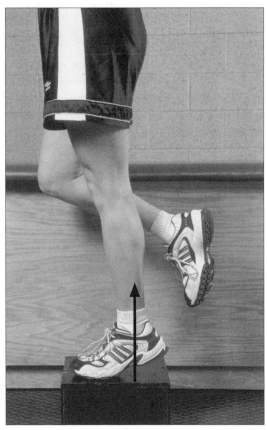

(s) Grade 4 and 5 test for plantar flexion: Full heel elevation should occur 20 times for normal strength. Watch for body rocking and knee flexion substitutions.

A thorough presentation of strength-testing positions and techniques for all grades of movement is available in various muscle-testing textbooks. Two suggestions are *Muscles, Testing and Function, Fourth Edition* (Kendall 1993) and *Muscle Testing: Techniques of Manual Examination, Third Edition* (Daniels and Worthingham 1972).

On rare occasions you may encounter a patient who does not offer a smooth resistance during the muscle strength test. The resistance is a series of catch-and-release tensions of the muscle as it goes through its range of motion. Called a **cogwheel resistance**, this response occurs in individuals who are not producing a maximal effort. Reasons for the response may include fear, pain, and malingering. When you see this form of resistance you should be aware that it is not a normal response, but rather a voluntary response that produces an inaccurate test result.

GRADATIONS OF MUSCLE ACTIVITY

▶ Muscles perform various gradations of muscle activity; from the least active to the most active, these are passive range of motion, active assistive range of motion, active range of motion, and resisted range of motion.

Just as there are grades of muscle strength, there are grades of muscle activity. The kind of muscle activity possible is, in part, determined by the muscle's strength.

Passive Range of Motion

Passive range of motion (PROM) is an activity that requires no active work on the part of the muscle. The motion is produced by an outside force, either a machine or another person. The intent is to maintain range of motion in situations in which either the muscle is incapable of moving voluntarily or it is desirable that the muscle not perform actively. Continuous passive motion machines, discussed in chapter 4, are sometimes used after surgery when motion is beneficial but active motion is not possible because of limitations such as pain, swelling, or spasm or because restricted muscle activity is desirable. The rehabilitation clinician can also perform PROM by moving the extremity through its motion without the patient's assistance.

Active Assistive Range of Motion

Active assistive range of motion (AAROM) is performed either when the muscle is incapable of producing the full motion without assistance, or when it is desirable for the individual to perform limited voluntary activity with assistance from an outside source to achieve the objective of the exercise. For example, if a patient has undergone reconstructive surgery on the shoulder, it may be desirable for him or her to perform actively through part of the motion, but not in the portions of the motion that may impose risk of shear stress or possible detachment of recently repaired tendons. Or a patient who has suffered a hamstring strain may not have full range of knee flexion because of weakness of the hamstrings. The hamstring is able to perform the motion through part of the range, but requires assistance from the clinician to complete the motion.

Active Range of Motion

Active range of motion (AROM) occurs when the patient is able to produce full range of motion of the segment, with no assistance. No resistance is applied. These types of exercises are also sometimes referred to as range of motion (ROM) exercises. Following surgery, the physician may permit a patient to perform full AROM exercises but may not want any outside resistance to be applied. These exercises are performed to maintain or increase range of motion and help reduce atrophy of the muscles involved in the motion.

Resisted Range of Motion

Resisted range of motion (RROM) falls into the broad category of dynamic exercises. Motion with resistance applied to the muscles is permitted. These types of exercise are commonly referred to as strengthening exercises or progressive resistive exercises. A later section of this chapter introduces the variety of progressive resistive exercise programs used in the rehabilitation of musculoskeletal injuries.

STRENGTH EQUIPMENT

▶ The primary methods of increasing strength include use of body weight, rubber tubing and bands, free weights, and isotonic and isokinetic machines. Each has its own advantages and disadvantages.

Many types of equipment are available to provide strength gains in both rehabilitation and conditioning programs. Most equipment can be used for both purposes. Cost varies greatly also—from very little to several thousand dollars. What you decide to use in your therapeutic exercise programs depends on your familiarity with the equipment, availability, budget, and the specific needs of the injured patients. Regardless of the amount or kind of equipment you have, you can design a very comprehensive, progressive, and appropriate therapeutic exercise program for every patient you treat. Your imagination and knowledge are ultimately the determining factors in the quality of the program you create.

The following sections deal with the most common items of equipment available on the market. Most are items you will become familiar with before you complete your curriculum.

Manual Resistance

Manual resistance equipment is the least-expensive therapeutic exercise equipment. The only requirement is you. Manual resistance exercise is an exercise in which the rehabilitation clinician applies manual force to produce either static or dynamic resistance. Manual resistance can be applied isometrically if movement is not desirable, if pain occurs with motion, or if the patient's muscle has a specific area of weakness within a range of motion.

Manual resistance can also be applied concentrically or eccentrically, through part of the motion or the full motion. It can be applied in a straight plane of movement or in a more functional diagonal plane.

Technique

Once you have assessed strength and identified deficiencies, you can determine how much resistance to apply during the exercise and whether you should provide additional special considerations such as an isometric activity at a specific point in the range of motion.

Before performing the exercise, the rehabilitation clinician explains to the patient the exercise, the sensations to be expected, the number of repetitions or qualifications for the duration of the exercise, and any necessary precautions. For example, I sometimes tell the patient that the goal is 15 repetitions or I'll state that we will continue the exercise until "one of us gets tired, or I start to sweat." If I want to deliver an isometric in the middle range, I tell the patient ahead of time to prepare him or her that at that point the motion will stop but the exercise will continue. As part of preparation it is also a good idea to take the extremity passively through the range of motion in the desired plane to let the patient know exactly what is expected during the exercise.

The resistance should be applied in a manner that permits the patient to perform the desired motion smoothly. The motion should not be jerky or uncontrolled. During the activity, the patient should produce a maximal effort and continue to breathe throughout. Occasionally, as already mentioned, a verbal reminder to breathe is necessary to prevent a Valsalva maneuver.

The rehabilitation clinician should watch carefully to see that substitution and unwanted movement patterns do not occur. It is important to correct the patient's motion if there is any substitution so the exercise is properly performed and facilitation of the appropriate muscle occurs.

Like in manual muscle testing, the force application should be near the joint distal to the joint being moved. If you cannot control the resisted movement because the patient's muscle is stronger than you are, as can be the case when you apply manual resistance to the hip, you can apply the resistance even more distally, at the ankle rather than the knee; this is permissible only if pain is not produced at the knee when the force is applied at the proximal ankle. The more distal application gives you a longer lever arm so you can do less work to offer the same amount of resistance to the hip. You can apply the same technique to shoulder exercises; in this case you offer resistance at the proximal wrist instead of at the elbow, but only if no pain occurs at the elbow. The exercise should be pain free and should offer enough resistance to produce the desired results.

Advantages

As already suggested, the greatest advantage of manual resistance is that it requires no equipment. It is also a good way to establish rapport with the patient, because a hands-on technique usually results in the patient's developing trust and confidence in the rehabilitation clinician. This often leads to a greater desire to work harder. It also gives you immediate feedback about the patient's progress. You assess the changes and improvements each time you perform the exercises, and you can make immediate changes according to the patient's response to a specific exercise. As the patient gets stronger, you can immediately increase the resistance or repetitions. The ability to modify the speed of the exercise within a set, the ability to change from concentric to eccentric activity or to include both, and the ability to incorporate isometric resistance into the weaker points of the motion are all unique to manual exercises. A progression of exercises is easily incorporated into a therapeutic exercise program by increasing either the manual resistance or the number of repetitions or sets.

Disadvantages

There are some unique disadvantages to the use of manual resistance. Because it requires one-on-one work with the patient, this method may be more time consuming than others and may not easily fit a situation that necessitates working with several patients at one time.

Another disadvantage is that manual resistance does not provide an objective measure for changes in strength. As a subjective method, it relies on performance by the same rehabilitation clinician to reflect the patient's strength changes.

In addition, if the rehabilitation clinician is not sensitive to the amount of force he or she is applying, judgment about the amount of force and about subsequent changes in the patient's condition may not be dependable. If you are more fatigued than usual on a given day, you may provide less force than on other days; without good awareness of how you feel you may incorrectly perceive a significant increase in the patient's strength.

Body Weight

Exercise using body weight also requires no equipment. The patient's own body weight provides the resistance. A variety of exercises for the upper and lower extremities and the trunk can be used, along with progressions, to offer an adequate system of therapeutic exercises.

Technique

You can provide a progression by increasing the amount of body weight used in an exercise, by prolonging the time of the exercise, or by increasing the number of repetitions or sets. For example, if a patient has a weak serratus anterior, a progression to increase the amount of body weight for a push-up exercise starts with a wall push-up, as seen in figure 7.28a and progresses to an incline, perhaps in a position with the hands on the back of a chair or a countertop (figure 7.28b), then to the hands on a chair seat (figure 7.28c). An even more advanced position is a modified push-up. As strength improves, the patient changes to a regular push-up position (figure 7.28d). If additional resistance is desirable, the patient can move to a decline push-up in which the feet are higher than the hands (figure 7.28e). The most advanced push-up is a handstand push-up. This is one example of a progression from easy to most difficult, providing the patient with a body-weight resistance exercise.

Figure 7.28 Body-weight resistance push-up progression: The easiest push-up is performed using a wall (a). Progression then moves to an incline (b and c), to the floor (d), to an inverted position (e). The positions shown in figures b-d increase difficulty by increasing the lever-arm length of the body. The position shown in figure e increases the difficulty by forcing the arms to bear more of the body's weight.

Examples of additional progressions include increasing the number of repetitions and/or sets the patient must perform, having the patient perform an isometric at the middle or end of the motion, and increasing the time of the hold as strength increases. A change of speed also changes the effort of the exercise.

You must impress on patients that performing an exercise through a full range of motion is necessary for maximal benefit. Partial range of motion execution provides for strength gains only in the portion of the motion being exercised. In the beginning, the patient should do the exercises slowly and in a controlled manner so that he or she executes them correctly without substitution of the wrong muscle. As strength and control improve, the speed of the exercise may increase to more correctly mimic functional activities.

It is also important to instruct the patient in correct execution of the exercise, providing information about common substitution patterns to avoid. This helps to minimize incorrect technique and to produce better results.

Once the patient has demonstrated the correct technique, he or she can perform the exercises without your assistance. This builds a sense of independence and control over the therapeutic exercise program and requires the patient to demonstrate initiative.

It is sometimes beneficial to give patients handouts illustrating these exercises. Such information serves as a reminder of correct exercise execution and also helps the patient comply with the therapeutic exercise program.

Pilates is a type of body weight resistance program that many people use for both conditioning and rehabilitation. Pilates is introduced in chapter 11 with the Feldenkrais Method and Alexander Technique, two other body awareness techniques.

Advantages

The most obvious advantage of body-weight resistance exercises is that they require no equipment. They can be performed anywhere, whether the patient is in the clinic, in the weight room, at home, or on the road. A related advantage is that there is no expense, although handouts provided to improve compliance may add minimal costs.

Another positive feature is that once the patient can perform the exercises correctly and continue them independently, treatment sessions can focus on other activities that require the expertise of the clinician, making optimal use of the treatment session.

Many weight-resistive exercises, such as the standing squat, are actually functional activities. They can be used as a progression of activities that naturally lead to those specific activities performed in the patient's sport.

Disadvantages

A disadvantage of body-weight exercises is that if the patient is performing them independently, there is no guarantee that he or she is doing them correctly or even doing them at all. On the other hand, it is not difficult to assess whether or not is complying with the home treatment program. If there are gains, chances are that the patient is complying; and, obviously, the converse is just as true.

Occasionally, a patient is unable to tolerate body-weight resistance exercises either because the area is too weak or because performing them is too painful. In this situation, it is better to begin with activities that provide less body-weight resistance—such as a wall push-up, or even independent isometrics. Once strength has improved, body-weight resistance activities can be incorporated.

Some areas of the body lend themselves better than others to body-weight resistance and progressive exercises using body weight. For example, the fingers and wrists are difficult to exercise with body resistance, especially in the beginning when the patient may not be able to perform an activity such as fingertip push-ups.

Rubber Tubing and Bands

Rubber tubing and bands provide dynamic resistance exercises. They are packaged in large and small rolls, so strips can be cut to varying lengths; they also come in a range of resistance levels, indicated by different colors. Although various companies market the bands with their own color indicators, the most familiar spectrum corresponding to resistance levels from lightest to heaviest is tan, yellow, red, green, blue, black, silver (gray), and gold (butterscotch). The color-coding scheme for tubing is similar.

Rubber tubing and bands provide resistance via the elastic elements of their makeup. The resistance provided is in direct relation to the amount the band or tubing is stretched (Page, Labbe & Tropp 2000). They can be stretched up to five times their original length; since most clinical use of rubber tubing and band does not stretch them more than 3 times their length, we can assume that as the band stretches, the resistance will change directly according to the amount of stretch is undergoes (Page 2003).

When selecting the length of a rubber band or tubing, it should be close to the length of the part being exercised. For example, if an elbow was going to be exercised, the length of the forearm to the hand should be measured, and rubber tubing or band of that length should be selected.

Technique

Rubber tubing and bands can be used both in straight-plane exercises and in functional patterns. Depending on the specific activity, the patient may use his or her own body to secure the band, or may use an object such as a door or table leg to secure it.

The bands and tubing can be used to mimic exercises performed with other equipment that is available in the clinic but not available for the patient at home. For this reason, tubing and bands are useful for home exercises.

Because of the variety of types of exercises that one can perform with tubing and bands, it is difficult to discuss specific application techniques. You should give the patient general guidelines, however, before providing bands or tubing to use for independent exercise. You should instruct the patient to perform the exercise slowly and in a controlled manner so the targeted muscles are used correctly. Going through a full range of motion is necessary for developing strength throughout the muscle's range. In addition, the area being exercised must be stabilized to ensure correct performance. Inadequate stabilization causes substitution and exercise of the wrong muscles.

To determine which color band or tubing to use, you will perform a MMT on the appropriate muscle. Trial and error may be necessary to become proficient at judging the correct resistance band to provide the patient, but after the test you should be able to narrow down the choice of colors. You have selected the appropriate color when the patient can perform the activity through an appropriate range of motion for the desired number of repetitions and feels that the muscle has been at least moderately exercised.

Once again, to ensure better compliance, it is advisable to give patients handouts that include drawings or photos along with providing oral explanations of the exercise. As mentioned in chapter 1, studies show consistently that if an individual receives both written and oral instructions, the likelihood of correct performance of the exercise and of compliance increases significantly.

Advantages

The cost of rubber tubing and bands is relatively low. In some clinics, it may be possible to recuperate the costs by billing the patient or the patient's insurance company. These items are easy to transport, because they weigh little and are not bulky, so patients can take them home or can easily pack them into suitcases and exercise almost anywhere.

Since exercises using bands or tubing are easily converted to home exercises, they need not be repeated in the treatment sessions. Treatment time can then be better spent on other activities that require the expertise of the rehabilitation clinician. This allows the patient to gain a sense of responsibility, independence, and control over the injury recovery process.

The color coded bands and tubing offers an easy-to-implement system of progression. As the patient's strength increases, you can provide additional colors to achieve greater resistance with the same exercise. Additional instruction is not necessary, because the exercise itself is the same.

Exercises that mimic functional motions can be used with the tubing and bands. This provides for strength gains in functional patterns. This method is especially convenient for upper extremity muscle groups that may not easily lend themselves to body-weight resistance and other exercise systems.

Disadvantages

Since the patient performs rubber-tubing and band exercises independently, you do not have control over compliance. It is the patient's responsibility to perform the exercises. This can be an advantage or a disadvantage, depending on the patient's attitude, dependability, and motivation.

Another disadvantage is that as the band or tubing stretches during the exercise, the resistance increases, causing more resistance to the muscle as it reaches its weaker point in the motion. The resistance is then greater at the end than at the beginning of the motion when the muscle is at a stronger physiological length. So although the band offers resistance to the muscle, the amount of resistance provided does not coincide with the muscle's ability to produce force.

If the clinic cannot recuperate the cost of bands and tubing, the expense can add up quickly. The heavier bands are more expensive than the lighter bands, so as a patient's strength increases, the cost of distributing the bands and tubing also increases. If a facility provides tubing and bands for patients but is unable to recover the costs, additional budget allowances are necessary.

Although it is possible to design exercises for the hip and knee using bands and tubing, the greater number of exercises using these items involve the upper extremities. Figure 7.29 provides examples of some rubber band exercises for the upper and lower extremity muscles.

Free Weights

When most people think of strengthening, they think of free weights. Free weights include cuff weights, barbells, and dumbbells. They come in a variety of sizes and styles. The weight is either attached to the body part or held by the patient during the exercises. Cuff weights typically cannot be changed in size. Some can be modified by the addition of preset weighted

Figure 7.29 Rubber band exercises: *(a)* hip internal rotator exercise; *(b)* shoulder horizontal extension (or bent-over row) exercise.

tubes or packets that are placed in a pocket on the cuff. The cuffs are attached to ankles or wrists.

Some dumbbells and barbells are adjustable: Various weights can be placed on the bar and are secured with collars. Other dumbbells and barbells are fixed and their weight cannot be changed. *Dumbbells* refers to weights that are used in one hand, are usually smaller, and are either fixed weights or adjustable. *Barbells* refers to a larger free-weight system that requires using both hands. Barbells are used for lower- and upper-body strengthening. The bars vary in length from 1.5 m to 2.1 m (5–7 ft). A bar that has become popular in the past several years for conditioning and later-stage rehabilitation is the standard Olympic bar, which weighs 20.5 kg (45 lb) and is about 2.2 m (87 in.) long. The collars used to secure the weight plates to an Olympic bar weigh 2.25 kg (5 lb) each. The sleeves on which the plates are mounted are larger than more conventional plates and rotate so that the plates do not stick to the bar when it is lifted. The plates are also larger in diameter than the traditional plates so that a patient who drops the bar is not crushed or otherwise injured by the weight.

Technique

As with any exercise, proper instruction in execution is necessary in order to achieve appropriate strengthening without substitution of activity by incorrect muscles. It may be helpful, especially in the beginning, to have the patient use a relatively light weight so that he or she can perform the technique correctly and learn what muscle should be performing the activity. Stabilization of the part being exercised is necessary and is more difficult with free weights than with machine weights. Once you are confident that the patient is able to perform the exercise correctly and understands the proper procedure, you can increase the exercise resistance.

The patient should have control of the weight throughout the full range of motion. A complete range of motion during the exercise is necessary to provide for strength gains throughout the motion. The patient should perform the activity in a slow, controlled manner. As the muscle's strength improves and more functional activities are appropriate, the speed of the motion may increase, depending on the goals of the exercise.

Free weight exercises are more difficult to perform than machine weight exercises, because while the weight is being lifted it must also be controlled. The exercising extremity must stabilize itself with the added weight and control the weight simultaneously. This requires work not only of the specific muscle being exercised, but also of the surrounding muscles.

One selects the exercise weight according to the strength of the muscle being exercised, while also considering the repetition and set goals. The weight should be heavy enough to challenge the patient yet light enough to allow him or her to accomplish the goals.

What determines the position in which the patient performs the exercise is the point in the motion where the greatest resistance is desired. For example, in an elbow curl, the greatest resistance in standing occurs when the elbow is at 90°. If the patient performs the exercise in supine, the greatest resistance is in the beginning of the exercise when the elbow begins moving into flexion from full extension. If a cuff weight is attached to a patient's ankle for a hamstring curl exercise, the maximum resistance occurs in the beginning of knee flexion if the patient is lying prone, but it occurs at 90° knee flexion if the exercise is performed in standing. This is so because the maximum resistance is determined by the relationship between the pull of gravity on the weight and the position of the segment being exercised. When the pull of gravity is perpendicular to the lever arm, the resistance is at its greatest. The rehabilitation clinician must determine where in the motion to place the primary emphasis for strength before selecting the proper position for the exercise.

When a muscle's position changes to attain a maximum resistance at a different angle, the stresses to the muscle change. For example, if a patient performs an elbow curl with 4.5 kg (10 lb) in a supine position, then changes to a sitting position, the weight tolerance will change. The maximum stress is applied in the middle of the motion in the seated position rather than at the beginning as it was in supine, so the muscles may not have the strength to lift 4.5 kg by the time the elbow moves to 90° in the seated position. One must consider this when determining the patient's exercise position.

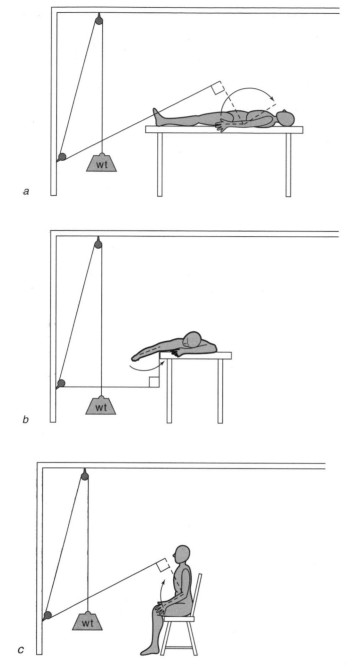

Figure 7.30 Different pulley angles for an elbow flexor strength exercise: *(a)* supine, *(b)* prone, and *(c)* seated. Maximum resistance occurs when angle of pulley cable to the arm is 90°.

A pulley system is a form of free-weight system. A pulley board or other unit includes a cable to which a weight is attached. The cable runs through at least one, or most often two, pulleys. The pulleys can be adjustable to provide more variety in exercise positions. The position of the pulley and rope determines where in the range of motion the greatest resistance is provided to the muscle. Maximum resistance occurs when the line of the rope from the pulley to the extremity forms a 90° angle with the extremity. Figure 7.30 demonstrates this concept.

Again, you can change the maximum resistance by changing the angle of the force. In this case, the angle of the force is determined not by gravity but by the pulley position. These lever arm concepts are presented in chapter 3.

The equipment should be secured before the patient is allowed to lift the weight. This means checking that the dumbbell and barbell collars are secure so the weight plates will not fall off during lifting. If the patient is using cuff weights, the straps should be in good shape and secured so that the weight will not fall off when the patient moves the extremity.

The amount of weight lifted must be adjusted as the patient's strength improves. Once strength improves, the weight's proportional resistance declines, the exercise becomes easier, and additional changes in strength do not occur unless the weight is increased. You must periodically reevaluate strength to determine whether or not the patient is ready for a weight increase.

Advantages

With free weights, the amount of resistance offered to the patient is not limited by the rehabilitation clinician's strength. This is the most obvious advantage of free weights over manual resistance.

There is a variety of free weight equipment on the market today, ranging from the plain, simple, and inexpensive to the complex, "gadgetized," and expensive. Selection depends on budget, space, needs, preference, and ability to use the equipment.

Free weights can be used in a number of ways to increase muscle strength, and they can be used in different positions to provide maximum resistance at varying angles. This can add variety to the therapeutic exercise program.

Another benefit is that free weights make it is easy to determine quantitative measures of strength and of improvement in strength. This gives the clinician an evaluative tool and provides the patient with an automatic motivating factor. The clinician can document objective improvements when the patient's weights change. The patient is motivated to increase the amount of weight lifted and feels a sense of accomplishment when achieving weight goals.

The cuff weights can be used in a functional activity when attached to the wrist or ankle. For example, an injured soccer player can add resistance to kicking during activity by attaching a weight cuff to the ankle.

Disadvantages

The greatest disadvantage of free weights is safety, which you must always consider when using this equipment. The risk of injury if the weight is too great or is not used properly is a consistent danger. The patient should be instructed to use the weights correctly and to return them to their proper place when finished with the exercise. A patient cannot control a weight that is too heavy. In this situation the patient may drop the weight or suffer an injury.

Because lifting free weights is an isotonic activity, the amount of weight lifted is no greater than that which the muscle is able to lift at the weakest part of its motion. The amount of resistance changes as the lever arm length changes when the segment moves through its motion.

Finally, lifting weights can be boring. Patients who are bored are less likely to work as hard during the exercise. It is also more difficult to become motivated if the exercise is not interesting, and compliance may be more difficult.

Isotonic Machines

In addition to free weights, a variety of machines can be used for isotonic exercises. Some have a fixed lever system that offers different amounts of resistance. Changes in resistance occur differently, depending on the machine. The most commonly used machines provide altered resistance with weights, resistance bands, or hydraulic pressure. This category of equipment includes a long list of machines made by many companies. A list of generic examples includes hydraulic devices, multiple-station units, individual freestanding stations, and rubber cord resistive machines.

Isotonic machines provide a constant load during an exercise. As with free weights, the load lifted is whatever the muscle at its weakest point is able to manage.

The design of some machines is such that you can control the allowable range of motion by placing a weight key at different positions on the weight's arm. This can change the excursion of the exercise and the weight lifted. For example, you can change a range of motion excursion on a bench press machine by first elevating the bench press arm and then inserting the key at the desired weight load.

Isotonic machines can also be used for isometric exercises. To use the machine this way, you place the weight key at a weight that is too heavy for the patient to lift, or lock the lever so that movement is not possible.

Other simple isotonic "machines" fall into this category because they offer isotonic activity against a mechanical resistance. This group includes a large variety of equipment such as the N-K table (named after its two designers R.B. Noland and F.A. Kuckhoff), hand putty, and grip exercisers.

Technique

As always, instruction in proper use of the equipment and proper execution of the exercise is necessary. You should not assume that patients are able to perform an exercise correctly merely because they state that they have done the exercise before. Patients often either perform an exercise incorrectly or, because of weakness, use the wrong muscles to perform an exercise that was easy before they were injured. You should first demonstrate the exercise for the patient and then have the patient do the exercise while you observe for correct execution.

It is important to watch the speed of the exercise to observe for and caution against muscle substitution. Educate the patient regarding the proper speed and performance. This is especially important if you intend to have the patient perform the exercises independently later in the program. Changes in speed can occur with strength advances. As indicated with other exercises, the patient should perform exercises through a full range of motion.

Advantages

The greatest advantage in the use of isotonic machines is safety. The weight is guided and controlled by the machine, so the chances of injury resulting from the weight's dropping or the patient's losing control of the machine are very slim.

The multiple-station units allow many patients to work simultaneously. You can easily establish a circuit program on the machine so that either one patient or several can exercise at one time.

Once the exercises have been established, the patient can exercise without assistance. The rehabilitation clinician can perform periodic reevaluation with increases in repetitions, sets, or weights. The treatment time can then be used for other, more directed activities.

It is easy to establish a machine exercise progression by changing the numbers of repetitions or sets, the speed of the exercise, or the resistance. Changing these parameters can also add some variety to a therapeutic exercise program.

Weight machines most often have either a specific weight indication or an arbitrary number indication on the plates. This permits an objective measure of improvement. Quantifying gains introduces a motivating factor and is an objective measure of progress for both the patient and the rehabilitation clinician.

Some pieces of equipment are not expensive; some can even be hand made and modified to fit specific clinic or individual needs. For example, a wrist exerciser can be made from a weight disk, dowel, and rope.

Disadvantages

Some of the disadvantages of isotonic machines are the same as for free weights. One is that the muscle's weakest point determines the maximum weight that can be lifted.

Using equipment can be boring. It may be difficult to motivate patients to perform daily exercises on the machines.

Additionally, some isotonic machines are very expensive and require considerable facility space. This is particularly true for the individual freestanding machines. The multi-unit machines may require less space, but they are also expensive, and many still require a relatively large space for installation and operation.

Figure 7.31 Isokinetic machine.

Isokinetic Machines

Isokinetic exercise machines have been available since the early 1970s. They were very popular during the 1970s and 1980s. Several manufacturers produced isokinetic equipment during the 1980s. Today, emphasis has moved away from isokinetic equipment, and the demand has dwindled drastically. Today, there are only two manufacturers—Biodex (Biodex Corporation, Shirley, NY) and Cybex (Henley Health Care, Cybex Medical Division, Sugarland, TX). A Biodex is shown in figure 7.31.

Isokinetic machines offer resistance at a constant speed, so the amount of resistance varies through the range of motion. This is sometimes referred to as *accommodating resistance*. To produce a constant speed, the machine offers a matching resistance when the patient attempts to push the arm of the machine as hard as possible. For an isokinetic exercise to produce the desired results, the patient must resist the machine with maximal effort.

Technique

Isokinetic machines today offer resistance concentrically, eccentrically, and isometrically. The type of exercise used depends on the settings established on the machine by the rehabilitation clinician. The settings are determined according to the specific goals and the type of exercise the rehabilitation clinician decides is the best method of achieving those goals.

The isokinetic machine's speed is preset before the exercise begins. Settings range from very slow (less than 30°/s) to very fast (over 300°/s). Even at the fastest settings, the speeds do not mimic the speeds of motion during functional activities. For example, forearm speeds greater than

9,000°/s occur with throwing a ball (Braatz and Gogia 1987). Even normal walking produces a tibial swing-through phase speed of about 48 kph (30 mph). One of the early claims of isokinetic advocates was that the isokinetic machines could mimic functional speeds; now that we can measure true joint speeds we know that this is not the case.

It is necessary to instruct the patient in proper exercise execution on the equipment. The exercise sensation is not necessarily one that the patient has experienced before, since other equipment provides a variation in resistance and speed whereas isokinetic equipment forces the patient's speed to remain constant throughout the motion.

Isokinetic equipment can be used at submaximal levels. This is particularly important if the patient's injury is recent or if the patient has too much pain to permit a maximal resistance output. It is important to explain to the patient the goal of the exercise if that goal is less-than-maximal output.

The equipment should be properly set before the exercise begins. Isokinetic machines can be placed in a variety of positions to be used on a variety of joints. Proper alignment of the machine's joint is necessary to avoid placing undue torque on the patient's joint. Correct machine lever arm length should also be determined before the beginning of exercise.

Instructions should include precautions about avoiding pain during the exercise and eliminating substitution by other muscle groups. Stabilization straps should be applied to ensure minimum substitution. If the patient experiences pain, changes in the exercise parameter settings are indicated.

Advantages

Isokinetic equipment provides a constant-speed, accommodating-resistance exercise to produce a maximum muscle resistance throughout the range of motion.

The machines can be used for maximal and submaximal muscle output. Less-than-maximal output can be controlled to permit exercise without increasing injury. Likewise, use of a maximal muscle output can provide increased stress to the muscle as healing progresses and the muscle's tolerance improve.

Diagonal patterns can be performed on the equipment to produce a more functional form of exercise. This can assist the muscles in relearning functional patterns of motion.

The machine produces measurable and reproducible results and can be used for testing as well as exercising. The machine's computer records the muscle's output throughout the range of motion and can correlate the strength with a specific degree within the motion.

The computer's visual readings provide immediate feedback to the patient and to the clinician. Goals can also be indicated on the screen. This information serves to motivate the patient as a goal is established and results of efforts toward it can be seen. The clinician also receives immediate information about the patient's effort, areas of weakness through the range of motion, and points at which there should be greater emphasis in other exercises.

Comparison of records between one session and another also provides feedback on progress. Maintaining a record reveals concrete and objective changes in the patient's progress.

The machine's speeds can be varied, so a patient can exercise at slower or faster speeds to work on fast-twitch and slow-twitch muscles in the same session. Exercises can be used to improve strength, muscle endurance, coordination, and speed of movement.

Disadvantages

Isokinetic machines have two primary disadvantages. One is cost: An isokinetic machine, with the equipment and computer, costs over $40,000. Many facilities find this price prohibitive. The other clear disadvantage is that the exercises are primarily OKC exercises. Since lower-extremity activities are primarily CKC, functional application is minimal.

Another disadvantage is that in performing evaluations, the rehabilitation clinician must remain consistent with respect to speed, settings, and positions from one session to another in order to obtain consistent results. Changing anything during the activity, even the motivating commands, can alter the results.

Some clinicians find the setup of the machine and the need to change its position and pieces of equipment too complicated and too time consuming to be practical. This is the case especially if the machine is used infrequently.

Isokinetic computers can offer a great deal of information on the patient's performance. This can be an advantage or a disadvantage. It can be advantageous if the rehabilitation clinician understands the information and its significance for the therapeutic exercise program. It is disadvantageous, however, if he or she does not understand the data and does not take time to learn their significance. In this case, the clinician may be frustrated and intimidated by the information so instead of using the machine, discards it as impractical.

If many patients are using the machine for therapeutic exercise, they may need to wait their turns. One patient may use the machine for several bouts of exercise or for various positions. This takes time and can prohibit its use by others for extended periods. In situations in which a clinician has limited time to spend with a patient, this may not be a piece of equipment that is available at the right time or convenient to use.

Other Equipment

Other accommodating-resistance machines provide variable resistance through the range of motion. One type of equipment, familiar in gyms, is known as Nautilus (Nautilus, Deland, FL)—so named because its cam resembles the cross section of the shell of the sea mollusk nautilus. Machines of this type offer a variable resistance through a cam system. The cam allows the lever arm length of the machine to change so that the amount of resistance changes. These changes are supposed to coincide with the change in the muscle's lever arm, so that as the muscle's strength changes, a concomitant change in the resistance is offered to it by the machine; however, because these machines are not designed for all body sizes, the machine's resistance may not match the individual's muscle-length changes through its range of motion. Smaller men and many women may find that the machines do not correlate with their extremity lengths. In these cases, using the machines may cause injury.

Other machines and exercise equipment are available for strengthening. Some of these devices are mentioned in other chapters in connection with such topics as proprioception. Nautilus and other machines may not be indicated for therapeutic exercise use, especially in the earlier stages of rehabilitation. The rehabilitation clinician must understand the functions, the weight minimums and increments, and the way in which each machine operates before determining whether or not a piece of equipment is appropriate for a patient's use. The patient's abilities, healing phase, size, injury limitations, and restrictions are all factors to consider before advocating the use of any machine.

PROPRIOCEPTIVE NEUROMUSCULAR FACILITATION

▶ Exercise techniques based on proprioreceptive neuromuscular facilitation use impulses from the afferent receptors in various parts of the body to stimulate the desired motion. One such technique, reversal of antagonists, is common in rehabilitation because it mimics daily and sport performance activities.

Sherrington, a neurophysiologist, provided the basic concepts that were used by Herman Kabat, MD, during the late 1940s and early 1950s to develop **proprioceptive neuromuscular facilitation (PNF)** exercise techniques. The underlying significance of this technique was in the use of combinations of primitive movement patterns performed with a maximum amount of resistance applied throughout the range of motion. The techniques were originally found to be useful in the treatment of neuromuscular disorders, but over time they have also proven beneficial for application to orthopedic disorders. Proprioceptive neuromuscular facilitation has been helpful in restoring flexibility, strength, and coordination of injured muscles and joints.

Facilitation

It is in this sense—restoration—that rehabilitation clinicians use PNF today. Proprioceptive neuromuscular facilitation incorporates the inhibitory and excitatory impulses from the afferent receptors of skin, muscle, tendon, visual, and auditory neurons that facilitate a response from the motor neurons, resulting in a desired action. For example, the rehabilitation clinician's hands on the patient's leg provide a stimulus from the skin receptors; a stretch force applied by the rehabilitation clinician on the muscle stimulates the muscle spindle and Golgi tendon organs; the patient's ability to see where the leg is going provides additional input to produce the desired motion pattern; and the verbal cueing and guidance of the clinician during the activity stimulate the patient's auditory receptors to send messages to increase or decrease muscle activity.

Each of these afferent stimuli influences the motor response. To see the significance of this point, you can easily perform a simple test. With a person lying supine, place one hand on the hamstring and one hand on the quadriceps. Ask the person to maximally resist you in a straight-leg raise, and judge the amount of resistance the person provides. Now place your hands only on the quadriceps and have the patient repeat the maximally resisted movement. You should experience greater resistance with both of your hands on the quadriceps surface and less resistance with one hand on the hamstrings and one on the quadriceps. With tactile input of both surfaces, the afferent stimulation is a mixed one, producing both facilitation in and inhibition to the anterior muscles. When both hands are on the same surface, facilitation to the muscles performing the action is provided without inhibition from sensory nerves of the hamstring surface.

A quick stretch provided in a PNF movement immediately before the exercise produces a stretch reflex from stimulation of the muscle spindles and Golgi tendon organs. This causes increased response from the muscle.

Taking the patient's leg passively through the activity before performing the actual exercise gives the patient the visual and proprioceptive feedback to realize the direction and pattern that the leg should traverse. If you do not do this before the exercise, you will find not only that the patient is confused about what to do, but also that the output of the muscle is significantly less. The more confidence the patient has about being able to perform the pattern correctly, the stronger the motion will be.

Verbal input is used commonly in athletic events. We do it when we cheer a team or player during competition. When we want a patient to perform an exercise at a maximal output, we use verbal cues to encourage him or her to do the most work possible. Verbal cues in PNF provide the same stimulus. They are also necessary for permitting the patient to correctly perform the pattern of activity desired. Cueing with brief, well-timed words and phrases facilitates an improved muscle response.

Patterns of Movement

The premise underlying PNF is that central nervous system stimulation produces mass movement patterns, not straight-plane movements. Natural motion does not occur in straight planes but in mass movement patterns that incorporate a diagonal motion in combination with a spiral movement. In other words, all major parts of the body move in patterns that have three components. These diagonal patterns include the components of flexion and extension. Because the patterns are diagonal, they also include motions either toward and across the midline (adduction) or away and across the midline (abduction). Rotation is the third component of PNF patterns. Figure 7.32 demonstrates these components. Although PNF can be used for the trunk as well as the extremities, discussion of PNF here is limited to the upper and lower extremities, since these are the areas primarily treated with PNF in musculoskeletal rehabilation.

The movement patterns are referred to as D1 and D2. D1 flexion and D1 extension patterns are moving into flexion and moving into extension, respectively. D2 patterns are divided in the same way.

This is easier to remember if you recall that in the upper extremity, lateral rotation always goes with flexion, and in the lower extremity, lateral rotation always goes with adduction. For example, in the upper extremity as the shoulder goes from extension to flexion it always laterally rotates whether the movement is adducted or abducted (figure 7.33a). So, when the arm goes into extension, the shoulder medially rotates, and the varying motion is either adduction in a D1 pattern or abduction in a D2 pattern.

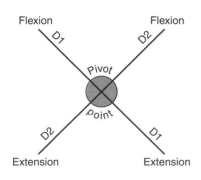

Figure 7.32 PNF patterns: Neural motion occurs in diagonal planes of component motions.

Figure 7.33 *(a)* Lateral rotation is associated with flexion while medial rotation is associated with extension in the upper extremities. *(b)* In the lower extremities, adduction and lateral rotation occur together as do abduction and medial rotation.

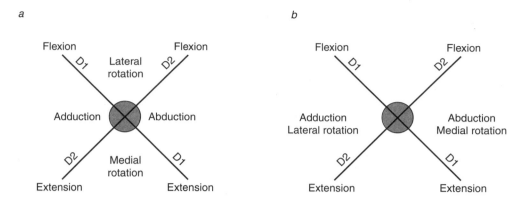

Because lateral rotation accompanies adduction in the lower extremity, when the hip is moved into flexion the movement also includes lateral rotation when it is adducted and medial rotation when it is abducted (figure 7.33b). Likewise, when the hip moves into extension, it also is laterally rotated if it is adducted (D2) and medially rotated if it is abducted (D1).

When you think about it, these are natural patterns that you see every day in sport and daily activities. For example, when throwing a ball overhand, the shoulder starts in abduction, flexion, and lateral rotation. As the ball is thrown, the follow-through ends with the shoulder in an extension, adduction, and medial rotation position. Kicking a soccer ball also demonstrates the PNF pattern: As the ball is kicked the leg moves from extension, abduction, and medial rotation to a follow-through position of flexion, adduction, and lateral rotation. When you sit in a relaxed position with your feet up and hands behind your head, the shoulder is in flexion, abduction, and lateral rotation, and your legs are extended in front of you, crossed, and in adduction and lateral rotation.

If you remember these natural positions, the patterns of movement for the part of the extremity beyond the shoulder and hip should make sense. Figures 7.34 and 7.35 diagram and illustrate the positions of the other joints in D1 and D2 patterns.

In each position, the joints go from one extreme to the other by the time the movement is complete. For example, if the patient begins with the shoulder extended, abducted, and medially rotated, the elbow extended, the forearm pronated, the wrist ulnarly extended, and the fingers and thumb extended, the end position will be the D1 flexion position—in shoulder flexion, adduction, and lateral rotation, elbow flexion, forearm supination, wrist radially flexed, and fingers and thumb flexed and adducted. Note that the elbow and the knee can be moved from flexion to extension or extension to flexion with any of the patterns. The position the elbow or knee is in at the end of the motion is the opposite of the joint's position at the beginning of the movement.

Essentially, all that has been written about PNF in recent years has been based on the works of Knott and Voss (1968). The patterns of movement, techniques, and principles most commonly used today center on the information these authors have provided to the medical community. For the best results, they advocate the use of basic principles in the application of PNF.

Principles

The principles of application incorporate the physiological facilitation and inhibition responses of the body to stimuli. Effective use of these responses produces an optimum result. The primary principles of application are the following:

1. *The clinician's hand placement is important for providing appropriate facilitation of the deep-touch and pressure receptors.* The hands should be placed on the surface side toward which the extremity is to move to stimulate those muscles. For example, if the patient's hip is moving into extension, the knee is flexing, and the foot is plantar flexing, the hamstrings and plantar foot should be the points of contact.

Joint	D1 flexion	D2 flexion
Shoulder:	Flexion	Flexion
	Lateral rotation	Lateral rotation
	Adduction	Abduction
Forearm:	Supination	Supination
Wrist:	Radial flexion	Radial extension
Fingers:	Flexion	Extension

Joint	D2 extension	D1 extension
Shoulder:	Extension	Extension
	Medial rotation	Medial rotation
	Adduction	Abduction
Forearm:	Pronation	Pronation
Wrist:	Ulnar flexion	Ulnar extension
Fingers:	Flexion	Extension

Figure 7.34 Upper-extremity PNF patterns.

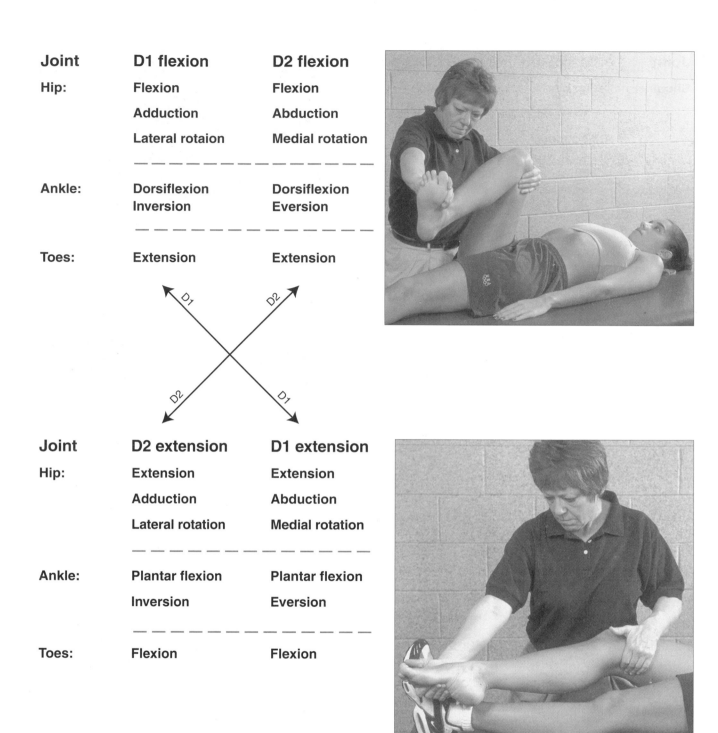

Joint	D1 flexion	D2 flexion
Hip:	Flexion	Flexion
	Adduction	Abduction
	Lateral rotaion	Medial rotation
Ankle:	Dorsiflexion Inversion	Dorsiflexion Eversion
Toes:	Extension	Extension

Joint	D2 extension	D1 extension
Hip:	Extension	Extension
	Adduction	Abduction
	Lateral rotation	Medial rotation
Ankle:	Plantar flexion Inversion	Plantar flexion Eversion
Toes:	Flexion	Flexion

Figure 7.35 Lower-extremity PNF patterns.

Manual contact using appropriately applied pressure also helps guide the patient's extremity in the correct direction. The contact should be firm and reassuring, not painful or hesitant.

2. *Verbal cues are given in a moderate tone if the patient is providing a maximal output.* If additional force is desired, a stronger, sharp verbal command is given. The wording should be one- or two-word phrases, simple and meaningful. For example, "push" or "pull," "hold" or "relax," and "rotate" or "across" are all simple commands that give the patient easy-to-understand, clear instructions. The commands should be timed correctly in relation to the activity.

3. *The technique should not be painful.* Pain will produce a reflex withdrawal and cause an inhibition of activity rather than facilitation.

4. *Proper instruction in the PNF pattern before the start of exercise is important if the muscles are to receive optimal facilitation.* The patient should receive simple instructions that include the sequencing of activities, the diagonal pattern, and appropriate speed of activity. If the patient knows before execution what is expected and understands the exercise, the patient is better able to perform the activity and elicit a stronger response from the muscle. The visual stimulation of seeing the movement before performance of the exercise provides additional feedback for the patient's increased facilitation of the muscles.

5. *Rotation is an important component of the diagonal motion.* It begins distally and progresses toward the proximal muscle groups as the patient continues through the motion. Rotation begins the pattern so by mid-ROM, rotation movement should be finished. Proper verbal cueing for correct distal-to-proximal movement assists the patient in proper execution of the exercise.

6. *Providing traction to separate the joint surfaces or approximation to compress the joint surfaces stimulates the joint's proprioceptive nerve endings.* As a general rule, traction is used in the pulling motions and approximation is used in the pushing motions. If a joint is very irritable, traction or approximation may aggravate it; one must use caution and good judgment before applying this technique.

7. *A quick stretch applied immediately before the beginning of the movement pattern uses the stretch reflex to facilitate the muscle into a stronger initial response.* In some injuries, a stretch may be contraindicated. Once again, caution and good judgment are needed before a quick stretch is applied.

8. *The motions are performed precisely and through a smooth range of motion.* The movement is not jerky. Isometric contractions should build until maximal output from the patient's muscle is achieved. No motion is produced by an isometric activity, and the rehabilitation clinician does not break the isometric hold.

9. *The clinician must use good body mechanics.* Application of manual resistance in PNF techniques requires that the rehabilitation clinician use his or her own body efficiently and safely and conserve energy. Proper body mechanics makes this possible.

Techniques

Stretching techniques of PNF, including hold-relax, contract-relax, and slow reversal-hold-relax, are discussed in chapter 5. The techniques used for strengthening are rhythmic stabilization, slow reversal, and slow reversal-hold. Whether a PNF technique is used to gain mobility or strength, the principles and movement patterns presented above hold true.

PNF techniques can be confusing if correct terminology is not understood. There are two patterns in PNF: agonistic and antagonistic. The *agonistic muscle pattern* occurs when the muscle is contracting toward its shortened state. The *antagonistic muscle pattern* occurs when the muscle is approaching its lengthened state. The location of the antagonistic pattern is diagonally opposite of the agonistic pattern of motion.

PNF Techniques

Stretching

Hold-relax
Contract-relax
Slow Reversal-Hold-relax

Strengthening

Rhythmic initiation
Rhythmic stabilization
Slow reversal
Slow reversal-hold

Rhythmic Initiation is used to increase a muscle's ability to initiate movement and stabilize. It includes voluntary relaxation, passive movement, and repeated isotonic activity in the agonistic pattern. The extremity is moved by the clinician to the shortened range of the antagonistic pattern. The patient is then asked to move the extremity through the agonistic muscle pattern. The exercise may start as an active-assistive exercise in a very weak patient and progress to resistive motion. In more advanced procedures, an isometric activity in the weaker portion of the motion can be incorporated within the isotonic movement. Athletes are usually at a higher level than patients who most benefit from this technique, so it is not used often with patients seen by rehabilitation clinicians working with athletes.

Reversal of Antagonists techniques are the ones most commonly used in rehabilitation. They most mimic normal activity because they incorporate the use of first one muscle group and then its opposing muscle group, much as daily activities and sport performance activities do. These techniques begin in the end range of the agonistic pattern with resisted motion occurring first in the antagonistic pattern of motion. This is immediately followed by resistance through the agonistic pattern. These techniques include rhythmic stabilization, slow reversal, and slow reversal-hold.

Rhythmic stabilization uses isometric activity of agonists and antagonists. The rehabilitation clinician offers resistance that does not break the isometric activity of the antagonist and then offers resistance to isometric activity of the agonist. This produces a co-contraction to improve stabilization. The technique is repeated several times without movement of the extremity with no pause between the contractions. It can be repeated at several points within the range of motion. Isometric contractions are first performed in an antagonistic pattern and then in an agonistic pattern.

Slow reversal is a technique that provides a maximum resistance in an antagonistic pattern from the rehabilitation clinician throughout a range of motion. This is followed by resistance in the agonistic pattern of motion. For example, if hamstrings were the weak muscle group, the clinician applies resistance to the lower extremity D1 pattern going into hip flexion-adduction-lateral rotation. At the completion of the antagonistic movement pattern, the rehabilitation clinician reverses hand positions on the patient's lower extremity to provide resistance to D1 going into hip extension-abduction-medial rotation moving into an agonistic pattern. In the *slow reversal-hold* technique, the procedure is the same except that an isometric hold is performed at the end of the motion.

These techniques can be applied individually or in combination. Their use is determined by the patient's deficiencies and needs.

▶ The rehabilitation clinician should be deliberate about when in a program to start strengthening exercises and should follow the principles of specificity, no pain, attainable goals, and progressive overload.

STRENGTHENING PRINCIPLES

When do strengthening exercises begin in a therapeutic exercise program? The answer depends on the severity of the injury, the tissue injured, healing time line, the physician's preference, and the patient's tolerance. Once a therapeutic exercise program starts, strengthening exercises at some level should begin. At first they may be no more than isometrics or exercises that concentrate on other areas or those adjacent to the injured site. Chapter 2 addresses the importance of rest and the importance of activity. The rehabilitation clinician makes a careful judgment and considers the variable factors to determine when the strengthening exercises should occur and how intense they should be.

The rehabilitation clinician should have a sound reason for using any strengthening exercise in a patient's therapeutic exercise program. Use of many exercises that have the same goal and that work the same muscle may be a waste of time unless the specific goal is to increase muscle endurance and provide variety to prevent boredom. The rehabilitation clinician should design a therapeutic exercise program specific to the needs of the patient as determined by analysis of the patient's deficiencies and knowledge of the demands of the patient's activities. A strengthening program may emphasize primarily strength or muscle endurance or a combination of these.

Progression of a patient in a therapeutic exercise program is individually determined. Each patient is different. Expectations based on other patients' progression or the rehabilitation clinician's hopes are unrealistic and unfair. You should periodically examine the injury during the treatment program so that you can accurately determine the response to treatment and maintain an optimal course of treatment.

A strengthening program is designed according to four principles. The acronym **SNAP** stands for the primary concerns in the establishment of any strengthening program:

Specific exercises
No pain
Attainable goals
Progressive overload

Let's look at each of these issues individually.

Specific Exercises

A therapeutic exercise program should contain specific exercises to achieve the long-term goal: the patient's return to normal activity or sport performance. This concept is often referred to as the **SAID** principle: **S**pecific **A**daptations to **I**mposed **D**emands (Wallis and Logan 1964). This means that the muscle will adapt and perform according to the demands placed on it. For example, if a patient lifts low weights for high repetitions, the muscle will gain endurance. If a patient wants to gain strength, resistance should be closer to his or her maximum resistance and consist of about six repetitions. The SAID principle also means that exercises should mimic stresses placed on a muscle during functional activities to produce appropriate strength gains. If a patient's sport calls for sustained activity, such as holding a pike position on the parallel bars in gymnastics, then the strength exercises for that patient should include isometric hip flexor and abdominal exercises. If the patient's sport is soccer, which does not demand sustained movements, the therapeutic exercise program for that patient requires more isotonic endurance and power-related activities.

Since a muscle's greatest recovery occurs in the first 30 to 90 s following exercise to exhaustion, the design of the therapeutic exercise program should take this into account (figure 7.36). As a muscle continues an activity, the maximal output declines as fatigue becomes more of a factor with more repetitions. Exercise sets should include a rest period of 30 to 60 s between each set. A rule of thumb is a 1:1 ratio between the time it takes to perform the exercise and the rest time. Later in the program the patient may need more or less rest, depending on the intensity of the exercise and the patient's goals.

a

b

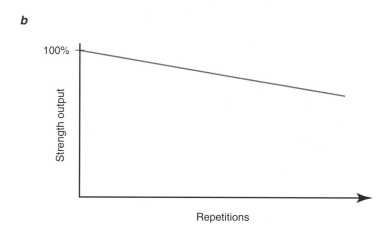

Figure 7.36 Effects of fatigue on strength and recovery: *(a)* recovery from fatigue, *(b)* maximal output declines with fatigue from repetitious activity.

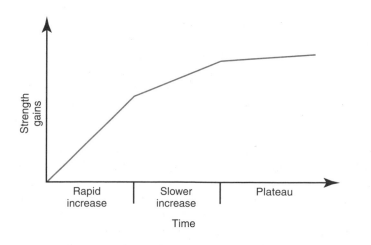

Figure 7.37 Rate of strength gains in a rehabilitation program.

In the early stages of a therapeutic exercise program, rapid gains in strength are commonly seen in a debilitated or deconditioned muscle. This occurs during the first three to five weeks of a therapeutic exercise program without a change in the muscle's atrophy (Moritani and deVries 1979). Many believe that these initial strength gains are primarily the result of neural adaptations within the muscle's neuromuscular system.

Reflex inhibition of the muscle occurs with injury or inactivity. Immediate weakness is present after surgery as well. These sudden declines in strength are attributable to decreased neural activity. Because neural adaptations occur quickly with injury, it is postulated that they are also affected with attempts to restore the injured part.

Strength is determined by both muscle fiber and neural control. The initial rapid gains in strength are attributed to improved neuromuscular recruitment, efficiency, coordination, and motor unit re-education. Many researchers believe that improved neural activation results in an increased activation of synergists with a better coordination and co-contraction of the synergists, an inhibition of the antagonists, and improved activation ability and sensitivity to facilitation of the prime movers. A learning factor also affects the neural element of muscle activity.

Evidence to date appears to be anecdotal only; clinical observation has indicated that the rate of strength gains decreases as a therapeutic exercise program advances in time and duration (Houglum 1977) (figure 7.37). Once the neural components have been retrained, the gains are primarily made through muscle fiber hypertrophy. The greatest gains in strength occur in the early stages of a therapeutic exercise program—presenting the probability that neural changes are more significant than muscle size changes, especially in rehabilitation. Primary hypertrophic changes occur more commonly in patients who have lifted weights over a longer period of time or who use drugs to enhance hypertrophy.

In the early stages of a therapeutic exercise program, especially in cases in which muscle inactivity has been prolonged, the initial exercise efforts should emphasize facilitation of the neural elements of the atrophied muscle. In addition to active exercise, electrical stimulation to assist in the facilitation of these neural pathways and in facilitation of proper muscle response may expedite recovery.

Refer to Denegar and colleagues' (2005) text, *Therapeutic Modalities for Musculoskeletal Injuries, Second Edition* in the Athletic Training Education Series, for specifics on the application of electrical stimulation for muscle facilitation.

If a therapeutic exercise program following severe injury or surgery is prolonged, you will see a sequence of rapid increase, slower increase, and plateau. These changes can occur over one cycle or more than one cycle. The pattern is individually determined and not predictable. If the patient reaches a plateau early in the program before achieving goals, you should explain that this is not unusual and that gains will come if the patient persists in the program. This situation can be difficult for the patient, since it may seem that no amount of effort produces gains. Patience and perseverance are key to maintaining a good motivation level during this time. Sometimes the psychological lift of having a day off from the therex program can have a rejuvenating effect.

No Pain

There should be no pain during strengthening exercises. Delayed pain or post-exercise pain should be avoided. Post-exercise pain accompanied by post-exercise edema is an indication that the exercises have been too severe. It is advisable to reduce the severity of the exercise or even postpone the application of a strengthening exercise if you observe these symptoms. Pain produces a reflex withdrawal of muscle activity so that the muscle will not produce a maximal output. Progression of strengthening exercises should be gradual and within the patient's tolerance. If you increase resistance too much too quickly, the patient's body may experience an inflammatory response. Increased edema and pain are key signs of inflammation.

Attainable Goals

Goals for the patient should be challenging but attainable. This means that it should be possible for the patient to move the selected weight for the required number of repetitions and sets and to perform the specific exercise. Most patients are goal oriented and are determined to achieve any goal set for them by themselves or by others. If goals are not achievable, the unrealistic expectations placed on the patient will serve only to frustrate both you and the patient. If you discover during the course of the exercise routine that you have set too high a goal, it is best to adjust the goal. Occasionally you may need to adjust goals according to the patient's response to the previous exercise session. This is more often the case early in the rehabilitation program when you may not yet know the patient's abilities, motivation level, and response to treatments. Realistic expectations are the key to a successful therapeutic exercise session.

Progressive Overload

Providing a **progressive overload** of exercises is key to muscle strengthening. To continue to produce strength gains, the load must be progressively greater. This concept is sometimes referred to as the **overload principle:** As a muscle's strength increases, the muscle must be overloaded. For example, if a biceps can lift 8 kg, it must lift more resistance than 8 kg in order to achieve increased strength. If the muscle lifts 8 kg repeatedly from one exercise session to the next, its strength will be maintained but will not increase. The weight must be greater than 8 kg, but still be possible to lift, in order to produce strength gains.

When it is not possible to actively exercise the injured area, **cross-training** can produce strength gains. Cross-training occurs when the contralateral part is exercised, resulting in strength gains on the opposite extremity. This form of training, sometimes also referred to as *cross-education*, has been around since the 1800s and has been used with varying degrees of success. The results depend primarily on the amount of resistance provided to the exercising extremity: The greater the effort of the extremity, the greater the results. This is a useful technique that you can apply in therapeutic exercise programs when the patient's injured area is restricted, perhaps because it is in a cast or splint, and exercise of the part is limited.

EXERCISE PROGRESSION

▶ Several commonly used progressive overload systems are available.

A progressive overload can be applied using various systems of progression. Several programs have been advocated by a number of professionals over the years and have been used rather widely in rehabilitation.

DeLorme and Watkins (1948) provided a system that would serve as a basis of progressive strengthening for many years. They used 10 RM as a maximum strength. They advocated the use of three bouts, or sets, of exercise, 10 repetitions each: The first set is at 50% of maximum, the second set at 75% of maximum, and the final set at 100% of the 10 RM (table 7.4).

Zinovieff, a physician who worked at England's United Oxford Hospitals, published a revision of the DeLorme program that he named the Oxford Technique (1951). Zinovieff found that with the DeLorme system his patients were too fatigued to complete the final set of 10 RM exercises. He suggested reversing the system, starting with the 10 RM on the first set of 10 repetitions and progressively reducing to 75% and then 50% on each successive set of 10 repetitions (table 7.5).

A number of authors have advanced a variety of other resistive exercise progressions. One of the more frequently used systems is the **DAPRE** (**D**aily **A**djusted **P**rogressive **R**esistive **E**xercise) technique (Knight 1985). This is a complex system of daily exercise (six days a week) progression that meets the individual's ability to tolerate increased resistance. Table 7.6 illustrates the establishment of an RM and number of repetitions along with the determination of the next session's exercise weight.

The essential element of DAPRE is that on the third and fourth sets of exercise, the patient performs as many repetitions as possible. The number of repetitions the individual can perform on the third set determines the amount of weight to be added for the fourth set of the day as well as for the next treatment session.

The intent of the program is to have the patient perform as many repetitions during the set as possible. The goal is 5 to 7 repetitions. If the patient does 8 to 12 repetitions, the weight change is minimal; but if the patient performs 15 to 20 repetitions, the weight change is significantly larger. This program continues until the strength of the injured part is within 10% of the strength of the noninjured counterpart. At that time the emphasis shifts to other deficiencies such as muscle endurance or coordination, and the DAPRE program is continued twice a week to maintain strength.

Most rehabilitation clinicians develop an exercise routine that seems to work best for them in achieving progression of a patient's strength. In the early stages of strengthening, the pro-

Table 7.4

DeLorme and Watkins Strength Progression

Set	Repetitions	Weight
1	10	50% of 10 RM
2	10	75% of 10 RM
3	10	100% of 10 RM

Table 7.5

Oxford Technique of Strength Progression

Set	Repetitions	Weight
1	10	100% of 10 RM
2	10	75% of 10 RM
3	10	50% of 10 RM

Table 7.6
DAPRE System of Strength Progression

Technique		
Set	**Repetitions**	**Weight**
1	10	50% of working weight
2	6	75% of working weight
3	As many as possible	100% of working weight
4	As many as possible	Adjusted from 3rd set*

*See Adjustment guidelines.

Adjustment guidelines		
Number of repetitions performed during prior set	**4th-set weight adjustment based on 3rd set**	**Next-day weight adjustment based on 4th set**
0-2	wt; redo set	wt; redo set
3-4	by 0-5 lb	Keep the same
5-7	Keep the same	by 5-10 lb
8-12	by 5-10 lb	by 5-15 lb
13 or more	by 10-15 lb	by 10-20 lb

The number of repetitions performed on the third set determines the weight used on the fourth set. The next treatment day's starting weight is determined by the number of repetitions performed on the fourth set of the previous treatment.

Based on Knight 1985.

gram I prefer has the patient lifting a weight that can be controlled for 6 to 15 repetitions for two sets. That weight is continued, with the patient attempting to perform as many repetitions as possible, until he or she is able to perform the exercise successfully for three sets of 20 to 25 repetitions each. At this point the weight increases and the patient reduces the number of repetitions. It is important, though, for the patient to perform as many repetitions as possible during each exercise session. The number of sets and repetitions depends on the demands of the patient's normal activity. Once the desired base-strength level is achieved, the number of sets, repetitions or exercise speed changes to meet the patient's sport demands.

As mentioned earlier in this chapter, Wathen (1994) advocates the use of three to six repetitions for strength gains, repeated for about three sets. Figure 7.38 shows the relative gains in muscle strength and endurance with varying numbers of repetitions.

The program that the rehabilitation clinician chooses depends on individual preferences, his or her judgment about which program would benefit the patient most, and time availability. All the programs we have considered have been shown to be beneficial for making strength gains. As you gain experience with many patients who have varied therapeutic exercise needs, you will find a system that seems to work best for you. Until then, I recommend that you keep an open mind, try different programs, and investigate the systems presented here as well as others to see what produces the best results for you. Whether you use an existing program or design one yourself, the key element for success is that it must be progressive; it must continue to stress the patient's muscles for continued improvement toward the specific rehabilitation goals. Experienced professionals often adjust programs according to what produces the best results.

Figure 7.38 Houglum progression.

SUMMARY

1. Describe the sarcomere and its function in muscle activity.

   The contractile element of a muscle fiber is the sarcomere. Actin and myosin filaments and their relationship to each other via cross-bridges determine the length of the sarcomere and its activity status. A complex system of biochemical processes and the stimulation of an action potential produce muscle activity through the release of calcium and ATP to cause a sliding of actin and myosin over each other, shortening the sarcomere's length.

2. Identify the elements of a motor unit.

   A motor unit consists of a number of muscle fibers and the nerve that innervates the fibers. When stimulated, a motor unit behaves according to the all-or-none law in that all muscle fibers of the motor unit contract.

3. Explain how an action potential is transmitted.

   The sarcoplasmic reticulum releases calcium to the muscle fibers through its T-tubules to the Z-disks where the calcium binds to the troponin on the actin filaments. This causes the tropomyosin on the actin filaments to shift and allow the head of the myosin cross-bridges to attach to the actin, shortening the sarcomere. The ATPase on the cross-bridges breaks down ATP for energy to allow the cross-bridges to re-cock and continue muscle activity. As long as calcium is present, the activity can continue.

4. Explain the differences between fast-twitch and slow-twitch muscle fibers.

   Compared to fast-twitch or type II fibers, the slow-twitch, type I fibers are smaller, are red, have a slower conduction velocity, have a lower recruitment threshold, have lower minimum and maximum firing rates, have slower-acting myosin ATPase, have a greater number of mitochondria, and function in endurance activities rather than in rapid, brief bursts of activity.

5. Discuss the relationship between muscle strength, endurance, and power.

   Muscle function includes strength, endurance, and power. Athletic activity involves all these factors to different degrees, depending on its specific demands. Muscle strength and endurance are closely related. Strength is the ability to produce force, and endurance is the ability to produce less forceful activities over a longer period of time; power is the strength output related to time.

6. Identify the various types of dynamic activity.

   Dynamic activity includes muscle tension with movement. Dynamic activity is divided into isotonic and isokinetic activity. Isotonic activity is further divided into concentric and eccentric activity.

7. Discuss the differences between open and closed kinetic chain activity.

   Open kinetic chain activity occurs when the distal aspect of the limb is not fixed; closed kinetic chain activity occurs when the distal aspect is fixed or anchored.

8. Identify the various grades of manual muscle testing.

   Muscle strength is rated from 5 (normal) to 0 (no function). A grade 4 muscle is one that offers some resistance beyond gravity but not normal resistance; a grade 3 muscle is able to lift the limb against gravity but unable to offer any additional strength; a grade 2 muscle is one that is able to move the limb through a full range of motion in a gravity-eliminated position; and a grade 1 muscle provides some voluntary activity but is unable to move the segment through a range of motion.

9. Discuss the types of muscle activity.

Passive motion is performed by an outside force without voluntary muscle activity; active assistive motion is motion that occurs through a combination of voluntary and assistive mechanisms; active motion occurs without the aid of any outside mechanism; and resistive motion occurs through a range of motion within which resistance to that motion is present.

10. List the PNF techniques commonly used in rehabilitaion and their purposes.

Rhythmic initiation, slow reversal, slow reversal-hold, and rhythmic stabilization are the PNF techniques most commonly used for strengthening. The techniques used to gain motion include hold-relax, contract-relax, and slow reversal-hold-relax.

11. Identify four principles of strengthening exercises.

Development of a therapeutic exercise program must include consideration of SNAP guidelines: specific exercise, no pain, attainable goals, and progressive overload.

CRITICAL THINKING QUESTIONS

1. If you provide manual resistance to a patient's shoulder flexors, will the position in which the patient has been placed make any difference? Why or why not?

2. What steps could you take to improve performance if a patient were unable to perform a straight-leg raise without assistance because of weakness? How would your selection improve the patient's performance? How would it enable the patient to perform a straight-leg raise independently?

3. Explain four techniques that you could use to change the resistance without changing the amount of weight in a shoulder flexion exercise.

4. For a patient who has weakness in the quads, explain three progressive open kinetic chain and three progressive closed kinetic chain exercises you could use to strengthen the quads. What, if anything, would determine whether you started with the open or closed kinetic chain exercises?

5. If a patient were unable to bear weight on the lower extremity, not because of medical restriction but because of apprehension, what progression of activities would you select so that the patient could progress to weight bearing? What obstacles would you have to overcome for the patient to gain confidence that the leg would support him or her?

6. Is a patient able to lift a heavier dumbbell in elbow flexion in a seated or supine position? Where in the motion is the weight the most difficult for the patient to lift? Why? Is it a good idea to have the patient perform an elbow curl in both positions? Why? What other elbow-curl exercise would be an adequate substitute for a dumbbell exercise?

7. List six progressive exercises you would give Kamryn in the chapter's opening scenario. What is your justification for each exercise, and what are your criteria for progression?

LAB ACTIVITIES

1. Have your lab partner lift 5 lb in shoulder flexion in a standing position, supine position, and prone position. Where in the range of motion for each exercise did the patient encounter the most difficulty? Why? Of what relevance is this to you in setting up a patient on a strengthening program?

2. With your lab partner in supine and one leg abducted and extension, place your hand on the top of her foot. Place your other hand on the calf and have your partner move the hip into flexion and adduction up and across the body. Instruct your partner to provide as much resistance moving into hip flexion as possible. Now repeat the resistive motion but remove your hand from the calf. What difference did you

detect in the amount of resistance offered by your partner? What do you think is the reason for this change in resistance?

3. Have your lab partner perform a lateral step up. Identify all the possible ways she could substitute and not use the muscles correctly for this exercise? For each error, indicate what suggestion you would provide the patient to perform the activity correctly.

4. Perform a step-up exercise and then return to the start position. What muscles are being used going up the step? What muscles are used going down? What type of muscle contraction is used to go up and to go down?

5. With your forearm on a table, grasping a bar with a weight at its end, move your forearm all the way from full pronation to full supination and back to the start position. Explain what muscle and what type of muscle contraction is occurring throughout the range of motion in both directions. How would this information influence a rehabilitation program for the elbow or wrist?

6. Have your lab partner lie prone and isometrically contract the hamstrings at 0, 45, 90, and 120° of knee flexion while you provide maximal resistance against your partner at each position. Compare the force production at each of these angles. Describe these differences. Consider the length-tension curve and the moment arm of the hamstrings. How does this information impact how you might set a patient on an early strength program?

7. Perform the following activities and identify the primary muscle(s) performing the activity and what part of the motion is concentric and what part is eccentric for that (those) muscle(s):

    a. Getting up from a chair

    b. Sitting down into a chair

    c. Doing a modified push-up

    d. Doing an abdominal curl

    e. Doing an elbow curl

    f. Doing a French curl

    g. Walking up stairs

    h. Walking down stairs

    i. Performing a vertical jump

   What realization has this given you regarding activity or performance? Of what relevance is this in establishing a strengthening program for a patient?

8. Identify how you could have a patient perform a quadriceps strengthening exercise using the following methods:

    a. Manual resistance

    b. Body weight resistance

    c. Rubber band or tubing

    d. Free weight

    e. Machine weight

    f. Isokinetics

9. A shot putter suffered a rotator cuff strain and has been undergoing a rehabilitation program. This will be his first day of strength exercises. How will you determine what exercises and number of repetitions he should start with today? Provide a justification for each exercise. What is the determining factor in the number of repetitions he will perform for all of his strength exercises? Indicate a progression of strength exercises for the rotator cuff for this patient. How will this patient's program differ from that of a baseball pitcher who has also suffered a rotator cuff strain and is at the same stage in his rehabilitation program? Why?

REFERENCES

Berger, R.A. 1962. Optimal repetitions for the development of strength. *Research Quarterly* 33: 334–338.

Billeter, H., and H. Hoppeler. 1992. Muscular basis of strength. In *Strength and power in sport*, ed. P.V. Komi. Boston: Blackwell Scientific.

Braatz, J.H., and P.P. Gogia. 1987. The mechanics of pitching. *Journal of Orthopedic and Sports Physical Therapy* 9:56–69.

Brown, D.R. 1980. *Neurosciences for allied health therapies.* St. Louis: Mosby.

Clarke, D.H. 1971. The influence on muscular fatigue patterns of the intercontraction rest interval. *Medicine and Science in Sports* 3:83–88.

Clarke, D.H. 1975. *Exercise physiology.* Englewood Cliffs, NJ: Prentice-Hall.

DeLorme, T.L., and A.L. Watkins. 1948. Technics of progressive resistance exercise. *Archives of Physical Medicine* 29:263–273.

Denegar, C., E. Saliba and S. Saliba. 2005. *Therapeutic modalities for musculoskeletal injuries.* 2nd ed. Champaign, IL: Human Kinetics.

Enoka, R.M. 1995. Morphological features and activation patterns of motor units. *Journal of Clinical Neurophysiology* 12: 538–559.

Feigenbaum, M.S., and M.L. Pollock. 1999. Prescription of resistance training for health and disease. *Medicine & Science in Sport & Exercise.* 31:38-45.

Hettinger, T., and E. Müller. 1953. Muscle strength and muscle training. *Arbeits Physiology* 15: 111–126.

Hislop, H.J. and J. Montgomery. 2002. *Daniels and Worthingham's muscle testing. Techniques of manual examination.* Philadelphia: WB Saunders.

Houglum, P. 1977. The modality of therapeutic exercise: Objectives and principles. *Athletic Training* 12:42–45.

Hortobagy, T., and F.I. Katch. 1990. Eccentric and concentric torque-velocity relationships during arm flexion and extension. *European Journal of Applied Physiology* 60:395–401.

Hunter, G.R. 1994. Muscle physiology. In *Essentials of strength training and conditioning*, ed. T.R. Baechle. Champaign, IL: Human Kinetics.

Johnson, E.W., and D. Wiechers. 1982. Electrodiagnosis. In *Krugen's handbook of physical medicine and rehabilitation*, 3rd ed., ed. F.J. Kottke, G.K. Stillwell, and J.F. Lehmann. Philadelphia: WB Saunders.

Kendall, F.P. 1993. *Muscles, testing and function*, 4th ed. Baltimore: Williams & Wilkins.

Knight, K.L. 1985. Guidelines for rehabilitation of sports injuries. *Clinics in Sports Medicine* 4:405–416.

Knott, M., and D.E. Voss. 1968. *Proprioceptive neuromuscular facilitation.* New York: Harper & Row.

Kottke, F.J. 1982. Therapeutic exercise to maintain mobility. In *Krusen's handbook of physical medicine and rehabilitation*, ed. F.J. Kottke, G.K. Stillwell, and J.F. Lehmann. Philadelphia: Saunders.

Lieber, R.L. 1992. *Skeletal muscle structure and function. Implications for rehabilitation and sports medicine.* Baltimore: Williams & Wilkins.

Lind, A.R. 1959. Muscle fatigue and recovery from fatigue induced by sustained contractions. *Journal of Physiology (London)* 147:162–171.

MacDougall, J.D., Elder, G.C.B., Sale, D.G., Moroz, J.R., and J.R. Sutton. 1980. Effect of training and immobilization on human muscle fibers. *European Journal of Applied Physiology* 43:25–34.

Moritani, T., and H.A. deVries. 1979. Neural factors versus hypertrophy in the time course of muscle strength gain. *American Journal of Physical Medicine* 58:115–130.

Muller, E.A. 1970. Influence of training and of inactivity on muscle strength. *Archives in Physical Medicine and Rehabilitation* 51:449–462.

Page, P. 2003. More than meets the eye. *Advance for physical therapists & PT assistants.* 14:47-48.

Page, P.A., Labbe, A. and R.V. Tropp. 2000. Clinical force production of Thera-bands®. *Journal of Orthopedic and Sports Physical Therapy.* 30:A47-A48.

Sinacore, D.R., Bander, B.L., and A. Delitto. 1994. Recovery from a 1-minute bout of fatiguing exercise: Characteristics, reliability, and responsiveness. *Physical Therapy* 74:234–244.

Stamford, B. 1985. The difference between strength and power. *Physician and Sportsmedicine* 13:155.

Stone, M.H., and M.S. Conley. 1994. Bioenergetics. In *Essentials of strength training and conditioning*, ed. T.R. Baechle. Champaign, IL: Human Kinetics.

Wallis, E.L., and G.A. Logan. 1964. *Figure improvement and body conditioning through exercise.* Englewood Cliffs, NJ: Prentice-Hall.

Wathen, D. 1994. Load assignment. In *Essentials of strength training and conditioning,* ed. T.R. Baechle. Champaign, IL: Human Kinetics.

Wilmore, J.H., and D.C. Costill. 2004. *Physiology of sport and exercise.* 3rd ed. Champaign, IL: Human Kinetics.

Zinovieff, A.N. 1951. Heavy-resistance exercises. The "Oxford Technique." *British Journal of Physical Medicine* 14:129–132.

The ABCs of Proprioception

© Empics

Objectives

After completing this chapter, you should be able to do the following:

1. List the afferent receptors involved in proprioception.

2. Identify the CNS sites that relay proprioceptive information to the motor system.

3. Discuss the ABCs of proprioception.

4. Identify the systems that control balance.

5. Describe the components involved in coordination.

6. Explain a progression of proprioceptive exercises for the lower or upper extremity.

259

■ **Anybody can grab a tiger by the tail. You only survive by knowing what to do next.**

Author unknown

Agility, balance, and coordination are united together to allow an individual to move accurately, quickly, and efficiently. These three parameters are a complex unit that is dependent upon strength and flexibility for its foundation. If a muscle is too weak to move a body part, it cannot be expected to control the movement of that part. Likewise, an extremity must have the flexibility and muscle endurance necessary to allow it to function and meet the demands of athletic activity. If a muscle has limited flexibility so that it lacks the full motion required for an activity, or if a muscle is unable to work long enough to perform an activity accurately, the muscle will be unable to coordinate the segment properly for that activity.

Agility, **B**alance, and **C**oordination are also controlled by what are collectively referred to as proprioceptors (figure 8.1)—which is why this chapter refers to the **ABC**s of proprioception. **Proprioception** is fundamental to correct performance, and correct performance requires good agility, balance, and coordination. In other words, proprioceptors play a vital neurosensory role in the patient's motor skills and are a key factor in the ability to perform tasks with dexterity, mastery, and proficiency. (Note, although proprioreception is important for most activities, this chapter makes more references to sports, athletics, and athletes than most other chapters.) It is certainly necessary for individuals to have good flexibility as well as muscle endurance and strength in order to perform well, but proprioception is crucial if the individual is to execute any skill with accuracy, consistency, and precision. To know how to influence proprioception in any performance, we must first understand what proprioceptors are and how they affect execution skill.

Proprioception is the body's ability to transmit position sense, interpret the information, and respond consciously or unconsciously to stimulation through appropriate execution of posture and movement. Neuromuscular control of proprioception is produced by the input received from receptors within skin, joints, muscles, and tendons. These proprioceptors play an important role in the maintenance of posture, the conscious and unconscious awareness of joint position, and the production of motion. Proprioception is what allows us to know what position our fingers are in without looking at them. It is what maintains our balance when we stand. It is what enables

Figure 8.1 Components of proprioception.

us to write smoothly. It is what enables us to jump, run, and throw. It is what permits us to change our delivery when we miss the goal on a jump, to move from an asphalt to a gravel surface, and to correct the overshoot of our target with our throw. Although we must first have the flexibility, muscle strength, and endurance to be able to perform these activities, it is proprioception that gives us the agility to change the direction of movement quickly and efficiently, the balance to maintain our stability, and the coordination to produce the activity correctly and consistently.

Proprioceptors are afferent nerves that receive and send impulses from stimuli within skin, muscles, joints, and tendons to the **central nervous system** (CNS). Some of these impulses transmit information regarding the tension of a muscle and the relative position of a body part to control muscular activity. Some of these proprioceptive elements, such as Golgi tendon organs and muscle spindles, have been discussed in previous chapters. Other afferent elements also provide input to the CNS and determine a patient's performance ability.

An individual's agility, balance, and coordination are determined by the reception, interpretation, and response that are initiated by proprioceptors. Proprioceptors can be classified according to their location. A brief look at these elements will enhance your ability to develop appropriate therapeutic exercise programs for patients.

NEUROPHYSIOLOGY OF PROPRIOCEPTION

▶ The major categories or proprioreceptors are cutaneous receptors, muscle and tendon receptors, and joint receptors. To varying degrees, they all influence proprioreception.

The proprioceptors are located in the skin, muscles, tendons, and joints. There are several different receptors that have unique abilities to respond to different stimuli (figure 8.2).

Cutaneous Receptors

Isolation of skin and subcutaneous proprioceptive **afferent receptors** has been primarily confined to investigations of the hand. The receptors in the skin are fast-adapting afferents, slow-adapting I afferents, and slow-adapting II afferents. The fast-adapting afferents are responsible for vibration sense, and the slow adapting I and slow adapting II afferents are responsible for sensory perceptions such as skin stretching. Most researchers believe that these receptors do not play a major role in proprioception. Evidence suggests that they provide cues regarding skin stretching and fingertip touching but do not have a major impact on joint proprioception in normal subjects (Grigg 1994). However, evidence does indicate that injured subjects have an increased reliance on cutaneous receptors for proprioception (Callaghan et al. 2002). This newer information suggests that although noninjured individuals do not utilize cutaneous receptors for proprioception, body segments that are injured rely on local cutaneous receptors to "take up the slack" for those joint and ligament proprioceptors that are damaged. Much like blind individuals who rely on other sensory feedback for information on their surroundings, cutaneous proprioceptors are called into action when normal proprioceptive receptors are damaged and unable to provide needed information on a joint's position.

Rapidly adapting receptors produce a rapid burst of impulses that is quickly eroded. These receptors detect sudden changes in speed and movement such as acceleration and deceleration. On the other hand, slowly adapting receptors produce a constant maintenance level of stimulation. They are responsible for providing information regarding joint and limb position and slow changes in position.

Muscle and Tendon Receptors

The **muscle spindles** and **Golgi tendon organs (GTOs)** are the primary afferent receptors of muscles and tendons. These sensory structures are discussed in chapter 7. They are complicated structures that produce complex neuromuscular responses not only from the muscles and tendons where they are located, but also in the corresponding **antagonistic** and **synergistic** muscles. The GTO detects tension within a muscle and responds to both the contraction and the stretching of a muscle. Its stimulation results in muscle relaxation. The muscle spindle, on the other hand, responds to the stretch of a muscle. Its stimulation leads to a contraction

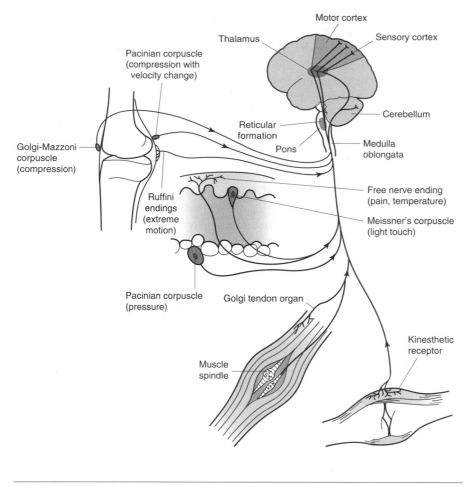

Figure 8.2 Proprioceptive afferent receptors.

of the muscle. Stimulation of these structures also causes facilitation to opposing muscles and to synergists to assist in accomplishing the desired movement. The GTO and muscle spindle are able to determine joint position because of their muscle length sensitivity. This capability also allows them to facilitate limb stabilization.

Joint Receptors

A variety of afferent receptors primarily lie within the connective tissue of a joint's capsule and surrounding ligaments and influence proprioception. They are divided into fiber type Groups II, III, and IV. Group II afferents are large-diameter axons that have high speed conduction and Group III and IV afferents are thinly myelinated or nonmyelinated, small diameter axons that have slower conduction of stimuli. The small diameter nerves do not conduct as fast as the large diameter nerves because they are not myelinated and/or their size offers more resistance to conduction than the larger diameter fibers.

The large diameter myelinated afferents are called Group II afferents. There are two types of nerve endings in this group, Ruffini endings and pacinian corpuscles. Both types are located in the joint capsule. Although the two types are sensitive to different stimuli, they both measure joint motion. The Ruffini endings, located in the joint capsule on the flexion side of the joint, are slowly adapting and respond more to loads on the surrounding connective tissue than to displacement of that connective tissue. These receptors are stimulated by extreme joint motion when the capsule is stressed in extension with rotation. They are thought to be limit-detectors and protectors of unstable joints.

Pacinian corpuscles lie throughout the capsule, joint, and periarticular structures. Because they are rapidly adapting receptors, they are thought to be compression sensitive, especially during high velocity changes when the joint accelerates or decelerates as it moves into its limits of motion.

Another afferent nerve ending, Golgi-Mazzoni corpuscles, are located in joint capsules. They are stimulated by joint compression but not by joint motion. Any weight-bearing activity stimulates these slowly adapting receptors. They do not appear to play a role in proprioception except in identification of joint compression.

The small diameter nonmyelinated axons are divided into Group III and Group IV afferents. Group IV afferents are C fibers and Group III afferents are small diameter A fibers. These are grouped together because they are both pain receptors and are called free nerve endings because of the appearance of their nerve terminals. Located throughout soft tissue and articular structures, these are **nociceptors** that are stimulated by pain and inflammation when a joint is placed in an end position. They do not play a role in proprioception, but can evoke a flexion response to cause a joint to unload and thereby protect it.

Other Receptors

Ligaments also contain receptors. Although receptors have been identified in knee and shoulder ligaments, the most thoroughly investigated ligament receptors are those in the knee's anterior cruciate ligament. These receptors are generally not active in the middle ranges of movement but become stimulated when the ligament is stressed. When stimulated by ligament tension, they produce an inhibitory response of the **agonistic** muscles.

As important as it is to realize that many different afferent receptors in many structures are affected by joint movement, it is also important to understand that they do not work independently (Strasmann and van der Wal et al. 1990). There are afferent nerves that collaborate with each other throughout the body. Local afferent nerves work together to produce a complete picture of joint position and motion for the CNS. Such input allows the CNS to process and interpret the input to produce an accurate response. To make this easier to understand, think about what it would be like to try to correct a baseball pitcher's delivery if you watched only the pitcher's hand. You could not accurately identify necessary changes in the delivery unless you had the complete picture of the pitcher's performance—by watching the entire delivery and analyzing all of the joint movements and positions. Similarly, the CNS cannot determine the position of an extremity unless it receives input from all sensory, motor, and joint receptors.

CENTRAL NERVOUS SYSTEM PROPRIOCEPTOR SITES

▶ After the afferent nerves send their input to the CNS, the body's motor response depends on which of three CNS sites has received the impulse—the spinal cord, the brain stem, or the cerebral cortex.

Once the afferent nerves have sent their input to the CNS, the body's motor response is determined by the location within the CNS that interprets the stimuli and initiates the efferent reaction. There are three areas within the CNS that will react to the stimuli: **spinal cord**, **brain stem**, and **cerebral cortex**.

Spinal Cord

If an impulse goes from a dorsal root afferent nerve either to an **internuncial** connecting nerve or directly to an efferent nerve in the spinal cord, and then immediately out the ventral root to the muscle, it is called a **spinal reflex**. This is a response in its simplest form. The reflexes that do not use an internuncial neuron produce a more rapid response than those that use an internuncial nerve. This is because of the additional time it takes to transmit from one nerve to another. The fewer the connections, the more rapid the reflex response. These proprioceptive reflexes are often used to protect an area through muscle splinting or rapid withdrawal motion. For example, a joint that is under excessive stress can be protected by the activation of the muscle's reflex flexion response to suddenly reduce the load on a joint. Reflexes are also used to provide joint stability, especially when there is a sudden change of direction or position. The joint proprioceptors, the muscle spindles, and GTOs all work together to produce a reflex response that provides the joint with stability to prevent injury.

Brain Stem

The brain stem is the primary proprioceptive correlation center. The proprioceptors relay information via interneurons in the spinal cord that connect to ascending pathways to the brain stem to maintain desired position or posture (figure 8.3). The brain stem also receives input from other areas such as the eye's visual afferent centers and the ear's vestibular afferent centers to assist in maintaining balance reflexively. The brain stem then sends excitatory or inhibitory efferent stimulation to produce an appropriate response. We will consider the importance of these sensory systems in the section "Balance."

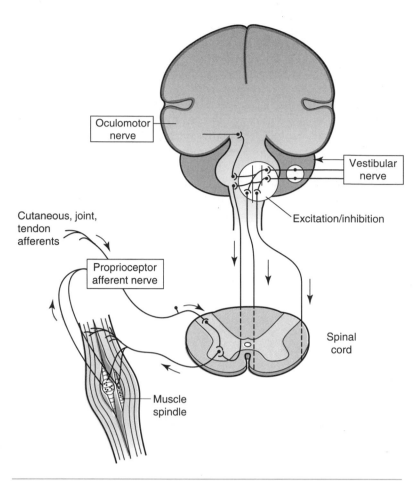

Figure 8.3 Balance pathways include oculomotor, vestibular, and proprioceptor pathways. These three neural pathways for balance result in inhibitory and/or excitatory stimulation to affect the body's motor response.

Cerebral Cortex

Sensory pathways travel to the cortex of the **cerebrum** (figure 8.3). This is the highest level of the brain and the location of conscious movement—the center of volitional control of movement. It is here that correct movement is learned and consciously controlled before it becomes an automatic response. To understand this process, think about how you learned to type. When you were first learning, you were very conscious of what your fingers were doing and where they were on the keyboard. Now, after several years of typing, you do not have to think about what you are doing because the activity has become automatic. You make fewer mistakes and perform the activity faster than you did as a beginning typist. This is what occurs with any activity that is practiced repeatedly; conscious performance becomes automatic performance, and cognitive awareness of the activity is not required.

The ABCs of proprioception include simple and complex functions. This is relative, though, since even the simplest function involves complex neuromuscular connections. Agility, balance, and coordination are all interrelated. This is the case simply because they have similar roots, the body's proprioceptors. These functions are discussed here in order of their complexity, beginning with the simplest and progressing to the more highly challenging functions.

BALANCE

▶ Balance involves three systems—the vestibular system, the oculomotor system, and the proprioceptive system. The rehabilitation clinician can perform simple tests to evaluate balance.

Balance is fundamental to most activities. Balance is required to perform a simple activity such as standing. Correct performance requires the maintenance of balance. An individual who does not have good balance is in danger of injury. If balance is not restored following an injury, the risk of re-injury significantly increases.

Balance is the body's ability to maintain equilibrium by controlling the body's center of gravity over its base of support. Balance is important in both static and dynamic activities. Standing and sitting are static balance activities. Examples of dynamic balance activities include walking, running, and dancing.

Balance is influenced by strength and by input from the CNS. It is because strength influences balance that strength is emphasized before proprioception in a therapeutic exercise program. As already mentioned, the brain stem receives sensory input from the vestibular system, the visual system, and the proprioceptors (figure 8.4). The combination of input from the ears, eyes, and proprioceptors is crucial to maintaining good balance and posture. If you have ever had an inner ear infection, you may remember the difficulty you had in maintaining balance. A simple test to highlight the importance of visual input for balance is to stand on one foot with your eyes open and then close your eyes. You will discover that without visual input, it is more difficult to maintain balance. So, too, when proprioceptors are damaged following surgery or injury, balance can be impaired.

Figure 8.4 Feedback system for coordination.

Other factors can influence balance, but they depend on the visual, auditory, and proprioceptive systems. For example, a patient's ability to focus on the task at hand is basic to the cognitive portion of the proprioceptive system, and a patient's ability to perform skills on different playing surfaces is directly related to the proprioceptive system.

Vestibular System

The **vestibular system** within the inner ear is responsible for sending messages to the CNS regarding vertical and horizontal position and motion. The vestibular system includes three semicircular canals within the inner ear that detect changes in position and aid the body in maintaining an upright posture. The inner ear also has two sacs. One sac, the saccule, regulates equilibrium; the other, the utricle, senses forward-backward head motion. Both sacs respond to gravity and are sensitive to head and body motions. The inner ear provides a vestibular ocular reflex. This allows the eyes to remain steady when the body is in motion.

Oculomotor System

Vision assists in providing feedback about the relative position of the body in space. This feedback system is referred to as the **oculomotor system.** As already noted, with your eyes closed it is more difficult to maintain good balance than with your eyes open. If you dive under water with your eyes closed or are in water in which vision is impaired, you can get disoriented and not know whether you are upright relative to the water's surface and bottom. If you sit in an environment that contains a lot of activity, the oculomotor and vestibular systems work together to determine whether you or the environment is moving. Sometimes the feedback is not interpreted correctly and you have a sense of moving when, in fact, you are staying still and it is the environment that is moving. This may occur when your car is stopped at a light but the car next to you is moving forward—you may have a sense that you are moving backward.

Patients who must perform activities requiring rapid change of position, such as ice skaters, gymnasts, or dancers, must learn to disregard the visual input in order not to get dizzy. The vestibular system provides rapid feedback about the change in position that occurs in these athletic events, but the athlete uses the technique of visual fixation, focusing on one object and disregarding other moving objects, in order to prevent dizziness and loss of balance.

Proprioceptive system

The proprioceptive system is sometimes referred to as the **somatosensory system.** We have already discussed the importance of a good proprioceptive system for balance. When proprioceptor nerves are damaged in injuries, the system's ability to function is impaired. Joint proprioceptors in the knee and ankle are commonly injured in sport, resulting in a reduction of balance and an increase in reaction time. If their function is not restored, the patient risks re-injury and impaired performance.

Balance must be restored and exercises must be included as part of the therapeutic exercise program if the individual is to have good stability and safety during performance. There are exercises that begin at a basic level and progress to more complex, functional activities as the patient's balance improves. These specific exercises and functional activities are discussed in later chapters.

Balance Evaluation

There are simple tests to determine a patient's balance deficiencies. The difficulty of these tests changes as the patient's ability improves, proceeding from static to dynamic and from simple to more complex. The simplest test is the **Romberg test,** in which the patient stands with feet together and eyes closed. No loss of balance is a normal response. Most individuals should be able to perform this test without difficulty. A slightly more difficult test is the stork stand, in which the patient stands only on the injured leg. The patient should be able to maintain this position for 30 s without touching the other foot to the floor or using hand support. If the patient is able to perform this test satisfactorily, you can use another test that is slightly more difficult, a stork stand with the eyes closed. The patient should also be able to perform this activity for 30 s. Difficulty with any of these static tests indicates a balance deficit and needs to be addressed in the therapeutic exercise program.

COORDINATION

▶ The components of coordination include perception of activity, feedback, performance adjustment, and repetition. Development of coordination involves progression of activities from simple to more complex, as well as repetition.

Coordination is another proprioceptive function fundamental to athletic activities. **Coordination** is the complex process by which a smooth pattern of activity is produced through a combination of muscles acting together with appropriate intensity and timing. Several muscles are involved in a coordinated activity. These muscles are connected by a complex neurological network of sensory receptors, internuncial neurons, ascending and descending corticospinal pathways, and efferent receptors. Some muscles are stimulated to provide an activity while others are inhibited to permit the activity, and still others are stimulated to provide synergistic or stabilizing responses to permit the desired motion to occur. Each muscle must provide an accurate response both in timing and in intensity in order for the activity to be coordinated. If a muscle is too weak to provide the appropriate response, the activity will be uncoordinated and undesirable. For example, if a volleyball player does not have an appropriate amount of strength in the scapular rotators, the arm is not in the correct position to hit and place the ball accurately. A soccer player who has weak hip abductors on the standing leg does not have the stability needed for holding the body firm and providing the base necessary to kick the ball well enough with the opposite leg. An archer does not have accuracy in shooting without the strength in the deltoids to control the weight of the bow or the pull on the string.

If muscles are weak, they must work harder to achieve a specific output. This causes an irradiation of stimulation, called **overflow,** to other muscle groups. We see this in a simple activity such as opening a jar. If the cover comes off with little effort, minimal activity of the hand and arm is required. However, if the cover is stuck and more effort is needed, the arm muscles tighten, the grip gets stronger, the jaw muscles contract, and the entire body tenses as we attempt to open the jar. Likewise, when the muscle is performing an activity but is not strong enough to provide the appropriate motion, it tries as hard as it can to perform the activity and in so doing stimulates otherwise inactive muscles to assist. This overflow causes an undesired motion. For this reason, it is important to have the patient achieve strength gains before you include coordination activities in a therapeutic exercise program.

Coordination Components

There are specific requirements for coordinated movement. Let's briefly look at them so that the logical progression of therapeutic exercises for improved coordination becomes clear.

Activity Perception

Probably the most basic of all elements within coordination is the awareness of **volitional** muscle activity. An awareness of joint position and movement is fundamental to the ability to perform activity. Proprioceptors are key to this awareness. Vision is also important, for it gives the patient feedback about the result of the activity: Has the activity been performed as desired? Vision slows down the response to activity, but especially in the beginning when a new activity is being learned and motor patterns are being established, vision is important to the development of accuracy of motion.

Feedback

The learning process involved in the development of coordinated movement is similar to programming a computer. An activity is performed; the CNS evaluates the quality of the performance; the body sends information to the CNS to make adjustments for undesired activity; and the activity is repeated with the adjustments made. The proprioceptors are the most important elements in this feedback process. The sensory afferents send information to the cerebrum where input of the activity is received, to the **cerebellum** where automatic adjustment of muscle position and length is made, and to the spinal cord for reflex adjustments (figure 8.4). Cognitive-response information is relayed to the brain stem where it is integrated with other response feedback and sent down the spinal cord to provide an adjusted performance.

Repetition

As the activity becomes more accurate with repetition and adjustments, the performance becomes more consistent. To visualize this, we could use an analogy from cross-country skiing. The more the tracks on a trail are used, the deeper they get and the easier it becomes to stay within them. Deviation from the tracks becomes less likely the more the trail is used.

Repetition is a requirement for development of accuracy and coordination. As the activity is repeated, the effort decreases and there is less chance of overflow to the wrong muscles. Eventually, an activity **engram** that can be repeated precisely and accurately is developed. An engram is an effect or performance that is impressed upon the CNS through repetition. At this point the coordinated activity becomes automatic and is no longer a conscious process.

Inhibition

In the development of coordination it is important to inhibit undesired muscle activity. **Inhibition** cannot be trained directly (Kottke 1982). It must be facilitated by precise, slow, and controlled activity until the engram is developed and the patient can increase speed of execution without producing unwanted muscle responses. In the early developmental stages of coordination, the activity should not be so difficult that the patient's performance causes an overflow and unwanted muscle responses. Given that early coordination requires cognitive awareness and conscious correction, it is best that the patient not be distracted with too many activities. Such distractions will lead to imprecise patterns of movement because the patient will not be able to concentrate adequately on any one activity. It is better to alternate attention if the situation calls for performance of more than one activity at a time.

Inhibition is part of the computer-like adjustment process that eventually results in coordinated activity. The patient should start with low-level, basic activity to eliminate the overflow to other pathways until a coordinated pattern is established. As the desired motion becomes an engram, the activity can become more difficult, because the capacity to inhibit undesired activity becomes greater with improved coordination.

Coordination Development

Precision of motion, speed of motion, and strength are fundamental to coordination in many sport activities. As previously mentioned, once strength is achieved, coordination development through repetition of activity is crucial. The patient needs to have activities that are simple in the beginning and become more complex as skill progresses. In the beginning, simple static exercises may be enough of a challenge. Coordination development progresses from static activities to dynamic activities. For example, once the patient is able to stork stand on an unstable surface such as a foam roller or trampoline, he or she can begin dynamic activities such as balance-board and jumping activities for the lower extremities or ball tossing at a target for the upper extremities.

Progression of coordination starts with simple activities and moves to more complex ones. Increasing the speed of the activity, increasing the force, and increasing the complexity are all ways to advance the difficulty of coordination exercises. All coordination activities require repetition. This means that any coordination exercise in a therapeutic exercise program should include many repetitions. This is especially important as the exercises progress to resemble the patient's sport activities.

Accuracy of performance is vital to coordination development. The rehabilitation clinician must be cognizant of this when the patient is performing therapeutic exercises. Once the patient begins to fatigue and coordination becomes less accurate, the activity should be discontinued. Continued execution of uncoordinated motions will engram undesired movement. This is also an important consideration with regard to the placement of coordination exercises within a therapeutic exercise session. The patient should perform coordination activities early in the treatment session when fatigue is not as much of a factor as it will be toward the end.

AGILITY

▶ Agility is an advanced skill that is built on flexibility, strength, and power first, followed by coordination and balance.

Agility is the ability to control the direction of a body or segment during rapid movement. Athletic agility requires a number of qualities: flexibility, strength, power, speed, balance, and coordination. It involves rapid change of direction and sudden stopping and starting.

Most sports require agility of the lower extremities. A football receiver must be able to cut suddenly to the left or right to evade a defensive player; a soccer forward must zigzag down the field to move the ball around an opponent; and a basketball player must sprint down the court and then suddenly stop to perform a jump shot. Upper-extremity agility is required of a piano player who moves the fingers rapidly across the keyboard, a water polo player who attempts to fake out an opponent and then score a goal, the hockey goalie who suddenly blocks a shot with his hands, and the racquetball player who moves quickly from a backhand to a forehand shot.

Agility is a highly advanced skill that requires a base of flexibility, strength, and power. Adequate flexibility provides a base for speed and power. Since power is needed for agility and power is force times distance divided by time ($F \times D/T$), one can increase power by increasing the distance through which the body part moves. Greater flexibility produces greater power. Power is important because the greater the power, the more quickly a patient is able to move.

Strength is also a component of agility. A patient who has good strength can control the inertia that forceful movement creates. If a 90-kg (200-lb) patient is unable to control his weight during movement, the movement will be of no value. Strength is a controlling factor in a patient's maneuverability.

In order to be effective, speed must be accompanied by coordination. Coordination, as we have seen, is important for proper execution of an activity.

As with coordination activities, therapeutic exercise for agility should begin with simple exercises and progress to more complex activities as skill level improves. The ultimate goal of agility exercises is for the patient to perform all agility activities involved in that patient's sport. Execution of simple activities, including simple drills, is used in the early stages of agility exercises. These activities are usually components of an athletic skill and are performed at slower-than-normal speeds. As the patient improves, the activity becomes more complex and the speed more closely resembles that of normal sport participation.

Activities that can test a patient's agility should resemble the patient's sport activities. It is your responsibility as a rehabilitation clinician to understand the demands of the patient's sport and the patient's position within the sport so you can provide appropriate agility exercises. For example, agility activities for a basketball player should include exercises such as lateral line running, figure-8 cone running, sudden-stop activities, and running backward. Agility exercises for a volleyball player may include sprint running forward and backward with sudden direction changes, lateral running drills, and run-and-stop-jump activities. Performance of these activities is graded by speed of the activity, ability to suddenly change direction, ability to use the injured and noninjured leg equally in all directions, and smoothness of execution.

THERAPEUTIC EXERCISE FOR PROPRIOCEPTION

▶ Therapeutic exercises for developing balance, coordination, and agility follow exercises for flexibility and strength gains. Exercises for the lower and upper extremities progress from simple to complex and emphasize accuracy through repetition.

Agility, balance, and coordination are parameters that naturally follow flexibility and strength within a therapeutic exercise program. It is often not possible to distinguish which exercises develop balance and which exercises develop agility except at the extreme ranges of the exercise spectrum. This is because balance and agility are often intimately related and can be difficult to distinguish except in very basic exercises that are elementary static balance activities and the more complex preparticipation agility exercises. What becomes difficult is distinguishing the exercises that are more complex than static balance and less complex than preparticipation agility exercises. Exercises that develop dynamic balance, improve coordination, and enhance early agility are not as easily categorized because they may involve any combination of agility, balance, and coordination.

There is a general progression of exercises for proprioception that is important whether you are working with upper- or lower-extremity injuries. Proprioception exercises should be a routine part of a therapeutic exercise program.

General Concepts

Some concepts related to exercise for proprioception have already been introduced but are important enough to be repeated. Balance is achieved first, followed by coordination, and finally agility. The order is important because agility depends on coordination and coordination depends on balance. Balance exercises start with static activities and progresses to dynamic activities as balance improves.

All exercises for proprioception progress from simple to complex. Simple exercises include activities in which the patient has only one or two items of concentration. Simple exercises also include activities that require only enough muscle activity to produce the desired result without overflow to unwanted muscles. Simple exercises involve activities performed slowly and deliberately in controlled situations and environments. Distractions should be avoided when a high level of concentration is required of the patient.

Progression from simple to complex occurs only after the patient has mastered the simple exercise. You can make the activity more complex by having the patient perform the simple activity at a faster pace or by requiring a more powerful output with control. Progression from simple to more complex can also include exercises requiring the patient to perform more than one task simultaneously. A task can become more complex when one of the feedback mechanisms is restricted, as when the patient performs the simple activity with eyes closed. Progression to exercises that mimic sport participation occurs as soon as the patient's abilities allow.

A goal in proprioceptive exercises is to have the patient perform the activity accurately. To encourage this, the difficult proprioceptive activities should come early in the therapeutic exercise session rather than later; when the patient is more fatigued and coordination is more difficult.

Repetition is always necessary to develop performance accuracy. Repetition is successful only if the patient is able to improve execution with repeated attempts. The rehabilitation clinician must carefully observe the patient for signs of fatigue to prevent an inaccurate engram from developing.

Lower-Extremity Progression

Although specific exercises are addressed in part IV as specific therapeutic exercise programs for the various areas of the body, a brief description of proprioceptive programs is presented here.

Static balance activities begin with the stork stand with eyes open. The patient stands on the foot of the involved leg with arms at sides. The goal is to stork stand for 30 s without touching the elevated foot to the floor. If a patient has difficulty with the stork stand, he or she can begin with stance in a tandem position with the toe of one foot touching the heel of the foot in front of it (figure 8.5a); this is more difficult with the injured leg in the back position. Without using arms to balance, the patient stands in this position 30 s with eyes open. The patient can progress to standing in a tandem position for 30 s with eyes closed. After

Figure 8.5   Static balance progression: *(a)* tandem stance balance, *(b)* stork stand balance, *(c)* stork stand on 1/2 foam roller.

accomplishing stork standing with eyes open for 30 s (figure 8.5b), the patient performs it with the eyes closed for 30 s. Balance activities progress from stork standing with eyes closed to stork standing on an unstable surface such as a mini-trampoline, foam rubber pad, or 1/2 foam roller, eyes open and eyes closed (figure 8.5c).

You can also create increased difficulty in stork standing by having the patient perform a distracting activity such as playing catch. This can become even more challenging if the ball is weighted.

The patient can also perform static balance activities in a sport-specific position. For example, a gymnast can perform the stork stand on a balance beam or with the hip in lateral rotation. A tennis player can perform static balance activities on the balls of the feet with hip and knee flexion. A wrestler can perform static balance activities on the unstable surface of a mat.

After having mastered static balance, the patient progresses to dynamic balance. These activities include sport-specific demands such as running, lateral movements, and backward movements. More advanced dynamic activities include jumping, cutting, twisting, and pivoting. They begin as low-level activities, performed at a slow speed with balance and control, and progress to faster speeds. Some activities, such as jumping, can begin with the use of both legs but then progress to unilateral activities as the patient gains skill and confidence in execution. Plyometrics can be incorporated into the later stages of proprioceptive exercises within a therapeutic program. Plyometrics is a specialized system of exercises used only in the final stages of a program when the patient has good strength, flexibility, and control. Plyometrics are discussed in chapter 9.

In the final stages of these dynamic movements, the exercises are advanced to mimic specific sport situations. These exercises represent the true agility activities required of the patient in sport participation. You must know the component activities and understand the stresses applied in the sport to be able to design this part of the therapeutic exercise program. These activities fine-tune the patient's agility skills and restore the patient's confidence in his or her ability to return to the sport. Many of these activities are called functional exercises and are discussed in chapter 10.

The use of braces, sleeves, and tape to enhance proprioception of ankle and knee injuries is still a matter of some dispute. There is evidence that proprioception input from skin and subcutaneous sensory receptors assists in perception of motion (Lephart et al. 1992). There is also evidence that proprioceptive function is improved with bracing (Surve et al. 1994). Other information indicates that the benefit of joint support is inversely proportional to the proprioceptive ability of the joint (Perlau, Frank, and Fick 1995). The proprioceptive influence of these devices on functional activities is controversial, but this may be because many of the studies have been performed on normal subjects. Recently, it has been demonstrated that individuals with proprioceptive deficient knees rely on their cutaneous proprioceptors more than noninjured individuals (Callahan et al 2002); it may be that tape or braces work by stimulating these cutaneous receptors to act as position sense monitors. Most studies on proprioception and kinesthesia have been able to demonstrate an improved awareness of the patient as to joint position or joint sense, but no evidence demonstrates that joint stability is enhanced during functional activities with use of such devices (Barrack, Lund, and Skinner 1994).

Without any strong evidence to support or discourage the use of braces and sleeves, you must decide about using them on an individual basis. If the patient feels more confident and better able to perform athletic activities, these devices may provide sufficient psychological benefit to warrant application.

Upper-Extremity Progression

Although most lower-extremity sport activities are closed chain activities, upper-extremity activities are both open and closed chain. The patient's sport requirements in relation to open or closed chain activities will determine the extent of the proprioceptive exercises to be used in the therapeutic exercise program. A well-rounded program should include both open and closed kinetic chain activities, but end-program emphasis is determined by the demands of the particular sport. For example, a pitcher's demands are open kinetic chain, so the majority of proprioceptive exercises for a pitcher should be of this type. A gymnast performs open and closed kinetic chain activities and thus should do a combination of open and closed kinetic chain proprioceptive exercises; but a cyclist performs closed kinetic chain activities, so the program for this patient should include primarily closed kinetic chain exercises.

Initial open kinetic chain proprioceptive exercises can include proprioceptive neuromuscular facilitation rhythmic stabilization. Rhythmic stabilization can progress to closed kinetic chain exercises. In a closed kinetic chain, the exercise can progress from co-contraction without movement, to movement on a stable surface, to movement on an unstable surface. For example, the patient can either be positioned on a Swiss ball and move his or her body with the hands on the floor, or be positioned with hands on the ball and the body supported on a table (figure 8.6). The activity can start with bilateral support and then advance to use of only the involved arm.

1. Patient lies prone on a Swiss ball with feet off the floor. Patient begins with both hands on the floor and then raises the uninvolved arm to balance for 30 s (figure 8.6a).

2. Patient lies prone on a table with lower extremities on the table and hands on the Swiss ball. The Swiss ball is rolled outward and the position is held for 30 s (figure 8.6b).

3. Progressions for both exercises can include the patient's moving the ball using only the arms to propel the ball forward and backward and from side to side.

4. Further progression can include resistance to movement, for example on a Fitter or with manual resistance (figure 8.7).

Active and passive repositioning can be useful for early proprioceptive gains. Passive repositioning occurs when the rehabilitation clinician passively moves the patient's uninvolved upper extremity into a position and the patient then moves the injured upper extremity into

Figure 8.6 Proprioception exercises for the upper extremity on the Swiss ball: *(a)* Patient is supported by Swiss ball only, and *(b)* patient is supported by a table while moving a Swiss ball.

Figure 8.7 Resisted proprioceptive exercise.

the same position. This activity can progress from eyes open to eyes closed. When a mistake occurs, the patient visually compares to correct the position and repeats the exercise.

In active repositioning, the rehabilitation clinician moves the injured arm into a position and then returns it to the starting position. With eyes closed, the patient then reproduces the position the arm was placed in.

Both these activities can be performed in straight plane and in functional positions. The best response will be achieved in functional positions near the end of the joint's range of motion.

Functional exercises can be easily incorporated into an upper-extremity program. Proprioceptive neuromuscular facilitation exercises using manual resistance, machines, and tubing provide for strength and proprioceptive gains. Proprioceptive exercises start slowly and increase in speed as the patient is able to maintain control of the arm throughout the activity.

Plyometric exercises for agility can also be used for the upper extremity. Plyometric exercises for the upper extremities can include the use of body resistance and medicine balls as discussed in chapter 9.

As with lower-extremity functional exercises, upper-extremity agility exercises should be designed with knowledge of the requirements of the patient's specific sport. For example, functional exercises for a throwing sport patient should progress from throwing activities that initially include short distances and easy throwing, to longer distances with an increase in speed, and finally a full speed throw for functional distances.

SUMMARY

1. List the afferent receptors involved in proprioception.

    Proprioception, an important part of therapeutic exercise programs, is determined by the input of several afferent receptors in skin, muscle, tendon, joints, and other areas.

2. Identify the CNS sites that relay proprioceptive information to the motor system.

    The afferent receptors transmit information to one of three CNS sites: the spinal cord, the brain stem, or the cerebral cortex. The most rapid reflexes involve quick transmission and response from the spinal cord. The slower responses are sent from the cerebral cortex where conscious execution of the response is initiated.

3. Discuss the ABCs of proprioception.

    The ABCs of proprioception are agility, balance, and coordination. Balance is fundamental to coordination and agility. A patient must have good balance, coordination, and agility to fully meet the demands of his or her sport. Specific exercises are used to restore these functions. These exercises can be initiated early in a program with simple activities and progressed to more complex activities as the patient advances in the therapeutic exercise program.

4. Identify the systems that control balance.

    Balance is influenced by three systems, the vestibular, oculomotor, and proprioceptive systems. These all provide input to the CNS to maintain both static and dynamic balance.

5. Describe the components involved in coordination.

    Coordination includes the process of perceiving an activity, getting feedback from the CNS about the result of the activity, and correcting the activity through a series of repetitions and alterations until the activity is performed correctly and without the need for cerebral cortex input.

6. Explain a progression of proprioceptive exercises for the lower or upper extremity.

    Therapeutic exercise for proprioception progresses from easy to difficult, from static to dynamic, from slow to fast, and from simple to complex. As a rehabilitation clinician you must understand the complexity and requirements of the patient's sport in order to include appropriate proprioceptive exercises that will eventually permit the patient to return to full sport participation.

CRITICAL THINKING QUESTIONS

1. If a patient stands on one leg with eyes shut, which balance system is eliminated? How can the other two balance systems be eliminated in a stork-stand activity?

2. Would you expect a patient with an ankle sprain to have difficulty balancing on one leg? Why? List three progressive exercises that you could use to improve balance. What would be your criteria for advancement from one exercise to the next?

3. Coordination exercises are more effectively performed in a therapeutic exercise program before the patient becomes fatigued. Why is this? When, during the day's program, would new coordination exercises make any difference in performance? Why?

4. Identify three criteria that should be met before a patient advances from balance to coordination activities, and from coordination to agility activities. You should be able to explain to the patient why you are setting these criteria.

5. List three agility exercises you would provide Tony on his first day of agility training in the chapter's opening scenario. Provide two progressions for each exercise and your criteria for each progression.

LAB ACTIVITIES

1. Use a five-exercise progression, beginning with the easiest and progressing to the most difficult, to challenge your lab partner's lower-extremity proprioception. The first exercise should be a static balance activity; subsequent activities should progress to the final exercise in agility. Grade your lab partner's ability to perform each exercise level as you would in a patient's note. Indicate with each exercise selection what makes the exercise more challenging than the previous exercise. How will you determine when the patient is ready to proceed to the next level?

2. Use a five-exercise progression, beginning with the easiest and progressing to the most difficult, to challenge your lab partner's upper extremity proprioception. Grade your lab partner's ability to perform each exercise level as you would in a patient's note. Indicate with each exercise selection what makes the exercise more challenging than the previous exercise. How will you determine when the patient is ready to proceed to the next level?

3. With your lab partner seated on the table's end, instruct your partner to keep his or her eyes closed and move the leg into 45° of knee flexion. Measure the knee with a goniometer and record the position. Repeat this activity three times. Now instruct your partner to move the opposite leg to 45° and hold the position for 5 sec. While keeping the eyes closed have him or her extend the knee to 45° again. Measure the knee with a goniometer and record the position. Repeat this activity three times.

4. Have your lab partner stand on one leg, the arms at the sides, and the NWB thigh hanging comfortably but not adducted to the WB extremity. With eyes open, have your partner stand for 30 sec. An error occurs if the arms come away from the sides, the NWB extremity moves either away from the body or the ankle wraps around the other leg, trunk moves out from alignment with the hips, or the NWB foot touches the ground. Count the errors. Repeat the exercise with the eyes closed. What is the difference between the two activities? Why? Identify two other ways the stork-stand exercise can be made more challenging for a patient. How would you determine when the patient is able to advance from one exercise to the next?

REFERENCES

Barrack, R.L., Lund, P.J, and H.B. Skinner. 1994. Knee joint proprioception revisited. *Journal of Sport Rehabilitation* 3:18–42.

Callagan, M.J., Selfe, J., Bagley, P.J., and J.A. Oldham. 2002. The effects of patellar taping on knee joint proprioception. *Journal of Athletic Training* 37:19-24.

Grigg, P. 1994. Peripheral neural mechanisms in proprioception. *Journal of Sport Rehabilitation* 3: 2–17.

Kottke, F.J. 1982. Therapeutic exercise to develop neuromuscular coordination. In *Krusen's handbook of physical medicine and rehabilitation*, ed. F.J. Kottke, G.K. Stillwell, and J.F. Lehmann. Philadelphia: Saunders.

Lephart, S.M., Kocher, M.S., Fu, F.H., Borsa, P.A., and C.D. Harner. 1992. Proprioception following ACL reconstruction. *Journal of Sport Rehabilitation* 1:188–196.

Perlau, R., Frank, C., and G. Fick. 1995. The effect of elastic bandages on human knee proprioception in the uninjured population. *American Journal of Sports Medicine* 23:251–255.

Strasmann, T., van der Wal, J.C., Halata, Z., and J. Drukker. 1990. Functional topography and ultrastructure of periarticular mechanoreceptors in the lateral elbow region of the rat. *Acta Anatomy* 138:1–14.

Surve, I., Schwellnus, M.P., Noakes, T., and C. Lombard. 1994. A fivefold reduction in the incidence of recurrent ankle sprains in soccer players using the Sport-Stirrup orthosis. *American Journal of Sports Medicine* 22:601–606.

CHAPTER 9

Plyometrics

Objectives

After completing this chapter, you should be able to do the following:

1. Identify the mechanical and neurological components of the neuromuscular principles involved in plyometrics.

2. Describe the factors involved in plyometric program design.

3. List three considerations for plyometric program execution.

4. List the precautions and contraindications for plyometrics.

5. Outline a progression of four plyometric exercises for either a lower- or an upper-extremity program.

Certified athletic trainer Larry Carrell has been recently hired by the local sports medicine clinic to head up its plyometric rehabilitation program. Once patients are sufficiently rehabilitated, Larry establishes the final phase of their sport rehabilitation program, the plyometric phase. Larry comes to the clinic with extensive experience and is well qualified to design and manage such a program to advance patients in this final portion of their rehabilitation.

Larry's most recent patient is his most challenging patient to date. Ed is a 70-year-old gold medal track patient who competes in the senior Olympics and has the endorsement of several companies. Ed strained his hamstrings several weeks ago and is now nearing the end of his rehabilitation program. Although Ed is energetic and enthusiastic, he also has a history of other lower extremity injuries and underwent cardiac bypass surgery eight years ago. The cardiac surgery and his postoperative recovery were what originally piqued his interest in track.

Larry sees Ed as an exciting challenge and is looking forward to designing a plyometric program to enable Ed to fully return to his competitive level of participation.

■ **Arriving at one goal is the starting point to another.**

John Dewey, American philosopher, psychologist, and educator, 1859-1952

Now that the patient has achieved goals in flexibility, strength, balance, coordination, and agility, the next step is to finely tune his or her abilities in preparation for specific sport skills and other activities. Most sports activities require explosiveness, rapid changes in direction and speed, and the ability to absorb and produce forces quickly—all performed automatically, economically, and efficiently. Goals established to successfully demonstrate these parameters must be achieved before the patient moves on to sport-specific activities. Athletic skills are the combined result of natural talent and proper training. An injured athlete possesses the same inherent talent he or she has always had, but the effects of training diminish following injury and inactivity. The capacity to perform athletic skills at pre-injury levels must be restored through therapeutic exercise and retraining before the patient is able to return safely to sport competition.

Execution of activities of this magnitude requires a relearning of the neuromuscular system. The relearning process utilizes what is commonly referred to as **plyometrics**. Plyometrics not only is a precursor to functional activities, but also can include specific functional sport activities. Plyometrics is the use of a quick movement of eccentric activity followed by a burst of concentric activity to produce a desired powerful output of the muscle. In other words, a plyometric exercise is one that facilitates a muscle to produce a maximum strength output as quickly as possible. It is a brief, explosive exercise. Power production is the ultimate goal in plyometrics. You will recall from previous discussions that power is force times distance divided by time ($F \times D/T$). The quicker the time, the greater the power. For example, if a patient weighing 80 kg (176 lb) jumps 0.6m (2ft) in the air and takes 1s to perform the activity, he produces 360 ft-lb of power ($180 \times 2 \div 1$). If, however, he is able to jump the same distance in half the time, he will produce 720 ft-lb of power ($180 \times 2 \div 0.5$).

Power is calculated as force divided by distance, over a given amount of time:

$$P = F \times \frac{D}{T}$$

The term *plyometrics* was not used until 1975 when an American track and field coach, Fred Wilt, originated the term (Chu 1992). Its Greek origins are *plio* and *metric*, which mean "more" and "measure," respectively. Before Wilt coined the term, plyometrics was referred to as "jump training." Although plyometric activities have been used since people first ran and jumped, plyometrics became popular in the late 1960s when people attributed the high performance abilities of Olympic athletes from the Eastern European countries to the jump-training exercises used by their coaches.

NEUROMUSCULAR PRINCIPLES

▶ Plyometrics works on the basis of specific mechanical and neurological components of the muscular system. The mechanical components are contractile and noncontractile elements; the neurological components are the muscle spindles and the Golgi tendon organs.

The theory of how plyometrics works is based on information about the neuromuscular system and its response to stress. Many of these principles have been discussed in previous chapters. Putting these principles into practical application in plyometrics helps the rehabilitation clinician understand the "whys" and "hows" of incorporating plyometrics into a therapeutic exercise program.

Plyometrics involves the technique of first lengthening, then shortening the muscle to produce an increased power output. This is referred to as **stretch-shortening** exercise. The stretch-shortening exercise is based on the stretch-shortening principles, which in turn are based on knowledge of the mechanical and neurological components of the neuromuscular system.

Mechanical Components

The mechanical components can be divided into contractile elements and noncontractile elements. Both are important elements that play a role in plyometrics and will be briefly presented here.

Contractile Components

The **contractile components** (CC) are the myofibrils. As discussed in chapter 7, the myofibrils contain the sarcomeres, the contractile element of the muscle. Muscle is the only structure in the body that actively shortens or lengthens to cause motion. The contractile elements of the muscular system control the noncontractile elements.

Non-contractile Elements

The noncontractile elements or components include the muscle's tendons and the connective tissue surrounding the muscle and its fibers. The noncontractile elements are divided according to their arrangement and include a **series elastic component** (SEC) and a **parallel elastic component** (PEC). The tendons, sheath, and sarcolemma are the primary structures that make up the SEC, and the muscle's connective tissue composes the PEC (Dean 1988).

Interaction of the Series Elastic Component, Parallel Elastic Component, and Contractile Component

When a muscle actively shortens, the component responsible for the muscle's ability to move the extremity or resist a force is the CC. As the muscle continues to shorten, a stretch is applied to the SEC.

When a muscle actively lengthens as in an eccentric activity, the components responsible for producing the force are the CC, SEC, and PEC. The SEC and PEC offer resistance to the movement as the muscle is elongated. The CC controls the speed and quality of the movement. When a muscle elongates, the contribution of the passive component force makes it unnecessary for the active component to produce the same total force as was produced during the shortening activity. To use a theoretical example, if a force of 4.5 kg (10 lb) is needed to lift a weight during a shortening activity, the active components must produce all 4.5 kg of force in order for the weight to be lifted. If the same weight is moved during a lengthening activity, only 3 kg (7 lb) of force needs to be produced by the active component, because

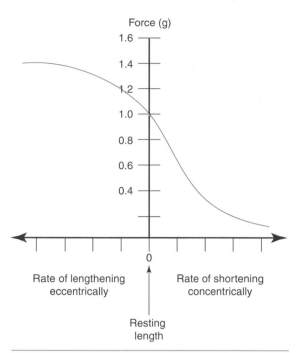

Figure 9.1 Concentric-eccentric force-production relationship.

Adapted from P.-O. Åstrand and Rodahl 1986.

1.3 kg (3 lb) is produced by the passive components. The muscle works less to produce the same force during the lengthening activity. Although the exact differences in eccentric and concentric forces vary depending on the muscle groups investigated, this example demonstrates that less active force is required by the muscle during eccentric activity than during concentric activity. (The numbers used in the example should not be interpreted as precise.) Whereas less work is required from active components during eccentric exercise, less energy is used during eccentric exercises—so if equal active muscle force is generated in concentric and eccentric activity, greater total force will be produced during eccentric activity.

As discussed in chapter 7, force production is different for concentric and eccentric activity (figure 9.1). At faster speeds of eccentric activity, a muscle is able to produce greater forces than at lower speeds, but the opposite is true for concentric activity. The importance of this principle will become apparent later in the discussion of specific plyometrics.

Neurological Components

The proprioceptors that play important roles in plyometrics are the muscle spindles and Golgi tendon organs (GTOs). The muscle spindle is stimulated by sudden changes in the muscle's length, as during an eccentric movement. It produces a stretch, or **myotatic reflex,** to facilitate a muscle shortening. The **stretch reflex** is the most basic sensorimotor response system because it does not involve an internuncial neuron, but instead goes directly from the afferent sensory nerve (muscle spindle) to the spinal cord where it makes contact with the efferent motor neuron to permit a rapid response by the muscle. Because no additional nerves are involved in the relay process, the stretch reflex is one of the fastest reflexes in the body. It is also referred to as a **monosynaptic response** because only one neural connection is involved.

The GTOs play an inhibitory role in muscle activity. As the muscle shortens, the GTOs are stimulated to send impulses to the spinal cord that relay, via an internuncial neuron, facilitation to limit muscle force production. Because of the internuncial neuron, this reflex is slightly slower than the muscle spindle reflex.

It is believed that during plyometric training, the GTO excitatory level is elevated so that more stimulation is necessary to facilitate a response from the GTO, and this allows for an increased tolerance for additional stretch loads in the muscle (Wilk et al. 1993). As the stretch loads are better tolerated, there may be the ability to create a stronger stretch reflex results in additional power during the concentric phase of motion (Lundin 1985).

PLYOMETRIC FORCE PRODUCTION

▶ Working together, the components of the mechanical and neurological systems that operate in plyometric activities increase strength and power output.

Force production during plyometric activity is facilitated through the mechanical and neurological systems that have been described. Combined, these produce the desired results of increased strength and power for athletic activity. The noncontractile, elastic elements are important in force production of stretch-shortening exercises. A simplified example of the way noncontractile elements work is a rubber band model: If the rubber band is stretched and then released, it shortens rapidly. The more it is stretched, the greater its force when the stretch is released. This is so because the greater the stretch, the greater the quantity of stored (potential) elastic energy there is within the rubber band. When the stretch is released, the stored elastic energy converts to kinetic energy to produce the rubber band's recoil.

Plyometric exercises provide for an increased output of power during concentric activity. This has to do with transfer of the elastic energy that is produced during eccentric activity immediately prior to concentric activity. In a muscle that moves eccentrically, the load that is produced in the muscle during its lengthening is stored as elastic energy in the noncontractile elements. As the muscle moves from eccentric to concentric activity, the elastic energy is released and assists in producing the force during the concentric action. It is believed that a muscle's increased power during plyometric exercise training may be the result of a combination of an increased level of muscle elasticity and the adaptations that occur in the neurological components (Wilk et al. 1993).

Another important factor in increased strength and power output is development of neuromuscular responses to the stresses applied. Raising the threshold of the GTOs permits a greater stretch of the muscle to provide for greater concentric activity. If a muscle is able to go through a greater range of motion, the ability to produce greater forces is improved. For example, the patient who squats to only 30° of knee flexion does not jump as high as when he or she squats to 90° of knee flexion prior to takeoff. Greater forces can be produced when greater lengthening prior to concentric activity is permitted.

Another factor in improved performance with plyometric activity is the improved neuromuscular coordination. As speed increases and the activity is performed more accurately, the strength to perform the activity is improved. Energy and movement are not wasted on ineffective activity. Neuromuscular training involves development of the engram as discussed in chapter 7. Better coordination permits greater power production since the activity can be performed more efficiently and in less time.

When speed and coordination of activity are improved, greater power can be produced, as follows from the force-velocity relationship of increased strength with increased speed during eccentric activity (figure 9.1). The greater the eccentric activity, the greater the concentric response will be; and the less time it takes a patient to perform an activity, the more power the patient will produce.

PLYOMETRIC EXERCISE PHASES

▶ Plyometric activities occur in three distinct phases. In the eccentric phase the muscle is prestretched; in the amortization phase it makes a transition to the third, or concentric phase; and in the concentric phase it produces the powerful outcome.

Plyometric exercises can be divided into three phases: the eccentric phase, the amortization phase, and the concentric phase. All three phases are important to plyometric performance. The eccentric phase prepares the muscle, the amortization phase transitions the muscle, and the concentric phase is the outcome.

Eccentric Phase

The eccentric phase occurs when the muscle is prestretched as it actively lengthens. The slack is taken out of the muscle, and its elastic components are put on stretch. This is the preparatory phase that "sets" the muscle as the individual gets ready to perform the activity. This phase utilizes muscle spindle facilitation so that the quality of the response is determined by the rate of the stretch. The muscle's activity directly correlates with the quantity of the stimulation: the greater the stimulation, the greater the muscle's response. The eccentric phase is the most important phase of plyometric activity because it increases the stimulation to provide for this increased muscle response.

The muscle spindle responds better to a rapid stretch and accommodates to a slow one. For this reason, the rate of the stretch is a more important factor than the amount of stretch. If a muscle lengthens quickly, it is able to produce more tension than if it is forced to elongate slowly (Koutedakis 1989). The best results occur when the eccentric phase is performed quickly and through a partial range of motion.

Amortization Phase

The eccentric phase is followed immediately by the **amortization** phase, which is simply defined as the amount of time it takes to move from eccentric to concentric motion. This phase should be quick. If too much time is spent here, the elastic energy is dissipated as heat and is wasted. A prolonged amortization phase also inhibits the stretch reflex. The concentric motion that results when the amortization is slow is weaker than intended. The amortization phase is the transition phase. The quicker the transition from eccentric to concentric activity, the more forceful the movement will be. The force produced is a result of the combination of the stretch reflex and the elastic energy released. The force produced is also influenced by the amount of time it takes to make the transition from eccentric to concentric activity, so the transition time must be quick for the plyometrics to produce maximum force.

Concentric Phase

The final phase, the concentric phase, is the result of the combined eccentric and amortization phases. The concentric phase is the outcome phase. If the eccentric activity has been quick and the amortization has occurred rapidly, the concentric phase will produce the desired powerful outcome (table 9.1).

If these phases are performed precisely, the end result should be an increased force production with a greater speed. Over time, with practice and neurological facilitation, this speed-strength production becomes more efficient because the plyometric exercises lead to an improved synchronous activity of motor units and an earlier recruitment of the motor units. Plyometrics bridges the gap between strength and explosive power by integrating the mechanical and neurological factors that influence these sport performance elements (Wilt 1975).

PREPLYOMETRIC CONSIDERATIONS

▶ Patients must have certain levels of strength, flexibility, and proprioception in order to participate safely in plyometric exercises.

Development of power is important in most sports. For example, it is an important element of basketball, volleyball, gymnastics, track and field, baseball, softball, and skating. Since power is crucial for sport performance and plyometrics promotes power development, plyometric exercises should be considered for patients who are returning to sport. Before plyometrics can become part of a therapeutic exercise program, however, specific parameters must be present, because plyometrics places great demands on the body.

Strength

Strength is basic to plyometric exercises. The patient should have enough strength to adequately control the activity. As the difficulty of the plyometric exercise increases, the patient needs to have even greater strength. One can minimize the potential for overuse injuries from plyometric activities with good preplyometric strength levels.

A greater strength provides for a better output during the plyometric exercise. Again, if $F \times D/T = P$, then the greater the force, the greater the power. Additionally, if a muscle has a greater cross section because of its hypertrophy following strengthening, it will have greater elastic elements to provide additional eccentric strength. Minimum strength requirement recommendations for plyometric exercises vary and depend on the severity of the plyometric exercise. For more severe lower-extremity plyometric exercises, the recommendation is that the patient be able to perform a squat with 60% of body weight for five repetitions within 5 s (Chu 1998). Less intense plyometric exercises such as skipping or hopping can begin earlier. Logic, common sense, and knowledge of the patient's strength and the stresses applied with any exercise are required of the rehabilitation clinician who is determining the use of plyometric exercises.

Table 9.1
Plyometric Phases

	Phase	Activity
1	Eccentric	Preparation
2	Amortization	Transition
3	Concentric	Outcome

Adapted from Åstrand and Rodahl 1986.

Flexibility

Flexibility is another preplyometric exercise requirement. As mentioned earlier, greater flexibility permits a greater lengthening of the muscle. A greater lengthening provides for a better eccentric phase that will lead to better concentric activity. A muscle that lacks good flexibility is unable to generate the forces for optimal plyometric results. The muscle is also at risk for injury because the reduced flexibility leads to a diminished level of force absorption, needed especially for impact and deceleration stresses. For example, the patient who is able to flex his knee to only 60° will be unable to absorb the forces imposed on him when he jumps from a 40 cm (16 in.) box; but the patient who is able to fully flex her knees can absorb the impact stresses much more effectively to prevent the forces from being transmitted up the extremity.

Proprioception

Another preplyometric consideration is the ABCs of proprioception as discussed in chapter 8. The patient must have agility, balance, and coordination to control the rapid and forceful movements in plyometric activities. The amount of control required depends on the complexity and severity of the plyometric activity. For example, a plyometric activity such as jumping rope is not as complex or as severe as the plyometric activity of bounding with vertical jumps. Although both activities require agility, balance, and coordination, the patient's abilities are more challenged with the bounding and vertical jump activities. For this reason it makes sense not to include even simple plyometric exercises in a therapeutic exercise program until the patient is able to perform some of the basic static and dynamic ABC activities discussed in chapter 8.

Because flexibility, strength, and proprioceptive elements are prerequisites to plyometric exercises, the progression of a therapeutic exercise program is important. As noted in chapter 1, each component is built on the previous one and serves as a foundation for the next one. Likewise, there are progressions within each parameter. Plyometrics is no different from any other type of exercise we have considered and must move in a progression from the simplest to the more difficult.

PLYOMETRIC PROGRAM DESIGN

▶ A plyometrics progression for a sport rehabilitation program uses a number of variables; intensity, volume, recovery, and frequency.

A plyometric program is designed to improve the patient's overall coordination, efficiency, speed, and power output in preparation for sport participation. Most sports require high power outputs and involve repetitive stretch-shortening muscle activity. Plyometric activities are the bridge between therapeutic exercise and functional performance. These exercises utilize the components of flexibility, strength, and proprioceptive elements that the patient developed in earlier exercise sessions and put these components to functional use through the further development of power, speed, coordination, and efficiency of movement. Whereas many plyometric exercises mimic functional sport skills, others serve as building blocks for progression from simple activities to functional skills.

Just as a patient with a 4/5 grade muscle strength cannot be expected to lift the same weights as a patient with a 5/5 grade muscle strength, a patient should not be expected to perform high-level plyometric exercises when beginning plyometric activities within the therapeutic exercise program. A progression is crucial to avoid injury and provide a successful outcome. The progression is from general exercises to more sport-specific activities, from simple to complex, and from low-stress to high-stress activities.

One can use a number of variables to provide a plyometric exercise progression: intensity, volume, recovery, and frequency.

Intensity

Intensity is the degree, extent, or magnitude of effort applied during an exercise or activity. In strengthening, it is the amount of weight used; in flexibility, it is the force applied to the stretch; in proprioception, it is the complexity of the agility, balance, or coordination activity. In plyometrics it is the stress of the activity. You can change stress in plyometrics by using weights during the activity, increasing the height of the vertical jump, increasing the distance of the horizontal jump or the throw, increasing the weight of the medicine ball, or increasing the speed of the activity. You can also increase stress by changing the complexity of the exercise. For example, hopping with one leg is more stressful than hopping with two legs, and hopping side to side is more stressful than hopping in place.

Volume

Volume is the total quantity of work performed during one session. Volume in lower-extremity plyometric exercises is measured in total number of foot contacts for jumping activities and in distance for bounding activities during the session. Volume in the upper extremity and in medicine ball exercises is measured in the total number of repetitions and sets. Selection of the volume of plyometrics depends on the intensity and goals of the session.

Although no guidelines have been established for therapeutic exercise, for normal athletic conditioning the lower-extremity guidelines for beginners at low-intensity levels are 60 to 100 foot contacts (Chu 1998). The rehabilitation clinician must have knowledge of the patient's ability and of the stresses applied by the activity, and must combine this knowledge with observation of the patient's performance quality, in order to determine the appropriate volume of plyometric exercises for the therapeutic exercise session.

Recovery

Recovery is the amount of rest time between sets or exercise groupings. The amount of rest time determines whether the plyometric exercises will be more effective in improving power or improving muscular endurance. The less rest time between exercise sets, the more the emphasis is on endurance; longer rest times will provide for more improvement in power. As a general guideline, rest periods of 45 to 60 s between sets or exercise groupings promote power increases (Chu 1998). This translates to a work-to-rest ratio of 1:5 to 1:10 (Chu 1998). For example, if an exercise set takes 5 s to perform, the recovery could be 25 to 50 s. If the exercise set takes 10 s to perform, the recovery could be 50 to 100 s.

If muscle endurance is a goal with plyometric exercise, the recovery time between exercise sets is less; the general guideline is 10 to 15 s. This amount of rest time does not allow an optimal recovery of the muscle, so muscle endurance improves.

Plyometric exercises can also be used to develop aerobic conditioning through use of a circuit program in which the patient performs various exercise groupings for 12 to 20 min with less than a 2 s rest between the exercises. A circuit program can develop aerobic, power, and muscle endurance levels.

Frequency

Another variable is the frequency with which plyometric activities are used in a therapeutic exercise program. Frequency depends on the exercise intensity and the patient's tolerance and ability to recover. As a rule of thumb, you should allow at least 48 h between plyometric exercise sessions. The research is very unclear about the time it takes healthy patients to recover from plyometric exercise, and is essentially nonexistent on frequency of plyometrics in therapeutic exercise programs. Your judgment, common sense, and knowledge of stresses and the patient's abilities are essential to determining frequency for an individual patient's program.

PLYOMETRIC PROGRAM CONSIDERATIONS

▶ A number of special considerations must enter into the decision whether and how to use plyometrics within a patient's therapeutic exercise program. Plyometrics in appropriate for patients with certain characteristics and not others. Plyometric activities require particular types of surfaces and footwear. Other considerations involve progression and goals for this type of exercise.

Because plyometric activities are generally more intense than other types of exercises, you must consider several special issues regarding their application in therapeutic exercise programs. If the patient has satisfied the preplyometric considerations and has the flexibility, strength, and proprioceptive elements required for plyometric activities, he or she must also meet other criteria in order to participate safely. In addition, plyometric exercises must be performed on an appropriate surface, and progression and goals must be determined appropriately.

Age

Although most children use plyometric activities in their everyday activities such as running, jumping, hopping, and skipping, one must use plyometrics carefully with children and youth from ages 8 to 13. Plyometric activities for prepubescent and early-pubescent patients should remain at low volume and low intensity. As an example, jumping with both feet and without the use of boxes or weights is low-intensity jumping. Children are at higher risk than older individuals for injury with plyometrics because their central nervous systems are not mature and their GTO activation threshold is lower than in adults. The proprioceptive feedback mechanism is unable to provide necessary safeguards against the high stresses of plyometrics. Muscles and bones of prepubescent patients are also not strong enough to tolerate the moderate and high stresses of more advanced plyometric exercises (Gambetta 1986). Because of variability in physical maturity, it may be a safe rule of thumb to restrict patients under age 16 from participating in moderate- to high-intensity plyometrics.

Body Weight

The design of a plyometric program must take into account the patient's weight. Patients weighing 100 kg (220 lb) or more are not able to participate in the same plyometric exercises as lighter patients (Allerheiligen and Rogers 1995). The stresses imposed on tendons and joints may be too great for safe participation by these patients in higher-intensity plyometric activities. For example, a 113-kg (250-lb) patient may perform single-leg hops for only half the distance that a 68-kg (150-lb) patient can. The intensity of plyometric exercises for heavier patients should be selected cautiously.

Competitive Level

Patients involved in competitive sports are more appropriate candidates for moderate- and high-level plyometric exercises than those in recreational activities are. The competitive patient has more advanced performance goals than the recreational patient and typically has more intense sport participation requirements. Although therapeutic exercise programs for all patients should include some level of plyometric exercises, only the competitive patients require higher-intensity plyometric activities.

Surface

The best surfaces for plyometric lower-extremity activities are those that have "give" to them. Although it can be indoors or outdoors, the surface should be one that yields to absorb some of the impact stress of the plyometric activity. Ideal surfaces include spring-loaded floors, Resilite mats, and grass. Harder surfaces such as asphalt, concrete, and carpet or rubber over concrete should be avoided. Although the surface should be able to absorb some of the impact forces produced during the activity, it should not be so yielding that it reduces the elastic recoil, the crucial element of plyometric activity. If the surface prevents sufficient amortization and impedes the individual's concentric phase, the surface is probably too soft. For the higher-stress plyometric activities, this becomes a key consideration.

Footwear

Shoes that offer good support and provide some cushion for shock absorption are the best shoes to wear for plyometrics. A shoe can offer too much absorption and thus be too spongy, causing instability instead of providing stability in landing. If this is the case, the individual may report a sense of instability or an inability to properly execute the exercise, or you may be able to observe instability at the foot landing or takeoff during the exercises. Shoes should be in good condition, not be excessively worn, be tied properly, and fit well.

Proper Technique

Technique is probably the most important among the special considerations. Foot position is an essential factor in jumping activities. The patient should land on the midfoot and then roll forward to push off from the balls of the feet (Gambetta 1986). The patient should not land on the balls of the feet or the heel, since these landing techniques increase the impact forces and thereby increase stress applied at the foot, ankle, and knee. The midfoot landing also allows a shorter amortization time so that a more powerful concentric motion can occur.

The trunk should remain upright with a straight back so that summation of forces from the back, abdominals, and arms can be utilized. The arms can contribute 10% of the force of the plyometric jump, so both timing of activities and posture are important factors (Gambetta 1986). Keeping the back straight will permit this transmission of forces and avoid back injuries.

The quality of the execution is important. As a rehabilitation clinician you must carefully observe the patient's quality of performance. As the patient fatigues, performance quality declines. This can result in two problems: risk of injury and development of an improper engram. It is important to know the proper exercise technique and to observe the patient's performance closely so that you can discontinue the exercise when performance begins to deteriorate.

Progression

A gradual progression from simple to difficult, from few to more, and from general to specific is vital to avoid injury in plyometric activities. The patient's body must be allowed time to adapt to new stress levels in order to avoid overstress injuries. As we have seen, there are a variety of ways to implement progression into a program. Changing the intensity, reducing the rest, and increasing the duration of the activity will all provide for a progression.

Goals

The program's goals are individually determined by the patient and the demands of the patient's sport. The specific exercises within the program are determined by the sport-specific requirements of each patient. For example, a long jumper will have a different plyometric jumping program than a basketball player, and a volleyball player will have a different jumping program than a wrestler. You must understand the stresses, skills, and demands of the patient's sport so that you can incorporate appropriate plyometric exercises into the therapeutic exercise program at the proper time.

You should assess the patient's plyometric performance at certain times during the therapeutic exercise program. Any time you initiate a plyometric activity, you should take initial measurements of the patient's performance. For example, in a standing jump, you should measure the jump height the first time the patient attempts the jump. As the patient progresses through the program, more intensive plyometric activities are introduced. Each time the patient performs a new activity, record initial performance values and establish new goals. Additional measurements can be taken either at specific intervals, such as every week, or when the patient is ready to advance to a more difficult activity. These recordings help the rehabilitation clinician maintain objective measures of improvement. They also provide additional motivation and goals for the patient.

PRECAUTIONS AND CONTRAINDICATIONS

▶ Precautions concerning the use of plyometrics relate to the time the patient spends on these activities and to vulnerability to post-exercise soreness. There are also a few frank contraindications to the use of plyometrics in a therapeutic exercise program.

As you realize, there are precautions for any therapeutic exercise program. Because plyometric activities can be vigorous, you must consider additional precautions before deciding to incorporate them into an individual's therapeutic exercise program:

- **Time.** Because plyometric activities place such high stresses on the body, they should not be performed for extended periods of time. They also should be performed in the early part of the therapeutic exercise session before the patient becomes fatigued and his or her strength, flexibility, and coordination are less than optimal. The time to perform the plyometric activities is after the warm-up but before fatigue increases and with it the risk of injury.

- **Post-exercise delayed onset muscle soreness.** It is important to caution the patient that because plyometric activities are more strenuous than other exercises, he or she may experience post-exercise soreness. Delayed onset soreness is common, especially at the time plyometric exercises are introduced into the program or when the intensity changes.

In addition, you must be aware of several clear contraindications to plyometric activity:

- **Acute inflammation.** Plyometric exercises should be avoided in acute inflammatory conditions. The intensity of these exercises can increase the inflammation.

- **Postoperative conditions.** Persons with immediate postoperative conditions should not engage in plyometric exercise. The tissues are unable to tolerate the stress of such exercises and are highly vulnerable to injury.

- **Instability.** Gross joint instability, until strength is sufficient to control the joint, is a contraindication. Strength is a prerequisite to any plyometric exercise. Strength permits the control necessary for safe and effective plyometric exercise execution.

EQUIPMENT

▶ Some plyometric exercises require no equipment, and others use a variety of items that are easy to obtain or to construct.

Equipment for plyometric activities need not be elaborate or expensive. In fact, most plyometric exercises require little or no equipment. In the following sections we review some of the most commonly used items.

Cones

Plastic barriers or traffic cones are used as jump obstacles or for sprint activities. Their plasticity makes them safe for patients to land on. These cones come in various sizes from 20 to 60 cm (8 to 24 in.) (figure 9.2).

Boxes

Boxes come in a variety of heights, ranging from 15 to 106 cm (6 to 42 in.), and various designs. The top should have a non-slip surface. The lower boxes are used for less intense activities and the higher ones for more intense activities (figure 9.3).

Figure 9.2 Plyometric cones.

Figure 9.3 Plyometric boxes.

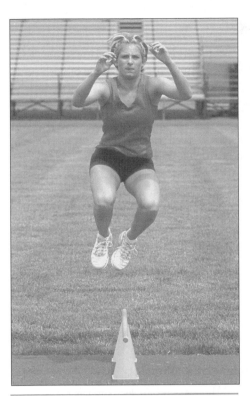

Figure 9.4 Plyometric hurdle constructed from cones and a dowel.

Hurdles

Hurdles are used for more advanced plyometric exercises. Some are adjustable within ranges of 15 to 100 cm (6 to 40 in.). A low hurdle can be easily constructed from two cones and a dowel (figure 9.4).

Medicine Balls

Medicine balls are useful in plyometric activities for the upper extremities and trunk, and also provide additional resistance for lower extremity plyometrics. They come in a variety of sizes, weights, and surfaces. The leather covered balls are limited to indoor use because moisture shortens the life of the cover. Balls should be of a manageable size and should have a surface that permits the patient to maintain an adequate grasp. If one-hand activities are required for the exercise, the ball should have a diameter that will accommodate the patient's hand size (figure 9.5).

Other Equipment

A variety of other equipment can be used for various plyometric activities. Jump ropes, stairs, and barriers are examples of items that are usually readily available. Their specific use depends on the goals of the exercise and the imagination of the rehabilitation clinician.

Figure 9.5 Medicine balls.

LOWER-EXTREMITY PLYOMETRICS

▶ Lower-extremity plyometric exercises use various types of jumps, as well as bounding and box drills, in various combinations to provide a progression of intensities.

Once the patient has the prerequisite strength, flexibility, and coordination, and the tissues have healed sufficiently to tolerate the stress of such activity without incurring damage or additional inflammation, plyometric exercises can become a part of the therapeutic exercise program.

Progression

A lower extremity plyometric exercise progression involves six types of exercises: jumps-in-place, standing jumps, multiple jumps and hops, bounding, box drills, and depth jumps (Chu 1998).

Jumps-in-Place

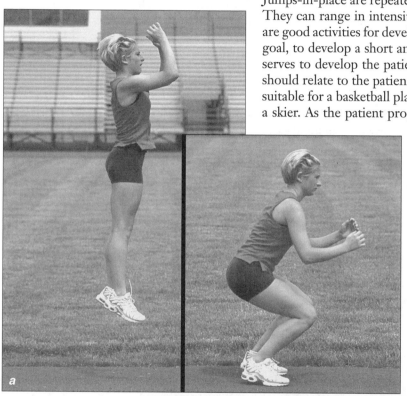

Jumps-in-place are repeated jumps that begin and end in the same place. They can range in intensity from low to high. The low intensity jumps are good activities for developing a brief amortization phase. The specific goal, to develop a short amortization phase with a rapid rebound, often serves to develop the patient's jump technique. Jump-in-place exercises should relate to the patient's sport. For example, a two-foot ankle hop is suitable for a basketball player, and a hip-twist ankle hop is well suited to a skier. As the patient progresses, he or she can perform more difficult jumps-in-place or can advance to another type of jump exercise.

Two-Foot Ankle Hop

Have the patient jump in place using only the ankles. The patient should jump as high as possible. The knees will bend, but only slightly (figure 9.6a). This exercise is particularly good for patients who play basketball.

Hip-Twist Ankle Hop

Have the patient, with feet together, jump and twist 90° to the left, return to start position, and then repeat to the right. The patient should twist from the hips, not the knees (figure 9.6b). This exercise is particularly good for patients who ski.

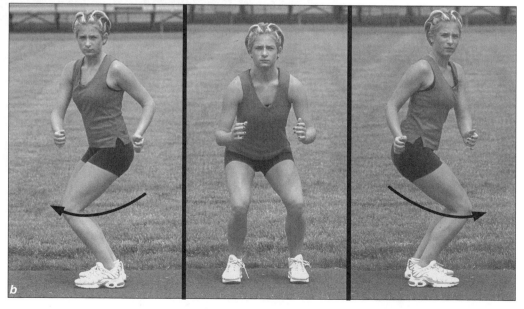

Figure 9.6 Jump-in-place plyometric exercises: (a) two-foot ankle hop; (b) hip-twist ankle hop.

Standing Jumps

Standing jumps are single jumps that emphasize a maximal effort with motion occurring either vertically or horizontally. Recovery between each attempt is necessary for a maximal effort each time. A progression of this type of jump could consist, for example, of beginning with a standing long jump, progressing to a jump over a cone, and advancing to a standing long jump with a sprint. Standing jumps can go forward or laterally and can involve barriers. Patients can combine standing jumps with multiple jumps, running, or sprinting in different directions.

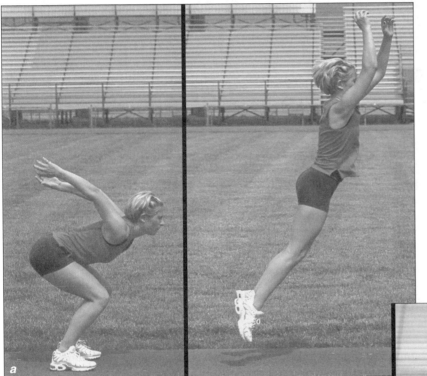

Standing Long Jump

The patient's feet are shoulder-width apart. Have him or her explode from semi-squat position to jump as far forward as possible. The patient should use arms to assist (figure 9.7a). This exercise is particularly good for patients who swim or participate in track.

Standing Jump over Barrier

Have the patient, with feet shoulder-width apart, jump upward and over cone, landing on both feet simultaneously. The patient should keep hips over knees and feet (figure 9.7b). You can add cones from 0.9 to 1.8 m (3–6 ft) apart for multiple jumps. This exercise is particularly good for patients who are figure skaters or basketball players.

Figure 9.7 Example of a standing jump progression: (a) standing long jump, (b) standing jump over barrier, and (c) standing long jump with sprint.

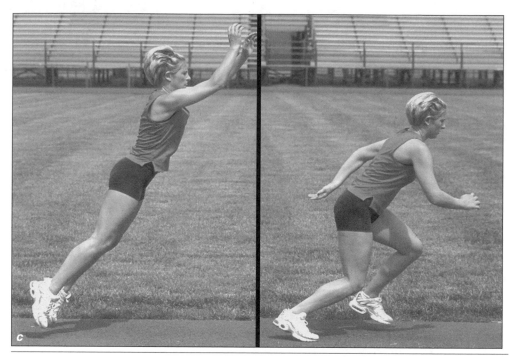

Standing Long Jump with Sprint

Using arms to assist, the patient should jump as far forward as possible. Immediately after landing, have him or her sprint forward as fast as possible for 10 m (figure 9.7c). Add sprints to left and right for additional activities. This exercise is particularly good for patients who play hockey, participate in track, or play football.

Figure 9.7 *(continued)*

Multiple Jumps and Hops

Multiple hops and jumps combine the skills of jumps-in-place and standing jumps. The patient attempts to jump maximally and repeats the jumps without resting. The total distance in each set of exercises is usually kept under 30 m (Chu 1998). The jumps can be performed with one or two legs, in a straight line or in multiple directions, with or without barriers. A front cone hop is an example of a simple multiple-hop exercise. The single-leg hop and a series of stadium-step hops are examples of more difficult multiple hops.

Single-Leg Hops

Have the patient jump from left leg, propelling as far upward and forward as possible, using arm movement to assist, and then land on the same leg. The patient should use forward movement of the right non-weight bearing leg to propel forward for the next jump, landing on right leg. Remind the patient to keep hips and knees directly over the landing foot (figure 9.8a).

> Refer to examples of plyometric jumping exercises for the lower extremities in Don Chu's *Jumping into Plyometrics, Second Edition* (1998). It is advisable for you refer to this book for additional suggestions for plyometric exercises and progression programs.

Stadium Hops

Have the patient jump one step at a time using both legs. The movement should be rapid, light, and continuous up the stairs, without stops or hesitation. The patient can progress to taking two steps at a time or using one leg and alternating (figure 9.8b). This exercise, as well as the single-leg hops on the previous page, is particularly good for patients who wrestle or play hockey.

Figure 9.8 Examples of multiple jumps or hops: *(a)* single-leg hops, *(b)* stadium hops.

Bounding

Bounding exercises are an exaggeration of the running stride. They are used to improve stride length and speed. These exercises are most commonly used for patients in track and field events. Distances usually exceed 30 m (Chu 1998). A simple bounding exercise is skipping; an advanced bounding exercise is single-leg bounding. Skipping and bounding are explosive activities with the patient exploding quickly from landing and jumping upward and forward.

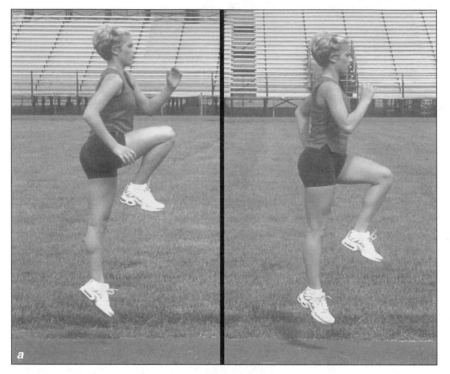

Skipping

Have the patient lift the right leg with the knee bent 90° while also lifting the left arm with the elbow bent 90°. Then the patient should alternate with opposite extremities (figure 9.9a).

Single-Leg Bounding

While on the right leg, the patient should move forward and upward as far as possible by using the momentum of the left leg and both arms to propel forward, landing on the right leg. Have the patient continue the forward and upward movement, this time landing on the left leg (figure 9.9b).

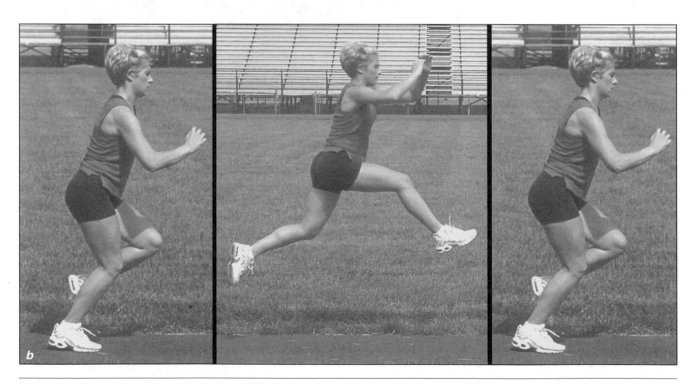

Figure 9.9　Examples of simple and more difficult bounding exercises: (a) skipping; (b) bounding.

Box Jumps

Box drills involve the more advanced skills required for multiple jumps and hops because the jumps and hops are performed onto and off boxes of varying heights. These exercises can be low or high intensity, depending on the box height. They use both vertical and horizontal jumps. Examples of box jumps are shown in figure 9.10.

Figure 9.10   Examples of box jumps: *(a)* front box jump; *(b)* pyramiding box jumps.

Front Box Jump

Begin with a box about 30 cm (12 in.) high. Jump onto the box with both feet. Step down and repeat. The difficulty can be increased by increasing the box height or using one leg, alternating left and right (figure 9.10a).

Pyramiding Box Hops

Place up to five boxes of increasing height about 0.6 to 0.9 m (2–3 ft) apart in a line. Jump onto the first box, onto the floor on the other side, and then onto the next box, repeating to the end of the row. Use the arms to assist in the motion (figure 9.10b).

Depth Jumps

Depth jumps are the most aggressive plyometric exercises. They are box jumps of greater intensity in that the patient is challenged by his or her own weight and the acceleration of gravity. The motion in depth jumps includes stepping off a box, dropping to the ground, and then rebounding immediately upward. These are intensive exercises that the patient must perform with caution. Jumping off the box is avoided in these exercises because a jump will increase the distance to the floor and significantly increase the stresses applied to the patient.

An example of progression using depth jumps consists of starting from a simple depth jump in which the patient steps down from a box and jumps vertically, using both feet, and advancing to a much more difficult depth jump—a single-leg depth jump in which the patient lands on one foot and jumps as high as possible from the one leg.

A more challenging progression can include using a higher box or using more than one box and jumping onto the second box from the ground.

Depth Jump

Have the patient step off a 30-cm (12-in.) box, landing on the floor with both feet. As rapidly as possible, the patient should jump upward as high as possible, using the arms to reach upward (figure 9.11a).

Single-Leg Depth Jump

Have the patient step off a 30-cm box, landing on the left leg only. The patient should spring upward as high as possible from the left leg. Then have him or her repeat the exercise with the right leg (figure 9.11b).

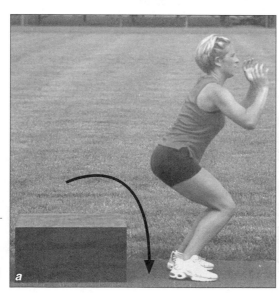

Figure 9.11
Examples of depth jumps: *(a)* depth jump; *(b)* single-leg depth jump.

Figure 9.11
(continued)

Box Height

You must select a box height for depth jumps carefully. If the height is too great, the risk of injury increases. A height that is too great also requires the muscles to absorb the impact of the drop, and the time required to absorb the force makes the amortization time too long to be effective.

Chu (1998) recommends determining a box height for depth jumps using the following procedure. The patient performs a standard jump-and-reach test, and the target point the patient achieves is marked. The patient then performs a depth jump from a 45-cm (18-in.) box and attempts to reach for the same point as attained on the test. If the mark is attained, the box height increases by 15-cm (6-in.) increments until the patient is unable to achieve the target point. The first box at which the patient is unable to achieve the target point is the depth-jump box height. If the patient cannot reach the target point from the 45-cm box, either the box should be lowered or the patient should not perform the activity until he or she has achieved greater strength.

Selection

Although all the types of plyometric exercises provide a progression of difficulty from low to high intensity, you must analyze the exercise to determine its relative intensity. For example, a high-level standing jump may be more intense than a moderate-level box jump.

The selection of exercise for a patient's program depends on the demands of the patient's sport and the level of participation of that patient. For example, you may give one patient appropriate plyometric exercises with varying intensities of multiple jumps and hops; another patient may be more appropriately stressed with box jumps and depth jumps. Two patients in the same sport, one at a recreational level and the other at an intercollegiate competitive level, have different requirements because of the different competitive demands. This is a prime consideration in exercise selection.

UPPER-EXTREMITY AND TRUNK PLYOMETRICS

▶ Plyometrics for the upper extremity and the trunk use tossing and throwing activities with medicine balls.

We will consider upper-extremity and trunk exercises together, because many of the upper-extremity exercises with medicine balls strongly influence the trunk muscles and vice versa. Some exercises are specific to either the upper extremity or the trunk, as indicated. Because the trunk plays a vital role in stabilization during upper-extremity activities, the strength of the muscle groups in the trunk is important to the strength of the upper extremity. The trunk muscles also perform trunk movement during upper-extremity activities.

Plyometrics for the upper extremity and trunk have essentially the same considerations as those for the lower extremity. The exercises should be specific to the sport demands, should provide a progression of difficulty so that there is a challenge and the patient makes the desired gains, and should be performed with controlled speed of movement.

You can provide progression by changing the intensity. This can be done by changing the weights of the medicine balls, the speed of the activity, and the distance the medicine balls are passed. Passing medicine balls includes tossing and throwing. Tossing is defined as passing a ball a short distance with the arm below 90° of shoulder flexion; throwing is defined as passing the ball a long distance with the arm above 90° of flexion (Chu 1989).

Passing exercises can be performed with either a partner or a rebounder—a trampoline inclined so that it permits return of the ball to the patient (figure 9.12).

Figure 9.13 provides examples of medicine ball plyometric exercises for the upper extremities and trunk. The chest pass photo shows the patient executing a chest pass from a distance of about 3 m (10 ft), using the forward movement of the legs to coincide with the snap of the ball. Follow-through should continue until the arms are fully extended in front of the body and the backs of the hands face each other. In the overhead throw, once again the patient uses leg movement to coincide with arm motion so that as the ball is released from behind the head. The patient moves from the back to the front leg. Follow-through is with the arms straight, upward, and forward. During both activities, the trunk muscles are kept taut and the back is held straight to allow force from the legs to be transmitted through the trunk to the arms.

As with lower-extremity plyometrics, upper-extremity and trunk plyometrics should be specific to the patient's needs. They should provide specific challenges that will permit the patient to make gains in the muscles most challenged by the patient's sport. The SAID principle is as important in plyometric exercises as it is in strength exercises. As was mentioned in chapter 7, the SAID principle is an acronym for **S**pecific **A**daptations to **I**mposed **D**emands and refers to the body's ability to adapt to stresses applied through exercise.

Figure 9.12
Rebounder and medicine balls.

Figure 9.13 Upper-extremity and trunk plyometrics: *(a)* chest pass; *(b)* overhead throw.

SUMMARY

1. Identify the mechanical and neurological components of the neuromuscular principles involved in plyometrics.

   Plyometrics involves the technique of first lengthening, then shortening the muscle to produce an increased power output. This type of exercise is based on the stretch-shortening principles. It is believed that a muscle's increased power during plyometric exercise training may result from a combination of an increased level of muscle elasticity and the adaptations that occur in the muscle spindle and GTO.

2. Describe the factors involved in plyometric program design.

   Every plyometric exercise includes three aspects—the lengthening or eccentric phase, the amortization phase, and the contracting or concentric phase. The lengthening phase prepares the muscles for the rapid change, or amortization, and allows for a greater contraction to produce greater results.

3. List three considerations for plyometric program execution.

   When designing a plyometric program, one must consider the patient's physical condition and the sport's demands. Specifically, the patient should have adequate flexibility, strength, and proprioception before beginning a plyometric program. Special considerations also include factors such as the patient's age, weight, level of competition, footwear, the surface, proper technique, progression, and goals.

4. List the precautions and contraindications for plyometrics.

   Precautions include factors such as the amount of time involved in plyometrics and the possibility of delayed-onset muscle soreness postexercise. Contraindications include an acute inflammation, postoperative conditions, and instability.

5. Outline a progression of four plyometric exercises for either a lower- or an upper-extremity program.

   A lower extremity plyometric exercise progression for a basketball player might begin with a two-foot ankle hop and progress to a single-foot ankle hop, side-to-side hops, standing jump-and-reach, long jump with lateral sprint, and box depth jumps.

CRITICAL THINKING QUESTIONS

1. If a plyometric jump is not executed quickly from the eccentric to the concentric phase, the patient is unable to jump as high during the concentric phase. What could the reasons be? What can be done if a patient does not understand the concept of a rapid change from eccentric to concentric and insists on pausing between the two phases? What cues or instructions can you provide to improve performance?

2. A patient with an ankle sprain is now ready for plyometric exercises. What are the criteria that he or she has to meet before these exercises can be added to the therapeutic exercise program?

3. A gymnast with a wrist sprain is ready for plyometric activities before returning to functional activities. Identify three plyometric activities that would prepare him or her for functional activities. What would your criteria be for progression from plyometric to functional activities?

4. The chief rehabilitation clinician of the college where you are working has asked you to write a sheet of instructions that the clinicians will hand out to patients before they begin the plyometric phase of their rehabilitation programs. What instructions will you include on the sheet? What precautions will you list? Are there any criteria that you will include for determining whether a patient is eligible for a plyometric program?

5. In the chapter's opening scenario, what precautions is Larry concerned about with Ed? What first-day plyometric activities would you recommend that Larry have Ed perform, and what should Larry look for when Ed performs them? How would you determine when Ed can progress in his plyometric program?

LAB ACTIVITIES

1. Have your lab partner perform each of the following jumps once, measure the height achieved with each jump, and record the results. Instruct your partner to begin each jump from the standing position. Allow a few practice jumps before doing the test jumps.

   a. Jump 1: Quickly bend the knees to approximately 60° and jump.

   b. Jump 2: Slowly bend the knees to approximately 60°, hold for 3 sec, and jump.

   c. Jump 3: Quickly bend the knees to approximately 120° and jump.

   d. Jump 4: Quickly bend the knees to approximately 120°, hold for 3 sec, and jump

   e. Jump 5: Step off a step stool or box, then immediately jump up.

   f. Jump 6: Jump up onto a box, then immediately jump off and jump upward.

   Which jump produced the greatest height? What is the physiological reason for your results? What is the importance of how these results relate to a plyometric rehabilitation program?

2. Have your lab partner perform a series of long jumps to determine the most advantageous body position and arm movement during the jump, as well as proper foot placement on landing for optimal force production. Repeat each jump from the preceding exercise, adding the conditions listed below. Perform three jumps using each condition. Record the subject's average jump height for each of the conditions. The jumps for each set should be performed rapidly with little or no rest between jumps.

   a. Condition 1: No arm movement; lands on the balls of the feet.

   b. Condition 2: Uses arm movement; lands on the balls of the feet.

   c. Condition 3: Uses arms and lands on the midfoot.

   Which jump produced the greatest distance? What is the physiological reason for your results? What is the importance of how these results relate to a plyometric rehabilitation program?

3. Have your lab partner select a sport he or she likes to play. Assume your lab partner is a patient who is now to the point where he is ready to perform plyometric exercises in the rehab program. Design a progression for the lower or upper extremity (using jumps in place, standing jumps, multiple jumps, box drills, and so on for LE; boxes, medicine balls, and so on for UE) to fit your individual patient's needs. Be sure to include how the patient would progress through the program and your outline of sets, reps, recovery, and intensity. Indicate your logic in why you selected these exercises, why you decided on this intensity level, and how you will determine when to advance the patient.

REFERENCES

Allerheiligen, B., and R. Rogers. 1995. Plyometrics program design. *Strength and Conditioning* 17: 26–31.

Chu, D. 1989. *Plyometric exercises with medicine balls.* Livermore, CA: Bittersweet.

Chu, D. 1998. *Jumping into plyometrics*, 2d ed. Champaign, IL: Human Kinetics.

Dean, E. 1988. Physiology and therapeutic implications of negative work. *Physical Therapy* 68: 233–237.

Gambetta, V. 1986. In Roundtable discussion: Blelik, E., Chu, D.A., Costello, F., Gambetta, V., Lundin, P., Rogers, R., Santos, J., and F. Wilt. Practical considerations for utilizing plyometrics. Part 1. *National Strength Coaches Association Journal* 8:14–22.

Koutedakis, Y. 1989. Muscle elasticity—plyometrics: Some physiological and practical considerations. *Journal of Applied Research in Coaching and Athletics* 4:35–49.

Lundin, P. 1985. A review of plyometric training. *National Strength Coaches Association Journal* 7: 69–74.

Wilk, K.E., Voight, M.L., Keirns, M.A., Gambetta, V., Andrews, J.R., and C.J. Dillman. 1993. Stretch-shortening drills for the upper extremities: theory and clinical application. *Journal of Orthopedic and Sports Physical Therapy* 17:225–239.

Wilt, F. 1975. Plyometrics. What it is—how it works. *Athletic Journal* 55:76–90.

CHAPTER 10

Functional Exercise

© Robert Bergstrom

Objectives

After completing this chapter, you should be able to do the following:

1. Explain the difference between functional exercise and functional testing.

2. Identify the contributions of functional exercise to a therapeutic exercise program.

3. Discuss the differences between basic and advanced functional activities.

4. List factors that can be varied in a progression of functional activities.

5. Identify precautions for functional exercises.

6. Outline a sample of functional progression for either the lower or upper extremity.

Casie Maran is a certified athletic trainer working with the college's tennis team. At the end of last season, Tim, the star singles player, underwent a shoulder capsular shift repair. He has progressed well through his rehabilitation program and is now ready to begin the process of returning to functional activities. It has been several months since Tim has swung a tennis racket, and he has a lot of apprehension about whether he will be able to return to competition. Casie is confident that he will do well once he has completed the functional rehabilitation phase of his program.

For the past few weeks Casie has had Tim get used to holding a tennis racket by having him bounce a ball on the ground and in the air with his elbow near his side. Now it is time for Tim to begin ground strokes. Casie has outlined the progression of the program she has designed for Tim, informing him that the program will move at his own pace and allow him and his shoulder to become accustomed to one level before advancing to the next level. Tim has confidence in Casie's ability and judgment because she has done an excellent job of bringing him this far along in his rehabilitation program. He knows that if she feels he can do an activity, he probably can do it.

> ■ Be such a man, and live such a life, that if every man were such as you, and every life a life like yours, this earth would be God's Paradise.

Phillip Brooks, American Episcopal bishop, 1835–1893

This chapter addresses an important but often forgotten aspect of therapeutic exercise: functional activities. Too frequently the injured athlete's program focuses on restoring flexibility, strength, power, and endurance, and the sport-specific demands are forgotten. During the later stages of the therapeutic exercise program it becomes important to prepare the injured athlete to withstand the specific stresses of his or her sport and meet the skill demands; it is also essential for the patient to have confidence that he or she can return to full participation.

Like the example in Reverend Brooks' quote above, most healthy individuals want to perform at exceptional levels. The presence of that preinjury attitude is critical if a patient is to return successfully to full participation. To restore that attitude, the rehabilitation clinician must include functional activities in the therapeutic exercise program. Functional activities are exercises that mimic the stresses, demands, and skills of the sport.

The rehabilitation clinician must understand and appreciate not only the patient's sport or occupation but also his or her responsibilities or activities. Offensive and defensive football players encounter different stresses and demands, just as the defensive lineman and defensive halfback position requirements are different. A volleyball setter and a volleyball hitter have different needs; a warehouse manager and a warehouse worker experience different stresses. The clinician should know the patient's specific sport or job requirements and also know how to incorporate those requirements into the therapeutic exercise program.

Once the basic parameters of flexibility, strength, endurance, and proprioception have been restored, specific exercises mimicking necessary skills are added to the program. This will restore the injured athlete's confidence in his or her performance ability and will also provide an avenue for renewing the skills lost following the injury.

DEFINITIONS, FOUNDATIONS, AND GOALS

▶ Functional exercise within a therapeutic exercise program encompasses exercise and evaluation. The goals of functional exercise are to attain full functional level of performance, restore the patient's confidence, and return the patient to sport participation.

Before we can discuss specific functional programs and activities, we must understand what functional exercises and evaluations are, and what their basis and goals are. Once you realize how a therapeutic exercise program progresses to its functional exercise portion, it will become clear when and how to apply functional exercises to this final phase.

Definitions

Functional exercise actually has two components in a therapeutic exercise program: exercise and evaluation. **Functional exercises** are activities that advance a patient to a safe return to full participation as soon as is feasible. These activities include exercises and skill drills in a progressive sequence that allows the patient to use the gains from one exercise to advance to the next level of exercise or skill drills.

Functional evaluation is performed throughout the program. **Functional evaluation** is an assessment of the patient's ability to perform an exercise or skill drill safely and accurately before he or she is allowed to advance to the next level. The final functional evaluation takes place before the patient resumes full participation. In order to safely advance to each therapeutic exercise level, the patient must pass the functional tests. The functional tests vary according to the patient's level within the therapeutic exercise program. Examples of these tests are discussed later.

Goals

Functional exercise has four goals. The first goal is to attain full functional levels of flexibility, strength, endurance, and coordination. The second is to achieve full functional ability so that normal speed, power, control, and agility are restored. The third goal of functional exercise is to restore the patient's self-confidence in his or her own performance as well as confidence in the injured body segment. The final goal is to return the patient to full participation safely and efficiently at a level at least equivalent to that of preinjury performance.

The first and second goals are achieved through the therapeutic exercise program for basic and advanced functional activities. These are discussed in the next section. The third goal is achieved through the advancement of functional exercises and the success the injured athlete experiences at each level. Success builds self-confidence, and failure makes self-confidence elusive; so it is important that the clinician provide exercise goals that are challenging yet achievable. Both being injured and being unable to participate in normal activities often cause an injured athlete to become unsure of his or her abilities. Not participating also leads to loss of some of the skills that were so natural before the injury. To reestablish in the patient a preinjury level of self-confidence in his or her athletic skills, it is necessary to incorporate into the therapeutic exercise program a progression of specific exercises that mimic the skills the patient will need to resume normal-level functions.

▶ Functional exercises contribute to the total rehabilitation process by imposing unique combinations of stresses on the injured athlete according to the individual's sport and position within the sport.

The final goal is achieved when all the other goals have been met. This goal is the end result and final goal of any therapeutic exercise program. To achieve it, the rehabilitation clinician must include both basic and advanced functional activities in the therapeutic exercise program. A final functional evaluation takes place before the patient returns to full participation, but it is the patient's ability to participate successfully in the normal activities that is the final test of a therapeutic exercise program.

CONTRIBUTIONS TO THERAPEUTIC EXERCISE

Functional exercises are a part of the total rehabilitation process. In that sense, they make a vital and unique contribution to the preparation and return to competition of the patient. They must place unique combinations of stresses on the patient to produce unique results. The following sections deal with eight of these demands and the corresponding results.

Normal Motion

Functional exercises are designed to reproduce the specific motions of the patient's normal activity. They are individually designed for the demands of each patient so that they mimic the normal activity that the patient will perform. Normal activity requires normal motion. If normal motion is lacking, the patient places undue stress on areas that must compensate for needed motion, and these areas are at risk for additional injury. For example, if a tennis player does not have the normal shoulder flexion and lateral rotation needed to serve, he or she may develop a low back injury by hyperextending the lumbar spine to hit the ball overhead.

Multifaceted Muscle Activity

Several different types of strengthening activities are used in functional exercises. They commonly include a mixture of isometric, concentric, and eccentric activities, because most functional activities include these types of movements. The muscle must have the strength, coordination, and control to quickly change from one type of movement to another and to effectively produce the summation of forces. Even in the simple activity of running, the lower-extremity muscles undergo a rapid change of concentric and eccentric activity in their roles as accelerators, decelerators, and stabilizers during different parts of the running cycle.

Multiplanar Motion and Multiple Muscle Group Performance

Functional activities are not performed in straight-plane movements. They involve the simultaneous use of all three planes of motion. They also include the use of many muscle groups that are recruited at one time to produce the desired activity. Functional exercises must mimic these functional activities by incorporating many muscle groups working in multiple planes.

Multiplanar motion is performed in a coordinated manner through the simultaneous facilitation and inhibition of many muscles. Even an activity like throwing a ball not only involves the shoulder, elbow, wrist, and hand muscles but also requires coordinated multiplanar motions from trunk and lower-extremity muscle groups.

Stabilization and Acceleration Changes

Functional motion requires that some muscles work to stabilize a part while other muscles work to either accelerate or decelerate or to change from stabilization to acceleration or deceleration quickly. If functional exercises are to mimic functional activities, muscles must be trained to perform these fluid functional changes that are part of even basic activities. To use the example of a throw, the trunk must be stabilized if the shoulder is to have a platform from which to propel the ball. Even during an activity such as walking, the hip and leg muscles stabilize and limit lateral movement as the body is propelled forward.

Proprioceptive Stimulation

Proprioception is the awareness of body movement and position. As discussed in chapter 8, proprioception is vital to performance. Proprioceptive skills, basic and advanced, must be finely tuned and must be prepared to meet the activity demands to which the patient will be returning. Performance of functional exercises requires the use of proprioception, and improvement of the patient's functional performance directly correlates to his or her proprioceptive development.

Agility and Power Development

Agility and power are essential requirements for most sports. Agility is necessary in order for the basketball player to dribble the ball downcourt, for the volleyball player to dive and pass the ball to the setter, and for the hurdler to time each jump correctly. Power allows the sprinter to reach the finish line before the other competitors, the football defensive lineman to sack the quarterback, and the crew team to sprint to the end of the race. Agility and power are required in a gymnast's floor exercise routine, an ice skater's triple-Lutz jump, and a water polo player's scoring a goal. Agility and power must improve as the patient increases his or her ability to perform functional activities. Progressive functional exercises steadily stress and, therefore, increase the patient's ability to perform at an agility and power level sufficient for appropriate skill execution within the sport and at the patient's level of competition.

Sport-Specific Skill Development

Functional exercises—from the basic exercises to the more advanced—have as their goal the injured athlete's return to sport participation. The advanced functional exercises used in the later stages of rehabilitation are specifically designed with this goal in mind. These functional exercises mimic the sport activities and place the same demands on the injured athlete that he or she will encounter when returning to participation. The specific skills needed to perform the rehabilitation exercises are the same skills that are needed to perform within the sport.

Confidence Development

As the patient succeeds in performing those functional exercises that mimic the demands of the sport, confidence returns. By the time the patient is ready to resume sport participation, he or she has demonstrated an ability to perform the skills that participation requires. This gives the individual the self-confidence to perform without hesitation and also to meet the demands of the sport with confidence in the injured part.

BASIC FUNCTIONAL ACTIVITIES

▶ The basic functional exercises that begin an injured athlete's therapeutic exercise program follow a progression to build the foundation for improvement in more specific skill activities.

In a good therapeutic exercise program, functional exercise and functional evaluation take place from the very beginning. The program starts with exercises for achieving basic parameter goals such as flexibility, strength, endurance, and proprioception. To some extent, these can be considered functional exercises because they are used to attain a goal that is necessary for functional performance. For example, in order to jump hurdles, a runner has to gain a functional degree of flexibility in the hamstrings. In order to compete, a wrestler must have full functional flexibility in the shoulders. A pitcher needs functional muscle endurance to pitch a game. A gymnast must be able to stork stand on the ground before he or she can stand on a balance beam.

Basic functional exercises have been discussed in previous chapters. At this point, the progression and sequence of the exercises should seem logical to you. Exercises for flexibility, strength, endurance, and proprioception follow a logical sequence. Each parameter requires a coherent progression of exercises that provides increasing stress as the area adjusts to and becomes able to tolerate greater stresses because of improvements already made.

Your functional evaluation tools utilize objective criteria. For example, gains in range of motion are evaluated by goniometry, and strength gains are evaluated by manual muscle testing or the use of objective tools such as isokinetic equipment or grip dynamometers. Once you have determined that a patient has reached specific goals, you advance the individual to the next goal. For example, once the patient has achieved 105° of knee flexion, he or she may exercise on a stationary bike. Once the patient is able to perform two sets of 15 repetitions of a biceps curl, you may either increase the weight or increase the repetitions. A patient should be able to stork stand on the ground before stork standing on an uneven surface. These are examples of functional progression of basic parameters.

ADVANCED FUNCTIONAL ACTIVITIES

▶ Advanced functional exercises build on fundamental skill functions that the injured athlete has already achieved and often include plyometrics and specific skill drills.

Functional progression of advanced parameters involves more specific skill activities. A patient must start with fundamental skill functions and progress to advanced skill functions after having mastered some of the basic skills. Advanced functional activities include plyometrics and specific skill-drill exercises. In addition to flexibility, strength, muscle endurance, and proprioception, they require the more advanced skills of agility, speed, power, and control. Depending on the requirements of the advanced skill, some advanced functional exercises can be started earlier in the program while the patient is still working to achieve proficiency of basic skill execution. For example, the patient can start basic coordination exercises such as bouncing a basketball before he or she has achieved full range of motion or full strength.

As with the evaluation of functional performance of basic exercises, evaluation of advanced functional exercises involves periodic examination and assessment and a logical progression. The patient should have good static and dynamic balance before performing plyometric exercises. He or she should be able to perform plyometric exercises before specific skill activities are incorporated into the therapeutic exercise program. These are all logical, commonsense concepts. The skill of the rehabilitation clinician is a factor in determining exactly when the progressions should occur and what they should be. This skill is based on knowledge about tissue healing; knowledge of the influences of the stresses applied by various exercises and activities; observation of the patient's reaction to the stresses; knowledge of an exercise sequence; and knowledge of the specific demands, skills, and requirements of the injured patient's sport or work tasks. The rehabilitation clinician's skill is also based on good judgment and common sense about how much stress to apply and when during the therapeutic exercise program to apply that stress.

Because the earlier chapters have addressed the progression of basic functional exercise and evaluation, this chapter focuses on progression of advanced functional exercise and evaluation.

ADVANCED FUNCTIONAL EXERCISE PROGRESSION

▶ Advanced functional exercises focus on the parameters of force and intensity, speed, distance, complexity, and support. Stresses are increased gradually and progressively according to the patient's ability to handle them, as well as other individual factors.

You may have noticed that some proprioceptive parameters are included in basic functional exercises and that agility is in the advanced functional exercises category. This is because proprioception is a transition parameter. Because of the wide range of complexity of proprioception, one of its simplest efferent results, balance, becomes a basic functional activity. Agility, however, requires a great deal of skill and is considered a more advanced functional activity.

Some basic functional exercises actually mimic advanced functional activities in that they are performed during a specific task. Examples of basic functional activities in various sports are stork standing in ice skating, standing on the unstable surface of the edge of a diving board, and walking on a gymnastics balance beam.

These examples of basic functional activities serve only as a reminder that it is sometimes difficult to draw the line between basic and advanced activities. It is a good idea to remember this as you think about progression of advanced functional exercises. You will also notice that some of the topics discussed here are similar to those presented in previous chapters on progression of exercises. The reason is that the same progression principles hold true, whether the topic is strength, plyometrics, or functional activity.

As with any progression in a therapeutic exercise program, the rate of increase should allow the body time to adjust to new levels of stress, should provide a continual overload stimulation to improve performance, and should involve systematic adjustments in parameters that influence the desired end of the progression—the return of the patient to competition. These parameters include force, speed, distance, complexity, and support.

Force and Intensity

Force and intensity are the amount of resistance that an activity provides. Forces and intensities vary in type depending on the specific activity and the outcome desired. The intent is to provide an overload in accordance with the SAID principle that has been described in chapter 7. The force or intensity starts light and increases as the patient is able to tolerate increased loads. For example, in an upper-extremity functional exercise such as a volleyball pass, the patient may begin with a medicine ball exercise using a 0.9-kg (2-lb) ball and increase to 1.8 kg (4 lb), then 2.7 kg (6 lb), and so on until the desired medicine ball weight is achieved.

Speed

Speed is the rate of a functional exercise. In the beginning, the speed is slower so that the patient can master correct execution of the exercise. As skill improves, the speed requirement increases. For example, an injured track athlete may begin running at half-normal speed for a specific distance but then increase the speed as his or her ability to handle increased stresses improves. In an upper-extremity exercise such as throwing, the patient may begin throwing at one quarter to one half normal speed and increase the speed of the throw as technique execution improves.

Specific speeds for initial functional exercises are individually established and are determined by a variety of factors. These factors include the length of time the patient has been out of full participation, the severity of the injury, the individual's competitive level, preinjury distances, motivation level, and goals for return to participation. As a rule of thumb, initial functional exercise speed may be one quarter to one half the normal or preinjury speed and progress to three-quarter speed and then to full speed. This is a very general rule, however, and you must always take into consideration the individual patient's condition and abilities, as well as the demands of the exercise.

Distance

Distances for functional activities range from short to long. The greater the distance, the greater the requirements of the activity. In the lower extremity, increasing distance may include increasing the patient's running distance or jumping distance. In the upper extremity it may include throwing or hitting a ball farther or swimming farther.

As in determining functional exercise speeds, one sets specific distances in initial functional exercises individually and according to the factors already discussed. A general guideline, though not a hard-and-fast rule, is to start with no more than one quarter to one half the preinjury distance. Initial distance, however, may be significantly less for a patient such as a marathoner who has been out of competition for four months and had a preinjury running distance of 16 km (10 miles) per workout, or for an outfielder who must throw a ball 55 m (180 ft). The rehabilitation clinician uses his or her best judgment and knowledge of healing and performance demands to determine the most appropriate distances for initial functional exercises. It is better to underestimate than to overestimate the patient's ability to withstand stresses. You can avoid aggravation of an injury when you underestimate but provoke it when you overestimate.

Complexity

Complexity of a functional exercise refers to how involved the activity is and how challenging it can be. Functional exercises progress from simple to complex. Each level of progression places more demands on the patient's ability and skill. For example, in the lower extremity, a jumping progression may begin with a simple standing jump activity and progress to multiple jumps-in-place, to a forward or backward jump, and to multiple forward or backward jumps. Upper-extremity functional exercises may begin with a simple activity such as bouncing a tennis ball into the air from the racket, and then progress to a forehand stroke, to a backhand stroke, to a combination of backhand and forehand strokes against a backboard, and to a combination of backhand and forehand strokes against another player across a net.

You can also increase complexity by having the patient perform a simple exercise and then progress to performing a number of simple exercises at one time. For example, a stork stand with eyes open becomes more complex when you have the patient catch a ground ball while stork standing. The progression continues when you have the patient catch the ground ball while stork standing on an uneven surface.

The rehabilitation clinician determines on an individual basis how complex the initial functional exercise should be and how quickly the complexity should increase. You must consider the factors already outlined and make the best judgment. Remember, it is always better to err on the side of caution when advancing the patient so that progression continues consistently forward, without regression.

Support

Support refers to the number of extremities that are bearing weight during the activity. In simple standing, support is bilateral; in a stork stand, support is unilateral. Unilateral stance is more difficult than bilateral stance. Jumping on one leg is a progression from performing the same activity on two legs. Throwing a ball with one hand overhead is more difficult than throwing a ball with two hands overhead; performing a push-up with one hand is more difficult than performing it with two hands.

The type of exercise is what determines whether the level of activity is basic or advanced. Once the exercise begins to mimic a specific skill or is a component of a skill, it is considered an advanced functional exercise. The progression of advanced functional exercises follows the same principles as for other types of exercises. For example, a common functional exercise progression for an injured track athlete may including starting with running a mile run at half speed, increasing distance or intensity until the patient has attained near-normal levels, and then increasing to three-quarter speed with the patient maintaining the previously achieved intensity and distance. Once normal speed and distance on level ground are achieved, hill work may proceed.

Throughout the progression, the exercises should be difficult enough to challenge the patient without causing failure. For this reason, the judgment and evaluative skills of the rehabilitation clinician are crucial in the decisions about the nature and pace of the progression of functional exercises. As the patient nears the end of the therapeutic exercise program and realizes that return to full participation is near, he or she must have self-confidence in performance ability, as well as confidence in the injured part, in order to be able to return to competition without hesitation or doubts. A progression of functional exercise to the final stages of advanced functional activities—essentially skill activities that mimic normal participation—must be severe enough to impose demands on the patient but simultaneously build the necessary self-assurance.

There may be several functional exercises that the patient is performing in one therapeutic exercise session. Some exercises may be at different demand levels than others. For example, one exercise may be at half-speed while another is at three-quarter speed. The session may include a simple exercise and also one that is much more complex. Selection of the level of each exercise is based on the individual's ability to execute each specific functional exercise.

▶ Because advanced functional activities increasingly challenge the patient's abilities, it is important to observe several important precautions within this part of the rehabilitation program. The patient must understand the exercise and avoid pain; the rehabilitation clinician must be aware of the patient's healing process and of his or her confidence and tolerance levels.

PRECAUTIONS

Advanced functional exercises are more complex, more challenging, and more rigorous than the basic functional exercises. This is generally so because multiple planes of motion, more muscle groups, more complex and simultaneous movements, and more agility are required for correct execution. Because of the increased demands such activities impose, there are also precautions that one must respect in assigning advanced therapeutic exercises to a patient.

Explain the Exercise to the Patient

Before executing the exercise, the patient should be made aware of how to perform the exercise, what its goals are, and what positions or movements to avoid. For example, the clinician demonstrates or else explains a stork stand on a trampoline by telling the patient that the eyes should remain open, that the arms are kept at the sides, and that the position should be maintained for 30 s. During execution, cues are given to correct the performance. The cues should be constructive and should include specific suggestions about how to improve the execution. Having the patient perform the exercise on the uninvolved extremity first may provide the individual with internal feedback of the correct performance. This is particularly helpful if the clinician tells the patient to note how the muscles feel when standing on the uninvolved leg and then try to attain the same feeling when standing on the injured leg. Instructing the patient to tighten the gluteal and thigh muscles may help to enhance stability.

Avoid Pain and Swelling

Residual pain and swelling, especially on the following day or evening, should be avoided. Any increase in pain or swelling indicates that the exercise level is too severe for the injured area. If this occurs, the patient should return to the previous level of exercise until the injured part is able to tolerate additional stress.

Any time a patient advances in a program, the rehabilitation clinician should observe for increases in pain and edema and instruct the patient to report any symptoms.

Understand Tissue Integrity

The rehabilitation clinician must be aware of the healing sequence and the time required for a specific tissue to complete the healing process. He or she must consider the tissue's structural integrity and understand the amount of stress involved in each specific functional exercise before including any functional activity in the therapeutic exercise program.

Know the Patient's Confidence Level

Performance of functional exercises requires the patient's confidence in his or her ability to perform the activity and in the ability of the injured part to tolerate the stress of the activity. If the patient is not prepared mentally or emotionally to handle a particular functional exercise, you should start with a less stressful, less complex activity that the person feels able to perform before advancing to more complex, more stressful exercises.

Be Aware of Progression Tolerance

Advanced functional exercises are introduced at lower-than-normal speed, intensity, and difficulty. Increases in these parameters are made one at a time until the exercise is equivalent to functional performance levels. The body must be allowed to adapt to increased levels of functional exercises before each change is are made. This will ensure that the patient's confidence can increase and that tissue overload is not excessive, thereby preventing additional injury.

▶ Step-by-step evaluation determines when the patient should advance to the next stage in the functional exercise program. The final functional evaluation, whose purpose is to determine whether the patient is ready to return to sport participation, is highly individualized.

FUNCTIONAL EVALUATION

Evaluation of function is an ongoing process. Throughout the therapeutic exercise program the rehabilitation clinician evaluates the patient's ability to perform both basic and advanced functional exercises. Advances in the program take place only after the patient is able to successfully perform to expected levels at each evaluation step. With the stork stand, for example, the patient does not progress until he or she is able to stork stand with eyes open for 30 s. Only after the patient passes that evaluation does the next phase of balance proceed. Then the patient may stork stand on an uneven surface or on the ground with eyes closed. The specific exercise used next depends on the demands of the patient's activity.

The final functional evaluation occurs before the patient is allowed to return to full participation. At this time the functional evaluation is highly individualized and is based on the specific demands of the patient's activity. The patient's performance in the evaluation determines his or her readiness to return to sport participation. Final functional examination includes highly specific drills and tests the person's performance skill. These functional examinations should be as objective as possible and mimic the individual's sport as much as possible. For a gymnast, the functional examination may include dismounts, tumbling skills, or apparatus skills. For a basketball player, the functional examination includes dribbling, shooting, cutting, or passing drills. For a football defensive lineman, the functional examination includes assessment of skills such as blocking, lateral or forward movements, agility, or quick changes of direction. Because specific functional activities vary greatly from job to job or sport to sport or positions within a sport, you must be familiar with the specific requirements for the patient. You may need to obtain the supervisor or coach's help in defining functional exercises and tests for some specific activities. It is the goal of the final functional examination, however, to demonstrate to the patient, the medical team, and the supervisor or coach that the individual is able and ready to withstand the stresses of full participation.

The functional tests for determining readiness to return to full participation must fulfill certain criteria, some of which have been previously mentioned. One criterion is that the examination tool should be as objective as possible. The tests should be repeatable so that it can be used both in initial examination and in final examination to measure changes and assess whether or not the patient has achieved the appropriate goals. The functional tests should provide useful information to the patient, and medical team about the progress and status of the patient's performance. They should also be able to show whether or not the functional exercise program is providing the advancement of parameters necessary for return to participation.

In the final functional examination, your observation and assessment of the patient's performance is critical. Any activity should be performed without hesitation, and the use of each extremity should be appropriate, with no favoring of the injured limb. The patient should move quickly, stabilize appropriately, and demonstrate self-confidence with all maneuvers. On the basis of the patient's performance, you should be unable to identify which extremity has been injured.

A LOWER-EXTREMITY FUNCTIONAL PROGRESSION

▶ A progression for lower-extremity function may begin with non-weight-bearing exercise and proceed to stork-standing exercises, dynamic movement activities such as lunges and jogging, and running activities. Lower-extremity functional testing should reflect the patient's sport activity as much as possible and should be as objective as possible.

This section presents functional exercises for the lower extremity and then describes functional testing that could be included as part of the assessment before the patient is allowed to return to unrestricted activity.

Functional Exercises

Any functional exercise should be preceded by a simple warm-up activity. Simple functional exercises for the lower extremity can begin relatively early with a non-weight bearing exercise such as proprioceptive neuromuscular facilitation. Partial weight bearing use of the BAPS board can also begin early in the therapeutic exercise program. As the patient becomes weight bearing, he or she can start to do stork standing, first with eyes open and then with eyes closed. This activity can progress from the floor to a BAPS board (figure 10.1), trampoline, 1/2 foam roller, or balance board (figure 10.2) and then to combining the balance activity with another activity such as ball catching. Stork-standing activities will then progress to dynamic movement activities such as lunges, step-ups and step-downs, walking, and jogging. Running activities begin with a forward jog on a flat surface, progress to increased speed and distances, and then move on to lateral runs and cuts and sudden changes in direction. In figure 10.3a, the patient pushes forward from the left foot to the right foot and then moves laterally to the left foot before retracing the steps to the starting position, moving from one position to the next as quickly as possible. Figure 10.3b shows W-sprints requiring the patient to sprint forward to the first marked spot or cone, then backpedal to the second marker, and then sprint forward to the next, repeating the series as illustrated to completion of the exercise. Figure 10.3c shows a figure-8 run, which uses markers or cones around which the patient runs in

Figure 10.1 BAPS board.

a figure-8 pattern. The exercise in figure 10.3d is similar to the W-sprint except that the patient runs straight ahead, pivots on the right outside leg to cut sharply to the left, runs straight ahead for a designated distance, and pivots on the left outside leg to cut sharply to the right until the end of the course. Each of these exercises can become more difficult if you require either a faster pace or smaller distances between the sudden motion changes.

Figure 10.4 shows examples of jumping exercises. In the jumping exercise in figure 10.4a, the patient faces a platform, places one foot on top of the platform, and then jumps as high as possible, switching foot placement so that the opposite foot ends up on the platform. This is a continuous and rapid jump-and-switch maneuver for a specified time or number of repetitions. A lateral jump is displayed in figure 10.4b; here the patient jumps from side to side over a dowel or other object, attempting to stay within the cones. Difficulty can be increased by spreading the outside cones and having the patient jump over the ball and toward the cones, or by placing a number of balls and cones in a line and having the person perform a series of lateral jumps in both directions.

A progression of jumping activities includes starting with jumping forward on a flat surface, then progressing to jumping backward and jumping laterally, first with both legs and then with only the involved leg. Jumping then can progress to box jumps, starting with low boxes and advancing to higher ones. Progressions for these lower-extremity and running activities are presented in figures 10.5 and 10.6.

Specific exercises are determined by the patient's activity demands. As much as possible, running and jumping exercises should mimic the activities that the patient will be performing once he or she returns to full participation.

Figure 10.2 Balance activities: *(a)* stork stand on ½ foam roller, *(b)* balance board.

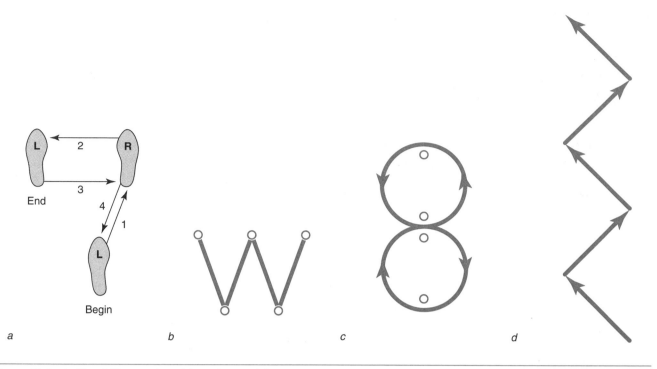

Figure 10.3 Agility drills, running: *(a)* 90° lunge, *(b)* W-sprint course, *(c)* figure-8 course, *(d)* Z-course (zigzag).

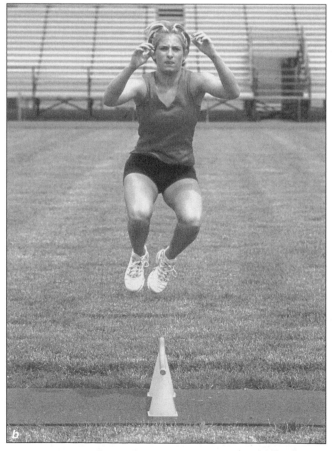

Figure 10.4 Agility drills: jumping.

Balance and Agility Progression Program

1. Beginning level
   a. Double-weight support for balance: static
      1) Stand with eyes closed, feet together, 30 s
      2) Stand in tandem-stance position, 30 s each
         — eyes open
         — eyes closed
   b. Single-weight support for balance: static
      1) Stork stand with eyes open, 30 s
      2) Stork stand with eyes closed, 30 s
      3) Stork stand with eyes open on unstable surface, 30 s each
         — trampoline
         — $\frac{1}{2}$ foam roller
      4) Stork stand with eyes closed on unstable surface, 30 s each
         — trampoline
         — $\frac{1}{2}$ foam roller
      5) Stork stand with complex activity
         — Stork stand on ground while playing catch
            – sport ball
            – medicine ball
         — Stork stand on uneven surface while playing catch
            – sport ball
            – medicine ball
2. Intermediate level: dynamic activities
   c. Two-leg support: balance board, wobble board
   d. One-leg support: trampoline jumping
   e. One-leg support: hopping
   f. Treadmill retrowalking
   g. BAPS board
   h. Fitter
   i. Step-up exercises
3. Advanced level
   j. Running activities (start at reduced speeds and distances, and progressively advance to normal speeds and distances)
   k. Jumping activities (bilateral support)
      1) Lateral jumping
      2) Forward-backward jumping
      3) Command jumping
   l. Hopping activities (unilateral support)
      1) Lateral hopping
      2) Forward-backward hopping
      3) Command hopping
   m. Cariocas
   n. Plyometric box jumping
4. Pre-injury level
   o. Sport-specific running, jumping, cutting activities at full speed
   p. Normal sport-specific drills
   q. Resumption of sport participation
   r. Mimic work activities (start at low reps, advance to more reps or more time)

Note: Jumping and hopping activities may start as exercises performed in place, but then can progress to line, target, and zigzag jumping and hopping exercises.

Figure 10.5 Example of a balance and agility progression program.

Lower-Extremity Functional Exercise Progression

1. Non-weight-bearing exercises
   - Proprioceptive neuromuscular facilitation
   - Joint reposition sense activities
2. Partial weight-bearing exercises
   - Aquatic exercises
   - BAPS board
   - Stationary bike
3. Full weight-bearing exercises
   - Lunges
     — partial depth
     — full depth (90°)
   - Running
     — running on level surface 50% maximum speed, $1/4$ normal distance
     — running on level surface 75% maximum speed, $1/4$ normal distance
     — running on level surface 100% maximum speed, $1/4$ normal distance
     — running on level surface 100% maximum speed, $1/2$ normal distance
     — running on level surface 100% maximum speed, full normal distance
     — running on incline surface 75% maximum speed, $1/2$ normal distance
     — running on incline surface 75% maximum speed, $3/4$ normal distance
     — running on incline surface 75% maximum speed, full normal distance
     — running on incline surface 100% maximum speed, full normal distance
   - Sprinting
     — sprinting on level surface 50% maximum speed, $1/4$ normal distance
     — sprinting on level surface 75% maximum speed, $1/4$ normal distance
     — sprinting on level surface 100% maximum speed, $1/4$ normal distance
     — sprinting on level surface 100% maximum speed, $1/2$ normal distance
     — sprinting on level surface 100% maximum speed, $3/4$ normal distance
     — sprinting on level surface 100% maximum speed, normal distance
   - Jumping/Hopping
     — jumping rope, both feet
     — jumping rope, one foot
     — jumping lines, both feet forward, backward
     — jumping lines, one foot forward, backward
     — jumping lines, both feet zigzag forward, backward
     — jumping lines, one foot, zigzag forward, backward
     — box jumps, 6-in. boxes, two feet, forward
     — box jumps, 6-in. boxes, two feet, sideways
     — box jumps, 6-in. boxes, one foot, forward
     — box jumps, 6-in. boxes, one foot, sideways
     — box jumps of increasing heights with sequences above repeated
   - Agility
     — cariocas, 50% speed, both to left and to right
     — cariocas, 75% speed, both to left and to right
     — cariocas, 100% speed, both to left and to right
     — circle-8s with same sequence as cariocas, starting with large circles and reducing the size to tight circles
     — zigzag sprints with same sequence as cariocas
     — command drills with sudden changes in direction of any agility exercise on command

   Note: Any of these exercises can be made more difficult by increasing distance or number of sets, or using weights with the exercise.

Figure 10.6 Example of a lower-extremity functional exercise progression.

Functional Testing

Several different tests for lower-extremity function can be used. The tests chosen should reflect the patient's sport activities as accurately as possible and should be as objective as possible. To measure gains in performance, you should use the same test to evaluate performance at the time the patient begins the functional exercise and before he or she returns to full activity.

Lower-extremity tests can be classified as running tests for time and distance, jumping tests for height and distance, and agility tests. The running tests can be sprints or can be timed long-distance runs, depending on participation demands.

Jumping tests can include a standing vertical jump, a step-and-jump, a repeated jump for distance, and a single jump for distance. A volleyball player's jump test is more functional if it is either a standing or a step-and-jump test, whereas a field athlete's test is more functional if it is a multiple or run-and-jump-for-distance test.

Agility tests use cariocas, zigzag runs, figure-8 runs, shuttle runs, and box runs, to name a few. Whatever activities are selected, the distances, angles, and sizes of the turns and circles should be the same on the pretest as on the posttest for accurate comparisons. Goals should also be predetermined. The specifics of these goals may be defined either with reference to established norms or by the athlete's pre-injury performance ability.

AN UPPER-EXTREMITY FUNCTIONAL PROGRESSION

▶ As with lower-extremity functional exercise, upper-extremity functional activities should resemble the activities of the patient's sport. Functional testing for the upper extremity varies greatly because use of the upper body differs markedly from one sport to another.

As in the discussion of the exercise program for the lower extremity, this section describes functional exercises and functional assessment for the upper extremity.

Functional Exercise

Like lower-extremity functional work, upper-extremity functional exercises may begin early in the program with proprioceptive neuromuscular facilitation (figure 10.7) and manual resistance for scapular stabilization. And again, upper-extremity exercises should be preceded by warm-up activities. Partial weight-bearing activities on a Swiss ball can sometimes be used early in the program as well. Closed kinetic chain activities such as weight-bearing exercises, first on a stable surface and then on an unstable surface, can be used once full weight bearing is permissible. A patient in a push-up position with hands on BAPS board or wobble board is an example of a closed kinetic chain activity on an unstable surface. Both hands are on the

Figure 10.7 Functional exercise progression for the upper extremity: *(a)* open kinetic chain, *(b)* closed kinetic chain.

board while the patient moves the board. In a push-up position, the patient can start with two arms and advance to one, while the hands move side to side by bouncing. In another example with the patient in a push-up position, the patient moves the Fitter platform side to side. All push-up positions can progress from a modified push-up position on hands and knees to a full push-up position on hands and feet. The patient must attain scapular muscle strength, rotator cuff strength, and large shoulder muscle and other upper extremity strength gains, along with proper range of motion, before beginning specific functional exercises. Having achieved proper stabilization, strength, range of motion, and control, the patient can progress to activity-specific functional exercises such as lifting, throwing, golf exercises, tennis exercises, or swimming exercises. A progression of throwing begins with shortened distances for reduced speed and with power throwing at reduced repetitions; it advances to increased distances, numbers of throws, and severity of throws. See figure 10.8 for an example of a throwing progression program.

Baseball/Softball Pitching/Throwing Progression Program

1. Beginning level
   a. 40–45-ft distance
       50% normal speed
       30 throws, 2 sets
   b. 40–45-ft distance
       50% normal speed
       30 throws, 4 sets
   c. 40–45-ft distance
       75% normal speed
       30 throws, 3 sets
   d. 40–45-ft distance
       75% normal speed
       30 throws, 5 sets
   e. 60-ft distance
       75% normal speed
       30 throws, 3–4 sets
   f. 60-ft distance
       75% normal speed
       30 throws, 5 sets

2. Intermediate level
   g. 60-ft distance
       100% normal speed
       30 throws, 3–4 sets
   h. 100-ft distance
       75% normal speed
       30 throws, 3–4 sets
   i. 100-ft distance
       75% normal speed
       30 throws, 5 sets
   j. 100-ft distance
       100% normal speed
       30 throws, 3–4 sets

   k. 100-ft distance
       100% normal speed
       30 throws, 5 sets
   l. 150-ft distance
       75% normal speed
       30 throws, 3–4 sets
   m. 150-ft distance
       75% normal speed
       30 throws, 5 sets
   n. 150-ft distance
       100% normal speed
       30 throws, 5 sets

3. Advanced level
   o. 180-ft distance
       75% normal speed
       30 throws, 3 sets
   p. 180-ft distance
       75% normal speed
       30 throws, 5 sets
   q. 180-ft distance
       100% normal speed
       30 throws, 3 sets
   r. 180-ft distance
       100% normal speed
       30 throws, 5 sets

4. Precompetition level
   s. Throw off mound
       100% normal speed
       30 throws, 3–4 sets
   t. Throw off mound
       100% normal speed
       30 throws, 5 sets

Note: All throwing sessions begin with a warm-up and end with a cool-down. Warm-up and cool-down throws are performed as light, arcing tosses. A rest of 3 to 5 min between sets is allowed. If the patient experiences pain with an increase to the next level, he or she should return to the previous level for another session. If the patient is not a pitcher, throwing progression follows the same routine as listed, but the distances vary according to the sport (e.g., discus, javelin, football) and are determined by the distances and weights used within the sport.

Figure 10.8 Example of a baseball or softball pitching/throwing progression program.

A golf progression may begin with the putter and short irons for putting and chipping activities and progress to longer irons, fuller swings, and then to the woods with a full swing. Each club the swing begins as a partial swing and increases to a full swing as the patient gains progressive control of the club. Repetitions also increase as the patient's endurance improves. See figure 10.9 for an example of a golf progression program.

Golf Progression Program

1. Beginning level
   a. Putts and chips
      20 putts, varying distances
      10 chips
   b. Putts and chips
      20 putts, varying distances
      20 chips
   c. Putts and chips
      20 putts, 3 sets
      20 chips, 2 sets
   d. Putts and chips
      20 putts, 3 sets
      20 chips, 3 sets

2. Intermediate level
   e. Short irons, no more than three clubs
      partial swing, 1   20 each
   f. Short irons, no more than three clubs
      partial swing, 2   20 each
   g. Short irons, no more than three clubs
      partial swing, 3   20 each
   h. Short irons, no more than two clubs
      full swing, 1   20 each
   i. Short irons, no more than two clubs
      full swing, 2   20 each
   j. Short irons, no more than two clubs
      full swing, 3   20 each

   k. Long irons, no more than three clubs
      partial swing, 1   20 each
   l. Long irons, no more than three clubs
      partial swing, 2   20 each
   m. Long irons, no more than three clubs
      full swing, 2   20 each
   n. Long irons
      full swing, 3   25 each
   o. All irons
      full swing, 1   20 each

3. Advanced level
   p. Woods
      partial swing, 2   20 each
   q. Woods
      full swing, 2   20 each
   r. Woods and irons
      full swing, 1   20–25 each

4. Preparticipation level
   s. Par-three course
   t. Nine-hole course
   u. Return to regular play

Note: All sessions begin with a warm-up and end with a cool-down. A rest of 3 to 5 min between sets is allowed. If the patient experiences pain with an increase to the next level, he or she should return to the previous level for another session.

Figure 10.9   Example of a golf progression program.

We have already briefly looked at a progression of tennis functional exercises. A simple stabilization exercise such as bouncing the ball on the floor with the racket can begin once the scapular stabilizers and rotator cuff are able to maintain proper control. This activity can advance to bouncing the ball in the air with the racket. More advanced exercises progress from a forehand to a backhand to overhead and serve strokes. See figure 10.10 for a general outline of a progression.

Tennis Progression Program

1. Ball bounce
   Bounce the tennis ball on the racket into the air. Start by grasping the racket on the neck and advance to the handle.
   - a. 50 bounces with a palm-down grip
   - b. 50 bounces with a palm-up grip
   - c. 50 bounces alternating between palm down and palm up

2. Forehand strokes
   Forehand strokes only against a backboard or wall
   - d. 50% power: 5   10
   - e. 75% power: 3   20
   - f. 100% power: 3   40

3. Backhand strokes
   Backhand strokes only against a backboard or wall
   - g. 50% power: 5   10
   - h. 75% power: 3   20
   - i. 100% power: 3   40

4. Alternate strokes
   Alternate between backhand and forehand strokes against a wall or backboard
   - j. 75% power: 5   15
   - k. 100% power: 3   30
   - l. 100% power: 4   40

5. Overhead serve
   Overhead serve against a wall or backboard
   - m. 50% power: 5   10
   - n. 75% power: 3   20
   - o. 100% power: 3   40

6. Game
   - p. Play one set of tennis
   - q. Play two sets of tennis
   - r. Play three sets of tennis
   - s. Play full game of tennis

Note: All sessions begin with a warm-up and end with a cool-down. The patient should attempt to hit a specific target or targets on the backboard or wall. If the patient experiences pain with advancement to the next level, he or she should return to the previous level for the next 2 to 3 sessions before returning to the higher level.

Figure 10.10   Example of a tennis progression program.

A swimmer's progression may begin with the use of a stroke for a short distance or with alternating strokes for short distances and performing the stroke for no more than half-normal speed. Distances and speed increase as tolerated. See if you can develop an example of a swimmer's progression program using these guidelines.

I want to emphasize that the progressive functional exercise programs presented here are only examples. Specific exercise progressions vary depending on the patient's needs, abilities, level of competition, length of time away from the activity, and degree of injury. The programs described in this chapter offer only general guidelines and are a means of demonstrating how to progress and change parameters of a functional exercise program.

Functional Testing

It is more difficult to examine the upper extremity and obtain objective and measurable criteria than for the lower extremity. This is because of the variety of uses of the upper extremity in activities. If a speed gun is available, it is relatively simple to measure the speed of a patient's throw. However, if you do not have a speed gun or the patient's activity does not involve throwing, measuring functional skill objectively is more difficult.

Functional goals are individually determined and based on the patient's preinjury performance. For a golfer, it may be his or her score on 18 holes of golf. For the swimmer, it may be the ability to perform a specific swim event within the same time he or she had in preinjury performances. For the tennis player, measurement using a speed gun for a serve is simple, but evaluating participation performance may be more difficult. Establishing goals such as hitting a specific target across the net on a given number of consecutive forehand and backhand shots, and using that number for pretest and posttest performance guidelines, may be a way of establishing an objective measure. When establishing any goal in this manner, it is important for you to consult with the supervisor or coach to arrive at realistic and achievable goals.

RETURNING THE PATIENT TO FULL PARTICIPATION

▶ Four criteria are used to determine that the patient has completed the rehabilitation program and is ready to return to sport participation. These relate to the status of the injury itself and to patient's functional levels, sport-specific skills, and degree of confidence.

Once the therapeutic exercise program, including advanced functional exercises, has been completed and the patient is ready to return to full participation, specific criteria must be fulfilled before the individual is actually allowed to return. The entire therapeutic exercise program has been designed and administered by the rehabilitation clinician for this very goal. The true test of the success of the program comes with the patient's return to his or her performance level.

In order for that to happen, the patient must meet four specific criteria:

1. The acute signs and symptoms of the injury have resolved, and no pain or edema is present.

2. The patient is able to demonstrate full range of motion; normal strength, muscle endurance, and cardiovascular endurance; and appropriate proprioception, agility, and coordination in relation to the required performance skills.

3. The patient is able to perform any and all activities at least as well as he or she could before the injury. As has been mentioned, you should be unable to identify the area that has been injured if the patient is performing the activities appropriately.

4. The patient has the confidence in both his or her own ability and the ability of the injured area to perform, without any hesitation or doubt, or any modification of performance or mechanics.

If these criteria are met and the patient is able to pass all functional evaluation tests, the rehabilitation clinician has accomplished the goals established at the start of the therapeutic exercise program.

SUMMARY

1. Explain the difference between functional exercises and functional testing.

   Functional exercises are used in a therapeutic exercise program from its early stages to its final stages. The early stages utilize functional exercises designed primarily to restore basic parameters such as flexibility, strength, endurance, and balance. In the later stages, more advanced functional activities gradually push the patient to the final level of functional activities, those that mimic normal activity. Functional testing uses activities or drills which are specific to the patient's sport demands and activities to mimic the maneuvers and movements that will be required when the patient returns to full participation. This testing assesses whether the patient is ready to resume normal activities.

2. Identify the contributions of functional exercise to a therapeutic exercise program.

   Functional exercises are used to ready the patient physically for the stress and demands of his or her activity and to prepare the patient mentally. The effects of successful execution of functional activities come through the patient's discovery that the injured segment is able to withstand normal stresses.

3. Discuss the differences between basic and advanced functional activities.

   Basic exercises begin early in the therapeutic exercise program to assist in achieving flexibility, strength, endurance, and proprioception. Advanced exercises, however, include specific skill activities that more closely resemble or even duplicate the demands of normal activity on the patient and the rehabilitated segment.

4. List factors that can be varied in a progression of functional activities.

   Functional exercises proceed from slow to fast, simple to complex, low force to high force, short distance to long distance, and bilateral support to unilateral support. A progression of functional exercises includes a steady change to allow for SAID principle advancement. Functional exercises include some characteristics unique to functional exercises and some characteristics common to most exercises.

5. Identify precautions for functional exercises.

   Some precautions are those discussed in prior chapters and include explaining the exercise to the patient, avoiding pain and swelling, considering tissue integrity when designing exercises, knowing the patient's confidence level, and being aware of the patient's progression tolerance.

6. Outline a sample of functional progression for either the lower or upper extremity.

   The specific progression and selection of exercises depend on the patient's specific task demands, especially as he or she nears the final stages of the program. A lower-extremity program may include a progression from non-weight-bearing use of the BAPS board that can start early in the therapeutic exercise program. As the patient becomes weight bearing, stork standing first with eyes open and then with eyes closed can begin. A progression of this activity can go from using the floor to using either a trampoline or a 1/2 foam roller or balance board to combining the activity with another activity such as ball catching. Stork-standing activities can then progress to dynamic movement activities such as lunges, step-ups and step-downs, walking, and jogging. Running activities begin with a forward jog on a flat surface, proceed to increased speed and distances, and then to lateral runs and cuts and sudden changes in direction.

CRITICAL THINKING QUESTIONS

1. On the basis of the scenario at the beginning of this chapter, what would you do to improve Tim's confidence in his tennis abilities? What activities would you have him do on the first day of his functional program? List three levels of progression and give your criteria for advancement. When would you have him start overhead activities and serves?

2. When would you decide that Tim is able to return to full participation? What would your criteria be for this, and why have you set these criteria?

3. A volleyball player who injured his knee and has completed the rehabilitation program up to the functional activities level is very anxious to return to full sport participation. You estimate that it will be another week before he has successfully completed the functional activities portion of the program. What will your first day's activities include, and how will you establish a progression of activities? What are your criteria for each level of progression? What specific activities must he be able to perform before he may resume full volleyball participation?

4. A cross country competitor is now ready for functional activities. She has been running short distances of no more than 2 min without difficulty. What distance, speed, and terrain progression will you give her over the course of the next two weeks? Write up a two-week progression of functional activities that will move her to full sport participation.

LAB ACTIVITIES

1. Design a functional upper-extremity program of five exercises for your patient who is a computer programmer. Identify the goals for each activity, have her perform the activity, and score the performance. Explain your scoring criteria and report your lab partner's score. Identify how you would know when to progress from one exercise to the next exercise.

2. Design a functional upper-extremity program for your lab partner who is a baseball outfielder. Identify the goals for each activity, have him perform the activity, and score the performance. Explain your scoring criteria and report his or her score. Identify how you would know when to progress from one exercise to the next exercise. How does this program differ from the one you set up for the computer programmer? Why?

3. Design a functional lower-extremity program for your partner who is a volleyball player. Identify the goals for each activity, have her perform the activity, and score the performance. Explain your scoring criteria and report partner's score. Identify how you would know when to progress from one exercise to the next exercise.

4. Design a functional lower-extremity program for your lab partner who is a 4 × 400m relay runner. Identify the goals for each activity, have him perform the activity, and score the performance. Explain your scoring criteria and report his score. Identify how you would know when to progress from one exercise to the next exercise. How does this program differ from the one you set up for the volleyball athlete? Why?

5. You are in the final phase of a rehabilitation program for a basketball forward who is recovering from a lateral ankle sprain. Design a progressive functional exercise program in preparation for return to play. Have your partner perform each exercise you include in the program to see if you have provided a progression of the exercises, moving from the easiest to the most difficult. Assuming no delays or backward steps in ability to perform the exercises, outline how you would progress her in the program and what criteria you would use to determine when to progress.

SUGGESTED READING

Cordova, M.L., and C.W. Armstrong. 1996. Reliability of ground reaction forces during a vertical jump: Implications for functional strength assessment. *Journal of Athletic Training* 31:342–345.

Kegerreis, S. 1983. The construction and implementation of functional progressions as a component of athletic rehabilitation. *Journal of Orthopedic and Sports Physical Therapy* 5:14–19.

Kegerreis, S., Malone, T., and J. McCarroll. 1984. Functional progressions: An aid to athletic rehabilitation. *Physician and Sportsmedicine* 12:67–71.

Kegerreis, S., and T. Wetherald. 1987. The utilization of functional progressions in the rehabilitation of injured wrestlers. *Athletic Training* 22:32–35.

Keskula, D.R., Duncan, J.B., Davis, V.L., and P.W. Finley. 1996. Functional outcome measures for knee dysfunction assessment. *Journal of Athletic Training* 31:105–110.

Lephart, S.M., Perrin, D.H., Fu, F.H., and K. Minger. 1991. Functional performance tests for the anterior cruciate ligament insufficient athlete. *Athletic Training* 26:44–50.

Tippett, S.R., and M.L. Voight. 1995. *Functional progressions for sports rehabilitation.* Champaign, IL: Human Kinetics.

III

General Therapeutic Exercise Applications

If you nurture your mind, body, and spirit, your time will expand. You will gain a new perspective that will allow you to accomplish much more.

Brian Koslow, author

As you progress through this text, you should continue to grow in your knowledge of therapeutic exercise and your appreciation of the complexity, expanse, and intricacy of the information that a rehabilitation clinician must possess. In reading part I, you obtained information vital to an understanding of the material in part II. Now that you have a basic knowledge of the physical and physiological concepts that underlie the principles of therapeutic exercise, we can investigate some general applications of this information. The remaining parts of this book, parts III and IV, will use the foundation established in these earlier chapters to provide you with the guidelines in the remaining chapters. These guidelines will allow you to develop and build a sound therapeutic exercise program for the patients you will encounter as an allied health professional.

Part III deals with general concepts that are important in themselves but also serve as the final foundational elements for the knowledge in part IV. Part III presents information on topics such as posture, body mechanics, and ambulation with and without aids. It also presents information on general therapeutic exercise programs that can be used with most injuries and for most body segments.

Chapter 11 presents information about posture and body mechanics. It is not unusual to find that posture abnormalities, the ways that people use the body in physical activity, and muscle imbalances are key to an injury or are the reason an injury does not respond readily to treatment. Learning about posture, body mechanics, and body awareness will help you become more knowledgeable about often undetected sources of injury.

Chapter 12 presents an overview of normal walking and running. This is followed by information on ambulation with assistive devices and correct methods of using the devices. You will also read about how to instruct the patient in the correct use of assistive devices, a critical topic for ambulation safety.

The next two chapters include information on commonly incorporated therapeutic programs using aquatics and aquatic equipment (chapter 13) and foam rollers and Swiss balls (chapter 14). Increasingly, therapeutic exercises include these items, so they are included as part of the total picture of therapeutic exercise.

The final chapter in part III, chapter 15, deals with therapeutic exercise for tendinitis. Tendinitis can affect several different parts of the body. Although it would have been possible to discuss tendinitis in part IV, which covers therapeutic exercise of specific body parts, I have chosen to devote a separate chapter to tendinitis. Tendinitis is a complex problem that can nag a patient for an extended time and delay resumption of full activity. Specific techniques and procedures can alleviate the problem. Considering the uniqueness of tendinitis in comparison to acute athletic injuries, I have given special attention to relevant principles, concepts, and precautions and to recent developments in the treatment of tendinitis.

Once you have completed part III, the remaining section, part IV, should simply be a matter of putting all the information gathered from parts I, II, and III together to create your own therapeutic exercise program. As you proceed through part III, continue to use your deductive reasoning skills, the knowledge that you have acquired from the previous chapters, and your common sense to see if you can anticipate the information presented in each chapter of part III. Although some of the material will be new, much of it will be based on what you have already learned.

Posture and Body Mechanics

Objectives

After completing this chapter, you should be able to do the following:

1. Identify the primary elements of proper alignment in standing from an anterior, posterior, and side view.

2. Discuss common postural faults and describe their causes.

3. Outline corrective exercises for common postural faults.

4. Explain the importance of good posture and proper body mechanics in athletics and physical activity.

5. List the basic principles of good body mechanics.

6. Discuss an example of the use of proper body mechanics by the rehabilitation clinician during a treatment program.

7. Explain the differences and similarities between the Feldenkrais Method and the Alexander Technique.

8. Identify concepts involved in Pilates exercise techniques.

> ■ **Great and noble are those scientific judgments that preserve the health and lives of their creatures.**
>
> Moshe ben Maimon (Maimonides), Rabbi, physician, and author, 1135-1204

This chapter opens the door on the topic of posture and body mechanics. Now that you have become familiar with basic concepts and therapeutic exercise program parameters, it is time to see how they can be applied. Part III begins with this chapter on posture and body mechanics because these factors can affect performance and risk of injury. If you are to improve an individual's posture or body mechanics, you must first identify what is normal. This chapter deals with normal standing and sitting posture, common causes and effects of pathological posture, and correct body mechanics. Body mechanics, as discussed here, relates to daily activities, sport activities, and activities that you as a rehabilitation clinician perform during your treatment sessions with patients. Two of the more commonly used body-awareness techniques will also be introduced. Pilates exercises will be introduced in this chapter since Pilates deals with balance of strength and flexibility to produce body control.

Once you have developed an appreciation for proper posture and correct body mechanics, it will become easier for you to examine injuries, especially chronic injuries, and develop the appropriate therapeutic exercise programs. Use of proper posture for you as the rehabilitation clinician is important if you are to conserve energy, prevent injuries for yourself, and provide efficient and effective manual therapy and manual-resistance applications.

POSTURE

▶ Posture, or the relative alignment of various body segments, includes standing alignment and sitting alignment. Anterior, posterior, and lateral views show whether alignment of the various segments of the body is normal.

Posture is the relative alignment of the various body segments with one another. When a person has good posture, the body's alignment is balanced so that stress applied to the body segments is minimal. When a person has poor posture, the body's alignment is out of balance, causing exaggerated stresses to various body segments. Over time this continual stress, even at relatively low levels, causes anatomical adaptations. These changes alter the individual's ability to perform and affect the body's overall efficiency.

Although people seldom stand still, static standing posture is used as the reference for posture evaluation. Static posture can reveal abnormalities in relative balance and alignment of body parts that can affect structure and function. Before we can discuss improper posture, we must identify normal posture.

Figure 11.1 Frontal posture view.

Correct Standing Alignment

Standing posture is assessed in three planes: sagittal, frontal, and transverse. A plumb line is used as a point of reference. This term is derived from the Latin word, *plumbum*, meaning "lead." A **plumb line** is a string with a weight (formerly a lead weight, but any weight object will do) at the end. When suspended, the string forms a vertical line. The patient stands behind the plumb line as posture is assessed.

Anterior View

From the anterior, or front, view, the plumb line bisects the body into symmetrical left and right sides (figure 11.1). The patient should stand so that the feet are equidistant from the plumb line. The arms should be relaxed with the palms of the hands facing the sides of the thighs. In this position, the line should bisect the nose and mouth and run through the central portion of the sternum, umbilicus, and pubic bones. The earlobes should be level with one another, as should the shoulders, fingertip ends, nipples, iliac crests, patellae, and medial malleoli. The patellae should point straight ahead with the feet straight or turned slightly outward. The knees and ankles are in line with each other, with the knees angled neither inward nor outward.

Figure 11.2 Posterior posture view.

Posterior View

The posterior, or back, view should demonstrate alignment similar to that observed from the front (figure 11.2). The plumb line should bisect the head and follow the spinous processes from the cervical through the lumbar spine. The earlobes, shoulders, scapulae, hips, posterior superior iliac spine, gluteal fold, posterior knee creases, and medial malleoli should appear level left to right. The scapulae should lie against the rib cage between the second and seventh ribs and about 5 cm (2 in.) from the spinous processes. The calcaneus should be straight and the calcaneal tendon perpendicular to the floor. Trunk muscles should appear balanced, with symmetrical development. The shoulders should be relaxed with the gap between the elbows and lateral trunk equal. Body weight should appear equally distributed over the two feet.

Figure 11.3 Lateral posture view.

Lateral View

From a lateral or side view, the patient stands with the plumb line slightly anterior to the lateral malleolus (figure 11.3). When the patient is positioned with the plumb line referenced at the ankle, observe the lateral alignment from the head down. The plumb line should pass through the external auditory meatus, the earlobe, the bodies of the cervical vertebrae, the center of the shoulder joint, and the greater trochanter. The plumb line should run midway between the back and chest and the back and abdomen, slightly posterior to the hip joint, and slightly anterior to the center of the knee just behind the patella. A horizontal line should connect the anterior superior iliac spine (ASIS) and posterior superior iliac spine (PSIS). The patient should remain relaxed with the body's weight balanced between the heel and the forefoot. The knees are straight but not locked. The chin is slightly tucked, and the chest is held slightly up and forward. There is a mild curve inward of the low-back and neck regions.

Correct Sitting Alignment

As in standing, correct sitting posture places the minimum amount of stress on the body. Students in high school and college and many individuals in the work force spend much of their day in chairs. Incorrect sitting posture can aggravate an injury and prolonged sitting can lead to injury.

In a correct alignment, the chair seat height must allow the individual's feet to rest comfortably on the floor with the knees and hips at 90°. The chair seat depth should be such that the edge of the seat does not press against the back of the individual's knees. The chair back should support the lumbar and thoracic spine and come to the lower border of the scapulae. A lumbar roll will contour to the curve of the lumbar spine and can provide additional low-back support. Higher-backed executive chairs should provide full thoracic support and permit the person to lean back comfortably. If the chair has arms, they should be at a level that provides for shoulder relaxation and permits the forearms to rest comfortably with the elbows at 90° (figure 11.4).

If the person is sitting at a desk, the chair height should be such that the person's forearms rest comfortably on the desk without hunching the shoulders up or down. If the chair height must be increased to achieve a correct position, a footrest may be necessary to maintain 90° knee and hip positions and still keep the feet flat on the floor. When the individual is using a computer keyboard, the forearms are at 90° or slightly less (0° is full extension), and the wrists are in a neutral position with the fingers resting on the keyboard.

All sitting postures should provide for good spinal alignment and normal spinal curves. The head should not be forward or the shoulders rounded forward.

Figure 11.4 Correct sitting posture with lumbar-roll support.

Pathological Alignment

Unfortunately, over time most people develop bad posture habits. The best posture can be observed in young children. Toddlers who are learning to stand and walk have good body alignment and move with straight posture. It is only as we get older that we develop bad habits that eventually lead to poor posture.

Good posture allows the individual to use his or her body efficiently and effectively. Bad posture, however, places abnormal stresses on the body and increases the demands during performance (Kendall, McCreary, and Provance 1993). Over time, bad posture habits develop, causing shortening of some structures and lengthening of opposing structures with secondary weakness of both shortened and lengthened structures. This change in strength with a change in relative muscle length is discussed in chapter 7 within the context of length-tension relationships. These changes can impair the individual's efficiency of movement. Inefficient movement burdens an already stressed area during performance, and over time, can cause injury. For this reason, the rehabilitation clinician should be aware of the common pathological postures. This knowledge can help the rehabilitation clinician develop an appropriate corrective therapeutic exercise program.

Abnormal alignment is usually recorded in terms of relativity. Rather than precise measurement, terms such as "mild," "moderate," and "severe" are used to identify and grade abnormal alignment. For example, a swimmer may have a mild forward-head posture, or a gymnast may have a severe lumbar lordosis.

Pelvis and Lumbar Area

Common posture faults in the pelvis and lumbar area include excessive lumbar lordosis, flat lumbar spine, and scoliosis. Scoliosis is discussed in the section "Thoracic Area." Often associated with a lumbar lordosis and flat lumbar spine is anterior pelvic tilt and posterior pelvic tilt, respectively.

A normal lumbar curve is slightly lordotic, but an excessive lumbar curve places undue stress on the lumbar spine and other segments (figure 11.5). An excessive **lumbar lordosis**, also referred to as "swayback," is accompanied by an anterior pelvic tilt in which the ASIS is rotated down in relation to the PSIS. It can be caused by tight hip flexors pulling on the lumbar spine and by weak low back extensors and abdominal muscles, especially lower abdominals. Over time, this abnormal postural alignment can result in tightness of lumbar fascia, increased stress to the anterior longitudinal ligament of the spine, narrowing of the vertebral disk spaces that will cause a narrowing of the intervertebral foramen, and approximation of the vertebral articular facets. These changes can result in nerve root compression, sciatica, joint inflammation, degenerative disk, and vertebral changes.

Figure 11.5 Lumbar lordosis.

In a flat lumbar spine, lumbar lordosis is reduced and there is a posterior pelvic tilt so that the PSIS are lower than the ASIS (figure 11.6). Abnormal hip extensor and rectus abdominis tightness is counterbalanced by weak hip flexors and lumbar extensor muscles. This posture reduces the lumbar spine's ability to absorb impact forces and increases the stress of the spine's posterior longitudinal ligament.

Figure 11.6 Flat lumbar spine.

Figure 11.7 Building-block alignment.

Figure 11.8 Kyphosis.

Thoracic Area

When you align building blocks, you find that if one block is not placed directly on top of the one below, the next block must be placed askew to compensate for the one that was poorly placed (figure 11.7). The body likewise compensates for malalignments by adjusting positions of adjacent structures in an attempt to keep the body balanced.

Therefore, in the thoracic region, the area can be excessively rounded or excessively flat, depending on the positions of the lumbar segments. It is common to see a **thoracic kyphosis,** or excessive rounding of the thoracic area (figure 11.8), in response to a lumbar lordosis. Chest muscles, including the intercostals and pectoralis major and minor are usually tight and are counterbalanced by weak thoracic erector spinae, rhomboids, and trapezius muscles. A thoracic kyphosis is typically associated with a round-shoulder posture. The scapulae will also be more than the normal 5 cm (2 in.) from the vertebral spinous processes.

A kyphotic posture can lead to **thoracic outlet syndrome,** which is discussed in chapter 16. Secondary cervical problems can result from excessive pressure placed on the cervical area by malalignment of the thoracic spine. People such as swimmers who place high demands on rhomboid and trapezius muscle groups can experience fatigue in these groups because of the muscles' lengthened and weakened status.

A flattening of the upper back, or a reduction of the thoracic curve, is not as common as a kyphotic posture. This flattening is characterized by an exaggerated attention posture that includes depressed scapulae and flat neck; it results in tightness in the thoracic erector spinae and scapular retractors with secondary weakness of the scapular protractors and anterior thoracic muscles. This posture can also lead to thoracic outlet syndrome because of the increased compression it produces between the first rib and clavicle.

Scoliosis is commonly seen in the thoracic or lumbar spine or in both areas. **Scoliosis** is a lateral curve of the normally straight spine and is classified as either a C-curve or an S-curve. A C-curve is usually indicated as either right or left according to its direction of convexity. A C-curve with a compensating secondary curve is called an S-curve (figure 11.9). In an attempt to keep the head level, the body compensates for a C-curve by developing a counterbalancing lesser lateral curve that results in an S-curve configuration. Scoliosis usually also includes a rotation of the vertebrae. If this occurs in the thoracic spine, an asymmetry of rib position can be observed from an anterior or posterior view, with one side of the rib cage more anterior than the contralateral side. If leg-length differences are the source of the scoliosis, the pelvic landmarks may not be level. Shoulders are often not level in scoliosis as well.

Common causes for scoliosis are congenital deformities of the spine, leg-length differences, and long-term unilateral activities. Tennis players, among others involved in physical activity, often may develop a scoliosis because of their participation in a unilaterally demanding sport. Tight soft tissue structures are found on the side of the concavity, while weaker structures are on the convex side of the scoliosis curve.

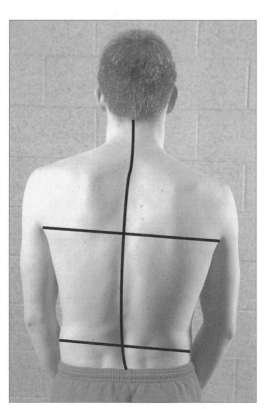

Figure 11.9 Mild scoliosis. Notice the uneven hips, unequal arm hang, and unequal shoulder and scapula heights.

Figure 11.10 Lateral shift. Notice the uneven hips with a shift of the trunk to the left. Hips and shoulders are not in alignment.

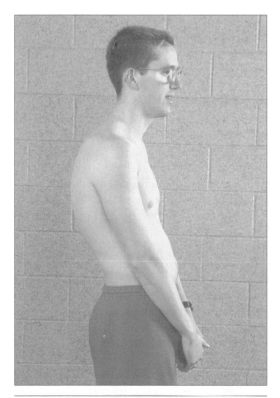

Figure 11.11 Cervical lordosis, thoracic kyphosis, and lumbar lordosis.

Scoliosis can cause muscle fatigue and increased ligamentous stress on the convex side because of weakness of those structures. Impingement of nerve roots with secondary nerve root pain can be seen on the concave side. If the scoliosis is caused by a leg-length discrepancy, the longer leg commonly has a lower longitudinal arch to compensate for the leg-length difference.

A scoliosis should not be confused with a lateral shift of the thoracic or lumbar spine. A shift is present when the pelvis and shoulders do not lie in the same frontal plane. Either the pelvis or the shoulders are shifted to the left or right of the midline of the body (figure 11.10). This shift can be caused by muscle spasm or pain from an impinged nerve root as the body attempts to move away from the source of pain. It is usually a temporary condition that is relieved when the cause is eliminated.

Head and Cervical Area

In response to the abnormal lumbar and thoracic alignment, the cervical spine develops a compensatory alignment. Most commonly, a forward positioning of the head occurs through either a flattening of the lower cervical curve or an exaggerated upper cervical lordosis. A cervical lordosis includes an increased flexion of the lower cervical and an increased extension of the upper cervical spine (figure 11.11).

Weakness in the lower cervical and upper thoracic erector spinae and anterior neck muscles is overpowered by tightness in cervical muscles including the levator scapulae, sternocleidomastoid, scalenes, suboccipitals, and upper trapezii. This imbalance encourages and perpetuates the abnormal cervical posture.

Many problems can result from prolonged poor cervical posture. Both the weak and the tight muscles can experience fatigue. The exaggerated cervical position can also increase cervical disk pressure, add irritation to cervical facet joints, increase nerve root pressure, and impinge on neurovascular bundles to increase the risk of thoracic outlet syndrome. Prolonged abnormal positioning also increases the stresses applied to the cervical spine's posterior and anterior longitudinal ligaments. Scholastic and collegiate athletes who spend their days in the classroom often sit with their elbows on the desk and their chins in their hands, and people in the work force spend their days at a computer sitting in a rounded-back and forward-head position; these positions exaggerate the cervical lordotic posture that places increased stress on the cervical spine. Prolonged posterior longitudinal ligament stress is marked by the formation of a "dowager's hump" at the base of the cervical spine in persons who have had long-term forward-head posture. In addition, temporomandibular joint stress can be exaggerated by abnormal cervical posture and lead to temporomandibular joint disorders.

Lower Extremities

Lower-extremity malalignment can begin in the feet, knees, or hips and often affects other structures along the closed kinetic chain. Common postural faults in the lower extremities include excessive flexion or extension, excessive abduction or adduction, and excessive medial or lateral rotation. The normal angle between the femoral neck and the femoral shaft in adults is 120° to 125° (figure 11.12). This angle is larger in infants and children, decreasing from 150° in a newborn to 133° in a teenager until it reaches 120° to 125° in the adult years. An

Figure 11.12 Femoral neck-shaft angles: *(a)* coxa valga causes increased femoral-joint pressure, *(b)* normal position, *(c)* coxa vara produces increased stress on femoral neck.

a *b* *c*

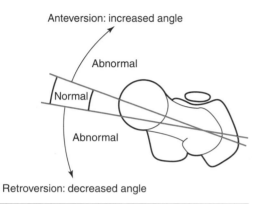

Figure 11.13 Relative position of the femoral neck and femoral condyles. Normal anteversion in an adult is 8° to 15°.

abnormally larger angle is referred to as **coxa valga,** and a smaller than normal angle is called **coxa vara.** As the neck-shaft angle increases with a coxa valga, there is an apparent lengthening of the limb. The opposite is true with a coxa vara, in which the limb shortens as the neck-shaft angle decreases. People with coxa valga have a higher propensity for eventual hip-joint arthritis, whereas those with coxa vara are more prone to femoral neck fractures.

In the transverse plane of the femur, there is a normal relative forward projection of the femoral neck relative to the femoral condyles. This angle decreases with age. A newborn's femoral neck-condyle angle is around 30° whereas in adults it is 8° to 15° (figure 11.13). **Anteversion,** an increased angle, results in greater hip medial rotation and causes squinting patellae and toeing-in during standing. A decreased angle, called **retroversion,** produces greater hip lateral rotation, and in standing the feet rotate outward. Anteversion decreases hip stability and places the hip at risk for dislocation, whereas retroversion increases the joint's stability.

The normal sagittal alignment of the femur and tibia at the knee is straight; an angling of the knees toward each another is called **genu valgus** or **genu valgum.** A bowing outward of the knees is called **genu varus** or **genu varum** (figure 11.14). These malalignments have a variety of causes. If they occur on one side, leg-length discrepancy may be the cause. Quadriceps weakness can produce genu valgus. Genu valgus deformities can be the source of excessive foot pronation, and varus deformities can be related to high arches.

In normal standing, the patellae faces forward with the feet positioned forward or slightly outward. The condition in which the patellae face toward each other is referred to as **squinting patellae** and may be related to medial hip rotation, hip anteversion, medial tibial rotation, or lateral rotation of the feet (figure 11.15). The condition in which the patellae face outward in relation to each other is referred to as **frog's eye** or **grasshopper eye.** This condition is often the result of lateral hip rotation or tibial rotation, and the feet often face inward in a pigeon-toed fashion.

In a side view, the knee is straight but not locked. If the line of gravity falls in front of the knee, the knee is hyperextended, a condition referred to as **genu recurvatum** (figure 11.16). Excessive stress is placed on the knee's ligamentous structures in this position. Genu recurvatum is commonly accompanied by excessive lumbar lordosis and anterior pelvic rotation.

Tibial torsion is present when the leg appears rotated in relation to the thigh. This is most evident when one looks at the positions of the patellae in relation to the positions of the feet. In an adult, the feet normally face approximately 12° to 18° from the sagittal axis of the body. In youth, this angle can be as small as 5° (figure 11.17). Excessive tibial torsion is usually a lateral torsion and is correlated with feet facing laterally when the knees face forward; when the feet point forward, the knees are medially rotated. To measure tibial torsion, place the patient in supine with the patellae facing directly upward. A line bisecting the

Figure 11.14 Knee alignment in the sagittal plane: *(a)* genu varus, *(b)* normal, *(c)* genu valgus.

Figure 11.15 Left squinting patella.

Figure 11.16 Genu recurvatum.

Figure 11.17
Normal adult foot position in weight bearing.

medial and lateral malleoli creates an angle with the plane of the tabletop; this is the tibial torsion measurement (figure 11.18). Normal values are less than 20° to 25° (Sahrmann 2002). Excessive lateral tibial torsion can increase patellofemoral stresses and lead to instability and fat-pad entrapment.

Medial tibial torsion is associated with genu varum, and lateral tibial torsion is associated with genu valgum. These conditions can become apparent with habitual use of poor sitting postures, especially in children, as seen in figure 11.19.

Foot position can influence knee and hip positions, and the converse is also true. One determines medial longitudinal arch height by drawing a line from the distal aspect of the medial malleolus to the weight-bearing surface of the first metatarsophalangeal joint. In both weight bearing and non-weight bearing, the navicular tuberosity should be on the line (figure 11.20). If the navicular tuberosity falls below the line, the arch is abnormally low; and if it falls above the line, the arch is abnormally high. A high arch is referred to as **pes cavus**. A low arch, **pes planus,** can be associated with excessive foot pronation and calcaneal eversion and accompanied by genu valgum and/or femoral anteversion. A pes planus is usually hypermobile, allowing for excessive rearfoot and forefoot motion during gait. This type of foot structure may not have the stability to create a strong base, and it places excessive stresses on soft-tissue structures and adjacent joints as the patient attempts to perform activities. The greater the foot's hypermobility, the greater the loss of its stability. Increased stress on foot and ankle structures can lead to injuries such as plantar fasciitis and Achilles tendinitis.

Calcaneal eversion with increased forefoot pronation can be identified from a posterior view of the ankle. In this position, the Achilles tendon appears to be at less than a 90° angle to the floor, and the calcaneus is in an everted position (figure 11.21).

Pes cavus, a higher-than-normal arch, is associated with a more rigid foot structure and produces less mobility of the joints within the rearfoot and forefoot. This type of foot has less ability to absorb stress than a foot with a normal arch position and is more prone to stress fractures. With reduced flexibility and associated diminution of stress-absorption capacity, increased stress is imposed on the joints of the foot. A high arch is often associated with hammertoes or claw toes and can be related to femoral retroversion.

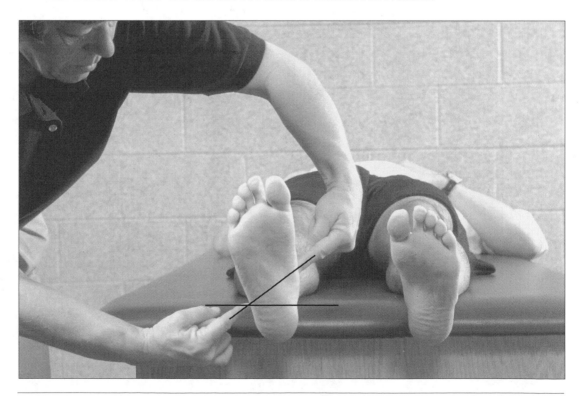

Figure 11.18 With the patella facing the ceiling, a line between the medial and lateral malleolus forms an angle with a line parallel to the tabletop for identifying the individual's tibial torsion.

Figure 11.19 Poor sitting posture for knees: *(a)* encourages lateral tibial torsion, *(b)* encourages medial tibial torsion.

Figure 11.20 Arch position: normal alignment.

Reprinted by permission from Richardson and Iglarsh 1994.

Figure 11.21 Pronation. Notice the everted position of the left calcaneus.

Toe positions are normally in a straight line. A positioning of the great toe laterally toward the other toes is called **hallux valgus.** A common cause is hypermobility of the foot. Over time, this additional stress on the first metatarsophalangeal joint causes it to become deformed (figure 11.22).

a   *b*   *c*

Figure 11.22   Toe deformities: *(a)* hallux valgus, *(b)* claw toes, *(c)* hammertoes.

Parts b an c reprinted by permission from Richardson and Iglarsh 1994.

Toes that become flexed or extended at the metatarsophalangeal joints or the interphalangeal joints are known as claw toes and hammertoes, respectively. **Claw toes** are extended at the metatarsophalangeal joints and flexed at the proximal and distal interphalangeal joints; **hammertoes** are extended at the metatarsophalangeal joints, flexed at the proximal interphalangeal joint, and extended at the distal interphalangeal joint. These conditions are usually accompanied by a high longitudinal arch and a rigid foot. Corns and calluses on the toes develop secondary to abnormal pressures as the elevated portion of the toes rubs against the inside of the shoe.

Upper Extremities

The primary area affected by bad posture in the upper extremity is the shoulders. If a person has a poor thoracic posture with rounded shoulders, the scapulae protract forward and downward around the rib cage. This positioning presents itself as an anterior rounding of the glenohumeral joint, and the dorsal hands will face forward, positioned in front of the anterior thigh rather than at the lateral thigh as they should (figure 11.23). This can lead to glenohumeral impingement, weakness of the scapular rotators, and tightness of anterior shoulder girdle muscles. These soft-tissue changes can cause inefficient use of the shoulder during upper-extremity activities and place the individual at risk for upper-extremity injuries.

Figure 11.23 Upper-extremity posture deviation.

MUSCLE IMBALANCES

▶ Improper posture is often perpetuated by muscle imbalances. Causes of muscle imbalance include overuse, loss of motion or flexibility in a muscle or muscle group, postural deviations, and injuries. It is necessary to determine the muscle imbalances involved before correcting postural deviations.

Muscle imbalances often impact posture. To correct posture, the rehabilitation clinician must be able to identify the muscle imbalances that perpetuate the patient's improper posture.

Causes

Poor posture results from an abnormal relationship between the forces that act on an area. Normal posture occurs when there is a balance of forces acting on bones and joints. Normal posture permits an efficient and effective use of the body to produce the desired motions.

When a body is in bad posture, the joints and muscles are already under stress, and activity increases that level of stress. In bad posture, muscles must work harder to produce desired motions and are not as efficient or as effective. Bad posture can also restrict muscles from performing optimally. For example, a freestyle swimmer with rounded shoulders has difficulty getting enough lateral rotation and abduction on the recovery phase of the stroke, so either hand entry into the water is premature or the swimmer has to compensate with an exaggerated body roll. The swimmer will also suffer an impingement injury of the shoulder because the scapula does not upwardly rotate and retract as it should. If this swimmer were to come to you with a rotator-cuff tendinitis and you did not correct the posture and muscle imbalances, your treatment success would be short-lived, for the injury would recur.

Sometimes pain in an area is the result of poor posture or muscle imbalances in another area. The site of pain is not always the source of the problem. For example, a gymnast who complains of back pain and has a lumbar lordosis may in fact be having back pain because of hip-flexor tightness, not a back injury. The hip flexors place abnormal stress on the lumbar vertebrae because tight hip flexors pull on the lumbar vertebrae, increasing low-back stress and making the area more susceptible to injury. The gymnast's back pain could also be related to hyperextended knees, which will tend to pull the pelvis forward, increasing lumbar lordosis. When combined with weak abdominals, especially weak lower abdominals, these factors can contribute significantly to low-back pain.

Commonly, the source of muscle imbalance is a loss of motion or flexibility in a muscle or muscle group, as well as lengthening and weakness from prolonged or sustained stretch of the opposing muscle or muscle group. If a muscle is shortened, its opposing muscle must be lengthened to compensate. It is this reciprocal activity that allows us to feed ourselves, walk, and perform most activities; when one muscle shortens, the opposing muscle lengthens to allow the activity. For example, when you perform a biceps curl, the biceps shorten and the triceps lengthen; or when you bend your knee, the hamstrings shorten and the quadriceps lengthen. When a lengthened or shortened position is sustained, a muscle's resting length changes over time. The sustained shortening of one muscle causes a loss of flexibility and strength, and the sustained lengthening of the opposite muscle causes a loss of strength and tone. One can compare the results of sustained lengthening to what occurs when a weight is hung on the end of a rubber band for a period of time. When the weight is removed, the rubber band has less tone than before, and less spring. So, too, a muscle that is positionally lengthened loses its spring and becomes weaker. If a patient performed only flexibility exercises to restore balance, the imbalance, caused by tightness of one muscle and weakness of its opposing muscle, would overpower the effects of stretching and would continue to encourage the imbalanced posture.

Some activities are more likely to cause postural deviations than others. For example, participants in sports that emphasize muscle activity on anterior more than on posterior body regions, such as swimming and boxing, are more likely than other athletes to develop postural deviations. Unilateral activities such as racket sports encourage muscle imbalance from left to right and can cause such postural deviations as scoliosis.

As the body ages, postural deviations become more pronounced. A mild forward-head posture in a young adult becomes a moderate forward-head posture in the middle-aged adult and becomes even more severe as the individual ages. As the muscle naturally weakens with age, it has increasing difficulty opposing tight structures, so pathological postures become even more apparent with aging—further increasing joint and muscle stresses.

Muscle imbalance can also result from joint abnormalities. These abnormalities run the spectrum from hypermobility to hypomobility. When joints are hypermobile, displaying an excessive amount of motion, the muscles must work harder to provide joint stability. This is true for a joint that is uniplanar or multiplanar. Joints that lack normal mobility—hypomobile joints—have less-than-normal motion and place additional stresses on muscles and joints. These conditions can also add stresses to other body segments. For example, the individual who has foot-joint hypermobility with excessive pronation may develop patellar tendinitis. This may be secondary to additional stresses on the patellar tendon when its insertion is rotated medially with the medial tibial rotation that occurs during prolonged pronation.

Injuries can also cause muscle imbalances. Scar-tissue adhesions following a ligament injury can cause the joint to become hypomobile, especially if the joint was immobilized immediately after the injury. The deleterious effects of immobilization are discussed in chapter 2. If the joint is not immobilized, ligamentous laxity can occur, making the joint hypermobile.

Another cause of imbalances is muscle strains. If the injured muscle is not properly rehabilitated, its normal strength is not regained. If adhesions within the muscle occur, the site can become tight, limiting flexibility and causing increased stress to the site or adjacent sites.

Treatment

It becomes important in any injury examination to assess the patient's posture and look for muscle imbalances that either may have contributed to the injury or may result from the injury. You should also look at the total body, not merely the injured site, because postural deviations from other locations may have contributed to the injury.

It is important to correct postural deviations not only to address the patient's current injury but also to prevent recurrence. As has been mentioned, if a postural deviation is either the source of an injury or a contributing factor, you must correct the postural deviation as part of the rehabilitation program in order to prevent recurrence of the injury. If you do not, the chance is good that the injury will recur.

In correcting postural deviations, the rehabilitation clinician must first identify the structure that has become tight and the opposing structure that has become overstretched. He or she can then give the patient exercises to correct the muscle imbalance—that is, to lengthen the short or tight structures and strengthen the opposing weak or lengthened structures. For example, if the freestyle swimmer's posture is a rounded-shoulder position, examination will show that the anterior chest muscles are tight; the downward scapular rotators are tight; and the upper back muscles, scapular retractors, and upward scapular rotator groups are weak and lengthened. The treatment program should include lengthening activities for the pectoralis minor, anterior deltoid, and pectoralis major and strengthening activities for the lower trapezius, middle trapezius, rhomboids, and posterior deltoid. It should also include activities that will recruit and retrain muscles to produce the desired activity correctly. It is useful to provide reminders that will facilitate correct postural alignment—for example, a visual cue such as a colored dot on the face of the patient's watch or on a fingernail can be used to remind the patient to think about and correct his or her posture. An example of a more direct reminder is tape applied between the shoulder blades to help the patient remember to keep the shoulders in correct alignment.

Conscious correction of posture is necessary for bad posture to improve. The patient must become aware of the abnormal posture and then make a deliberate effort to alter the habitual posture; otherwise, posture does not change. As the patient continues to improve muscle balance through proper exercises and to correct bad postural position, and maintains a proper posture more and more frequently, the posture eventually will improve.

It is more difficult in the initial stages than it will be later for the patient to change posture, for two primary reasons. The first one is habit. Habit, whether good or bad, is easy and comfortable and thus difficult for anyone to change. The second reason is the relationship between the weak and tight muscles. The tight muscles overpower the weak and lengthened muscles, making it difficult for the patient to maintain a proper posture when attempting correction. But as the muscle imbalance is reduced, the task becomes easier. Conscious effort is vitally important throughout the process if the patient is to achieve the ultimate goal of improved postural alignment.

Posture- and Muscle Imbalance-Related Injuries

To make it easier to understand the process, let's look at a couple of examples of injuries and their relationship to improper posture and muscle imbalance.

Lower Extremity

Iliotibial band (ITB) friction syndrome is a common problem in injured athletes, particularly in runners. The pain occurs along the ITB and is typically located along the superior-lateral aspect of the knee or toward the hip. The patient reports that the pain worsens with hill running. The examination reveals a tight ITB, and the patient stands with the leg in more medial rotation than normal. Muscle testing demonstrates weakness of the quadriceps and hip lateral rotators, and probably weakness of the gluteus maximus as well. Examination of the soft tissue along the ITB reveals tenderness in areas of soft-tissue thickness.

Treatment includes softening the ITB-restrictive areas with deep friction massage techniques, along with lengthening the tight ITB and strengthening the lengthened, weak gluteus maximus, hip lateral rotators, and quadriceps muscles. Instructions to the patient include conscious positional correction: keeping the leg in only slight lateral rotation alignment when standing or walking. The use of a modality, such as heat, prior to friction massage allows for better massage results by making the soft tissue more pliable.

Upper Extremity

A common upper-extremity problem in patients who participate in upper-extremity sports such as tennis, golf, swimming, and gymnastics is shoulder impingement. This often appears as rotator-cuff tendinitis, and the patient complains of pain with movements such as shoulder elevation, putting the hand behind the back, and resisted activities. He or she experiences pain through the middle arc of shoulder range of motion, and the impingement tests produce a positive sign. The rotator-cuff tendons are tender to palpation at their insertion on the greater tubercle. Examination of muscles reveals tightness of the pectoralis minor, anterior deltoid, latissimus, and pectoralis major. The rhomboids and levator scapulae may also be tight. Weakness is apparent in the lower and middle trapezii, infraspinatus, and teres minor. The capsule may have areas of restriction. The scapulae may not rotate fully into an upward and retracted position because of weakness of the upward rotators and tightness of the downward rotators.

Effective treatment of this condition must include correcting the faulty posture, strengthening weak muscles, and stretching tight muscles. Balance between muscle length and strength of opposing muscle groups is the goal that will lead to reduced impingement in the shoulder. It is important to make the patient aware of the proper posture of the shoulder and thoracic area so that he or she can work at improving posture and alignment. Exercises should include stretching of the anterior capsule, pectoralis minor, pectoralis major, and latissimus. Strengthening exercises should include appropriate exercises for the lower and middle trapezius muscles, the infraspinatus, and teres minor. Restoring the balance between scapular upward and downward rotators, protractors and retractors, and elevators and depressors must be part of the rehabilitation program for resolution of postural defects and muscle imbalances to occur. Because weakness of the lengthened posterior muscles is one of the sources of shoulder impingement, retraining the depressors, retractors, and upward rotators to provide the appropriate movement of the scapula during shoulder movement is vital to reducing impingement of the rotator cuff.

A Challenging Example

Let's look at one more example and outline an appropriate program. A basketball player comes to you with complaints of pain around the patella, especially when jumping for a rebound. He also has pain going down stairs, and in the weight room he has pain on the leg extension and squat machines. When he stands in front of you, the patellae face forward and the feet are in a laterally rotated position. In weight bearing, the longitudinal arches are low. When he performs a step-down exercise, you notice that he lacks full control of the knee and that there is slight knee wobble medially-to-laterally as he lowers himself. Range-of-motion testing shows tightness of the ITB, but range of motion of the knee is normal. Strength testing indicates weakness of the vastus medialis oblique (VMO), and you can see some atrophy of the VMO compared to that in the contralateral knee. With the patient in long sitting, the patella is positioned with the medial side higher than the lateral side. When he contracts the quadriceps, you observe that the patella tracks primarily laterally. What is the cause of this individual's pain, and what treatment plan would you provide for him? Think for a moment before you read on, and identify the types of corrective exercises and the progression you would recommend to resolve this problem.

The cause of the patient's pain is a malalignment and maltracking of the patella. This in turn is caused by a combination of weakness of the VMO, tightness of the ITB, and malalignment of the feet. Lower-than-normal arches can result in a tibial torsion to increase stresses on the patella. You should check hip rotation to eliminate tightness of the lateral rotators. The patella is not tracking normally because of weakness of the VMO and tightness of the ITB overpowering the VMO pull. There may also be an imbalance between the vastus lateralis and the VMO that would add to the lateral tracking. Tightness of the ITB can also be responsible for the lateral tilt of the patella.

Treatment for this patient should include stretching exercises for the hip and ITB and progressive strengthening exercises for the VMO, such as terminal knee-extension exercises, squats, step exercises, and lunges; these exercises should be pain free and should increase in intensity, repetitions, and number of sets as the patient's strength increases. Taping the patella may also reduce the pain. If inspection of the feet reveals excessive pronation, taping the arch and limiting rearfoot motion may be beneficial.

The exercises you select should be designed to increase flexibility of the tight muscles and increase strength of the weak muscles to provide for a restoration of balance between muscles. If modalities are the only treatment technique used or if flexibility is the only type of exercise included, the rehabilitation program will not succeed in relieving the patient's complaints and permitting a full and successful return to sport participation and normal activity.

BODY MECHANICS

▶ Proper body mechanics is fundamental to proper posture. Important principles include keeping the spine straight, lowering the center of gravity, and keeping the base of support broad. Patients need to perform daily activities using correct body mechanics, and the rehabilitation clinician should also pay attention to his or her own body mechanics.

Body mechanics is related to posture in that proper body mechanics is easier to perform with good posture. **Body mechanics** refers to the way the body is positioned and used during activity. Incorrect body mechanics increases stresses placed on various body segments, but correct body mechanics makes the most effective use of the body's forces and lever systems. Body mechanics is briefly discussed here because an awareness of good body mechanics is important to the rehabilitation clinician from both a personal and a treatment perspective. From a personal perspective, use of proper body mechanics makes you more efficient in the application of manual therapy and exercises. It conserves your energy and makes the most effective use of your body.

From a treatment perspective, knowledge of correct body mechanics in the execution of specific sport activities allows you as a rehabilitation clinician to provide the patient with proper exercises. Such exercises will enhance the patient's performance and include corrective techniques to further prepare the individual for returning to competition.

Basic Principles

A few basic concepts are important to remember regardless of the activity that is being performed. The first principle is that the spine should remain straight. A "straight spine" is one that has the natural curves with the pelvis in neutral. A straight spine has slight lumbar lordosis, thoracic kyphosis, and cervical lordosis. In this position, each vertebra is in correct alignment with the adjacent vertebrae (figure 11.24). Pelvic neutral is present when the pelvis is in a mid-position between an anterior and a posterior pelvic tilt. In this position the stress on the pelvis is minimal, and the vertebrae should be balanced. This position is sometimes referred to as **neutral spine** or **pelvic neutral.**

Figure 11.24 Proper spinal alignment is a "straight spine."

Maintaining a neutral spine is important if forces from the lower extremities are to be properly transmitted to the trunk and upper extremities. It is easier to understand this concept if you think of the legs, trunk, and arms as three sections connected in series. When the sections are all rigid, forces are transferred easily; but if the middle section, the spine, is a spring rather than a rigid structure, it is more difficult to transfer forces from one section to another. When the middle segment is not rigid, the forces produced in the lower segment are dissipated and the upper bar, the arms, must develop their own forces—a far more difficult and strenuous method of delivering force for desired activity.

For this reason, it is important for athletes to have a straight back during activities, especially those activities that require force transmission. For example, a football lineman squats with the back straight to utilize the driving force from the legs; the warehouse worker keeps the back straight in a squat to transfer the lifting force from the legs to the arms; and the golfer's back is straight so that the summation of forces from the legs and trunk can drive the ball down the fairway. The rehabilitation clinician must also maintain a straight back so the power of the legs, not the arms, is the primary source to deliver manual resistance forces for therapeutic exercises.

If the back is not kept straight, transfer of forces from the lower extremities to the trunk and upper extremities is not possible. To illustrate the significance of this, have a friend bend over from the waist so that his or her back is not straight, and then push on the friend's shoulders to move the person off balance. Now have your friend bend at the hips but keep the back straight as you again push his or her body off balance. You will find that with the back straight, the power of the legs will provide increased stability and better resistance to outside forces.

When lowering the body to sit or to lift an object, the back should remain straight so less stress is applied to the spine. It is not enough just to bend the knees. The knees must bend, but the hips are also pushed back while the chest is kept up. If the hips are not pushed back, the bend occurs in the back, not the hips, and the lower back will round, losing the back's proper alignment. If the chest is lowered, the spine will round and lose its proper straight position (figure 11.25b).

Lowering the center of gravity increases the body's stability. This is important if resistance to outside forces is needed. For example, if you push your friend while he or she is standing fully upright, it will be easier for you to move the person than if he or she squats down to reduce the body's center of gravity. This is one reason linemen in football or rugby get into a squat position.

Figure 11.25 Keeping back straight when bending: *(a)* Knees and hips are flexed, hips are pushed backward, and lumbar curve is maintained, chest is held up. *(b)* Leg and lower back positions are maintained properly, but the head and chest are lowered. *(c)* Leg and chest positions are maintained, but lumbar curve is lost and hips are not pushed backward.

Broadening the base of support is another method of providing increased stability. If your friend stands with feet together, it is much easier to push him or her off balance than if the feet are positioned apart. A broader base of support produces a larger area for the center of gravity to move within before balance is lost. When you move an object, a broad base of support will increase your stability.

Another principle of good body mechanics is to stand in the direction of force application. This allows the use of force transfer from the legs. For example, when you throw a ball forward, your feet should be in a backward-forward straddle. This permits transfer of forces from the back leg to the front leg as your trunk is rotated and your arm is brought through the throwing motion. To see this concept, throw a ball with your feet in a side-by-side stance and then with your feet in a backward-forward straddle stance. You will find that the ball goes farther with the straddle stance. If it is necessary to transfer an object or exert a force from one side of the body to the other, the best stance is a side-by-side stance with the feet in line with the shoulders. For example, if you are resisting a patient's straight-leg raise with the patient supine on the table, your stance should be side by side as you face the table. This way, as the patient raises his or her leg, your weight can transfer from the leg you have positioned next to the patient's foot (lower) to the one you have positioned next to the patient's hip (upper). You will be able to use a body-weight shift from your lower-positioned leg to your upper-positioned leg as the patient's leg moves.

Abdominal strength is important for force transfer from the lower to the upper extremities. Strong abdominals provide the support needed to keep the back straight, help to diffuse the forces applied to the back, and assist in the transfer of forces from the legs to the arms. Arm and leg movement must be assisted by stabilization of the spine for the arms and legs to produce the desired activity. You can see this if you have someone resist your shoulder flexion-to-extension movement. You should feel your abdominals tighten as you extend the arm against his or her resistance. You should also feel the abdominals tighten when hip flexion is resisted. An injured individual's therapeutic exercise program should include abdominal strengthening exercises.

The Patient's Daily Activities

Performing daily activities using correct body mechanics is important because it conserves energy, makes for efficient and effective use of the body, and reduces stress on the back and other segments. Knowledge of these techniques enables you to instruct patients, especially those with back injuries, to minimize stress to the injured area.

Patients routinely lift and carry objects such as book bags, backpacks, boxes, athletic gear, and athletic bags. The way an object is lifted depends on its size and weight. It is important to test the weight of the object before it is lifted. If an object is heavy, the proper way to lift it is to approach it front on. This means facing the object, standing as close to the object as possible and standing so that when the back is straight and the person is flexed at the hips and knees, the arms fall directly over the object. As the individual bends the knees to lift the object, the knees should never be higher than the hips. Positioning the knees greater than 90° imposes a great deal of stress on the knee's meniscus. Additional lowering of the body is achieved by pushing the hips backward, bending the knees as far as possible but bending the knees to no more than 90°, and keeping the chest up and the back straight. With the abdominals tightened, the person lifts the object by straightening the legs while moving into a standing position (figure 11.26). The object should be kept close to the body to reduce its force (force equals weight times distance). The farther away from the body the object is, the more force is required to lift it.

To push or pull an object, the individual places his or her legs in the direction of movement (side by side if the object is being moved left to right; backward-forward if the object is to be moved toward or away from the person). The person then moves the object by transferring the body's weight from one leg to the other. If the object is to be moved from the right side of

Figure 11.26 Proper lifting technique.

Figure 11.27 Proper pushing technique.

Figure 11.28 Proper sit-to-stand position.

the body to the left, the individual positions the legs in a side-by-side stance, grasps the object, and moves the body weight from the right to the left leg. If the object is to be moved from a position in front of the person to one farther away, the individual begins in a backward-forward stance, grasps the object, and moves the body weight from the back leg to the front leg to move the object. The legs, not the arms, provide the force to move the object.

While carrying objects in only one hand, it is best to periodically shift the object from one side to the other, especially when carrying an object for more than a short period of time. Keeping the object close to the body and no higher than waist level will help to minimize the load.

The easiest way to push or pull objects is to keep the back straight, lower the center of gravity, and use a wide forward-backward stance position. Keeping the center of gravity low will assist in using the lower-extremity forces to move the object (figure 11.27). Pushing is easier than pulling because it is better use of the body's weight is made in pushing.

Rising from a chair is performed according to the same principles as bending. As figure 11.28 shows, the back is kept straight; the bend occurs at the hips and knees; and the chest is kept up.

The proper technique for getting down on the floor is to go down first on one knee then the other before placing the hands on the floor in a quadruped position. From there, the person walks the hands out to get into a prone position, and then rolls into either a sidelying or a supine position. The technique is performed in reverse to return to a standing position.

Athletic Events

Athletic activities, like daily activities, demand a straight back for the optimal transmission of forces from the lower extremities to the upper extremities. Abdominal strength is also important for transmitting these forces. Maintenance of pelvic neutral and straight back is important for force production, injury prevention, and efficiency of movement.

It is beyond the scope of this text to describe proper body mechanics for execution of all activities. However, on the basis of the information presented regarding body mechanics, the rehabilitation clinician should have a concept of the proper posture and position for the execution of many activities. For example, a canoeist must have a straight spine with pelvic neutral to transmit forces from the legs to the arms and move the canoe quickly and forcefully (figure 11.29); a gymnast must be in pelvic neutral as she goes into a kip on the uneven bars; a weightlifter's back must be straight as he lifts the weight overhead (figure 11.30); and a shot-putter must transfer the lower-extremity forces to the upper extremity by keeping the back straight to propel the shot for the desired distance.

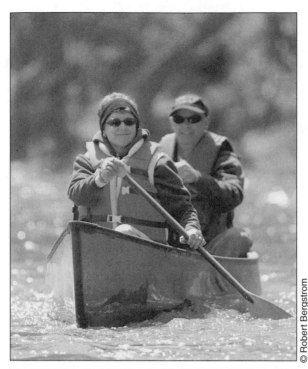

Figure 11.29   Canoeists with proper technique.

© Robert Bergstrom

The Rehabilitation Clinician's Daily Activities

Just as the patient needs to use the body efficiently and effectively, the rehabilitation clinician must use his or her body correctly in order to be effective, competent, and proficient in the application of rehabilitation techniques.

This means that the rehabilitation clinician must use good body mechanics. It is important that your body weight be equally distributed over both feet, that your feet be positioned in a correct alignment depending on the direction of the forces you are applying to the patient, and that the force you use is from the legs rather than the arms. Remember to keep the back straight so leg strength rather than arm strength is used. Moving from right to left foot and back again as you move or resist the patient's extremities through a range of motion reduces the demands on your body and conserves energy. Keeping the upper extremities relaxed but in proper alignment makes it easier for you to achieve the transfer of forces from the lower to upper extremities. Figure 11.31 demonstrates using proper body mechanics when working with patients.

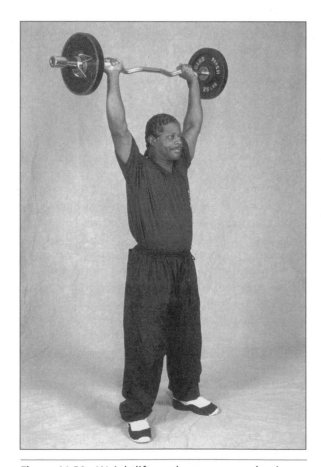

Figure 11.30   Weightlifter using proper mechanics.

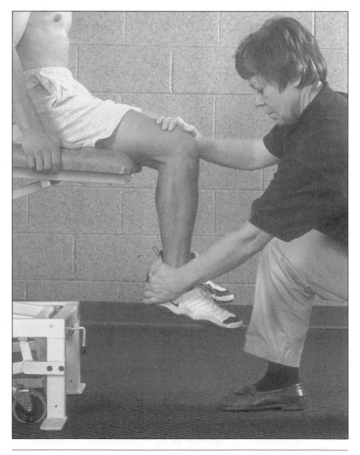

Figure 11.31   Rehabilitation clinician with proper body mechanics.

Proper body mechanics includes keeping the spine in a neutral position so that you can use your body as effectively and efficiently as possible; a neutral spine allows the powerful lower-extremity muscles to be used as the source of strength. Keeping the back straight, bending the knees, and transferring body weight with movement help to minimize risk of injury and maximize body forces. This is true for the athlete during sport participation, for the rehabilitation clinician during execution of therapeutic exercises, and for employees in daily work activities.

BODY-AWARENESS PROGRAMS

▶ Body-awareness programs, which focus on self-improvement through awareness of movement patterns and abilities, include the Feldenkrais Method, the Alexander Technique, and the Pilates Method.

Over the years, many programs have been developed to improve body awareness through body movement. Three of these programs are introduced here. The intent is to familiarize you with the various kinds of approaches that body-awareness programs use. The two basic premises common to all these programs is that the techniques produce self-improvement through increased body awareness and that a strong body-mind interaction exists that determines an individual's movement patterns and abilities. The whole body, not just the area of pain or dysfunction, is addressed. Some athletes use these programs to enhance their athletic skill and performance. Others find the programs useful in treating injuries that impede normal body function.

Feldenkrais Method

Moshe Feldenkrais (1904–1984) was a Russian-born Israeli who obtained a doctorate in physics from the Sorbonne in Paris. He held a black belt in judo and was a recognized judo instructor. An old soccer injury of the knee became painful and crippling in Feldenkrais's later years. Physicians were unable to provide a satisfactory medical treatment, so he taught himself medicine, anatomy, therapeutic exercise, and body mechanics. His mechanical and electrical engineering background was an asset as he developed what became known as the Feldenkrais Method. He taught himself to walk pain free using this method. By the 1950s he had given up his career as a research scientist and had begun to devote his work to teaching and using the Feldenkrais Method.

> For more information about the Feldenkrais method, see the Feldenkrais Guild of North America's Web site at www.feldenkrais.com.

Dr. Feldenkrais believed that an individual develops inefficient movement patterns for a variety of reasons—that cultural influences, illness, injury, and other factors can cause limited movement leading to inhibition of normal movement ability. In the Feldenkrais Method, movement patterns and habits are assessed before a treatment program is initiated. Feldenkrais believed that a person's unconscious pattern of movement is influenced by several factors, including the unconscious sensorimotor relationship that affects muscles and joints and their associated motor skills and abilities; the individual's perception of balance, space, and gravity; self-image; and kinesthetic awareness. His approach for changing these components to improve movement involves engaging the whole person in the treatment regimen, promoting self-esteem, and improving learning skills.

Pain is avoided in the Feldenkrais Method. Pain encourages the unfavorable muscle movement patterns that the person has established. Movement is usually performed slowly through an easy direction of motion. Slow and easy movement allows the individual to become sensitive to motions and positions, allows muscle relaxation, and permits a change of position through a new and more correct movement pattern.

As the individual progresses, the movements become more advanced in their complexity, speed, size, and trajectory of motion. This process permits an increased awareness of kinesthesia and coordination and causes a decrease in pain.

The Feldenkrais Method encompasses two approaches to this somatically based reeducation. One is "Awareness through Movement" and the other is "Functional Integration." Awareness through Movement includes the use of active motion either with the individual or with a group. In 45- to 60-min sessions the instructor guides patients through a series of active movements using imagery and focused attention. Through the guidance, the patients become aware of their somatic reception and the influence it has on their movement. Imagery and visualization help them to develop this awareness and movement perception. The goal is for patients to become aware of their bodies and how their bodies move, of the relationship between one segment and another during movement, and of the influences that affect their movement.

The lessons often include developmental movements such as rolling, crawling, and standing up. They also include somatic awareness, visualization, and imagery for functions such as posture, breathing, and simple movements. The exercises are not vigorous but rather are explorations of the somatopsychic connections that increase self-awareness and facilitate an assessment of sensory-based movement. The movements often start as very small motions with emphasis on ease of movement, comfort, and development of an awareness of the way the muscles and bones are integrated with the individual's somatosensory system and personality. Small movements progress to more complex, larger, and faster ones until the movements are functional and can be put to daily use. Imagery and verbal suggestion guide the patient toward incorporating the new movement patterns into daily activity.

Functional Integration uses individualized sessions designed to meet the person's specific needs to improve movement. As with Awareness through Movement, Functional Integration is a learning-based method of improving movement efficiency, coordination, awareness, and self-control. Movement awareness and response are facilitated through the use of touch, imagery, repetition, and guidance. A new awareness and perception of movement are created and integrated into the individual's motions through the instructor's guidance, much as one dance partner is guided by the other, until the new neuromuscular patterns become ingrained and translate into a change in the injured patient's active performance.

An Example of the Feldenkrais Method

As an example of the Feldenkrais Method, a simple 2-min activity experiment from Alon (1990) is reprinted here. It is designed to improve and refine an individual's ability to look up. Take a couple of minutes to go through it and note any changes you experience. To perform the activity, go through the following steps:

In a sitting position, raise your head upward and try to see the ceiling. Make a note how this movement works for you. At what point in your reach do you have a feeling of difficulty? What happens to your breathing? Now, shift your attention to the feet. Take off one shoe and extend that foot forward, as far as you can; the sole stays flat on the floor. Begin to slowly flex your toes downward, dragging them along the floor closer to your heel. In this position, lift the ball of the foot from the floor and decrease the angle of bending in the ankle. All this time, the heel is still anchored to the floor. This is an unusual combination of movements involving the foot. Allow the foot to return to its comfortable place on the floor, and repeat the whole sequence several times.

In the next step, place your foot in full contact with the floor again, but this time bend the toes upward, raising them into the air while the ball of the foot stays on the ground. Alternate several times between the two movements, from bent ankle to outstretched ankle, with the heel planted all the time on the floor. The toes point to the floor when the foot comes up, and they are turned to the ceiling when the ball of the foot rests on the floor. See if you can reduce the amount of effort you invest in bending the ankle and the toes. Notice that to design a strange arrangement that is perhaps totally new to you, you have to use a device other than direct physical power. Identify within yourself this quality of listening and clarification—it is this quality which makes the difference between exercise and learning.

Now, bring the foot back to its usual place, and again lift your head so as to look at the ceiling. Has your scan of the ceiling now been made a bit easier than it was earlier?

The Feldenkrais Method is a complex system that takes time to learn. There are several classifications of Feldenkrais-trained professionals. Awareness-through-movement Feldenkrais teachers must have a minimum of 2 years of instruction; Feldenkrais practitioners have a minimum of 4 years of instruction; assistant trainers have a minimum of 7 years of activity; and trainers must have at least 11 years in the area. The Feldenkrais Guild in Albany, Oregon, is the accrediting body for the Feldenkrais Method.

Alexander Technique

Frederick M. Alexander (1869–1955) was an Australian-born actor who owned his own theater company and performed readings of Shakespeare. Before the invention of microphones, voice projection was vital to an actor's livelihood. After many fruitless attempts by physicians to cure the projection difficulty that Alexander had, he discovered that his problem lay in his body posture and movement. He discovered how faulty posture, incorrect movement patterns, and inefficient movement could affect health, movement, and body function. He eventually abandoned his theatrical career and studied the human body and techniques to improve its efficiency of movement. In the early 1900s he moved from Australia to England, where he taught his techniques.

Alexander discovered that posture is complex and that it involves not just sitting or standing straight, but also supporting and balancing against gravity during all daily activities. Children, he noticed, have good posture and good mechanics; but as people become older, the stresses and strains of life increase muscle tension and affect posture, as well as the way they use the body. Alexander believed that daily stresses over time cause increased muscle tension. This increased tension causes people to use their bodies inefficiently and ineffectively, eventually leading to injury and poor performance. For this reason, Alexander advocated unlearning, rather than learning. He felt that once we discarded the old, incorrect way of performing activities, the body would move naturally and easily.

For more information about the Alexander Technique, see http://alexandertechnique.com, www.life.uiuc.edu/jeff/alextech.html, or www.ati-net.com.

The Alexander Technique involves the self-examination of functions such as posture, breathing, balance, and coordination. It is an educational process that includes an increased perception of kinesthesia and balance, self-awareness, and natural, stress-free movement. The Alexander Technique is also used to improve functional activities for fine-arts performers and athletes. As an individual's awareness, kinesthesia, and performance improve, pain is relieved and movement becomes more efficient.

The Alexander Technique includes first becoming aware of and releasing the tension that has become habitual over many years of improper movement; it then focuses on re-education to new ways of standing, sitting, and moving that are easier, more efficient, and less stressful to the body. The final phase of the technique includes development of new ways of handling the stresses encountered in daily living so that unnecessary muscle tension does not return. Changing behavior is vital to creating an effective and permanent alteration in body movement. Alexander's method of body awareness, re-education, and self-awareness is designed to allow the individual to make choices that ultimately influence movement. His intent was to create a re-education process that provides a stronger awareness of inner and outer self.

Alexander discovered that the body works as a whole, not in parts. He saw that a painful body part may be influenced by another area that may be the actual site of the pain or dysfunction. He also discovered that an individual produces the same reaction repeatedly until the abnormal motion becomes habitual and feels natural, even though it is abnormal. To correct these problems, he inhibited old motions, encouraged new and more correct motions, and had the individual repeat the corrected motions until the new task became natural. He would use light touch, verbal cueing, and self-awareness techniques until the individual did not need the touch and verbal cueing to perform the task correctly.

Alexander Technique sessions usually last 30 to 60 min and involve group classes or individual lessons. These lessons are a cooperative effort between the participant and the instructor. As the participant receives feedback, he or she gradually feels a lightening sensation. Normally, no more than about eight sessions are needed.

Alexander thought that there were two levels of control or "direction," primary and secondary. The primary control, according to Alexander, stems from the core of the body—the head, neck, and back. If freedom of this primary direction is not managed first, secondary control is not possible. Alexander's primary directions include release of neck, head, and back tension. Releasing the neck is necessary before releasing the tension in the head, and both those sites must be released before the back tension can be released.

Once the primary directions have been applied, the secondary directions can follow. These directions are more numerous and involve the extremities. Depending on where tension is, the secondary release areas may include the shoulders, hips, hands, knees, or other sites. For example, to release tension in the feet, the individual may be instructed to think of the feet spreading onto the ground as the toes lengthen. To release the tension in the upper chest, the person may be instructed to allow the shoulders to release away from one another.

An Alexander Technique Experiment

Try this experiment reprinted from Barlow (1977) on yourself:

Lie down on the floor with a book under your head, your hips and knees bent with your feet flat on the floor. Find a quiet place so you won't be disturbed, and don't succumb to additional stimuli such as wriggling, scratching, and irrelevant thought patterns.

Think, "neck release, head forward and up." As you give this sequence thought, at first you won't "realize" what the direction means, but as you continue you will begin to associate it with an awareness you've had in the past. By "awareness" is meant that what should be a normal sense of "being in yourself," as opposed to the state of mind-body split that is so often present in adults. While you are still preserving by direction this awareness of the head and neck—an awareness in which your verbal order [of the words and directions] will be part and parcel of the actual perception as the organizing component of it—add on the verbal direction, "lengthen and widen your back." Your lessons will already have made you familiar with the meaning of this phrase, and it is likely that fresh meaning and fresh simplification will accrue as you run over the sequence to yourself. For example, you may realize that the whole of the back is lengthening in one unit instead of thinking of the upper back as separate from the lower back; or perhaps you may suddenly notice that widening of the back includes releasing the shoulder blade and upper arm. At this point, your interest in the new realization may have caused you to "lose" the head direction, and it will be necessary to reinforce it before returning to the lengthening and widening direction.

The process of adding together the direction to the head and the direction to the back may take several minutes or even longer; indeed, if it seems to take less time, you almost certainly have been making a muscular change by direct movement, instead of sticking to realizing the meaning of the orders. Remember that in this process we do not move our bodies in the same way as when we pick up an external object, a brush or pen or pail. To move our forearm is not the same as to move a spoon. Moving ourselves and bits of ourselves—as opposed to moving external objects—is always a question of allowing movement to take place, rather than of [making movement take place by] picking up and putting down somewhere else. Allowing the movement, say, of an arm will involve a total general awareness of the body; the active process involved in this particular movement is small compared with the active process of awareness that is going on in the whole of the body all of the time. Similarly, a movement of standing up after sitting down—a movement which involves mainly a leg adjustment—does not require only the leg activity, but primarily a maintenance of the awareness of the rest of the body while allowing the necessary leg movement to take place.

The Alexander Technique is one of thought rather than of action. It emphasizes the individual's thinking of the release rather than actually performing the activity. Attempting to produce the action often increases muscle tension instead of relieving it. The individual must practice following the directions several times so that he or she becomes very familiar with them and can feel a change in control. Awareness of actions and performance makes one better able to control those actions and change performance.

Alexander Technique instructors must obtain a minimum of 1,600 hours or three years of experience and education before they can become certified. The American Center for the Alexander Technique is headquartered in New York City.

It will be helpful to consider a couple of athletic activities and incorporate into them the Alexander Technique of improved awareness and conscious correction with assistance. The common activity of running requires an inefficient expenditure of energy if it is not performed correctly. The Alexander Technique teacher uses gentle touch and verbal instructions to correct the runner's movements until the runner is able to perform the technique using self-awareness and self-correction.

The Alexander Technique as used in soccer can also be used to improve kicking technique. The Alexander Technique teacher can provide instruction to permit the soccer player to release unwanted muscle tension, become aware of muscle activity, and correct the kicking technique to permit a more effective and efficient movement.

Pilates Method

Joseph H. Pilates (1880-1968) was born in Germany. He was a sickly child, suffering from asthma, rickets, and rheumatic fever. Determined to overcome his illnesses, he underwent self-study and practice in a combination of yoga, Zen, and ancient Greek and Roman physical conditioning regimens. Prior to World War I he was living in England and working as a performer and boxer. During the war he was interned with other German nationals in a camp where he began instructing his fellow camp members in his exercise routines. From England he moved to New York City where he opened a studio and used his techniques with dancers.

Pilates called his exercise regimen "Contrology." He defined it as the art of control. He believed that our will should control our muscles. He was a firm believer that movement starts from our core: the abdominal, lower back, buttock, and hip muscles. The body's balance and stability originated in these muscles. He called these muscles the "powerhouse" of our bodies.

His method was based on a philosophy that integrated body awareness with conditioning. The goal was to improve flexibility, coordination, strength, tone, muscle control, and mental conditioning to improve the whole person. Pilates was also concerned with the process, so he advocated continuous movement through a natural evolution: moving from one exercise to the next to ultimately build strength from the inside out and rebalance the body. He believed that balance was the factor to be sought, and since everyone is different, each person's program must be individually designed. Because of this belief, he often did not teach the same exercise from one day to the next but rather adjusted to meet the individual's needs.

Although different pieces of equipment have been designed for the Pilates Method, it is not necessary to use equipment to perform Pilates exercises. During his life, Joseph Pilates designed 500 exercises. This is probably because he designed programs to meet the needs of the individual. He did not organize or form an organization to carry on his techniques and methods; for this reason, there are many different instructors, companies, and businesses today that have created programs based on the Pilates Method and various versions of it. Pilates classes can be found around the country in workshops, private sessions, health clubs, hospitals, clinics, and gyms.

The Pilates Method revolves around a few basic principles. Most advocates list eight to nine principles. The first principle is *relaxation*. Relaxation allows the body to release tension and stress and provides a nice balance for body and mind. Many people use relaxation at the beginning of their Pilates workout to rid themselves of the day's stress and allow themselves to concentrate better on the session. Relaxation enhances correct firing patterns to improve posture and breathing. The next principle is *concentration*. Since the mind is used to reeducate the muscles, Pilates exercises should be performed in an environment without distractions to achieve the necessary level of concentration. Focusing your mind on your movements enhances the sense of where your body is in space. *Control* is learned using concentration and practice of each exercise. Exercises start simple and become more complex as control improves. Another principle is *breathing*. Using the diaphragm and other respiratory muscles encourages both flexibility and strength of the rib cage and its muscles. This allows for optimal use of breathing during exercises to both prepare for movement and aid in the exercise and recovery. *Centering* is the fifth principle and deals with the idea that motion and energy begins

---

A Pilates Method Example

The following example of a progression of the Pilates Method is based on a program outlined in Siler's *The Pilates Body* (2000). Outlined below is a description of sequential exercises for beginners; each exercise is performed 3 to 5 times:

1. Lie down on a floor mat on your back with your hips and knees flexed and feet comfortably on the floor; the arms are extended along the sides. Tighten your buttocks, squeeze the knees together, pull your navel to your spine, inhale, and roll up slowly, starting with moving your chin to your chest and moving your shoulders and trunk up and forward. As your body comes up into a sitting position, you exhale and the legs are simultaneously stretched forward into extension. As you move sequentially through this motion, imagine a progression of lifting from the beginning with your chin lifted to your chest, your chest lifted over your ribs, your ribs lifted over your abdomen, and your abdomen lifted over your hips. To return to the starting position, breathe in, squeeze the buttocks, tuck your coccyx, and pull your navel to your spine as you start to flex your knees. Reverse the roll-up sequence, and exhale as you feel your back begin to unroll onto the mat. By the end, your head and arms should be resting on the mat.

2. Begin in the starting position of the first exercise. Pull your navel to your spine and extend one leg to the ceiling with the hip in lateral rotation. Maintain the navel-to-the-spine position and perform a hip circle, inhaling and beginning the movement in an adducted position, circling down, around, and breathe in as you move the leg up to the start position; the circle should be large enough to maintain control and prevent the leg from wobbling and not permit the buttocks to lift off the mat. Once you have completed the 3 to 5 repetitions, perform the exercise in the opposite direction, and then repeat the exercise with the other leg. Return to the starting position.

3. In a sitting position with the hips and knees flexed, placed a hand under each distal thigh and lift the feet off the floor until you are balancing on your coccyx. Become round like a ball by tucking your chin to your chest and moving your elbows away from your sides. Pull your navel to your spine, inhale, and roll backward, maintaining your arm and leg positions relative to each other and to your chest. Exhale as you return to the starting position but do not touch the feet to the floor. Create the movement from your abdominals, not your neck, shoulders, or legs.

4. Lie on your back with your knees pulled toward your chest. Grab one shin with your hands and extend the other leg to the ceiling. Place the outside hand on the flexed leg's ankle and the other hand on the flexed leg's knee; both shoulders should remain depressed throughout the exercise. Pull your navel to your spine and lift your head and neck to reach your chin toward your abdomen. Exhale and hold the position. Keeping your navel to your spine, inhale and switch arm and leg positions, maintaining a flat back to the mat. Squeeze the buttocks as you switch leg positions.

5. Sit in a long-sitting position with your knees flexed slightly and your feet separated wider than your hips. Flex the shoulders to 90° with the elbows extended in front of you and your scapula depressed. In this position, flex your ankles and inhale to extend your trunk longitudinally. As you bring your chin to your chest, roll downward and bring your navel to your spine. Keeping your hips stable, exhale and move your upper body forward while resisting the stretch forward by pulling back with your abdominals. Now inhale and reverse back to the chin-tucked position. Then exhale as you return to the tall seated starting position. At the very end you should be sitting tall with your back flat and your scapulae depressed.

in the center or the core and branches outward to the periphery. Using the core muscles as stabilizers produces effective and safe body movements. *Postural alignment* is important for safety during exercises and correcting muscle imbalances. A correct posture will encourage proper muscle activation and coordination. *Fluidity of movement* means moving slowly and gracefully with control. Slow movements allow you to monitor your posture and muscle activity to assure correct activation patterns. The exercises are performed with the individual moving from one exercise to the next, flowing gracefully through the exercise routine. Since Pilates movements are executed with precision, motions should be slow to more accurately assess them as you perform them. Finally, *stamina* is achieved as you progress in the program. As motion becomes more efficient, endurance improves. Your body becomes less tired with activities you found previously exhausting because your body moves with less stress and more energy conservation.

The advantage of Pilates is that anyone at any level of fitness may begin the program. It is not meant to increase bulk, but its goal is to create total body awareness and control through a coordinated effort between the mind and body. The exercises should be pain free. The method can be used for general health, rehabilitation, and sport-specific training.

For more information about the Pilates Method, see www.pilates.com or www. pilates.net.

SUMMARY

1. Identify the primary elements of proper alignment in standing from an anterior, posterior, and side view.

In an anterior position, a plumb line should bisect the nose and mouth and should run through the central portion of the sternum, umbilicus, and pubic bones. The earlobes should be level with one another, as should the shoulders, fingertip ends, nipples, iliac crests, patellae, and medial malleoli. The patellae should point straight ahead, with the feet straight or turned slightly outward. The knees and ankles are in line with each other with the knees angled neither inward nor outward in relation to each other.

From a side view, the plumb line should pass through the external auditory meatus, the earlobe, the bodies of the cervical vertebrae, the center of the shoulder joint, and the greater trochanter. The plumb line should run midway between the back and chest and between the back and abdomen, slightly posterior to the hip joint, and slightly anterior to the center of the knee just behind the patella. A horizontal line should connect the ASIS and PSIS. The patient should remain relaxed with the body's weight balanced between the heel and the forefoot. The knees are straight but not locked. The chin is slightly tucked and the chest is held slightly up and forward. There is a mild curve inward of the low back and neck regions.

In the posterior view, a plumb line should bisect the head and should follow the spinous processes from the cervical through the lumbar spine. The earlobes, shoulders, scapulae, hips, PSIS, gluteal fold, posterior knee creases, and medial malleoli should appear level left to right. The scapulae should lie against the rib cage between the second and seventh ribs and about 5 cm (2 in.) from the spinous processes. The calcaneus should be straight, and the calcaneal tendon should be perpendicular to the floor. Trunk muscles should appear balanced, with symmetrical development. The shoulders should be positioned down and relaxed. Body weight should appear equally distributed over both feet.

2. Discuss common postural faults and describe their causes.

A muscle strength imbalance or shortening of a muscle or group can cause common postural faults. These changes usually occur over time and can cause any number of postural changes, depending on the specific area. Some examples of common postural faults include anterior-posterior or lateral spinal deformities such as scoliosis, lordosis, and kyphosis; hip anteversion and retroversion; winking or frog-eye patellae, genu recurvatum; genu and ankle varus and valgus; pes cavus and pes planus; and hammertoes, claw toes, and bunions.

3. Outline corrective exercises for common postural faults.

Once the cause of the fault has been determined, corrective exercises are used to reduce or relieve the fault. In many instances, strengthening of weak muscles combined with stretching of tight structures is fundamental and vital to correction, especially the strengthening of the weak muscles. In addition, the individual must make a conscious effort to correct postural faults in order to stop poor habits and establish new, correct ones.

4. Explain the importance of good posture and proper body mechanics in athletics.

Good posture is vital to good execution of sport activity because it improves efficiency and reduces the risk of injury. Imbalances that occur because of poor posture and mechanics place the body at risk of injury because of already increased stresses on structures. One area must compensate for the deficiencies in another area, causing the body to perform less efficiently and effectively.

5. List the basic principles of good body mechanics.

Maintain a "straight" spine so that forces from the legs can be transferred upward; reduce the height of the center of gravity for increased stability; widen the base of support for more stability; stand in the direction of movement or force application; and maintain good strength in the abdominals and lower-extremity muscles.

6. Discuss an example of the use of proper body mechanics by the rehabilitation clinician during a treatment program.

When providing manual resistance, the rehabilitation clinician stands close to the patient, uses leg strength to deliver the manual resistance, keeps the back straight, and stands with the feet in the direction of the resisted movement.

7. Explain the differences and similarities between the Feldenkrais Method, the Pilates Method, and the Alexander Technique.

All methods are based on correction of the dysfunctional somatic feedback system and use of self-awareness, reeducation, and repetition as part of the correction process. The Feldenkrais Method improves movement through changing awareness of movement; it engages the entire person in the treatment program by promoting self-esteem and improving learning skills. The Pilates Method controls body movement through a balance between mind and body. The core muscles serve as the "powerhouse" from which movement is initiated, and movement follows a smooth flow from one motion to the next. The Alexander Technique emphasizes the unlearning of old and improper habits and establishing new habits based on self-evaluation and increased perception of kinesthesia and natural movement.

CRITICAL THINKING QUESTIONS

1. You are working in an industrial clinic where back injuries are frequent. In an effort to be more efficient, you design a handout for these back patients that will include instructions for proper lifting and sitting. What items will you include in the handout? Will you include any precautions? What about general information on back anatomy and mechanics? Why would you or would you not include this information?

2. A shoulder patient you are treating has poor upper-back and cervical posture. You feel that this is complicating the shoulder injury and that you must correct the patient's posture before you can effectively impact the shoulder. How can the thoracic and cervical posture affect the shoulder? What will you do to improve this posture? What cues and instructions will you provide the patient?

3. The secretary for your department spends most of her day at the computer and on the phone. She is complaining about upper back and neck pain and has asked you to help her. On what areas will your examination be focused? What is the probable cause for her complaints, and what can she do to alleviate the problem?

4. A patient with plantar fasciitis has some postural deviations in the lower extremities. In addition to excessively pronated feet, she also has tibial torsion and squinting patellae. What other deviations in the hips would you expect, given these abnormalities?

5. Based on the opening scenario for this chapter, what instructions would you give Russell on proper lifting mechanics? What precise lifting instructions would you give him? What types of lifting activities would you include in his program?

6. When you are providing lower-extremity proprioceptive neuromuscular facilitation to a patient who is lying on the table, what correct body mechanics would you use? What would be the position for your base of support? How would you transfer your body weight? Where would your body be positioned to offer the best resistance on hip extension? On hip flexion?

LAB ACTIVITIES

1. Perform a posture analysis on a lab partner. Identify all areas of malalignment or deviations from normal. Evaluate her posture from all three angles. Identify if there are any corrective causes for these postural deviations. What exercises would you provide to correct or reduce these deviations.

2. If you have a digital camera, take photos of your friends of family members who have postural deviations. Identify which deviations each has and if the deviation is mild, moderate, or severe.

3. In a group made up of three or four people, go around campus and take digital photos of as many postural deviations as you can find. After a specific time established by your instructor, report (along with the other teams) the types and numbers of postural deviations you have captured. The team with the greatest number or types of postural deviations is the winner.

4. Have your lab partner lie supine on the treatment table. If you are going to provide manual resistance to your lab partner's hip flexion and hip extension motions, how are you going to stand and move as he moves the hip through the range of motion? What is the best position for your body? Where is the best placement of your hands on your partner's leg for your mechanical advantage? How do you move your body to allow the resistance to be easier for you? Where is your arm offering the resistance in comparison to where your body is throughout the exercises? What have you learned from this activity?

5. Have your lab partner sit on the end of a treatment table. Offer her manual resistance to knee extension. How are you going to position your body to make the activity easiest for you? Where is your body in relation to your lab partner's leg? How does your body movement change as the leg goes through its range of motion? What must you do to continue to make the manual resistance exercise an easy activity for you? What is the significance of this activity?

6. Have your lab partner perform an athletic activity such as a tennis serve, basketball free-throw or layup, soccer kick, volleyball serve or net block, football pass or front line block, or baseball toss. What instructions are you going to provide that will allow your partner to perform the athletic activity using good body mechanics? Have him repeat the performance using your instructions; how was the performance this time? What additional tips and instructional points do you need to provide for your partner to perform with better body mechanics? What are the basic principles that your lab partner must remember to perform the activity correctly? Once your partner is able to perform the activity using good body mechanics, how did the actual performance change (in terms of distance thrown or kicked, force produced, or speed of delivery)? Why?

REFERENCES

Alon, R. 1990. *Mindful spontaneity: Moving in tune with nature: Lessons in the Feldenkrais Method.* New York: Harper & Row.

Barlow, W. 1977. *The Alexander Technique.* New York: Knopf.

Kendall, F.P., McCreary, E.K., and P.G. Provance. 1993. *Muscles: Testing and function.* 4th ed. Baltimore: Williams & Wilkins.

Sahrmann, S.A. 2002. *Diagnosis and Treatment of Movement Impairment Syndromes.* St. Louis: Mosby.

Siler, B. 2000. *The Pilates Body.* New York: Broadway Books.

SUGGESTED READING

Hislop, H.J. and J. Montgomery. 2002. *Daniels and Worthingham's muscle testing. Techniques of manual examination.* Philadelphia: WB Saunders.

Ambulation and Ambulation Aids.

Objectives

After completing this chapter, you should be able to do the following:

1. Discuss the general concepts of gait.
2. Identify the range-of-motion changes during the gait cycle.
3. Explain the muscle activity involved in ambulation.
4. Describe the general mechanical differences between walking and running.
5. Discuss one abnormal gait commonly seen following a musculoskeletal injury.
6. Outline the various types of gait with assistive devices.
7. Explain the technique involved in stair climbing with assistive devices.
8. Identify the safety measures involved in ambulating with assistive devices.

When Michelle, a 38-year-old competitive soccer player, first injured her ankle, she was unable to walk on it. The second-degree sprain was conservatively treated with a cast for two weeks and then placed in a splint for four weeks. By the time Andrew Williams, certified athletic trainer, saw Michelle, she was out of the splint and off crutches but was still not able to walk normally. Andrew analyzed her gait to evaluate for deficiencies in range of motion and strength before performing specific motion and strength tests. Because she was not walking normally, he did not have her run, but he knew that one day he would analyze her running gait as well.

Since Michelle was still limping severely, he instructed her in how to walk with a cane. She didn't want to use crutches any longer, but saw the cane as a compromise until she could walk normally without it. Andrew was careful to provide her with precautions about using the cane and would not allow her to use it on her own until she demonstrated proper use on the floor, carpet, and stairs.

■ **Walking is the best possible exercise. Habituate yourself to walk very far.**

Thomas Jefferson, (1743-1826), third president of the United States (1801-1809); author of the Declaration of Independence

People have been walking long before Mr. Jefferson advocated it as exercise. Watching how a patient moves during ambulation, from the feet all the way up to the shoulders, can yield important information to the rehabilitation clinician. To know whether or not a patient ambulates normally, you must understand what normal gait is. Before you can instruct a patient in how to use assistive devices during ambulation, you must first understand the mechanics of those assistive devices and the desired gait with the devices.

Ambulation is a normal activity that most of us perform every day without thinking about it, about what it involves, or about how we do it. We just do it. When an injury prevents normal ambulation, the activity becomes difficult and energy consuming. It no longer is something we take for granted, and it is no longer is automatic.

This chapter introduces the mechanics of walking and addresses the differences between walking and running. We will consider normal ambulation, common pathological gaits, and ambulation with assistive devices. Topics include the mechanics of assistive device applications, various gaits with different types of assistive devices on different surfaces, and methods of selecting assistive devices for the patient.

NORMAL GAIT

▶ Elements of gait include the gait cycle, the center-of-gravity pathway, gait kinematics, and ground reaction forces. Lower-extremity injuries can lead to abnormalities of these elements and are reflected in the patient's pathological gait.

Ambulation, or walking, is the locomotion method we use to move our body from one place to another. The way we walk is called gait. Although each person's gait is slightly different from everyone else's, all normal gaits have basic similarities. In fact, considering how many body types and sizes there are among human beings, it is surprising how little normal gait differs from one person to the next. Major differences commonly result from postural variations, weaknesses, structural abnormalities, and soft-tissue length alterations, some of which are discussed in chapter 11. Knowledge of normal gait is essential to the rehabilitation clinician so that he or she can correct abnormal gait following injury and understand the use of assistive devices.

Gait Cycle

One gait cycle is the time from the point at which the heel of one foot touches the ground to the time it touches the ground again. A gait cycle is divided into two phases, the stance phase and the swing phase. The stance phase occurs when the foot is in contact with the floor and the extremity is bearing partial or total body weight. The stance phase is subdivided into three parts. Heel strike (foot strike) occurs when the heel or foot first comes in contact with the floor. Foot flat, as the term implies, occurs when the foot is flat on the floor. Just as the heel may not be the first part of the foot to strike the ground in runners and some pathological gaits so that "foot strike" is more appropriate than "heel strike", some believe that the term "foot flat" should be replaced with the term "reversal of fore shear to aft shear" since the foot may not achieve a flat position in some pathological gaits (Chambers & Sutherland 2002). The midstance phase occurs when the foot is directly under the body's weight and the entire foot is in contact with the floor. Because the body weight is transferred entirely to the one supporting leg and the other leg is in the middle of its swing phase, this is also referred to as single-leg support. Heel-off occurs when the weight begins to transfer to the front of the foot, and the heel is lifted off the floor. Partial weight remains on the extremity as the other extremity is now in contact with the floor again. Toe-off occurs when the foot comes off the floor and the swing phase begins. This is also referred to as *push-off*, since the extremity now propels the body forward and the leg continues into the second phase of gait.

The second phase, swing phase, occurs when the foot is not in contact with the floor and no weight is borne on the extremity. The swing phase begins with toe-off and is divided into early-, mid-, and late-swing phases. Immediately after toe-off, the leg begins its early swing, or acceleration, as momentum is increased in its non-weight-bearing propulsion forward. The mid-swing of the swing phase is called swing-through. The leg continues its swing-through until just before heel strike when it goes through the late swing, or deceleration, to slow its forward propulsion, make a smooth contact with the floor, and begin a new gait cycle. Alternative terminology can also be used and is often seen in research reports on gait. With this nomenclature, the initial heel strike with the floor is termed initial contact, and as the foot progresses to increased weight bearing, it goes from initial contact to loading response (foot flat), then midstance (single-leg support). In this terminology, heel-off is referred to as terminal stance and progresses to preswing (toe-off). The swing phase begins with toe-off and is divided into initial swing (early swing/acceleration), midswing (swing-through), and terminal swing (late swing/deceleration). Some researchers and clinicians prefer this terminology because the terms provide for greater consistency and descriptor accuracy in reporting analysis and results.

Clinicians vary in the terminology they use. Clinicians' choice of terminology for gait analysis most often depends on the method they were taught and on what is most intuitive for them. Both groups of terms are presented here so you can become familiar with each. The alternative terms are used interchangeably throughout this text.

If one gait cycle from the beginning of stance phase to the end of swing phase is 100%, stance phase is 62% (usually rounded off to 60%) of the gait cycle. Within the stance, heel strike to foot flat covers 0% to 12% of the gait cycle; midstance occurs over the next 12% to 30%; heel-off begins at 30% and continues until toe-off at the start of the swing cycle (figure 12.1). The remaining 38% (usually rounded off to 40%) of the gait cycle occurs during the swing phase. As speed of the gait increases, the percentages between the stance and swing phases become more equal. In running, the percentage becomes greater for the swing phase than for the stance phase.

During the first and last 10% of stance in walking, the body is supported by both lower extremities (Ounpuu 1994). This occurs at the beginning of the stance phase during heel strike for one leg and at the end of the stance phase, just before toe-off, for the other. This part of stance is referred to as double-limb support.

Figure 12.1 *(a)* Single-leg gait cycle, *(b)* double-leg gait cycle.

Center-of-Gravity Pathway

During ambulation, the body's center of gravity is propelled forward. Its relative position also changes because of the associated changes in position of the joints and extremities during ambulation. Before we can understand the changes that occur and their importance, we must clarify some terms.

Stride length is the distance from heel strike of one foot to heel strike of the same foot in one gait cycle. Step length is the distance from heel strike of one foot to heel strike of the other foot in one gait cycle. Although stride length depends on the individual's height, an average stride length is 156 cm (61 in.) (Lehmann & DeLateur 1990).

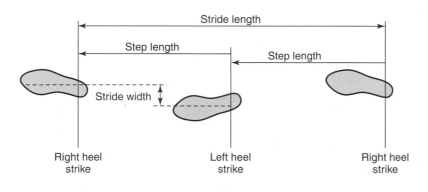

Figure 12.2 Stride length and stride width.

The body's side-to-side movement as weight is shifted from one lower extremity to the other is called stride width (figure 12.2). It is the distance between the midline of one foot at midstance and the midline of the other foot at midstance. Stride width also has individual determining factors such as body size and weight, but the average stride width ranges from 5 cm (about 2 in.) (Chambers & Sutherland 2002) to 8 cm (about 3 in.) ± 3.5 (Lehmann & DeLateur 1990).

There is large variation in the rate at which individuals walk. Reports of what is normal walking speed vary. The range is from just under 60 strides per minute (Murray et al. 1964; Lehmann & DeLateur 1990) to 101 to 122 steps per minute (Winter 1987). Stance and swing phases are directly influenced as cadence increases to jogging, running, and sprinting speeds. We will consider the mechanics of running in the section "Normal Running Gait" later in this chapter.

As the body is propelled forward, it attempts to create motion that is as efficient as possible. Keeping the center-of-gravity movement to a minimum is how we achieve efficiency of movement. Short of the lower extremities being wheels instead of legs, a multijoint system is the best way to propel the body forward efficiently. Although a wheel system would move the body very efficiently over flat surfaces, movement over uneven surfaces would become quite difficult. Using a number of joints from the pelvis to the foot, the body minimizes center-of-gravity pathway changes by changing the position of the joints as the body moves, and also allows for adjustment to varying types of surfaces and terrain.

In order for propulsion of the body to be smooth and efficient, the body must produce enough force to move forward but also control the movement and momentum so that the body remains stable as its positions change; it must also absorb the impact shock of moving weight from one leg to the other. All these capabilities must be present and must be controlled if movement is to be efficient and effective. Loss of one of the contributing factors can result in poor quality of movement, high energy requirements, or injury.

Since the body does not move on wheels, its bipedal system causes an efficient sinusoidal motion of the body's center of gravity that rises and falls an average of about 4 cm (1.6 inches) (Chambers & Sutherland 2002). Moving the body's center of gravity in a wavelike fashion conserves energy and reduces impact forces (figure 12.3).

Determinants of Gait

The body accomplishes a sinusoidal movement in both vertical and horizontal directions during locomotion through six determinants of gait. (Saunders et al 1953). If any of these movements are restricted, the patient's gait will be inefficient and lack the smoothness of motion seen in normal gait.

Figure 12.3 Sinusoidal motion.

Pelvic Rotation

Pelvic rotation occurs around a horizontal axis in the transverse plane. As one leg swings forward, the pelvis rotates forward to increase the length of the leg's step. The pelvis attains its maximum rotation on one side, 4°, at the point of double-leg support. With lengthening of the leg, the center of gravity is prevented from dropping lower than it otherwise would (figure 12.4). This motion reduces the center-of-gravity vertical movement by 3/8 in. The pelvis rotates 4° on the opposite side as that leg rotates forward during the same process. The total pelvic rotation is 8°, or 4° on each side.

Figure 12.4 Pelvic rotation causes an increase in the length of the leg's step to reduce the center of gravity's vertical displacement.

Pelvic Tilt

During midstance the pelvis tilts downward from the stance leg so that the hip on the swing-leg side is lower than that on the stance-leg side (figure 12.5). The hip abductors of the stance leg control this movement. Because the center of gravity is midway between the hips, it is lowered when the swing leg is lowered. This movement depresses the center of gravity during midstance by 5° and decreases the vertical displacement of the center of gravity by 3/16 in.

Figure 12.5 Pelvic tilt decreases vertical displacement of the center of gravity.

Knee Flexion at Midstance

At heel strike the knee is in extension, but immediately afterward it begins to flex until it flexes to 15° by midstance (figure 12.6). This knee flexion reduces the center of gravity's vertical excursion by 7/16 in. when it is at its highest point of the sinusoidal curve.

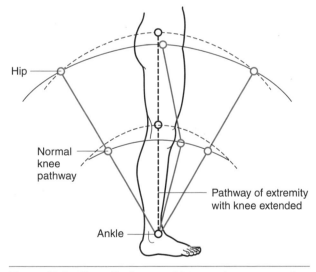

Hip

Normal knee pathway

Pathway of extremity with knee extended

Ankle

Figure 12.6 Knee flexion at midstance decreases vertical displacement of the center of gravity at midstance.

Ankle Motion

The center of gravity of the ankle joint is highest at heel strike and toe-off and lowest at midstance. This is the opposite of what happens with the knee joint, as seen in figure 12.7. These combined motions help to reduce the vertical excursion of the center of gravity and smooth out its sinusoidal curve.

The combined effects of pelvic rotation, pelvic tilt, and knee and ankle motions during stance are responsible for reducing vertical excursion of the center of gravity by 2.5 cm (1 in.) so that the overall vertical displacement is less than 5 cm. This becomes significant in terms of energy expenditure since the less movement, the less energy expended.

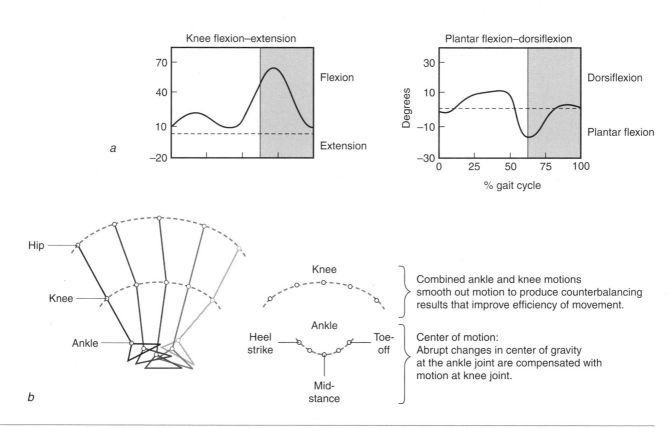

Figure 12.7   Knee and ankle motions in gait. The opposite motions occurring at the ankle and knee reduce vertical excursion of the center of gravity.

Lateral Motion of Pelvis

In order for a person to stand with stability, the center of gravity must be over the base of support, the feet. When we stand on two feet, the center of gravity is between the feet. To stand on one leg, the center of gravity must shift so that it is over the supporting leg. If the thighs were arranged in a parallel fashion, a maximum shift of 15 cm (6 in.) of the pelvis would be needed to transfer the center of gravity from one supporting leg to the other during single-limb support (figure 12.8). Because the femurs are not straight but angled medially to place the knees in a slight valgus position, the lateral shift required of the pelvis to move from one leg to the other is 4.3 cm (1.7 in.) for an adult. This lateral sway of less than 5 cm (2 in.) is also a sinusoidal curve, making the movement from one leg to the other during gait as smooth as possible.

The maximal position of the left-to-right sinusoidal curve occurs during midstance of each leg and is at the midline during double-limb support. The maximal height of the sinusoidal curve in vertical displacement also occurs during midstance of each leg and is at its lowest point during double-limb support.

Gait Kinematics

The sinusoidal curves of motion that occur during ambulation are caused by changes in the joints' ranges of motion. Some of these changes are not large but are important for smooth, energy-efficient motion. Movement occurs in the sagittal, coronal, and transverse planes. If movement in one plane is restricted, smooth gait will not occur. Therefore the clinician needs to understand the sequence, degree, and timing of joint motion so that when deficiencies exist, he or she can correct them.

a   *b*

Figure 12.8   Hip and knee alignment in lateral pelvic shift. Adducted thigh alignment reduces lateral sway during gait. *(a)* If thighs were parallel, it would require a lateral movement of 15 cm during ambulation. *(b)* Normal hip angulation minimizes lateral pelvic motion during ambulation to less than 5 cm.

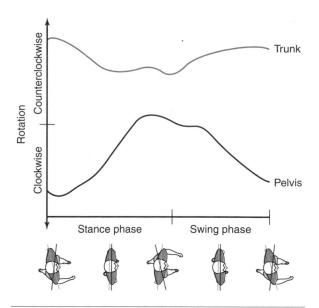

Figure 12.9 Trunk and pelvic rotation.

Adapted by permission from M.P. Murray, A.B. Drought, and R.C. Kory 1964.

Trunk and Upper Extremities

Throughout all cycles of normal gait, the trunk is held in an erect and neutral position. This is necessary to maintain the center of gravity over the base of support. Trunk movement is coordinated with pelvic movement so that as the pelvis rotates in one direction, the trunk rotates in the opposite direction (figure 12.9). The swing momentum of the arms assists the trunk in its rotation, so trunk muscle activity and energy requirements for trunk movement are reduced. This coordinated movement between the pelvis and trunk aids in making the gait smooth, stable, and efficient.

Pelvis

Pelvis movement is defined in terms of iliac crest movement. Forward motion of the iliac crest produces an anterior pelvic tilt, and backward motion produces a posterior pelvic tilt. Pelvis motion in the coronal, sagittal, and transverse planes is seen in the graphs in figure 12.10.

Heel Strike to Midstance

As the heel hits the ground at heel strike, the pelvis remains level and is in a 5° forwardly rotated position in the sagittal plane; as the body progresses toward midstance, the pelvis reduces its anterior tilt. In the coronal plane it is elevated 4° at heel strike and begins to drop after initial contact has been made. As the leg goes from heel strike to midstance, the pelvis medially rotates 4°.

Midstance to Toe-Off

By the time the leg is reaching the end of stance phase, the pelvis has moved into a posterior rotation position of about 5°. In a coronal plane during midstance to toe-off, the pelvis continues to drop until it reaches a total of 8° of lateral movement. During the final moments of stance phase, the pelvis rotates laterally, 8° from the initial position of 4° medial rotation to an ending stance position of 4° lateral rotation.

Early Swing

In early swing, the pelvis is level and in a posterior rotation of 5° moving toward anterior rotation. In the coronal plane it begins to move from a downward to an elevated position. Rotation in the transverse plane is gradual from 4° of lateral rotation to 4° of medial rotation by late swing.

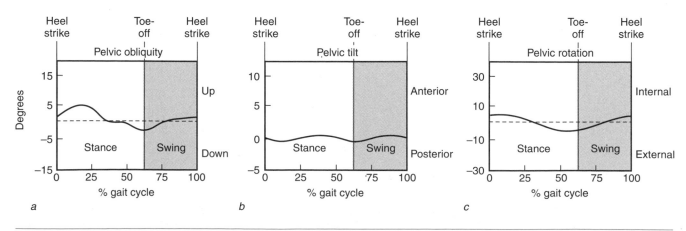

Figure 12.10 Pelvic motion in (a) coronal plane, (b) sagittal plane, (c) transverse plane. Pelvic motion is a triplanar event.

Late Swing

The pelvis continues to be level throughout the gait cycle, moving in the sagittal plane from an anterior position at the middle of the swing phase to a posterior position by the end of late swing. Coronal plane movement continues from its maximum downward position during early swing on its way toward an elevated position such that it is slightly elevated by the end of swing. Rotation also continues to progress in a medial direction as swing phase is terminated.

Total motions of the pelvis during a gait cycle are 4° of anterior-posterior tilt, 8° of lateral tilt, and 8° of rotation.

Hip

Hip motion also occurs in three planes of movement: the coronal, sagittal, and transverse planes (figure 12.11).

Heel Strike to Midstance

At heel strike the hip is in 30° of flexion, slight adduction of 2° to 6°, and near-neutral rotation at 5°. As the leg advances in the stance phase, the hip becomes less flexed, becomes less adducted, and goes from slight medial rotation to slight lateral rotation.

Midstance to Toe-Off

In the last half of the stance phase, the hip goes from 10° of extension at heel-off to ~5° to 0° extension at the time of toe-off. The hip is at neutral in the coronal plane at heel-off and goes into 4° of abduction at toe-off. After midstance the hip moves from medial rotation to neutral at heel-off until it reaches 4° of lateral rotation at toe-off. Part of the apparent hip extension that occurs from midstance to toe-off is actually the result of a posterior rotation and downward tilt of the pelvis.

Early Swing

In its initial swing, the hip continues to flex to 15° to 20°, reaches its maximum abduction of an average of 5°, and continues to have slight lateral rotation.

Late Swing

Frontal plane movement continues to advance to ~30° just before the end of swing. Coronal plane movement continues to advance from maximal abduction just after the start of early swing toward the midline until a neutral position is achieved just before heel strike. Transverse plane movement oscillates from medial to neutral to lateral rotation then back to slight medial rotation just before heel strike.

Total hip motions occurring during the gait cycle include 43° in the sagittal plane from flexion to extension, 13° of abduction-adduction in the coronal plane, and 8° of rotation in the transverse plane.

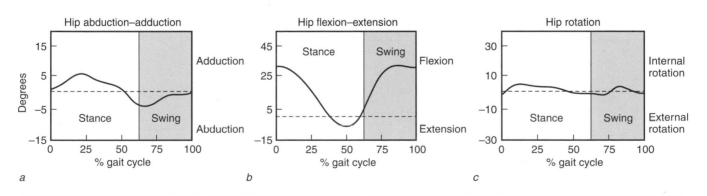

Figure 12.11   Hip motion in the *(a)* coronal plane, *(b)* sagittal plane, *(c)* transverse plane. Hip motion is triplanar with the greatest movement occurring in the sagittal plane and the least occurring in the transverse plane.

Knee

The knee performs the greatest amount of motion during the swing phase of the gait cycle. Rotation of the knee occurs through the gait cycle and is probably affected by a combination of tibial rotation and hip rotation occurring synchronously.

Heel Strike to Midstance

At heel strike the knee is in or close to full extension. The tibia is laterally rotated 8° to 10°. As weight acceptance on the leg increases, the knee is flexed to 15° and tibial rotation begins to occur in a medial direction (figure 12.12).

Midstance to Toe-Off

By the time the leg reaches midstance, the knee has achieved its maximum degree of flexion in the stance phase and begins to move into full extension at heel-off. After achievement of maximal tibial medial rotation just before midstance, a return to lateral rotation occurs during the later half of stance until maximal lateral rotation is achieved immediately before toe-off. Immediately before toe-off, the knee is passively flexed to 35° by the active movement of the ankle as it goes into plantar flexion and forces the knee to flex.

Early Swing

The knee continues to progress to a maximum of 60° of flexion; this occurs so that the foot clears the ground during the swing phase. In the body's attempt to conserve energy, foot clearance from the floor during swing is only a mere 0.87 cm (.3 in.) (Rodgers 1988). That small clearance leaves little room for error from fatigue or restricted motion. The tibia begins moving from the maximum laterally rotated position that it was in at toe-off toward inward rotation, although it continues to be positioned in lateral rotation throughout swing.

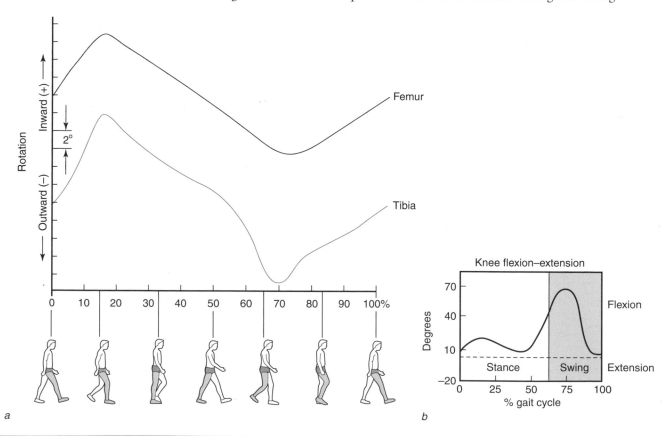

Figure 12.12 Knee motion: *(a)* Maximum medial rotation of hip and knee occur prior to midstance, and maximum lateral rotation occurs at the end of stance and into early swing phase. *(b)* Maximum knee extension occurs after midstance, whereas maximum knee flexion occurs in swing phase.

Late Swing

After achieving 60° of flexion in the first half of swing, the knee moves progressively and steadily toward extension until it is at 0° just before heel strike. Total knee range of motion in the sagittal plane is 60°, and tibial rotation is 18°. Maximum knee flexion during the stance phase occurs during midstance, and maximum knee flexion during the swing phase occurs during midswing. Maximum knee medial rotation occurs between heel strike and midstance in what researchers call the loading response, and maximum lateral rotation occurs at toe-off.

Ankle

The ankle and foot work together during gait and provide for needed balance as the body moves over uneven ground. The ankle joint is responsible for forward motion and stability, and the foot joints are responsible for medial and lateral adjustments. The foot and ankle are complex structures and are highly variable in structure and function from one individual to the next. As with other measurements indicated here, the values given are averages.

Heel Strike to Midstance

At heel strike, the ankle and toes are in neutral (figure 12.13). As weight is borne on the leg, the ankle moves into 15° of plantar flexion before midstance. The subtalar joint moves into pronation to accept the forces of impact. The toes remain in a neutral position through midstance. Once the leg moves into midstance, the ankle moves into 10° of dorsiflexion. This 10° permits a smooth glide of the limb as the body moves over its support. A lesser amount of motion causes the body to lurch as it moves into midstance. Once heel strike occurs, the calcaneus everts to cause subtalar pronation. This pronation permits the midtarsal area to remain flexible and to adapt to varying terrains. Pronation also allows the foot to act as a shock absorber. The subtalar joint remains in pronation until just before midstance when it begins to supinate. The longitudinal arch passively lengthens from heel strike until it reaches its maximum length at midstance. At heel strike the foot makes contact with the ground on the posterior aspect of the heel, slightly lateral to the midline. As the body moves forward and more weight is borne on the leg, the weight is transmitted distal to the heel in the midtarsal foot area.

Figure 12.13 Ankle motion.

Midstance to Toe-Off

Following midstance, the ankle moves quickly from 10° of dorsiflexion to about 20° of plantar flexion by the time of toe-off. The calcaneus inverts and causes the subtalar joint to move into supination so the foot will become stable for propulsion at toe-off. The longitudinal arch begins to shorten, and the metatarsophalangeal joints extend to 30° after midstance until reaching maximum extension of about 60° at toe-off. The interphalangeal joints remain in neutral throughout the stance and swing phases of gait. As stance progresses, the body's weight is advanced forward on the foot (figure 12.14). At midstance it is located just behind the metatarsal heads, and at toe-off the weight is primarily over the first and second metatarsophalangeal joints.

Key

1 = Initial contact (heel strike)

2 = Loading response (foot flat)

3 = Midstance

4 = Terminal stance (heel-off)

5 = Preswing (toe-off)

Figure 12.14 Weight transmission during walking: Initial contact at heel strike occurs in the posterior-lateral heel and advances forward on the foot through the stance phase. At midstance the body's weight is just behind the metatarsal heads and at toe-off the weight is primarily over the first and second metatarsal heads.

Early Swing

Once toe-off occurs, the ankle begins a dorsiflexion movement until it reaches a neutral position. By the time of middle swing, the ankle and toes are in a neutral position.

Late Swing

The ankle and toes remain close to neutral throughout the remaining part of the swing phase. The subtalar joint remains in pronation through the swing phase.

Total movement from plantar flexion to dorsiflexion in the sagittal plane is 30°. A great deal of motion in the lower extremities occurs during one stride. Figure 12.15 presents a summary of the joints' motions during ambulation. The motion is usually

Normal Gait

	Stance 60%					Swing 40%		
	Heel strike (initial contact)	Foot flat (loading response)	Midstance	Heel-off (terminal stance)	Toe-off (preswing)	Early swing (initial)	Midswing	Late swing (terminal)
Trunk	Erect Neutral	Erect Neutral	Erect Neutral	Erect Neutral	Erect Neutral	Erect Neutral	Erect Neutral	Erect Neutral
Pelvis	Level Forward rotation	Level 5° forward rotation Upward lateral rotation	Level Neutral rotation	Level 5° posterior rotation Downward lateral rotation	Level Posterior rotation Downward lateral rotation	Level Posterior rotation moving forward Lateral position is down	Level Neutral lateral rotation moving up	Level 5° forward rotation
Hip	30° flexion Slight adduction Near-neutral rotation	30° flexion Slight adduction Slight rotation	Extends Slight adduction Slight medial rotation	10° hyper-extension Slight abduction	5° Neutral Extension Slight medial rotation 4° Abduction	20° flexion Slight lateral rotation 5° Abduction	Flexing Lateral rotation	30° flexion Mild lateral rotation going to medial rotation
Knee	Full extension Tibia in lateral rotation	15° flexion Tibia in medial rotation	Moves toward extension	Full extension	35° flexion	Cont. to 60° flexion Tibial lateral rotation	Begin to move to 30° flexion Tibial lateral rotation	Cont. to extend
Ankle	Neutral	15° plantar flexion Pronation	10° dorsi-flexion Starts to supinate	Moving into plantar flexion Supinating	20° plantar flexion	Moving to neutral	Neutral	Neutral
Toes	Neutral	Neutral	Neutral	MTP: 30° extension IP: Neutral	MTP: 60° extension IP: Neutral	Neutral	Neutral	Neutral

Figure 12.15 Summary of kinetics and kinematics for the hip, knee, and ankle in the sagittal plane through the gait cycle. Movement is a smoothly flowing change of range of motion in each joint throughout the gait cycle.

Hip

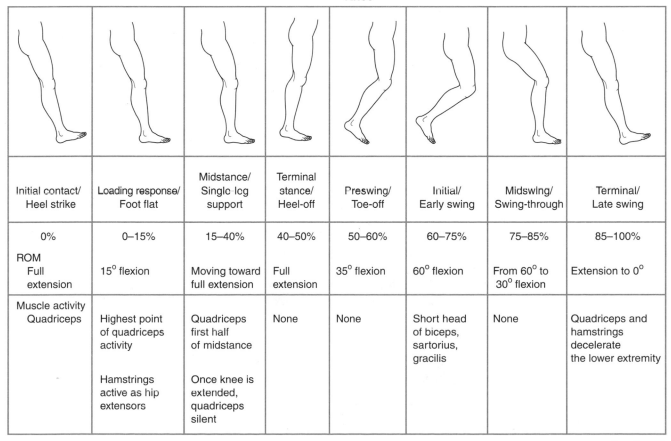

	Initial contact/ Heel strike	Loading response/ Foot flat	Midstance/ Single-leg support	Terminal stance/ Heel-off	Preswing/ Toe-off	Initial/ Early swing	Midswing/ Swing-through	Terminal/ Late swing
	0%	0–15%	15–40%	40–50%	50–60%	60–75%	75–85%	85–100%
ROM	Flexion 30° neutral abduction, adduction rotation	30° flexion	Full extension	10° hyper-extension	Neutral extension	20° flexion	Flexion from 20° to 30°	30° flexion
Muscle activity	Gluteus maximus, medius, tensor fascia lata, and hamstrings	Gluteus maximus, gluteus medius, tensor fascia lata, and hamstrings	Gluteus medius, tensor fascia lata	Hip flexors to prevent further extension	Hip flexors to initiate swing	Hip flexors	Hip flexors	Hamstrings to decelerate hip

Knee

	Initial contact/ Heel strike	Loading response/ Foot flat	Midstance/ Single-leg support	Terminal stance/ Heel-off	Preswing/ Toe-off	Initial/ Early swing	Midswing/ Swing-through	Terminal/ Late swing
	0%	0–15%	15–40%	40–50%	50–60%	60–75%	75–85%	85–100%
ROM	Full extension	15° flexion	Moving toward full extension	Full extension	35° flexion	60° flexion	From 60° to 30° flexion	Extension to 0°
Muscle activity	Quadriceps	Highest point of quadriceps activity; Hamstrings active as hip extensors	Quadriceps first half of midstance; Once knee is extended, quadriceps silent	None	None	Short head of biceps, sartorius, gracilis	None	Quadriceps and hamstrings decelerate the lower extremity

(continued)

Ankle

Initial contact/ Heel strike	Loading response/ Foot flat	Midstance/ Single-leg support	Terminal stance/ Heel-off	Preswing/ Toe-off	Initial/ Early swing	Midswing/ Swing-through	Terminal/ Late swing
0%	0–15%	15–40%	40–50%	50–60%	60–75%	75–85%	85–100%
ROM Neutral	15° plantar flexion	Neutral to 10° dorsi-flexion	Heel-off Prior to heel contact, opposite foot Moving into plantar flexion	20° plantar flexion	10° plantar flexion moving to neutral	Neutral	Neutral
Muscle activity Dorsiflexors maintain neutral position	Dorsiflexors control amount of plantar flexion, prevent foot slap	Plantar flexors control advance of tibia	Plantar flexors control tibia, restrict dorsiflexion	Dorsiflexors begin activity	Dorsiflexors active for toe clearance	Dorsiflexors maintain neutral position	Dorsiflexors maintain neutral position

Figure 12.15 *(continued)*

rapid, and some motions are difficult to detect visually without a video camera or similar device that can slow the motion so visual detection is possible. If visual recording devices are not available, it is useful to have the patient walk on a treadmill at a comfortable pace while you observe the gait from anterior, lateral, and posterior views. It is best to take an overall perspective first and notice any gross abnormalities in stride-length differences, stride width, and cadence. The next focus is on individual segments one at a time to discover any abnormalities in each of the joint's movements. These may include pelvic obliquity, premature heel-off or toe-off, knee position during various phases of gait, and calcaneal position during weight bearing. It makes little difference if your segmental observations begin proximally or distally, but whatever routine you select is best performed consistently in the same manner so you don't overlook any segment.

Gait Kinetics

Movements that occur during ambulation are the result of forces acting on the body. These forces include primarily those produced by the muscles, ground reaction forces, gravity, and momentum.

Muscles

The muscles function in gait to produce acceleration, deceleration, and stabilization. Acceleration is needed to propel the body or segment forward to produce motion. Acceleration is generally the result of the muscle's concentric activity. Deceleration is used to slow down momentum of the segment or body to produce a smooth and controlled motion during ambulation. Deceleration is most commonly produced by eccentric activity. Muscles that act as stabilizers are used as guy wires to hold a segment stable during movement. Stabilization is frequently produced by isometric activity. Some muscles are used at some times during gait as accelerators and at other times as decelerators. Other muscles are used primarily for stabilization of the body or segment.

Obviously, not all muscles are being used all the time during gait. The cyclic activity of a muscle in gait provides periods of rest for a muscle. Brief periods of peak muscle activity followed or preceded by less activity or periods of rest give the muscle enough recovery time so that an activity such as walking can continue for extended durations if necessary. Because walking is the means by which we move our body from one location to another, it matters quite a bit that locomotion does not require continuous muscle activity.

The greatest energy requirement of muscles is present during the stance phase; less energy is required during the swing phase. The times of the greatest amount of muscle activity are in the first 10% of the stance phase and the last 10% of the swing phase. Periods of relative inactivity occur during midstance and the swing phase. The times of greatest muscle activity are during periods of acceleration and deceleration. The swing phase is a relatively quiet time of muscle activity because the momentum produced during the final stages of stance carries the leg forward. As the muscles prepare the leg for heel strike during the final stages of swing, their activity increases.

Let's take a brief look at the specific muscles that produce ambulation. Once you know what muscles are important for gait, it becomes easier to establish corrective gait training and therapeutic exercises for gait deficiencies after a musculoskeletal injury.

An easy way to look at muscles for gait is to divide them into categories according to their function. These categories include shock absorbers, stabilizers, accelerators, and decelerators. Some categories overlap because, for example, shock absorption requires deceleration. It is helpful to further divide categories according to the various body segments the muscles influence. Refer to figure 12.16 for a summary of the muscle activity described in the following sections.

Shock Absorbers

During the first 15% of stance from initial contact to loading response, the quadriceps are working as shock absorbers to reduce impact forces. They do this by eccentrically flexing the knee. At initial contact the foot extensors, also working eccentrically as shock absorbers, prevent the foot from slapping down onto the ground. The quadriceps group decelerates knee flexion and controls the amount of knee flexion that occurs during the first 15% of the gait cycle. At the instant the heel makes contact with the floor, the foot dorsiflexors are at their peak output as they work to keep the forefoot off the floor; they then immediately act to control the lowering of the foot to the floor, functioning as a decelerator and shock absorber so that the movement is smooth.

Stabilizers

The hip extensors and torso muscles act as stabilizers to maintain the trunk in an erect position as the weight is transferred from one leg to the other, preventing excessive side tilting of the pelvis or trunk. The gluteus maximus stabilizes the spine to prevent a forward lean of the trunk during weight bearing and weight transfer from left to right; the gluteus medius, gluteus minimus, and tensor fascia lata stabilize the pelvis laterally on the femur; and the erector spinae muscles balance the head, arms, and trunk on the pelvis. These groups reach their peak levels of activity during the beginning and late stages of stance when weight is transferred from one leg to the other. The tensor fascia lata also works during initial swing phase to stabilize the pelvis and prevent a lateral tilt.

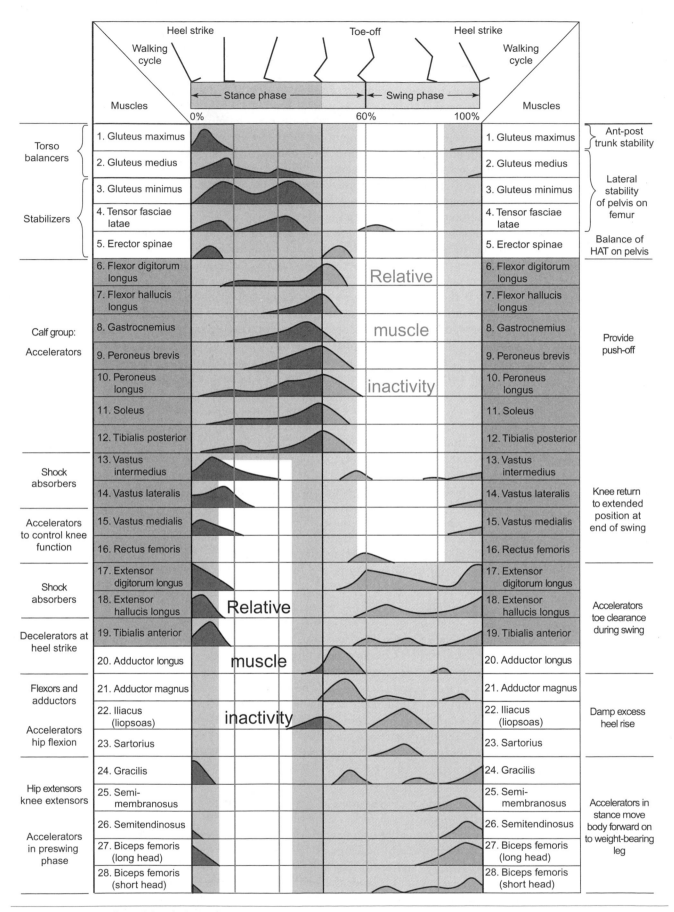

Figure 12.16 Muscle activity during gait.

*Peaks indicate periods of highest activity on each graph.

Adapted from J. Perry 1990

Accelerators

Accelerators in the leg and thigh have peak outputs at various times during gait. The posterior calf accelerators have their peak activity during the end of stance phase as they accelerate the leg forward, providing for a push-off to produce an accelerated passive momentum of the leg during swing phase. The posterior calf muscles begin activity during the middle portion of the weight-bearing phase as they provide control and balance during weight bearing. This is especially true of the lateral muscles, the ankle inverters and everters. Since the peroneals and tibialis posterior work through the majority of the weight bearing phase, it is easy to appreciate how tendinitis may develop if their workload is increased because of poor foot mechanics as seen in an excessive pronator.

During swing, the foot and toe dorsiflexors are working to lift the foot and toes to clear the floor and prepare the foot for the right position at heel strike.

The thigh accelerators work primarily in the early and middle stages of swing to increase hip flexion to clear the foot from the ground. They also adduct the thigh to keep it close to the support leg to reduce the energy requirements for holding the trunk erect during single-leg stance on the opposite leg.

Decelerators

During swing phase, the hamstrings work as decelerators of the knee to slow the swing of the lower leg so that initial contact occurs smoothly. The hamstrings also act as accelerators in the very early portion of stance phase to bring the body forward onto the weight-bearing leg.

Note that the shock-absorbing activity of the quadriceps group, mentioned earlier, is also categorized as a decelerating activity. Shock absorption is provided through the deceleration of the muscles. This is also true for the dorsiflexors during the early portion of stance phase.

Ground Reaction Forces

Ground reaction forces are the forces exerted between the body and the ground during ambulation. Since the foot hits the ground at an angle, there is a combination of vector forces. One is a shearing force that is parallel to the ground, and the other is a impact force that is perpendicular to the ground. Shear forces occur in fore-aft and lateral-medial directions. At initial contact the fore-aft shear force is a forward force, and during preswing it is a backward force. If you step on ice and lose your footing at initial contact, the forward force causes your leg to slip forward. The reverse is true if you lose your footing during preswing; your foot slips backward.

Shortening stride length reduces fore-aft shear forces but increases vertical forces (figure 12.17). This is why it is safer to walk on ice with a shortened stride length: There is less forward force to slip the foot forward at initial contact and less backward force to slip the foot backward during preswing.

Fore-aft, or anteroposterior, forces are indicative of the deceleration forces that slow the body during initial contact and the acceleration forces that speed up the body before preswing. The medial-lateral shear force is predominantly a medial shear force through initial contact; it moves to a lateral shear force as weight is transferred to the front of the foot. The medial-lateral shear forces are indicative of how the body weight is being transferred from side to side.

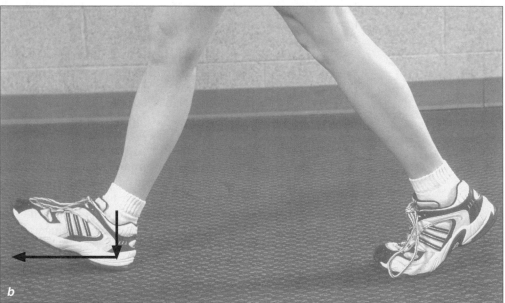

Figure 12.17 Shortened stride reduces fore-aft shear force. *(a)* Shortened stride produces a greater perpendicular force vector than fore-aft force vector. *(b)* A longer stride produces a greater fore-aft force vector than perpendicular force vector.

Vertical forces applied to the foot during weight bearing are the effects of the body's weight. The amount of vertical force varies through the gait cycle and reflects shock absorption and deceleration during heel strike and acceleration as the body prepares to push off and move into the swing phase. The greatest vertical force occurs during push-off as the body is accelerating to propel itself forward and off the ground. Vertical forces are at minimal levels when the body weight is shared with the other lower extremity during double-limb support (figure 12.18).

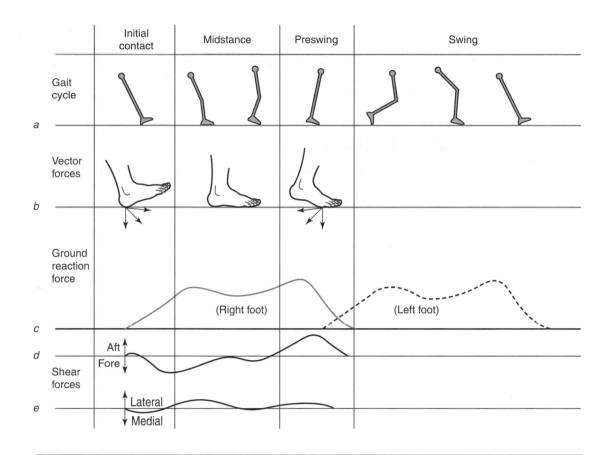

Figure 12.18 Ground reaction forces in walking.

Adapted from D.E. Klopsteg and P.D. Wilson 1954.

Awareness of ground reaction forces is important in examination of gait and musculoskeletal injury. Some of the greatest forces applied to the foot occur during acceleration. This can be crucial information when you are treating a patient who is a runner or a jumper or who participates in any activity in which ground reaction forces impact performance. For example, a pitcher who is experiencing first metatarsophalangeal joint pain will have difficulty during ball release and will require treatment of the toe, since ground reaction forces applied to the painful joint significantly impact the follow-through.

PATHOLOGICAL GAIT

▶ Pathological gait is a reflection of injury, weakness, loss of flexibility, pain, or bad habits. As with normal gait, observation of pathological gait begins with an overview assessment and proceeds with segmental assessment.

When a segment does not move as it should during ambulation because of injury, weakness, loss of flexibility, pain, or bad habit, a pathological gait results. The body attempts to continue to ambulate, but it must make adjustments to accommodate for the loss of normal function. This places stress on other segments and promotes weakness, and if the situation continues it can cause additional injury. Here we consider a few typical pathological gaits that result from musculoskeletal injuries.

When examining gait, you should have the patient walk while you observe the entire body's movements. First, gain an overview and note any obvious abnormalities that would indicate the need for a more detailed examination of any area. Part of the overview examination includes observation of stride length, stride width, cadence, trunk lean, and arm swing. The arms normally swing in time with the opposite lower extremity. An unequal arm swing may indicate either a leg-length discrepancy or tissue shortening on one side. After this, the observation proceeds either from proximal segments down or from distal segments up, looking at one joint or region at a time. Head position, shoulder position, shoulder movement relative to pelvis movement, knee alignment, and foot and heel positions during stance are examined from anterior and posterior views. Side-view examination includes observations of knee position at heel strike, midstance, and heel-off; head, trunk, and hip alignment; swing-through motion of the lower extremity; arm swing; pelvis motion; and timing of heel strike, heel-off, and toe-off. You should examine any observed segmental deviation for possible causes. Following are some common gait deviations seen in musculoskeletal injuries.

Gluteus Medius Gait

If an individual sustains an injury that necessitates prolonged non-weight bearing on an extremity, or if he or she directly injures the hip, the gluteus medius can become weak. Once the patient resumes full weight bearing, the gluteus medius is too weak to maintain a level pelvis during single-leg stance. What is typically seen is a drop of the pelvis on the uninvolved side. This drop occurs from initial contact on the involved side through to initial contact on the uninvolved side. This is referred to as a Trendelenburg, or gluteus medius, gait.

When the gluteus medius is weak, the pelvis drops on the opposite, non-weight-bearing side because the pelvis does not have the muscular support it needs to remain level. To compensate for this, a patient may move the trunk laterally over the weak hip. This forces the erector spinae and quadratus lumborum of the opposite side to contract and lift the pelvis and reduces strength required of the gluteus medius by reducing the body weight's lever arm length.

Quadriceps Gait

Surgery or severe injury to the knee or quadriceps can leave the quadriceps very weak and unable to function properly during ambulation. Even after strengthening the quadriceps, the patient can continue to ambulate with a pathological gait because of bad habits established during ambulation when the muscle was too weak to be used properly. With a quadriceps gait, the patient keeps the knee extended at heel strike and through the stance phase. If the quadriceps is very weak, a lurch immediately after heel strike can occur as the individual forces the femur backward and the trunk forward to passively lock the knee. The hip extensors then stabilize the knee to keep it locked after heel strike.

Ankle Tightness

If an individual sustains an ankle sprain and subsequently suffers a reduced range of motion in dorsiflexion, a pathological gait develops. During midstance when the ankle should move suddenly from plantar flexion to dorsiflexion, the person lurches forward over the foot, experiences increased knee extension, and moves quickly toward heel-off in an attempt to shorten the time requirement for dorsiflexion. There will be a rapid movement from initial contact to loading response if the ankle does not have dorsiflexion to 0°, and the patient may either hike the involved hip upward or increase knee and hip flexion in an attempt to clear the toes from the floor during the swing phase.

Painful Knee

When an individual incurs an injury and ambulates with pain, you can observe a typical, obvious pathological gait. The patient attempts to reduce the time spent on the painful extremity to minimize the stresses placed on it during gait. The stride is shortened and asymmetrical; initial contact is replaced by direct movement to loading response or initial contact by the distal foot to minimize impact stress; knee flexion during midstance is usually exaggerated if the knee has increased edema; and the knee motion is minimized during the swing phase. To compensate for the lack of motion during the swing phase the patient either hikes the hip up, goes up on the toes of the uninvolved leg during midstance, or uses a circumduction swing, all in an attempt to clear the foot from the floor.

NORMAL RUNNING GAIT

▶ Running gait differs from walking gait in several major ways—stride length and rate, joint motions, ground reaction forces, and kinetics.

Running and walking differ, just as running differs at different speeds. Running differs from walking in that the stance phase is shortened, the swing phase is lengthened, there is no time of double support, and there is a nonsupport phase in which neither leg is weight bearing. The nonsupport phase in running, also referred to as the double float phase, occurs during the early-initial swing phase of one leg and the end of terminal swing for the other leg (figure 12.19). Since gait characteristics also change with a change in running speed, categories of running must be defined.

A variety of factors affect running mechanics, including speed, age, somatotype, fatigue, surface, footwear, and skill level. Researchers who compare running speeds vary considerably in their categorizations. In one study, for example, slow runners are defined as those who run 4 m/s (4.4 yd/s), or are able to run a mile in 6:42 (6 min, 42 s). A fast runner is defined as one who runs 8 m/s (8.7 yd/s) or 91 m (100 yd) in 11.4 s. A sprinter is able to run 10 m/s or 100 yd in 9.1 s (Dillman 1975). In another study, a runner is defined as someone moving at 19.3 kph (12 mph; slightly less than a 5-min mile), and a sprinter is one who is able to run 27.6 kph (17.1 mph; 109 m in 12.2 s) (Mann and Hagy 1980). Whereas the average walking speed is approximately 1.4 m/s (1.5 yd/s), ranges in running speeds vary from 2 to 5.5 times the speed of walking (Perry 1990). These variations make analysis and comparison of results difficult at best.

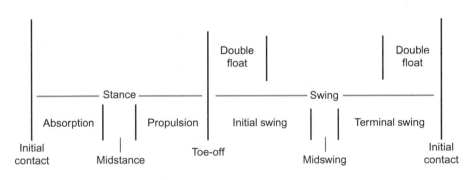

Figure 12.19 Model of one running stride: Double float is unique to running and occurs when there is nonsupport of either extremity.

Adapted by permission from Ounpuu 1994.

Figure 12.20 Stride length and running speed.

Adapted by permission from K.R. Williams 1985.

In most instances, terminology used for walking is the same as for running. A few additional terms are used for running, however. A running stride is from toe-off of one foot to toe-off of the opposite foot, and one running cycle includes two running strides. Because runners do not always impact the ground at the heel, initial contact is called foot strike rather than heel strike. Cycle time, or stride time, is the amount of time it takes to perform one step length. Stride rate is the inverse of stride time. As mentioned previously, the nonsupport phase is the time when there is no weight bearing. The stance phase is sometimes referred to as the support phase for consistency with the term "nonsupport phase."

Stride Length and Stride Rate

Although researchers differ in their definitions of running speeds, the information available on running yields several basic observations. Stride length and cadence increase with an increase in velocity. Cycle time decreases with an increase in speed. After about 7 m/s (7.6 yd/s), stride length does not increase remarkably, but stride rate does (figure 12.20).

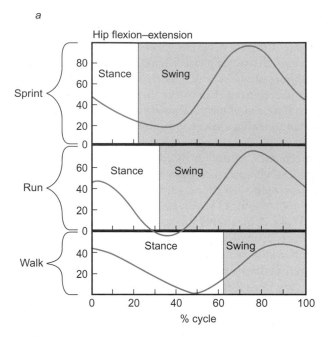

Joint Motions

Generally, as speed increases, the body tends to move its center of gravity lower by increasing the degree of hip flexion, knee flexion, and ankle dorsiflexion during the early stages of the stance phase.

The hip increases its flexion during midswing with increases in speed, but hip position changes little with speed variations during weight bearing except in sprinting when the hip never reaches full extension. Overall, hip motion increases as speed increases (figure 12.21).

The knee motion changes with changes in speed. There are greater degrees of knee flexion and there is less extension with greater speeds. During sprinting, the knee does not extend; it continues through the gait cycle in varying degrees of flexion. Some evidence indicates that at higher speeds the trend is toward extension at toe-off, although full extension is not achieved (Williams 1985). During the swing phase, knee flexion has been recorded at more than 120°

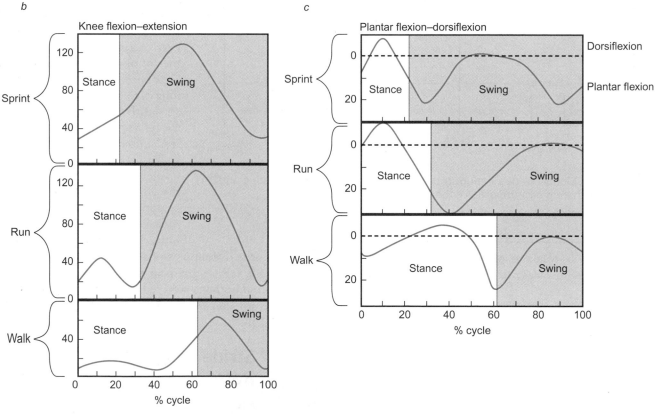

Figure 12.21   Range of motion during running. As locomotion speed increases, the swing phase (nonsupport phase) time increases and joint range of motion changes.

Adapted by permission from Mann and Hagy 1980.

(Williams 1985). Increased knee flexion provides for additional shock absorption, but it also requires greater quadriceps output. This topic is discussed later in the section "Kinetics."

Ankle plantar flexion at toe-off has been recorded in ranges between 59° and 75° (Williams 1985). Which part of the foot makes initial contact with the ground depends on the angles of the hip, knee, and ankle. Runners most often land on the midfoot. As a general rule, faster runners tend to land at the midfoot, and slower runners land at the rearfoot (Williams 1985).

Although an erect trunk is thought to be the best position for running form, most reports indicate that runners use a forward trunk lean throughout the running cycle (Williams 1985). The amount of trunk lean increases from 4° to 7° in runners at speeds up to 7 m/s (7.7 yd/s) and to 11.6° in sprinters running at 9.2 m/s (10.06 yd/s).

Ground Reaction Forces

As speeds increase, ground reaction forces also increase. In running and walking, ground reaction forces reach two peaks. The first is at impact during initial contact. This peak, which occurs very quickly with running impact, is referred to as the impact peak. The second peak occurs during the last half of support and is referred to as an action peak because of muscles influences on it during acceleration prior to toe-off (figure 12.22).

Vertical impact forces encountered during running are mathematically combined with joint positions to determine joint moments. Joint moments are the stresses applied to the joints. During running, the knee encounters flexor moments 7.7 times greater than those encountered during walking. The hip and ankle flexion demands during running are double those during walking (Perry 1990).

Body weight, surfaces, shoes, speed, and where on the foot the runner lands all influence the impact peak forces. Softer surfaces can eliminate the impact peak. A good running shoe has a lower impact peak than a poorly constructed shoe. Runners who land on the midfoot or forefoot have a significantly reduced impact peak compared to those landing on the rearfoot; and runners landing on the rearfoot have a single peak whereas runners landing on the midfoot have a biphasic peak impact. Faster runners have greater ground reaction forces than slower runners.

 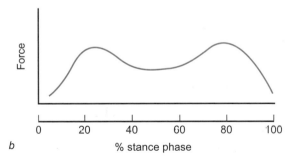

Figure 12.22 Ground reaction forces in (a) running and (b) walking. The impact ground reaction force in running occurs very quickly. (a) Running, (b) walking.

Adapted by permission from Ounpuu 1994.

Kinetics

Specific activity varies greatly, depending on running speeds and on the investigation, but a general conclusion is that muscle activity increases with increased running speeds, as seen in figure 12.23.

Hip

There is an increase in hamstring activity from heel strike and throughout stance as the hamstring assists concentrically in hip extension. The semimembranosus is at a particular advantage to provide hip extensor force since it is 1.4 times larger than the biceps femoris (Perry 1990). The hamstrings also play a concentric and stabilizing role during trunk lean. The rectus femoris is more active at foot strike, but this activity diminishes by the end of support. The rectus femoris is also active during hip flexion in the early swing phase. The hamstrings and hip extensors in the late-swing leg act eccentrically to slow hip flexion and prepare the leg for the support phase.

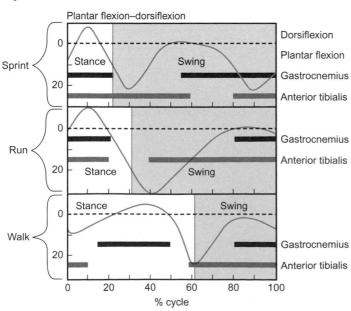

Figure 12.23   Muscle activity with range of motion during walk, run, and sprint.

Adapted by permission from Mann and Hagy 1980.

Knee

The quadriceps, especially the vastus lateralis and vastus medialis, are extremely active at foot strike; they continue to be active along with the rectus femoris during the early portion of support. High demands are placed on the quadriceps muscles during most of the stance phase. Their activity diminishes as the leg continues to the end of support, but increases again just prior to foot strike in preparation for its impact-loading response. As running speeds increase, the amount of time the quadriceps are active in both the stance and swing phases increases.

The hamstrings begin their aggressive activity in the last half of swing phase to prepare the knee to land in the stance phase. The hamstrings continue their activity halfway through stance and may be an active restraint against anterior tibial shear. During the last half of stance, the hamstrings and quadriceps are in co-contraction, presumably for additional knee support.

Ankle

At foot strike the tibialis anterior and triceps surae group co-contract to stabilize the foot at impact. The contraction of the posterior muscle group through most of the stance phase may provide tibial stability for improved quadriceps function. If the runner's foot strike occurs at the heel, the tibialis anterior immediately eccentrically contracts to control foot pronation. The triceps surae concentrically contracts to provide thrust for propulsion of the body into the nonsupport phase. This is especially true for faster speeds (Williams 1985).

MECHANICS OF AMBULATION WITH ASSISTIVE DEVICES

▶ The rehabilitation clinician should understand several issues regarding the use of assistive devices for ambulation. These include proper fitting, correct gait patterns, proper use on various types of surfaces, and safety instructions and precautions.

Now that you have an understanding of normal gait mechanics, you will more easily appreciate the intricacies of ambulation with assistive devices. Assistive devices are used either to provide additional stability during ambulation or to reduce or eliminate weight bearing on a lower extremity. They can permit the patient to walk safely and unassisted by others. As a general rule, assistive devices are used during weight bearing if the patient is unable to walk normally. The purpose is to prevent the added stresses of abnormal gait from causing additional injury.

Fitting

Before a patient can use any assistive device, the device must be properly fitted to the individual's height. Axillary, or underarm, crutches are measured with the crutch tips flat on the ground and approximately 15 cm (6 in.) lateral to and 15 cm in front of the foot (figure 12.24). There should be a two- to three-finger space between the top of the axillary pad and the patient's axilla. The handgrip should be at a level such that there is a 20° to 30° bend in the elbow with the crutch at the correct length as the patient stands with the crutches 15 cm laterally and 15 cm anterior to the feet.

Forearm crutches are adjusted so that the handgrip is at the level of the greater trochanter and the forearm cuff is just distal to the elbow. This should provide for about a 30° elbow bend during weight bearing. Cane measurements are made with the arm in a relaxed resting position at the side and the cane next to the leg. The top of the cane handle should be at wrist level.

Gait Patterns

A basic concept in the use of assistive devices is to keep the center of balance within the base of support. A person is more stable when using assistive devices because the base of support is increased (figure 12.25). Gait patterns are generally designated according to the number of support points in contact with the floor. These contacts include the assistive devices and the feet.

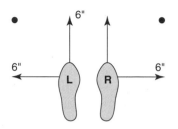

Figure 12.24 With the crutches 15 cm (6 in.) lateral and anterior to the feet, and the shoulders relaxed, proper crutch height should allow two to three fingers between the axilla and axillary pad. Elbows should be flexed 20° to 30°.

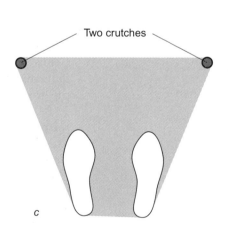

Figure 12.25 Base of support with *(a)* no assistive devices, *(b)* one cane or crutch, *(c)* two crutches. The base of support area is increased when assistive devices are used. As long as the patient's center of gravity falls within the base of support, the patient is stable.

Three-Point Gait

A three-point gait is so termed because there are three points of contact with the floor—two made by the assistive device and one made by a foot. This gait is used when the patient is unable to bear weight on one extremity. It is also called a right (or left) non-weight-bearing gait. For young, healthy individuals who have been injured, underarm crutches are the most frequently used assistive devices. Forearm crutches or a walker can also be used in a three-point gait.

In a three-point gait, while remaining non-weight bearing (NWB) on one leg, the patient advances the crutches simultaneously in front of the body along with the non-weight-bearing leg; he or she then bears weight on the crutch handles and lifts the weight-bearing leg by pushing down on the crutch grips to move it either to or in front of the crutches (figure 12.26).

A gait in which the individual swings the weight-bearing leg to the crutches is called a swing-to gait. If the weight-bearing leg is advanced far enough to land in front of the crutches, the gait is a swing-through gait. The swing-through gait is more difficult and requires more self-confidence than the swing-to gait does. A patient who is hesitant about using the crutches uses a swing-to gait initially; as the individual gains confidence and it is safe to do so, he or she advances to a swing-through gait. The swing-through gait is faster than the swing-to gait, but requires

Swing-to

Swing-through

Figure 12.26 In a three-point gait, the patient places the crutches in front of the body *(a)* and advances the weight-bearing leg either to the crutches *(b)* or in front of the crutches *(c)*. Weight is borne entirely by the hands during the swing-to or swing-through phase of this gait.

Figure 12.27 A four-point gait is used when partial weight bearing is permitted. The crutches are used with the involved extremity with partial weight on the crutches and partial weight on the lower extremity.

Key
1 = Lever-arm length of body weight
2 = Lever-arm length of cane support

Figure 12.28 Ambulation with single support allows reduced force application to the involved lower extremity.

more balance and control.

Four-Point Gait

A four-point gait is used when partial weight bearing (PWB) is allowed on the involved extremity. The injured leg continues to move with the crutches, but some body weight is placed on the injured extremity. The amount of weight permitted is dictated by the patient's pain or the physician's prescription. In this gait, the crutches and involved leg advance simultaneously. Partial body weight is placed on the extremity, and the remaining weight is placed on the hands (figure 12.27). The uninvolved leg is then advanced forward in a normal stride, passing the opposite leg as it swings through.

A modification of the four-point gait may be seen in individuals who use crutches for assistance with bilateral lower-extremity involvement. This involves using one crutch with each lower extremity. The most stable method, although the slowest, is advancing the left crutch with the right leg and the right crutch with the left leg. This type of four-point gait is not common in the younger population when only one extremity is involved.

Single Support

When a single device, either a cane or a crutch, is used, it is placed in the hand on the side opposite to the leg injury. Single devices are used primarily for stability, not weight-bearing support, because only about 25% of the body's weight can be borne on a cane or on one crutch (Lehmann 1990).

Single support is essentially a second-class lever system. It is designed to be efficient so minimal force from the upper extremity is required to produce the desired effect of support for the involved leg. The injured lower extremity's hip is the fulcrum from which the cane or crutch leverage is applied. The head, arms, and trunk (HAT) are the resistance force that is positioned between the fulcrum and the cane or crutch (figure 12.28). If the cane or crutch were placed in the hand on the same side as the injured leg, it would provide no assistance for weight distribution, and the patient would have to lurch over the outside of the involved leg to place the HAT weight between the cane and the injured leg.

In a single-support gait, the cane or crutch moves with the injured leg so the two advance together. As the patient bears weight on the injured leg and swings the uninvolved leg forward, some weight is also applied to the single-support device. This gait is used when minimal support for balance is required or when the patient is able to bear weight on the extremity but displays an abnormal gait because of pain, loss of motion, or weakness.

Assistive Devices on Various Surfaces

The patient will be ambulating with assistive devices on varying surfaces such as stairs and ramps, so he or she needs to receive instruction before being allowed to use the assistive devices without supervision. Risk of injury and falling is significant until the patient is safe on all surfaces.

Stairs

When maneuvering stairs with a railing, the patient should use the handrail. A railing is more secure than crutches and will provide more safety going up and down stairs. If the person is using two crutches, both are placed in the same hand, the one away from the railing. If the stairs have a handrail on each side, it is easiest if the patient is positioned to place the hand of the uninvolved side on the railing when going up or down the stairs.

Stair climbing involves two basic concepts. One is that the uninvolved leg advances up the stairs first and the involved leg advances down the stairs first. This can be confusing, so you can use a simple reminder. "The good go up to heaven and the bad go down to hell," is a reminder that most patients find easy to recall.

The second concept is that the assistive device always goes with the involved leg. In other words, the crutches go on the same step as the injured extremity. For example, when descending stairs, the patient grasps the railing with one hand and holds both crutches in the opposite hand (figure 12.29a). The crutches advance down a step (figure 12.29b); then the involved extremity is lowered to the same step (figure 12.29c). The patient bears weight on the arms and involved leg, if weight bearing is permitted, and then lowers the uninvolved leg to the same step. For ascending steps the process is the reverse; the uninvolved leg is advanced first (figure 12.29d), and then the crutches and involved leg are raised to the same step.

Figure 12.29 How to ambulate on stairs with crutches: *(a)* Use the rail if one is present and place both crutches in one hand. *(b)* Advance the crutches to the lower step and move the rail hand to keep the hands even. *(c)* Lower the body to the step, bearing weight on the hands as the involved leg is lowered before the uninvolved leg. *(d)* When going up stairs, the uninvolved leg leads, and the crutches remain on the lower step with the involved leg until the uninvolved leg is secure on the higher step.

If the stairs do not have a railing, the patient must use the crutches in both hands in lieu of a railing. This is less safe and requires more concentration, especially in the first few attempts; but navigation is feasible according to the same concepts as with a railing. Curbs are essentially stairs without railings and are managed the same way.

Ramps

Ramps may have varying degrees of incline, but the principle for ambulating on them with assistive devices is the same in any case. The most important concept on ramps is that, as with stairs, the crutches and involved leg are kept together. The other important additional concept is that the individual must take shorter steps going up and down for safety. The tendency is to take larger steps going down a ramp, but this can be dangerous and lead to falls. The patient should also remember to maintain an upright posture going down ramps since the natural pattern is to lean forward. This can lead to falling, but a reminder to take shorter steps can reduce this risk.

Transfers

Getting up and down from a chair when a patient is using assistive devices can be treacherous. Using the correct technique will ensure greater safety. If using crutches, the individual places both crutches in one hand, holding the handgrips with the hand, and places the crutches in a vertical position near the chair but in front of it and to its side. The other hand is placed on the arm of the chair or on the seat if there are no chair arms. The patient pushes from the crutch handgrips and chair simultaneously to gain assistance in standing. He or she then places a crutch under each arm before proceeding. This technique is used with two crutches, one crutch, or a cane. The steps are reversed to move from standing to sitting.

Safety Instructions and Precautions

Walking with assistive devices can be energy consuming and poses a risk of falling, especially if the activity is performed incorrectly or with faulty equipment. Precautions should be taken at the outset to minimize these factors.

Equipment

Crutch tips, handgrips, and axillary pads should be inspected to make sure that they are not excessively worn or damaged. Lack of tread on a crutch or cane tip can cause the assistive device to slip when weight is applied to it. Cracked or damaged handgrips and axillary pads can cause the pads to become loosened during use and put the patient at risk of falling.

If the crutches are adjusted with screws, the screws should be secured and in working order. Wing nuts should be firmly in place.

Environmental Factors

Throw rugs are among the environmental factors that pose a risk to people using assistive devices. The patient must take care not to trip when walking on rugs of this type. Removing them until the person is able to ambulate without the assistive device may be the safest thing to do.

Extra caution must be taken in rain, ice, or snow. A slippery surface increases the patient's risk for falling. Instructions to ambulate more slowly and use smaller steps should be given. If the crutches are advanced too far forward, the fore-aft shear force, discussed earlier, has a greater forward than downward component, causing the crutch to slip forward and putting the person at risk for falling.

To avoid someone accidentally tripping over or kicking the assistive device, the patient should keep the crutches or cane to his or her side rather than in front, but not so far out as to present an obstacle for another person. An exaggerated outward position also places too much pressure on the patient's sides if axillary crutches are being used. The devices should be advanced far enough forward to provide for an economical gait but not so far as to endanger the patient's balance and increase the risk of falling.

Axillary Crutches

The patient should be instructed in proper use of axillary crutches. The purpose of the axillary pad is not to allow the patient to rest the axilla but rather to serve as a cushion against the lateral chest wall so that the crutch does not slip out from under the arm. Resting the axillae on these pads poses a risk of radial nerve damage from pressure on the nerve as it runs through the axillae. The patient's weight should be borne through the hands, not the axillae.

SUMMARY

1. Discuss the general concepts of gait.

    The gait cycle is divided into two phases, stance and swing. The stance phase is divided into initial contact, or heel strike; loading response or foot flat; midstance; heel-off, or terminal stance; and preswing, or toe-off. The swing phase is divided into initial, or early swing; midswing; and terminal swing. In normal walking, the stance phase constitutes about 60% of the gait cycle. Double support occurs during loading response and preswing.

2. Identify the range-of-motion changes during the gait cycle.

    At initial contact, the hip is at 30° flexion, the knee is at full extension, and the ankle is in neutral. By midstance the hip is extending, the knee has moved from 15° flexion toward extension, and the ankle has moved from 15° plantar flexion to 10° dorsiflexion. At toe-off the hip has moved from 10° extension to neutral, the knee is in 35° flexion, and the ankle is in 20° plantar flexion. During swing, the hip moves from 20° to 30° flexion, the knee moves into 60° flexion and progresses to full extension, and the ankle remains in neutral.

3. Explain the muscle activity involved in ambulation.

    Muscles are divided into groups: shock absorbers, accelerators, decelerators, and stabilizers. Muscles act in cyclic fashion, with the greatest activity occurring during early and late stance and early and late swing as muscles prepare to change activity.

4. Describe the general mechanical differences between walking and running.

    In running there is a double-float portion in the gait cycle during which the body is not supported by either lower extremity. The stance phase is divided into initial contact, midstance, and toe-off. The swing phase becomes longer than the stance phase, the stride length increases in a curvilinear fashion in relation to running speed, and ranges of motion for all joints increase with increased running speeds.

5. Discuss one abnormal gait commonly seen following a musculoskeletal injury.

    Prolonged knee extension is an example of a common gait following knee injury and subsequent quadriceps weakness. It occurs because the quadriceps lack control of the knee, and keeping the knee locked prevents the knee from buckling during weight bearing.

6. Outline the various types of gait with assistive devices.

    A three-point gait is used with two crutches when weight bearing on the involved extremity is prohibited. A swing-to or swing-through gait can be used with a three-point gait. A four-point gait is used when partial weight bearing on the involved extremity is permitted. The involved extremity is placed between two crutches; some weight is borne by the crutches and some by the extremity. When a cane or single crutch is used, it is placed in the hand opposite the involved extremity, and weight is simultaneously borne by the involved extremity and the cane.

7. Explain the technique involved in stair climbing with assistive devices.

When going up stairs, the patient places the uninvolved extremity on the upper stair, places weight on the crutches or the crutches and handrail, and hops up. Going down stairs, the individual places the involved extremity and crutches on the lower stair before lowering the uninvolved leg.

8. Identify the safety measures involved in ambulating with assistive devices.

The assistive device should be adjusted for proper fit; crutch tips, pads, and grips should be inspected for wear before use. Proper instruction in the use of assistive devices on various surfaces and in proper transfer techniques should be provided before the patient is permitted independent use. Instructions should cover use on slippery surfaces, avoiding axillary pressure with crutches, and proper weight bearing on the involved extremity. Scatter rugs should be removed from the patient's environment, and the person should receive instruction about keeping the assistive device close to the body to avoid tripping or falling.

CRITICAL THINKING QUESTIONS

1. If the patient you are treating has limited range of motion in dorsiflexion and plantar flexion, what kind of gait deviation would you expect to see? How would it alter the timing of the knee and ankle motions? Would the patient have normal knee motion during weight bearing? If not, why not? What possible substitutions might the patient use to compensate for the loss of ankle motion?

2. If a patient has weak quads, there will be full knee extension during midstance. Why will this occur? What must be done before normal knee flexion during midstance occurs?

3. If hip flexors are tight, what changes in gait will occur? What changes in pelvic rotation can occur? Will tight hip flexors cause an apparent short-leg syndrome? Why?

4. If the hip abductors are weak, what type of abnormal gait would you expect to see? Identify what can be used to correct this type of gait, and explain the mechanics of how the correction works.

5. You are developing a handout for instructions on gait with crutches. Assuming that the instructions will be for conditions that are non-weight bearing on one extremity, what instructions will you include? What precautions will you include? What surfaces will you deal with in your instructions?

6. Based on the chapter's opening scenario, what instructions should Tony give Mary Ann for ambulation with a cane? What precautions should he also include? What criteria should he use to determine when Mary Ann can begin running?

LAB ACTIVITIES

1. In groups made up of three or four students, evaluate each person's gait. Evaluate gait from anterior, lateral, and posterior views. Identify any gait deviations for each person. List the deficiencies that are causing the gait deviations and identify corrective exercises for each one.

2. In your same group, go to the campus mall or student union and watch people walking. How many gait deviations can you identify? Is there a common one or are there many various gait abnormalities? Can you identify the source of the gait deviation?

3. Measure your lab partner for axillary crutches. Measure your partner for a cane. Instruct him or her in a gait with the crutches with NWB on one leg. Instruct him or her in a gait using PWB on one leg. Practice rising from and lowering to a chair, ambulation on a flat surface, up and down ramps, and up and down stairs.

4. Using a three-point gait, walk around campus with crutches. What were the most difficult aspects of walking around campus with crutches? What surprised you the most? How did you find people around you responding to your crutches? What precautions did you take or fears did you find yourself feeling?

REFERENCES

Chambers, H.G. and D.H. Sutherland. 2002. A practical guide to gait analysis. *Journal of the American Academy of Orthopaedic Surgeons.* 10:222-273.

Dillman, C.J. 1975. Kinematic analyses of running. *Exercise & Sport Sciences Reviews.* 3:193-218.

Klopsteg, D.E. and P.D. Wilson. 1954. *Human limbs and their substitutes.* New York: McGraw-Hill.

Lehmann, J.F. and B.J. DeLateur. 1990. Gait analysis: Diagnosis and management. In *Krusen's handbook of physical medicine and rehabilitation,* ed. F.J. Kottke and J.F. Lehmann. Philadelphia: Saunders.

Mann, R.A., and J. Hagy. 1980. Biomechanics of walking, running, and sprinting. *American Journal of Sports Medicine* 8:345–350.

Murray, M.P., Drought, A.B., and R.C. Kory. 1964. Walking patterns of normal men. *Journal of Bone and Joint Surgery* 46-A:335–360.

Ounpuu, S. 1994. The biomechanics of walking and running. *Clinics in Sports Medicine* 13:843–863.

Perry, J. 1990. Gait analysis in sports medicine. *Instructional Course Lectures* 39:319–324.

Rodgers, M.M. 1988. Dynamic biomechanics of the normal foot and ankle during walking and running. *Physical Therapy* 68:1822–1830.

Saunders, J.B.deC.M., Inman, V.T., and H.D. Eberhart. 1953. The major determinants in normal and pathological gait. *Journal of Bone and Joint Surgery.* 35-A:543-558.

Williams, K.R. 1985. The biomechanics of running. *Exercise & Sport Sciences Reviews.* 13:389–441.

Winter, D.A. 1987. *The biomechanics and motor control of human gait.* Waterloo, ON, Canada: University of Waterloo.

CHAPTER 13

Aquatic Therapeutic Exercise

Objectives

After completing this chapter, you should be able to do the following:

1. Identify and discuss the physical properties of water that affect the ability to exercise in water.

2. Define and explain the difference between assistive and resistive aquatic equipment and give examples of each.

3. List precautions and contraindications for aquatic exercise.

4. Identify three advantages of aquatic therapeutic exercise.

5. List three aquatic exercises for each body segment and identify their purposes.

Before Misty Dawn became a certified athletic trainer she had been a swimming instructor at the local beaches during the summer. She was well aware of the physical properties of water and of ways it can be used to either assist a body in water or resist it. In her current job as aquatic rehabilitation clinician at the city's largest sports medicine facility, she felt her position was a perfect match for her since it combined her sports medicine knowledge with her love for the water.

Misty's patients had various kinds of injuries and were at different levels within their rehabilitation programs. Misty enjoyed this situation because it allowed her to make use of the various pieces of exercise equipment and the various water properties. With some patients she used the water to eliminate weight bearing for ease of lower-extremity activities. With others she used the water to resist movement in strengthening activities. Still other people were in the water to stress their cardiovascular systems. Some weight-bearing patients were in shallow water so that they would encounter greater weight-bearing forces, while others were in the deeper end for activities that were less weight bearing. Some patients could use water dumbbells for resistance activities, whereas others were challenged simply by the water's drag and viscosity. Several of the patients were just beginning their rehabilitation work and using the water to gain motion, while others were in the final phases, letting the water provide them with an aggressive exercise program.

■ Common sense is genius dressed in its working clothes.

Albert Einstein, physicist, 1879-1955

Common sense in the application of knowledge is what makes a skillful clinician. It also is a key to good judgment. Decisions about what therapeutic exercises to apply, when to use them, and how best to deliver them are based on a healthy mixture of knowledge and common sense.

This chapter includes information that you will apply in a systematic manner on the basis of your newly gained knowledge of exercise and your common sense. General concepts and principles of aquatic exercise are introduced first. On this foundation, examples of exercises for the trunk, lower extremities, and upper extremities are then presented.

Water-based treatment has been in existence for a long time. The ancient Greeks and Romans used water therapeutically. The development of whirlpools and Hubbard tanks promoted the use of water in the early 1900s. Recently there has been a resurgence of interest in aquatic therapy, emphasizing its use in exercise rather than its more traditional effects. This chapter addresses the therapeutic exercise use of aquatic therapy rather than its use as a thermal modality.

For additional information on aquatic modalities, refer to *Therapeutic Modalities for Musculoskeletal Injuries, Second Edition* by Craig Denegar, Ethan Saliba, and Susan Saliba (2005).

Aquatic therapeutic exercise is the application of therapeutic exercise that takes place in water. Exercise in water is advantageous when the patient is unable to perform land-based exercises, allowing the individual to begin exercises sooner than would otherwise be possible. It also provides a means of exercise while the patient is non-weight bearing on an injured lower extremity. Aquatic therapeutic exercise (aquatic therex) can offer the patient a total exercise program that includes activities for cardiovascular conditioning, flexibility, strength, and muscle endurance. It can be instituted early in a rehabilitation program and can continue past the time when the patient is able to perform land-based exercises.

PHYSICAL PROPERTIES AND PRINCIPLES OF WATER

▶ Several major physical properties of water, including specific gravity, buoyancy, center of buoyancy, and hydrodynamics, affect the way people exercise in water.

An understanding of how water affects the body's ability to move and exercise is necessary before one can apply water exercises. Although some of these properties can be specifically determined by formulas, we will not focus on the precise mathematical applications here. It is important only to appreciate that one can acquire an understanding of the impact of these properties on the body exercising in water by gaining a thorough knowledge of these mathematical formulas.

Specific Gravity

Specific gravity is also called **relative density**. It refers to the density of an object relative to that of water. It is, then, a ratio of an object's weight to the weight of an equal volume of water. The specific gravity of water is 1. If an object has a specific gravity greater than 1, it will sink in water since its relative weight per volume is more than that of water. If an object has a specific gravity of less than 1, it will float in water. If the object's specific gravity is 1, it will float just below the water's surface.

Specific gravity for the human body varies from one individual to another and from one body segment to another within the same individual. The individual's specific gravity depends on the body's composition of lean and fat mass and the distribution of body fat. The specific gravity of fat is 0.8, bone is 1.5 to 2.0, and lean muscle is 1.0 (Hay 1993). The average range of specific gravity for the human body is 0.95 to 0.97 (Davis and Harrison 1988). Since the specific gravity of the average human body is less than 1, people will most often float. Women usually have more body fat than men, so women float better than men. A lean, muscular person may have a specific gravity of 1.10; an obese individual may have a specific gravity of 0.93 (Edlich et al. 1987). These wide variations in individual specific gravities lead to a wide range of abilities to float. Patients who are more muscular and have less fat mass may have a difficult time floating and may require flotation devices during aquatic therex.

Buoyancy

Archimedes' principle of buoyancy states that a body partially or fully immersed in a fluid will experience an upward thrust of that fluid that is equal to the weight of the fluid the body displaces. Buoyancy and specific gravity are closely related in that a body with a specific gravity of less than 1 will float because the weight of the water it displaces is less than the weight of the full body. For example, if a person has a specific gravity of 0.95, 95% of the body will be submerged and 5% of the body will float above the water's surface. The amount of water displaced is 95% of the body weight. Specific-gravity values, in essence, indicate the amount of the body that floats and the amount that is submerged; and the weight of the body or part of the body submerged is equal to the weight of the water it displaces.

Center of Buoyancy

Center of buoyancy is the center of gravity of the displaced fluid and the point at which the buoyant force acts on the body. In water, two opposing forces act on the body. Buoyancy is the upward force, and gravity is the downward force. Each has a center point of balance. When a floating body is in equilibrium, the center of buoyancy and the center of gravity are in vertical alignment with each other (figure 13.1). In this position, the body is balanced. If the center of buoyancy and the center of gravity are

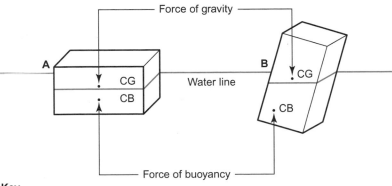

Key
CG = Center of gravity
CB = Center of buoyancy
 A = Body in equilibrium with CB and CG in vertical alignment
 B = Body out of equilibrium with CB and CG out of alignment

Figure 13.1   When the center of buoyancy and the center of balance are not in vertical alignment, a person must actively work to keep from rolling in the water.

Reprinted from Bates and Hanson 1996.

not in vertical alignment with each other, the body is out of equilibrium and will tend to roll or turn. For example, if you place a kickboard between your knees, the center of buoyancy will cause your lower extremities to float upward.

Hydrodynamics

The fluid's resistance to movement, the size and shape of the object moving, and the speed of the object govern movement through water. Some of the factors that impact a body's movement through fluid are interrelated.

Viscosity

Viscosity is the resistance to movement within a fluid and is caused by the friction of the fluid's molecules. Additional factors include physical properties such as cohesion (the attraction of water molecules to adjacent water molecules), adhesion (the attraction of water molecules to the individual's body), and surface tension (the attraction of water molecules on the surface to each other). Movement within the water is resisted by the adhesion and cohesion of water molecules to the person in the water and to other water molecules, respectively. Surface tension provides a resistance when an individual attempts to break the water's surface with the body or a body segment.

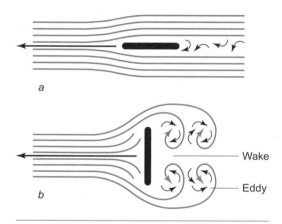

Figure 13.2 Form drag: *(a)* laminar flow, *(b)* turbulent flow. Form drag is caused by turbulence behind an object moving through a fluid.

Reprinted from Bates and Hanson 1996.

Drag

Drag is the water's resistance to a body that is moving through it. There are three types of drag: form drag, wave drag, and frictional drag (Koury 1996).

Form Drag

Form drag is the resistance that an object encounters in a fluid and is determined by the object's size and shape. A larger object has more drag than a smaller object. A broad-shaped object has more drag than a streamlined object. Form drag is directly related to turbulence. The greater the form drag, the greater the turbulence. Turbulence produces a low-pressure area behind the object that tends to pull the object backward (figure 13.2).

A streamlined object moving through water produces a laminar flow—a smooth movement of water that causes a minimal amount of resistance to movement. There is less form drag because of less turbulence. The water molecules all travel at the same speed past the body. Friction of the fluid is minimal because the water molecules separate easily, moving smoothly behind the object.

On the other hand, a broad-shaped object produces a turbulent flow as it moves through the water. The object has more form drag because of the greater turbulence created behind it. The layers of the water move irregularly as they run into the object and rush to move past and behind it. This causes a circular movement of the water layers as they rejoin behind the object. This circular motion of water layers pulling against the moving object is called an **eddy**. Because of the disturbance caused by the eddy, a wake or trail is left in the water (seen as either bubbles behind the body or white water, depending on the amount of turbulence created).

Form drag can be used in an aquatic therex program as a means of altering resistance to exercises. A change in the position of the body or body segment can increase or decrease form drag. For example, moving the arm horizontally in the water with the palm down causes less form drag than with the hand in a vertical position. Shortening or lengthening the body's extremity decreases or increases the form drag, respectively, since the longer lever arm pushes more water than a shorter one. Adding equipment such as hand paddles increases the surface area of the hand, and other equipment such as long paddles increases the lever-arm length; both provide additional form drag to increase the resistance of an exercise.

Wave Drag

Wave drag is the water's resistance because of turbulence. The greater the speed of an object, the greater the wave drag. Wave drag is reduced if movement remains under water. The amount of water wake is an indication of wave drag. Swimming pools often have a splash gutter around the periphery to reduce wave drag for swimmers.

Exercises performed in calm water produce less resistance than those performed in turbulent water. The individual can create wave drag during an exercise by changing positions frequently and rapidly. Increasing the speed of an exercise also increases the wave drag that the exercise causes. For example, walking in water provides the body with 5 to 6 times the resistance that walking in air does. Running water, however, increases the resistance to more than 40 times that of air (McWaters 1988).

Frictional Drag

Frictional drag is the result of water's surface tension. This is not a factor in therapeutic exercise, but it becomes an important element for the competitive swimmer. Frictional drag can add crucial milliseconds to a race time, and swimmers can reduce it by shaving body hair before competition. Recently, custom-made bodysuits constructed from unique, new fibers have been designed to reduce frictional drag.

Hydrostatic Pressure

Pascal's law states that pressure from a fluid is exerted equally on all surfaces of an immersed object at any given depth (figure 13.3). The more deeply the object is immersed, the greater the pressure it encounters. Atmospheric pressure at the surface is 14.7 psi (pounds per square inch). For every foot of submersion, water pressure increases by 0.43 psi (Edlich et al. 1987). Hydrostatic pressure can positively affect edema both by reducing postinjury edema and by allowing exercise without the risk of increasing edema.

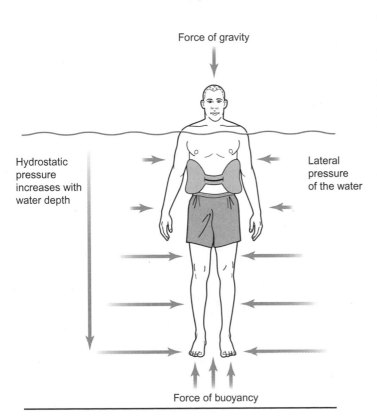

Force of gravity

Hydrostatic pressure increases with water depth

Lateral pressure of the water

Force of buoyancy

Figure 13.3   Pascal's law.
Adapted from Bates and Hanson 1996.

Weight Bearing in Water

Since buoyancy and gravity are opposing forces on a body in water, the more deeply the body is submerged in water, the less weight is borne by the lower extremities (figure 13.4). Because a male's center of gravity is lower than a female's, the specific percentage of body weight borne at different depths varies slightly from female to male. For example, with the body immersed to the xyphoid process, females bear 28% of their weight whereas males bear 35% of their weight (Thein and Brody 1998).

These percentages are useful information, especially in the early stages of rehabilitation. For example, an injured basketball player who is partial weight bearing to 50% on the left lower extremity can perform therapeutic exercises for the left leg in water that is at hip level. As the patient is permitted to bear more weight on the leg, he or she can perform the exercises in shallower water.

Changing walking speed in the water will change the weight-bearing forces in the water (Harrison, Hillman, and Bulstrode 1992). Generally, the faster a person walks in the water, the higher the weight-bearing percentages. For example, if you walk at a slow pace, you must walk in water that is at a level below the axilla in order to be 50% weight bearing. If you walk at a fast rate, 50% weight bearing occurs in water above the axilla level.

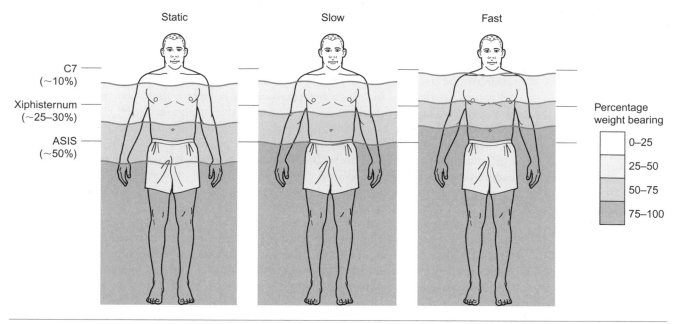

Figure 13.4 Weight bearing in water.

Adapted by permission from R.A. Harrison, M. Hillman, and S. Bulstrode 1992.

EQUIPMENT

▶ Major categories of aquatic equipment include safety equipment and exercise equipment. Equipment for exercising in the water comprises many types of assistive devices, which help to stabilize or support the patient in the pool, and resistive devices that increase the difficulty of an exercise.

In recent years, more and more manufacturers have produced more types and varieties of aquatic exercise equipment. Aquatic equipment can be divided into safety equipment and exercise equipment. Exercise equipment is used and classified as assistive or resistive.

Safety Equipment

The specific safety equipment required at a pool depends on the size of the pool and on state regulations. Safety equipment includes various rescue equipment such as ring buoys, the shepherd's crook, and rescue tubes. Ring buoys are useful in towing and in-water rescues; the shepherd's crook is used for rescue of victims from the side of the pool. A rescue tube has an attached towrope and can support one or more persons. It is flexible enough to wrap around a body.

Spine boards should be among the items of safety equipment at a pool (figure 13.5). These are made of wood, plastic, or fiberglass and have neck and head straps and/or supports. Transport litters or stretchers should be readily available.

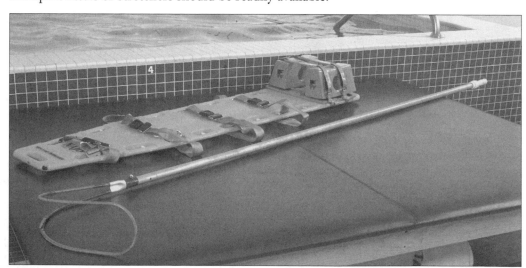

Figure 13.5 Safety equipment. A shepherd's crook or other retrieval equipment and a spine board should be readily available.

Secondary safety equipment should include a basic first-aid kit. In addition to the routine first-aid items, the kit should contain items such as rubber gloves, earplugs, nose plugs, and waterproof bandages.

Exercise Equipment

Exercise equipment most often comprises items that are portable but may also include installed or fixed equipment. Rails and benches are examples of fixed equipment. Portable items may range from simple kickboards to elaborate in-water gym equipment. The selection of specific items depends on the budget and on the sophistication of the pool exercises incorporated into a rehabilitation routine.

Figure 13.6 Flotation cuffs.

Assistive Devices

Assistive exercise equipment helps to stabilize or support the patient in a desired position while in the water; this may be upright, supine, or prone. Flotation devices are used to maintain buoyancy in these positions. They can also serve to assist in the motion of an exercise and often are used to provide additional motion of a joint. The following sections deal with some of the more commonly used devices.

Flotation Cuffs

Flotation cuffs are worn on the upper arms or on the ankles to provide buoyancy for the arms or legs (figure 13.6). When used on the ankles, they can facilitate gait activities or provide buoyancy for range-of-motion activities.

Pull Buoys

Pull buoys are usually Styrofoam devices that are held between the thighs to provide flotation for the legs and lower body during arm exercises (figure 13.7).

Vests and Belts

Vests and belts are used to maintain buoyancy for the trunk during deep-water arm or leg exercises. They are also used for deep-water running and prone- or supine-position exercises (figure 13.8). They should fit comfortably and snugly so they do not ride up. They should also fit well enough not to impede arm or leg movement.

Kickboards

Kickboards provide buoyancy for the arms, legs, head, or trunk. They are available in soft or hard materials and can be used in a vertical, supine, or prone position. They can be used on the water's surface or under the water (figure 13.9). A disadvantage of using kickboards with the arms is that prolonged positioning can cause shoulder fatigue.

Figure 13.7 Pull buoy.

Water Dumbbells

Water dumbbells resemble regular dumbbells; but they are made of Styrofoam, and the bar is padded (figure 13.10). The dumbbell can be placed under the axillae or under the knees to provide buoyancy. Dumbbells offer buoyancy to the arms without adding to the stress of the shoulders the way kickboards can. The bars come in different lengths: The shorter lengths are used under the axilla or held in each hand, and the longer lengths are used under the knees or held with both hands.

Figure 13.8 Flotation belt.

Figure 13.9 Kickboard.

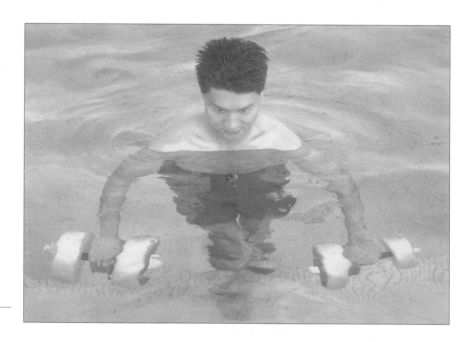

Figure 13.10 Water dumbbells.

Other Buoyancy Equipment

Other buoyancy equipment encompasses items such as inner tubes, water mattresses, ski belts, and cervical float collars. Facilities with restricted budgets may use empty plastic gallon containers as flotation devices.

Resistive Devices

Resistive devices can advance the difficulty of an exercise to increase muscle strength or endurance. They increase exercise difficulty by increasing a body segment's surface area, requiring increased speed of movement, or adding buoyancy or weight.

Lower Extremity

Lower-extremity resistive devices are designed to increase resistance to lower-extremity movement. They do this by either increasing the friction during ambulation in the water or increasing the form or wave drag of the lower extremity.

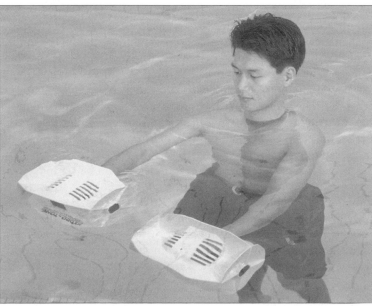

Water shoes are used when the patient is in shallow water and able to touch the bottom of the pool. They are not used during swimming or kicking. They increase the weight of the lower extremity and increase the leg's drag in the water. Their rubberized soles make them good for providing traction during walking, running, or jumping activities. The surface of the sole results in an increase in friction to increase resistance as well as providing stability during these activities.

Fins, which come in a variety of styles and lengths, increase resistance because of the increase in drag they produce. The shorter fins are more appropriate for patients with limited ankle range of motion. Shorter fins are more manageable in the water, offer less resistance than longer fins, and allow the patient to perform a more normal kick while swimming. Any fin that is used should fit the patient well and not pinch, as pinching can cause blisters or cramping.

Boots covering the feet and ankles increase form and/or wave drag during the exercise (figure 13.11). Extension panels on the front or sides of the boot cause turbulence of the water during movement to increase the extremity's form and wave drag. Boots can be used for exercise or during walking or running activities to increase difficulty.

Upper Extremity

Upper-extremity resistive devices, like those for the lower extremity, are designed to increase extremity resistance by increasing form or wave drag or turbulence.

Webbed gloves are the least-resistive devices for the arms. They can be used earlier in the aquatic exercise program than some of the other devices. The gloves are made of Lycra, nylon, or neoprene, so they are soft and pliable. They thus permit the patient to close or open the hand to reduce or increase the water resistance during an exercise.

Figure 13.11 Boots and bells.

Paddles either are handheld or are attached to the hand with straps. They come in a variety of sizes and shapes. The larger the size, the more resistance the paddles produce by increasing form and wave drag. Some paddles look like dumbbells except that they are flat and their disks can be open-vented or close-vented to reduce or increase resistance. Typically made of rigid plastic, paddles offer more resistance than gloves.

Bells provide greater resistance to the arms than the other devices and so are appropriate in the later stages of an aquatic exercise program. Like the boots, they offer resistance by providing turbulence and form and wave drag. They are similar in structure to the boots (figure 13.11) and have either side panels or hollow cores.

Cardiovascular Devices

Cardiovascular devices are available either as separate aquatic containers or as treadmills that can be immersed in swimming pools. The separate containers offer resistance by providing turbulence against an individual who is walking. These devices are costly, but they may be an aquatic exercise solution for facilities without swimming pools. They do require substantial space and some maintenance but obviously not as much as a regular swimming pool.

INDICATIONS, ADVANTAGES, PRECAUTIONS, AND CONTRAINDICATIONS

▶ One major advantage of aquatic therex, among others, is that exercise in the water is feasible for patients who are not yet weight bearing. Precautions and contraindications relate to the use of medications, various medical conditions, and illness.

Although aquatic exercise has the advantage that it can begin early in a rehabilitation program when other forms of exercises are contraindicated, aquatic exercise is not for everyone. Before deciding to use an aquatic therapeutic exercise program, the rehabilitation clinician must be aware of the indications, as well as the limitations and dangers, of this type of system.

Indications

An aquatic therapeutic exercise program is indicated when the patient has many of the typical signs and symptoms associated with musculoskeletal injuries. These include pain, edema, muscle spasm, loss of motion, weakness, limited endurance, or restricted weight-bearing status. Aquatic exercise can also serve as a method of maintaining cardiovascular conditioning or normal status of the uninvolved extremities.

Advantages

The indications lead naturally to advantages of the use of aquatic exercises. This type of exercise can be particularly beneficial when the patient is non-weight bearing on the injured extremity. While the patient may be restricted in activities on dry land, he or she may perform a wide range of activities in the water. The warmth of the water causes a relaxation of muscles. The buoyancy reduces joint compressive forces to allow movement and positioning with reduced pain. The warmth of the water also reduces pain sensation by bombarding the sensory system with temperature input and decreasing the painful noxious input that travels the same pathways. This relief of spasm and reduction of pain assists in breaking down the pain-spasm injury cycle discussed in chapter 2.

Reduction of joint compressive forces and relaxation of muscles permit better movement of the injured area. Buoyancy equipment can help even further in reducing stress to the area's muscles and permit greater ease of movement. Reduction of gravitational forces on the body allows activity when weight bearing is not permissible. Walking in water with reduced weight bearing makes it possible for muscles to function properly for the gait sequence. This encourages the maintenance of muscle tone and balance. Weight bearing can be progressive if the patient walks in water of decreasing depths; the lower the water level, the greater the weight bearing.

Instituting exercises early helps the patient maintain or develop a healthy attitude, promotes body awareness and balance, and stresses newly forming tissue without overstressing it. The healing process is advanced because of the greater exchange of nutrients and metabolites that occur with improved circulation in the injured site. Movement in water can often relieve or reduce pain due to immobilization or edema. If pain and edema can be reduced to affect the pain-injury cycle, the healing rate may be accelerated so that recovery occurs more readily.

The patient's ability to begin exercises sooner also helps to prevent the deconditioning that can play a part in delaying the return to full participation.

Precautions

As with any exercise, the rehabilitation clinician must be aware of precautions and must take special care to administer the aquatic rehabilitation program with these in mind. In the presence of any doubt or question about the patient's ability to perform an aquatic program, it is essential to consult the physician in advance.

Fear of the Water

A patient's fear of water often calls for encouragement and patience. It is advisable to use a vest, even in shallow water, for reassurance. The patient should begin in shallower water if the injury permits. As a rehabilitation clinician, you may have to give the patient assistance and physical support through a hands-on approach, especially until he or she becomes more comfortable in the water. Any patient who experiences an excessive fear of the water should not be forced into an aquatic exercise program.

Medications

Some medications that affect heart rate, blood pressure, or respiration, or any other medication that may alter cardiorespiratory function, may impact the patient's ability to exercise in the water. The rehabilitation clinician should check with the patient's physician or pharmacist before permitting the individual in the water.

Ear Infections

If the patient has a tendency toward chronic ear infections, he or she should apply proper protective ear devices before entering the water. Exercises should be designed so that the head is kept above the water to reduce the risk of an infection.

Specific Conditions

Patients with certain systemic or compromising diseases such as diabetes, cardiovascular disease, or seizure disorders should be carefully monitored while in the water. If the person is sensitive to the pool chemicals, it is essential to observe for unwanted side effects.

No patient should ever be in the pool alone, even if he or she is a good swimmer. Someone should always accompany patients during aquatic exercise.

Contraindications

Under certain conditions or in certain situations, patients should not be allowed in the pool for aquatic therapeutic exercises. These are absolute contraindications that, if ignored, could lead to serious consequences.

Illness

A patient who has a contagious infection and is at risk of transmitting the infection to others should not be allowed in the water.

A severe cold or the flu warrants keeping the patient out of the water until he or she has recovered. Any urinary tract infection should be resolved before the patient is allowed in the water. If the patient has a temperature of 100°F, aquatic exercise must be postponed. Not only is the temperature a problem in that it indicates an illness; it may rise further because of the temperature of the water and the exercise.

Open Wounds

Open wounds should be healed before a patient is allowed into the pool. After surgery, the healing time is usually about seven days. However, if any portion of the surgical scar is open, the patient should remain out of the water.

Other Medical Conditions

Some conditions are not usually found in the young population but need to be mentioned as a point of information. Conditions that are absolute contraindications for an individual's participation in an aquatic exercise program include tracheostomy, severe kidney disease, presence of a nasogastric tube, fecal incontinence, radiation treatments within the past three months, and a history of uncontrolled seizures.

AQUATIC THERAPEUTIC EXERCISE PRINCIPLES AND GUIDELINES

▶ The rehabilitation clinician moves the patient through a sequence of water-based exercises in accordance with the principles of progression for other forms of exercise.

As with therapeutic exercises on land, aquatic therapeutic exercises follow a system of progression. They begin with range-of-motion and flexibility exercises, progress to strength and endurance exercises, and then advance to coordination and agility activities before the patient begins doing activity-specific functional activities. It is also recommended that an exercise session begin with a warm-up and end with a cool-down.

The length of the warm-up depends on the temperature of the water. Therapeutic pools used exclusively for exercise are often set at 92° to 98° F (33-37° C). Swimming pools are set at a lower temperature, 80° to 85° F (27-30° C). The cooler the pool temperature, the longer the warm-up should be.

A cool-down is particularly important if the exercise session has included cardiovascular activities. Cool-down activities can include walking, easy treading water, or sculling in deep or shallow water. It is important to remind the patient to rehydrate following exercises in the pool. Because of the warm water temperature, the patient will perspire and not realize it.

Principles Related to Water Properties

The rehabilitation clinician determines the primary portion of the aquatic exercise session on the basis of specific findings and gears the session toward correcting the deficiencies observed. The same principles of advancement are used for aquatic exercises as for dry-land exercises.

Additionally, because of the properties of water discussed earlier, other factors enter into the selection of specific exercises. These factors include hydrostatic pressure, drag and turbulence, and buoyancy.

Hydrostatic pressure can affect the edema of a segment. It is more advantageous to exercise a swollen extremity in deep water than in shallower water because of the greater hydrostatic pressure at greater depths.

A longer lever arm increases form drag. The straighter the arm, the greater the resistance. It is best to start with a shorter lever arm and progress to longer ones as strength improves. You can make additional changes in lever-arm length by changing the position of the resistive equipment. The farther away from the body's core the resistance is, the greater it is.

Resistance can be provided for a segment using the properties of water. Increasing the speed of the activity causes increased resistance to movement. Moving objects toward the surface of the water, increasing the surface area by using the equipment discussed earlier, and using floats can all increase water resistance to provide for additional strength gains. Exercising in differing depths of water will also change the weight bearing and resistance.

Buoyancy can make an exercise easier or more difficult, depending on the relative position of the center of buoyancy and center of gravity. Buoyancy becomes a greater factor for the body in deeper water.

Aquatic Exercise Progression

Although we have noted that an aquatic therex program can serve to maintain cardiovascular conditioning and status of the uninvolved extremities, we will not consider such exercises in detail. The emphasis here is on the injured segment. Keep in mind that cardiovascular activities are generally performed in the deep water unless in-water treadmills are used. Deep-water cardiovascular exercises include activities such as running, treading water, and swimming. If it is desirable to exercise the uninjured extremities, the more advanced exercises that are presented later in this chapter can be used.

Early-Phase Exercises

The early portion of an aquatic therex program includes gait-training activities in appropriate-depth water, range-of-motion exercises, and perhaps early strengthening activities, if these are indicated and tolerated. Gait training emphasizes the correct manner of ambulation, proper posture, and good balance. The rehabilitation clinician should rely on knowledge of proper posture and proper gait timing and sequencing as discussed in chapters 11 and 12 to assist and instruct the patient in correct posture and gait techniques. The goals in this phase are to achieve normal gait in water and restore normal range of motion.

It is beneficial to use buoyancy equipment in range-of-motion exercises. Buoyancy equipment allows the extremity to come to the water's surface, where range-of-motion gains are easiest to achieve. At the surface, the drag is kept to a minimum, so movement is made with less effort. Resistance exercises in the beginning are low level and are provided without resistive devices. Use of the body segment's own drag in the water is sufficient in the early stage of strengthening activities. Speed of movement is kept slow initially so that less resistance is offered by the water. Koury (1996) recommends limiting initial bouts of resistance exercises to one to two sets of 10 to 15 repetitions, but the specific numbers of sets and repetitions are individually determined and based on the patient's level of fitness, tolerance, and ability and on the program goals. Increasing the repetitions or increasing the sets makes the exercise progressive. The method selected to provide progression specifically determined by the individual's tolerance, normal activity demands, rate of healing, and fitness level.

Middle-Phase Exercises

As the patient progresses, restoration of muscle strength and endurance—the goal of the middle phase—receives more emphasis.

Viscosity-producing drag and buoyancy-permitting motion are now used to provide resistance to increase strength. Speed of motion and lever-arm length are other variables that change the resistance. Deeper water offers additional resistance because it increases pressure on the extremity and increases stability requirements.

Progression with resistive equipment includes starting with short objects and progressing to longer objects. Using lower-profile objects is less difficult than exercising with higher-profile objects. The more drag an object provides, either because it increases the water's resistance or because its profile is made larger, the greater the resistance. The more turbulence the object produces, the greater the resistance. The farther along the extremity the object is placed, the greater the resistance it offers. Each of these ways of increasing resistance creates an additional level of difficulty.

As was done in the early-phase exercises, you can increase the intensity of an exercise by increasing the repetitions or sets. This will help improve endurance more than strength, but there will also be strength gains at a lower rate. This principle is discussed in chapter 7.

Advanced-Phase Exercises

The later stages of the aquatic therex program present a progression toward achieving the goal, normal restoration of the ABCs of proprioception—agility, balance, and coordination. This prepares the patient to withstand the stresses that will be applied during land-based activities.

Gait-training activities can now include walking at a faster pace or running, side-stepping, cariocas, and retrograde walking. Hopping, jumping, squatting, and other sudden changes in direction are also appropriate in this phase. Coordination exercises with eyes open and eyes closed can be included as well.

Strength activities can continue to increase in intensity if the rehabilitation clinician uses more aggressive resistive equipment, increases the speed, requires more than one activity simultaneously, increases repetitions and sets, or changes the shape or size of the resistive equipment.

Land-based exercises may have started during this phase or during the middle stage. Whether or not the aquatic therex program continues depends on the patient's interest in the program, the rehabilitation clinician's preference, rehabilitation goals, and equipment and pool availability.

End-Phase Exercises

If a patient continues in the pool for therapeutic exercises, this is the final stage of aquatic-based exercises. Because of involvement of land exercises, aquatic exercises constitute a fraction of the time of the total therapeutic exercise program; however, some patients may prefer to continue in the water because of satisfaction they receive from their workout. The goal in this phase is to prepare the patient for the specific demands of his or her activity.

Exercises during this phase mimic the skill demands of the patient's sport; include aggressive coordination, agility, and speed activities; and reinforce performance of specific skills using proper posture. High-demand activities can include plyometrics such as box jumping drills and bench stepping. Activity-specific activities can include the use of equipment such as a golf club, tennis racket, or baseball bat in the water.

Progression Guidelines

Progression requires close observation by the rehabilitation clinician and accurate reporting by the patient to the clinician. You should observe the patient's response to the exercise program and the quality of performance. If the patient is able to perform the required exercises correctly, swiftly, and without difficulty, he or she should advance to the next level of difficulty. You must also examine the patient's range of motion, strength, and balance in order to note improvements or changes. This examination is based on both observation and specific objective testing.

The patient must communicate to the rehabilitation clinician any increases in pain or swelling or other symptoms following an exercise session. In the absence of any injury aggravation, he or she can progress to the next level.

It is essential to advance the patient at a rate that will provide for a continued overload, but not so quickly that his or her body is unable to adapt to the stresses and incurs an injury.

DEEP-WATER EXERCISE

▶ Important benefits of exercise in deep water include the absence of weight bearing and the lack of impact forces on the body of the patient.

Even patients who are unable to swim can exercise in deep water. Because of its advantages, deep-water exercise warrants special attention in this chapter. We will look briefly at the benefits of this type of exercise.

The most obvious benefit of deep-water exercise is that it involves no weight bearing and no impact forces on the body. This is particularly important if the patient wants to exercise but either is unable to tolerate impact forces or needs to remain non-weight bearing. For example, a basketball player with patellar tendinitis that is sufficiently intense to restrict ground running may be able to tolerate running in deep water. This activity can help keep the individual's cardiovascular fitness level and strength intact during the rehabilitation process. A runner with a stress fracture is another example of a patient who can benefit from deep-water running.

Since gravity is opposed by buoyancy in deep water, the forces of gravity on a submersed body are minimal. If weights are applied to the ankles, a slight traction force is produced by the force of gravity and the counterbalance force of buoyancy. This can be important for a patient who has low-back pain secondary to either facet irritation or intervertebral disk compression.

Deep-water exercises are essentially concentric. Trauma to inflamed tendons, muscles, or bones is reduced without eccentric activity, yet good strengthening can be provided with deep-water exercises.

Some Recommendations for Optimal Benefits

Figure 13.12 Correct vertical alignment.

During deep-water exercises, the body should remain in good alignment to keep stresses reduced and to use muscles effectively. The head should be out of the water and in proper alignment with the rest of the body. There should be no forward positioning of the neck or upward positioning of the chin to produce an excessive cervical lordosis. The lumbar and thoracic spine should be in correct alignment as discussed in chapter 11 in relation to proper standing posture (figure 13.12). Buoyancy vests or belts help the patient maintain a good postural alignment in deep water. If the spine is not in a neutral position, the center of gravity and the center of buoyancy will not be in a vertical alignment. It becomes more difficult for the patient to maintain a vertical position in deep water when the spine is not in good alignment.

To keep the spine in a good alignment, the patient should attempt to keep the chest lifted and to maintain some tension in the abdominals and gluteals. This preserves good spinal alignment in the water just as it does on land.

Arm activity during deep-water exercises should occur from the shoulders, not the elbows. The arms, as in land running, are used in a pumping activity, with initiation of the activity occurring at the shoulders.

Correct   Incorrect

As in ground running, hip flexion and extension coincide with knee flexion and extension. The ankle goes into plantar flexion during leg extension motion and into dorsiflexion as the hip moves into flexion.

Throughout deep-water running, the spine remains in neutral with a slight forward inclination (figure 13.13). The movement through the water is produced by the extremities, not the trunk. It is necessary for the trunk muscles, the abdominals and the back extensors, to act as stabilizers of the trunk as the body is propelled through the water by the arms and legs.

Figure 13.13 Position for deep-water running.

AQUATIC THERAPEUTIC EXERCISES

▶ Many water-based therapeutic exercises are similar to exercises that patients do on dry land. As with dryland exercise, most aquatic exercises for the spine and the lower and upper extremities can be made more demanding to provide a progression.

The sections that follow present a variety of aquatic exercises for the spine, the lower extremities, and the upper extremities. First, though, a few special points relevant to water-based exercise deserve mention. The first concerns refraction in water and its effect on observation. When light rays move from the air through water, they bend as a result of the lower density of water compared to that of the air. This bending of the light rays makes the bottom of the pool appear closer to the surface than it actually is. It also makes the submerged portion of the patient's body appear distorted (figure 13.14). The submerged body segments appear to be flexed at a different angle than the body segments that are not in the water. This can make it difficult for someone standing at poolside to accurately judge the position of the body or body segment. At times it may be necessary for the rehabilitation clinician to get into the water

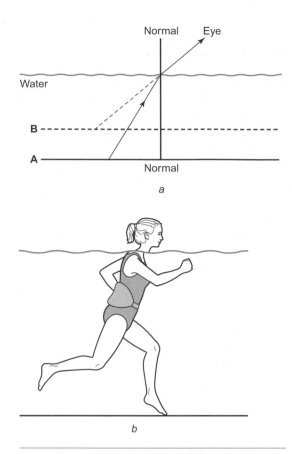

Figure 13.14 *(a)* Refraction of light causes rays reflected from the true bottom of the pool **A** to appear at a false bottom **B**. *(b)* Refraction can create illusions in alignment of body segments.

with the patient to make sure the positioning is correct, especially if the patient has difficulty with proprioception and is unable to align him- or herself correctly without tactile guidance.

The patient should wear a vest or ski belt while performing deep-water exercises. The use of fins can make deep-water exercises more difficult, so goals of the exercise should be determined before the decision to use them is made.

Another point relates to exercises in shallow water. It is advisable for a patient exercising with the feet on the bottom of the pool to wear aquatic shoes. These will enhance balance and provide friction resistance, as well as protecting the patient's feet from abrasions.

The exercises described here are intended only as suggestions and are presented in a progressive series. The discussion is far from all-inclusive. Indeed, the range of possible exercises is limited only by the patient's abilities and your imagination and knowledge. If you know the goals of the therex program, understand the injury limitations, know the patient's abilities, and have an appreciation of the water's physical properties, you can incorporate any appropriate exercise into the aquatic therex program that your ingenuity allows.

A final point is that you should determine the depth of the water for the exercise according to the patient's confidence in the water, weight-bearing status, and the goals for the treatment session.

Some of the exercises are presented, along with their purposes, in the following sections. For many of the strengthening exercises, however, the discussion does not specify which muscles the activity is designed to strengthen. Using your knowledge of kinetics and aquatic principles, attempt to identify the muscles each exercise is intended for.

Exercises for the Spine

An important concept to remember about aquatic spine exercises is that the patient should maintain a neutral spine during all activities. This keeps the vertebrae in good alignment, places minimal stress on the spine, and uses the spine and trunk most efficiently, effectively, and correctly. If the patient is unable to maintain a proper spinal alignment during an exercise, the intensity, complexity, or demand level should be decreased and the patient should concentrate on a lower-level exercise until he or she has mastered spinal alignment at that level. If an individual has difficulty identifying correct spinal alignment with even the basic exercises, it may be necessary for the rehabilitation clinician to get into the pool and use tactile stimulation to provide sensory feedback. This feedback will help the patient identify and learn correct neutral spine alignment.

You will see that many of the exercises described here are similar to dryland exercises. When patients perform them in warm water, the activity is often easier and more comfortable.

Spine Exercises in Shallow Water

The following sections describe only a few of many exercises that could be suggested for the spine. They begin with the cervical spine and move to the pelvis and advance from easiest to most difficult.

Neck Stretches. To stretch the lateral neck, the patient holds the right arm down and across the front of the body and then side-bends the neck to the left, as seen in figure 13.15a. Reverse neck and arm position to stretch the left lateral neck. Figure 13.15b shows an alternative stretch in which the left hand is over the head. In this position, the patient provides a gentle stretch with the left arm while keeping the opposite arm behind the back. In the neck flexion stretch in figure 13.15c, the patient places both hands on the back of the head and performs a gentle pull of the head forward and downward with the hands as the chin is tucked toward the chest. The levator scapula stretch (13.15d) is similar to that seen in figure 13.15b except that the neck is rotated slightly.

a

b

c

d

Figure 13.15 Neck stretches, shallow water: *(a)* active lateral neck stretch, *(b)* stretch to right lateral neck with assistance of left arm, *(c)* stretch to posterior neck muscles using weight of both arms to assist, *(d)* right levator scapula stretch.

Figure 13.16   Spine: *(a)* flexion, *(b)* extension.

Spine Flexion-Extension. Standing with hands on the pool wall and feet shoulder-width apart, the patient keeps the arms straight throughout the exercise (figure 13.16). The hips are pressed forward toward the wall, then backward. During the move forward, the chest is lifted upward; when moving backward, the patient attempts to make the spine rounded.

Figure 13.17
Lateral trunk
stretch.

Lateral Stretch. With the feet shoulder-width apart, the patient raises one arm overhead and reaches upward and across the body (figure 13.17) feeling a stretch on the arm-elevated lateral trunk side.

Figure 13.18   Pelvic roll.

Pelvic Roll. With the back against the pool wall, the patient supports him- or herself by holding on to the edge of the pool as seen in figure 13.18. With the lumbar spine kept flat against the pool wall and the abdominals tensed (pulling the naval to the spine), the legs are lifted until the knees and hips are at 90°. In this position, the patient slowly lifts the pelvis off the wall by increasing the tension of the lower abdominals. The pelvis is rolled back to the wall before the legs are lowered.

a   b

Figure 13.19 *(a)* Standing crunches, *(b)* rotational crunches.

Standing Crunch. The patient stands with a flotation device or a ball against the chest (figure 13.19). The abdominals are contracted to flex the spine, and the position is held for at least 5 to 10 s. A pelvic tilt should be maintained throughout the exercise. This exercise can be modified to include rotational crunches as seen in figure 13.19b. The trunk is rotated about 10° to one side before the crunch is performed. The motion is repeated to the opposite side.

Figure 13.20 Trunk rotation.

Trunk Rotation. In a neutral standing position with the abdominals tightened, the patient rests the arms on a kickboard that is floating in the water. Slowly and in a controlled manner, he or she rotates to one side and then to the other maintaining tension in the abdominals throughout the movement (figure 13.20). The motion should not cause any pain. If pain is present, the motion should be restricted to a pain-free range. The exercise can be advanced through increasing the surface area of the resistance device.

Figure 13.21 Wall push-off.

Wall Push-Offs. The wall push-off strengthens the thoracic spine. Standing away from and facing the pool wall, the patient keeps the spine straight and does not bend at the hips or the back during the exercise (figure 13.21). The feet are kept in the same position throughout the exercise. The patient begins the exercise with the hands on the pool wall and the arms straight. He or she then leans forward by dorsiflexing the ankles and bends the arms until the chest comes close to the pool wall, and finally pushes away from the wall until the arms are straight.

Pull-Downs. With the feet shoulder-width apart, the knees slightly bent to relieve stress to the low back, and the spine in neutral, the patient moves arm bells from in front of the body downward toward the sides (figure 13. 22). The elbows are kept in flexion and the spine in neutral throughout the motion.

Figure 13.22   Pull-down.

Spine Exercises in Deep Water

The patient must have good trunk control in order to perform the spine exercises. An individual who has difficulty with the exercise should perform it in waist-high or chest-high water first.

Double-Leg Lift. With flotation devices in the hands or under the arms, the patient maintains a neutral spine as he or she lifts the legs to a 90° hip flexion position with the knees extended (figure 13.23). The abdominals must remain tight throughout the exercise. If it is too difficult for the patient to maintain a neutral spine position during this exercise, have the person either begin with a single-leg lift or bend the knees so that the hips and knees are at 90° at the top of the motion.

Figure 13.23   Double-leg lift.

Trunk Rotations. Using a flotation tube, the patient maintains a vertical position in the water (figure 13.24). The hips and knees are flexed, and the oblique muscles are used to rotate the hips first in one direction and then to the opposite side. The exercise is more demanding if the knees are fully extended.

a   b

Figure 13.24   Trunk rotations.

Lateral Flexion. Using a flotation tube or other flotation device, the patient flexes the hips and knees to 90° (figure 13.25a). He or she maintains this position while lifting both hips laterally toward the left ribs and then lifting both hips laterally toward the right ribs. The back should not twist or arch during this exercise. You can make this exercise more difficult by having the patient supine in the water with a flotation device at the waist and a small flotation tube or bells at the feet (13.25b).

Figure 13.25 *(a)* Lateral flexion and *(b)* added resistance with flotation device at feet.

Exercises for the Lower Extremities

Exercises in this section begin with the simpler exercises in shallow water and advance to deep-water exercises. Keep in mind that the patient may progress to some deep-water activities while still needing to continue with some shallow-water activities. The primary determinants of the time to move from shallow to deep water are your determination of the patient's ability to perform an exercise, the goals, and the patient's comfort in water.

Ambulation and Balance Activities in Shallow Water

The following are examples of shallow-water exercises. You can increase difficulty by increasing the depth of the water in which the patient performs the activity. As previously discussed, the patient should maintain control of the body throughout each exercise.

Forward walking. This is useful as a gait-training exercise. Encourage the patient to maintain a correct gait pattern, as outlined in chapter 12, while in the water. Look for correct trunk stability. In the beginning, if necessary, the patient may use buoy lines or may walk along the side of the pool, holding on for balance.

Backward walking. This exercise works particularly on the extensor muscles of the trunk and legs. It is good for balance and coordination as well. Emphasize normal stride backward with a good toe-to-heel pattern, normal and equal stride length, and proper weight shifting. The patient should maintain proper trunk alignment.

Toe walking. The patient walks on his or her toes. This exercise is good for strength and proprioception.

Heel walking. The patient walks on the heels. This is a strengthening exercise for the dorsiflexors and is a proprioceptive exercise as well.

a

Single-leg balance. The patient stands on the involved leg, moves the other leg forward, and holds that position for 30 s (figure 13.26). To advance this exercise, you can have the patient stand on the involved leg while moving the uninvolved leg forward and backward or sideways. This exercise focuses on static balance improvement.

Lunges. The patient performs a forward lunge by taking a large step forward and then bringing the back leg up to meet the front leg. This activity is good for increasing strength and range of motion of the hip and knee. Good trunk alignment is necessary throughout the exercise. The patient can also do backward lunges and side lunges to increase hip extension and hip abduction, respectively. These exercises are good for balance and strength as well.

Grapevine. The grapevine is also referred to as a carioca or braid step. The patient first steps to the side with the first leg, then in back (crossing behind the first leg) with the second leg, out to the side again with the first leg, then in front (crossing in front of the first leg) with the second leg. This exercise is good for improving proprioception through improving coordination and balance.

b

Figure 13.26 Single-leg balance: (*a*) Static, (*b*) with contralateral leg movement. The trunk should remain stable and erect throughout the exercise, with tension maintained in abdominal and gluteal muscles.

Running. Analogously to walking in the water, water running should imitate the technique of land running as much as possible. The patient should use the arms to keep an upright posture and should avoid the tendency to lean forward. Running forward, running backward, and cutting can all be performed in shallow water as a prelude to land running.

Hip Exercises in Shallow Water

Good trunk stability is important during all of the following hip exercises. You should instruct the patient to maintain vertical trunk alignment and to maintain tension in the abdominals to assist in this activity. If the patient is unable to demonstrate good trunk alignment, it may be necessary to work on the previously presented trunk activities in addition to the lower-extremity exercises here.

Hip extension. This activity can be used to stretch the hip flexors and strengthen the hip extensors (figure 13.27). The patient stands in a backward-forward straddle position with the involved leg behind. The spine is kept in a neutral position throughout the exercise. Keeping the abdominals tense will help ensure a correct spinal alignment. The involved knee is kept straight and the hip is pushed forward while the heel stays on the floor. The gluteals are tightened during the exercise.

Figure 13.27 Hip extension.

Figure 13.28   Hip adductor stretch.

Hip adductor stretch. In this activity for stretching the hip adductors, the patient stands in a side-straddle position (figure 13.28). The uninvolved knee is flexed as the weight is shifted to that side. The involved knee is kept straight, and the trunk is kept in an upright position.

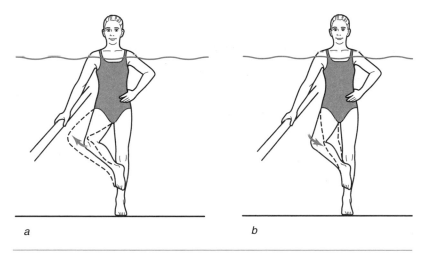

a   b

Figure 13.29   Hip rotation: (a) Medial rotation, (b) lateral rotation.

Hip medial-lateral rotation. These exercises can be used to stretch one group as they strengthen the opposing muscle group. The patient may need to hold on to the pool wall or rail. The knee and hip of the involved leg are flexed, with the sole of the foot on the shin of the opposite leg (figure 13.29). The knee of the involved leg is then rotated outward as far as possible to stretch the medial rotators. To stretch the lateral rotators, the knee is moved inward toward the opposite leg. The trunk should remain in neutral throughout the exercise, and the pelvis and back should not rotate.

Figure-8s. This alternative to the rotation exercise just described offers resistance more than increases in range of motion. The patient draws figure-8s in the water with the entire leg, initiating the movement from the hip, not the knee or ankle. Progressions from this exercise can include proprioceptive neuromuscular facilitation patterns in the water and breaststroke kicking.

Knee Exercises in Shallow Water

The first two knee exercises that follow are flexibility exercises; the others are strengthening exercises. The initial strengthening exercises should use only the limb as the source of resistance. As the patient's strength and control improve, you can add drag equipment to the activity or can have the patient perform the exercise faster as long as he or she maintains control of the limb.

Quadriceps stretch. This stretch is similar to the land exercise in which the patient grasps the ankle of the involved leg, which is positioned behind, and attempts to pull the foot toward the buttock. The knee should remain pointing downward, and the trunk should remain in a neutral position.

Hamstring stretch. The patient places the involved foot on the pool wall or on a step. The knee is slightly flexed, and as the stretch is applied, the knee is extended (figure 13.30). Good trunk alignment is maintained throughout the exercise with trunk forward lean coming from the hip, not the back.

Figure 13.30   Hamstring stretch.

Figure 13.31 Single-leg bicycle.

Single-leg bicycle. The patient flexes and extends the involved hip and knee in a cycling pattern while holding on to the side of the pool (figure 13.31). The trunk remains in neutral and does not move. This exercise is more difficult if the patient performs it without holding on to the side of the pool.

Figure 13.32 Step-up.

Squats. With the feet shoulder-width apart, the patient slowly bends the knees until the thighs are almost parallel to the pool floor. The spine should remain in a neutral position throughout the exercise. You can make this exercise more difficult by having the patient perform it without holding on to the side of the pool or perform it only on the involved leg. In a further progression, the patient performs a jump squat so that he or she lifts off the pool floor.

Step-ups. The involved leg is placed on the top of a box or platform. The patient steps onto the box by lifting his or her body upward, using the knee and hip muscles (figure 13.32). The trunk remains in a neutral position throughout. The patient should avoid trunk lean or hip hike. This exercise can be performed with the patient standing in front of, behind, or at the side of the box for forward step-ups, reverse step-ups, or lateral step-ups, respectively.

Ankle Exercises in Shallow Water

The ankle exercises outlined here are similar to those frequently performed on land, but the water is an ideal place to begin these exercises when weight bearing on the extremity is limited. In these situations, the patient begins in deeper water and progresses to shallower water as more weight bearing is permitted.

Gastrocnemius-soleus stretch. The patient stands facing the pool wall and places the involved leg behind him or her and the uninvolved leg in front. The heel of the involved leg is kept in contact with the pool floor; the knee is kept extended; and the body weight is moved forward onto the hands and front leg. This stretches the gastrocnemius. For stretching the soleus, the leg is brought forward slightly; the involved knee is bent; and the heel is kept on the pool floor as the weight is moved forward.

Heel raises. To perform this activity the patient may need initially to hold on to the side of the pool for stability. The patient slowly rises up onto the toes while the knees remain straight. The body should not lean or move forward. This exercise becomes more difficult if the patient does not hold on to the side of the pool. It is also more difficult if he or she stands only on the involved leg or moves to shallower water.

Ankle walking. The patient walks first on the toes, then on the heels, then on the lateral side of the feet, finally and on the medial side of the feet. Progressions include increasing the stride length, increasing the speed, moving to shallower water, and using resistive equipment.

Figure 13.33 Hopping.

Hopping. The patient jumps forward, using the arms to assist but keeping the spine in neutral (figure 13.33). The knees bend to absorb the impact landing forces. Progression of this exercise includes going from using both legs to one-legged hops, moving to shallower water, increasing the repetitions or sets, and increasing the speed.

Ambulation Activities in Deep Water

The following activities are appropriate when weight bearing is restricted. Cycling and running in deep water can also serve as cardiovascular activities, as well as lower-extremity exercises.

Stride walking. Stride walking is the use of exaggerated strides that are initiated from the hips. The spine should remain in neutral during the exercise.

Cycling. Cycling is performed with the patient in a vertical position. The patient mimics a bicycle motion with exaggerated hip and knee movement. The motion can be either forward or backward.

Running. Running in deep water, as with walking activities, is a good exercise for patients who must remain non-weight bearing. Running in deep water can include jogging or sprinting. The form is as close to dryland running as possible. The trunk should remain in neutral throughout the running phase.

Figure 13.34 Cross-country skiing.

Cross-country skiing. The patient performs a reciprocal motion of the arms and legs, similar to the cross-country skiing action, while maintaining a neutral spine position as seen in figure 13.34.

Hip Exercises in Deep Water

Deep-water exercises are more difficult than shallow-water exercises because in addition to staying afloat, the patient must also work to maintain an upright posture and stable trunk during the lower extremity exercise. Instructions to keep abdominal muscles tense and the chest elevated can be useful cues. Use of a flotation belt can assist the patient in the early phases of deep-water exercise.

Jumping jacks. The elbows and knees are kept straight, and the spine is in neutral (figure 13.35). The arms begin in an abducted position. As the hips are abducted, the arms are adducted, and vice versa.

Figure 13.35 Jumping jacks.

Figure 13.36   Double-knee lift.

Double-knee lift. The patient lifts both legs together, bringing the knees toward the chest while the spine remains in neutral (figure 13.36).

Figure 13.37   Hip flexion with lateral rotation.

Flexion with lateral rotation. The patient is in a vertical position with the spine in neutral (figure 13.37). The legs are moved together, simultaneously into hip flexion and lateral rotation, and are then returned to the starting position.

Figure 13.38   Hip abduction: (a) front view, (b) side view.

Hip abduction. In a vertical position, the patient keeps the knees extended and the spine in neutral. The hips are abducted at the same time and then returned to the starting position. This exercise is more difficult if the patient performs abduction with the hips in a 90° flexion position, as seen in figure 13.38.

Flutter kicking. Flutter kicking prone or supine, with two legs or with one, is useful for the hip. Be sure that the patient initiates the movement from the hip, not the knee.

Figure 13.39   Double-knee bend.

Knee Exercises in Deep Water

The knee exercises suggested here become more difficult if you have the patient perform them with both legs simultaneously or with resistance attached to the feet. Trunk and hip control should be maintained throughout the exercises.

Double-knee bend. In a vertical position with the spine in neutral, the patient simultaneously flexes the knees while keeping them pointing directly downward (figure 13.39).

Figure 13.40   Seated knee extension.

Seated knee extensions. With the hips flexed to 90° and the thighs together, the patient extends the involved knee to full extension (figure 13.40). A vertical position is maintained throughout. To make this exercise more difficult, have the patient extend both knees simultaneously.

Exercises for the Upper Extremities

Keep in mind that just as with the lower-extremity exercises, the following exercises for the upper extremities do not constitute a complete list but are merely some suggested activities for use in therapeutic exercise. Although weight bearing is not the issue for the upper extremity that it is for the lower extremity, aquatic exercises can provide the patient with another way of rehabilitating the arm. Diversification of activities can help to maintain the patient's interest in the therapeutic exercise program, and the variety can be enjoyable for the rehabilitation clinician as well.

Shoulder Exercises in Shallow Water

Presentation of upper-extremity exercises will start with the shoulder and progress through the upper extremity, beginning with stretches and advancing to strengthening exercises.

Pectoralis stretch. In water above shoulder level, and with the arms elevated to shoulder level with elbows extended, the patient horizontally abducts the arms, squeezing the shoulder blades together. The palms should be facing upward.

Capsule stretch. With the involved arm at shoulder level, the patient grasps the elbow of the involved arm with the uninvolved hand and pulls the involved arm across the chest to stretch the posterior capsule (figure 13.41a). To stretch the anterior capsule, the patient grasps the hands behind the back and attempts to lift the hands upward (figure 13.41b). Figure 13.41c demonstrates the inferior-capsule stretch with the patient's hands overhead. The back should not be arched or out of a neutral spine position for any of these stretches.

a   b   c

Figure 13.41   Capsule stretches: (a) Posterior, (b) anterior, (c) inferior.

a   b

Figure 13.42   Lateral rotator stretch, (a) active, (b) passive.

Lateral rotator stretch. For this stretch of the lateral rotators, the patient places the involved hand on the low back (figure 13.42a). Keeping a neutral spine and erect posture, the patient flexes the elbow and reaches upward as high as possible with the hand. In an alternative stretch, the patient grasps a bar or stair rung behind the back and attempts to bend the knees (figure 13.42b).

Medial rotator stretch. The patient stands with the involved side near the pool wall. The elbow is flexed to 90° and the palm is on the wall (figure 13.43). The patient rotates the trunk away from the wall while keeping the hand in contact with the wall surface and the elbow at his or her side. This exercise stretches the medial rotators.

Figure 13.43   Medial rotator stretch.

Figure 13.44 Shoulder press-down.

Figure 13.45 Shoulder flexion-extension.

Figure 13.46 Elbow extensor stretch.

Shoulder press-down. This is a shoulder-strengthening exercise. Using dumbbells or another flotation device, the patient allows the arms to elevate under the water until the upper arms are at shoulder level and in an abducted position (figure 13.44). The patient then pushes the dumbbells downward until the elbows are extended.

Shoulder abduction-adduction. Using resistive devices and keeping the elbows extended, the patient abducts the arms until the hands are at shoulder level and then returns to the starting position. The trunk remains in a neutral position.

Shoulder flexion-extension. This exercise is similar to the preceding one, but the arm moves from flexion at shoulder level to hyperextension with the hand moving past the hips (figure 13.45).

Horizontal abduction-adduction. In this exercise the patient keeps the arms at shoulder level and the elbows straight. The spine is kept in neutral. With resistive devices in the hands, the patient moves the arms through horizontal abduction and horizontal adduction.

Medial rotation-lateral rotation. With the elbow at the side, the spine in neutral, and a resistive device attached to the hand, the patient moves the arm into lateral rotation and medial rotation. If only one direction is desired, on the return to the starting position the hand is rotated so that the hand's profile in the water is reduced.

Elbow Exercises in Shallow Water

Stretching exercises are often more comfortable when performed in water. The elbow can be particularly uncomfortable to stretch and may be better stretched in the pool than on land. Strength exercises can also be useful when performed in the pool. Consider the following activities:

Elbow extensor stretch. To increase the range of motion of the elbow in flexion, the patient bends the elbow as far as possible, and then applies additional force by using the uninvolved hand to increase the motion of the involved elbow (figure 13.46).

Forearm curl. Using a resistive device, the patient flexes the elbow as the shoulder is abducted and the arm is brought toward the water's surface. The shoulder and trunk should be maintained in a stable position throughout the exercise.

Supination-pronation. With the elbow at the side and flexed to 90°, the patient holds on to a resistive device with the hand. The hand is slowly moved from a palm-up position through a full range of motion to a palm-down position, and then to the starting position, while the trunk and shoulder are maintained in stable positions.

Elbow extension. With the elbow kept at the side and a resistive device in the hand, the patient moves the elbow from a fully flexed to a fully extended position. The hand should remain in a palm-down position.

Figure 13.47 Bent-arm pull.

Upper-Extremity Exercises in Deep Water

Because so many of the deep-water exercises for one upper-extremity joint simultaneously work the other upper-extremity joints, we will consider all the upper-extremity exercises together.

Bent-arm pull. With the body maintained in a vertical position, the patient keeps the arms at approximately shoulder level (figure 13.47). As one arm is brought back with the elbow bent, the other arm moves forward until the elbow is fully extended. This motion occurs in a reciprocal fashion with the other upper extremity.

Figure 13.48 Straight-arm pull.

Straight-arm pull. With the body in a vertical position, the elbows kept straight, and the trunk stable and erect, the patient alternately swings the arms forward and then backward into hyperextension (figure 13.48). As the arm is brought forward, the hand faces upward; as the arm is brought backward, the hand faces downward.

Figure 13.49 Arm circles.

Arm circles. In a vertical position, the patient places the arms at shoulder level (figure 13.49). With the elbows kept straight, the arms are moved in circles, clockwise and counterclockwise. Changing the size of the circles, changing the speed of movement, or attaching resistive devices to the hands can alter the resistance.

Figure 13.50   Shoulder press.

Breaststroke. With the body in a vertical position, the patient keeps the arms at shoulder level. The arms begin in a horizontally adducted position and are moved into full horizontal abduction as during a breaststroke.

Shoulder press. In a vertical position, the patient pushes both arms forward at shoulder level from the chest as in a shoulder-press exercise with weights (figure 13.50). To increase the resistance of this exercise, you can add resistive devices, increase speed, or increase the number of repetitions.

Figure 13.51   Elbow press.

Elbow press. In a vertical position, the patient flexes and extends one elbow, alternating the motion with the opposite arm (figure 13.51). The movement occurs in an up-and-down motion in front of the body.

Wave. In a vertical position, the patient places the arms at shoulder level away from the sides. The elbows are kept straight throughout the exercise. The wrists are alternately flexed and extended through their full range of motion.

SUMMARY

1. Identify and discuss the physical properties of water that affect the ability to exercise in water.

    The physical properties of water, including specific gravity, buoyancy, center of buoyancy, and hydrodynamics, influence the way a patient is able to exercise in water. Water has a specific gravity of 1. If a body's specific gravity is less than 1, the body will float; but if the specific gravity is more than 1, the body will sink. Buoyancy occurs when the specific gravity is less than 1. In order for a body to remain upright while floating, the center of buoyancy must be in line with the center of gravity; otherwise the patient must work to maintain an upright position. Resistance to movement in water is called drag; the greater the drag, the more resistance there is. We can influence drag by increasing the speed of movement, turbulence, surface area being moved, and depth of the water.

2. Define and explain the difference between assistive and resistive aquatic equipment and give examples of each.

> Assistive devices in the water provide the body support to aid in buoyancy; examples are the kickboard and the flotation belt. Resistive equipment in the water increases the drag and makes it more difficult for a body to move; examples are paddles and boots.

3. List precautions and contraindications for aquatic exercise.

> The most common precaution relates to the patient's fear. Other precautions relate to certain medications that can compromise the patient's situation, to ear infections, and to certain medical conditions. A patient who has epilepsy, for example, may be endangered in a pool and must be closely observed. Contraindications include illness, open wounds, and medical conditions that may be dangerous for either the patient or others in the pool; in these cases the individual must not be allowed in the pool.

4. Identify three advantages of aquatic therapeutic exercise.

> Aquatic exercise can begin early in the therapeutic exercise program; patients with non-weight-bearing conditions can begin water exercises before land exercises. Aquatic therex can relax muscle spasm and pain, and provides for diversity and variety in the patient's rehabilitation program.

5. List three aquatic exercises for each body segment and identify their purposes.

> An example of a trunk exercise is the lateral stretch in shallow water, used to improve flexibility. An example of a lower-extremity exercise is step-ups in shallow water, which increase strength of the knee muscles, especially the quadriceps. An upper-extremity exercise is the shoulder press-down with water dumbbells, used to strengthen the shoulder depressors.

CRITICAL THINKING QUESTIONS

1. Why is it that some of the patients you place in the pool have no trouble floating while others must work to keep their heads above water? What principle does this phenomenon involve?

2. If the patient you are rehabilitating is non-weight bearing on an injured ankle but wants to perform cardiovascular activities in the pool, what program will you design for him? What water depth should he be in for resistive exercises?

3. The softball player with whom you have been working to rehabilitate her shoulder is fearful of going into the water. You would like to have her in the pool, since water activity would help increase her shoulder motion and strength. What would you do to encourage her to get into the pool and relieve her fears? What would be your initial exercises with her, and at what water depth would you place her?

4. You are using the pool to rehabilitate a gymnast with a hip strain until she has less pain with land activities. Her motion is good, but her strength is limited in all hip motions, especially abduction. List resistive exercises that you will include in her pool program, and provide a progression for each one.

5. Identify a simple core stabilization exercise that you would use for a patient with a recent back injury, and include a four-step progression for the exercise. What would your criteria be for advancement from one level to the next?

LAB ACTIVITIES

1. While standing in waist-deep water, move your hand through the water in the following manners:

    a. With the fingers together and the hand parallel to the water surface

    b. With the fingers together and the hand perpendicular to the water surface

    c. With the fingers apart and the hand perpendicular to the water surface

    d. With the hand grasping a paddle and perpendicular to the water surface

    Rate the movements from easiest to perform to most difficult. Which one was easiest and which one was most difficult and why?

2. Walk across the pool in waist-high water. Walk across the pool in chest-high water. Walk across the pool in neck-deep water. Which depth was the most difficult to walk in? Why? At which depth did you feel the most weight applied through your feet? Why?

3. Now run across the pool at the same depths in question 2. Which depth was the most difficult? Why?

4. While maintaining pelvic neutral in chest deep water, perform a single knee to chest exercise, alternating legs. Now repeat the activity in deep water. Which was the more difficult exercise and why?

5. While maintaining pelvic neutral in chest-deep water, perform a shoulder flexion-extension exercise, alternating arms. Now repeat the activity in deep water. Which was the more difficult exercise and why? What do the results of this activity and the one in question 4 teach you in terms of rehabilitation exercises in the pool?

6. Create an exercise program for a lower-extremity injury beginning with NWB and progressing to partial then full weight-bearing activities. Don't forget to design exercises to include pelvic stabilization during lower-extremity exercises.

7. Create an exercise program for an upper extremity injury. Don't forget to design exercises to include pelvic stabilization during lower extremity exercises.

REFERENCES

Davis, B.C., and R.A. Harrison. 1988. *Hydrotherapy in practice.* New York: Churchill Livingstone.

Denegar, C., E. Saliba, and S. Saliba. 2005. *Therapeutic modalities for musculoskeletal injuries.* 2nd ed. Champaign, IL: Human Kinetics.

Edlich, R.F., Towler, M.A., Goitz, R.J., Wilder, R.P., Buschbacher, L.P., Morgan, R.F., and J.G. Thacker. 1987. Bioengineering principles of hydrotherapy. *Journal of Burn Care and Rehabilitation* 8:580-584.

Harrison, R.A., Hillman, M., and S. Bulstrode. 1992. Loading of the lower limb when walking partially immersed: Implications for clinical practice. *Physiotherapy* 78 (3):164-167.

Hay, J. 1993. *The biomechanics of sports techniques.* 4th ed. Englewood Cliffs, NJ: Prentice-Hall.

Koury, J.M. 1996. *Aquatic therapy programming.* Champaign, IL: Human Kinetics.

McWaters, G. 1988. *Deep water exercise for health and fitness.* Laguna Beach, CA: Publitec Editions.

Thein, J.M., and L.T. Brody. 1998. Aquatic-based rehabilitation and training for the elite athlete. *Journal of Orthopaedic and Sports Physical Therapy* 27:32-41.

CHAPTER 14

Swiss Balls and Foam Rollers

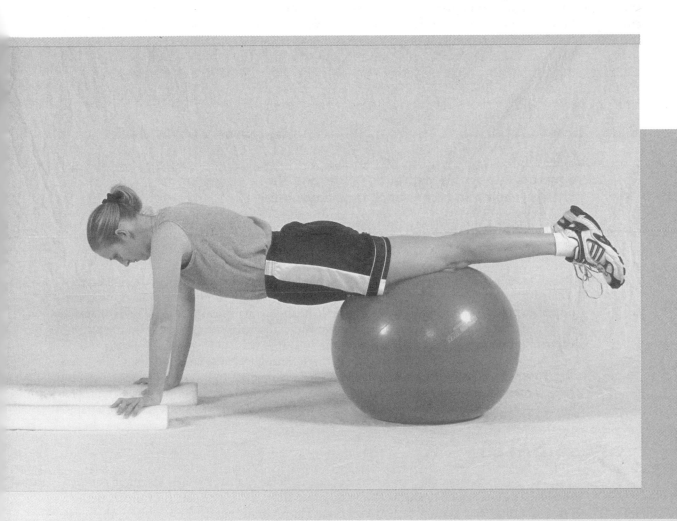

Objectives

After completing this chapter, you should be able to do the following:

1. Explain how Swiss balls and foam rollers can increase the challenge of a traditional exercise.

2. Identify the rehabilitation parameters that are benefited by the use of Swiss balls or foam rollers.

3. Discuss safety factors, precautions, and contra-indications relating to the use of Swiss balls and foam rollers.

4. Explain how to properly fit a Swiss ball.

5. List one exercise each for the trunk, upper extremity, and lower extremity using a Swiss ball, and identify its purpose.

6. List one exercise each for the trunk, upper extremity, and lower extremity using foam rollers, and identify its purpose.

Of all the exercise equipment in the sports medicine facility where Donald Richards worked, he enjoyed the Swiss balls and foam rollers the most. He believed that these items could provide a challenging and interesting rehabilitation program for any of his patients. In his opinion, no other piece of equipment challenged the trunk muscles as well as the foam roller. Don routinely placed all his patients on it, since not only back injuries, but also upper- and lower-extremity injuries, could benefit from the challenge of the foam roller.

As much as he liked foam-roller rehabilitation, Don also liked the Swiss ball for its versatility in upper- and lower-extremity and trunk rehabilitation. Whenever possible, he liked to include both of these items in a patient's program. He would often provide patients with a Swiss ball and foam roller so that they could continue their rehabilitation programs at home.

The beauty of the foam roller and Swiss ball, Don thought, was that the rehabilitation exercises could be easy or difficult; patients could perform them initially in the clinic and then progress to a home program; they weren't expensive; and they made what might otherwise be a boring weight program fun and interesting for those patients with whom he worked.

■ **Progress is impossible without change, and those who cannot change their minds cannot change anything.**

George Bernard Shaw, dramatist and critic, 1856-1950

Rehabilitation and the treatment of musculoskeletal injuries have changed over the years. Many techniques we use today were unknown 20 years ago. Among the changes in therapeutic exercise techniques is the use of Swiss balls and foam rollers. These are both relatively new items in the orthopedic and rehabilitation arena that are commonly used in therapeutic exercise programs today.

This chapter presents information about how to introduce Swiss balls and foam rollers into the rehabilitation program, techniques to use, and examples of exercises that patients can perform with them. We also consider indications, precautions, and contraindications that represent crucial guidelines for the use of Swiss balls and foam rollers in therapeutic exercise programs.

▶ Swiss balls can be used in a progression of exercise to challenge flexibility, strength, muscle endurance, balance, coordination, and joint- and body-position awareness. Ball size is chosen according to the patient's height. Safety factors include avoidance of bouncing in combination with spine movements and being aware of several contraindications.

SWISS BALLS

The Swiss ball, a large vinyl ball, was developed by an Italian toy manufacturer and first produced in 1963 under the name Gymnastik, and later, Gymnic. Using the Bobath method, Dr. Elsbeth Köng, a Swiss pediatrician, and Mary Quinton, an English physiotherapist, developed pediatric neurological rehabilitation programs using Swiss balls. In the 1960s, Dr. Susan Klein-Vogelbach, a physical therapist in Switzerland, began using the Swiss balls as an instructional tool in classes for adult orthopedic and other medical problems.

The term **Swiss ball** refers to the large vinyl balls because U.S. physical therapists who introduced the balls in this country first saw them used in clinics in Switzerland (Posner-Mayer 1995). Although Swiss balls were introduced in the United States during the early 1970s, they did not begin to catch on until the late 1980s. Today, many facilities use them for a wide range of orthopedic activities, including spinal stabilization, upper- and lower-extremity strengthening and flexibility, balance and coordination, and body awareness.

Swiss-Ball Challenges

Most patients enjoy exercising with balls. Balls provide a diversion from uninteresting and boring exercises. Swiss-ball activities can also be more challenging than regular exercises. The use of the Swiss ball in therapeutic exercises can stimulate interest, offer activity complexity, and motivate the patient to perform more diligently.

The Swiss ball can provide challenges within a variety of rehabilitation parameters. Swiss-ball exercises can increase flexibility, strength, muscle endurance, balance, coordination, and joint- and body-position awareness. They can be used for open and closed chain activities. They can provide for a progression of difficulty to continually challenge the patient as parameters improve. Swiss balls can be used throughout a therapeutic exercise program to offer the patient a number of stimulating activities.

A simple activity becomes more complex and challenging when it incorporates additional elements. For example, standing on the ground is a relatively simple activity for a patient, but standing on a boat that is moving through water, or standing on skis while moving downhill, is more challenging. Sitting on a chair at a desk requires little balance; sitting on a Swiss ball requires more balance. Lying on a table is no challenge, but lying prone on a Swiss ball with only one hand in contact with the ground requires effort.

Activity on a Swiss ball requires more effort because the surface is unstable—the instability challenges balance. Coordination is more difficult on a Swiss ball because more than one body segment and more than one system must participate simultaneously to maintain position or balance during an activity. Coordination is additionally tested if the patient is required to perform more than one activity while on the Swiss ball.

Body weight can be used in a variety of positions to offer resistance during activity. Using weights during exercises on the Swiss ball makes the exercise more stressful. The unstable surface requires a greater effort by the exercising muscles, as well as effort by a greater number of muscles, to perform the exercise. Increasing repetitions, sets, and difficulty of the exercises on the Swiss ball can each improve muscle endurance and strength.

Flexibility can also be improved on the Swiss ball. Many people find the ball a comfortable surface on which to perform stretching exercises. The Swiss ball can also provide a comfortable and relaxing gravity-assisted method of stretching (figure 14.1).

When the body performs an activity, it receives feedback on the accuracy and quality of the performance in the form of sensory information from visual, auditory, vestibular, and somatosensory systems. Adjustments in performance are made based on the feedback received and interpreted at various neural levels as discussed in chapter 8. Joint- and body-position awareness is facilitated in Swiss-ball exercises because there is a continual change of position, and the body must adjust and adapt to those changes appropriately, while performing the activities correctly.

Figure 14.1 Gravity-assisted Swiss-ball stretch.

Figure 14.2 Reduced base of support from two arms *(a)* to one arm *(b)* on Swiss ball increases the activity's difficulty.

Figure 14.3 Increased lever-arm length on Swiss ball increases the activity's difficulty. Ball is moved from the thighs *(a)* to the lower legs *(b)*.

Increasing Swiss-Ball Challenges

Whether your goal is to increase strength, balance, coordination, or flexibility, there are several ways you can make Swiss-ball activities more challenging. The obvious modification is the addition of resistance equipment such as weights, rubber tubing/bands, pulleys, or the use of manual resistance to increase strength gains.

Other modifications include decreasing the base of support. For example, if a patient is balancing on the ball with both hands on the floor, a narrower placement of the hands will make the activity more difficult. This activity becomes even more difficult if you have the patient perform it with only one hand on the ground, or perform movement on the ball while supporting the body with one hand on the floor (figure 14.2).

Increasing the lever-arm length makes the activity more difficult. For example, a push-up performed on the Swiss ball will increase in difficulty if the ball is moved from under the thighs to under the shins (figure 14.3).

Increasing the distance traveled is another way to make the exercise more difficult. Going through a greater range of motion requires recruitment of more muscle fibers, so the muscle must work harder. For example, the difficulty of a squat exercise with the Swiss ball is increased if the range of motion of the squat is increased (figure 14.4).

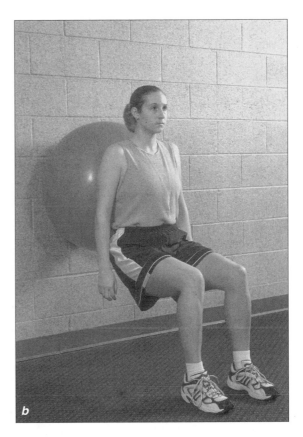

Figure 14.4
Moving through a greater ROM on the Swiss ball requires greater muscle activity. *(a)* Slight squat motion, *(b)* full squat.

As with many other exercises, increasing the speed of movement and requiring the same amount of control as with the slower speed will increase the difficulty of the exercise on a Swiss ball.

Equipment and Exercise Area

There are currently several manufacturers of vinyl Swiss balls. Gymnic and Physioball are well-known Swiss-ball names. These balls are durable enough to withstand an individual's weight. The Gymnic ball will hold 454 kg (1,000 lb), while the Physioball resists loads up to 299 kg (660 lb).

Swiss balls come in various sizes. Each company makes balls in different colors corresponding to different sizes; but because the colors vary among the companies, you should select balls according to size, not color. Ball size is indicated by diameter. The size to select for a particular patient is determined by the patient's height. Table 14.1 lists appropriate Swiss-ball sizes for individuals of varying heights. When the patient is sitting on the ball, the hips and knees should be at 90°. If the patient's height is between the heights listed in table 14.1, use the larger-sized ball and underinflate it to fit the patient.

The floor surface should be firm and smooth but not slippery. Firm mats, linoleum, hardwood, and low-pile carpet are good surfaces. Surfaces should not be rough or uneven. Swiss balls should not be used outdoors because of the unevenness of the surface and because objects on the ground, such as pebbles or debris, can puncture them. The area where a patient exercises with a Swiss ball should be spacious enough to allow moving and rolling without danger of hitting furniture or other objects that could cause injury.

Safety Factors

The rehabilitation clinician should keep some safety factors in mind when beginning an exercise session that uses a Swiss ball. The patient's clothing should be free of objects such as belt buckles that may puncture the ball. The patient should wear rubber-soled shoes that

Table 14.1
Swiss-Ball Sizes

Patient's height	cm	in.
Under 5 ft	45	18
5 ft to 5 ft 7 in.	55	21Aw
5 ft. 8 in. to 6 ft. 2 in.	65	25
6 ft 3 in. to 6 ft. 10 in.	75	29 Aw
Over 6 ft 10 in.	85	33 Aw

provide traction. If the shoes are worn outdoors, the soles should be inspected for pebbles that could fall off and puncture the ball.

The patient's clothing should be proper athletic wear that allows freedom of movement. If the individual will be on the floor on the knees, he or she should wear sweatpants or warm-up pants that will protect the skin from abrasions. Pants of these types will also prevent the skin from sticking to the ball and reduce restriction of movement or skin discomfort.

When performing exercises on the Swiss ball, patients should not combine bouncing on the ball with bending and twisting or rotating the spine. This can cause injury to the spine. The exercises should be performed with control and not so quickly that the motions are incorrect.

The patient's hair should be restrained if necessary, so that it does not impede the exercise, hamper vision, or get in the way.

Contraindications

▶ Swiss-ball exercises can improve trunk stabilization, flexibility, and strength; there are also many Swiss-ball exercises for strengthening the upper and lower extremities. The upper-extremity exercises become more challenging if the Swiss ball is used in combination with such devices are rubber bands or tubing and weights.

Although contraindications are not commonly seen in the young population, the rehabilitation clinician should be aware of them. An individual who has a fear of using or falling off the ball, and who cannot be reassured, should not use the Swiss ball. Increased pain, dizziness, or any other undesirable symptom is an indication to stop the exercises. Any disease or injury that is contraindicated for specific exercises should be avoided. For example, a patient who is non-weight bearing should not use the feet to stabilize while sitting on the ball.

SWISS-BALL EXERCISES

Many Swiss-ball exercises are used for trunk stabilization, but a number of these can be used to strengthen the upper and lower extremities as well. The activities described here by no means represent all Swiss-ball exercises and are examples only. As with many other therapeutic exercises, specific Swiss-ball activities are limited only by the rehabilitation clinician's knowledge and imagination and the patient's restrictions.

Trunk Exercises

For all Swiss-ball exercises, the patient should be instructed to maintain a pelvic-neutral posture throughout the activity. To maintain this position, the patient must know where his or her pelvic neutral is located and must keep some tension in the muscles controlling the position, especially the abdominals.

Swiss-Ball Care

As mentioned earlier, the Swiss ball should not be used outdoors. A Swiss ball can be easily damaged by pebbles or other sharp or hard objects on the ground. The balls should be kept away from excessive or prolonged heat sources such as lamps, heat ducts, and direct sunlight.

Swiss balls should be inflated when at room temperature. They can be inflated with an air compressor, air-mattress pump, or gas-station air compressor or pump with a trigger nozzle attachment. A bicycle pump will not work well because of the large volume of air the ball requires—using a bicycle pump will simply take too long. A ball is maximally inflated when it is firm; but as already indicated, less-than-maximal inflation is appropriate when a patient's height requires a slightly smaller ball.

Warm, soapy water and a cloth are used to clean the ball. Abrasive or chemical cleaners may cause damage and should be avoided.

Figure 14.5 Bounce and kick.

Bounce and Kick

This is a stabilization exercise. The patient sits on the ball in pelvic neutral. Without rotating the spine or hips, the patient bounces on the ball. While bouncing, he or she alternates kicking out one leg and then the other, one kick for each bounce (figure 14.5). This becomes more difficult if the patient simultaneously raises the opposite arm.

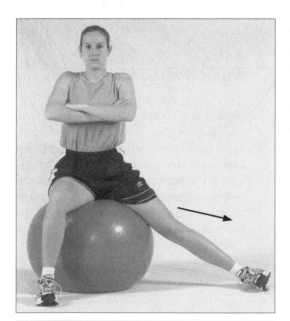

Figure 14.6 Side foot reach.

Side Foot Reach

This is also a stabilization exercise. The patient sits on the ball in pelvic neutral. The arms are crossed (figure 14.6). As the patient bounces on the ball, he or she extends one leg out to the side and then brings it back to the starting position. Movements should coincide with the bounces. The opposite leg is then moved to the other side in similar fashion. This is more challenging if arm movements are added, with the same-side arm extending sideways simultaneously with the leg.

Lateral Glide

The lateral glide is for pelvic flexibility. The patient sits on the ball in pelvic neutral (figure 14.7). The pelvis is rolled out to one side and then the other, then returns to pelvic neutral. The patient uses the trunk muscles to perform the exercise, not the legs.

Figure 14.7 Lateral glide to the right.

Pelvic Circles

This exercise is for pelvic flexibility. The patient sits on the ball in pelvic neutral and rotates the pelvis first clockwise and then counterclockwise (figure 14.8). The pelvic and trunk muscles are used to produce the motion, not the legs. The legs and shoulders should move minimally.

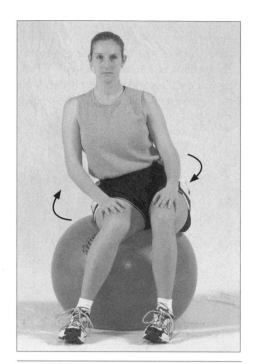

Figure 14.8   Clockwise pelvic circles.

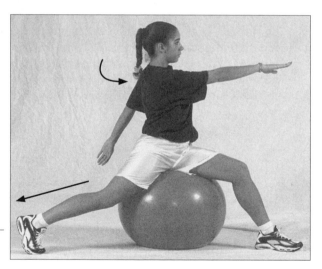

Figure 14.9   Trunk rotation in sitting.

Trunk Rotation in Sitting

This exercise is for trunk flexibility. The patient sits on the ball in pelvic neutral with the arms abducted to 90°. The trunk is rotated to the left, and the right arm reaches in the direction of the trunk rotation as the right leg is extended behind the person (figure 14.9). The patient returns to the starting position and repeats the motion to the right.

Trunk Rotation in Supine

This is a variation of the exercise just described. The patient lies supine on the floor with the knees and hips bent, holding the ball in the hands with the arms straight and directly overhead. Keeping the abdominals tight to stabilize the spine, the individual moves the ball to the right as the hips are rotated to the left (figure 14.10). The hip movement is initiated from the low-back and oblique abdominal muscles.

Figure 14.10
Trunk rotation in supine.

Figure 14.11   Stretch in kneeling.

Stretch in Kneeling

This stretch for the back can be used for the shoulders also. The patient kneels on the floor with his or her hands on the ball, which is in front of the person. The patient bows forward and lets the ball roll out (figure 14.11). The elbows are extended as the patient attempts to lower the upper trunk toward the floor.

Figure 14.12   Lateral stretch.

Lateral Stretch

This stretch is for the lateral trunk. The patient kneels beside the ball and lies sideways on the ball to touch the lower hand to the floor (figure 14.12). The upper arm is extended overhead.

Thoracic Stretch

The patient sits on the ball with the feet about shoulder-width apart. He or she then lies back on the ball as it rolls up the back until the buttocks are toward the floor and the shoulder blades are on the ball (figure 14.1, p. 427). The patient then raises the arms overhead and pushes the ball backward with the legs so that the head moves closer to the floor and the knees are straight.

Supine Leg Lift

This exercise strengthens the back extensors. The patient sits on the ball and walks out until the head and shoulders are supported on the ball (figure 14.13). While the individual maintains pelvic neutral, he or she alternately lifts the legs off the floor in a marching sequence. There should be no rolling of the trunk or hips, and the pelvis should not drop. This becomes more difficult if performed with the arms overhead.

Figure 14.13   Supine leg lift.

Figure 14.14   Hip rotation.

Hip Rotation

This hip rotation exercise strengthens the abdominal oblique muscles. The patient lies supine on the floor, with the lower legs on the ball and arms at the sides (figure 14.14). The individual rolls the knees from side to side as far as possible without falling off the ball. The abdominals, kept tightened, initiate the movement of the hips. The back should not arch, and the shoulders should remain on the floor throughout the exercise.

Bridging

This exercise, which strengthens the back extensors, can be performed in two positions. In one variation, the patient is positioned supine on the ball so that the scapulae are on the ball and the feet are on the floor about shoulder-width apart (figure 14.15, a and b). The pelvis is in neutral and

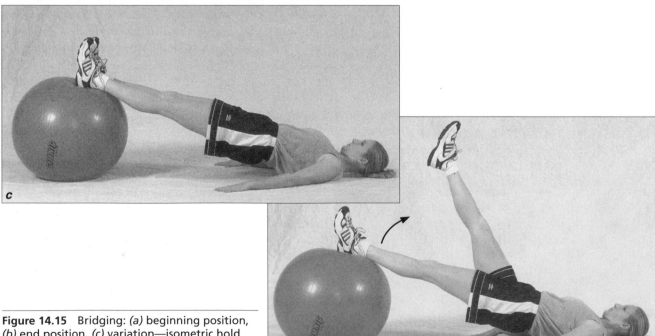

Figure 14.15   Bridging: *(a)* beginning position, *(b)* end position, *(c)* variation—isometric hold with feet on ball, *(d)* variation—alternate leg raise while maintaining trunk position.

the abdominals are tight as the patient lifts the buttocks and extends the hips. The movement is initiated at the buttocks, and the pelvis is kept in neutral throughout. This exercise is more challenging if the patient marches in place while maintaining pelvic neutral.

The other variation of the bridging exercise is with the patient lying supine on the floor and the feet on the Swiss ball. Keeping pelvic neutral, the individual lifts the hips off the floor as the buttocks and abdominals are tightened (figure 14.15c). You can make this exercise more difficult by having the patient alternate leg lifts off the ball (figure 14.15d). The exercise also becomes more challenging if you have the patient change the arm positions, from arms extended away from the body, to arms across the chest, to hands behind the head.

Back Extension in Prone

This exercise strengthens the back extensors. The patient lies prone on the ball; the ball is under the lower abdomen and pelvis, and the balls of the patient's feet are on the floor. The trunk is flexed forward with the pelvis in neutral (figure 14.16a). The patient lifts the trunk by squeezing the gluteals and the lower back paraspinal muscles. The arm positions change to increase the difficulty of the exercise, beginning with the hands behind the back and progressing so that the hands are out to the sides (figure 14.16b) and then overhead (figure 14.16c). To create an additional level of difficulty, the patient places his or her feet on a chair as seen in figure 14.16, d through f.

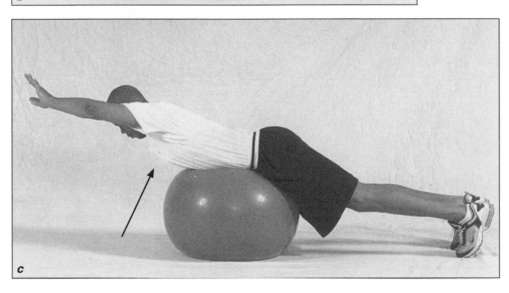

(continued)

Figure 14.16 Back-extension progression. Changes in arm placement change the exercise's difficulty by moving the center of gravity.

Figure 14.16 *(continued)* Additional levels of difficulty of the back-extension progression.

Figure 14.17 Prone leg lift.

Prone Leg Lift

This leg lift strengthens the trunk extensors. The patient lies prone on the ball with the hands and the balls of the feet on the floor. The Swiss ball should be positioned under the lower abdomen and pelvis. The patient squeezes the buttocks to raise the legs, keeping the pelvis in neutral and the knees straight (figure 14.17).

Swimming

This exercise strengthens the midback region. With the ball placed under the patient's abdomen and the knees extended, with only the balls of the feet on the floor, the patient places one arm straight out in front and the other behind, by the hip (figure 14.18a). The patient maintains a neutral spine as the arms reverse positions (figure 14.18b). Weights can be added to increase the difficulty of the exercise. The trunk should not rotate as the arms move.

Figure 14.18 Swimming.

Figure 14.19   Seated abdominal strengthening: *(a)* with arms forward, *(b)* more difficult with alternating arms overhead.

Seated Abdominal Strengthening

The patient sits on the Swiss ball in pelvic neutral. The feet are shoulder-width apart. Maintaining pelvic neutral, the person leans back on the ball, moving from the hips, not the spine (figure 14.19a). Changing the arm positions changes the difficulty of the exercise. The least-difficult variation is with the arms outstretched. As the arms move upward toward the head, the exercise increases in difficulty. The activity can stress the oblique muscles if the patient places the arms overhead and alternately lowers each arm to the opposite knee as seen in figure 14.19b.

Ball Lift

The purpose of this exercise is to strengthen the lower abdominals. The patient lies supine on the floor and maintains pelvic neutral. The ball is picked up between the ankles, and the hips are maintained at 90° flexion (figure 14.20a). With the lower abdominals kept tight, the knees are flexed and extended at 90°. The progression for this exercise is from flexing & extending the knees with the hip position maintained to lowering the legs toward the floor and extending the knees as the legs are lowered (figure 14.20b). It is important that the lower abdominals remain tight throughout this exercise and that the lower back maintains contact with the floor.

To increase the difficulty, the patient rotates the legs, bringing one in front of the other and then reversing positions. Again, the pelvis should remain in neutral, and the lower spine remains in contact with the floor as seen in figure 14.20c.

Figure 14.20   Ball lift: *(a)* Hips are at 90° and knees are extended, *(b)* legs are lowered while back remains flat, *(c)* legs are rotated with spine in neutral.

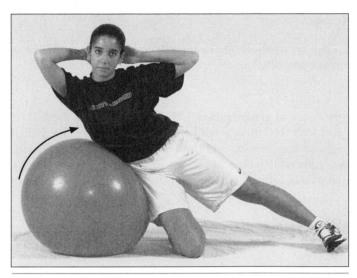

Figure 14.21 Side sit-up.

Side Sit-Ups

This sit-up strengthens the obliques. The patient kneels on the floor beside the ball. The individual then lies sideways on the ball, with the lateral hip and trunk in contact with the ball and the outer knee extended out to the side (figure 14.21). The patient then lifts sideways off the ball.

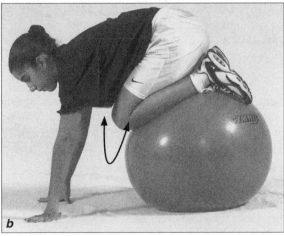

Figure 14.22 Prone walk-out: *(a)* beginning position, *(b)* ending position. The ball can be rolled from side to side for an additional level of this exercise (see arrow).

Prone Walk-Out

This exercise strengthens the abdominals. The patient walks forward until the ball is at the shins and the arms support the weight of the trunk in a push-up position as shown in figure 14.22a. Pelvic neutral is maintained while this position is held on a timed basis.

A variation of this exercise is to have the patient maintain pelvic neutral while bringing the knees up toward the chest (figure 14.22b). You can add difficulty by having the patient roll the ball to one side and then to the other so that the side of the thigh comes in contact with the ball while the legs remain in the position seen in figure 14.22b. This variation also exercises the oblique muscles.

Lower-Extremity Exercises

Some of the trunk exercises also can be used for the lower extremities. A few additional exercises for the lower extremities are described here.

Reverse Squats

This squat strengthens quadriceps, calf, and gluteal muscles. The patient places the ball on the wall and leans prone on the ball with the ball at waist level (figure 14.23a). The patient remains on his or her toes throughout the exercise, and the feet are shoulder-width apart. The individual squats down to a comfortable level and returns to the start position (figure 14.23b). This exercise is substantially more difficult when performed in a unilateral leg stance position.

Figure 14.23
Reverse squats: *(a)* start position, *(b)* end position.

Side Leg Lift

This exercise strengthens hip abductors. The patient kneels and lays sideways on the ball in a position similar the side sit-up position shown in figure 14.21. The top leg is lifted toward the ceiling with the knee extended and the leg in line with the trunk. The raised leg should not move into the flexion plane.

Half Squat

This exercise strengthens the quadriceps. The patient stands with the ball on the wall and with the ball placed in the low back. The feet are positioned shoulder-width apart, and far enough in front of the person so that when he or she squats, the knees do not bend more than 90° (see figure 14.4, p. 429). Additional knee flexion places too much stress on the patellofemoral joint. A patient who has knee pain during this exercise should place the feet farther out or reduce the depth of the squat.

Hamstring Curl

This exercise strengthens the hamstrings. The patient lies supine on the floor with his or her feet on the Swiss ball. The hips are kept off the floor so that the trunk and legs form a straight line, as illustrated in figure 14.15a. While maintaining a hip-elevated position, the patient flexes the knees to move the ball closer to the hips, and then extends the knees to the starting position. A progression includes starting with the arms on the floor and then moving them to the chest and overhead. In another progression the patient first uses both legs, then crosses the uninvolved over the involved leg, and finally uses only the involved leg.

Sidelying Ball Lift

This exercise strengthens the hip and trunk muscles. The patient lies on his or her side with the knees and hips extended; one arm is overhead, and the other is across the front for stabilization as shown in figure 14.24a. The ball is grasped between the legs, and the pelvis is maintained in neutral. Both legs are lifted off the floor as high as possible, with the legs and spine kept straight (figure 14.24b).

Figure 14.24 Sidelying ball lift: *(a)* start position, *(b)* upward lateral movement of the legs.

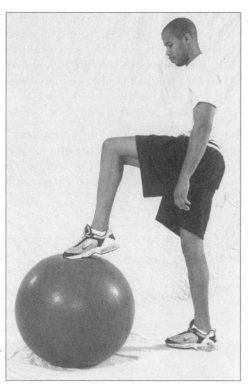

Figure 14.25 Ankle motion exercise.

Ankle Motion Exercise

This is a balance exercise for the lower extremity. The patient stands in pelvic neutral with the uninjured foot on top of the ball; he or she then writes the alphabet with the uninjured foot, using the ball as a base of support (figure 14.25).

Upper-Extremity Exercises

As with the lower-extremity exercises, some of the upper-extremity exercises were described earlier in the section on trunk exercises. Although they are not mentioned here, many upper-extremity exercises using rubber tubing and rubber bands, as well as medicine-ball exercises, become more difficult when performed on the Swiss ball.

Figure 14.26 Prone flys.

Prone Fly

This exercise is used to strengthen scapular retractors. The patient lies prone on the Swiss ball with the ball under the lower abdomen or upper thighs. The legs are straight, with the balls of the feet in contact with the floor. The patient's arms are anterior to the chest and resting on the floor, and elbows are flexed (figure 14.26). The patient lifts the elbows toward the ceiling while keeping the shoulders elevated to about 90° and squeezes the scapulaes together. Weight is used to provide resistance.

Triceps Extension

The patient is reclined with the ball supporting the low back or midback as illustrated in figure 14.15a or seated on the ball. The abdominals are kept tight to maintain pelvic neutral. The arms are overhead with the elbows flexed and hands behind the head. Keeping the arms above the head, the patient extends the elbows.

Push-Ups

The patient lies prone on the ball with hands on the floor and feet elevated. The ball is placed under the lower abdomen or pelvis (figure 14.27a). With the hands positioned as close together as possible and still complete the exercise, the patient performs a push-up, keeping good spinal alignment throughout the motion (figure 14.27b). Progressions of this exercise include placing the ball under the thighs, placing the ball under the legs (figure 14.27c), and reversing the body position so the hands are on the ball and the feet are on the floor (figure 14.27d).

Figure 14.27 Push-up progression: *(a-c)* Progression is provided by increasing the lever-arm length; *(d)* progression is provided by using an unstable base for the arms.

Figure 14.28   Scapular retraction.

Scapular Retraction

This exercise uses the Swiss ball with rubber bands or tubing. The patient sits on the ball, with the feet on a foam roller for a more difficult exercise or on the floor for a less difficult exercise. While maintaining balance on the Swiss ball, the patient pulls the bands and squeezes the scapulae together, keeping the elbows below shoulder level (figure 14.28). Upper-extremity exercises using rubber tubing, medicine balls, and other equipment become more challenging with the patient on a Swiss ball.

FOAM ROLLERS

▶ Foam rollers help to improve joint- and body-position awareness, balance, proprioception, flexibility, and strength. Precautions relate to various skin conditions and various types of hypermobility, and the rehabilitation clinician should keep in mind several contraindications.

Moshe Feldenkrais was one of the first to use rollers as a therapeutic tool. He used rollers in his Feldenkrais Method, discussed earlier in this text (chapter 11). Feldenkrais used wooden rollers until 1972, when he was introduced to **foam rollers** while in the United States.

In recent years, the use of foam rollers has become commonplace within rehabilitation in neurological, orthopedic, and sports medicine facilities. Several annual professional workshops and seminars in foam roller use take place across the country.

Foam rollers are used in therapeutic exercise to improve body awareness and joint-position sense, enhance balance and proprioception, aid in muscle reeducation, and to promote flexibility and strength. Because of its cylindrical shape, the foam roller provides little contact with the floor and moves quickly and easily; standing on the roller challenges the patient's balance reaction. As with the Swiss ball, the roller presents an unstable surface and thus a more challenging platform for performing what are normally easily managed activities. The use of foam rollers offers the patient a diversion from routine exercises and still accomplishes many of the same goals that more traditional exercises do. Rollers are relatively inexpensive and can be used in the treatment facility and at home.

Foam-Roller Design

Most foam rollers are made of Ethafoam, which is a polyethylene product; others are made of polyurethane. They all are cylindrical and come in a variety of lengths, circumferences, and densities. Diameters are 7.6, 10.0, and 15.2 cm (3, 4, and 6 in.). The lengths vary from 30 cm to about 180 cm (1-6 ft). Rollers can also be cut in half longitudinally with a bread knife to form a half roll so one side is flat and the other is a half circle.

The Ethafoam rollers are dense rolls that can support up to 159 kg (350 lb). Because of their buoyancy, patients can also use them in aquatic therex programs. Their density makes them effective for use in soft-tissue and joint mobility exercises, and they are firm enough for muscle strengthening. The Ethafoam rollers can also help to improve proprioception. The softer polyurethane rolls offer more stability. They can be more comfortable to lie on than the Ethafoam rollers, but they tend to lose their shape more quickly and become difficult to roll.

Precautions and Contraindications

Before the rehabilitation clinician uses a foam roller, he or she must observe several precautions and must examine the patient for existing contraindications. If an individual has contusions, acne, or other skin disturbances, the rehabilitation clinician should observe for responses that aggravate the condition.

Patients experiencing temporary conditions of vertigo brought on by ear infections or other disorders should either postpone using a foam roller or should use the roller under careful supervision and be sure to perform slow, controlled, and adequately supported movements.

Hypermobility of joints, postpartum hypermobility, and acute fractures are conditions that require caution in the use of foam rolls. Performing some activities on a foam roller can aggravate these types of hypermobility.

A patient showing signs of nausea, light-headedness, pallor, or shortness of breath should be taken off the foam roller. The few outright contraindications for the use of foam rollers are commonsense ones. Any symptoms of increased pain, dizziness, nausea, or tinnitus are contraindications, as are full-weight-bearing restrictions on segments. Other contraindications not commonly seen in young adults include osteoporosis, connective-tissue disorders such as fibromyalgia and rheumatoid arthritis that are in a flare-up condition, current use of anticoagulant medication, and tumors.

FOAM-ROLLER EXERCISES

▶ Patients can perform foam-roller exercises for the trunk, lower extremity, and upper extremity with or without other equipment such as Swiss balls and rubber tubing and bands.

As with the Swiss-ball exercises, the foam-roller exercises described here do not represent an entire program but serve only as examples. The exercises suggested may give you ideas for others. You can use foam rollers with equipment such as the Swiss ball, rubber tubing and bands, and other exercise equipment. The following exercises are presented according to body segments.

Trunk Exercises

Some of the exercises described here for the trunk may also be used for upper and lower extremities. Some are stretching exercises, some are for strengthening, and others are self-massage techniques.

Quadratus Massage

This exercise relaxes the quadratus lumborum to increase range of motion. The patient lies on a horizontally positioned foam roller with the roller in the small of the back (figure 14.29). The individual rolls to his or her side and gently rolls back and forth over the foam roller to relax the quadratus.

Figure 14.29   Quadratus massage.

Thoracic Massage

This exercise massages the thoracic area to relax muscles and improve range of motion. The patient lies supine on a foam roller positioned perpendicular to the line of the body. The roller is placed under the thoracic region (figure 14.30). The patient supports his or her head in both hands and keeps the buttocks lifted off the floor and the feet flat on the floor. He or she rolls gently up and down from the lower ribs upward to the shoulders.

Low-Back Mobilization

The purpose of this exercise is to improve low-back flexibility. The patient stands with feet shoulder-width apart; the foam roller is hooked under the elbows and across the low back. The patient arches the back into the roller.

Cat Stretch

This is a back-flexibility exercise using two foam rollers. The patient is in a kneeling quadruped position, with both knees on one roller and both hands on another roller. The patient arches the back up as high as possible by tightening the abdominals and then relaxes the back toward the floor.

Quadruped Balance

This exercise develops balance and pelvic stabilization. The patient kneels on one roller and places the hands on a second roller, as in the cat stretch just described. Keeping pelvic neutral throughout the exercise, the patient first lifts one leg and the opposite arm and then reverses the position (figure 14.31).

Figure 14.30
Thoracic massage.

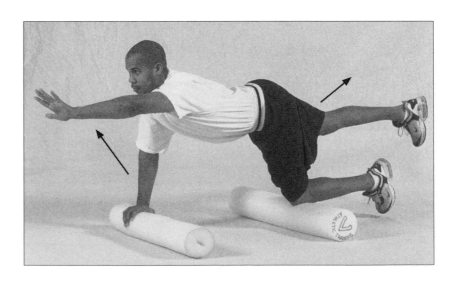

Figure 14.31
Quadruped balance using two foam rollers.

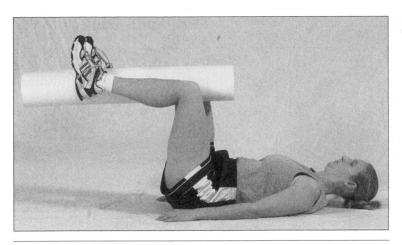

Figure 14.32 Supine lower-abdominal exercise.

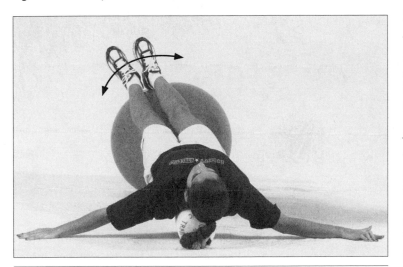

Figure 14.33 Oblique exercise.

Supine Lower Abdominal Exercise

This exercise strengthens the lower abdominal muscles. The patient lies supine with the knees flexed. The roller is placed between the knees (figure 14.32). The patient tightens the lower abdominals and lifts the knees toward the chest, keeping the back flat on the floor. The back should not arch at any time during this exercise.

Supine Oblique Exercise

This exercise strengthens the obliques. The patient lies supine on the foam roller and places the feet on a Swiss ball (figure 14.33). While keeping the knees extended, the patient rolls the ball from side to side. The back should not arch.

Abdominal Crunch

This exercise strengthens the abdominals. The patient assumes a kneeling position; the roller is under both knees, and the hands are flat on the floor. The patient pulls the knees up toward the chest as the foam roller moves down the legs. This exercise becomes more difficult if the patient begins the exercise in a prone position (figure 14.34a) and moves to the same end position as in the easier exercise (figure 14.34b).

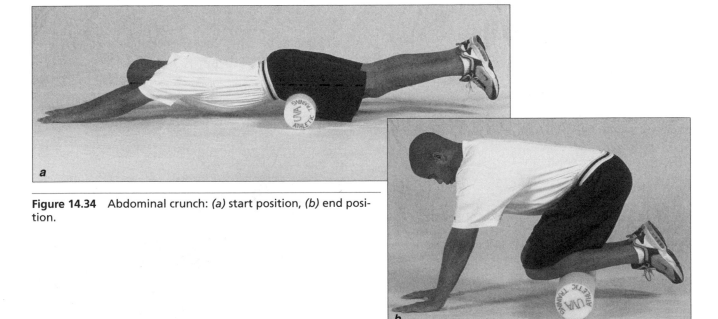

Figure 14.34 Abdominal crunch: *(a)* start position, *(b)* end position.

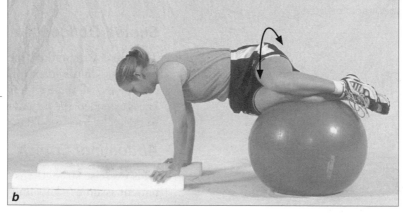

Rotational Crunch

This exercise strengthens the obliques. The patient lies prone on a Swiss ball with the thighs on the ball and each hand on one of two ½ rollers, flat side down (figure 14.35a). The patient brings the knees toward the chest and then rotates the hips, first to one side and then to the other, so that the bottom lateral thigh rests on the ball (figure 14.35b). A pelvic neutral position is maintained throughout the exercise. This exercise becomes more difficult with the half rollers placed flat side up.

Figure 14.35 Rotational crunch: *(a)* start position, *(b)* with knees up, patient rolls side to side from one hip to the other.

Bridging

This exercise strengthens hamstrings, hip extensors, and back extensors. The patient lies supine on the floor with the feet placed on a horizontally positioned foam roller (figure 14.36a). The patient lifts the hips upward and rolls the roller toward the buttocks. This activity becomes more difficult if the individual performs it with only one leg at a time (figure 14.36b). A pelvic neutral position should be maintained throughout.

Figure 14.36   Bridging: *(a)* start position, *(b)* end position.

Figure 14.37 Quadratus lumborum strengthening.

Quadratus Lumborum Strengthening

The patient lies supine longitudinally on the foam roller. The knees are flexed and the feet flat on the floor. The shoulders and elbows are at 90° in a goalpost position. The patient brings the right elbow and the right rear pocket toward each other without changing the arm position and then repeats the movement to the opposite side (figure 14.37).

Lower-Extremity Exercises

Foam-roller activities for the lower extremities can include techniques for massage, flexibility, strengthening, and proprioception.

Iliotibial-Band Massage

This exercise massages the iliotibial band (ITB) to increase flexibility. The patient lies on his or her left side with the left elbow flexed. The roller is placed under the left thigh, and the left leg is positioned under and in front of the right leg (figure 14.38). The patient gently moves the roller from the knee to the hip. Reverse position to massage the right ITB. Areas of tenderness will be areas of soft-tissue restriction. This massage causes no discomfort in non-restricted areas.

Figure 14.38 Iliotibial-band massage.

Quadriceps Massage

This exercise massages the quadriceps to increase flexibility. The patient lies prone on the floor with the roller in a horizontal position under and across the thighs. The individual then places his or her upper-body weight on the hands and pulls the body back and forth with the arms, allowing the roller to gently move up and down the anterior thighs.

Figure 14.39
Standing balance.

Standing Balance

This exercise improves balance. The patient stands with both feet on a horizontally positioned foam roller (figure 14.39). To prevent falling, the patient needs to mount the roller using both hands to grasp a support structure, such as a table, handrail, or spotters, and must be secure before letting go with the hands. It may be necessary for the clinician to assist with additional manual support in the initial attempts to balance. If this exercise is too difficult, the patient can begin by standing on one or two half rollers with the flat side up, that is, by using either one half roller for each foot or only one half roller for both feet. You can make this exercise more difficult by having the patient stand only on one leg. Standing in a forward-backward tandem position on the roller is also more advanced.

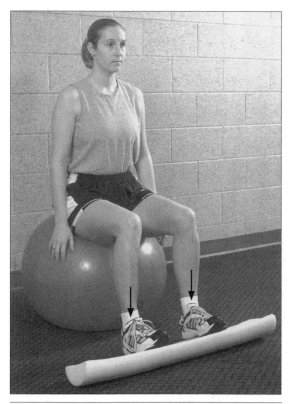

Figure 14.40   Sitting soleus stretch.

Anterior Tibialis Stretch

The patient kneels on the floor. The foam roller is on the ground behind the body and crosswise with the body. The dorsum of the distal feet are placed on top of the roller. The patient then leans back to sit on his or her heels while keeping the distal feet on the roller.

Gastrocnemius Stretch

The patient stands on the flat portion of a half roller, with the balls of the feet on the roller and the heels on the floor. The knees are extended but not locked, and the body leans forward slightly while the patient places the hands on the wall or other structure for balance and support.

Soleus Stretch

The patient sits in a chair and places the balls of the feet on a half roller, flat side up (figure 14.40). He or she then pushes the heels to the floor.

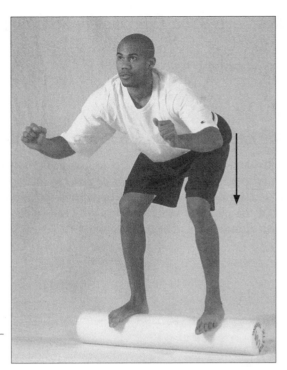

Figure 14.41
Squats.

Squats

The patient stands on the roller, with the roller in a horizontal position and the feet about shoulder-width apart. The patient squats and raises the arms in front to maintain balance (figure 14.41). This is an advanced exercise that requires good balance and postural control. The patient may need stabilizing assistance from a spotter or need to use one hand on a stable object until balance is maintained.

Upper-Extremity Exercises

Upper-extremity exercises on the foam roller can begin early in a therapeutic exercise program in the form of flexibility exercises and then progress to open and closed kinetic chain activities as the patient improves.

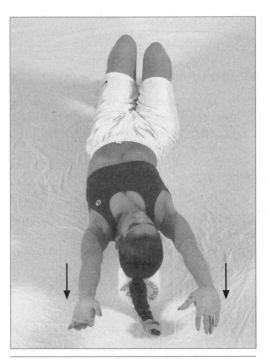

Figure 14.42 Arm stretches.

Arm Stretches

The patient lies supine longitudinally on the roller with the knees flexed and feet flat on the floor. The patient then moves the arms into 90° abduction, then 135°, and then overhead (figure 14.42). During each of these movements, he or she attempts to pull the arms to the floor.

Push-Ups

The patient kneels on the floor, places the hands shoulder-width apart on the roller, and then performs a push-up. With the hands on the roller, the progression for this exercise is from the modified position on the knees, to the regular position, to a position in which another roller is placed under the knees, and finally to a position in which either an additional roller is placed under the shins or the legs are placed on a Swiss ball.

Figure 14.43 Resistive-band exercise in standing.

Resistive-Band Exercises in Standing

Isolated or combined movement patterns using rubber tubing or bands can be performed on foam rollers. The beginning-level exercise is performed on half foam rollers, flat side up (figure 14.43), and the more advanced exercise is performed with the patient's standing on a full foam roller.

Resistive-Band Bench Press in Supine

The patient lies in a supine hooklying position with the knees flexed and the feet flat on the floor. The resistive band is secured under the roller at chest level. The patient pushes the hand toward the ceiling until the elbow is in full extension. This exercise can be performed with either one arm or both (figure 14.44).

Figure 14.44 Resistive-band bench press in supine.

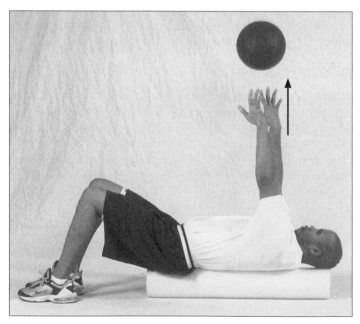

Ball Toss in Supine

The patient lies in a supine hooklying position on the roller with the knees flexed and feet flat on the floor. He or she then tosses a ball, either a Swiss ball or a medicine ball, toward the ceiling (figure 14.45).

Triceps Press

The patient sits on the floor with the knees extended out in front. One roller is placed under the ankles, and a small roller is placed on each side of the body near the hips. The patient places his or her hands on the rollers next to the hips and presses down to straighten the elbows and lift the buttocks off the floor. The shoulders should depress as much as possible.

Figure 14.45 Ball toss in supine.

SUMMARY

1. Explain how Swiss balls and foam rollers can increase the challenge of a traditional exercise.

   Swiss balls and foam rollers provide an unstable surface for an exercise. They can be used for open and closed chain activities. They can provide a progression of difficulty to continually challenge the patient as parameters improve. Swiss balls can be used throughout a therapeutic exercise program to offer a number of stimulating challenges to the patient.

2. Identify the rehabilitation parameters that are benefited by the use of Swiss balls or foam rollers.

   Flexibility, strength, muscle endurance, balance, coordination, and joint- and body-position awareness are all stressed with Swiss ball and foam roller activities.

3. Discuss safety factors, precautions, and contraindications relating to the use of Swiss balls and foam rollers.

   For safety, the patient's clothing should be proper athletic wear to allow freedom of movement and should be free of objects such as belt buckles; shoes should have rubber soles to provide traction; bouncing on the ball should not be combined with bending and twisting or rotating of the spine; long hair should be restrained; and exercises should be performed with control and not too quickly. Precautions for the rehabilitation clinician to observe include carefully explaining and demonstrating the exercise before having the patient attempt it, taking proper care of the equipment, fitting the ball correctly, and not using the equipment if you have any doubt about an patient's ability to handle it. Contraindications include fear of falling off the ball or roller, use of any medication that poses a danger, and complaints of increased pain or dizziness.

4. Explain how to properly fit a Swiss ball.

   With the patient sitting on the ball and the feet flat on the floor, the hips and knees should be at 90°.

5. List one exercise each for the trunk, upper extremity, and lower extremity using a Swiss ball, and identify its purpose.

   A bridge is an exercise for strengthening the back extensors; hip rotations in supine are used to gain flexibility and strength of the hip muscles; and a push-up with the feet on the ball can serve as an early upper-extremity strengthening exercise.

6. List one exercise each for the trunk, upper extremity, and lower extremity using foam rollers, and identify its purpose.

   Lying on the foam roller and lowering the knees from the chest is a lower abdominal strengthening exercise; lying sideways on the roller and rolling the lateral thigh along the foam roller is a massage technique for the ITB; and lying with the foam roller down the spine with the arms out to the side is a stretch for the anterior shoulder.

CRITICAL THINKING QUESTIONS

1. Because the Swiss ball can be used early in rehabilitation, you decide to use it in stabilization exercises for weak scapular muscles. Identify three low-level stabilization exercises that would incorporate the Swiss ball. What would be a more rigorous Swiss-ball stabilization exercise? Identify a Swiss-ball exercise that can also be used for the trunk.

2. You have decided to give a Swiss ball to a patient with a back injury. You feel that she is now ready to continue the Swiss-ball exercises on her own at home. You want to limit the number of exercises to 10 so that the patient will be more likely to perform all of them. Identify no more than 10 exercises that you would give this patient, and justify each one.

3. A patient wants to buy a Swiss ball to use at home during the semester break but does not know what size to buy. What guidance would you give him?

4. A patient with weak abdominals is going home for the summer and wants to take with her either a Swiss ball or foam roller, but not both. Which one would you advise her to take with her and why? List four exercises on the piece of equipment you have selected for her to take.

LAB ACTIVITIES

1. Measure your lab partner to select a Swiss ball that is the correct size for her.

2. Of the following Swiss ball exercises, select five trunk exercises to instruct to your lab partner. Be sure to have your "patient" maintain pelvic neutral throughout each exercise. As your partner is performing each exercise, use verbal cues to correct for any errors in his or her performance. Identify the purpose of each exercise.

    a. Bounce and kick
    b. Side foot reach
    c. Lateral glide
    d. Pelvic curls
    e. Trunk rotation in sitting
    f. Trunk rotation in supine
    g. Stretch in kneeling
    h. Lateral stretch
    i. Thoracic stretch
    j. Back extension in prone
    k. Supine leg lift
    l. Hip rotation
    m. Bridging
    n. Prone leg lift
    o. Swimming with 5-lb weights
    p. Seated abdominal strengthening
    q. Ball lift
    r. Side sit-ups
    s. Prone walk-out

3. Of the following Swiss ball exercises, select three lower extremity exercises to instruct to your lab partner. Be sure to have your "patient" maintain pelvic neutral throughout each exercise. As your partner is performing each exercise, use verbal cues to correct for any errors in his performance. Identify the purpose of each exercise.

    a. Side leg lift
    b. Half squat
    c. Reverse squat
    d. Hamstring curl
    e. Sidelying ball lift
    f. Ankle motion exercises

4. Of the following Swiss ball exercises, select three upper extremity exercises to instruct to your lab partner. Be sure to have your "patient" maintain pelvic neutral throughout each exercise. As your partner is performing each exercise, use verbal cues to correct for any errors in his performance. Identify the purpose of each exercise.

   a. Prone flys

   b. Triceps extension

   c. Push-ups

   d. Scapular retraction

5. Create an original Swiss ball exercise that isn't included in your text for the trunk, upper, and lower extremities. Identify the purpose of each exercise.

6. Of the following foam roller exercises, select five trunk activities to instruct to your lab partner. Be sure to have your "patient" maintain pelvic neutral throughout each exercise. As your partner is performing each exercise, use verbal cues to correct for any errors in her performance. Identify the purpose of each exercise.

   a. Quadratus massage

   b. Thoracic massage

   c. Low-back mobilization

   d. Cat stretch

   e. Quadruped balance

   f. Supine lower abdominal exercise

   g. Supine oblique exercise

   h. Abdominal crunch

   i. Rotational crunch

   j. Bridging

   k. Quadratus lumborum strengthening

7. Of the following foam roller exercises, select three lower extremity activities to instruct to your lab partner. Be sure to have your "patient" maintain pelvic neutral throughout each exercise. As your partner is performing each exercise, use verbal cues to correct for any errors in his performance. Identify the purpose of each exercise. You may use either half rollers or full rollers for the exercises.

   a. Iliotibial band massage

   b. Quadratus massage

   c. Standing balance

   d. Anterior tibialis stretch

   e. Gastrocnemius stretch

   f. Soleus stretch

   g. Piriformis stretch

   h. Squats

8. Of the following foam roller exercises, select three upper extremity activities to instruct to your lab partner. Be sure to have your "patient" maintain pelvic neutral throughout each exercise. As your partner is performing each exercise, use verbal cues to correct for any errors in his or her performance. Identify the purpose of each exercise.

   a. Arm stretches

   b. Push-ups

   c. Resistive-band exercises in standing

   d. Resistive-band exercises in supine

   e. Ball toss in supine

   f. Triceps pass

9. Design an exercise for the trunk, lower extremities, and upper extremities using a combination of the Swiss ball and foam roller. Indicate the purpose of each exercise and the muscle(s) it is working.

REFERENCE

Posner-Mayer, J. 1995. *Swiss ball applications for orthopedic and sports medicine*. Denver: Ball Dynamics International.

SUGGESTED READING

Craeger, C.C. 1996. *Therapeutic exercises using foam rollers*. Berthoud, CO: Executive Physical Therapy.

Institute of Physical Art. 1991. *Integrating function: The foam roll approach*. Steamboat Springs, CO: Author.

Therapeutic Exercise for Tendinitis

Objectives

After completing this chapter, you should be able to do the following:

1. Define tendinitis.
2. Discuss various etiologies of tendinitis.
3. Explain the inflammatory response of tendons.
4. Identify parameters governing the initial treatment for tendinitis.
5. Outline the progression of a tendinitis treatment program.

> **D**uring his career, Troy Roberts had seen many athletes with tendinitis. As much as he urged athletes to report early onsets of tendinitis, it seemed that they consistently waited until the problem became much more difficult to treat than it would have been if the athlete had been seen in the early stages of the condition.
>
> Troy knew that tendinitis could not be treated like acute injuries, especially in the beginning. He enjoyed the challenge of treating cases of tendinitis because he had to be a detective to discover the cause and reduce the risk that the tendinitis would return later. As much as he enjoyed the challenge, he often became frustrated with the frequently slow progression of the treatment program. Of course, each patient responded differently to the treatment; but Troy realized that if the injury were treated early, improvements could occur much sooner than they would when the patient delayed reporting the injury, thinking it would go away on its own. If only there were some way he could impress on athletes the importance of early intervention.

■ Leaders don't create followers, they create more leaders.

Tom Peters, *Fast Company*

Although tendinitis can affect many body segments, it is worthwhile to discuss this condition in a separate chapter rather than including it in chapters on specific body segments. Looking at tendinitis separately makes sense because treatment of tendinitis differs from treatment of acute conditions, yet treatment of tendinitis in one area is similar to treatment of tendinitis in other areas.

TERMINOLOGY

▶ Tendinitis is the global, abeit inaccurate, term used to identify an inflammation in a tendon area.

There are many variations of tendinitis, and various terms are used to describe these conditions. These terms relate to the specific tissue involved. They can be confusing, so we will clarify them briefly here. **Tenosynovitis** is an inflammation of the synovial sheath that surrounds a tendon. **Paratendinitis** is an inflammation and thickening of the paratenon sheath of tendons that do not have synovial sheaths. **Tendinitis,** also spelled **tendonitis,** is the global term used to identify an inflammation of a tendon. **Tendinosis** involves microscopic tears of the tendon caused by repeated trauma. Whereas it is nearly impossible for the rehabilitation clinician to differentiate between a tenosynovitis and tendinitis and because the symptoms and treatment are similar, the global term, tendinitis, is commonly used in referring to inflammations involving tendons or their sheaths. Although terms such as tendinopathy or tendon stress syndrome would be more accurate, the term tendinitis is the generally accepted, albeit incorrect, term used to describe inflammation of tendinous origin.

TENDON STRUCTURE

▶ The basic structure of a tendon consists of collagen bundles containing fibroblasts and extracellular matrix. When a load is applied to a tendon it becomes stiffer and is subjected to stress-strain principles.

To develop an appreciation of tendinitis and its treatment, you must first understand the structure and function of a tendon. The specific structure varies somewhat from one tendon to another, but all tendons contain certain basic components. Normal tendon is composed of collagen bundles that contain fibroblasts and an extracellular matrix. The extracellular matrix is composed primarily of water, type I collagen, and ground substance. Type I collagen is a tendon's primary fiber component. Tendons are viscoelastic because of glycosaminoglycans, glycoproteins, and other substances in the ground substance that form a gel-like structure that supports the extracellular matrix. Because tendons are viscoelastic, they take on all the properties of viscoelastic tissue discussed in chapter 5. The tendon's blood vessels and nerves are contained in the paratenon, the loose areolar tissue that surrounds the collagen bundles. Synovial sheaths surround tendons that are subjected to greater than normal friction stresses, such as the Achilles and biceps tendons. If a sheath is present, it contains the primary blood supply for the tendon. Sheaths also normally contain a very small amount of fluid and serve to reduce friction in these high-stress areas.

In normal resting, a tendon has a crimped or wavy appearance, but as a load is applied to the tendon it becomes stiffer and is subject to the stress-strain principles discussed in chapter 5. A tendon's tensile strength is determined by how well it resists the stress applied to it. One estimate is that a tendon's tensile strength is about four times the maximal force produced by its muscle (Elliot 1965). Because tendon tensile strength is so much greater than muscle force generation, there must be factors other than tensile strength that enter into tendinitis injuries. Exactly what these additional factors are has yet to be determined.

ETIOLOGY

▶ The fundamental cause of any form of tendinitis, including conditions resulting from repetitive stress and those resulting from acute trauma, is excessive stress on the tendon.

Although tendinitis may have several causes, the consequence is the same: too much stress applied to the tendon. Excessive stress may take the form of cumulative trauma typically seen in overuse injuries, or may take the form of acute trauma such as a direct blow. Most cases of tendinitis are considered overuse injuries. In overuse injuries, cumulative trauma results in a breakdown of otherwise normal tissue. In traumatic tendinitis, the tendon suffers a sudden severe injury and does not have sufficient time to recover before additional loads are applied to it, so breakdown occurs. Pain, swelling, and reduced function are the clinical manifestations of tendinitis.

One of the most difficult problems for the rehabilitation clinician in dealing with overuse tendinitis is identifying where the tendon is in the healing process. This is not the case for traumatic tendinitis, because this condition results from a specific incident and the healing process is easy to identify. The injured individual's symptoms and response to the first treatment may be the best means of identifying the healing stage for overuse tendinitis. An injury's healing stage is important to pinpoint because this is what determines the treatment course, as outlined later in this chapter.

Tendinitis can occur in the upper and lower extremities. Rotator cuff tendinitis, bicipital tendinitis, and lateral and medial epicondylitis are common upper-extremity tendinitis conditions. Common lower-extremity tendinitis sites include the patella, posterior tibialis, peroneal, and Achilles tendons. Although most believe that tendinitis occurs because of chronic overload situations, the specific types of stress and the load magnitudes that lead to tendinitis are still mysteries.

Common etiology for tendinitis includes loading errors; technique and execution errors; structural abnormalities; inappropriate equipment, play or work conditions, and training or standing surfaces; and muscle imbalances. Loading errors include excessive increases in the progressive overload, excessive durations or distances, and excessive increases in speed. Examples are increasing hill-running workouts in speed, distance, or incline; increasing the intensity of jump workouts; throwing too far, too hard, too fast, or for too many repetitions; and typing at a computer too long without a break. Any type of loading error can be the problem, but they all essentially increase the workload to a level greater than the tendon is able to tolerate. As a rule of thumb, an increased workload of 10% to 15% a week is usually safe and tolerable.

Technique and execution errors can place additional stress on a tendon. For example, if a tennis player hits a backhand late, extensor tendons on the lateral epicondyle suffer significant increases in stress.

Inappropriate equipment and standing or training surfaces can alter forces placed on the body. For example, if the tennis player's racket grip is too large, the athlete must grip harder to hold onto the racket. This increases the stresses applied to the elbow where the tendons insert. If an athlete ties his or her shoes too tightly, the foot's extensor tendons incur increased pressure and tendinitis can develop. Playing basketball on a vinyl-covered concrete floor rather than a force-absorbing suspended wood floor can make a player susceptible to patellar tendinitis. Using a too-short computer desk chair can lead to carpal tunnel syndrome.

Structural abnormalities and muscle imbalances are intrinsic factors that place additional stresses on tendons. If a patient excessively pronates when running, the medial Achilles and posterior tibialis tendons are placed on excessive stretch during the activity. If the rotator cuff is weak, the humerus does not glide into the inferior aspect of the glenoid during shoulder motion so soft tissues become subject to impingement, especially during arm elevation activities.

Two additional factors that may lead to tendinitis are circulation and friction. Reduced circulation is a major detriment to a tendon's health. Two tendons particularly prone to tendinitis, the Achilles and the supraspinatus tendon, both have areas of reduced circulation that are frequent sites of tendinitis. Tendons that are compressed against bone or retinacular pulleys and tendons that are subject to high-friction forces are susceptible to tendinitis. For example, the biceps tendon's common site of inflammation is the point at which the transverse ligament holds the tendon in the bicipital groove.

Overload may include not only exaggerated tensile stresses, but also an accumulation of internal and external forces, producing stress during activity. These stresses cause the tendon to alter its behavior in an attempt to adapt to them. As with muscle, bone, and other structures, tendons respond to overload stresses by hypertrophying and remodeling. However, before their strength increases, they undergo a period of breakdown that leaves them weaker than normal. Although it is not known how long this process takes, one postulate is that if the tendon is overloaded again before it is permitted to remodel and adapt, breakdown can occur (Archambault, Wiley, and Bray 1995).

How much stress is enough to cause hypertrophy of the tendon, without overloading it to cause breakdown, becomes the question—a question that researchers have not yet answered. From a clinical standpoint, the best answer in the absence of definitive research conclusions must come from the observational skills of the clinician. Monitoring the patient's tendon responses to stress and adapting the therapeutic exercise program accordingly is the best method, at present, for determining appropriate load applications. Increase in pain, crepitus, or edema are clinical signs that overload has been excessive.

TENDON RESPONSE

▶ Tendinitis involves changes within a tendon such as thickening of the tendon's sheath, areas of fibrosis and tissue thickening, and formation of nodules. Tendons break down when they incur stresses that are too great or when they are not given enough time to recover from a stress.

When a tendon becomes inflamed, a number of changes occur. The magnitude of these changes is governed by the extent of the inflammation. At the macroscopic level, the tendon's sheath is thickened. Additionally, areas of fibrosis and connective tissue thickening can often be palpated. Nodules can be palpated on superficial tendons, and adhesions can be present. At the histological level, chronic inflammatory cells and chemicals, discussed in chapter 2, are prevalent, including myofibroblasts, fibroblasts, fibronectin, and fibrinogen. Additional changes include a reduction in vascularity, a fraying and splitting of collagen fibers, and the presence of type III collagen. As you will recall, type III collagen has less tensile strength than type I collagen.

How a tendon responds to stresses depends on its circulation, its ability to withstand stresses, and the quantity of load applied. Healthy tendons that receive appropriate stress loads are able to increase strength through matrix adaptations. If loads are excessive and time for recovery is insufficient, the tendon eventually breaks down (figure 15.1) and symptoms occur. Rehabilitation intervention then becomes necessary for the tendon's recovery and ability to restore normal function.

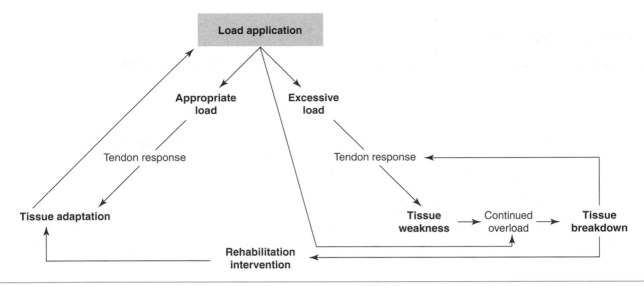

Figure 15.1 Load application and tendon response: When applied tendon loads are excessive without sufficient recovery time, tissue breakdown occurs. Healing tendons are maintained when load applications permit adequate tissue adaptation.

GENERAL TREATMENT

▶ Guidelines for treatment that relate to all forms of tendinitis include two critical components: identifying the cause of the condition and modifying the causative factor. Selection of treatment depends on where in the healing process the tendon is.

Treatment of tendinitis includes the identification and modification of those factors causing the patient's tendinitis. This aspect cannot be overemphasized. If the rehabilitation clinician does not correct the causative factor, the treatment will be in vain. The patient will be plagued with recurrent episodes of tendinitis and ultimately develop a chronic condition that will be frustrating for both the patient and clinician.

To identify the cause, the rehabilitation clinician must take a thorough history, rely on the patient, coach, or supervisor for information about load changes and poor technique; personally observe the patient's execution; investigate equipment use and play or work surfaces; and evaluate for muscle imbalances and structural abnormalities. To prevent the tendinitis from recurring, each causative factor must be changed before the patient can be safely returned to full participation.

The initial treatment decision is the most difficult. The goal is to help the patient progress without aggravating the injury. Lacking knowledge of where in the healing process the tendon is makes accomplishing this goal challenging. Before therapeutic exercises can be instituted, the inflammatory process must be brought under control. The intensity of the symptoms can sometimes guide you in determining early treatments. Because pain is a highly subjective symptom, it can be difficult to accurately assess the intensity and stage of the inflammation. In these situations, it is better to err on the side of caution and do less treatment than to provide more treatment and increase the irritation. The accuracy of this trial-and-error approach to initial treatment depends on your knowledge of the patient's injury responses and tissue healing phases, skill in observation and history taking, and good judgment. If the tendon becomes more irritable because of your treatment, you know that the tendinitis is now acutely inflamed, and you can gear future treatment accordingly. If the first treatment either improves the symptoms or has no effect, treatment can advance to the next level.

Although most chronic tendinitis is in the remodeling stage of healing, this is not always the case. As already noted, the symptoms serve as the primary guidelines for determining the intensity of the inflammation: The more intense and prolonged the symptoms, the more severe the inflammation. General guidelines based on work by Stanish et al (2000) can help you ascertain the intensity of the inflammation and select an appropriate initial treatment (table 15.1). For example, if the patient has Achilles tendon pain while walking to class, you know the inflammation is acute and the patient will be able to tolerate little exercise. On the other hand, if the individual has Achilles pain only while running, the initial treatment can include therapeutic exercises.

Table 15.1

Tendinitis Classifications

Intensities	Level	Pain occurrence	Activity restriction
Mild	1	No Pain	No restriction
	2	Pain with extreme exertion that stops when activity stops	No restriction
Moderate	3	Pain with extreme exertion that lasts 1-2 h afterward	Can limit extreme exertion but has little effect on normal workouts
	4	Pain with moderate exertion that lasts 4-6 h afterward	Inability to perform at normal level or to perform some activities
Severe	5	Pain with any exertion that rapidly increases in itensity and lasts 8-24 h	Inability to perform any sport or work activity
	6	Pain during even daily activities	Inability to perform any sport or work activity and possible difficulty with some daily activities

Adapted from Curwin and Stanish 1984.

It is important to continually monitor the tendon's response to treatment throughout the rehabilitation program. Pain and swelling are key signs of inflammation that should be respected and regarded with care. Any increase in symptoms indicates an increase in the inflammation and is the result of recent activity. Thermal or electrical modalities and medication, as well as a reduction in activity can be used to relieve symptom exacerbations.

Therapeutic exercises are a critical aspect of tendinitis treatment, but they must be provided only when appropriate; otherwise they can aggravate the condition. When exercises are used, flexibility exercises are usually a chief component. Concentric and eccentric strengthening exercises stress the tendon and play a vital role in preparing the tendon to for normal functional activities.

SPECIFIC TREATMENT

▶ Components of specific treatment programs for tendinitis may include relief of pain and inflammation in addition to exercises in a progression that is consistent with the phases of the condition.

A tendinitis rehabilitation program follows a logical progression that is carefully designed to allow the patient to advance to full participation and normal activity. Figure 15.2 depicts this rehabilitation progression for tendinitis. The progression consists of five phases that are determined by the tendon's healing stage and its response to the treatment parameters within each phase. Despite this outline of phases, each patient's progression from one phase to another must be individually decided. At no time do you want an exacerbation of symptoms from one treatment session to the next. If this happens, it is essential that you return the patient to the previous level and allow the tendon time to adapt to that stress level before advancing the person to the next level.

Early tendinitis rehabilitation is similar to early rehabilitation of other injuries. In addition to maintaining the patient's cardiovascular conditioning level and the parameters of the uninvolved segments and extremities, the rehabilitation clinician uses techniques to relieve the pain and inflammation. The physician may have prescribed anti-inflammatory medication. Modalities that can be used to relieve the pain and inflammation include pulsed ultrasound, iontophoresis, phonophoresis, and electrical stimulation.

See Craig Denegar, Ethan Saliba, and Susan Saliba's (2005) text, *Therapeutic Modalities for Musculoskeletal Injuries, Second Edition,* for more specific information on modalities most appropriate for treatment of tendinitis.

Figure 15.2 Tendinitis treatment phases and rehabilitation: Emphasis in phase I is on reducing the inflammation. Phase II begins with flexibility exercises once the inflammation subsides. As the patient's injury improves, phase III includes the addition of strength exercises. Phase IV begins with agility activities and eventually progresses to phase V, where functional activities are added in preparation for return to full participation.

Adapted, by permission, from P.A. Houlgum, 1986, "A clinical view of causes and cures for Achilles tendinitis in runner," *Topics in Acute Care Trauma Rehabilitation* 1(2): 55–56.

	Start of program				End of program
Functional activities					
Agility					
Strength					
Endurance					
Flexibility					
Modalities					
Exercises for uninvolved areas and cardiovascular					
Phases	Phase I Tendinitis classification levels 5, 6	Phase II Tendinitis classification levels 3, 4	Phase III Tendinitis classification levels 2, 3	Phase IV Tendinitis classification levels 2, 3	Phase V Tendinitis classification levels 1, 2

Cross-friction massage, described in chapter 6, helps to release adhesions between newly formed collagen and adjacent structures. These adhesions can cause continued discomfort by preventing normal tissue mobility and irritating the local tissue when movement is attempted. The cross-friction massage can also exert tensile force on the tendon by causing a bowstring effect (Gross 1992).

As the tendon is able to tolerate additional stress, therapeutic exercises begin. The tendon should be at least in the proliferation phase. Exercises should certainly begin if the tendon is in the remodeling stage. In the inflammation phase, passive motion is useful because it does not stress the tissue but does assist in tissue organization. Loss of flexibility, a contributing factor to tendinitis, is seen in many cases. Flexibility exercises should usually be a part of the program and should start in phase II.

Strengthening exercises can apply stress to a tendon. Low-load, high-repetition exercises can be useful for increasing muscle endurance and strength as discussed in chapter 7. Endurance activities put less stress on the tendon and still permit strength gains, but the patient's response to these activities should be carefully monitored. The patient begins strengthening with endurance exercises and he or she can often advance relatively rapidly to exercises that emphasize strength. How quickly this occurs depends on the tendon's response to the activities.

Initial strength activities may include concentric activities. Eccentric exercises, however, are an important part of most therapeutic exercise programs for tendinitis. Stanish et al. (2000) advocate using three sets of 10 repetitions of eccentric exercise, beginning with a slow movement and progressing to a moderately fast and then to a fast motion as the tendon tolerates. Such a program for Achilles tendinitis, for example, starts with three sets of 10 heel raises at a slow speed on days 1 and 2, progresses to a moderate speed on days 3 and 4, and then progresses to a fast speed on days 5 and 6. This cycle is repeated when additional resistance is provided on day 7 (table 15.2). The patient performs stretching exercises before and after the resistance series. If pain occurs during the first two sets, the stress is too much for the tendon, and the patient should return to the preceding level. Stanish et al. (2000) suggest that if pain occurs during the last set, the exercise is at an appropriate level for the tendon.

This progression is based on the force-velocity relationship of muscle, discussed in chapter 5; according to this principle, the faster the eccentric activity, the greater the force exerted. The tension on the tendon is increased when the speed of the eccentric movement is increased. This progression allows for a gradual buildup in overload and increases strength output as the tendon's tolerance improves.

Table 15.2
Eccentric Exercise Progression

Day	Speed of movement	Reps	Sets
1	Slow	3	10
2	Slow	3	10
3	Moderate	3	10
4	Moderate	3	10
5	Fast	3	10
6	Fast	3	10
7			

Increase resistance

Adapted from Curwin and Stanish 2000.

During the last half of Phase III, when strength is the primary emphasis and the tendon is tolerating eccentric and concentric exercises, the patient can progress to plyometric exercises. These should be low-level and low-impact exercises and should progress as the patient tolerates.

Within this period the patient transitions to Phase IV, agility becomes the primary focus. Strength and flexibility exercises continue, but the activities become more strenuous as the patient is prepared for the final phase in which functional activities are the primary thrust. It bears repeating here that if symptoms return or become exaggerated during any progression, the patient should remain at the lower level for a couple of days more to allow the tendon additional time for adaptation to stress at that level.

EXAMPLES OF TENDINITIS CASES

The best way to demonstrate rehabilitation for tendinitis injuries is to provide examples. This section presents two examples, one for the lower extremity and one for the upper extremity. For one final example, you will be asked to outline an appropriate rehabilitation program.

Lower-Extremity Case

A 20-year-old collegiate cross country runner, Sally, presented with complaints of right Achilles pain that had begun about three months earlier. She usually ran about 65 km (about 40 miles) a week on varying terrain. At first she had pain only when running hills, but at the time she came to the clinic she was experiencing pain even when walking across campus. She finally sought treatment because the intensity of the pain made it impossible to run.

Examination

On examination, Sally had a mildly antalgic gait. She had prolonged pronation in the stance phase of gait. She was unable to hop on the right leg because of pain. Although Sally said that she performed stretching exercises, her ankle dorsiflexion was 0° when the rearfoot was stabilized in subtalar neutral. Palpation revealed swelling along the Achilles tendon and a painful nodule about 8 cm (3 in.) above the tendon's distal insertion.

Treatment

Sally was instructed to stop running for the time being. She was advised to continue her cardiovascular conditioning either in a pool or by performing stationary cycling using only the left leg. She could continue any weight exercises with the upper extremities, left lower extremity, and trunk, but was instructed not to use the right leg for any exercise.

Sally was given crutches and instructed in partial weight bearing on the right. Right lower-extremity weight bearing was allowed only to the extent that her gait was pain free. Sally's first treatment included the use of phonophoresis, ice, and strapping to reduce her excessive pronation.

On the next day Sally returned, feeling better. The phonophoresis treatment was repeated. Cross-friction massage was used, first in nontender areas and then on the nodule and in other tender areas as Sally was able to tolerate. The strapping helped to reduce the pain, so Sally was measured for orthotics as a permanent correction for her excessive pronation. Ice was applied as a final treatment.

By her third visit Sally was able to walk around campus without pain, so the use of crutches was discontinued. She was instructed in proper stretching exercises for the gastrocnemius and soleus. She was also started on a progressive isotonic exercise program of three sets of 20 repetitions of bilateral heel raises, then unilateral heel raises, then heel raises with weights. Each level of isotonic exercise began with slow repetitions and advanced to medium then fast repetitions before progressing to the next isotonic exercise. She continued with the phonophoresis for one more week. She was taught how to self-administer cross-friction massage.

Exercises were then advanced to include trampoline jumping activities, rapid heel drops on a step, lateral-movement exercises, and fast walking. Fast walking progressed to alternately walking and jogging, then jogging, then running on flat surfaces, and finally running hills.

Upper-Extremity Case

Tom, a 24-year-old, right-handed baseball pitcher, was seen because of pain in the right shoulder. He reported that the pain was located over the deltoid tubercle and that it sometimes radiated down the lateral arm to the elbow. He was unable to sleep on his right side. The pain had started about two months before, in the beginning of the season after Tom had pitched seven long innings in a game. He usually had pain during the last two innings that he pitched, especially with curve balls; the pain would last for about 2 or 3 h after he had finished pitching. He was pitching more during the current season than he had the year before. In the off-season, he had fallen while skiing, landing on his right shoulder but did not think at the time that the shoulder was injured. It was just sore for a couple of days, and he did not seek any medical attention. During preseason, the flu kept Tom out of most of the regular preseason conditioning program.

Examination

Active range of motion and overpressure of the neck were normal. Shoulder range of motion was normal for a pitcher, but Tom had pain during the middle arc of shoulder elevation, especially abduction. Weakness was present, and Tom complained of pain with resisted manual muscle tests to lateral rotation and abduction in the scapular plane. He had shoulder tenderness when he put his hand behind his back and raised it upward along his back. There was tenderness to palpation of the greater tubercle. The findings were consistent with a tendinitis of the supraspinatus. Tom's history indicated that the irritability of the tendon was moderate.

Treatment

Because the injury was in the moderate irritability stage (according to Stanish et al. [2000] tendinitis classification system), Tom was able to begin exercises on the first treatment. The first treatment included concentric exercises consisting of manual resistance to the rotator cuff. Scapular rotator muscle exercises were also started. All exercises were performed in a pain-free range of motion. Ice application ended the treatment session. Home exercises included three sets of 20 repetitions with rubber bands for lateral rotation and abduction in a pain-free range of motion. Tom was told that he could also do scapular rotator exercises, such as push-ups, seated push-ups, and flys, as long as they were pain free.

The rotator cuff exercises progressed with the shoulder at 90°. Agility and plyometric exercises with medicine balls and rubber tubing, as well as body-weight-resisted exercises, were added.

A throwing progression similar to the one outlined in chapter 10 was given Tom. He began with tosses, progressed to throwing, and increased the speed and distance of the throws as he was able to tolerate.

A Challenging Case

Joe, a 19-year-old, right-handed tennis player, complains of right elbow pain. The pain is located over the lateral elbow and sometimes radiates down the dorsal forearm. It began about four months ago, about three weeks after Joe had bought a new tennis racket and started playing in two leagues. He stopped playing for a month until he was pain free, but when he went back to playing, the pain returned. He plays or practices tennis daily. He has noticed that the elbow especially bothers him on his tennis backhand, when he attempts to lift heavy objects, and when he shakes hands.

Examination

The right elbow and forearm have full range of motion in all planes. The neck and shoulder also have normal motion. There is pain to resisted wrist extension. Joe's grip strength on the right is 8 kg (17.6 lb) weaker than that on the left. Palpation of the lateral epicondyle reveals swelling over the epicondyle and tenderness to even light palpation. There is some tenderness to palpation extending into the proximal wrist extensor muscle bellies in the forearm.

Questions for Analysis

1. What will you include in your first treatment session?

2. What instructions will you give Joe about what he should and should not be doing at home?

3. How will you advance him in his program?

4. What exercises will you include?

SUMMARY

1. Define tendinitis.

   Tendinitis is an inflammation of a tendon, its paratenon, or its synovial sheath. Unless visualized in surgery, the precise structure involved is difficult to determine.

2. Discuss various etiologies of tendinitis.

   Tendinitis can occur as a traumatic or an overuse condition. The most common cause is excessive or repetitive stress: The tendon breaks down because cumulative trauma is applied without an opportunity for the tendon to recover before additional stress is applied. Abnormal stress resulting in tendon breakdown occurs most commonly because of loading errors; technique and execution errors; inappropriate equipment, play or work conditions, or training or working surfaces; structural abnormalities; or muscle imbalances.

3. Explain the inflammatory response of tendons.

   The inflammatory response in tendinitis reduces the tendon's tensile strength because the quantity of type I collagen normally present is reduced through damage, and type III collagen becomes a significant structure of the tendon. This makes the tendon susceptible to tears when tendinitis is present.

4. Identify parameters governing the initial treatment for tendinitis.

Identifying the stage of the tendinitis is fundamental to deciding what should be included in the first treatment. The identification is based on the patient's history and complaints of pain and restriction of activity. The stage of the tendinitis determines the treatment; the more advanced the tendinitis, the more careful the rehabilitation clinician needs to be and the more conservative the course of treatment should be.

5. Outline the progression of a tendinitis treatment program.

Treatment for tendinitis is divided into five phases. In addition to correcting the cause and maintaining the conditioning status of unaffected segments, treatments should address restoration of flexibility, muscle endurance, strength, agility, and functional performance. These goals are accomplished by careful progression of the program, beginning with modalities if the tendon is very inflamed and progressing to cross-friction massage and exercises as tolerated. Observation by the rehabilitation clinician and reports by the patient regarding the tendon's response to treatment determine the rate of progression. If the tendon responds negatively to the treatment, the rehabilitation clinician should return the patient to the previous exercise stress level and resume modalities as indicated. To reduce the chance of recurrences, it is important that the rehabilitation clinician identify and correct the underlying precipitating factor.

CRITICAL THINKING QUESTIONS

1. A patient with Achilles tendinitis has advanced nicely over the past three weeks of treatment. He has responded well to all therapeutic exercises. Today, however, he returns for additional treatment, complaining that since yesterday's treatment he has experienced the same pain that he had at first. Yesterday you increased the number of repetitions of the exercises he had been doing. What will your treatment today include? What will your criteria be for again attempting the program you tried yesterday?

2. A tennis player reports that she has tennis elbow for the second time this season. Last year she experienced the condition toward the end of the season, but with rest it went away. She wants to know what you will do for her, why this problem is recurring, and how it differs from a forearm strain she had two years ago. Explain how you will answer her questions.

3. A basketball player who has been unable to run for the past six weeks because of peroneal tendinitis has responded well to your rehabilitation program. He is now ready to start running. What will the first day's running program be, and how will you have him progress to normal running activities?

LAB ACTIVITIES

1. Perform the following heel raise exercises on a stair ledge:
   a. Slow-speed drop of the heels from the top of a heel raise, 3 × 10; rest 2 min.
   b. Moderate-speed drop of the heels from the top of a heel raise, 3 × 10; rest 2 min.
   c. Fast-speed drop of the heels from the top of a heel raise, 3 × 10; rest 2 min.

   When during each set of exercises did you begin to feel a burn in your calf? At which speed did the exercise seem the easiest? Why?

2. If you are treating a patient with an Achilles tendinitis, explain ways you could increase the progression of an eccentric exercise program other than increasing speed.

3. Perform the following wrist extension exercises using a 5 lb. or 8 lb. weight, 3 × 20, with the wrist hanging over the edge of a table top:

   a. Slow-speed drop into full wrist flexion from full wrist extension

   b. Moderate-speed drop into full wrist flexion from full wrist extension

   c. Fast-speed drop into full wrist flexion from full wrist extension

   Where did you feel the burn occur? Did the repetition at which the burn began vary for each speed? At which speed did the weight seem the lightest? Why?

3. If you are treating a patient with tennis elbow, explain ways you could increase the eccentric program's progression other than increasing speed.

REFERENCES

Archambault, J.M., Wiley, J.P, and R.C. Bray. 1995. Exercise loading of tendons and the development of overuse injuries. *Sports Medicine* 20:77-89.

Stanish, W.D, Curwin, S. and S. Mandel. 2000. *Tendinitis: Its etiology and treatment.* New York: Oxford University Press.

Denegar, C., E. Saliba, and S. Saliba. 2005. *Therapeutic modalities for musculoskeletal injuries,* 2nd ed. Champaign, IL: Human Kinetics.

Elliot, D.H. 1965. Structure and function of mammalian tendon. *Biological Reviews* 40:392-421.

Gross, M.T. 1992. Chronic tendinitis: Pathomechanics of injury, factors affecting the healing response, and treatment. *Journal of Orthopaedic & Sports Physical Therapy* 16:248-261.

Specific Applications

Imagination is only intelligence having fun.

George Scialabbe

Parts I, II, and III have established the groundwork for this final part of the book. Having acquired the information from the earlier parts, you are now prepared to fully understand and appreciate the information presented in part IV. Part IV is where you will put all the information and knowledge you have gained in the other parts into whole therex programs. Part IV consists of therapeutic exercise programs for each body segment. The programs are not divided by activity, for an ankle sprain is an ankle sprain regardless of whether it occurs in basketball, volleyball, or at work, and regardless of whether it is incurred by a teenager, college student, or other individual. The only point when a treatment program for an injury will deviate from one individual to another is in the final stages of therapeutic exercise, when the patient begins specific functional exercises that will allow return to a specific activity.

Part IV is also not a cookbook for rehabilitation of injuries. A cookbook is not necessary, nor is it practical. Now that you have the information from parts I, II, and III, you have the tools to design your own rehabilitation programs. Because each patient must have an individualized program, a cookbook approach is irrelevant and useless. The information in part IV provides suggestions for exercises and treatment techniques; but for application, you will depend on the knowledge you have gained throughout this text to put those suggestions together in an appropriate and formidable program for each patient you work with.

By now it should be clear that the rehabilitation clinician is a detective, problem solver, innovator, and educator who follows laws of knowledge, skill application, logic, and common sense to achieve the final goal of returning a patient to full participation as efficiently and safely as possible. Detective work involves examination of the injury's status, determination of the underlying causes of the injury to correct these causes and reduce the chance of reinjury, and continual reassessment of the patient's response to the treatment so that the results are positive.

As a problem solver, the rehabilitation clinician must be able to adjust treatment programs, exercises, and progression sequences when a patient does not respond according to expectations. The program is always individualized, so the rehabilitation clinician must be alert to problems and must be able to adjust the program as needed for each patient.

As an innovator, the rehabilitation clinician attempts to achieve treatment goals and still make the program interesting and stimulating for the patient to help ensure compliance in the therapeutic exercise program. If equipment is limited, innovation becomes an even more important element, because making the program interesting using minimal materials presents an even greater challenge to the rehabilitation clinician's imagination. This situation of limited resources can make a therapeutic exercise program as interesting and challenging for you to design as it is for the patient to perform.

Throughout a therapeutic exercise program, the rehabilitation clinician is an educator. The patient is educated regarding the "dos and don'ts" following an injury—what activities are important to perform and what activities should be avoided to prevent further harm. The patient is educated about what to do to protect the injury and to promote an uneventful healing process. The patient is educated with regard to the injury, the rehabilitation program process, the rationale for specific exercises, and the importance of home exercises; each of these is vital to assuring the patient's compliance and the program's success. The rehabilitation clinician educates the patient throughout the program as the injury changes and the program evolves.

The rehabilitation clinician's knowledge, understanding, observation skills, evaluation skills, application skills, and ability to apply common sense and logic all contribute to the success of the rehabilitation process. Rehabilitation involves applying all these elements to provide a balanced program for the patient—one that provides appropriate stresses with the right degree of protection to advance the patient efficiently and effectively toward the goal of safe return to participation as soon as possible.

Along with all of these caveats on putting a rehabilitation program together, the final one is that the rehabilitation clinician should make the program fun for both the patient and clinician.

The clinician with a good imagination can combine that imagination with all the knowledge and skills that have been learned to create a rehabilitation program to not only achieve the program's goals but stimulate the patient to perform at his or her best in rehabilitation and make the treatment something to look forward to each day.

PROGRAM CONSIDERATIONS

The specific elements and the complexity of a rehabilitation program are determined by a variety of factors. These include the magnitude of the injury, the type of injury, the body segment involved, the patient's activity, the patient's response to the injury (physical, emotional, and psychological), and the patient's goals. All must be considered in the injury examination design and rehabilitation program execution.

Examination

Before providing treatment in a rehabilitation program, the rehabilitation clinician must examine the injury to determine where in the healing process the injury is and how irritable it is. If the injury is very irritable, regardless of healing stage, the treatment must begin gently and include primarily modalities to calm the area. If the patient had reconstructive surgery three days ago, the initial treatments are not aggressive with strengthening activities. If, on the other hand, the injury is not very irritable and is well into the healing process, the rehabilitation clinician can be more aggressive in the first treatment. Whatever the initial treatment includes, careful observation for responses to the treatment is necessary, both during the first treatment session and before the next. The current treatment course is always determined by the injury's response to the previous treatment session.

Modalities

A total rehabilitation program includes the use of modalities to modulate pain and enhance the healing process. Modalities serve as preliminary adjuncts to the total program and should not be considered the primary means of returning the patient to full participation. Once pain modulation and healing are under way, therapeutic exercises become the primary emphasis in the rehabilitation process. Since this text includes information specific to therapeutic exercise, you should keep in mind as you read the following chapters that although a rehabilitation program may include pain-modulating modalities and efforts to manage and promote the healing process, these are not included in this text. *Therapeutic Modalities for Musculoskeletal Injuries, Second Edition,* by Craig Denegar, Ethan Saliba and Susan Saliba (2005) covers modalities used in rehabilitation.

An injury does not have to become entirely pain free before exercises begin. In fact, most of the time it is not desirable to wait until the patient is completely pain free before starting exercises. Pain and swelling, however, are monitored throughout the rehabilitation process, especially in the first half of the therapeutic exercise program when the newly forming tissue is more susceptible to overstress from exercise than it will be later. Both pain and edema act as neural inhibitors, reducing the patient's rehabilitation output and ability to perform therapeutic exercises.

Remember the advice of Hippocrates: "Do no harm." If you are unsure as to whether you should advance a patient's program, do not until you are sure it is appropriate to do so. If you have any doubt about whether an exercise may cause edema or increased pain later, it is advisable to apply ice following the exercise session to reduce the risk for these deleterious effects. As you obtain a more accurate impression of the patient's ability to tolerate the stresses applied during the therapeutic exercise program, and as the injury advances in the remodeling phase, application of ice after a session becomes optional and relates more to the patient's preference or comfort level than to any physiological benefit.

Maintenance of Conditioning Level

Throughout this book I have emphasized the importance of maintaining cardiovascular health and conditioning levels of noninjured body segments. Although this is a vital aspect of a total therapeutic exercise program, it is not addressed in the chapters in part IV; however, you should always include exercises for these parameters in a rehabilitation program. The exercises discussed in this part of the book include only those relevant to the injured segment.

CHAPTER SEGMENTS

Each chapter in part IV includes specifics on various aspects of topics that have been covered in earlier chapters. The first portion of each chapter in part IV includes general considerations and specific techniques corresponding to concepts, theories, and applications presented in part II: soft-tissue and joint mobilization. The next portion deals with the usual progression of therapeutic techniques for achieving goals of normal range of motion, strength and muscle endurance, and coordination and agility. Once you are familiar with these elements, you will learn to apply them in the next section of the chapter, "Special Rehabilitation Applications." These sections address injuries that require special program considerations, precautions, or unique therapeutic exercise applications, followed by case studies. Specific answers are not given for the questions in these case studies because the studies are meant to stimulate discussion between students and instructor. There is no right answer for each question, because the answer is driven by the particulars of the case and is to some extent flexible, as dictated by the rehabilitation clinician's preferences and the equipment available. Of course, you must take into consideration specific precautions, contraindications, healing time line, and injury-unique information when creating a program for each case study.

Soft-Tissue Mobilization

You may want to refer to earlier chapters that deal specifically with these techniques to review technique application. Soft-tissue mobilization techniques in the chapters to follow do not include the full range of soft-tissue techniques discussed in chapter 6. The primary techniques discussed are myofascial release and trigger point release. You should realize that these specific techniques or other soft-tissue mobilization techniques may or may not be indicated in individual situations; you must examine the patient's injury to decide whether they may be appropriate. The intent of the discussion of these techniques is to provide examples to help you appreciate the important role that soft-tissue mobilization can play in the total rehabilitation process.

The soft-tissue pain-referral patterns discussed in these chapters are based on the extensive work of Travell and Simons (1983, 1992). Other pain-referral patterns are based on common neurological patterns.

Joint Mobilization

As discussed in chapter 6, joint mobilization is a complex technique entailing either accessory movements or physiological movements. When using joint mobilization, the rehabilitation clinician should remember that the movement is produced not by the rehabilitation clinician's hands but by his or her body; this produces a better perception of the movement by the clinician and a more comfortable sensation for the patient. The hands are the vehicles through which the rehabilitation clinician's body produces the joint motion.

Joint mobilization is not used in all conditions. Positive results in mobilization should usually occur within four to five days (Maitland 1990). As discussed in chapter 6, joint mobilization is appropriate for treatment of pain using I and II grades of movement or treatment of joint stiffness using grade III or IV. These movements can be oscillatory motions or sustained. Please refer to chapter 6 for review of these techniques if necessary.

Most of the joint mobilization techniques presented in part IV are based on Maitland's work. Various scholars have developed a number of variations and techniques. At the back of this book is a listing of suggested readings that you can refer to for specific instruction in joint mobilization techniques.

Therapeutic Exercise Phases

The therapeutic exercise phases differ slightly from the rehabilitation phases outlined in chapter 2. The primary difference is that the therapeutic exercise program does not include very early aspects of rehabilitation. I recommend that you refer to *Therapeutic Modalities for Musculoskeletal Injuries, Second Edition* (Denegar, Saliba, and Saliba 2005) for information regarding the use of modalities in rehabilitation. Of course, the emphasis in the early stage of rehabilitation is to get the inflammation under control and protect the healing process, as dealt with in earlier chapters. Although the rehabilitation clinician must know what constitutes a total rehabilitation program and know how to administer such a program, only therapeutic exercises and manual techniques are addressed in the following chapters.

The therapeutic exercise portion of a rehabilitation program can be divided into three phases: early, middle, and late. In administration of a program, the exercise progression is not specifically dictated; but the components of the progression are distinguished here to make the progression easier to comprehend and identify.

Early Phase

The early therapeutic exercise phase includes achieving gains in range of motion through joint and soft-tissue mobilization techniques, as well as range-of-motion exercises. Beginning-level strength and proprioception activities may also be included at this time. If exercises start in early proliferation or late inflammation, range of motion may be the only exercise possible. Once tissue is stable, strength and proprioception exercises may be permitted. The closer to early healing the injury is, the more cautious the clinician should be in the amount of stress applied to newly developing tissue. In some cases, exercises may not be permitted until three weeks after injury. "Early phase" here refers to when exercises in the rehabilitation program are initiated.

In the early phase, flexibility and range of motion are deficient. Weakness and loss of agility and coordination are also readily apparent when one compares the injured segment to the opposite side.

The intent of the early phase of therapeutic exercise is to achieve significant gains in range of motion and flexibility, to begin early strengthening activities, and to initiate low-level proprioception activities. Range-of-motion and flexibility gains are acquired with soft-tissue and joint mobilization techniques. Passive, active, and assistive exercises can also be used to improve range of motion. Early strengthening exercises vary depending on the severity of the injury and include a range of activities, such as isometrics and concentric, concentric-eccentric, and/or eccentric exercises. Isometric exercises are often performed in either multiple angles, midrange, or in an anatomic position, depending on mobility and medical restrictions for motion. Strength exercises are usually performed in a straight plane, not progressing to diagonal or functional positions until the patient has achieved sufficient strength in straight-plane movement to control the extremity through a functional motion. It is not unusual for strength exercises to begin with high repetitions and low weights. This reduces stress on joints that may not be strong enough to tolerate the shear forces produced by heavy resistance. Proprioception exercises begin at a simple level and do not advance to more complex exercises until the patient demonstrates an ability to perform the lower-level activity well.

Middle Phase

By the time the patient progresses to the middle phase, range of motion is nearly or completely normal. Edema and pain have come under control. Strength and muscle endurance have improved but remain at a significant deficit.

The middle phase includes primarily strength and muscle endurance exercises along with low- and middle-level proprioception exercises. Flexibility exercises should continue in this phase to prevent a loss of motion since continued contraction occurs because of the myofibril activity during the healing process. If flexibility is not yet normal, stretching exercises are a requirement during this phase. This is the time the patient begins more aggressive exercises, as discussed in chapter 1, including a progression of exercises that continue to work on range of motion and also advance strength, muscle endurance, and proprioception. Strength exercises here are in transition. In the beginning of this phase, patients may perform the strength exercises primarily in a straight plane; but as the patient continues through this phase, many exercises advance to diagonal, functional patterns of movement. This is possible because the muscle strength improves to a level that allows the patient to maintain extremity control while moving the segment.

Proprioception exercises become more complex in this phase. They may include multiple tasks, and the aim is to help prepare the patient for the stresses of functional activities in the next phase.

Late Phase

The middle phase readies the patient for the late phase, when power, strength, and coordination are jointly stressed in agility activities. By the time the patient reaches the final phase, flexibility, strength, and muscle endurance are all at near-normal levels; so the patient is ready for more advanced activities that further stress the injured area in preparation for return to normal activities. At this point the only real deficit lies in the patient's functional performance level. Flexibility and strength activities are now at a maintenance level, and the major emphasis is on finely-tuning the patient for a smooth transition and return to full

Therapeutic Exercise Continuum

```
        Early                        Middle                      Late

Start |--------------------------------------------------------------| End
ROM:
      |PROM|
      |AAROM--|
        |AROM------|
        |Soft-tissue mob------------------------------|
         |Joint mob-----------------------------------------|
          |Active stretches-------------------------------- →Maintenance
          |Passive stretches--------------------------|


Strength/Endurance:
               |Isometrics
                  |Progressive isotonics ----------------------  →  Maintenance
                          |Isokinetics ----------|
ABCs:
           |Balance-----|
             |Coordination-------------------|
                    |Agility---------------------|
                      |Progressive plyometrics----|


Functional & sport-specific:
                 |Easy functional---------|
                   |Complex functional----------|
                       |Sport-specific-|
```

participation. Although these chapters mention functional activities, they do not fully address activity-specific exercises because these are so numerous and so varied in their demands. You must remember, though, that functional activities are a vital part of the final phase and must always be part of a therapeutic exercise program. Functional activities should include a progression of activity-specific exercises. These begin with less stress, speed, force, and distance and continue to increase these parameters as the patient's body adjusts to the stresses and the patient acquires better skill and ability to execute the specific activities appropriately.

Exercise Continuum

The exercises for each phase can be placed on a rehabilitation continuum. On the continuum are all the parameters that have been discussed, as well as exercises corresponding to the phases as seen in the figure on p. 474. The diagram outlines the progression of a therapeutic exercise program according to parameter and divides those parameters according to the early, middle, and late phases of a program. The progression is a continuum in that exercises in a therapeutic exercise program flow from one level to the next. It is sometimes difficult to determine whether an exercise corresponds to the early or middle phase or to the middle or late phase, and a particular exercise can correspond to one phase with one injury and another phase with another injury. That is the essence of a continuum.

PUTTING IT ALL TOGETHER

The purpose of the phases and exercise continuum is less to delineate a specific program and progression for a patient than to give you a mental image that helps you identify how to advance a patient in a therapeutic exercise program. knowing to which phase an exercise corresponds is not as important as recognizing the progression and level of difficulty of the exercise and identifying when the patient is able to move from one level to the next.

To make the rehabilitation program progression even less clear cut and more confusing, a patient may be in the early phase with one parameter and in the middle phase with another parameter. For example, the patient may have good range of motion and grade 4/5 strength, indicating that he or she is in the middle phase of a therapeutic exercise program, but the balance ability of that patient may still be in the early phase. Each segment must be stressed to its capacity as long as this does not overly stress other segments. As an example, a patient with a shoulder impingement and weakness of the scapular rotators should not be advanced to open chain exercises in the higher elevations of motion if such exercises will worsen the injury; if the scapular muscles lack sufficient strength, they will not be able to hold the scapula properly to prevent impingement. In that case, although coordination abilities of the patient may be able to advance, his or her strength remains deficient, so attempting to advance the coordination parameter before strength improves will aggravate the injury.

THERAPEUTIC EXERCISE INDIVIDUALIZATION

As has been mentioned throughout this book, it is important to design the patient's therapeutic exercise program for the individual patient. Even though two patients have ankle sprains, they will not necessarily progress at the same rate, so expectations of a specific time line of advancement are not appropriate. These patients may even have different exercises within their programs. The individual's injury and the body's response to the injury, the patient's abilities and goals, and the way the patient responds to both the program and the clinician all determine the exercises selected, the rate of progression, and the final outcome of the therapeutic exercise program. Expecting an individual to progress on the basis of any other guidelines leads to frustration for both the patient and the rehabilitation clinician.

The clinician should continually assess the patient's performance; examine outcomes before, during, and after treatment to see whether the treatment has had the desired effect; and be ready to alter treatments if undesirable effects are seen. It is essential to obtain information from the patient regarding post-treatment responses in order to further assess the effects of the treatment program. If increased pain, swelling, and other deleterious effects are recorded after treatment, the program has been too stressful on the injured part and needs to be revised to a less intense exercise level. *Progress without regression* should be the rehabilitation clinician's creed. In other words, the program should challenge the patient enough to improve all parameters without overstressing the injury to increase symptoms.

CHAPTER PROGRESSION

Part IV begins with the spine (chapter 16) and then moves to the upper extremities (chapters 17-19); the final chapters (20-22) include therapeutic exercise programs for the lower extremities. The material has been arranged this way because many upper- and lower-extremity problems can be related to the core, the spine. The spine is also an important consideration in rehabilitation of upper and lower extremities, because core strength is vital for both upper- and lower-segment stability and performance.

It would be nearly impossible to list all the exercises in a therapeutic exercise program. Those outlined in these chapters include more commonly used activities, as well as some that are unique for each parameter. As always, the clinician's knowledge of injury healing, appreciation of the patient's abilities, the facilities and equipment available, and his or her own imagination are the only limiting factors of a therapeutic exercise program. A therapeutic exercise program can be fun and challenging for the patient as well as the rehabilitation clinician. The clinician can be imaginative in providing stimulating exercises for the patient so both enjoy the rehabilitation process. So as you read through these next few chapters, see whether you can think of exercises in addition to those presented that would challenge and stimulate a patient in a therapeutic exercise program.

CHAPTER 16

Spine and Sacroiliac

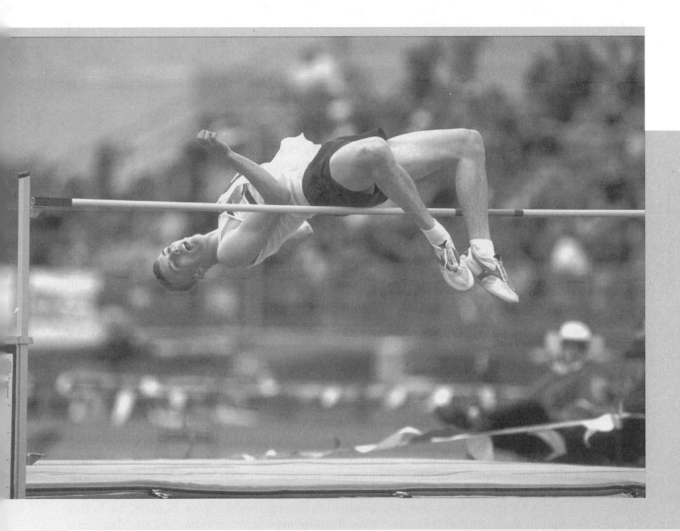

Objectives

After completing this chapter, you should be able to do the following:

1. Explain three flexibility exercises for the cervical spine and lumbar spine.

2. Explain three strengthening exercises for the cervical spine and lumbar spine.

3. Identify three progressive spinal stability exercises.

4. Identify three sacroiliac muscle energy release techniques and the indications for their use.

5. Outline a therapeutic exercise program for a cervical sprain.

6. List precautions for a therapeutic exercise program for disk lesions.

7. Discuss the difference in therapeutic exercise programs for a lumbar strain and a facet injury.

About half the patients Rita sees have back injuries. Joey, a high school athlete she is currently rehabilitating, is one of these. While practicing his high jump maneuver last week, he slipped during his approach and injured his back. Now that the muscle spasms are resolved, Rita is improving Joey's soft-tissue mobility with myofascial release (MFR) across the lumbar area. His sacroiliac became malaligned when he slipped, so Rita used muscle energy techniques and home exercises to correct the problem. Her initial examination revealed significant weakness of the trunk muscles, so she plans to develop Joey's abdominal and back strength. Rita is confident that this will not only protect Joey's back from further injury but may also improve his high jump.

> ■ Both science and art enable us to see more deeply into the mystery of existence. . . . their greatest similarity is that they are both means of furthering our personal awareness, of expanding consciousness.
>
> John Eichinger, PhD, Professor

This chapter begins the fun part of therapeutic exercise, applying the science that we have been discussing and letting our imaginations create therapeutic exercise programs. We will start the true blending of science and art in rehabilitation. We now have the opportunity to apply our scientific knowledge in an artful manner to provide patients with a complete, stimulating, and challenging therapeutic exercise program that will allow those patients a safe and speedy return to full participation and normal activity.

The spine and sacroilium (SI) are composed of several different segments. Any segment can have separate injuries that do not affect the other spinal regions. They also can have injuries that affect or are affected by other regions. Since the spine and SI are interrelated, we are considering the spine and sacroilium together.

There are both similarities and unique characteristics among regions of the spine. For example, in the thoracic region, each vertebra is joined with a rib; the cervical spine has the atlas and brachial plexus; and the lumbar region has the lumbar plexus, larger vertebral bodies, and is connected to the sacrum. Examples of similarities are that vertebrae in the three regions have spinous and transverse processes and are separated by disks.

This chapter addresses general rehabilitation concepts for the spine. Some of the factors unique to the spine that influence a rehabilitation program are also introduced. Many texts are devoted to spine anatomy and function, so this chapter by no means deals with all there is to know about the spine. The aim is to present key information that will enable you to treat most spine and spine-related injuries that you will encounter as a rehabilitation clinician.

Catastrophic injuries that include spinal cord injury resulting in paralysis are not among injuries seen for therapeutic exercise with the goal of returning the patient to sport participation, so they are not addressed here. Emergency treatment of these injuries is covered in *Examination of Musculoskeletal Injuries, Second Edition* (Shultz et al. 2005), which readers should consult for information on this topic.

The spine is a complex structure that is often neglected in education programs because of its uniqueness in comparison to the upper and lower extremities. Rather than approach the spine as another segment that is subject to injury and in need of treatment, many approach the topic with apprehension because of ignorance and fear: ignorance because the spine seems to be a mystifying body segment that is far too complex to understand, and fear because its complexity gets in the way of appreciating its simplicity.

The spine is complex. So is the shoulder. So is the knee. There are many segments of the body that we still have much to learn about and understand, yet we do not hesitate to deal with injuries to these segments. The spine is like any other segment in that, regardless of its complexity, it is often injured and needs to be addressed. This chapter deals with common spinal injuries and outlines typical therapeutic exercise programs for them.

By the end of the chapter, you should view the spine not as a body segment to shy away from, but rather an area that you can approach with an appreciation of both its simplicity and its complexity.

GENERAL REHABILITATION CONSIDERATIONS

▶ Treatment of spine injuries has changed greatly in the last few years. A therapeutic exercise program for the spine typically has many components, including instruction on posture and stability as well as exercises for flexibility, strength, and muscle endurance.

As recently as 10 years ago, conservative treatment of spine injuries, especially low-back injuries, involved bed rest for extended periods of time. As medical professionals realized how detrimental immobilization and extended rest were and noticed that those individuals who did not rest improved faster than those who did, the standard of care for spine injuries changed. Current treatment applications include minimal rest and progression into activity as quickly as is appropriate for the individual and the specific injury.

For many years, Williams flexion exercises were the accepted back-exercise regimen. Williams flexion exercises are a series of exercises that emphasize flexion and include activities such as the pelvic tilt, single and double knees-to-chest, and straight-leg raise. More recently, extension exercises became the exercises of choice because flexion exercises made many patients with disk injuries worse. Extension exercises, advanced by Robin McKenzie, a New Zealand physiotherapist, emphasize trunk extension aimed at relieving posterior pressure on disks. Many rehabilitation clinicians today do not advocate a purist attitude of either flexion or extension exercises for spine patients. Rather, a program is individualized on the basis of the problems and needs of the patient.

A complete rehabilitation program for the spine typically involves modalities, therapeutic exercise, manual techniques, and patient education. Manual techniques include soft-tissue and joint mobilization. Spinal injuries respond well to Swiss ball, foam roller, and aquatic exercises. As you have learned, it is easy to incorporate these into a therapeutic exercise program.

It is important for spine rehab programs to include cardiovascular exercises. The specific injury dictates the requirements for each program. The rehabilitation clinician must identify the patient's deficiencies before deciding on a precise therapeutic exercise program.

In addition to cardiovascular activities, a therapeutic exercise program for the spine should routinely include spinal stability instruction, posture correction, and body mechanics instruction. It should also include flexibility exercises, strengthening exercises, and muscle endurance activities. Hip tightness, especially in the lateral rotators, is often correlated with low-back pain; so the program should include flexibility activities for those hip muscles that have been assessed as having restricted motion. The abdominals (transverse, abdominus, and obliques) and spine extensor muscles are key muscle groups that provide support and stability to the spine, so strength exercises for these groups should also be included.

If one segment of the spinal column is hypomobile, it is common for an adjacent segment to be hypermobile. One must carefully examine each vertebra's mobility before applying joint mobilization. Random joint mobilization to any segment in the absence of an examination of its mobility may increase, not decrease, the patient's symptoms. If you are ever in doubt whether to use joint mobilization, do not use it.

Although approaches to the various spinal segments have many similarities, and although the symptoms and treatment from one segment to an adjacent segment frequently overlap, this chapter deals with the segments separately to make it easier to identify and discuss treatment for each. You should keep in mind, however, that one segment and its injury are often intimately related to another segment. For example, painful symptoms at T4 are often associated with cervical dysfunctions, and pain in the low back can be related to sacroiliac dysfunctions.

REHABILITATION TECHNIQUES

▶ Rehabilitation techniques for the various segments of the spine include soft-tissue mobilization, joint mobilization, and exercises to improve parameters such as flexibility, postural and pelvic stablility, strength, and agility.

Soft-tissue mobilization techniques are presented here before joint mobilization techniques; other types of exercises focusing on flexibility, stability, strength, and agility and coordination are presented in subsequent sections. Because there are so many types of soft-tissue mobilization techniques, only a couple are described. Keep in mind, however, that other soft-tissue mobilization techniques may be more appropriate than those presented here, depending on the individual and the specific injury.

Vertebral Artery Compromise

Prior to treating cervical injuries, the clinician should examine the patient for possible vertebral artery involvement. Although such a problem is rare in young athletes, injury to the cervical spine or poor posture may create vertebral artery compromise. Treating patients with such a condition has the potential to create serious complications such as brainstem ischemia.

To identify patients with vertebral artery compromise, static and dynamic tests should be performed prior to cervical treatment. These tests are particularly important if the patient reports any symptoms of vertebral artery involvement; these symptoms include dizziness, light headedness, nausea, blurry vision, tinnitus, headaches, or facial sensory deficiencies.

The five static tests are passive and can be performed with the patient sitting, standing, or supine. The clinician maximally rotates the patient's head and neck to the left, to the right, maximally extends the patients neck with exaggerated lordosis in the mid-cervical region, maximally rotates and extends to the left, and repeats both movements to the right. Each position is held for 10 seconds during which time the clinician observes the patient's eyes for either changes in pupil size or nystagmus, and asks the patient to report any symptoms.

The two active tests are performed with the patient sitting or standing and the clinician behind the patient. In the first test the clinician stabilizes the patient's shoulders and has the patient rotate the head and neck maximally to the left and to the right, holding each position for about 10 seconds. In the second test, the clinician holds the patient's head stable while the patient rotates the body repeatedly to the left and right for about 10 seconds. If the patient reports symptoms in the first test but not the second test, the problem is related to the vestibular system. Symptoms produced with the second test may indicate vertebral artery compromise. A positive test should be reported to the physician, and the patient should avoid positions in cervical rotation until further examination is provided.

Soft-Tissue Mobilization

Although various techniques are available for soft-tissue mobilization as discussed in chapter 6, the techniques emphasized here are trigger point release and myofascial release. If the rehabilitation clinician observes pain-referral patterns identified with these muscles, he or she should use some of these techniques. Trigger points, referred pain, and release techniques presented here are based on the work by Travell and Simons (1983).

The upper trapezius, levator scapulae, sternocleidomastoid, scalenes, spleni, and posterior cervical muscles are the primary cervical muscles that often have soft-tissue restriction. The following sections cover treatment of these muscles.

Upper Trapezius

This muscle commonly refers pain to the posterolateral neck, the mastoid process, the temple and posterior region of the head, occiput, and angle of the jaw (figure 16.1a). One or more of these areas may be a site of pain.

With the patient in supine, the clinician places the muscle on slight slack by having the patient move the ear toward the shoulder on the pain side. The rehabilitation clinician can then either grasp the muscle at the juncture between the neck and shoulder portion of the muscle, or apply a caudally-directed pressure over the area (figure 16.1b). If direct pressure is used, it is held until palpation reveals muscle relaxation and the patient's pain subsides. The pressure applied may be uncomfortable but tolerable. An alternative treatment method is to use either the ice-and-stretch technique with the patient sitting, or a deep massage with the patient supine while the clinician

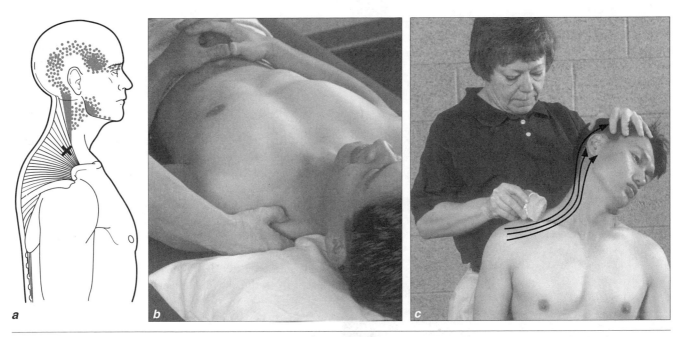

Figure 16.1 Upper trapezius: *(a)* pain pattern (x indicates trigger point), *(b)* myofascial release, *(c)* ice-and-stretch.

Pain pattern *(a)* adapted by permission from Simons, Travell, and Simons 1999

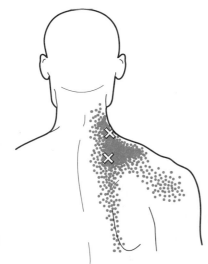

applies a mild stretch by rotating the head to the opposite side and flexing the neck (figure 16.1c). The direction of the ice strokes is upward from the acromion process toward the base of the skull.

Levator Scapulae

The site of most intense referred pain from the levator scapulae occurs at the angle between the neck and the shoulder with occasional referral along the vertebral border of the scapula or to the posterior shoulder (figure 16.2a). Trigger point release is performed as the patient is supine or sidelying with the clinician's fingers on the trigger points, indicated in figure 16.2b, either at the distal insertion of the levator scapulae on the vertebral angle of the scapula or at the angle of the neck. Ice-and-stretch is performed with the patient in sitting, the same-side arm anchored, and the head tilted forward and to the opposite side (figure 16.2c). A steady stretch is applied while the ice is stroked from the base of the skull downward along the path of the muscle.

Figure 16.2 Levator scapulae myofascial release: *(a)* pain pattern (x indicates trigger point), *(b)* trigger point release, *(c)* ice-and-stretch.

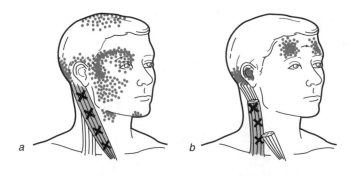

Sternocleidomastoid (SCM)

Both the sternal and clavicular heads can refer pain into the face and head. The most common areas are in and behind the ear, around the eye, the forehead, cheek, teeth, tongue, pharynx, and the upper aspect of the sternum. There are multiple trigger points along this muscle as seen in figure 16.3, a and b. With the patient in supine and the head tilted to the same side, the rehabilitation clinician can either use a pincher grasp on the muscle at the trigger point or apply vertical pressure to it (figure 16.3c).

Ice-and-stretch is applied with the patient sitting, the same-side arm anchored, and the neck positioned in extension and rotation to the opposite side if the clavicular head is being treated (figure 16.3d). If the sternal head of the muscle is being treated, the neck is rotated to the same side and extended (figure 16.3e). The ice strokes are swept from the clavicle upward toward the head.

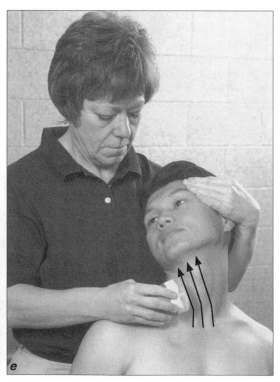

Figure 16.3 Sternocleidomastoid myofascial release: *(a-b)* trigger point pain-referral patterns (x = trigger point), *(c)* release of clavicular head, *(d)* ice-and-stretch of clavicular head, *(e)* ice-and-stretch of sternal head.

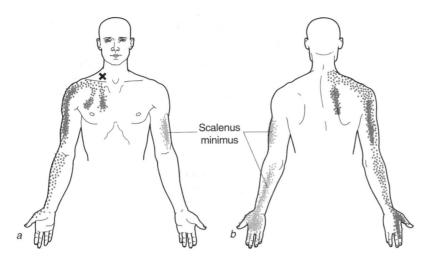

Scalenus
minimus

Scalenes

We will consider the scalene muscles—anterior, medius, and posterior—together. Trigger points of these muscles are seen in people with a forward-head posture. The pain-referral patterns for the scalenes include pain along the anterior chest, lateral shoulder and arm, vertebral border of the scapula, radial forearm and hand, posterior thumb and index finger & metacarpal, and interscapular areas (figure 16.4, a and b). The trigger points for these muscles are located and treated with the patient in supine (figure 16.4c). The posterior sternocleidomastoid is first located cephalad to the clavicle. The scalenes lie just lateral to the sternocleido-

Figure 16.4 *(a)* Trigger point pain-referral pattern for scalene anterior and medius. *(b)* Trigger point pain-referral pattern for scalene posterior. *(c)* Scalenes myofascial release: With the two fingers of the left hand on either side of the anterior and medius scalenes, the right thumb is on the groove between these two muscles. *(d)* Ice-and-stretch for scalenes.

mastoid. The rehabilitation clinician identifies the external jugular vein and applies pressure to observe its expansion. This vein usually crosses over the anterior scalene. The anterior scalene's trigger point is just below the external jugular vein. The scalene medius is deep; it is found just lateral to the anterior scalene and just above the clavicle. The subclavian artery lies between the medius and anterior scalenes and can be palpated as it passes over the first rib behind the clavicle. The cervical transverse processes can be palpated when pressure is applied to the scalene medius. Trigger point treatment applied to these muscles often causes referral into the

shoulder or arm. The rehabilitation clinician must take care to avoid applying pressure over the blood vessels in this area.

Ice-and-stretch is applied with the patient in sitting, the arm anchored (figure 16.4d). The neck is positioned in extension with the head rotated away from the side being treated. Ice stroking is applied from the cephalad insertion of the muscles downward and along the shoulder and arm.

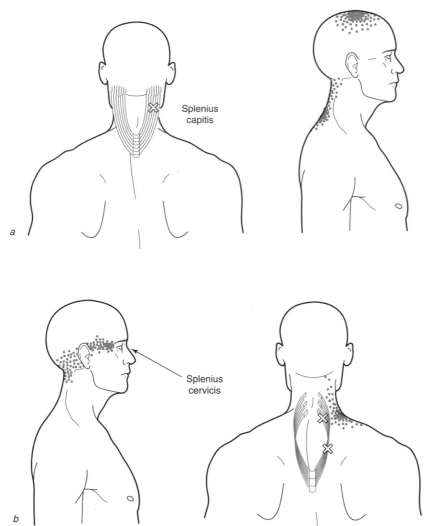

Spleni Muscles

As with the scalenes, we will look at treatment of the capitis and cervicis—the spleni group—together. These muscles also are frequent sites of trigger points in individuals with a forward-head posture. The spleni muscles refer pain to the top of the head, behind the eye, to the base of the neck, and along the side of the head (figure 16.5, a and b). Trigger point treatment is performed in supine or sitting. The splenius capitis trigger point is located just distal to its mastoid attachment (figure 16.5c).

The cervicis lies posterior to the lower cervical transverse processes and is located by laterally flexing the neck to the same side to relax the upper trapezius and levator scapula. The cervicis is palpated over the lower cervical transverse processes. Its trigger point is located between the upper trapezius and SCM.

Ice-and-stretch is performed with the patient in sitting. The neck is rotated and laterally flexed to the opposite side, with the ice sweeps directed from the base of the neck upward and downward (figure 16.5d).

Figure 16.5 Splenius myofascial release: (a) trigger point pain-referral pattern for splenius capitis, (b) upper and lower trigger point pain-referral patterns for splenius cervicis, (c) trigger point release, (d) ice-and-stretch.

Layer	Muscle	Fiber direction
1	Trapezius	
2	Splenii	
3	Semispinalis capitis	
	Semispinalis cervicis	
4	Multifidi	
	Rotatores	

Posterior Cervical Muscles

There are two groups of muscles in the posterior cervical region, one superficial and the other deep. The more superficial group is referred to as posterior cervical muscles and include the semispinalis capitis, semispinalis cervicis, multifidi, and rotatores (figure 16.6a). Beneath the semispinalis muscles are several additional smaller muscles, termed the suboccipital muscles. These include the major and minor rectus capitis muscles and the superior and inferior oblique capitis muscles. The posterior cervical muscles commonly refer to the base of the neck and upward into the suboccipital area, down the neck to the vertebral border of the scapula, and in a horizontal band to the temple on the same side of the head (figure 16.6, b-f). The suboccipital muscles refer to the occiput, the eye, and the forehead. They often give the injured patient a sensation of pain inside the skull; sometimes the patient describes either a vague headache or a pain that is all over the head on one side.

Figure 16.6 Posterior cervical muscles (a) myofascial release. Pain-referral patterns for subocciptal muscles (b), posterior cervical muscles (c), multifidus (d), semispinalis cervicis (e), and semispinalis capitas (f). Trigger point release for posterior cervical muscles (g). Ice-and-stretch to posterior cervical rotator muscles (h).

(a) Adapted by permission from Simons, Travell, and Simons 1999.

(continued)

For trigger point release, the patient is positioned in supine with the rehabilitation clinician at his or her head (figure 16.6g). The finger pads are applied over the trigger points.

Ice-and-stretch is applied in sitting. Head and neck position depends on the specific muscle being treated. The parallel semispinalis muscles can be treated bilaterally in a forward-head position. The rotator muscles that are angled from their distal to their proximal insertion are treated with the neck flexed forward and side-ward and rotated to place the muscle on stretch (figure 16.6h). The ice is applied from the base of the neck upward toward the head.

Figure 16.6
(continued)

Thoracic and Lumbar Spine

Often the muscles treated with soft-tissue mobilization in the thoracic area are the shoulder and scapular muscles. Those are discussed in chapter 17. Some of the cervical muscles, as you have just seen, can refer into the scapular area; so if a patient describes pain around the scapula without any frank injury to the shoulder or thoracic region, you should examine the neck as a possible source of the pain. Likewise, some lumbar pain is referred from the thigh and gluteal muscles; these areas are discussed in chapters 21 and 22.

Because thoracic muscles commonly refer pain into the lumbar area, and because many lumbar and thoracic muscles are extensions of the same muscles, the thoracic and lumbar muscles are discussed together. It is often very difficult to separate the two regions from each other. Treatment also often overlaps from one area to another, so it is logical to consider the two areas at the same time.

Muscles in the thoracic and lumbar regions that can refer pain into the thoracic, lumbar, and sacral areas include the thoracic and lumbar paraspinals, the quadratus lumborum, and the serratus posterior. The following sections cover their referral patterns, trigger points, and ice-and-stretch treatments.

Paraspinals

This group of muscles includes deep and superficial paraspinal muscles. The superficial group, the iliocostals and longissimus muscles, are collectively referred to as the erector spinae. The deep muscles include the rotatores, semispinalis, and multifidi; of these, the multifidi group most commonly produces pain.

Midthoracic superficial paraspinals can refer pain into the scapula or anterior chest area (figure 16.7, a and b); the lower thoracic superficial paraspinals can refer pain upward into the scapula (figure 16.7c), anteriorly to the lower abdomen (figure 16.7d), or downward to the low back and buttock (figure 16.7, e and f).

Thoracic multifidi refer pain to the spinous process near the trigger point (figure 16.7, g and h), while the lumbar multifidi can also refer pain into the abdomen (figure 16.7i). Multifidi at S1 can refer into the coccyx (figure 16.7h).

(continued)

Figure 16.7 Paraspinal pain-referral patterns (x indicates trigger point sites): *(a-f)* superficial paraspinals.

Figure 16.7
(continued) *(g-i)*
deep paraspinals, *(j)*
myofascial release,
(k) ice-and-stretch.

Treatment of the trigger points can be performed with the patient in sidelying or prone, if the neck can be comfortably positioned (figure 16.7j). To perform an ischemic compression treatment, the clinician applies pressure to the trigger point site that reproduces the patient's pain. Ice-and-stretch is applied in a sitting position with the patient in a trunk flexion position (figure 16.7k). The ice is applied in a cephalad-to-caudal motion from the head to the sacrum. If the deep paraspinals are being treated, the stretch must involve rotation and flexion while the ice stroking is performed at an angle.

Deep   Superficial

a

Quadratus Lumborum

The quadratus lumborum pain-referral pattern often gives the false sign of a disk syndrome and is neglected as a source of low back pain (Travell and Simons 1992). The pain, which can be intense, can accompany deep inhalation or make walking painful.

Typical quadratus lumborum pain can be either a deep ache or a sharp pain. The superficial fibers can refer pain along the iliac crest or greater trochanter or can wrap around to the outer groin. The deep fibers refer down to the sacroiliac joint or lower buttock (figure 16.8a).

For treatment, the patient should be positioned on the uninvolved side. If the area is not too tender, he or she can lie with the top arm overhead to elevate the lower ribs, and the top thigh and knee flexed with the knee on the table to lower the ilium (figure 16.8b). If the area is too tight or painful for the patient to lie in this position, the top knee should be placed on the bottom ankle or on a supportive pillow to reduce the stretch of the muscle. The superficial trigger points are located laterally, just cephalad to the iliac crest or distal of the 12th rib. The deep trigger points are located just lateral to the paraspinal muscles.

Ice-and-stretch treatment is applied with the patient in a position similar to that for trigger point release, but with the top leg forward of the bottom leg and distal thigh and leg positioned off the table to provide a stretch (figure 16.8c). The ice strokes are swept in a cephalad-to-caudad motion.

b

Figure 16.8 Quadratus lumborum: *(a)* pain-referral pattern, *(b)* trigger point release, *(c)* ice-and-stretch.

c

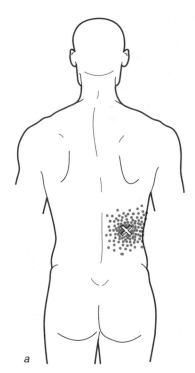

Serratus Posterior Inferior

This muscle causes an annoying ache in the posterior lower rib area in the site of its locale, from the posterior ninth rib medially to the L2 spinous process (figure 16.9a). Pain in this muscle usually remains localized and does not refer to other sites.

Trigger point treatment is performed with the patient in sidelying or prone. The trigger point is located in the lateral region of the muscle close to its rib insertion (figure 16.9b). Ice-and-stretch is performed with the patient in a sitting position. The trunk is flexed and rotated, and the ice is applied in upward and outward sweeps from the spine to the lateral trunk (figure 16.9c).

Figure 16.9   Serratus posterior: *(a)* trigger point (x) with pain referral pattern, *(b)* trigger point release to right serratus posterior inferior, *(c)* ice-and-stretch to left serratus posterior inferior.

Figure 16.10 Tennis ball release. The patient relaxes and lies down so body weight pushes balls into trigger point or area of restriction.

Self Soft-Tissue Mobilization

This is a soft-tissue mobilization technique that you can instruct the patient in and that does not require assistance. It uses either one or two old tennis balls that have lost their compression. If two balls are used, they can be either taped together (figure 16.10) or placed together in a sock. The patient lies on the tennis balls, which are placed under a restricted soft-tissue area. The patient lies on the tennis balls until the tenderness is gone and he or she feels only the pressure of the tennis balls. The balls are then moved to another location of restriction and discomfort and the technique is repeated. This technique can be performed in the thoracic and lumbar areas; it can also be used in other soft-tissue restricted areas of the body such as the hip and thigh.

Joint Mobilization

Obviously, the degree of movement in spinal joint mobilization accessory motion is very different from that in peripheral joints. Before you acquire the ability to determine normal movement, you will have evaluated many different vertebral movements on many different patients of varying ages and with various conditions. Normal accessory movement in the lumbar spine is different from that in the cervical spine, and joint accessory movement in a 19-year-old patient is different from that in a 40-year-old. You must recognize and consider these normal variations when assessing and treating a patient with joint mobilization.

Joint mobilization is used to reduce pain or improve mobility. Since it is common to find a hypermobile vertebral joint adjacent to a hypomobile joint, each spinal level should be assessed prior to joint mobilization application. The hypermobile joint should not be mobilized, but treatment will be necessary to improve motion of the restricted joint.

It is necessary to outline some basic principles of application before discussing specific application techniques. When the cervical spine and head are in normal alignment, the lower cervical and lower lumbar spines are curved slightly anteriorly. Because the best position for joint mobilization is an open-packed position, these areas of the spine should be placed in slight flexion to place the joints into a midposition before mobilization is performed. Rotating the head to the nonpainful side opens the vertebral foramen of C2 to C7. You can also open these by laterally tilting the patient's head away from the painful side. Mobilization techniques differ for the upper and lower cervical spine.

The clinician should use body weight and weight transfer as the force source, not the force from the fingers, thumbs, or hands. Using the body as the source of force permits a finer sense of touch for joint movement; is more comfortable for the patient; imposes less stress on the fingers, thumbs, and hands; and conserves the rehabilitation clinician's energy.

Initial mobilization techniques should be gentle. There should be no increase in symptoms because of the treatment. Examination before, during, and after the application is necessary in order for you to decide the appropriate depth of treatment. The primary factors restricting the depth of mobilization application are muscle spasm and pain. Frequently, muscle spasm will not permit grades III or IV mobilization because of the increased pain that results from the pressure. When this occurs, gentle mobilization may be used. Mobilization that exacerbates distally referred pain should be modified to include reduced amplitude or discontinued. Refer to chapter 6 for joint mobilization indications, precautions, and contraindications.

Although there are several mobilization techniques for use in the spine, only a few for each area of the spine are discussed here. The primary techniques to be described include central posterior-anterior (PA) and unilateral PA mobilization. The symbols used to record these techniques are ↓ for central PA and ⌐ or ⌐ for right or left unilateral PAs, respectively. The symbols used to record rib mobilization are ⌐ for right-rib and ⌐ for left-rib mobilizations. In this section we will consider additional techniques for some specific sites. I recommend that once you begin practice as a qualified health care provider, you participate in continuing education courses to develop an understanding and appreciation of more complex maneuvers.

Cervical Spine

Description of these techniques will primarily emphasize hand placement. The specific grade to apply is determined by the patient's condition and the treatment goals. Refer to chapter 6 for a review of joint mobilization.

Longitudinal Movement

Longitudinal movement is a relaxing technique that can help you to gain the patient's confidence. It is often the technique used to initiate mobilization treatments. With the patient in supine, the head is grasped and supported with one of the rehabilitation clinician's hands behind the head, and the thumb and fingers at the occiput. The other hand is placed under the chin (figure 16.11). While maintaining the position of the upper extremities, the clinician leans back to produce a gentle longitudinal pull of the neck. The hand on the chin is for positioning only; no force is directed into the chin.

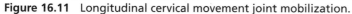

Figure 16.11 Longitudinal cervical movement joint mobilization.

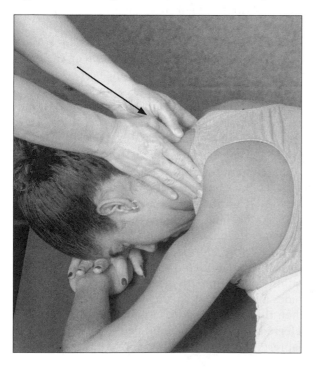

Central PAs

This technique can be used for midline or unilateral pain and spasm. The patient lies prone with his or her hands under the forehead and the chin slightly tucked. The rehabilitation clinician stands at the head and places the thumbs on the spine with the fingers relaxed, along the sides of the neck (figure 16.12). C1 and C3 are usually too difficult to palpate; but C2, C4, C5, C6, and C7 can usually be readily identified. The clinician applies PA pressure with the thumbs through movement of his or her trunk over the hands. The pressure should be gentle initially; adjustments are made using I and II grades according to the patient's response.

Figure 16.12 Central PA cervical mobilization.

Figure 16.13 Unilateral cervical mobilization.

Unilateral PAs

The technique described here can be used for the lower cervical spine and for unilateral neck pain. The patient lies prone with the hands under the forehead and the chin slightly tucked. The rehabilitation clinician stands on the side that is to be treated. The thumbs are placed on the articular pillar and angled about 30° medially (figure 16.13). The pressure is applied at the thumbs in a PA direction with a constant medially directed pressure to maintain position on the articular pillar. The head may nod slightly, but there should be no rotation motion if the pressure is applied correctly.

Thoracic Spine

Look at the bony arrangement on a skeleton to see how the position and relative alignment of the spinous processes change from the cervical to the lumbar spine. The angle of the joint mobilization force must change to produce a force in the plane of the joint. This is a crucial point to keep in mind as you perform mobilization techniques along the spine.

Central PAs

This technique can be used for central or unilateral symptoms. The patient is prone with the hands under the forehead and the chin slightly tucked. The specific thoracic segment being treated determines where the rehabilitation clinician stands. His or her position is at the head (figure 16.14a) if the upper segments are treated and at the side (figure 16.14b) if the middle and lower segments are treated. The thumbs are placed directly over the spinous process, with the fingertips spread across the back to act as a stabilizer for the thumbs. The pressure is applied at an angle perpendicular to the surface, so the position will change slightly as the hands move along the thoracic spine. The force is transmitted from the trunk through the arms to the thumbs. The fingers should remain relaxed.

Figure 16.14 Central PA thoracic mobilization: *(a)* Thumbs are placed over the spinous process. One thumb can be used to reinforce the other thumb. *(b)* Upper thoracic mobilizations are most easily performed while standing at the patient's head. *(c)* Lower and middle thoracic mobilizations are performed while standing at the patient's side.

Figure 16.15   Unilateral PA thoracic mobilization.

Figure 16.16   Unilateral costovertebral PA mobilization.

Unilateral PAs

This technique can be used for unilateral symptoms. The patient lies prone with the head turned to the side being treated. The arms hang over the side of the table. The rehabilitation clinician stands on the side being treated and places his or her hands on the patient's back, with the thumb pads on the transverse process and the fingers buttressed over the back (figure 16.15). The clinician's shoulders and arms are directly over his or her hands; the force is directed perpendicular to the surface. Movement occurs as a result of trunk, not thumb, movement.

Unilateral Costovertebral PAs

This technique can be used for painful or restricted ribs. The patient lies prone with arms at his or her sides or hanging over the table. The rehabilitation clinician stands on the side being treated. The ulnar border of the rehabilitation clinician's hand is placed along the line of the patient's rib over the costovertebral joint, with the other hand placed on top of the second metacarpal and digit (figure 16.16). Placement of the ulnar border is approximately two finger-widths from the spinous process. The pressure is applied perpendicular to the joint surface from the trunk through the shoulders and into the hands.

Lumbar Spine and Sacroiliac

Like the cervical and thoracic areas, the lumbar spine can be treated with central and unilateral PA movements. In addition, rotation mobilizations can be performed as a gross technique affecting the lumbar spine as a whole rather than treating individual levels.

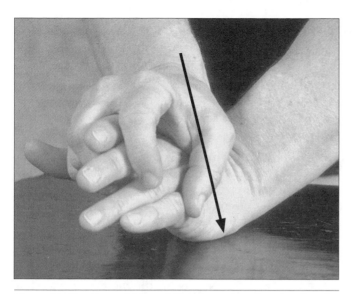

Figure 16.17 Central PA mobilization using the ulnar border of the left hand with reinforcement from the right hand.

Central PA Mobilization

This technique can be used for hypomobility and central and unilateral pain and derangements. Lumbar spine PA movements can be applied using the pisiform area of the hand as the point of force application (figure 16.17). The patient lies prone and the rehabilitation clinician stands to the side. Pressure is applied perpendicularly to the joint surface through the shoulders from the trunk.

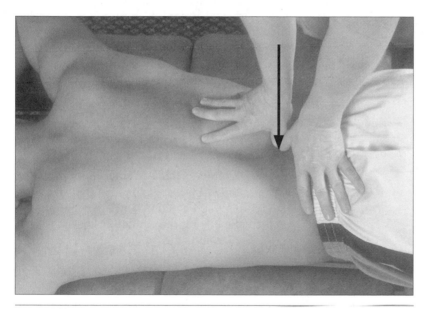

Figure 16.18 Unilateral lumbar mobilization.

Unilateral PA Mobilization

This technique can be used for unilateral pain. The patient lies prone with the head turned to one side. The rehabilitation clinician stands on the side to be treated and places the thumbs just lateral to the spinous process, at the level being treated, with the fingers spread across the back (figure 16.18). The clinician's shoulders are placed directly over his or her hands, and the pressure is applied directly perpendicular to the joint surface through the shoulders. The fingers remain relaxed; no pressure is applied through them.

Figure 16.19 Unilateral lumbar mobilization: *(a)* grade I and II rotation, *(b)* grade III rotation, *(c)* grade IV rotation.

Rotation

This technique can be used in unilateral restriction of movement or unilateral back or leg pain. The patient lies on the unaffected side with a pillow under the head. The top shoulder is near the side, and the elbow is flexed with the forearm resting on the side. The lower-extremity position depends on the grade of pressure being applied. For grades I and II, the hips and knees are flexed with the top leg slightly more flexed than the bottom leg. The lumbar vertebrae are positioned in midrange flexion-extension by the amount of hip flexion. The rehabilitation clinician places his or her hands on the pelvis and creates a gentle rocking motion of the pelvis (figure 16.19a).

In grade III, the top shoulder is rotated slightly more posteriorly so that the chest faces the ceiling and the torso is in a three-quarter position. The bottom leg is more extended than in grades I and II; the top leg is flexed with the medial femoral condyle on the table or just off the edge, and the ankle is hooked around the bottom leg. The rehabilitation clinician places one hand on the patient's shoulder and the other on the pelvis with the fingers pointing forward. If the desired motion is more into extension, then the hand is placed over the iliac crest with the clinician standing near the shoulder (figure 16.19b); but if the desired motion is flexion, the hand is placed over the greater trochanter with the clinician standing near the pelvis. The movement is caused by the hand at the pelvis, not the shoulder. Grade IV motion is produced with the top leg more extended and off the table (figure 16.19c). The clinician may need to kneel on the table behind the patient or lower the table so the force can be directed more easily from the shoulders to the hand on the pelvis. The clinician's knee behind the patient's back can also assist in stabilization. Motion for each grade should be a rotatory motion of the pelvis, not posterior to anterior or inferior to superior.

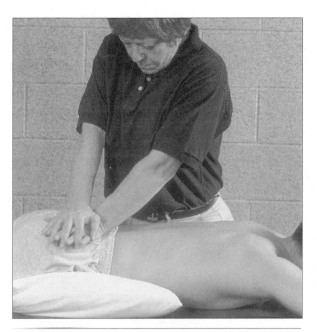

Figure 16.20 Sacroiliac posterior-anterior mobilization. The rehabilitation clinician is shown on the opposite side from the side being treated; this is only to allow better visualization of the technique.

Sacroiliac Posterior-Anterior Pressures

These techniques can be applied centrally or unilaterally. The patient lies prone with the rehabilitation clinician standing on the side to be treated. The lateral aspect of one hand is reinforced with the other hand on top of it and is placed over the upper sacrum. Posterior-anterior pressure is applied at the S1 level and gradually continued distally to the distal end of the sacrum (figure 16.20). Because of the complexity of the SI joint, the PA pressure can be applied in a cephalic, caudal, medial, or lateral direction or in any combination of these.

Flexibility Exercises

Because the lower cervical spine is related to the upper thoracic spine and the lumbar spine is related to the lower thoracic spine, sacrum, and hips, some of the flexibility exercises for cervical and lumbar regions of the spine overlap into these respective areas. Unless otherwise indicated, the stretch is held for about 20 s and repeated four to five times.

Cervical Spine

The description of each flexibility exercise in this section includes the correct manner of execution and common incorrect substitutions that should be avoided. These substitutions occur as the patient attempts to produce as much motion as possible. You should watch for these patterns carefully and correct them as they occur to prevent the patient from stretching ineffectively.

Axial Extension

This exercise helps the patient restore normal cervical alignment and correct posture. The patient lies supine on a firm surface, such as a tabletop or the floor. A pillow is not used. The patient places the fingertips of one hand on the cervical spinous processes and the other hand under the chin (figure 16.21a). The neck is then pushed into the fingertips as the patient pushes the tucked chin back with the front hand. As the patient finds this activity easier to perform, he or she can perform it in sitting. The patient places the index finger and thumb of one hand on the chin and the fingertips of the other hand along the upper cervical spine. With the chin tucked, the patient pushes the chin back with the chin hand and feels with the other hand as the cervical spine is pushed into that hand (figure 16.21b). In the common substitution for this exercise, the patient extends the cervical spine and presses the head backward rather than extending the cervical spine. If this occurs, have the patient tuck the chin first, then press the cervical spine into the fingertips.

Figure 16.21 Axial extension in *(a)* supine and *(b)* sitting.

Cervical Retraction

Also called the turtle exercise because of its motion, this exercise is used to stretch the posterior cervical muscles and improve posture. It can be performed in sitting or supine. The chin is tucked, and the head is pulled back while the chin stays at the same level (figure 16.22). The head does not tilt up or down during this activity. The common substitution for this exercise is cervical extension and lifting of the chin. Instruct the patient to keep the chin tucked if you observe the substitution.

Figure 16.22 Cervical retraction: (a) forward, starting position; (b) retracted, end position.

Figure 16.23 Cervical flexion.

Cervical Flexion

This exercise stretches the posterior cervical spinal muscles. With the chin tucked, the patient bends the head forward, attempting to touch the chin to the chest. Slight overpressure can provide additional stretch: The patient places his or her hands on top of the head and relaxes the shoulders. The weight of the arms will provide sufficient stretch, so instruct the patient not to pull the head but to let the arms relax and the elbows hang down (figure 16.23). The common substitution for this exercise is not to curl the neck but to use the lower cervical spine as a fulcrum while the upper cervical spine stays straight. If this occurs, instruct the patient to unwind the neck, beginning with the upper spine and moving downward. Remind the patient not to pull with the arms since this will provide unnecessary force to the posterior neck.

Upper Trapezius Stretch

This stretch isolates the upper trapezius muscle. In sitting, the patient grasps the wrist of the side to be stretched and pulls it across the body. The head is tilted away from the shoulder (figure 16.24a). Leaning the head to the opposite side can increase the stretch. Common substitutions for this exercise are allowing the shoulder to shrug upward, rotating the neck, or bending the head forward, rather than directly sideways. If these substitutions occur, correct the patient by instructing him or her to stabilize the shoulder by sitting on the hand, and to keep the nose in a forward position. Sometimes it may be necessary to start the patient in a supine position so that rotation and forward bending are minimized.

An alternative stretch uses a stretch strap that is draped over the treated shoulder. The opposite foot's toes are used to anchor the strap to the floor (figure 16.24b). The patient aligns the strap from the anchoring toes to beneath the elevated heel and takes up the slack with the hands in front of the body. A towel or other pad is placed under the strap on the shoulder for comfort. The heel is then moved to the floor so that the strap becomes taut, applying pressure on the upper trapezius. In this position, the neck is laterally flexed until the patient feels a stretch on the strap side of the neck.

Figure 16.24 Upper trapezius stretch: *(a)* active stretch, *(b)* with stretch strap.

Scalene Stretch

Because the scalenes have three different parts, there are three positions to stretch them. These stretches can be performed in sitting or supine. The arm on the side being stretched is anchored under the hip in all positions, and the opposite hand is placed over and across the top of the head and above the ear on the stretch side. For stretching the posterior, the face is turned to the opposite axilla (figure 16.25a). To stretch the medius, the face is kept looking forward while the head is tilted laterally (figure 16.25b). To stretch the anterior, the face is turned to the side being stretched and the patient looks to the ceiling (figure 16.25c). The hand over and across the top of the head applies a gentle stretch that produces a stretch sensation without discomfort or pain. The common substitution for this exercise is to move the shoulders or lean sideways during the stretch. If this occurs, have the patient perform the exercises in supine, and make the patient aware of the substitution.

Figure 16.25 Scalene stretch: *(a)* posterior, *(b)* medius, *(c)* anterior.

For additional information about physiotherapy, see www.physio-net.com/aboutphysio/.

Figure 16.26 Stretch to middle pectoralis.

Pectoral Stretch

This exercise stretches the pectoral muscles, a common source of poor cervical posture. The patient stands in a doorway with the forearms on the doorframe and elbows at shoulder level. With one foot in front of the other, the patient attempts to push through the doorway (figure 16.26). This exercise can also be performed in a corner, although empty corners are often difficult to find. The common substitution for this exercise is rotating the body toward the tight shoulder, especially if patients are small and the doorframe is too wide. If this occurs, have the patient keep both arms at the same level on the doorframe. Using a corner instead of a doorframe also helps improve execution of the exercise.

Sternal Raise

This exercise for the cervical and upper thoracic spine assists in improving posture. The patient elevates the sternum while moving the scapulae downward toward the back pockets. A common substitution for this exercise is to hyperextend the lumbar spine rather than elevate the sternum. You can limit the substitution if you instruct the patient to simultaneously contract the abdominals to stabilize the lumbar spine.

Thoracolumbar Spine

Because the ribs restrict mobility of the thoracic spine, thoracic motion is possible but limited. Abnormally limited motion in the thoracic ribs or spine can reduce shoulder motion and lung inhalation.

For links to a wide range of sports medicine resources, see *The Physician and Sportsmedicine* Web site at www.physsportsmed.com/links.htm.

Figure 16.27   Spinal twist stretch.

Spinal Twist

This exercise stretches the middle and low back and buttocks. It can be performed sitting on the ground or in a chair. On the ground, the patient crosses one leg over the opposite outstretched leg so that the crossing foot is placed on the outside of the outstretched leg. The elbow on the outstretched-leg side is placed on the outside of the bent knee, and the opposite arm is placed behind the body with the elbow straight. The patient then twists the body around toward the straight arm. If performing this exercise in a chair, the patient uses a straight-backed chair without arms. The feet are firmly planted on the floor, and the trunk is rotated toward the back of the chair. With one hand placed on the chair back, the other hand is placed on the outside of the knee as shown in figure 16.27. The patient uses the hands to pull around and provide the stretch. The thighs should not move but should remain in place during the stretch. A common substitution for this exercise is to allow the hips to rotate with the stretch. Instruct the patient to apply a hand on the outside of the thigh during the chair-twist stretch. To correct substitution in the stretch when it is performed on the floor, the patient should use the hand on the thigh to apply additional stabilizing force.

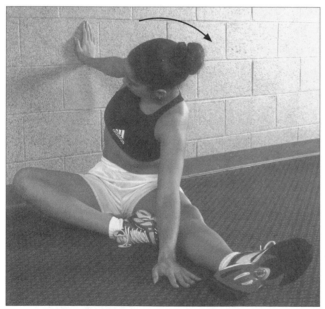

Figure 16.28   Quadratus lumborum stretch.

Quadratus Lumborum Stretch

This exercise stretches the quadratus lumborum and latissimus dorsi. The patient sits on the floor. One thigh is parallel to the wall and flexed at the knee so that the sole of the foot of that leg is placed on the inner thigh of the opposite leg, which is extended out to the side and close to perpendicular to the wall (figure 16.28). The arm farther from the wall is in front of the ipsilateral leg and the hand nearest the wall is placed on the wall to push the trunk away from the wall. The hips remain on the floor. In an alternative position that offers more stretch, the patient places the wall arm over the head in lateral rotation and full abduction and leans toward the opposite side. The patient should maintain pelvic neutral during the stretch. A common substitution for this stretch is to move out of pelvic neutral and flex the trunk. Instruct the individual to maintain pelvic neutral and lean only as far as possible while in pelvic neutral.

Figure 16.29 Prolonged sidebending stretch.

Prolonged Sidebending

This exercise stretches out the lateral trunk area. It can also be used to open up a facet joint. Depending on the position, it can be used to stretch out the middle or lower thoracic area or the lumbar area. The patient is in sidelying with the tight region on the top and a rolled towel or pillow supporting the portion of the trunk that is directly under the tight region. The top arm is placed overhead, and the top leg is straight in extension (figure 16.29). Increasing or decreasing the size of the rolled towel or pillow can alter the degree of stretch. Trunk flexion is the common substitution for this exercise. The patient must remain in a straight-aligned position of the trunk relative to the pelvis to attain maximum results.

Lumbar Rock

This exercise stretches the low back and hips. The patient is positioned on hands and knees with elbows straight, hands shoulder-width apart, knees under the hips, and hands under the shoulders. The back is arched, and the hips are pushed back toward the ankles as the shoulders go down toward the floor (figure 16.30, a and b). Without moving the hands or knees, the patient then moves forward to the starting position and continues forward until he or she is in a press-up position (figure 16.30c). A common substitution is to move the hands rather than keeping them stationary. If you observe this, remind the patient to maintain hand positions.

Figure 16.30
Lumbar rock stretch: (a) start position, (b) end position for lumbar flexion portion of the lumbar rock, (c) end position for lumbar extension of the lumbar rock.

Bent-Over Stretch

This exercise stretches the lumbar and thoracic spine. The patient sits in a chair with feet flat on the floor and apart. Starting from the neck, the patient slowly flexes forward and continues to bend the spine as the body flexes forward. The patient can wrap the hands around the ankles from inside the legs to outside the ankles and pull in order to give an extra stretch. When returning to the starting position, the patient places the hands on the knees and pushes with the arms to move upright rather than using the trunk muscles. Bending from the hips is the most common substitution for this exercise. Instruct the patient to roll and feel each segment moving as he or she curls to the end position.

Knees-to-Chest

This exercise stretches the low back and hips. The patient lies supine with the knees flexed. For a single knee-to-chest exercise, the patient first tightens the abdominals to stabilize the pelvis, and then lifts one knee to the chest. The knee is held to the chest passively by the arms. In the more aggressive double knee-to-chest stretch, the patient stabilizes the pelvis by tightening the abdominals, and then raises one knee to the chest. While keeping the knee up, the patient raises the other knee to the chest and pulls both knees to the chest with the arms. In a double knee-to-chest stretch, one leg at a time is raised and lowered to prevent the back from arching.

Lateral Trunk Stretch

This exercise stretches the lateral lumbar area. The patient is in supine with the knees flexed, feet flat on the floor, and arms outstretched. One knee is crossed over the other, and the top leg pulls the bottom leg toward the top-leg side while both shoulders remain in contact with the floor (figure 16.31). A common substitution is to allow the ipsilateral shoulder to come off the floor so less stretch is applied. Remind the patient of the importance of shoulder stabilization if you observe this error.

Figure 16.31 Lateral trunk stretch.

Thomas Hip Flexor Stretch

This exercise stretches the hip flexors. The patient sits on a table so that the thigh is halfway off the table. The patient lies supine with both knees to the chest. One thigh is grasped behind the knee, and the leg being stretched is lowered. The thigh of the leg being stretched (the lowered leg) should be kept in alignment with the body's midline, without hip rotation or abduction and with knee flexion to 90° (figure 16.32). If the patient has normal flexibility, the thigh should rest comfortably on the table with the back in full contact with the table. A common substitution for this exercise is hyperextension of the lumbar spine. If you observe a lift of the lumbar spine, have the patient bring the nonstretch leg up closer to the chest.

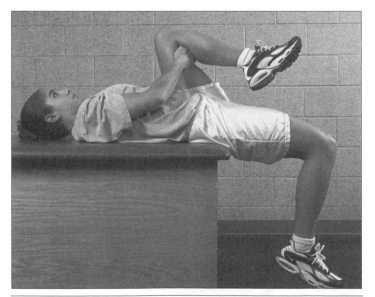

Figure 16.32 Thomas hip flexor stretch.

Figure 16.33 Hamstring stretch.

Figure 16.34 Piriformis stretch: *(a)* supine, *(b)* quadruped.

Straight-Leg Raise

This exercise stretches the hamstrings. Hamstring tightness can contribute to low-back inflexibility. Although a variety of methods are available to stretch the hamstrings, this exercise places minimal stress on the spine. In supine, the patient places the hands behind the thigh of one leg while the other leg remains extended. The patient then straightens the knee of the leg that the hands are on until he or she feels a stretch in the posterior thigh or behind the knee (figure 16.33). The common substitution for this exercise is to flex the opposite hip to relieve the stretch. The patient should keep the other leg in a fully extended position throughout the exercise.

Piriformis Stretch

This exercise stretches the lateral hip rotators, a common source of low back pain. The patient lies supine with the knees flexed and feet flat on the floor. The knee of the involved leg is crossed on top of the other, and both knees are brought to the chest. The patient grasps the lower knee and pulls both knees toward the chest (figure 16.34a). A common substitution is to provide less rotation of the stretched hip. The knees should be adequately crossed to aim the knee toward the opposite shoulder when the knees are brought to the chest.

In an alternative piriformis stretch, the patient is on hands and knees with the uninvolved leg crossed over the involved leg and behind the involved hip. The patient moves the hips backward, keeping the uninvolved leg straight and bending the knee of the involved leg (figure 16.34b). A common substitution is moving the hips toward the extended leg rather than keeping the weight equally distributed over both hips. Instruct the patient not to rotate but move straight back if you observe this substitution.

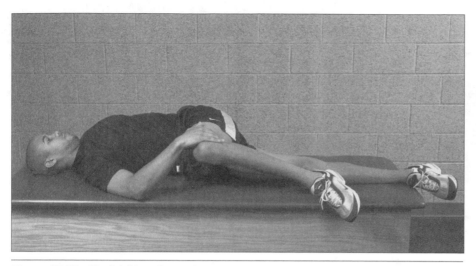

Figure 16.35   Iliotibial band stretch.

Iliotibial Band (ITB) Stretch

This exercise stretches the lateral thigh. Tightness in the ITB can affect the low back. The patient lies supine with the knees straight. The leg to be stretched is crossed over the other so that the foot of the crossed-over leg lies on the outside of the opposite knee. The hand on the opposite side grasps the crossed-over knee and pulls it toward the floor (figure 16.35). The common substitution for this exercise is to lift the ipsilateral shoulder off the floor. Instruct the patient in proper stabilization of the trunk for this exercise.

Lateral Shift

This exercise is used to correct a lateral shift. The patient stands next to the wall, with the side that has the lumbar lateral shift farthest from the wall. Keeping the shoulders level, the patient shifts the pelvis laterally to the wall (figure 16.36a). The common substitution for this exercise is a tilting of the shoulders away from the wall, or a leaning of the hips into the wall, or both. If this occurs, either have the patient perform the exercise in front of a mirror or place your hands above the shoulders, but not touching them, and instruct the patient to perform the exercise without letting the shoulders touch your hands.

To perform this stretch passively, the rehabilitation clinician stands facing the patient's side with the shift. The clinician then encircles the patient's waist and clasps his or her hands together on the opposite hip (figure 16.36b). The rehabilitation clinician stabilizes the trunk with his or her shoulder into the patient's waist while pulling the pelvis toward him- or herself.

Figure 16.36   Lateral shift: *(a)* independent, *(b)* assisted.

Standing Extension

This exercise increases trunk extension and relieves tension after prolonged sitting or forward bending. The patient stands and places both hands in the small of the back. The patient then leans backward, leading with the head and keeping the knees and hips extended. A common substitution is moving the hips posteriorly and bending the knees, leaning back from the knees. If this occurs, have the patient perform the exercise with his or her back against a countertop to stop the hips from moving backward.

Posture and Pelvic Stabilization Exercises

Any patient who has a spinal injury should be examined for posture. Posture plays a vital role in both recovery from and prevention of injuries. If a patient has poor posture and nothing is done to correct it, the poor posture will continue to exacerbate the injury and make recovery difficult. Instruction in techniques to maintain proper posture and use of proper body mechanics should also be a part of the rehabilitation program. Refer to the discussion of posture in chapter 11 as necessary.

Pelvic Neutral

Essential to good posture is strength of the trunk and hips to provide pelvic stability. Individuals without good strength in these areas are at risk for injury and impaired performance. A stable pelvis serves as a platform from which the arms and legs are able to perform their activities. Pelvic stability is also referred to as *lumbar stability, trunk stability, core stability, spinal stability,* or *lumbosacral stability.* These various terms will be interchanged throughout this section so you may become accustomed to their use. Pelvic stability relies on the strength and control of several trunk muscles: abdominal obliques, transverse abdominis, and multifidus, and the gluteal muscle group. The quadratus lumborum and latissimus dorsi also play a role in stability.

It is important that the clinician design a program that strengthens these core stabilizing muscles before performance activities are initiated. The stabilization muscles are generally the muscles more central to the body while the peripheral muscles are used to move the body segment. For example, the abdominal muscles most important for stability are the transverse abdominis and obliques while the rectus abdominis is used to flex the trunk. Likewise, the multifidus is a back stabilizing muscle while the longer and more superficial erector spinae muscles are the movers of trunk extension.

Before an individual can have good pelvic stability, he or she must be able to maintain a *pelvic neutral* position. **Pelvic neutral** is a position where the least amount of stress is placed on the lumbar spine. Sometimes the position is called *lumbar neutral*, or *neutral spine*. Pelvic neutral can be difficult to find for someone who is not accustomed to being in this position. I have found the best position for the patient to be in for instruction on how to achieve pelvic neutral is sitting. With the patient sitting, have the patient place his or her fingers on the left and right ASIS. Instruct the patient to rock the pelvis as far as possible posteriorly and note the end position, and then rock the pelvis as far as possible anteriorly, noting the end position. Now the patient rocks between each extreme, moving through a progressively smaller range of motion until he or she is balanced in the mid-position between the ends of motion. This is the patient's pelvic neutral; it is the center of pelvic motion where the spine should be balanced over the pelvis.

Once the patient is able to find and hold pelvic neutral, it is important to explain and emphasize to the patient the need to maintain this position during all activities. Maintaining this position will require some contraction of the stabilizing muscles. The exercises presented on the next few pages can be used in the early phase when the patient has difficulty maintaining pelvic neutral with arm and leg motions. The intent of these exercises is to have the patient perform arm and leg motions while maintaining pelvic neutral. Careful attention must be paid to the patient's performance so correction of erroneous performance can be made and encouragement is given for correct performance.

Stabilization Exercise Progression

A progression of exercises designed to assist the patient in spine stabilization includes exercises in the supine and quadruped positions. The intent is to strengthen the lower back and abdominal core stabilization muscles to provide spinal stability during arm and leg motion. These exercises constitute the initial step toward movement without stress to the spine and should be a part of the rehabilitation program if a patient is unable to identify and maintain good spinal alignment during activities.

Early supine exercises are often referred to as "bug exercises" or "dead-bug exercises," presumably because of the position they are performed in and the arm and leg movement that occurs. The supine and quadruped exercises are outlined here from the easiest to the more difficult. Progression from these can be made to standing exercises using rubber band resistance for either upper or lower extremity activities while the patient maintains a pelvic neutral position.

Core stabilization progresses from these basic exercises to more functional activities. It is important that the patient maintains good trunk stability during all activities. This protects the spine and allows the patient to perform physical activities more skillfully and with greater force, because with good pelvic stability the lower-extremity forces can be more readily transmitted to the upper extremities. Activities in the final phase of pelvic stabilization include performance of skill drills while in pelvic neutral.

It is important to remember that pelvic stability must be maintained throughout each of these exercises. The hips should not roll; the lumbar spine should not flex or extend; and there should not be an anterior or posterior pelvic tilt. If the patient is unable to maintain stability during any exercise, it may be necessary to return to exercises at the previous level of difficulty before advancing. The abdominal and buttock muscles should be tensed in each of these exercises to provide the stabilization necessary for correct performance. You should instruct or remind the patient regarding this until he or she can perform the exercise without verbal cueing. Before using any of these exercises, you should instruct the patient in how to find and maintain a pelvic neutral position. Once the patient can find pelvic neutral and know how recruit and use the transverse abdominis and multifidus, the exercises can begin.

Transverse Abdominis and Multifidus Recruitment

Even healthy patients may have a difficult time performing these exercises, so time is required to establish the basics in core stability before the stabilization exercises are started. The patient must be able to recruit both the transverse abdominis and multifidus muscle groups before correct execution of spinal stabilization exercises is possible.

Transverse Abdominis Recruitment Activities. With the patient in a supine hooklying position, a blood pressure cuff is placed comfortably beneath the patient's low back. The cuff is inflated to 40 mmHg. The patient moves into a pelvic neutral position and is instructed to, "Pull your navel to your spine." This abdominal tension should be produced without changing the pelvic neutral position. The clinician is able to monitor whether the patient has successfully performed the activity by monitoring the blood pressure cuff gauge. If the pressure jumps significantly, then the patient has also lost pelvic neutral and gone into a posterior pelvic tilt; if the pressure decreases significantly, the patient has moved into an anterior pelvic tilt. Allow the patient to see the blood pressure gauge as a feedback mechanism. Palpation of the abdominals may also assist the patient in correct muscle recruitment. Once the patient is able to pull the navel to the spine without more than a 3- to 5-degree change in blood pressure gauge reading, correct recruitment of the transverse abdominis has occurred.

Multifidus Recruitment Activities. The multifidus is too deep to palpate, so it may be difficult to determine whether or not the patient is using the muscle correctly. However, we do know that the multifidus is activated when pelvic floor muscles are used. In order to activate the pelvic floor muscles, the verbal cue that is provided to the patient is, "Tighten muscles as if you were stopping urination at mid-flow." Although you will not palpate the multifidus directly, you may be able to feel it tighten indirectly if you place your finger tips adjacent the patient's lumbar spinous processes as you provide the verbal cue. If the muscle is weak, it may feel like a very light pressure into your fingertips.

With the patient in a hooklying supine position and in pelvic neutral, provide the verbal cue, "Tighten muscles as if you were stopping urination at mid-flow." Once again, the blood pressure cuff inflated to 40 mmHg placed in the lumbar region provides feedback to the clinician and patient as to the patient's quality of performance. As with the transverse abdominis exercise, if the pressure increases or decreases substantially, the patient has lost pelvic neutral. Tension in the muscle should be produces without changing the position of the pelvis.

Combining Transverse Oblique and Multifidus Activity

Before the patient moves into dead-bug exercises, he or she must be able to perform simultaneous activation of the transverse abdominis and multifidus muscles. Once each muscle is able to be activated individually, the clinician now instructs the patient to both, "and now pull your navel to your spine. Tighten your muscles as if stopping urination mid-flow." The patient is able to perform these activities correctly if there is no change in the blood pressure gauge.

Once the patient is able to recruit the transverse abdominis and multifidus muscles, progression to the dead-bug exercises can be made. Dead-bug exercises should be performed, at least in the early stages, with the blood pressure cuff to provide the patient with feedback on his or her performance. If the patient's pressure gauge indicates a big jump during any of the exercises, it may be necessary to start with a smaller range of movement; the patient should perform an exercise only in the range of motion where pelvic stability is maintained. As greater control is achieved, a greater range of movement will be possible.

Dead-Bug Exercises. Not all patients with back injuries need to perform these dead-bug exercises and some may be able to progress rapidly through the earlier-stage exercises. For all patients performing these exercises, rehabilitation clinician should determine the patient's ability to maintain pelvic neutral throughout the exercises. Any difficulty the patient has with any of these exercises indicates that pelvic stabilization is limited, and that the patient should do the exercise until he or she is able to perform it correctly.

Once the patient masters one exercise, he or she can progress to the next one. These may seem to be simple exercises, but if you try them, you quickly realize that when they are performed correctly they may not be as simple as they look. These exercises can be made more difficult with the patient lying on a foam roller during their execution.

Each exercise is prefaced with the verbal cues from the rehabilitation clinician to, "Pull the navel to the spine," and "Tighten muscles as if stopping urination mid-flow." Once the patient sets the transverse abdominis and multifidus muscles, the exercises are performed.

Each of these dead-bug exercises can be made more difficult by having the patient perform arm and/or leg motions in a diagonal pattern rather than straight-plane motions. This alteration will require recruitment of the oblique muscles.

Supine Stabilization with Arm Movement. This exercise provides arm resistance to pelvic stabilization. The patient lies supine with the knees flexed. Cues are given to the patient to position and maintain a neutral spine position. One arm is raised overhead, and then the other, in an alternating fashion (figure 16.37). The trunk is stabilized, with no movement occurring in the spine or pelvis while the arms are moving. The patient must maintain pelvic neutral and breathe while performing the movement.

Figure 16.37 Spine stabilization with arms.

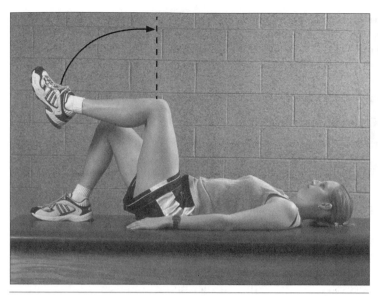

Figure 16.38 Spine stabilization with legs.

Supine Stabilization with Leg Movement. This exercise strengthens the lower abdominals and provides increased resistance to pelvic stabilization. The patient lies supine with the legs flexed. While in a neutral spine position, the patient raises one knee up toward the chest and then extends the leg from the knee without moving the hips as the abdominals are contracted more tightly to maintain pelvic neutral (figure 16.38). The hips should not rise up or rotate, and the back should not arch. The motion should be smooth. The patient returns the leg to the starting position and repeats the movement with the opposite leg.

Supine Stabilization with Arm and Leg Movement. This exercise is designed to strengthen the abdominals and stabilize the spine while the arms and legs move independently of the spine. The patient lies supine with the knees bent and the spine in a neutral position. One arm and the opposite leg are raised simultaneously and then lowered while pelvic neutral is maintained (figure 16.39). The movement is repeated with the contralateral arm and leg. The movement should be smooth, and no trunk motion should occur. The pelvis is maintained in neutral throughout. The back should not roll from one side to another and should not arch off the floor.

Figure 16.39 Spine stabilization with arm and leg movement.

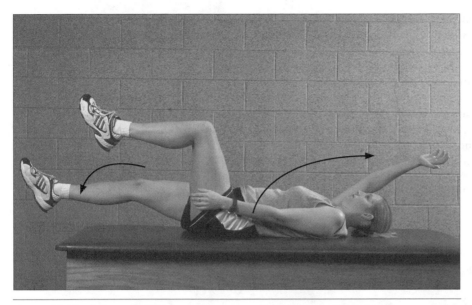

Figure 16.40 Spine stabilization with arms and unsupported legs.

Supine Stabilization with Arms and Unsupported Legs. This is a more severe exercise for strengthening the abdominals and maintaining pelvic neutral during independent arm and leg movement. The patient lies supine with the knees bent and the spine in pelvic neutral. The neck and shoulders should remain relaxed throughout the exercise. The abdominal muscles remain tightened as the patient lifts the arms and legs off the floor. The patient gradually extends one leg while flexing the arm on the same side then reverses the position with the extremities on the opposite side (figure 16.40). The back should not lift off the floor, and the hips should not roll.

Quadruped exercises

When the patient is able to perform the supine stabilization exercises, progression can be made to exercises in a quadruped position. As with the dead-bug exercises, the quadruped exercises are presented in a progressive manner, from easiest to most difficult. As with the dead-bug exercises, these exercises can be further advanced by having the patient perform arm and/or leg motions in a diagonal pattern rather than straight-plane motions to not only make the exercise more difficult but also recruit the oblique muscles.

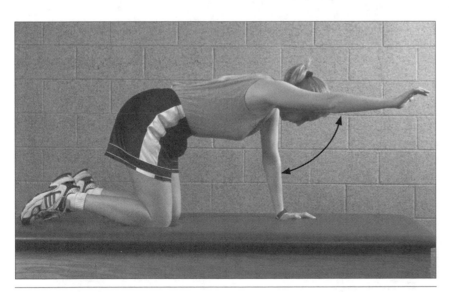

Figure 16.41 Quadruped arm raise.

Quadruped Arm Raise. This exercise is for spinal stabilization. The patient is in a quadruped position and in pelvic neutral. One arm is raised and lowered, and the movement is then repeated on the opposite side (figure 16.41). The hips and back should not move throughout the exercise. A good feedback technique to help the patient detect hip motion during these exercises is to place a 0.9-to 1.2- m (3- to 4-ft) stick or dowel across the low back. The dowel should be balanced on the back. If the patient sees the stick drop on one side during the exercise, he or she knows that the hips have rotated and that pelvic neutral has not been maintained.

Quadruped Leg Raise. The purpose of this exercise is to enhance pelvic stabilization. The patient is in a quadruped position with the pelvis in neutral. The patient extends one leg, rather than an arm, and moves it backward by tightening the buttocks and hamstrings. No movement of the pelvis, trunk, or back occurs throughout the motion. The extremity motion should be smooth and steady. As with the arm exercises, a stick placed across the lumbar spine can provide the patient feedback on unwanted pelvic movement.

Quadruped Arm and Leg Raise. This exercise enhances stabilization and strengthens the spinal extensors. With the patient in a quadruped position and the abdominals tightened to stabilize the spine in neutral, the patient lifts one arm and the opposite leg and then repeats the motion with the other arm and leg (figure 16.42). The shoulders, hips, and back should not move throughout the exercise. The hip should not drop or lift, and the back should not roll. Use of the stick on the low back is useful with this exercise.

Figure 16.42 Quadruped arm and leg raise.

Additional Activities

Once the patient is able to perform the stabilization exercises presented above, he or she should attempt maintaining pelvic neutral in other positions such as standing position, and then progressing to maintaining pelvic neutral during functional activities like walking, jogging, jumping, upper extremity exercises and movements, and other functional activities.

More advanced exercises for trunk stabilization include strength exercises for the abdominals and back extensors. These exercises are discussed in the next unit on strengthening exercises. Careful attention must be given by the clinician to the patient's performance of all activities to assure the patient is able to maintain a pelvic neutral position throughout his or her performance.

Strengthening Exercises

These exercises are used in the muscle strength and endurance component of the therapeutic exercise program. We begin with the mildest and proceed to more challenging exercises, first for the neck and then for the lower back. Keep in mind that other exercises you can use for strengthening include the aquatic exercises discussed in chapter 13 and the Swiss-ball and foam-roller exercises discussed in chapter 14. The patient should maintain a pelvic neutral position throughout each of these exercises.

Cervical Exercises

Distinct advantages of isometric exercises are that they can be initiated early in the therapeutic exercise program and that the patient can perform them independently throughout the day.

Cervical Isometrics

Each isometric exercise is held for 10 s. These exercises are performed in either an anatomical or a midrange position. In the forward flexion exercise, the patient places the palms of the hands on the forehead and attempts to touch the chin to the chest while providing resistance to the motion with the hands on the forehead (figure 16.43a). In the extension exercise, the patient places both hands behind the back of his or her head while attempting to tilt the head backward, resisting the motion with the hands (figure 16.43b). To perform lateral flexion, the patient places one hand near the ear, resisting the motion of bringing the ear to the shoulder on the same side (figure 16.43c). The exercise is repeated on the opposite side. In isometric rotation, the patient places one hand on the side of the face and resists the movement of rotating to look over the same-side shoulder (figure 16.43d). The exercise is repeated on the opposite side. A common substitution for each of these exercises is to perform them out of cervical alignment. Each exercise should be performed with the head and neck in correct postural alignment. If the patient has difficulty identifying correct postural alignment, he or she should perform the exercises in front of a mirror until correct alignment can be maintained during the exercises.

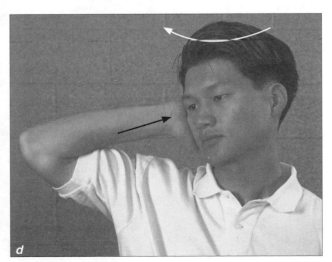

Figure 16.43 Cervical isometric exercise: *(a)* flexion, *(b)* extension, *(c)* lateral flexion, *(d)* rotation.

Figure 16.44 Prone cervical retraction.

Prone Neck Retraction

This exercise strengthens the posterior cervical muscles and encourages correct cervical spine alignment. The patient lies prone with his or her head and neck off the table. Keeping the chin tucked, the patient lifts the posterior head toward the ceiling (figure 16.44). The scapulae can also be squeezed together. At the top of the movement, the position is held for 5 to 10 s. This exercise is often incorrectly performed with the neck in extension and the head tilted upward. Instructing the patient to keep the chin tucked and describing the activity as, "like opening and closing a drawer," may give the patient a visual image that will help.

Sidelying Head Lifts

This exercise strengthens the lateral neck muscles. The patient is in sidelying with the head hanging down to the table or off the table. The individual then lifts the head toward the top shoulder, going through a full arc of motion. An incorrect performance often seen is with the neck in a forward-head position. Correct posture should be maintained throughout the exercise.

Resisted Cervical Exercises

These are more aggressive exercises for strengthening the cervical muscles. They can be performed with rubber tubing, pulleys, or machines applied to the head. It is important to be careful using the machine exercises, because if applied inappropriately, they can place too much stress on the cervical spine and increase the risk of injury. Proper cervical alignment must be maintained throughout the exercises with movement occurring at each segment—the lower cervical spine should not be used as a fulcrum.

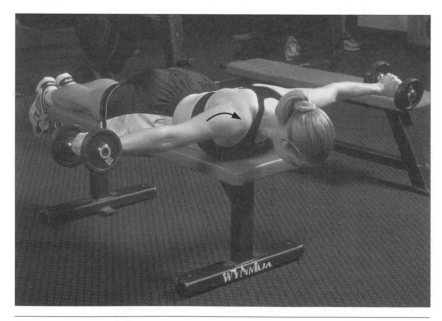

Figure 16.45 Prone flys.

Upper-Back Exercises

Many upper-back exercises are also shoulder exercises, because many of the shoulder muscles are located in the upper-back region.

Prone Fly

This exercise strengthens rhomboids, middle trapezius, and cervical and thoracic spine extensors. The patient lies prone on a bench with the arms hanging down to the floor. The patient lifts dumbbells toward the ceiling while squeezing the scapulae together (figure 16.45). People often perform this exercise incorrectly by raising the arms but not squeezing the scapulae together. The patient should be instructed to go through the full scapular retraction motion.

Figure 16.46
Upright row.

Upright Row

This exercise strengthens the upper back, trapezius, and deltoids. The patient uses pulleys, weights, or rubber tubing with hands close together while standing erect. With the abdominals tightened to maintain a pelvic neutral position, the patient lifts the device upward toward the chin, keeping the elbows higher than the wrists (figure 16.46). Keeping the elbows down rather than up provides less resistance for the deltoids and rotator cuff.

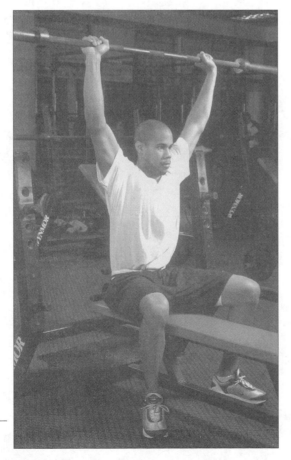

Figure 16.47
Upright press.

Upright Press

This exercise strengthens the deltoids and trunk stabilizers. It is also called a seated press or a military press. The patient can be standing or seated. The weight is grasped in the hands; with the elbows bent, the weights start at shoulder level. The abdominals are tightened to maintain trunk stability and prevent the back from arching as the patient lifts the weight straight up and overhead toward the ceiling (figure 16.47). The patient should also be instructed not to shrug the shoulders or arch the back, common errors in execution of this exercise.

Bouhler Exercises

These exercises strengthen the middle back muscles and lower trapezius. The patient stands with the back to the wall, arms overhead with elbows next to the ears, and elbows straight. In the first exercise the patient pushes the thumbs to the wall, holds the position for 5 s, relaxes, and then repeats (figure 16.48a). In the second exercise, the patient, positioned with the thumbs facing each other, repeats the movement of the hands moving to the wall (figure 16.48b). In the third exercise, the arms are positioned at a 45° angle from the horizontal and then pushed backward to the wall, with the elbows straight and the scapulae retracted together (figure 16.48c). In each position the patient must tighten the abdominals to stabilize the trunk and prevent the back from arching. A progression of these exercises is to position the patient in prone to perform the exercises (figure 16.48d) or to add weights while in prone. Common errors in execution include arching the back and standing too far from the wall. Good lumbar stability helps to ensure correct execution.

Figure 16.48
Bouhler exercises: (a) thumbs to wall, (b) thumbs facing each other, (c) 45° angle, (d) prone.

Lower-Back, Abdominal, and Pelvic Exercises

You may recall the abdominal and trunk exercises using the Swiss ball and foam roller (chapter 14) and the medicine ball (chapter 9). It is easy to incorporate these exercises into a progressive strengthening exercise program for the abdominals and lower back. You must be able to judge the degree of difficulty of each of these exercises and incorporate them at an appropriate time in the strengthening program. Most of the exercises listed in this section are useful for pelvic or lumbosacral stabilization.

Posterior Pelvic Tilt

This exercise strengthens the abdominals and gluteals and encourages the patient to maintain a pelvic neutral. It can also increase pelvic mobility. The patient lies supine with the legs extended, or with hips and knees flexed and feet flat on the floor, and arms relaxed at the sides. The patient tightens the abdominals, tightens the buttocks, and pushes the back to the floor. The pelvis should roll posteriorly (figure 16.49). Once the patient is able to perform this exercise in supine, he or she can also perform it in sitting and standing. Common errors include using the legs to move the pelvis rather than the abdominal and back muscles, arching the back rather than performing a pelvic tilt, and pushing the abdomen outward rather than tensing the abdominal muscles to pull the navel toward the spine.

Figure 16.49 Posterior pelvic tilt.

Trunk Curl

This exercise strengthens the upper rectus abdominis and obliques. The patient lies supine with legs extended and hands on top of the head. The chin is tucked to the chest and the upper trunk is slowly curled toward a sitting position (figure 16.50). The end position is not a full sitting position. The abdominal muscles should be tensed so that the umbilicus moves toward the spine. A curl should occur throughout the movement. Holding the top of the position for several seconds or holding weights in the hands makes the exercise more difficult. The feet are not anchored in this exercise because this would permit the hip flexors to perform the exercise instead of the abdominals. Hips and knees should be extended to prevent hip flexor activity during the curl; tensing the gluteus maximus can assist in holding the leg position. The patient should curl the upper spine rather than lift the trunk from the hips.

Figure 16.50 Supine trunk curl.

Figure 16.51 Abdominal crunch.

Crunch

This exercise strengthens the upper abdominal muscles. The patient lies supine with the knees bent, feet flat on the floor, and hands behind the head. The abdominals are tightened, and the head and shoulders are lifted upward toward the ceiling. There is no curling movement. The position is held for 10 to 20 s at the top of the motion (figure 16.51). The exercise becomes more difficult if the patient has the legs in an unsupported position with the feet off the floor. This exercise can serve as a progression toward abdominal crunch exercises combined with medicine-ball tosses as introduced in chapter 9. The patient is performing this exercise incorrectly if he or she moves toward the knees rather than toward the ceiling. The elbows should remain back with the scapulae retracted as the patient lifts the upper trunk upward. If the patient complains of low back pain during the exercise, it is likely that he or she is either too weak or performing it incorrectly and not maintaining enough tension in the abdominals.

Oblique Abdominal Curl

This exercise strengthens the oblique muscles. The patient lies supine with knees bent and feet flat on the floor. The patient rotates the hips to one side so that he or she is lying on the back while on one hip and the other hip is facing the ceiling (figure 16.52). With hands on shoulders, or in the more difficult position, on top of the head, the patient curls toward the top hip, attempting to lift the head and shoulders upward and forward as much as possible. So that the obliques, not the hip muscles, perform the exercise, the feet are not anchored. A common error is beginning the rotation at the end of the motion rather than beginning the rotation at the onset and continuing through the range of motion. An alternative method is for the patient to lie supine and rotate one elbow toward the opposite knee while performing a crunch. Difficulties with this method are that hip rotation can be easily substituted for trunk rotation, trunk rotation can begin too early or too late in the motion before the patient lifts the shoulders upward, or the rotation can be performed with too much momentum.

Figure 16.52 Oblique abdominal curl.

Supine Leg Exercises

These exercises strengthen the lower abdominal muscles and facilitate maintenance of pelvic neutral. The patient lies supine with the knees bent and feet flat on the floor. The arms should be across the stomach, but if the patient has difficulty with the exercise, initial performance may be with arms at the sides; however, this position should be changed to the correct arm position before the exercise is advanced. The spine is kept in neutral throughout the exercise. One hip is flexed with the knee extended, foot pointing toward the ceiling. The leg is slowly lowered to the floor (figure 16.53a). The back should not arch or roll, and the abdominals should not push outward during the movement. As the patient gradually lowers the leg, he or she must progressively tighten the abdominals to maintain a pelvic neutral position.

The patient can progress in this exercise by performing leg thrusts. With the spine in a neutral position, the patient has both knees and hips flexed and the feet off the floor. One leg is thrust outward into extension and returned to the starting position. The other leg then performs the same exercise (figure 16.53b). In the more advanced version of this exercise, the patient alternately moves one leg out into extension while bringing the other leg toward the starting position so that both legs are moving simultaneously in opposite motions without touching the ground.

In the next progression of this exercise, the patient is in supine with both legs raised toward the ceiling and knees straight. As with the other exercises, the abdominals must control and keep the spine in a neutral position. The patient slowly lowers the legs to the floor without letting the low-back arch (figure 16.53c).

A final progression includes the V-sit-up (figure 16.53d). It is important that the patient maintain pelvic neutral and have control of the low back—that there is no arching of the back. If the patient is unable to maintain a pelvic neutral position and arches the low back, the person should return to the preceding exercise level until he or she achieves greater strength and control.

Figure 16.53 Supine leg exercises: *(a)* leg lowering, single; *(b)* leg thrusts; *(c)* leg lowering, bilateral; *(d)* V-sit-up.

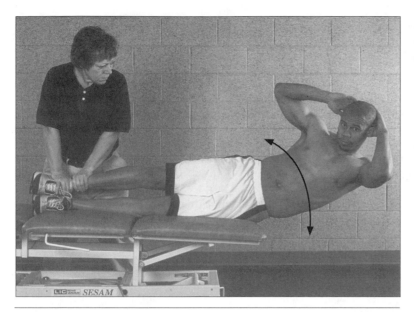

Figure 16.54   Sidelying sit-up.

Sidelying Sit-Up

This exercise strengthens the quadratus lumborum and the obliques. The patient is in sidelying with the feet anchored. The hands are placed across the chest or in the more difficult position behind the head. The patient curls sideways toward the top hip as much as possible, attempting to curl rather than just lift from the hips (figure 16.54).

Figure 16.55   Bridging progression: *(a)* bridging, *(b)* leg lift.

Bridging

This exercise strengthens the abdominals and back extensors and emphasizes trunk stabilization. The patient lies supine with the knees bent and feet flat on the floor. The abdominals are tightened and the spine is in neutral. The gluteals are tightened to lift the hips off the floor until the thighs and trunk form a straight line (figure 16.55a). This position is held for 15 to 60 s.

The next progression of this exercise is to perform the bridge and then lift each leg to march in place while maintaining the bridge in pelvic neutral. The patient must use the abdominals and buttocks while performing this exercise to maintain a straight line from the trunk to the supporting thigh.

A more advanced version of this exercise has the patient in the same bridging position, keeping abdominal, buttock, and lower-back muscles in good tension to maintain the position. The patient first brings one knee into full extension without moving the hips, then lowers it, and then performs the motion with the other leg (figure 16.55b). The hips should not drop or roll throughout the exercise. A stick placed across the hips and parallel to the floor will notify the patient of any change in pelvis position during the activity. If the stick either falls off or dips on one side, pelvic stability has not been maintained.

Figure 16.56 Lateral trunk rotation: start position—hips and knees flexed with knees together.

Lateral Trunk Rotation

This exercise strengthens the obliques and quadratus lumborum. The patient lies supine with knees bent. Rubber tubing or a pulley system is secured around both knees. The feet can be up on a stool or flat on the floor. The patient lets the pulley or tubing pull the knees downward to the side and then brings the knees upright by tilting the pelvis to flatten the back onto the floor, initiating the movement from the abdominals and back muscles rather than from the knees (figure 16.56).

Lunges

This exercise strengthens the abdominals, thigh, and gluteal muscles. It also facilitates correct trunk stability during lower-extremity activities. The patient begins in a standing position with the spine in neutral. Keeping the abdominals tightened and the back straight, the patient moves to a lunge position, going down smoothly, and then returns to a standing position (figure 16.57).

In the reverse lunge, the patient starts in the same position with the spine in neutral and the abdominals tightened. He or she steps backward and lowers the trunk in one smooth motion, keeping an upright position, and then returns to standing. The trunk should not tilt or rotate during either a forward or reverse lunge exercise. People often perform these exercises incorrectly with trunk rotation or flexion. The hips and shoulders should remain in the same plane throughout the exercise.

Figure 16.57 Lunge.

Figure 16.58 Prone trunk extension: *(a)* with assist on a table, *(b)* independently on Roman chair. Movement comes from the hip with the contraction of the gluteus maximus. The back should remain straight throughout the exercise, regardless of position of equipment on which it is performed. Dot indicates point from which movement occurs.

Prone Trunk Extension

This exercise strengthens the lower-back extensors and buttock muscles. The patient lies prone over the seat of a chair, a table, a Roman chair, or a Swiss ball. The feet are anchored either by another person (figure 16.58a) or by equipment (figure 16.58b). The easiest position is with the hands placed behind the back or at the sides; the exercise is more difficult with the hands placed farther away from the body's center of gravity to increase the lever-arm length for additional resistance. Weights can be placed in the hands with the arms overhead for the most difficult position. The patient begins in a slightly downward position, flexed approximately 30° at the hips. The gluteals are then tightened to lift the patient upward without curling backward. The lift is a straight lift from the hips and not a backward roll from the spine; and the patient should not start in a full trunk flexion position, because this can put unwanted stress on the intervertebral disks.

Once the patient has mastered the straight-plane extension exercises on the Roman chair, a progression can include trunk rotation during extension exercises. The patient can perform this exercise similarly to a rotational abdominal curl but in reverse motion, or the exercise becomes more difficult if the patient uses a medicine ball, rotating with the ball in the hands while going into extension. Patients cannot perform this exercise until they have good strength in the abdominals and trunk extensors; they must also be able to perform side sit-ups and trunk rotations in standing with a medicine ball without difficulty or pain.

Figure 16.59   Prone leg lift. Dot indicates point from which movement occurs.

Prone Leg Lift

This exercise strengthens the back extensors, abdominals, and buttocks. With the patient in a position that is the reverse of the position for the prone trunk lift, the trunk is supported on the table or a Roman chair, and the legs hang downward to the floor. The buttocks are squeezed to lift the legs until they are parallel with the floor. The pelvis must be positioned on the support structure, and movement occurs at the hips, not at the back (figure 16.59).

Figure 16.60   Latissimus pull-down.

Latissimus Pull-Down

This exercise is used to strengthen the latissimus dorsi. The latissimus dorsi is important in providing stabilization to the thoracolumbar spine because the muscle originates from the lower thoracic spinous processes, lumbar fascia, and iliac crest and has interdigitations with the external oblique muscles. The exercise uses an overhead pulley bar, with the patient's hands positioned shoulder-width or slightly farther apart and the elbows extended. The abdominals remain taut throughout the exercise and the pelvis is neutral. The patient brings the bar downward toward the thighs while keeping the elbows in near-extension (figure 16.60). Common errors are flexing the elbows too much, shrugging the shoulders, or flexing the lumbar spine. You should instruct the patient in proper technique before he or she performs the exercise and correct the execution as needed.

Agility and Coordination Exercises

Once patients have mastered the strengthening exercises, they should be ready for the trunk rotation and plyometric exercises that involve higher forces, quicker movements, and functional multiplanar motions. Pelvic stability should always be maintained throughout execution of any of these exercises.

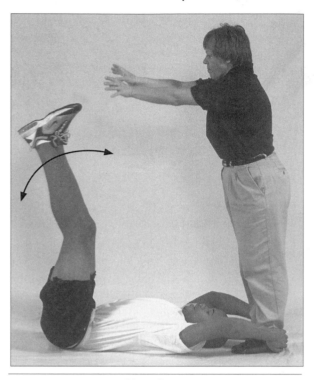

Figure 16.61 Resisted leg lifts.

Resisted Leg Lifts

This exercise is performed with the patient supine on the floor and the rehabilitation clinician standing at the patient's head. The patient's knees are extended, and the hips are flexed to approximately 90°. The patient attempts to lift the legs upward as the clinician attempts to push them back down (figure 16.61). This exercise is performed quickly but with control. It is important that the patient maintain pelvic neutral and that the back not arch throughout the exercise.

Medicine-Ball Exercises

Many of these medicine-ball exercises are listed in chapter 9. As a reminder, figure 16.62 depicts some of them. These exercises include activities such as ball passing low or high, trunk rotations, and abdominal curls with ball catching.

Figure 16.62 Medicine-ball exercises: *(a)* Trunk rotations. *(b)* Medicine-ball toss can be performed in straight plane to body or rotationally to facilitate oblique activity.

Many other exercises can be used to increase agility and resistance. Additional exercises include ball tossing on the Roman chair to increase trunk extension activity and adding rotation with the medicine ball to the Roman chair exercise.

SPECIAL REHABILITATION APPLICATIONS

▶ Specific types of back injuries call for particular kinds of exercises. Back problems that the rehabilitation clinician often encounters include sprains and strains; spondylosis, spondylolysis and spondylolisthesis; disk lesions; fact injuries; sacroiliac joint injuries; and thoracic outlet syndrome.

Before we look at specific injuries and the corresponding programs, let's use our artillery of exercises and progressions to put together a generic outline of a spinal rehabilitation program. We should keep in mind that modalities might be required initially to provide pain modulation and control inflammation. Soft-tissue mobilization and joint mobilization, if appropriate, are also part of the program. Flexibility exercises to improve range of motion of deficient areas are usually incorporated in the early days of the program, with instructions to perform the exercises frequently throughout the day. Instruction in pelvic neutral, pelvic stabilization exercises, and body mechanics must be part of the early portion of the program. Once the patient is able to maintain pelvic neutral in simple dead-bug exercises, he or she can progress to pool exercises and trunk-strengthening exercises. Early trunk-strengthening exercises include abdominal crunches and curls, oblique exercises, and bridging exercises. The latissimus pull-down is included as part of the strengthening exercises. As the patient is able to maintain a proper pelvic-neutral position, he or she performs lower extremity-strengthening exercises. Swiss-ball exercises such as crunches, bridges, leg lifts, side sit-ups, and progressions of strengthening exercises for the abdomen and trunk can begin in the middle phase of the program once the patient demonstrates good pelvic stability during arm and leg movements.

More aggressive strengthening exercises for the trunk begin when the patient is able to demonstrate good pelvic control and strength with the Swiss-ball and weight exercises. Examples of these more aggressive exercises include trunk and leg extension exercises on the Roman chair and abdominal crunches and standing trunk rotations using the medicine ball.

The final aspect of the program includes incorporation of drills that mimic sport-specific activities. The patient should be able to maintain good spinal stability and alignment throughout the activities. When the individual is pain free, has good strength and flexibility, and is able to perform functional activities without difficulty, return to full sport participation is indicated.

The spine is subject to a few unique injuries that require special consideration in an injury-specific therapeutic exercise program. The following sections present these injuries and therapeutic exercise programs to address them.

Sprains and Strains

Sprains and strains are among the most common back injuries. If they are not appropriately evaluated and treated, sprains and strains become frustrating and aggravating injuries because they can linger and cause lasting disability.

Program Considerations

The resulting pain and muscle spasm from acute sprains and strains must first be resolved with modalities and mild stretching exercises. Sometimes these conditions respond to grade I and II mobilization, but early response will depend on the severity of the pain and spasm and on the effectiveness of the modalities in relieving these problems.

Acute conditions require primarily modalities in the initial treatment phase along with limited activity and stretching exercises. As spasm and pain are reduced, soft-tissue mobilization is indicated if restriction is noted with palpation. Joint mobilization may be useful if the restriction is the result of joint hypomobility.

As with all spinal injuries, posture and body mechanics should be assessed and corrected as needed. Spasm will persist if the muscles are required to work more than they should because poor posture or body mechanics is present.

A progression of strengthening exercises should begin once the pain and spasm are under control. The muscles requiring the greatest emphasis are the pelvic stabilizers, abdominals, especially the obliques, lower abdominals, trunk extensors, and gluteals.

Case Study

A javelin thrower injured his back last week in practice when he attempted to throw the javelin and felt a sudden pain in the right low-back area. He comes to you stating that he applied ice to the injury when it occurred. The pain is now better than it was last week, but he still has pain when he rotates his trunk to the left and to the right. He has pain when he gets up from a chair and when he gets out of bed in the morning. His pain is worse at the end of the day. He has been taking it easy for a couple of days but is still unable to practice because of the pain. His pain is located on the right side of his low-back area. He has no radiation of symptoms into the lower extremities, but he does get pain in the right buttock. When you examine him you find that he is unable to forward bend because of pain; sidebending to the left is too painful to perform, but sidebending to the right is better. Trunk rotation is more painful to the left than to the right. His spine has a lateral shift to the right in the lumbar region. Palpation reveals muscle spasm with tenderness in the right paraspinals and quadratus lumborum muscles. Pressure over the multifidi reproduces his buttock pain.

Questions for Analysis

1. What stage of the healing process is he in? How severe is the injury?

2. How irritable is his injury? What is the nature of the injury?

3. What is your first treatment?

4. What is your treatment progression and what guidelines will you use to advance this patient from one level to the next?

5. What are some examples of specific exercises, including functional activities you should use before the patient's return to full participation?

Spondylosis, Spondylolysis, and Spondylolisthesis

Before presentation of the case study is a brief outline of considerations to keep in mind in a therapeutic exercise program for spondylosis, spondylolysis, and spondylolisthesis.

Program Considerations

Although these three conditions differ from one other, they all most often involve the lower lumbar spine and become irritated with extension movement. Patients with any of these conditions should be taught to maintain a posterior pelvic tilt and should attempt to avoid hyperextension movements as much as possible. It is vital that these patients establish and maintain pelvic stability in more of a posterior-tilt position and strengthen the abdominals. In spondylolisthesis, the most severe of the three conditions, there can be a forward displacement of the vertebrae.

Case Study ✓

A gymnast has seen an orthopedic physician because of persistent complaints of low-back pain that did not resolve after two weeks of modality treatments and reduced activity. The physician's diagnosis is a spondylolysis. The patient needs a rehabilitation program before she can return to competition.

Questions for Analysis

1. What exercises would you have this patient avoid?

2. What progression of exercises and activities should her therapeutic exercise program include to return her to full participation?

Disk Lesions and Sciatica

Disk lesions can be unnerving conditions for both a patient and the rehabilitation clinician. You should be familiar with the factors identified here and consider them before establishing care.

Program Considerations

A protruding or herniated disk can be a serious problem and most often cause radiculopathy down one or both extremities, depending on the location of the protrusion. The mere presence of pain or symptoms down the leg does not mean that there is a disk herniation, but you should consider this a possibility until it has been ruled out. Other conditions such as facet injuries, muscle spasm, and myofascial restriction can also cause pain referral down the leg.

Patients who have been diagnosed with disk lesions should avoid those positions and motions that aggravate or produce the sciatica symptoms. These motions most commonly are forward flexing or flexing and twisting in the direction that further compresses the disk protrusion.

Patients who have disk lesions must learn to find and maintain pelvic neutral and must strengthen the abdominals, obliques, back extensors, and gluteal muscle groups. They should learn correct body mechanics and posture and should eventually progress to performing all physical activities in a neutral spine position.

Although not all authorities agree on its importance, some advocate the centralization of pain for disk lesions. What this means is that if the treatment is appropriate, the patient will experience a gradual and progressive retreat of the sciatic pain distally to proximally until the only pain remaining is localized to the back. It is the goal of treatment to also relieve this central pain. Most often, the use of extension exercises, flexibility and strengthening activities, and pelvic-neutral exercises will accomplish this goal. Exercises progress at the patient's own rate. Progression depends on the treatment results and the patient's feedback regarding the pain. If the pain is receding, the progression of exercises can continue; but if the sciatic pain worsens, you must reevaluate the most recently performed exercises and activities, first for possible incorrect execution and secondly for appropriateness. It may be too soon for the patient to tolerate the severity of the exercise. Use of the wrong exercises or failure to correct body mechanics and posture may aggravate the disk lesion. It is vital that the clinician have a good understanding of the exercises and stresses that occur with each exercise.

Those patients who have undergone microdiscectomies follow a course of treatment similar to that for patients who have disk pathology but have not had surgical correction. In a typical time line, treatment begins about one week postoperatively and follows a progression, including pain modulation, flexibility exercises, pelvic stabilization, and strength exercises of increasing difficulty as already outlined. If post-surgical muscle tightness and soft-tissue restriction are present, they are treated with soft-tissue release and modalities.

Case Study

A football lineman injured his back in a game four weeks ago. He was referred to an orthopedic surgeon because of continued low-back and right lower-extremity pain. Magnetic resonance imaging (MRI) revealed that he has a disk bulge of 3 mm at L4-5. The physician indicates that this patient is not a surgical candidate because the problem may be resolved with rehabilitation, corticosteroid injections, or Medrol dose pack. The patient has had two of the three injections and reports significant relief of back and leg pain. He is now coming to you for a rehabilitation program. He moves pretty well when he enters the examination room. He does not appear to hesitate to walk or get up from a chair. When he moves around the room, however, you notice that he has very poor body mechanics, bending from the back to sit down and bending and twisting sideways to retrieve his backpack. His examination reveals a straight-leg raise to 50° on the right and 55° on the left, and his medial hip rotation is 20° bilaterally. In a forward bend, he is able to touch his fingers to his knees; in a sidebend he can touch 10 cm above his knee; and in backward bending he has normal motion. Forward bending produces some discomfort. You notice that when he bends, most of the motion occurs in the thoracic spine, with the lumbar spine remaining essentially flat. The neurological examination reveals no deficiencies in sensory, motor, or reflex innervation. The patient's gluteal muscles and abdominals each test at 4/5 strength. He is unable to perform a side sit-up on the right side. The paraspinals, quadratus lumborum, and hip lateral rotators are all tender to palpation, especially on the right; and you are able to palpate restriction of soft-tissue mobility in those tender areas. There is some restriction of joint mobility to PA tests in the lower lumbar spine.

Questions for Analysis

1. What precautions would you observe in treating this patient?

2. What would your initial treatment program include?

3. What techniques would you include in your first three treatment sessions?

4. What progression of exercises would you select for this patient, and what criteria would you use for progression from one level to the next in the program?

Facet Injuries

Facet injuries can be frustrating to treat, especially if you do not consider the factors listed here. Facet injuries can also be difficult to identify. The rehabilitation clinician must use his or her deductive tools if there is a possibility of facet injury.

Program Considerations

Facet restriction can occur from an impingement following a traumatic event. The position the facet is held in is called *positional dysfunction*. A *motion restriction* is what the facet is unable to do. A positional dysfunction will always be contralateral to a motion restriction. A facet can be restricted in either flexion or extension. A facet joint in flexion is considered *open* since the two facet surfaces comprising the facet joint are apart; a facet joint in extension is considered *closed*. If a facet is restricted in opening (flexing), it the facet is stuck in extension and has motion restriction in opening; extension is the positional dysfunction and flexing is the restricted motion. Since rotation and sidebending are coupled with each other, they will also have motion restrictions in positional dysfunctions. In a positional dysfunction of *(stuck in) extension*, rotation and sidebending will be limited on the *opposite side of the problem facet*.

For example, if a left facet has a postural dysfunction of (stuck in) extension, rotation left and sidebending left, the motion restriction will be flexion, right rotation, and right sidebending. On the other hand, if the positional dysfunction of *(stuck in) flexion* is present, restricted motion in sidebending and rotation will be *ipsilateral*. For example, if a patient had a positional dysfunction of (stuck in) flexion because the left facet will not close, the stuck position will be flexion, rotation left and sidebending left with motion restricted in extension, right rotation and right sidebending. Other signs include radiating pain mimicking dermatomal distribution, tenderness of spinous processes, and reflex muscle spasm.

More trauma causes sprains rather than impingement so tissue injury is greater. A more conservative treatment approach is needed. Additionally, soft tissue around the joint may also have been injured, and swelling and muscle spasm are common. A cervical collar may reduce pain. A forward-head position is seen because extension is painful. If motion loss occurs, a unilateral capsular pattern may develop. The capsular pattern for facets is limitation of rotation to the involved side and sidebending to the opposite side. For example, if a left cervical or lumbar facet has a capsular pattern, left rotation and right sidebending will be restricted but right rotation and left sidebending will be free. Gentle ROM in pain-free movements and joint mobilization following modalities can relieve muscle spasm, pain, and edema. Later, grades III and IV joint mobilization is used for facet mobility.

Case Study

A diver landed poorly in a dive during practice four days ago. She has had a stiff neck since that time. This morning she awoke and could not turn her head to the left. She presents to you with her head laterally flexed about 20° to the right and is unable to look straight ahead. Her head is rotated to the right about 15°. It is painful for her to attempt to place her head in an upright and straight position, but she has no difficulty turning her head all the way to the right and looking over her right shoulder. Your palpation reveals tenderness over the C5 and C6 spinous processes, and there is some tightness in the muscles in the same area.

Questions for Analysis

1. What do you believe her problem is; what side of her cervical spine is the location of her problem?

2. Outline your treatment program, sequencing your treatment in a logical progression.

Sacroiliac Joint

Although the impact of the SI joint on low back pain is controversial, most clinicians agree that the SI is a complex structure. There is some evidence to indicate that the SI should be an important consideration in low back pain, and back can refer pain into the SI joint (Cappaert 2000). The SI and hip can also refer pain to each other. An examination of the SI should be part of the examination of any patient who complains of back or hip pain.

As you learned in biomechanics, as the spine flexes forward, the sacroilium rotates posteriorly in extension, and the opposite occurs when the spine is extended. During ambulation, the sacrum rotates posteriorly on the same side as heel strike and anteriorly on the same side as toe off. This will assist in also causing a rotation around a diagonal axis. The pubic bones correspond to iliac motion during walking. You may remember from anatomy that the sacrum has an inferior lateral angle (ILA) at its base. It is located most easily by first locating the cornua, the inferior facet of the sacrum that connects to the coccyx. The right and left ILA are located just lateral to and on either side of the cornua (figure 16.63). The sacrotuberous ligament connects the ischial tuberosity to the inferior sacrum. It is located at about a 45° angle

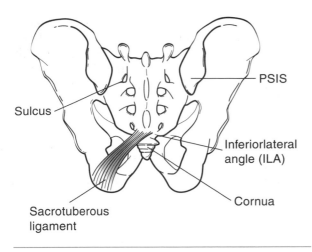

Figure 16.63 Sacroilium.

superior and medial from the ischial tuberosity between the ischium and inferior-lateral sacrum. You will need to identify each of these structures during an SI evaluation.

Patients who have excessive lumbar lordosis with an exaggerated sacral forward tilt can place excessive stress on the SI joint and cause pain in the area. Patients are susceptible to SI injuries if they have a leg-length discrepancy, fall on the side or buttocks, misstep off a curb while running, run while twisting, or bend and twist the lumbar spine. The patients most susceptible to SI injuries because of the stress of their sports are soccer, basketball, and football players; gymnasts; wrestlers; and track and field athletes.

Sacroiliac malalignments can occur with imbalances caused by injury or secondary spasm, weakness, or loss of mobility. Some SI joint injuries result from classic types of injuries. Upslips, inflares or outflares, and pubic subluxations can occur when there is a sudden, sharp jolt to the leg as a person steps off a curb or steps down and does not realize that there is another step. Landing on the buttock can lead to sacral flexion, pubic subluxations, and up-slip injuries. Trunk rotation and bending activities can cause sacroiliac dysfunctions. Knowing the history will help to identify the problem.

Sacroiliac Examination

Before treatment is initiated, an examination to determine the areas of malalignment must be made. A complete sacroiliac examination includes an investigations of posture, alignment, and lumbar range of motion. There are specific factors that are also examined when sacroiliac pathology is suspected. These factors are used to determine either relative alignment or quality and quantity of motion. The three special tests used to determine quality and quantity of motion include the standing forward bend test (StFBT), kinetic test (KT), and seated forward bend test (SitFBT). The relative alignment tests are performed with the patient in supine and prone positions; the supine tests include examination of left and right iliac crest height, leg length (Leg L), distance of the ASIS to umbilicus and the ASIS height (ASIS), and height and springiness of the symphysis pubis (Pube ht, Pube Spring). The prone tests include examination of positions of the sulcus (Sulcus), inferior lateral angle (ILA), and sacrotuberous ligament (St. Lig).

Standing Forward-Bend Test

The standing forward-bend test is sometimes called the Piedallus test and is performed with the clinician facing the patient's back and placing each thumb on the patient's PSIS and the hands on the iliac crests. The patient then bends forward (figure 16.64). If the SI joint is normal, the thumbs will move inferiorly as the patient bends forward; if there is a lesion, the thumb on the side of the lesion will either move upward or not move as the other thumb moves inferiorly. This test only identifies the side of the lesion; it does not identify the kind of lesion.

Seated Forward-Bend Test

The seated forward-bend test is performed with the clinician's hands as indicated in the standing forward-bend test. The patient is in a seated position with the knees apart and higher than the hips (figure 16.65). The patient bends forward; in normal movement, the thumbs should move as they do in the standing forward bend-test. If a thumb either does not move or moves superiorly, the patient has a sacroiliac lesion on that side.

Kinetic Test

In the kinetic test (also called the Norwegian test), the patient stands with his or her back to the clinician. To evaluate the left, the clinician places one thumb on the left PSIS and the other thumb at the same level on the mid-superior sacrum (figure 16.66). The patient then lifts the left knee toward the chest; if the SI joint is normal, the left thumb moves inferiorly, but it stays at the same level if motion is restricted. This test checks for left iliosacral motion. With the thumbs and patient in the same start position, the patient then lifts the right knee toward the

Figure 16.64
Standing forward
bend test.

Figure 16.65 Seated
forward bend test.

Figure 16.66
Kinetic test.

Figure 16.67   Leg-length difference.

chest; if the SI is normal, the right thumb moves inferiorly, but motion is restricted if the thumb stays at the same level; this test checks for left sacroiliac motion. The clinician then places the thumbs in a reverse position with the right thumb on the right PSIS and the left thumb on the mid-superior sacrum and repeats the two tests; lifting the right leg and watching right thumb movement assesses right iliosacral motion, and lifting the left leg while watching left thumb movement assesses right sacroilial motion.

Pain with pressure on each palpation point during supine or prone tests is a positive sign. Before performing the supine tests, the patient performs a bridge then moves both hips and knees into extension. Leg length is assessed by comparing levels of medial malleoli; if leg length discrepancy is present secondary to SI dysfunction, the difference will be readily apparent (figure 16.67).

The clinician then determines iliac crest (figure 16.68) and ASIS height (figure 16.69a); each ASIS should be equal in height when compared to each other. If one ASIS is more posterior than the other, it will appear more superior. The distance between each ASIS and navel should be determined by placing a thumb on each ASIS and rotating the hands to place the index finger at the navel (figure 16.69); obvious differences between the distances will be approximately 1 to 2 inches, if present. Springiness of the pubic bones is tested by first locating the pubic symphysis by placing the palm of the hand on the patient's abdomen and moving the hand caudally until the heel of the hand contacts the superior portion of the symphysis pubis. Once located, the clinician's index fingers are then positioned about 2 cm (<1 in.) laterally from the superior symphysis pubis to the pubic tubercles. The clinician then presses down

Figure 16.68 Iliac crest height test.

on the left then the right pubic tubercle (figure 16.70); pain or restricted mobility is a positive sign. Differences in height between the right and left pubic bones is assessed by placing a finger or thumb on each bone and noting differences.

Prone examination is made of the position of the right and left PSIS (figure 16.71a); they should be of equal height to each other. Prone examination is also made of the position of the left and right sulcus (figure 16.71b). The left and right sulcus are located immediately medially and about 30° caudally from the left and right PSIS, respectively (figure 16.72); the position of each should be equal, but if one is more posterior or anterior, it should be noted since this is abnormal (figure 16.71b). The height of right and

Figure 16.69 ASIS (*a*) height and (*b*) to-navel tests.

Figure 16.70 Pubic symphysis test. (*a*) Locating symphysis pubis and (*b*) testing for springiness sand height sof left and right.

Figure 16.71 (a) PSIS examination and (b) location of right and left sulcus.

Figure 16.72 Sulcus and PSIS. The middle fingers indicate the location of the left and right PSIS and the index fingers show the location of the left and right sulcus, 30° medial and inferior to their respective PSIS.

left ILA are then evaluated (figure 16.73). To locate the ILA, the cornua or the very end of the sacrum as it meets the coccyx, is palpated; the ILA are about 1.5 to 2 cm lateral on either side of the cornua. The ILA should be level with each other, but if one is more anterior or more posterior than the other, this should be noted. There should be no pain with palpation or pressure of any of these landmarks; pain is an abnormal response.

Additional examinations include trunk range-of-motion tests for quality and quantity of motion and pain during any motion. If lateral flexion is limited and accompanied with signs of SI dysfunction, the problem is probably of sacroiliac origin. If flexion-extension motion is limited, the problem may be iliosacral in origin.

The pathological patterns that can develop occur because either the sacrum is malaligned on the ilium or the ilium is malaligned on the sacrum. When the sacrum is malaligned on the ilium, it is called sacroiliac dysfunction; the sacrum can become malaligned between the two iliac bones to result in either bilateral or unilateral restriction of motion. The dysfunctions with their common causes and symptoms are listed in table 16.1. The iliosacral pathologies are listed in table 16.2a and the sacroiliac pathologies are listed in table 16.2b. Once you have examined a patient for possible SI lesions, compare your results with tables 16.2a and 16.2b. If your patient has a SI lesion, your findings should correlate with the findings of one of the pathologies in these tables. The iliosacral and sacroiliac pathologies are listed along with the examination results for each condition. Treatment is directed toward relieving and correcting the SI joint alignment, stabilizing the joints, and correcting posture or faulty techniques. The techniques used to correct alignment are referred to as muscle energy techniques. The specifics of theory and application for these are presented in chapter 6. The muscle energy techniques discussed here are treatments for specific SI dysfunctions.

Figure 16.73 The clinician (*a*) locates the cornua and (*b*) moves thumbs laterally to palpate the ILA.

Table 16.1

Dysfunctions and Symptoms

Type of Dysfunction	Dysfunction	Common Cause	Signs and Symptoms
Iliosacral	Pubic subluxation	Soccer; after pregnancy and delivery	Groin pain, buttock pain; may have only low-back pain
	Iliac inflare	Direct blow; soccer	Groin pain; may or may not have leg pain
	Iliac outflare	Falls; direct blow; soccer	Groin pain; may or may not have hip pain or leg pain
	Anterior iliac subluxation (R Upslip)	Past history of falling on buttock; sudden step off curb; hockey; basketball; motor vehicle accident (MVA)	Always on right (right upslip); pain often on opposite side; leg pain; low-back pain; coccygeal pain; nerve-root pain
	Posterior iliac subluxation (L Upslip)	Same as anterior iliac subluxation	Always on left (left upslip); often occurs with other spinal problems that haven't responded to treatment; often occurs with spinal flexion.
	Anterior iliac rotation	Usually occurs with other lesions	Long leg on side of lesion; should be the last to treat
Sacroilial	Sacral flexion	Occurs with bending and twisting activities or push-pull activities; MVA	Pain is often on opposite of lesion; patient may report feeling as if back popped at the time of injury
	Forward torsion: same letters (1st letter = sacral motion; 2nd letter = axis)	Bending with twisting motion; getting out of car quickly	Most common SI injury. Back or leg pain. Buttock pain. Pain may be on opposite side of lesion. Indicated as a right on right (RonR) or left on left (LonL) forward torsion.
	Backward torsion: opposite letters (1st letter = sacral motion; 2nd letter = axis)	Bending with twisting motion	Doesn't occur as often as the forward torsions. Patient is bent in flexion 2° to pain and waddles like a duck; painful in extension; may appear to be a disc lesion or may have pain in the buttock and L/S; indicated as a right on left (RonL) or a left on right (LonR) backward torsion.

Table 16.2a
Illiosacral Pathology

Pathology	Sit FBT	St FBT	KT	Leg L.	Pube Ht	Pube Spring	ASIS	Sulcus	ILA	St Lig
R Superior Pubic Subluxation	Neg	Pos R	Pos R	Short R	R Superior	Pain R				
R Iliac Inflare	Neg	Pos R	Pos R		R Ant	Pain R	↓ Dist R ASIS to umbilicus			
R Iliac Outflare	Neg	Pos R	Pos R		R Post	Pain R	↑ Dist R ASIS to umbilicus			
R Upslip: Ant Iliac Subluxation (Always on Right)	Neg	Pos R	Pos R	Short R	R Sup	Pain R	R Superior	Varies	Shorter R	R Slack with high R Isch T
L Upslip: Post Iliac Subluxation (Always on Left)	Neg	Pos L	Pos L	Short L	L Sup	Pain L	L Superior	Varies	Shorter L	L is slack
R Ant Iliac Rotation	Neg	Pos R	Pos R	Long R	R Inf	Pain R	R Inferior			

Table 16.2b
Sacroiliac Pathology

Pathology	Sit FBT	St FBT	KT	Leg L	Pube Ht	Pube Spring	ASIS	Sulcus	ILA	St Lig
L Sacral Flexion	Pos L	Pos L	Pos L	L Long	Varies	Varies	Varies	L Deep	L Post	
Forward Torsion L on L (same)	Pos L	Pos L	Pos L				L Inferior	R Deep	L Post	
Backward Torsion L on R (opp)	Pos R	Pos R	Pos R				L Inferior	R Deep	L Post	

Muscle Energy Treatment Techniques

Muscle energy techniques are a form of manual therapy that lend themselves well to the sacroiliac region. As was mentioned in chapter 6, muscle energy techniques can be used for either the spine or the extremities. Isometric contractions are used with spinal techniques while isotonic contractions are used for the extremities. Muscle energy techniques for the SI will be presented here.

When muscle imbalances occur, malalignments result and cause restriction of movement. These issues have been previously discussed. These restrictions are referred to in the muscle energy terminology as *barriers* to movement. A barrier is not an end of movement but rather a resistance to movement. The objective of muscle energy is to relieve these barriers and restore balance. Muscle energy allows the patient to control the muscle contraction but the clinician must first place the patient's segment in the correct alignment and correctly instruct the patient to produce a specific muscle contraction in a specific direction to promote optimal results. Common errors are made by the clinician to reduce optimal outcome of the treatment. These errors include: not controlling the joint position or direction of movement, not applying a counterforce to the patient's force in the correct direction, not allowing enough time between the contractions to achieve complete muscle relaxation prior to moving the segment to a new barrier, and not providing the patient with sufficient instructions for him or her to perform the activity correctly. On the other hand, patients also make errors in their muscle energy performance. Some of the patient errors include: using too much force, not contracting in the correct joint or segment position, not holding the contraction long enough, and not completely relaxing after the contraction.

Application of muscle energy techniques involves some very precise applications. The clinician must remember and perform these correctly for optimal results. An isometric contraction is held for 3 to 10 s and the amount of the contraction is only 2 ounces of force. Typically, the patient attempts to produce a maximal contraction, but the clinician must establish the importance of a light resistance force application by the patient. Once the contraction is relaxed, the clinician should pause to allow full relaxation of the muscle before applying the stretch. As the segment is moved, the clinician pay attention to where the new barrier is felt, for motion goes only to that point and not beyond. Once the new barrier is reached, the process is repeated for 3 to 5 times.

Listed here are a few muscle energy techniques. These techniques are used to treat some of the more common SI lesions.

Anterior Iliac Subluxation: UpSlip

This treatment is for an iliosacral lesion—an upslip of the ilium whereby the ilium on the right is higher than the one on the left. This injury can occur when someone falls on the buttock or steps down off a curb. It is also seen in sports such as basketball and hockey. Although it always occurs on the right, the pain is sometimes on the left. Pain can also be located in the low back or coccyx or can mimic nerve root pain. The right leg appears shorter than the left leg, and the right iliac crest is higher. When palpated, the right sacrotuberous ligament feels slack compared to that on the left side.

The muscle energy treatment is to have the patient lie prone with the right leg in 30° of abduction and extension. The rehabilitation clinician grasps the tibia and fibula above the ankle to maintain the leg position and takes up the slack of the leg. The patient takes in a deep breath and blows it out as the rehabilitation clinician takes up the slack of the leg again (figure 16.74). This is repeated three or four times. On the last repetition, the clinician has the patient cough twice and simultaneously provides a quick pull on the leg along the long axis of the leg.

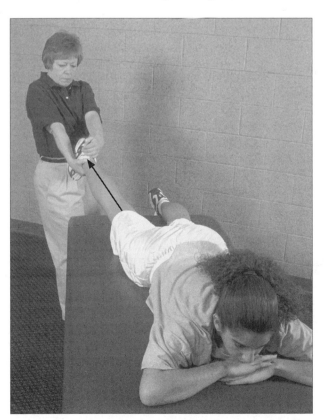

Figure 16.74 Anterior iliac subluxation: upslip treatment.

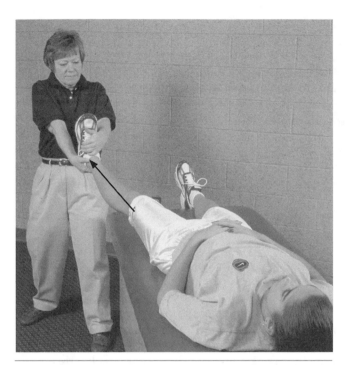

Figure 16.75 Posterior iliac subluxation: upslip muscle energy treatment.

Posterior Iliac Subluxation: UpSlip

This treatment is for an iliosacral lesion. This upslip always occurs on the left. It commonly occurs with other spinal problems and should be investigated if the pain does not respond to treatment. The left leg is the short leg this time, and the left sacrotuberous ligament is slack when palpated. The left iliac crest appears higher than the right.

Treatment is performed with the patient in supine and the left leg held by the rehabilitation clinician, proximal to the ankle in 30° of abduction and flexion (figure 16.75). The slack is taken out of the leg, and the patient is instructed to take a deep breath in and then let it out as the clinician takes out additional slack. After the final repetition, the patient is asked to cough, and simultaneously with the cough the clinician provides a quick longitudinal pull on the leg.

Sacral Flexion

This treatment is for a sacroiliac lesion that can occur with a bending-and-twisting activity. Push-pull activities can also cause a sacral flexion injury. This injury is more commonly seen on the left than on the right, but it can occur on either side. The pain may sometimes be on the side opposite the injury. If the injury is on the left side, the left sulcus will appear deeper (more anterior) than the right, and the left inferior lateral angle of the sacrum (ILA) is palpated more posteriorly.

Treatment is to have the patient lie prone with the leg in 30° abduction and medially rotated. The patient's thigh is stabilized on the thigh of the rehabilitation clinician, whose hand applies pressure to the left ILA (if the injury is on the left) (figure 16.76). The patient takes a deep breath in and holds it, then breathes out while the clinician continues to exert constant pressure over the left ILA. The pressure is maintained as the patient breathes in again. This technique is performed three times. Sometimes a click can be palpated or heard on the maneuver.

Figure 16.76 Sacral flexion muscle energy treatment.

In an exercise that can accompany this treatment, the patient lies with both knees to the chest. This facilitates sacral extension because the sacrum moves in the opposite direction of the lumbar spine. As the lumbar spine moves into flexion, the sacrum should extend; and as the spine extends, the sacrum flexes.

Forward Torsion

A sacroiliac lesion of a forward torsion occurs primarily on the left and is more common than a backward torsion. Simultaneous bending and twisting is the most common mechanism for this injury. The pain may be present in the back, buttock, or leg, and it may occur on the opposite side. Because this is a torsion injury, one side of the sacrum is twisted on the other. For example, if the torsion is on the left, the left ILA is more posterior than the right; but the right sulcus lies deeper than the left. The left piriformis is tight.

Treatment is delivered with the patient lying on the side of the injury, usually the left, with the knees and hips flexed to 90°. The patient then pushes up with his or her top hand to lift the trunk off the table and places the bottom arm behind the back. The patient then lies back down with the top arm hanging over the table toward the floor. The rehabilitation clinician places a hand in the L5-S1 joint space to monitor and maintain the spine in neutral (figure 16.77). The patient's thighs are supported on the table to the knee, and the lower legs are off the table. The clinician provides light resistance at the distal legs as the patient produces an isometric lift of the feet toward the ceiling. The muscles relax, and the clinician lowers the patient's legs to the floor until a new barrier is felt.

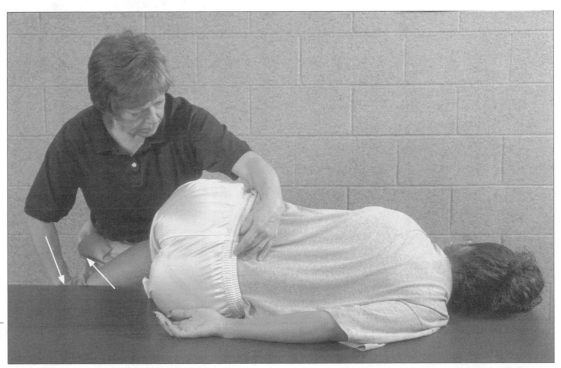

Figure 16.77 RonR Forward torsion muscle energy treatment.

The exercise that helps correct a forward torsion is similar to the treatment. The patient assumes a sidelying position; the bottom arm is behind the trunk and the top arm hangs to the floor while the knees and hips are flexed to 90° with the lower legs over the edge of the bed or table. This position is held for 5 to 10 min. This exercise is performed until the area is stable.

Backward Torsion

This treatment is for a sacroiliac impairment that has classic signs. The patient is unable to stand upright because extension is too painful. He or she may waddle like a duck and is unable to walk normally. Pain may be in the low back or buttock or may mimic nerve root pain. Treatment for this injury has the patient standing facing a table and leaning onto it with the anterior superior iliac spine (ASIS) on the edge of the table. The trunk is supported on top of the table. The rehabilitation clinician applies firm pressure on the sacrum, with the heel of the hand at the base and the fingers pointing toward the sacral apex (figure 16.78a). The pressure should be downward and firm throughout the motion. The patient then walks with the hands on the table to a standing position (figure 16.78b). The movement may be uncomfortable, but the patient should be encouraged to continue to the end of the motion.

Figure 16.78 Backward torsion muscle energy treatment: *(a)* start position, *(b)* end position.

The exercises that the patient should do to promote correction of the backward torsion are press-ups or standing trunk extensions. If standing extensions are too painful, start with press-ups. If press-ups are too uncomfortable, the patient can begin by lying prone on a pillow (figure 16.79a), progressing to lying prone without a pillow (figure 16.79b), and then progressing to lying prone on elbows (figure 16.79c) before advancing to a press-up (figure 16.79d).

Figure 16.79
Extension progression: *(a)* prone with pillows, *(b)* prone without pillows, *(c)* prone on elbows, *(d)* press-ups.

Figure 16.80 Right anterior iliac rotation muscle energy treatment.

Anterior Iliac Rotation

The dysfunction known as anterior iliac rotation usually occurs with other lesions. It is an iliosacral lesion and is sometimes called an anterior innominate lesion. It usually occurs on the right, and the patient can complain of cervical or lumbar symptoms. The iliac crest may be low on the same side as the injury, whereas the posterior superior iliac spine (PSIS) is high and the ASIS is low.

For treatment of this injury, the patient lies prone on the table with the leg of the involved side positioned over the side of the table and the foot on the floor. The rehabilitation clinician places his or her thumb in the sacral sulcus to monitor the SI joint. For control of the leg, the foot is placed on the clinician's thigh and the knee is grasped (figure 16.80). The patient's 3 to 10 s isometric contraction toward extension is resisted. The patient is instructed to relax, and the leg is moved into flexion until its barrier is felt. This exercise is repeated three to five times.

The exercises used to facilitate correction are a pelvic tilt and both knees to chest.

Posterior Iliac Rotation

This iliosacral lesion is also called a posterior innominate lesion. It commonly occurs on the left side and is seen following a fall or sudden hamstring contraction. The patient may use an antalgic gait and walk with reduced hip extension movement. Patients with this injury usually complain of a lot of pain that can be located in the buttock or knee. The ilium is posteriorly rotated, and the ASIS, PSIS, and iliac crest can appear high. There may also be a short-leg appearance on the same side.

For treatment, the patient is placed in a prone position. The rehabilitation clinician places one hand on the ilium to monitor stability of the joint and the other on the anterior thigh proximal to the knee. The hip is extended while the pelvis maintains neutral until the barrier is felt (figure 16.81). The barrier occurs when the monitor hand feels ilium movement as the hip is extended. The patient is instructed to attempt to push the thigh to the table isometrically for 3 to 10 s. The patient then relaxes, and the thigh is passively moved into extension to its next barrier. The procedure is repeated three to five times.

Exercises that accompany this technique include press-ups and hip-flexor stretches.

Figure 16.81 Left posterior iliac rotation muscle energy treatment: *(a)* Start position—patient is prone; rehabilitation clinician's monitor hand is on the ilium and the movement hand is under the patient's knee. *(b)* Once relaxed after isometric hip flexion, the thigh is passively moved into extension to the new barrier.

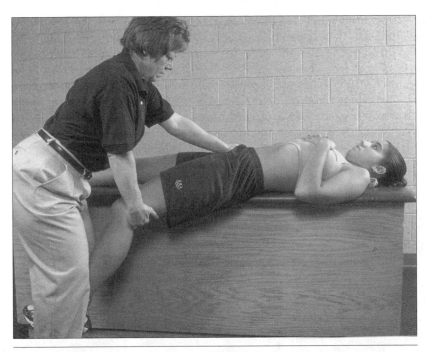

Figure 16.82   Left superior pubic subluxation muscle energy treatment.

Figure 16.83   Inferior pubic subluxation muscle energy treatment.

Pubic Subluxation

This is an iliosacral lesion that occurs in soccer players. It occurs also during pregnancy or delivery of a child. These lesions are commonly found in combination with other SI lesions, especially up-slips, or low back injuries. The patient may complain of only low-back pain or may have groin or buttock pain. Pushing down on the left or right pubic bones produces pain (spring test). If it is a superior lesion, the leg will appear shorter, but if it is an inferior lesion, the leg will appear longer.

Treatment depends on whether the pubis is superior or inferior and involves a contract-relax-stretch technique. For a superior subluxation, the patient lies supine with the leg over the edge of the table. The rehabilitation clinician supports the hanging leg under the patient's thigh and stabilizes the ASIS on the opposite side (figure 16.82). The patient performs isometric hip flexion for 5 to 10 s against the clinician. The leg is relaxed and the hip is then passively moved into extension to its new barrier.

For an inferior subluxation, the patient lies supine with the hip in flexion while the clinician places a hand under the ischial tuberosity to monitor its stability. The patient performs isometric hip extension against the clinician's hand on the proximal lower leg (figure 16.83). A passive movement into hip flexion to the new barrier is performed after the patient has relaxed the muscles.

Occasionally, a treatment technique specific to superior subluxations or one specific to inferior pubic subluxations can be successful for either problem. The patient is supine with the hips and knees flexed and the feet on the table. The patient performs a series of isometric abduction exercises of both legs simultaneously as the rehabilitation clinician resists the movement (figure 16.84a). This is followed by a series of isometric adduction exercises with the clinician's forearm placed between the patient's knees during the isometric exercise (figure 16.84b). Sometimes a pop of the pubic bones may be heard.

Exercises the patient should perform for superior pubic subluxation include a Thomas stretch. The inferior pubic subluxation exercise is a single-knee-to-chest stretch.

Figure 16.84 Inferior or superior pubic subluxation muscle energy treatment: *(a)* isometric abduction, *(b)* isometric adduction.

Inflares and Outflares

Inflares and outflares are also referred to as innominate medial and lateral rotations, respectively. These iliosacral conditions often produce groin pain. Leg and hip pain may or may not be present as well. They occur in soccer players and can result from a direct blow on the ilium. In an inflare, the distance from the ASIS to the umbilicus is shorter on the affected side. In an outflare, the distance is greater on the affected side than on the opposite side.

Treatment for an inflare is to have the patient lie supine with the leg of the involved side flexed and the foot flat on the table. The rehabilitation clinician's hand is on the medial malleolus, with the forearm against the lower leg. The patient's knee rests against the rehabilitation clinician's hip (figure 6.85). The clinician's other hand is used to stabilize the opposite ASIS. The patient performs an isometric hip adduction exercise for 5 to 10 s. When the muscle relaxes, the patient's leg is passively moved into hip abduction until the new barrier is felt. When the exercise series is complete, the patient's leg is passively moved into extension.

The exercise position for an inflare is supine with the leg flexed at the hip and knee and the foot on the table. In this position, knee is dropped out to the side to move the hip into abduction.

An outflare is treated with the patient in supine and the knee of the affected side brought toward the opposite shoulder. The rehabilitation clinician places his or her hand on the sulcus of the involved side. The hip is medially rotated. While maintained in this position, the patient performs a series of isometric exercises in hip flexion, adduction, and medial rotation (figure 16.86). The leg is returned passively to full extension when the series is complete.

To perform the exercise for this dysfunction, the patient moves the knee to the opposite shoulder and produces a series of hold-relax techniques.

Figure 16.85 Inflare muscle energy treatment.

Figure 16.86 Outflare muscle energy treatment.

Program Considerations

When the SI is being treated, the low back and hip areas should also be addressed to eliminate other sites of injury or referral. Muscle energy techniques are used in combination with flexibility and strengthening exercises. The cause, if it was not a traumatic injury, should also be corrected to prevent a recurrence.

If the SI joint is the source of pain, muscle energy techniques are usually very effective in relieving or reducing the pain. If the problem has not been long-standing, the patient experiences significant resolution within a few treatments, in many cases.

Case Study

In last week's game, a basketball player was going in for a layup when she collided with an opponent whose knee hit her on the front of the left hip. She had an initial bruise over the anterior ilium but since then has noticed persistent left groin pain. She also has pain that goes into the left leg. Examination shows that she has normal lumbar range of motion. There is no spasm or pain in the low back area. In supine, the distance from the umbilicus to the ASIS is 0.5 cm (1/5 in.) longer on the left than on the right.

Questions for Analysis

1. What do you suspect this patient has, and what is your treatment program?

2. What exercises would you include in her home program?

Thoracic Outlet Syndrome

Thoracic outlet syndrome (TOS) can be classified as a cervical injury or a shoulder injury. The classification depends on your orientation. Because the syndrome can be caused by structures in the neck region, some feel it is related to the cervical spine. Many of the structures contributing to it, however, are shoulder based; and certainly many of the exercises used to correct the problem are shoulder exercises. It is logical to include TOS in a discussion of either cervical or shoulder injuries. The syndrome is discussed here, but you should keep in mind that examination of shoulder injuries and development of shoulder rehabilitation programs should also include consideration of possible TOS manifestations, particularly if the patient does not respond as expected to a shoulder rehabilitation program.

Program Considerations

Although the diagnosis of TOS can be difficult and the signs and symptoms complex, the treatment program is simple. Symptom control is the first goal; this should include the use of modalities as needed and instruction in positions that relieve the tension or compression on the brachial plexus. The position that best relieves TOS in a supine sleeping position is with the scapula in protraction and elevation and the shoulder in medial rotation and adduction. Pillows should be used to support and position the shoulder and scapula as seen in figure 16.87. In severe cases, it may be necessary for the patient to wear a sling during the day. In less severe cases, the patient can obtain relief during the day by placing his or her hand in a front pant pocket or in the waistband when standing and by supporting the arm when sitting.

Soft-tissue mobilization of the cervical spine and scapular muscles—especially the upper trapezius, scalenes, pectoralis minor, and occasionally the cervical paraspinal muscles—is often effective in relieving pain and tenderness if the muscle tension in these muscles is contributing to the symptoms.

Improving joint mobility of the first rib may also help to relieve symptoms if the rib is restricted and impinging on the brachial plexus. If the rehabilitation clinician is comfortable with spine mobilization techniques, he or she should perform cervical spine and thoracic spine mobilization if areas of restriction are present.

Figure 16.87 Resting position for TOS.

Once the inflammation has subsided, flexibility and strengthening exercises should begin. The brachial plexus is stretched using the upper-limb tension tests (ULTT) described in chapter 6. These are reviewed in figure 16.88. These stretches are performed to the point of pain, not beyond, because pushing into the pain may reinflame the nerve.

Flexibility exercises for the cervical and thoracic spine should also be included. Axial extension and cervical retraction exercises (figures 16.21 and 16.22) are simple beginning exercises. Additional flexibility exercises include cervical extension, lateral flexion, and forward flexion exercises. Cervical extension is performed with the neck maintained in a slightly retracted position as the patient extends the neck beginning from the upper spine and moving through the lower spine. If tolerated, overpressure with the hand on the chin can be added (figure 16.89). Lateral flexion is essentially an upper trapezius stretch as seen in figure 16.24. The patient may find it more comfortable to perform the lateral flexion exercise in supine, but it is also effective when performed either in sitting or supine.

Figure 16.88 Brachial plexus stretches for TOS: *(a)* ULTT with elbow extended, *(b)* ULTT with elbow flexed, *(c)* ULTT with elbow flexed into a corner.

Figure 16.89 Cervical extension with overpressure.

Because thoracic mobility can influence cervical range of motion, flexion and extension flexibility exercises of the thoracic spine should also be part of a program for TOS. These are performed in sitting with the hands clasped behind the neck. A rolled towel can be placed around the neck at the restricted level and pulled downward from the front with the hands as the neck is extended. For extension, the elbows are raised toward the ceiling and the patient looks upward (figure 16.90). For flexion, the patient lowers the elbows toward the chest with hands clasped together at the base of the neck. The movement should come from the thoracic spine without pressure on the neck from the hands.

Because brachial plexus mobility can be restricted by shoulder positioning and associated scapulothoracic and glenohumeral soft-tissue tightness, shoulder flexibility exercises should also be included in a TOS program if there are deficiencies in the shoulder motions of lateral rotation, medial rotation, or flexion or scapulothoracic motions of retraction, rotation, and elevation. Stretches for these muscles are presented in chapter 17.

Figure 16.90 Thoracic extension with overpressure.

Figure 16.91
Poor posture associated with TOS.

Correction for posture and body mechanics is vital to correcting and preventing recurrence of TOS. A typical posture held by persons with TOS is a forward-head, round-shoulder posture as seen in figure 16.91. The patient should be made aware of his or her current posture and receive instruction in how to correct it. It may be difficult for the patient to assume normal posture initially because of pain, habit, reduced flexibility of muscles, and weakness of opposing muscles; however, it is important for the individual to gain posture awareness and begin posture correction early in the program.

Strength exercises are designed to restore correct muscle balance of the neck and upper back so that normal movement of the brachial plexus and related soft tissue can occur and stress is reduced. The clinician should assess balance of respiratory muscles by determining how the patient breathes. It is common for patients with TOS to breathe using primarily upper respiratory muscles, the sternocleidomastoid and scalenes. These patients should be taught how to do diaphragmatic breathing or belly breathing in addition to using a combination of upper and lower respiratory muscles.

Other strengthening and muscle balance activities include exercises for the rotator cuff, especially lateral rotators; rhomboids, and middle trapezius for scapular retraction; and cervical and thoracic extensors. These are commonly the weakest muscle groups in patients with TOS and should be strengthened to create a balance with their opposing muscles.

Case Study

A 20-year-old wrestler reports that for the past week he has had trouble sleeping at night. He awakens with severe numbness and tingling in the right hand and a feeling of pressure in the forearm. The problem has been getting progressively worse since it started. He has pain if he carries a lot of books between classes, but feels all right when he is sitting in class. He does not recall any specific injury. He has been wrestling for eight years and lifts weights during the preseason. His shoulder weight program includes bench press, military press, push-ups, flys, and biceps curls. Your examination confirms the doctor's diagnosis of TOS; although the Military brace and Allen tests are negative, you can reproduce his hand's tingling symptom when you perform an Adson test. His posture is one of forward-head and round-shoulder alignment. He has limited shoulder range of motion in elevation and lateral rotation, and he is unable to move his elbow behind his shoulder in horizontal extension without discomfort in the chest. He has well-pronounced pectoralis and anterior deltoid muscles, but his rhomboids appear diminished and his rotator cuff muscles are weak.

Questions for Analysis

1. What instructions on posture will you give this patient?

2. What flexibility exercises will you give him, and what guidelines will you use in determining when to begin them?

3. What are his strength deficiencies and muscle imbalances, and what exercises will you use to restore muscle balance?

SUMMARY

1. Explain three flexibility exercises for the cervical spine and lumbar spine.

    Cervical flexion: Bring the chin down to the chest, attempting to move one cervical level at a time. Rotational stretch: While sitting in a chair, reach behind to grasp the back of the chair with the near hand, and use the opposite hand to keep the legs stable. Both knees to chest: In a supine position, bring one leg to the chest, then the other leg; return to the starting position by reversing the procedure.

2. Explain three strengthening exercises for the cervical spine and lumbar spine.

    Isometrics: In a proper posture, place the right hand along the right side of the head; push the head against the hand while not allowing any movement. Prone leg lift: Lying prone in a neutral spine position, squeeze the buttocks and lift the legs upward. Abdominal crunch: in a hook-lying supine position with hands behind the head, lift the chest and head toward the ceiling.

3. Identify three progressive spinal stability exercises.

    Dead-bug, quadruped, and abdominal exercises.

4. Identify three sacroiliac muscle energy release techniques and the indications for their use.

    Upslip: Upslip is always on the right and often accompanies other spinal problems. A leg pull is performed with the patient in prone and the leg positioned in 30° abduction and extension. Forward torsion: This occurs primarily on the left and occurs with twisting and bending motions. With the patient lying on the involved side, the legs are off the table, where resistance is provided to leg movement toward the ceiling. Posterior iliac rotation: This occurs primarily on the left side because of a fall or sudden hamstring contraction. With the patient prone, the hip is passively extended; the isometric force occurs in hip flexion.

5. Outline a therapeutic exercise program for a cervical sprain.

    The program should begin with modalities for pain and spasm, soft-tissue mobilization, and joint mobilization if there is soft-tissue or joint restriction. Range-of-motion exercises begin with active motion within a pain-free range of motion. Overpressure can occur as the tissue continues to heal. Isometric exercises can be initiated after pain and spasm are relieved. Other exercises can include strengthening exercises such as machine resistance and manual resistance through a full range of motion. Strengthening exercises should address the abdominals, trunk extensors, and gluteals for a foundation for the cervical spine. Agility and coordination exercises with medicine balls for the upper extremity and abdominals are included once strength and endurance are good. Functional exercises are the final phase of the program and depend on the patient's specific activity requirements.

6. List precautions for a therapeutic exercise program for disk lesions.

    Avoid positions that aggravate the sciatica; rule out other causes of sciatica; strengthen abdominals, gluteals, and back extensors; have the patient maintain a pelvic neutral position during activities; exercises should progress at the patient's own pace; and the rehabilitation clinician should have a good understanding of the exercises and the stresses that are imposed by each exercise.

7. Discuss the difference in therapeutic exercise programs for a lumbar strain and a facet injury.

    Facet injury treatment includes gentle rotation and side-bending in a pain-free range of motion, as well as avoiding extension activities (pain will occur in rotation to one side and sidebending to the opposite side). Extension exercises do not have to be avoided in lumbar strains; rotation and sidebending are painful in the same direction and should occur in pain-free motions.

CRITICAL THINKING QUESTIONS

1. Regarding the scenario presented at the beginning of this chapter, identify a myofascial release technique Rita probably used on Joey. Why did you select the this technique?

2. What exercises would you give Joey to strengthen his trunk muscles? What progression would you include for each exercise, and what are your criteria for progression?

3. With reference to the example of the gymnast with spondylolysis mentioned in the chapter, extension exercises should be avoided. How can you strengthen her back muscles without aggravating her injury? Will your attempts to strengthen her abdominals irritate the spondylolysis? Why or why not?

4. A football lineman who has been diagnosed with a disk herniation is attempting conservative rehabilitation to avoid surgery. What will your program of therapeutic exercises include? What will you avoid in the exercises? Does body mechanics impact his injury, and if so, how?

LAB ACTIVITIES

1. Have your lab partner lie prone; be sure to have him or her positioned comfortably and in a neutral position from the cervical to the sacral area. Start at the cervical spine and palpate each the spinous process to the L5. Locate L4; first examine your partner's joint excursion at L4-5, and then apply grades 1, 2, 3, and 4 PA joint mobilizations to the joint. Determine mobility of each joint throughout the spine. Where is there laxity and where is there restriction? Now examine another lab partner and repeat the process. How do they differ or are they similar? Have each person on whom you performed a joint mobilization examination stand and forward bend while you observe the spine from a posterior view. Do the areas of restriction you found during joint mob examination correlate with the range of motion restrictions you see during active physiological motion? What does this indicate for you in terms of patient motion related to joint mobility?

2. Locate the trigger points for the following muscles on your lab partner:
   a. Upper trapezius
   b. Levator scapulae
   c. Sternocleidomastoid
   d. Scalenes
   e. Spleni
   f. Quadratus lumborum
   g. Lumbar multifidus

   Where were your partner's most sensitive trigger points? Perform an ice-and-stretch technique on the most sensitive areas after you have determined for active range of motion of the muscle. After the treatment, have your partner repeat the active range of motion so you can determine the effectiveness of your treatment. How did the AROM change from before to after the treatment? Why?

3. Demonstrate two flexibility and strength exercises for each of the muscle or muscle groups listed below:
   a. Scalenes
   b. Upper trapezius
   c. Sternocleidomastoid
   d. Quadratus lumborum
   e. Erector spinae
   f. External obliques

4. Find your pelvic neutral position while sitting. Now find pelvic neutral while supine, and then while standing. Perform a progression of supine lumbar stabilization exercises outlined in the chapter. Now attempt the lumbar stabilization exercises in a quadruped position. Perform a sit-to-stand motion while in pelvic neutral. While your lab partner observes you, maintain pelvic neutral while you walk and then while you perform a jump. If you are unable to maintain pelvic neutral during these activities, have your partner provide you with cues and instructions that will improve your performance.

5. Examine your partner's sacroiliac joint for proper alignment using all the examination techniques outlined earlier in the chapter. Be sure to locate each landmark appropriately.

6. Perform the following muscle energy techniques:
   a. Anterior iliac subluxation
   b. Sacral flexion
   c. Forward torsion
   d. Anterior iliac rotation
   e. Pubic subluxation
   f. Inflare
   g. Outflare

   What will the malalignments be for each of these conditions? What home exercise will you provide a patient who presents with these problems? How will you know if your treatment has been effective?

7. Case Study: A 21-year-old male discus thrower began having left low back pain after a long workout last week. He presents to you today with complaints of left low-back pain that goes into his left buttock. He does not remember a frank injury. Your examination reveals a deep sulcus and a posterior left ILA. He is tender to palpation of the left sulcus. What do you suspect is his problem? What will your treatment with him today include? What home exercise will you give him? What therapeutic exercises would you provide as part of his treatments? What other things would you include in his rehabilitation program?

REFERENCES

Shultz, S.J., Houglum, P.A., and D.H. Perrin. 2005. *Examination of musculoskeletal injuries*. 2nd ed. Champaign, IL: Human Kinetics.

Travell, J.G., and D.G. Simons. 1983. *Myofascial pain and dysfunction. The trigger point manual*. Vol. 1. Baltimore: Williams and Wilkins.

Travell, J.G., and D.G. Simons. 1992. *Myofascial pain and dysfunction. The trigger point manual*. Vol. 2. Baltimore: Williams and Wilkins.

SUGGESTED READING

Cappaert, T.A. 2000. The sacroiliac joint as a factor in low back pain: a review. *Journal of Sport Rehabilitation*. 9:169-183.

Cibulka, M.T. 1992. The treatment of the sacroiliac joint component to low back pain: A case report. *Physical Therapy* 72:917-922.

Corrigan, B., and G.D. Maitland. 1989. *Practical orthopaedic medicine*. Boston: Butterworth-Heinemann.

Erhard, R.E., Delitto, A., and M.T. Cibulka. 1994. Relative effectiveness of an extension program and a combined program of manipulation and flexion and extension exercises in patients with acute low back syndrome. *Physical Therapy* 74:1093-1100.

Foster, D.N., and M.N. Fulton. 1991. Back pain and the exercise prescription. *Clinics in Sports Medicine* 10:197-209.

Hodges, P.W., and C.A. Richardson. 1997. Contraction of the abdominal muscles associated with movement of the lower limb. *Physical Therapy* 77:132-144.

Hopkins, T.J., and A.A. White. 1993. Rehabilitation of athletes following spine injury. *Clinics in Sports Medicine* 12:603-618.

Johannsen, F., Remvig, L., Kryger, P., Beck, P., Warming, S., Lybeck, K., Dreyer, V., and L.H. Larsen. 1995. Exercises for chronic low back pain: A clinical trial. *Journal of Orthopaedic and Sports Physical Therapy* 22:52-59.

Kaltenborn, F. M. 2003. *Manual mobilization of the joints. Vol II. The spine.*4th ed. Minneapolis: OPTP.

Kuzmich, D. 1994. The levator scapulae: Making the con-NECK-tion. *Journal of Manual and Manipulative Therapy* 2:43-54.

Lee, H.W.M. 1994. Progressive muscle synergy and synchronization in movement patterns: An approach to the treatment of dynamic lumbar instability. *Journal of Manual and Manipulative Therapy* 2:133-142.

Maitland, G.D. 1990. *Vertebral manipulation.* Boston: Butterworth-Heinemann.

Oliver, J. 1994. *Back care. An illustrated guide.* Boston: Butterworth-Heinemann.

Saudek, C.E., and K.A. Palmer. 1987. Back pain revisited. *Journal of Orthopaedic and Sports Physical Therapy* 8:556-566.

Smith, K.F. 1979. The thoracic outlet syndrome: A protocol of treatment. *Journal of Orthopaedic and Sports Physical Therapy* 1:89-99.

Tan, J.C., and M. Nordin. 1992. Role of physical therapy in the treatment of cervical disk disease. *Orthopedic Clinics of North America* 23:435-449.

Walker, J.M. 1992. The sacroiliac joint: A critical review. *Physical Therapy* 72:903-916.

Watkins, R.G. 1996. *The spine in sports.* St. Louis: Mosby.

Shoulder and Arm

Objectives

After completing this chapter, you should be able to do the following:

1. Explain how knowledge of the mechanics of sport performance impacts the establishment of a therapeutic exercise program.

2. Discuss the importance of stability in shoulder rehabilitation.

3. Explain the role of scapular stabilization in shoulder function.

4. Describe two soft-tissue mobilization techniques for the shoulder.

5. List three joint mobilizations for the shoulder.

6. Identify three strengthening exercises for the scapula and three for the glenohumeral muscles.

7. Discuss the general progression of strengthening exercises for the shoulder.

8. List precautions for a therapeutic exercise program following a rotator cuff repair.

9. Outline key factors for a program for a biceps rupture.

Bob George, certified athletic trainer for the local baseball farm team, sees several shoulder injuries each season. He is very familiar with the shoulder rehabilitation process, having successfully treated many players over the years.

His latest patient, P.G. Pamaloo, is one of the more promising pitchers Bob has seen in recent years. P.G. began having shoulder pain as a result of scapular muscle weakness and fatigue. Although he didn't have any capsular tightness in the shoulder that would have necessitated joint mobilization techniques, he did have the lateral rotator tightness that pitchers often acquire. Bob has provided P.G. with a good rehabilitation program that has resolved the shoulder's motion and strength deficits, and P.G. is about to begin a plyometric exercise program before beginning throwing activities.

Bob likes to make the rehabilitation program interesting for the baseball players. On different days he provides different exercises that can produce the same result. He uses rubber bands, manual resistance, and medicine balls instead of machine weights or dumbbells, because he feels that his patients find these more interesting and fun than weights.

■ **Time isn't a commodity, something you pass around like cake. Time is the substance of life. When anyone asks you to give your time, they're really asking for a chunk of your life.**

Antoinette Bosco

The purpose of the shoulder is to position the hand for function. The shoulder provides the impetus for propelling objects from the hand; it also places the hand in a position that enables you to catch or propel an object or to make contact with an object or surface. For these activities to occur, the entire shoulder complex, including its related joints and muscles, must operate with precise timing, intensity, positioning and speed of movement.

The shoulder has more mobility than any other joint in the body. Differentiated into one-degree increments, there are approximately 16,000 different possible shoulder positions (Perry 1978). The shoulder is designed for large ranges of motion, making thousands of hand placements possible. People who participate in overhead sports, such as baseball; softball; golf; football; swimming; volleyball; racket sports; and field events including javelin, discus, and shot put, utilize the shoulder's expansive mobility repetitively throughout each day of practice and participation. Overhead sports entail the use of tremendous forces to produce great upper-extremity velocity. During the acceleration phase of pitching, for example, arm movement at a velocity of around 7,500°/s has been recorded (Pappas, Zawacki, and Sullivan 1985). Rotational velocity in a tennis serve is 1500°/s, and hand speed at ball impact has been clocked at 75.6 kph (47 mph) (Kibler 1995). These velocities are generated from the shoulder starting essentially at rest in the cocking phase of a movement, accelerating to these top speeds and then suddenly decelerating in the follow-through, all in the space of less than 180° of rotation and milliseconds of time. For the shoulder to withstand these repeated stresses, the joints and muscles must all work as a highly synchronous, well-balanced unit. If a joint fails to move correctly or the muscles are imbalanced, an injury is sure to occur.

The risk of injury makes it vital for the rehabilitation clinician to understand the mechanics of normal shoulder motion and to have the knowledge, wisdom, and good judgment for appropriate rehabilitation progression. Before presenting specific therapeutic exercises for the shoulder, this chapter introduces the mechanics of overhead activities and basic considerations that are unique to the shoulder. As a clinician you must be aware of these elements to design an appropriate rehabilitation program for an injured shoulder.

MECHANICS OF OVERHEAD SPORT ACTIVITIES

▶ Overhead motions, such as those that athletes perform in baseball, tennis, swimming, and golf, place particular types of stresses on the shoulder.

All overhead activities impart stress to the shoulder and other upper extremity segments. An appreciation of these stresses and of the biomechanics in overhead sports can help you develop suitable rehabilitation programs.

The muscles to be discussed in relation to each motion include only those that have been investigated by researchers. Even though the research on shoulder biomechanics and muscle activity is extensive, we still have much to learn before we will have a complete picture of the shoulder in overhead activities. Meanwhile, you need to realize the importance of your own observations, understanding of shoulder function, and knowledge of the muscles that produce those functions. Even though research may not have yielded all the answers you need, your clinical skills, knowledge, and observations will help you identify and correct a patient's deficiencies to permit a safe return to full participation.

Baseball Pitching

Pitching has been investigated more thoroughly than any other overhead activity, with the shoulder most often the primary focus. It is recognized that the baseball pitcher uses the entire body in the pitching motion, beginning with the lower extremities and advancing to the trunk, shoulder, elbow, wrist, and hand. An alteration in any segment of this chain can affect the outcome. Consistent accuracy through repetition of coordinated high-velocity activity is the key to successful pitching. It is also the source of injury.

Pitching is a smooth, continuous motion that occurs during a relatively brief period. It can be divided into four segments--windup, cocking, acceleration, and follow-through (figure 17.1).

Windup

Windup, the setting phase of the pitching motion, occurs when the individual positions the body such that the glove (nonthrowing) side is facing the target. In the beginning of windup, the two hands are together and near the chest. As the movement begins, the athlete takes a step toward the target with the foot opposite the throwing arm. This phase is a minimally demanding portion of the pitching motion. Speed, energy expenditure, and forces generated are all at low levels.

Cocking

Cocking begins when the hands separate and ends when maximum lateral rotation and abduction of the shoulder have been achieved. Cocking is divided into early cocking and late cocking according to the contact of the forward foot on the ground. In early cocking, the scapula is

Figure 17.1 Throwing motion: *(a)* windup, *(b)* late cocking, *(c)* acceleration, *(d)* follow-through.
Reprinted by permission from Jobe and Ling 1988.

retracted and the humerus is abducted, laterally rotated, and horizontally extended. The elbow is flexed, and the forward leg advances toward the target almost directly in front of the back leg. At the time of foot contact, both arms are elevated about 90° and in line with each other along the plane of the shoulders. Anterior stress on the glenohumeral joint is predominant at this time, with the body in front of the arm. The deltoid is strongly active during early cocking. When maximum shoulder lateral rotation and abduction to 90° occur, the static stabilizers of the shoulder, the glenohumeral capsule and ligaments, serve to limit further motion. Active stabilizers, including the forward flexors, lateral rotators, the subscapularis, pectoralis major, and latissimus dorsi, act as additional restraints to control motion. Scapular stabilizers such as the pectoralis minor and serratus anterior are also active in late cocking. Reciprocal inhibition of the other rotator cuff muscles, the teres minor, supraspinatus, and infraspinatus, is also taking place as these muscles attempt to resist the superior subluxating forces that occur when the trunk is in a forward lean and the shoulder is maximally laterally rotated. The supraspinatus and infraspinatus are particularly active in late cocking. By the end of this phase, the shoulder medial rotators are on maximum stretch, the body is 'wound' optimally for the elastic energy transfer, and the legs and trunk begin their acceleration for energy release.

Acceleration

Acceleration starts with maximum shoulder lateral rotation and abduction and ends when the ball leaves the fingers. The movements in this phase include scapular protraction, humeral horizontal flexion and medial rotation, and elbow extension. At ball release, the shoulder is still at about 90° abduction. This helps to reduce impingement during acceleration. During this phase the speed of the arm has increased significantly in a relatively brief period, beginning from almost 0°/s at the end of cocking to 7,500°/s by the end of acceleration (Pappas, Zawacki, and Sullivan 1985). The serratus anterior and pectoralis major are strongly active during this phase as the arm moves forward and the scapula protracts. The subscapularis and latissimus dorsi are contracting concentrically as the arm is moved into medial rotation during acceleration.

Follow-Through

Follow-through occurs from the point of ball release to the completion of the motion. It is divided into early and late follow-through according to the point of maximal shoulder medial rotation. Early follow-through is completed rapidly, in less than 0.1 s (Moynes et al. 1986). Trunk rotation and scapular motions occur and are diminished to a varying extent from one style to another, depending on the individual thrower. The deltoid is strongly active during early follow-through. The rotator cuff, especially the lateral rotators, must decelerate the arm after ball release and work against the momentum distraction forces occurring at the shoulder. The biceps is also working eccentrically to reduce distraction forces at the elbow. It is during the follow-through that injuries to the posterior shoulder occur. The body must now dissipate the energy that has been developed to accelerate the ball. This is one reason it is important for the body to continue to move after the ball is released. An abrupt stop in arm motion will prevent this energy dissipation and cause these tremendous forces to be absorbed primarily by the shoulder. Flexing the trunk, extending the supporting knee, and allowing the arm to continue along its path of movement across the body and to the opposite leg all assist in dissipating this energy and reducing distraction forces on the shoulder.

Tennis

The repetitive motions and forces applied to the shoulder in tennis are a frequent cause of tennis injuries. Overhead serves and hits require more muscle activity of the shoulder than other motions and are the leading cause of shoulder injuries in this sport. The three main strokes in tennis are the serve, the forehand groundstroke, and the backhand groundstroke. Each deserves a brief discussion because the rehabilitation clinician must understand the motions involved and the demands placed on the shoulder to effectively and safely advance the patient in a functional therapeutic exercise program.

Serve

The serve is divided into four phases-windup, cocking, acceleration, and follow-through (figure 17.2).

Windup

Windup, the setting phase of the serve, takes place when the athlete prepares for the motion. The serve stance is taken in preparation for the ball toss. The body is perpendicular to the service line, with the weight on the back leg and the front leg facing the target. The shoulder muscles are relatively quiet. The shoulder is in slight abduction, extension, and lateral rotation. The trunk is slightly laterally flexed and rotated, and the legs are rotated.

Cocking

Cocking begins with ball release from the opposite arm and continues to the point at which the racket shoulder is at maximum lateral rotation. The scapula is upwardly rotated and adducted, the shoulder is abducted and laterally rotated, and the elbow is flexed. The supraspinatus, infraspinatus, and subscapularis muscles are very active, stabilizing the humerus in the glenoid and positioning the shoulder. The subscapularis also works to decelerate lateral rotation in preparation for acceleration. The serratus anterior is active to stabilize the scapula on the thoracic wall and simultaneously rotate the scapula into the correct position to serve as a platform from which the glenohumeral joint moves (Ryu et al. 1988). The posterior deltoid and trunk lean produce shoulder abduction. Biceps activity is moderately high during this phase so that the racket is held in the correct position with the elbow flexed overhead.

Acceleration

Acceleration begins with medial rotation movement of the shoulder and ends with ball contact. Glenohumeral medial rotation is rapid and forceful, occurring with shoulder adduction, elbow extension, and trunk flexion. It is the quickest and briefest phase of the serve. The subscapularis is very active to produce medial rotation. The pectoralis major and latissimus dorsi adduct the arm. Scapular stabilizers, performing a critical function, are active as they continue to maintain good scapular positioning and stabilization on the thoracic wall. The biceps is eccentrically controlling elbow extension and pronation.

Follow-Through

The last phase of the serve, follow-through, occurs from ball impact to the end of the motion. As with pitching, the rapid change from acceleration to deceleration places tremendous stress

Figure 17.2   Tennis serve: *(a)* windup, *(b)* cocking, *(c)* acceleration, *(d)* follow-through.

on the shoulder and causes the scapular and glenohumeral muscles to work at moderate to high levels primarily to decelerate and protect the shoulder. Most of these muscles work intensely in the early part of follow-through, their activity declining as the motion continues. The latissimus dorsi and pectoralis major decelerate forward shoulder motion; the rotator cuff muscles work eccentrically to provide deceleration of the forward momentum and distraction pull on the humerus in the glenoid; the serratus anterior (the most thoroughly investigated scapular rotator) is active eccentrically; and the biceps continues its eccentric control of the elbow.

Forehand Ground Stroke

The forehand ground stroke is divided into three phases—racket preparation, acceleration, and follow-through (figure 17.3).

Racket Preparation

The racket preparation phase begins with the shoulder turn and ends with the initiation of weight transfer onto the front foot. The trunk and hips are rotated away from the front foot. The arm is positioned into abduction and lateral rotation, and the weight is on the back foot. The shoulder positioning is primarily the result of hip and trunk rotation; little muscle activity occurs in the shoulder.

Acceleration

This phase begins with weight transfer onto the front foot and ends at ball impact. During this phase the body and racket are moved forward, and the hips and trunk begin to rotate. A rapid medial rotation of the shoulder and adduction occur. Medial rotation results from strong concentric contraction of the subscapularis; adduction occurs because of the pectoralis major. The serratus anterior also works actively to continue protraction and scapular stabilization. The biceps works to keep the elbow slightly flexed.

Follow-Through

Follow-through occurs from ball contact to the end of the motion. The serratus anterior, biceps, infraspinatus, and supraspinatus are highly active as during other follow-through motions.

Backhand Ground Stroke

The backhand ground stroke is similar to the forehand ground stroke in having three phases: racket preparation, acceleration, and deceleration (figure 17.4).

Racket Preparation

This phase begins with shoulder turned to place the racket shoulder to the net and ends with weight-transfer initiation to the front foot. The trunk and hips are rotated with the weight primarily on the back foot, the shoulder is in medial rotation and adduction, and the elbow is flexed. As with other preparatory phases, shoulder muscle activity is relatively quiet.

Figure 17.3   Forehand ground stroke: *(a)* racket preparation, *(b)* acceleration, *(c)* follow-through.

Figure 17.4 Backhand ground stroke: *(a)* racket preparation, *(b)* acceleration, *(c)* follow-through.

Acceleration

Acceleration begins with weight transfer to the front foot and ends with ball contact. The hips and trunk begin rotation; and as the weight is transferred, the scapula retracts, the shoulder abducts and laterally rotates, and the elbow extends. This movement occurs with strong, forceful shoulder lateral rotation caused by the rotator cuff (supraspinatus, infraspinatus, and teres minor). The middle deltoid is also active as the shoulder is abducted. The serratus anterior, acting as a scapular stabilizer, and the biceps, working as an elbow decelerator, are also active during this phase.

Follow-Through

Follow-through takes place from ball contact to the end of the stroke. The most active muscles during this phase are the middle deltoid, biceps, supraspinatus, and infraspinatus.

Swimming

Shoulder pain is common in swimmers. The shoulder provides the propulsive force to permit use of the hand as a paddle for moving the body through the water (Perry 1983). The legs provide less propulsion than the arms in swimming, and they are important for smoothing out the stroke and making it more efficient. The legs also provide a base for body roll during the stroke, so therapeutic exercise programs for injured swimmers should include lower-extremity exercises.

Each of four primary swimming strokes—the freestyle, the backstroke, the breaststroke, and the butterfly—has unique characteristics, but they all have two phases of motion, pull-through and recovery (figure 17.5a). With the exceptions of the backstroke and the recovery phase in the breaststroke, which are performed out of the water, all are performed in a prone position. Because most shoulder injuries in swimming are seen with the freestyle stroke, we will consider this stroke here.

Pull-Through

The pull-through phase is the propulsive phase of the freestyle stroke and is similar to the acceleration phase in throwing. In contrast to the acceleration phase in throwing, though, pull-through is the longest phase in swimming. This requires sustained activity of the muscles producing the movement. Pull-through occurs during 65% to 70% of the freestyle stroke (Nuber et al. 1986). The shoulder begins in lateral rotation and abduction at hand entry into the water and ends medially rotated and adducted just before leaving the water. The elbow moves from flexion to extension. The body rolls to a maximum of 40° to 60° from horizontal, and the shoulder is at 90° abduction and neutral rotation during the middle of the pull phase (Richardson, Jobe, and Collins 1980). In the early portion of pull-through, the arm reaches forward underwater with the hand lateral to the head, but medial to the shoulder,

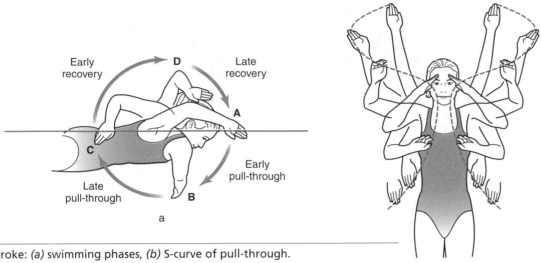

Figure 17.5   Swim stroke: *(a)* swimming phases, *(b)* S-curve of pull-through.

Adapted by permission from Pink et al. 1991.

and becomes positioned for the pulling aspect of the phase. The fingers enter the water first. Pulling begins after the arm is positioned in the water and continues until the hand is near the thigh, before the hand exits the water. During the most propulsive portion of the pull-through phase, the arm moves in an S-shaped curve: The hand moves across the chest as the shoulder adducts, then moves laterally as it passes by the pelvis. Before lifting the hand out of the water, the shoulder medially rotates to turn the palm to reduce drag (figure 17.5b). During hand entry and early pull-through when the hand crosses the body, the shoulder is in adduction, flexion, and medial rotation; this position can produce mechanical impingement on the biceps tendon and the supraspinatus tendon.

Muscles active during the early pull-through phase include the upper trapezius to upwardly rotate the scapula, the rhomboids to retract the scapula, and the supraspinatus and anterior and middle deltoids to work as a force couple to stabilize the humerus. During later pull-through, the pectoralis major and latissimus dorsi act as the propulsive muscles; the deltoids lift and place the arm in preparation for hand exit from the water; the serratus anterior stabilizes the scapula and the teres minor and the subscapularis both stabilize the humerus in the glenoid and provide humeral motion; the teres minor assists with shoulder extension, and the subscapularis medially rotates the humerus. The rhomboids downwardly rotate the scapula as the shoulder moves into extension (Pink et al. 1991).

Recovery

The recovery phase begins when the arm leaves the water and continues until hand entry. This phase, used as a preparation for the pull phase, is equivalent to the cocking phase in pitching. During recovery, the shoulder abducts and is in medial rotation but moving into lateral rotation as the elbow is lifted and the body rolls to the opposite side, as during early pull-through (Richardson, Jobe, and Collins 1980). It is during this time that impingement can occur. This is especially true if weakness prevents the swimmer from lifting the elbow out of the water first or if weak rotator cuff and biceps muscles prevent adequate humeral head depression. By mid-recovery, the shoulder is abducted to 90° and in lateral rotation. The body roll reaches its maximum of 40° to 60° as the athlete breathes. By the time the hand enters the water, the shoulder is maximally laterally rotated and abducted, and the body roll is back to a neutral position.

Early recovery is initiated by the muscles abducting and rotating the humerus (middle deltoid and supraspinatus, respectively) and rotating the scapula (trapezius and serratus anterior). As recovery progresses, the rhomboids retract the scapula; and the subscapularis medially rotates the shoulder from a maximally laterally rotated position at middle recovery and assists the infraspinatus in depression of the humerus in the glenoid before hand entry.

The subscapularis and the serratus anterior are essentially active throughout the entire swimming stroke (Pink et al. 1991). The range of activity varies according to the arm position and the activity occurring, but the sustained activity of these muscles is significant and should be taken into account in the design of a therapeutic exercise program. Therapeutic exercise programs for these two muscles must include both high-endurance and strength exercises to provide proper shoulder positioning during swimming and to prevent fatigue.

Golf Swing

There are four phases of the golf swing: take-away, forward swing, acceleration, and follow-through (figure 17.6). Research on the golf swing has been limited. The information presented here is based primarily on the work of Jobe, Moynes, and Antonelli (1985). These investigators looked only at the supraspinatus, subscapularis, infraspinatus, latissimus dorsi, pectoralis major, anterior deltoid, middle deltoid, and posterior deltoid.

The shoulders do not elevate in golf as they do in other overhead sports. For this reason, the deltoids do not play as important a role in golf as they do in throwing, tennis, and swimming. The major muscles in golf, according to the investigation by Jobe, Moynes, and Antonelli (1985), include the rotator cuff (especially the subscapularis), latissimus dorsi, and pectoralis major. Keep in mind that the researchers did not investigate all the muscles surrounding the shoulder complex. Other muscles not investigated may play an important role in the golf swing, injury etiology, and treatment.

Take-Away

This phase begins when the golfer addresses the ball, and it ends at the top of the backswing. The body is positioned with the front leg and arm facing the direction the ball is to be hit. During take-away, the front shoulder has low-level activity except in the subscapularis. The primary activity of the back shoulder is in the supraspinatus.

Forward Swing

This phase begins at the end of backswing and continues until the club becomes horizontal. The front arm has moderate activity of the subscapularis and latissimus dorsi, whereas the back arm has more activity of the other rotator cuff muscles—the infraspinatus and subscapularis—and less of the supraspinatus. The pectoralis major and latissimus dorsi of the back arm also increase their activity.

Figure 17.6 Gold swing: *(a)* take-away, *(b)* forward swing, *(c)* acceleration, *(d)* follow-through.

Acceleration

Acceleration occurs from the time the club becomes horizontal to the time of ball contact. The front and back arm muscles that are highly active at this time are the same; these include the pectoralis major, latissimus dorsi, and subscapularis.

Follow-Through

Follow-through begins with ball contact and continues to the end of the stroke. The front shoulder's subscapularis continues at high activity levels, but the activity of the pectoralis major and latissimus dorsi subsides. The infraspinatus produces increased activity during this phase. In the back arm, the subscapularis, pectoralis major, and latissimus dorsi continue high activity output.

GENERAL REHABILITATION CONSIDERATIONS

▶ To function normally, the should must have stability, scapular muscle strength, and balance within force couples. Other elements affecting shoulder function include the relationship between the shoulder and the other body segments, as well as posture.

The shoulder is a unique area that is composed of several joints: the sternoclavicular, acromioclavicular, scapulothoracic, and glenohumeral joints. Not only must these joints possess appropriate mobility and provide stability, but also the muscles that surround and control these joints must all work synchronously to provide normal shoulder function and timing of movement.

Stability

Fundamental to normal joint function is stability. When an injury occurs, normal joint stability is compromised, and full recovery is threatened unless the stability is restored. Joint stability is provided by static and dynamic factors. Static stability is provided by the inert structures. In the shoulder, these inert structures include the joint capsule, ligaments, and glenoid labrum. Dynamic stability is the responsibility of the nerves and muscles, providing appropriate input from the afferent receptors to the central nervous system to impart timely support through balanced muscle activity as discussed in chapter 8. When the joint's ligaments are injured, the afferent receptors located in those ligaments are unable to provide adequate sensory input. This creates insufficient neural input and, in turn, inappropriate muscle responses. The result is a deficiency in static stability because of the injury itself, and a secondary dynamic instability caused by the damage to the afferent receptors. These conditions set up a continuous injury cycle in which continued dynamic and static instability causes functional instability. The cycle continues and leads to progressive injury (figure 17.7).

Dynamic instability results if muscles surrounding the shoulder are imbalanced. If the agonist and antagonist groups are not balanced, there is loss of proprioceptive and kinesthetic control, leading to dynamic instability. Muscle imbalance, if not corrected, can be the primary cause of shoulder injury.

The rehabilitation clinician is able to break this cycle by designing a rehabilitation program to restore dynamic stability. Rehabilitation programs include reeducation of the neuromuscular system and exercises to reestablish balance between agonists and antagonists. Sometimes, this is enough to restore the patient to full sport participation. When the static instability is too great, surgical intervention is necessary. Rehabilitation of dynamic stabilizers is just as important after surgical correction of static instability as it is in cases without surgical intercession.

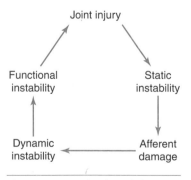

Figure 17.7 Joint instability cycle.

Scapular Muscles

Fundamental to all shoulder rehabilitation is rehabilitation of the scapular stabilizers. These muscles control scapular motion. Their strength and control are crucial to the shoulder because the scapula serves as a platform from which the shoulder moves. Weak scapular muscles will produce insufficient scapular stabilization for shoulder movement. The difference between a stable and an unstable scapula for the shoulder is similar to the difference between running on firm ground and running on a suspended wood-and-rope footbridge. The ground provides the runner with a stable base from which to move the body forward smoothly and efficiently. Running on an unstable footbridge places high energy demands on the individual's leg muscles, causes incoordination and inefficiency of movement, and increases risk of injury. So, too, a shoulder with an unstable scapula moves inefficiently and is at risk for injury. With an unstable scapula, the glenohumeral joint tends to migrate superiorly. This leads to impingement and biceps or rotator cuff tendinitis. It is imperative, then, that all therapeutic exercise programs for the shoulder include exercises for the scapular stabilizing muscles.

Fatigue of scapular muscles can also affect shoulder motion and performance. The scapular muscles' role as a stabilizer is disrupted when the muscles are fatigued. This disruption occurs because of changes in normal scapulohumeral rhythm with fatigue of the scapular muscles, as shown by McQuade, Dawson, and Smidt (1998). The results of their study point to the importance of endurance activities in a therapeutic exercise program.

Because scapular muscle strength is so important to the function and stability of the shoulder, exercises for these muscles should begin early in the rehabilitation program, even after surgical repair. You can start strengthening exercises for these muscles without stressing the glenohumeral joint by using manual resistance to all scapular motions. In many cases, the upper trapezius and levator scapulae muscles are not weak, but the other scapular muscles are and, therefore, need reeducation and rehabilitation. Scapular depression, protraction, retraction, and upward and downward rotation are all motions that can and should be manually resisted early in the rehabilitation process.

If the upper trapezius and levator scapulae are weak, of course, strengthening of these muscles is in order. Often, however, these muscles overpower weak shoulder muscles during scapular rotation so muscle imbalances become more pronounced when deficiencies are left uncorrected. If the rotator cuff is weak, the upper trapezius may work with the deltoid to elevate the shoulder, enhancing muscle imbalances, encouraging incorrect mechanics, and aggravating the shoulder injury. Two techniques that can be used to control and retrain the upper trapezius are biofeedback and taping. Biofeedback can be used to either facilitate rotator cuff activity or reduce upper trapezius activity during shoulder elevation exercises (figure 17.8). The specific application depends on the electrode placement, machine settings, and motions desired. Refer to Denegar and colleagues (2005) for specific applications.

Figure 17.8   Biofeedback: electrode placement for upper trapezius inhibition to *(a)* decrease activity, and *(b)* for infraspinatus facilitation to increase activity.

Scapular taping can be useful in cases of secondary impingement in which faulty positioning of the scapula during overhead movements causes impingement of the rotator cuff tendons. The taping must be accompanied by retraining exercises to reeducate the scapular muscles so that they position the scapula correctly during shoulder motions. The taping technique was introduced by Jenny, an Australian manipulative physiotherapist. Limited research McConnell has demonstrated that tape application inhibits upper trapezius and facilitates middle and lower trapezius activation (Morin, Tiberio, and Austin 1997). This can improve scapular stability by facilitating muscle balance during motion to permit arm movement without impingement pain; it can also enhance muscle reeducation for normal scapular alignment and positioning (Host 1995). Two types of tape are used together: a protective stretch tape called Cover-roll stretch, and a support tape, Leukotape P (both distributed by Beiersdorf, Inc., Norwalk, CT). Two to three strips of the protective stretch tape are applied to the skin over the shoulder from the clavicle anteriorly and across the upper trapezius to below the scapula toward the lower thoracic spinous processes posteriorly. With the patient in a proper posture position, the support tape is applied in several strips from the middle clavicle in a direction downward and medially to the inferior angle of the scapula (figure 17.9). As the tape is pulled downward, the rehabilitation clinician supports and lifts the shoulder from under the axilla so that the upper trapezius stays relaxed during the tape application. The tape should be snug but still permit scapular motion during shoulder elevation.

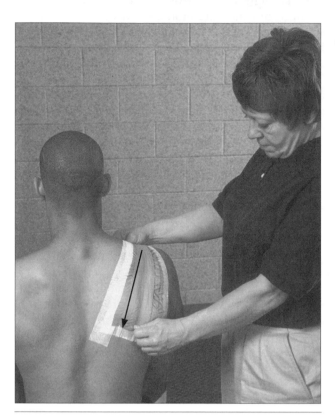

Figure 17.9 Scapular taping support.

Force Couples

Force couples are two equal forces acting in opposite but parallel directions to produce rotatory motion. The shoulder has several force couples that function during arm movement. It is important that the muscles within each of these force couples are balanced to provide optimal function. In the glenohumeral joint, the infraspinatus and teres minor form a force couple with the subscapularis, and the rotator cuff forms a force couple with the deltoid. Scapular force couples include the upper and lower trapezius and serratus anterior, which work together to upwardly rotate the scapula, and the pectoralis minor, levator scapulae, and rhomboids working together to downwardly rotate the scapula. The muscles within each force couple must work cooperatively in timing and level of intensity to produce the desired activity. For example, if the deltoid overpowers the rotator cuff, the glenohumeral joint becomes unstable during elevation. If the upper trapezius is stronger than the lower trapezius and serratus anterior, the scapula is not positioned correctly during arm elevation, and impingement of the rotator cuff occurs.

Relationship Between Trunk/Hip and Shoulder

Just as scapulothoracic stability and strength are important for glenohumeral function, trunk and lower-extremity stability and strength are important for scapular function. The trunk must have the strength to maintain a stable base for the functioning of the scapula. The legs and trunk provide 51% to 55% of the total kinetic energy and total force for overhead activities (Kibler 1995). The shoulder contributes 13% to the total energy production and 21% of the total force. For this reason, exercises for hip rotators, extensors, and abductors, as well as transverse abdominis, obliques, and multifidus, should all be included in a shoulder rehabilitation program.

The forces generated from the legs, hips, trunk, shoulder, and arm are delivered through summation via the body's kinetic chain and are ultimately delivered to the hand and transferred to the object within the hand. These forces must be timed, directed, and applied in a specific sequence if the body is to work efficiently and effectively. This requires a balance of muscle strength throughout all the delivery systems involved.

Posture

Any patient with a shoulder injury should have a posture examination. Correct posture is crucial to shoulder balance and function. If a patient has a forward-head posture with a thoracic kyphosis, the shoulders are drawn forward and medially rotated (figure 17.10). This causes a protraction of the scapula and medial rotation of the humerus with weakness of the scapular retractors and shoulder lateral rotators and tightness of the scapular protractors and shoulder medial rotators. These deficiencies prevent full elevation of the shoulder and lead to subacromial impingement to cause rotator cuff tendinitis. A forward-head posture causes a muscle imbalance: shortening the anterior muscles and lengthening and weakness of the posterior muscles. Posture must be corrected if the rehabilitation program is to be successful.

Cervical Influence

There is an intimate relationship between the cervical spine and shoulder. Patients who complain of shoulder pain without a frank shoulder injury should be examined for cervical involvement. Cervical disk pathology can refer pain along the medial border of the scapula, into the shoulder joint, or down the arm. If shoulder symptoms increase with movement, palpation, or joint mobilization of the spine, the cervical spine may be the source of shoulder pain. It is sometimes difficult to determine whether the cervical spine or the shoulder is the primary source of pain. A quick quadrant test can rule out the possibility of cervical involvement. If the test is negative, the neck may not be the source of pain; however, if the patient does not respond to shoulder treatment, reassessment of the cervical spine is in order. Reproducing the patient's pain is a key component of the rehabilitation assessment for determining the origin of the patient's complaints.

Thoracic Influence

Shoulders lacking full range of motion may have joint mobility restriction in the ribs and thoracic spine. If a patient lacks full elevation of the glenohumeral joint and the shoulder complex has been mobilized with good results, the thoracic spine and costothoracic joints should be examined for hypomobility. Restricted costothoracic and thoracic spine mobility can restrict the shoulder's movement by limiting the expansion of the trunk that is necessary for full shoulder motion. This is particularly true if the patient has habitually poor posture. Application of posterior-anterior movements of the thoracic spine or rib mobilization techniques, or both, should restore normal shoulder mobility when thoracic hypomobility is a factor in a patient's difficulty achieving the last few degrees of glenohumeral motion.

Scapular Plane

It is important to exercise the rotator cuff in the scapular plane. This is a position about 30° forward of the coronal plane. In this position, the arm is in line with the scapula as it lies on the ribs. It is a functional position for the rotator cuff. Often, exercises for the rotator cuff performed in the coronal plane are too uncomfortable for the rotator cuff and encourage impingement of its tendons. Placing the arm in a scapular plane reduces this possibility and is generally more comfortable for the patient.

Figure 17.10 Forward-head, kyphotic posture.

Figure 17.11 Using a rolled towel under the arm helps to position the shoulder in the scapular plane during medial and lateral rotation exercises.

When medial and lateral rotation exercises are performed, a roll should be placed between the arm and the ribs (figure 17.11). This positions the shoulder in a scapular plane. This position also reduces the tension on the supraspinatus tendon, lessening irritation to the tendon (Kelley 1995). In addition, this position may improve the subscapularis alignment to more effectively depress the humeral head.

Exercise Plane and Height Progression

Strength exercises may begin as isometrics and progress to concentric and eccentric exercises. When agonists are weak and are imbalanced with their antagonists, the exercises should be initially performed in straight-plane motions. As strength and control of motion improve, the exercises progress to diagonal, multiplane, functional motions. Patients should not perform diagonal motions until they have adequate muscular strength in straight planes, because the complexity of the shoulder's motions requires good control. Good straight-plane strength permits the patient to perform functional activities without aggravating the shoulder or using inappropriate muscles to produce the motion.

Exercises should be kept to less than 60° elevation in the initial strengthening stages; since little scapular motion occurs in the first 60° of glenohumeral motion, scapular muscles exercised below 60° work primarily as stabilizers, not scapular movers. Elevation higher than 90° is an unstable position for the glenohumeral joint, and scapular muscle strength in the early stages is not adequate to keep the shoulder stabilized. The scapular muscles are also not strong enough in their shortened range to provide the scapular stabilization necessary for glenohumeral motion above 60° elevation. Once scapulothoracic and glenohumeral muscles have adequate strength to control shoulder motion and provide the stabilization necessary for activity at 80° to 110°, progression of exercises to the fully elevated ranges is appropriate after strength in mid-range elevation is achieved.

REHABILITATION TECHNIQUES

Soft-Tissue Mobilization

▶ Two rehabilitation techniques for the shoulder are soft-tissue mobilization and joint mobilization. Trigger point release and ice-and-stretch are soft-tissue mobilization techniques used to improve parameters in the rotator cuff muscles, the scapular muscles, and the large glenohumeral muscles. The rehabilitation clinician uses joint mobilization techniques to improve mobility in the glenohumeral joint, the scapulothoracic joint, and the clavicular joint.

Because of the intimate relationship between the cervical spine and the shoulder, some of the muscles discussed in the preceding chapter are also relevant here. Refer to chapter 6 for details on soft-tissue mobilization theory, physiology, and application. Trigger point release and ice-and-stretch techniques are the primary treatment approaches discussed here. These techniques and the pain referral patterns described here are based on the work of Travell and Simons (1983).

Rotator Cuff Muscles

Each rotator cuff muscle has distinct pain-referral patterns. The rehabilitation clinician should be aware of these differences to make an accurate differential diagnosis and correctly treat the patient's injury.

Supraspinatus

The muscle and the tendon have trigger points and can refer pain into the arm. The referred pain pattern is a deep ache that occurs around the lateral shoulder in the middle deltoid area down to the deltoid insertion (figure 17.12, a and b). The pain can also be referred to the elbow's lateral epicondyle.

Trigger point treatment can be performed with the patient in sidelying on the opposite side or sitting. The medial trigger point is often the more sensitive site. With the patient's arm in a relaxed position, sustained pressure is applied over the trigger point site just above the clavicular spine, 2 to 3 cm (0.8-1.2 in.) lateral to the vertebral border (figure 17.12c). The clinician should palpate an expansion, tightening, or nodule within the soft tissue over the trigger point site.

Ice-and-stretch is applied with the patient in sitting and the forearm behind the waist. Ice strokes are swept from the proximal supraspinatus insertion, across the muscle and acromion, over the deltoid, and down the arm to the elbow (figure 17.12d). The clinician applies the stretch by raising the patient's hand behind the back upward toward the opposite scapula.

Figure 17.12 Supraspinatus: *(a-b)* pain-referral pattern, *(c)* trigger point release, *(d)* ice-and-stretch.

Subscapularis

The subscapularis refers pain to the posterior wrist and in the inferior aspect of the posterior shoulder region where the arm meets the trunk. It can also occasionally refer pain into the scapula, down the posterior arm to the elbow, and circumferentially around the wrist (figure 17.13, a-b).

Trigger point release is performed with the patient supine and the arm abducted comfortably away from the body to about 60° to 90°. The clinician supports the patient's arm while applying traction to keep the scapula away from the ribs, then moves his or her fingers past the teres major and latissimus dorsi and palpates the anterior surface of the scapula. A sustained pressure in a cephalic direction toward the spine is applied once the trigger point has been located (figure 17.13c).

Ice-and-stretch is applied with the patient supine and the arm in partial abduction and lateral rotation. Ice sweeps start at the side and move over the axilla and along the posterior arm. As the sweeps are repeated, the arm is moved into more abduction and lateral rotation until it is positioned overhead in full abduction and lateral rotation (figure 17.13, d-e).

Figure 17.13   Subscapularis: *(a-b)* pain-referral pattern, *(c)* trigger point release, *(d)* ice-and-stretch in moderate stretch position, *(e)* ice-and-stretch in full stretch position.

Teres Minor

The teres minor muscle refers pain to the upper posterior arm, proximal to the deltoid attachment and about 5 cm (2.0 in.) in diameter (figure 17.14a). The pain is frequently described as deep and sharp. The spillover area of pain referral remains in the proximal aspect of the posterior upper arm and the lateral arm from the acromion downward.

Trigger point release is performed with the patient in sidelying on the opposite side with the arm comfortably supported. The trigger point is located in the teres minor muscle belly along the lateral scapular border between the teres major inferiorly and the infraspinatus superiorly (figure 17.14b).

Ice-and-stretch is applied with the patient in sidelying on the opposite side. The ice sweeps begin low on the side and move along the lateral border of the scapula over the teres minor and along the posterior arm. As the ice is applied, the arm is moved overhead and medially rotated (figure 17.14c).

a

Figure 17.14 Teres minor: *(a)* pain-referral pattern, *(b)* trigger point release, *(c)* ice-and-stretch.

Infraspinatus

The infraspinatus refers pain most often to the anterior shoulder, to the anterior arm, to the wrist, and to the radial fingers (figure 17.15, a-b). On occasion, vertebral border scapular pain or pain at the base of the skull can also occur. Pain can be felt deep in the anterior shoulder as well.

The most commonly irritated trigger points are in the superior aspect of the muscle inferior to the scapula spine. Trigger point release is performed by application of sustained pressure over the muscle with the patient in sitting or sidelying on the opposite side. The trigger point sites are easily located as tender bands within the muscle (figure 17.15c). Ice-and-stretch is applied with the patient in sidelying on the opposite side or sitting. The muscle can be progressively stretched by moving the arm either behind the back with the shoulder in medial rotation, or horizontally in front and across the body with medial rotation. The ice is applied from the vertebral border upward to the shoulder and then either up to the head or down the arm (figure 17.15d).

Figure 17.15
Infraspinatus: pain-referral patterns *(a)* anterior and *(b)* posterior; *(c)* trigger point release, *(d)* ice-and-stretch.

Scapular Muscles

Although the scapular muscles refer pain primarily to the upper back, they can also refer pain to the chest and upper extremity. As with the rotator cuff muscles, the scapular muscles have pain-referral patterns that are unique for each muscle.

Upper Trapezius and Levator Scapulae

Trigger points and treatment of these muscles are described in chapter 16. Refer to figures 16.1 and 16.2 for details.

Serratus Anterior

This muscle refers pain laterally to the midchest area or to the inferior angle of the scapula (figure 17.16, a-b). Spillover referral pain can also be experienced as abnormal breast sensitivity, pain down the anteromedial forearm to the palm and ulnar digits, or pectoralis major pain. Trigger point release is performed with the patient in supine and the arm positioned slightly extended behind the lateral trunk. Sustained pressure is applied over the level of the fifth or sixth rib just anterior to the midaxillary line at the nipple level (figure 17.16c).

Ice-and-stretch is performed with the patient in sidelying. Ice stroking is applied from the trigger point outward anteriorly and posteriorly over the muscle (figure 17.16d). The progressive stretch is applied with backward and downward pressure on the arm. An additional stretch can be applied to the muscle if the patient takes a deep breath and holds it during the stretch.

a   *b*

c   *d*

Figure 17.16   Serratus anterior: *(a-b)* trigger points and referral points, *(c)* trigger point release, *(d)* ice-and-stretch.

a

Rhomboids

These muscles have pain-referral patterns similar to those of the levator scapulae except that there is no neck component. The pain-referral pattern is along the vertebral border of the scapula, with some pain possible into the medial supraspinatus area (figure 17.17a).

Trigger point release is performed with the patient in prone or sitting. The area of restriction is often palpated as tender bands in the muscle along the vertebral border. Sustained pressure over this area should be maintained until the pain subsides (figure 17.17b).

Ice-and-stretch is applied with the muscle on stretch. The patient is in a relaxed sitting position with the thoracic spine flexed and the arms hanging forward or across the chest to protract the scapula. Ice sweeps are made in parallel strokes across the back in the direction of the muscle's fibers from the vertebral border and upward to the shoulder (figure 17.17c).

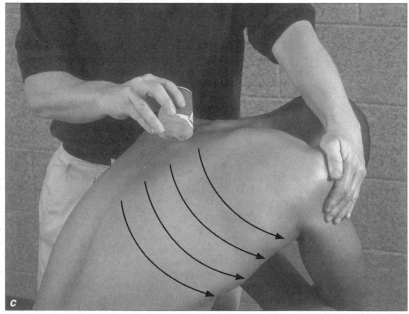

Figure 17.17
Rhomboids: *(a)* pain-referral patterns, *(b)* trigger point release, *(c)* ice-and-stretch.

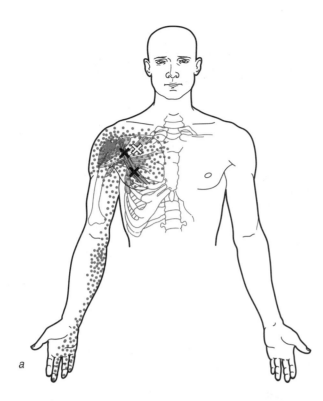

Pectoralis Minor

This muscle refers pain over the anterior deltoid with some spillover into the subclavicular area, entire pectoral area, and ulnar aspect of the arm, forearm, palmar hand, and fingers (figure 17.18a).

Release of the active trigger point can be performed with the patient supine. The forearm should be supported on the abdomen or relaxed overhead to keep the pectoralis major lax. The rehabilitation clinician counts the ribs down from the concave aspect of the clavicle to the third and fourth ribs. The cephalic trigger point or taut band in the pectoralis minor should be palpated in this region (figure 17.18b). The more distal trigger point is located one rib down and slightly medial to the cephalic trigger point.

Ice-and-stretch is performed with the patient seated or supine with shoulder over table edge. The arm is abducted, and the shoulder is pulled posteriorly in horizontal extension and lateral rotation to elevate and retract the scapula to put the pectoralis minor on stretch. Ice sweeps are made from the anterior chest region upward to the anterior shoulder, along the medial upper arm and forearm to the ulnar fingers (figure 17.18c).

Figure 17.18 Pectoralis minor: *(a)* pain-referral patterns and trigger points, *(b)* trigger point release, *(c)* ice-and-stretch.

Large Glenohumeral Muscles

Some of the large glenohumeral muscle pain-referral patterns can closely resemble those of other shoulder muscles, including the rotator cuff and scapular rotators. Careful observation and testing are necessary in order to focus in on the proper muscle to treat.

Latissimus Dorsi

A constant aching in the inferior angle of the scapula and midthoracic area is typical of a pain referral with this muscle. Spillover pain referral can also occur in the posterior shoulder, down the posterior or medial arm and forearm, and to the ulnar hand and fingers (figure 17.19a-c).

Release of this trigger point can be performed with the patient supine and the arm abducted to about 60° to 90°. The clinician can palpate myofascial bands by grasping the muscle a couple of centimeters below the top of the arch of the posterior axillary fold at the midscapular level (figure 17.19d).

Ice-and-stretch is performed with the patient in supine or sidelying on the opposite side. Ice sweeps are performed in parallel strokes, from the distal insertion of the muscle upward over the axilla and along the arm and ulnar aspect of the forearm to the hand (figure 17.19e). The muscle is stretched upward so that the arm is eventually placed behind the ear.

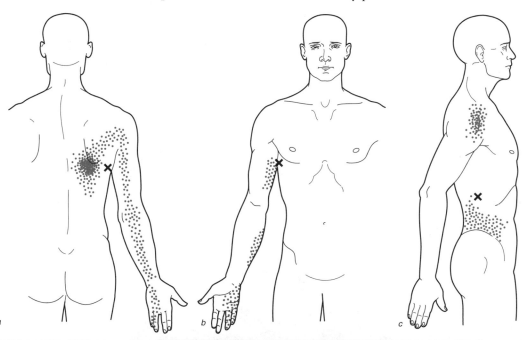

Figure 17.19
Latissimus dorsi: *(a-c)* trigger point and pain-referral patterns, *(d)* trigger point release, *(e)* ice-and-stretch.

Teres Major

The teres major refers pain over the posterior deltoid, over the triceps long head, and occasionally into the posterior forearm (figure 17.20, a-b).

Trigger point release is performed with the patient in supine and the arm abducted to 90°. The groove between the lateral lower edge of the scapula and the axillary fold is palpated; the muscle is grasped by the thumb and index finger, whose web space surrounds the latissimus dorsi. A tender, taut band can usually be palpated. When the patient is in sitting or sidelying, the muscle is located near the scapula's lateral border approximately at midscapular level and released with pressure using the thumb or finger pad (figure 17.20c).

Ice-and-stretch is performed with the patient supine or sidelying and with the arm overhead in shoulder abduction and lateral rotation and elbow flexion. Ice strokes are swept from the lateral inferior border of the scapula along the triceps as the arm is moved into medial rotation (figure 17.20d).

Figure 17.20 Teres major: *(a-b)* pain-referral patterns and trigger points, *(c)* trigger point release, *(d)* ice-and-stretch.

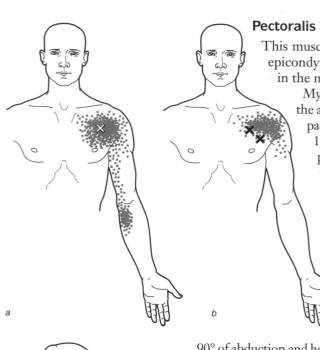

a

b

c

Pectoralis Major

This muscle refers pain to the anterior chest, anterior deltoid, medial epicondyle, sternum, and breast. Overspill referral pain can also occur in the medial arm and ulnar digits (figure 17.21, a-c).

Myofascial release of the pectoralis major can be performed with the arm in 90° abduction. Consistent upward pressure with a finger pad is applied to the muscle between the fifth and sixth ribs (figure 17.21d). The site is located by first finding the tip of the xiphoid process and drawing a horizontal line laterally that intersects with a vertical line imagined between the lateral sternum and nipple; the point of intersection of these two lines is the site of a common trigger point. Other areas of localized tenderness can be treated in the trigger point regions of the muscle identified by "x" in figure 17.21a-c. Some trigger points in the sternocostal area can be treated with a pincer grasp rather than flat finger pressure.

Ice-and-stretch is applied with the patient either supine or sitting. The various heads of the pectoralis major are stretched in different positions. The clavicular portion is stretched with the patient in sitting, with the shoulder in 90° of abduction and horizontally extended (figure 17.21e). The sternocostal portion is stretched in sitting or supine, with the shoulder in abduction and lateral rotation moving into full flexion. If the application is performed with the patient supine, care must be taken to keep the scapula unimpeded during the treatment. Ice strokes are swept from the sternum to the shoulder, along the medial arm, to the ulnar aspect of the hand as the stretch is applied. Traction should be applied to the arm throughout the treatment.

d

e

Figure 17.21 Pectoralis major: *(a-c)* pain-referral patterns and trigger points, *(d)* trigger point release, *(e)* ice-and-stretch, clavicular portion.

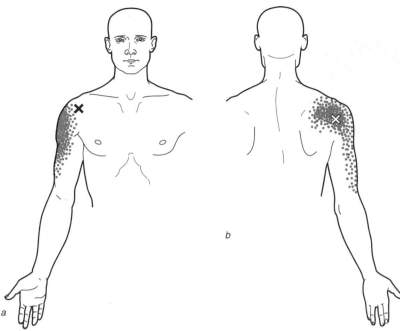

Deltoid

The anterior and posterior deltoid portions can refer pain over the anterior, posterior, and middle deltoid locations with some spillover into adjacent areas of the arm (figure 17.22, a-b). The taut bands and trigger points can be treated with the arm in 30° to 90° of abduction. Pressure is then applied to the trigger point areas (figure 17.22c). Since the deltoid trigger point pain pattern can be similar to rotator cuff muscle pain referral patterns, care should be taken to eliminate those muscles as potential sources of referred pain before treating the deltoid.

Ice-and-stretch is applied with the patient in sitting. The arm is positioned in horizontal flexion and medial rotation to stretch the posterior deltoid, and in horizontal extension at 90° abduction and lateral rotation to stretch the anterior deltoid (figure 17.22d). As the muscle is being stretched, the ice strokes are swept from the origin of the specific muscle portion, and over the shoulder and arm along the pain referral pattern. For the posterior deltoid ice strokes, move from posterior to anterior; reverse the direction for the anterior deltoid.

Figure 17.22 Deltoid: *(a-b)* trigger points and pain-referral patterns for the anterior and posterior deltoid, *(c)* trigger point release, *(d)* ice-and-stretch of posterior deltoid.

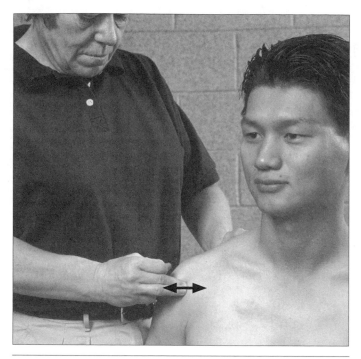

Figure 17.23 Cross-friction massage to supraspinatus tendon.

Supraspinatus Friction Massage

This massage technique is used to treat supraspinatus tendinitis. The patient is in sitting with his or her hand behind the back to expose the supraspinatus tendon. The rehabilitation clinician's index finger is reinforced by the middle finger and placed on top of the tendon about two finger-widths inferior to the acromion. Cross-friction pressure is applied to the tendon for 1 to 2 min or until the tenderness subsides (figure 17.23).

Myofascial Stretch: Arm Pull

This technique is a general myofascial stretching technique for stretching or mobilizing soft tissue. With the patient in supine, the clinician grasps the patient's hand to apply a longitudinal traction. While traction is applied, the arm is passively placed in lateral rotation, and a gradual, passive movement of the arm into abduction occurs (figure 17.24). When the clinician feels a barrier to motion, the position is held until a release is felt.

This procedure is repeated with the arm in horizontal adduction. For the horizontal adduction pull, the scapula is protracted, and the patient rolls to the side.

A final arm-pull technique is performed with the patient supine. As traction is applied to the arm, the arm is medially rotated and adducted. For each pull, the clinician moves the arm until the barrier is felt and holds that position until the barrier releases before moving to into a greater range of motion.

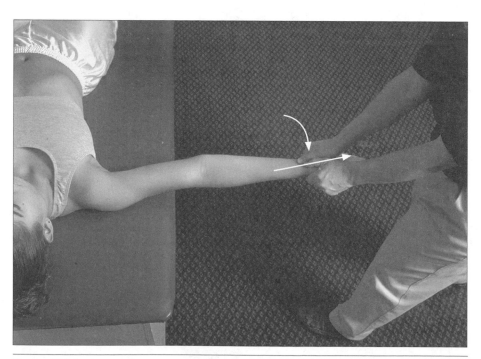

Figure 17.24 Arm pull.

Joint Mobilization

Joint mobilization can be performed on all joints of the shoulder complex. Findings from the initial examination will determine the specific joints requiring mobilization treatment. Shoulder joint mobility is also influenced by the mobility of the ribs and thoracic spine. As mentioned earlier in this chapter, if a shoulder lacks full range of motion and appears to have good mobility in its joints, examination of rib and thoracic spine mobility may demonstrate restriction of these joints. If this proves to be the case, thoracic and rib mobilization techniques discussed in chapter 16 for these areas may be helpful in restoring full shoulder motion.

Capsular restriction of the glenohumeral joint follows a capsular pattern: more restricted motion in lateral rotation than in abduction, more restricted motion in abduction than in flexion, and more restricted motion in flexion than in medial rotation. For example, if a patient's shoulder has 100° flexion, 90° abduction, and full lateral rotation, the joint capsule is not the primary structure limiting full motion. However, if the joint measures 100° flexion, 90° abduction, and 60° lateral rotation, the joint capsule is probably restricting full motion. If a patient's shoulder presents with this loss-of-motion profile, the capsule is restricted, and joint mobilization is needed to restore glenohumeral motion. If a shoulder does not demonstrate this capsular pattern, capsule tightness is not the primary cause for the patient's loss of motion.

Initial glenohumeral mobilizations should be applied with the joint in resting position—55° flexion and 20° to 30° horizontal abduction. As additional mobility is achieved but full mobility is still lacking, the joint may need to be mobilized out of its resting position and in other loose-pack positions. The extreme close-packed position for the glenohumeral joint is full abduction with full lateral rotation.

While applying joint mobilization, the rehabilitation clinician should always use proper body mechanics. The hand applying the force should be positioned as close to the joint as possible. The mobilization force should be directed from the legs, not the arms.

The rehabilitation clinician needs to remember the principles of glide, roll, and spin so that the force application is proper for the desired movement. The humerus is a convex surface moving on the glenoid fossa's concave surface, so the convex-concave rule applies. The joint mobilization techniques presented here are the most commonly used techniques. As with any joint mobilization procedure, it is important for the clinician to visualize the joint surfaces and apply the mobilization force parallel or perpendicular to the plane of the surface. As the arm is moved into different positions, the plane of the glenoid changes; you must consider this as you determine the angle of force application.

Precautions and contraindications should be respected. The time line for tissue healing and the status and strength of new tissue must be considered when one is deciding whether to apply joint mobilization and how much force to use. Joint mobilizations applied to hypermobile joints can increase instability and cause further damage, and is contraindicated. Improper technique, incorrect force application, excessive force, and inappropriate timing of application can all result in unnecessary injury or damage to the joint's structures.

Glenohumeral Joint

During some mobilization techniques for the glenohumeral joint, a sustained joint distraction force is applied in addition to the mobilization force. The techniques are usually named according to the direction of the mobilization force.

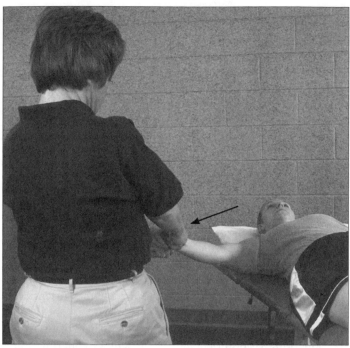

Figure 17.25   Joint mobilization: distraction with oscillation.

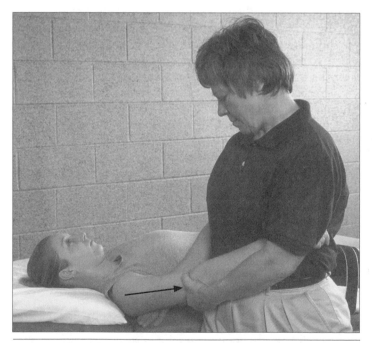

Figure 17.26   Joint mobilization: longitudinal distraction.

Distraction with Oscillation

This type of mobilization, a relaxation technique, is a good way to begin and end mobilization treatment; it relaxes the joint before and after treatment. The patient lies supine, and the rehabilitation clinician grasps the patient's distal forearm and wrist with two hands. The shoulder should be in the resting position, about 55° of flexion and 30° of horizontal abduction. The clinician applies mild distraction force perpendicular to the glenohumeral joint plane while performing oscillations (figure 17.25).

Longitudinal Distraction

The resting position, the most comfortable position for the glenohumeral joint, is the position used for longitudinal distraction. This is a good beginning technique for improving inferior capsule mobility. The patient is supine with the involved shoulder as close to the edge of the table as possible. For a right shoulder, the rehabilitation clinician places his or her right hand in the axilla to stabilize the glenoid. The left hand grasps just above the elbow joint and applies a distraction force to the humerus (figure 17.26). Although a prolonged force is more effective, an oscillation can also be used.

Inferior or Caudal Glide

This technique is used to improve inferior capsular mobility and glenohumeral abduction by stretching the inferior capsular pouch. The patient lies supine with the involved shoulder as close to the edge of the table as possible. A stabilization strap may be placed around the chest to stabilize the scapula. The clinician places the stabilizing hand on the proximal humerus and places the mobilizing hand on superior aspect of the humerus as close as possible to the acromion. The mobilizing hand web space should be over the superior humeral head. The stabilizing hand maintains the shoulder in a resting position with some distraction as the mobilizing hand applies a glide force in a caudal direction parallel to the joint's surface (figure 17.27a). The arm can be abducted to a maximum of 60°, but initial glides should be performed in the resting position.

Once approximately 120° of flexion has been attained, an inferior glide can be performed with the arm in an elevated position. As the shoulder's position changes, the glenoid joint surface changes; likewise, the mobilization force direction changes as the joint plane changes: the force is directed inferiorly (figure 17.27b).

Figure 17.27 Joint mobilization—inferior glide: *(a)* initial position, *(b)* advanced position.

Alternative Caudal Glide

As with the previous technique, this technique is useful for improving inferior capsule mobility and is another way to apply an inferior or caudal glide to the glenohumeral joint. The patient lies supine with the involved shoulder flexed to 90°. The rehabilitation clinician's hands grasp the humerus as close as possible to the shoulder joint. The patient's upper arm rests on the rehabilitation clinician's shoulder. The clinician then applies an inferior force to the proximal humerus (figure 17.28). A prolonged or oscillation technique can be used.

Figure 17.28 Joint mobilization: caudal glide.

Figure 17.29   Joint mobilization: lateral glide.

Lateral Glide

This technique is used to increase all motions of the glenohumeral joint. The patient lies supine with the involved shoulder as close to the edge of the table as possible. A strap may be needed to stabilize the scapula. The clinician faces the patient at shoulder level and grasps the patient's humerus as proximally as possible with the patient's shoulder flexed to 90° and the patient's upper arm resting on the rehabilitation clinician's shoulder. A lateral force is applied to the humerus (figure 17.29).

Posterior or Dorsal Glide

This technique is used to improve flexion and medial rotation motions by improving posterior capsule mobility. The patient lies supine with the shoulder as close to the edge of the table as possible. A towel roll or wedge is placed under the scapula for stabilization. The clinician abducts the patient's arm; standing between the patient's arm and trunk, the clinician places the stabilizing hand at the elbow and the mobilizing hand just distal to the acromion, as close to the humeral head as possible. The mobilizing hand applies a downward and slightly lateral force, and the stabilizing hand applies slight traction of the patient's glenohumeral joint at the patient's elbow (figure 17.30a). An alternative technique is performed with the patient's shoulder in medial rotation to gain additional motion in that direction (figure 17.30b). An advanced flexion technique can be performed with the patient's shoulder flexed to 90° and adducted with the elbow flexed. In this position the rehabilitation clinician stabilizes the arm with a hand on the proximal humerus. A downward mobilization force is applied with the mobilizing hand on the patient's elbow and the clinician's forearm in line with the patient's arm (figure 17.30c).

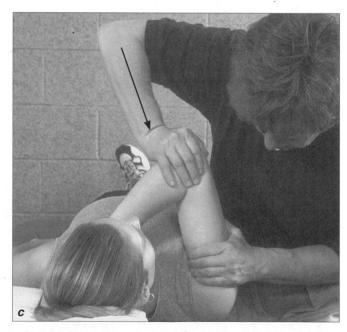

Figure 17.30   Joint mobilization: *(a)* posterior glide, *(b)* posterior glide with medial rotation, *(c)* advanced posterior glide with flexion.

Anterior or Ventral Glide

This technique is used to increase anterior capsule mobility for improving extension and lateral rotation. The patient lies prone with a towel or wedge support under the anterior clavicle and coracoid process to stabilize the shoulder. The glenohumeral joint is off the edge of the table, and the arm is placed in the resting position. The rehabilitation clinician stands between the patient's arm and side, facing the shoulder, and places the stabilizing hand on the distal humerus and the mobilization hand on the posterior aspect of the humeral head just distal to the acromion. As the stabilizing hand applies a distraction force, the proximal mobilizing hand applies an anterior and slightly medial mobilization force (figure 17.31a). As additional motion is achieved but restriction in the anterior-inferior capsule remains, an alternative position for mobilization is with the arm in elevation (figure 17.31b). An alternative technique can be used to increase lateral rotation by positioning the arm in additional lateral rotation during the mobilization. With another technique, one that is less comfortable for the clinician, the patient is supine and a force from the posterior aspect of the shoulder is applied (figure 17.31c).

Figure 17.31   Joint mobilization—anterior glide: *(a)* initial position, *(b)* alternative position, *(c)* supine position.

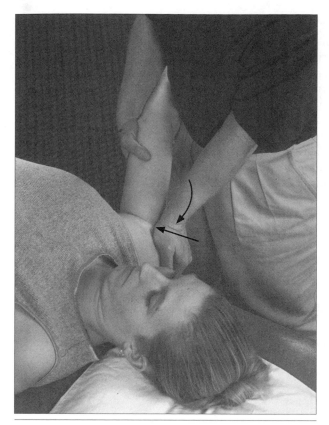

Figure 17.32   Joint mobilization: lateral rotation.

Lateral rotation

This technique is used to improve lateral rotation motion. The patient lies supine with the arm abducted in the scapular plane. The rehabilitation clinician places the distal hand over the distal humerus and the heel of the proximal hand over the humeral head. As the distal hand stabilizes the arm in lateral rotation, the proximal hand applies a simultaneous lateral rotation and inferior glide force (figure 17.32).

Scapulothoracic Joint

These mobilization techniques for the scapulothoracic joint are possible only if the patient remains relaxed. If a patient is not relaxed, the rehabilitation clinician will be unable to position his or her hands between the scapula and ribs to apply the techniques.

Scapular Distraction

This technique is used to improve scapulothoracic mobility. The patient is in sidelying with the involved arm on top. The rehabilitation clinician positions his or her lower hand between the patient's arm and rib cage and grasps the inferior angle of the scapula. The upper hand grasps the scapula's upper vertebral border. For personal comfort and professional consideration, a pillow should be placed between the patient and the clinician. As the shoulder is stabilized by the clinician's abdomen against the anterior shoulder, both hands apply a force to tilt the vertebral border of the scapula posteriorly away from the ribs (figure 17.33a). An alternative position is with the patient prone. The patient's arm is extended alongside the body, supported on the table. The clinician stands beside the patient, facing the patient's head, and cups one hand around the anterior humeral head and places the other hand under the inferior angle of the scapula as shown in 17.33b. The hands are moved simultaneously toward each other, the hand under the humerus lifting upward and medially, and the hand under the scapula moving laterally under the scapula.

Figure 17.33   Joint mobilization—scapular distraction: *(a)* in sidelying, *(b)* alternative technique in prone.

Figure 17.34   Joint mobilization: scapular inferior glide.

Scapular Inferior Glide

This technique is used to improve downward mobility of the scapula. The patient is in sidelying, and the rehabilitation clinician faces the patient. The rehabilitation clinician's cephalad hand is placed over the superior scapula, and the caudad hand is positioned with the web space cradling the inferior angle of the scapula. As the superior hand pushes the scapula in a caudal direction, the inferior hand moves under the inferior angle of the scapula (figure 17.34).

Clavicular Joints

Because clavicular motion contributes 60° to glenohumeral motion, it is important for clavicular joint mobility to be intact. After shoulder immobilization, these joints may become restricted and should be mobilized if hypomobility is present.

Four mobilization techniques are used at the sternoclavicular and acromioclavicular (AC) joints: inferior, superior, anterior, and posterior glides. The force is applied with the thumb pad of one hand, reinforced with the other thumb.

The resting position for the AC and sternoclavicular (SC) joints is called the physiological position; it is the position the joints are in when the arm is resting at the side. The close-packed position for the sternoclavicular joint is with the arm in full elevation overhead. The close-packed position for the AC joint is with the arm abducted to 90°.

Figure 17.35   Joint mobilization—AC glides: *(a)* anterior glide, *(b)* posterior glide.

Acromioclavicular Glides

These techniques are performed either with the patient supine and the arm supported on the table, or with the patient sitting. When the patient is supine, the rehabilitation clinician stands at the head for inferior (caudal) glides, and at the side for posterior (dorsal) glides. To perform anterior (ventral) glides with the patient sitting, the clinician is behind the patient (figure 17.35a) and in front of the patient for posterior glides (figure 17.35b). With each technique, the rehabilitation clinician applies a force on the end of the lateral clavicle, parallel to the joint-surface plane.

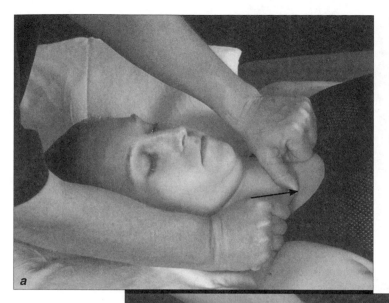

Sternoclavicular Glides

For these techniques, the patient is supine, and his or her arm is supported on the table. The rehabilitation clinician stands at the patient's waist for superior glides, at the head for inferior glides (figure 17.36a), and at the side for posterior glides. The force is applied parallel to the joint surface on the medial end of the clavicle.

Figure 17.36 Joint mobilization—sternoclavicular glides: (a) inferior glide, (b) posterior glide.

FLEXIBILITY EXERCISES

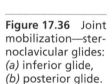

▶ Flexibility exercises for the shoulder include pendulum exercises, active and assistive stretches, wand exercises using the uninvolved extremity, and pulley exercises.

The stretch force for all flexibility exercises should be sufficient to produce a stretch sensation without pain. Pain indicates that the stretch force is too aggressive and should be reduced. Stretches can be either short term or prolonged. Recent injuries with newly formed scar tissue can be effectively treated with short-term stretches. Injuries that occurred several months before treatment and contain scar tissue that is more mature will benefit from prolonged stretches.

Pendulum Exercises

These exercises can be performed in the early rehabilitation phase to distract the glenohumeral joint, relax the muscles around the shoulder, and provide pain modulation. They are also called Codman's exercises. A cuff can be applied to the wrist. It is important that muscles are relaxed, so the patient should not hold on to the weight with the hand; it should be passively secured to the wrist.

Codman's exercises are performed with the patient flexed forward at the waist with the involved arm hanging in a resting position away from the body; the body weight is supported by the uninvolved arm on a table. Involved arm motion is initiated from the hips, not the shoulder. The arm should remain relaxed throughout the motions. Passive flexion-extension motion of the shoulder occurs with the patient's legs in a forward-backward straddle position; body weight is transferred from the front to the back leg to provide momentum for arm movement (figure 17.37a). Horizontal flexion-extension movement occurs with the patient standing in a side-to-side straddle position, and body weight is transferred from the left leg to the right leg to produce sideward arm motion (figure 17.37b). Circular motion of the shoulder is produced by the hips as the patient moves the body in a circular direction while the arm hangs passively, swinging with momentum produced from the hips. Circular motion can occur in a clockwise or counterclockwise direction. It is important that all shoulder motion occurs passively during these exercises.

Figure 17.37 Codman's exercises: (a) flexion-extension, (b) horizontal flexion-extension. Passive motion of the shoulder occurs because of weight transfer back and forth between the left leg and the right leg while the arm remains relaxed.

Figure 17.38 Flexibility exercise: inferior capsule stretch.

Active Stretches

Selection of these stretches is based on areas of the capsule that are tight. These exercises are often used in conjunction with joint mobilization.

Inferior Capsule Stretch

This exercise increases inferior capsular mobility to improve shoulder elevation. The patient positions the arm overhead with the elbow flexed and the forearm behind the head. The uninvolved hand, placed on the elbow, pulls the elbow behind the head (figure 17.38). A common substitution with this exercise is lateral trunk lean away from the shoulder being stretched. If this occurs, the patient should perform the exercise in front of a mirror to monitor and correct trunk position. The patient should not shrug the shoulder as it is stretched.

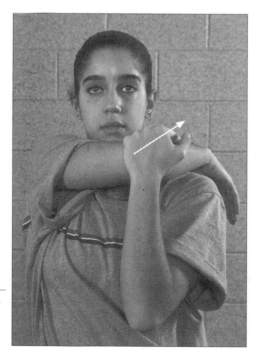

Figure 17.39 Flexibility exercise: posterior capsule stretch.

Posterior Capsule Stretch

This stretch, used to gain medial rotation and horizontal flexion, is for the posterior rotator cuff. The patient positions the involved arm at shoulder level and grasps the elbow with the opposite hand. The patient pulls the arm across the body, attempting to place the hand of the involved shoulder behind the opposite shoulder and the elbow close to the chin (figure 17.39). A common error is to rotate the trunk rather than pull the arm across the body. The patient may also tend to lower the elbow below shoulder level. The clinician uses verbal cueing to correct for proper execution. If necessary, the patient can also stand in front of a mirror to receive visual feedback.

Figure 17.40 Flexibility exercise: anterior capsule stretch: *(a)* upper, *(b)* lower.

Anterior Capsule Stretch

This stretch is used to gain horizontal extension and lateral rotation. It stretches the anterior capsule and pectoralis major. The patient stands in a doorway with the elbows and forearms on the door jamb. To stretch upper pectoralis fibers, the elbows are positioned below the shoulders (figure 17.40a). To stretch middle fibers, the elbows are positioned at shoulder level. To stretch lower fibers, the elbows are positioned above the shoulders (figure 17.40b). With one foot placed in front of the other, the patient pushes from the back foot to lean through the doorway and feel a stretch in the anterior chest area. Common substitutions include arching the back, moving the elbows off the door jamb, and keeping the involved shoulder behind the uninvolved shoulder so that the trunk is at an angle to the doorway. Verbal cueing for proper technique should be used to correct these substitutions. This stretch can also be performed in a corner, but it is often difficult to find an available corner that is not occupied with furniture or other difficult-to-move objects.

Figure 17.41
Flexibility exercise: superior capsule stretch.

Superior Capsule Stretch

This exercise increases superior capsule mobility. The patient places a rolled towel under the arm and positions the elbow next to his or her side. With the uninvolved hand, the patient pulls the elbow toward the side (figure 17.41). A common error is to use a roll that is not large enough to provide adequate stretch. Applying the stretch force too high on the arm delivers less stretch force.

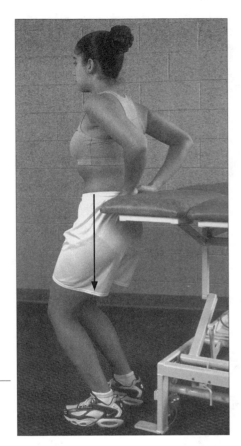

Figure 17.42 Flexibility exercise: medial rotation stretch.

Medial rotation Stretch

This exercise increases medial rotation and stretches the capsule. The patient stands with his or her hands behind the back and grasps the countertop. The feet are shoulder-width apart. The patient squats down while maintaining a grasp on the countertop (figure 17.42). The hands may start in a shoulder-width grip, but the patient should move the hands closer together as flexibility is gained until one hand is on top of the other. The most common substitutions are bending over at the waist, looking down at the floor, and flexing the wrist. The wrist should remain straight, and the patient should maintain an erect position. Giving the patient a verbal cue to keep the head up or to look at the ceiling will help correct the posture.

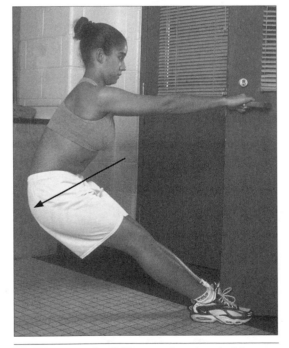

Figure 17.43 Flexibility exercise: rhomboid stretch.

Rhomboid Stretch

This exercise stretches the rhomboids and posterior capsule. The patient stands facing the edge of an open door, with the feet placed on either side of the door and the hands on the doorknobs. With the legs straight, the patient pushes the hips backward. The arms should remain straight and relaxed as the body weight moves backward (figure 17.43). A common error is not allowing the body weight to stretch the shoulders. If this error occurs, instruct the patient to relax the arms and let the hips move backward and downward, attempting to sit on the floor while the legs are kept straight.

Figure 17.44 Flexibility exercise: supraspinatus stretch.

Supraspinatus Stretch

This stretch increases supraspinatus flexibility and superior capsular mobility. The patient positions the involved arm behind the body with the elbow flexed and grasps a chair back with the hand. The patient then leans away from the hand. An alternative technique is to grasp the hand behind the back with the opposite hand and pull the involved arm toward the uninvolved side (figure 17.44). A common substitution is twisting the body. Bending the trunk rather than leaning is also a substitution.

Assistive Stretches

These stretches require the assistance of the clinician. They can be combined with contract-relax-stretch techniques to give the stretch a neuromuscular facilitation element. Improper technique and substitutions should be corrected so that the intended structures are appropriately stretched.

Supraspinatus Stretch

This exercise increases supraspinatus motion and superior capsular mobility. The patient's arm is placed behind the low back with the elbow flexed similarly to as shown in figure 17.44. The clinician pulls the arm across the body and maintains medial rotation of the shoulder. The trunk should not be permitted to laterally flex toward the shoulder that is being stretched. To prevent this movement, you can place a hand on the contralateral shoulder to stabilize the trunk.

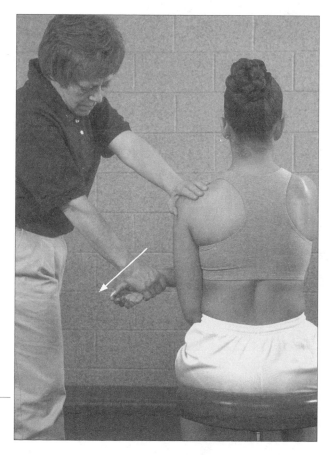

Figure 17.45 Assistive infraspinatus stretch.

Infraspinatus Stretch

This stretch increases infraspinatus flexibility and posterior capsular mobility. The patient's arm is positioned in medial rotation and in front of the body. The clinician grasps the elbow and pulls the arm across the body while maintaining medial rotation (figure 17.45). To prevent trunk rotation and lean, place a stabilizing hand on the patient's shoulder.

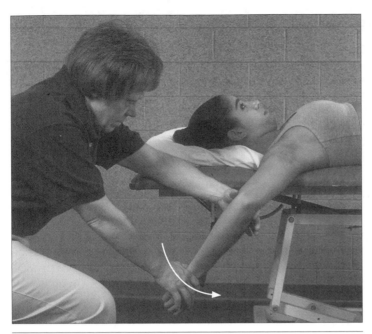

Figure 17.46   Assistive subscapularis stretch.

Subscapularis Stretch

This stretch increases subscapularis flexibility and improves inferior capsular mobility. The patient lies supine, and the clinician moves the arm into abduction and lateral rotation (figure 17.46). A stretch force is applied into lateral rotation. The back and chest should remain flat on the table. Care must be taken to avoid excessive elbow stress.

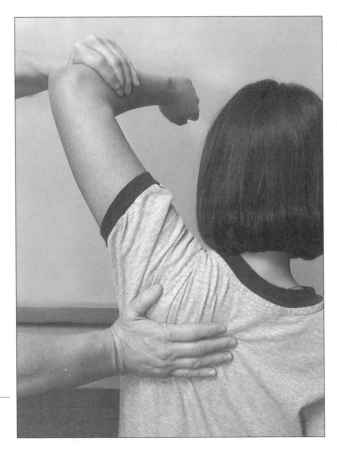

Figure 17.47
Assistive teres
minor stretch.

Teres Minor Stretch

This stretch increases teres minor flexibility and stretches the inferior capsule. The patient is sitting with the arm abducted away from the body. The arm is then medially rotated (figure 17.47). The clinician stabilizes the scapula to isolate teres minor movement as the medial rotation stretch is applied. An alternative position can be used with the arm overhead in end-range abduction with medial rotation; the scapula must be stabilized by the clinician in this stretch.

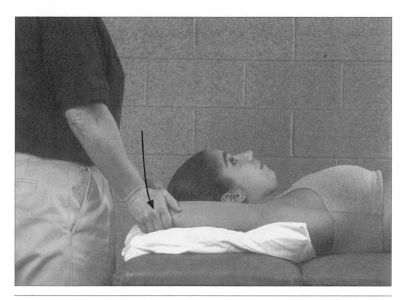

Figure 17.48 Assistive teres major stretch.

Teres Major Stretch

The teres major is stretched with the patient supine and the arm overhead in flexion and lateral rotation. The clinician applies the stretch force in flexion and lateral rotation (figure 17.48). The thoracolumbar spine should not rise up from the table. Instruct the patient to lie with the hips and knees flexed with the back flat on the table if spine hyperextension occurs.

Latissimus Dorsi Stretch

This stretch increases latissimus dorsi flexibility. The patient lies prone with the arm overhead. The clinician grasps the forearm and then distracts and laterally rotates the shoulder as the arm is lifted toward the ceiling (figure 17.49). The trunk should not rotate, and the elbow should remain extended. If the patient has a history of elbow or wrist injury, the force should be applied just proximal to the elbow joint.

Figure 17.49 Assistive latissimus dorsi stretch.

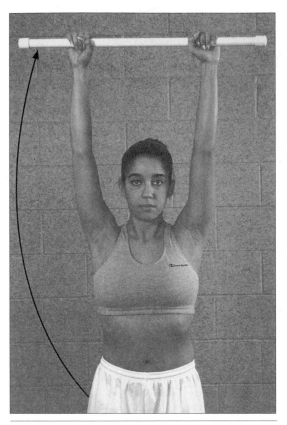

Figure 17.50   Wand flexion.

Wand Exercises

These exercises, performed with a wand, use the uninvolved contralateral arm to provide the stretch force. Commercial wands and T-bars can be used; but a 2.5-cm (1-in.) diameter dowel, broom handle, cane, and other similar items are readily available, inexpensive, and easy to use.

The patient uses the uninvolved arm to guide the wand in the desired direction to provide the stretch force needed to increase motion. He or she holds the end position 5 to 10 s and repeats each motion several times. The advantage of these exercises is that the patient can perform them independently several times throughout the day.

Wand Flexion

This wand exercise increases flexion motion. The patient can perform this exercise in sitting, standing, or supine; but because strength may be a factor in the sitting and standing positions, supine is the recommended position. The patient grasps the wand in each hand, with the hands shoulder-width apart. He or she moves the arms overhead, keeping the elbows straight throughout the exercise (figure 17.50). Substitutions include arching the back, bending the elbows, and hyperextending the wrists.

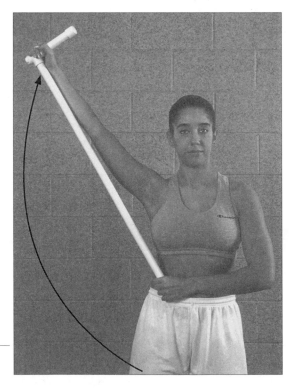

Figure 17.51
Wand abduction.

Wand Abduction

This exercise increases shoulder abduction. The patient can stand or lie supine. He or she grasps the end of the wand with the involved hand and places the uninvolved hand toward the other end of the wand. The uninvolved arm pushes the involved arm upward into abduction (figure 17.51). Substitutions include leaning sideways, moving the shoulder into the flexion plane, and bending the elbow.

Wand Lateral rotation

This exercise increases lateral rotation. The patient lies supine with the involved hand on one end of the wand and the uninvolved hand toward the other end. The involved elbow is kept next to the side at 90° flexion throughout the exercise. With the wand, the patient pushes the involved hand away from the body to laterally rotate the shoulder (figure 17.52a). Common substitutions here include extending the elbow as the wand is pushed laterally, and abducting the involved shoulder.

A more advanced lateral rotation exercise can be performed with the hands shoulder-width apart on the wand. The patient raises the wand overhead and then bends the elbows to attempt to place the wand behind the neck (figure 17.52b). Neck flexion, trunk flexion or rotation, elbow extension, and wrist hyperextension are common substitutions with this exercise.

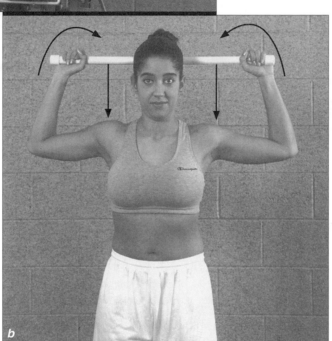

Figure 17.52 Wand lateral rotation: *(a)* supine, *(b)* advanced.

Medial rotation

This exercise increases shoulder medial rotation. The patient stands with the wand behind the waist; hands are placed shoulder-width apart. The bar is raised along the back as high as possible (figure 17.53a). Common substitutions include excessive wrist flexion and trunk lean.

An alternative stretch is with the wand placed vertically behind the back. The involved hand is at the waist, and the uninvolved hand is at the top of the wand. The wand is pulled upward with the top hand (figure 17.53b). Trunk flexion is a common substitution with this alternative stretch.

Figure 17.53 Wand medial rotation: *(a)* initial position, *(b)* alternative position.

Horizontal Flexion-Extension

This exercise increases horizontal movements. The patient lies supine with the hands overhead, shoulder-width apart on the wand, and the elbows straight. The uninvolved arm pushes the involved arm away from the body as far as possible, and then pulls the arm across the body as far as possible (figure 17.54). Throughout the exercise the hands remain at shoulder level and the elbows remain straight. Common substitutions include elbow flexion, trunk rotation, moving the arms into extension, and shoulder rotation.

Figure 17.54 Wand horizontal flexion-extension.

Figure 17.55 Pulley: shoulder flexion.

Pulley Exercises

These exercises can be performed with a pulley, rope, or stretch strap. They are easy to incorporate into a home exercise program that the patient can perform independently. The patient must be careful to avoid driving the humeral head into the glenoid socket, especially when using the pulleys for frozen-shoulder exercises. The patient should be instructed to maintain the scapula in a depressed position throughout the motion.

Shoulder Flexion

For this exercise, an overhead rope and pulley or a stretch strap and hook are attached in a doorway or on a wall. The patient sits with his or her back to the door or wall. The hands are positioned with the thumbs facing upward. The uninvolved arm pulls the rope or strap down to elevate the involved arm into flexion as high as possible. The involved arm is lowered and the motion is repeated several times.

One alternative stretch uses a stretch strap placed over the top of a door. The patient reaches up as high as possible on the strap, and then bends the knees to lower the body and apply the stretch force to the shoulder. Another alternative position is with the patient supine and the pulley attached to the wall or doorjamb (figure 17.55).

Shoulder Abduction

This exercise is similar to the shoulder flexion exercise except that the arm is raised in abduction from the side of the body.

STRENGTHENING EXERCISES

▶ Exercises for strengthening the shoulder begin with isometric activities and straight-plane isotonic exercises, then progress to multiplane and diagonal exercises.

These exercises incorporate a broad spectrum of degrees of difficulty and of stresses applied to the shoulder. They are presented here from easiest to more advanced exercises, beginning with early-phase isometric exercises and progressing to later-phase plyometric exercises. As the exercises become more difficult, they advance from straight-plane to diagonal exercises. We will consider the diagonal exercises, which combine movement planes to stress muscles for all the shoulder joints, in terms of their function and goals within a therapeutic exercise program. The rehabilitation clinician should note and correct substitution patterns to achieve optimal strengthening of intended muscles and facilitate appropriate muscle firing patterns.

Isometrics

Isometrics begin early in a rehabilitation program when the patient is limited in shoulder mobility and strength. They are used to minimize atrophy during times when use or motion of the shoulder is limited. They are performed in a pain-free position and may be performed at multiple angles of a motion, if motion is permitted. If motion is limited, the exercises are performed in nonaggravating, acceptable positions. Each isometric contraction is gradually increased to a maximum contraction, held at the maximum, and then decreased gradually until the muscle is relaxed. The patient must be instructed to avoid sudden maximal contractions to avoid injury or undue strain of the muscle. The patient should maximally contract only if no pain is produced. If pain occurs, effort should be limited to a submaximal contraction until the greater force is nonirritating. Each isometric is held for 5 to 10 s and repeated 10 times. These exercises are performed frequently throughout the day.

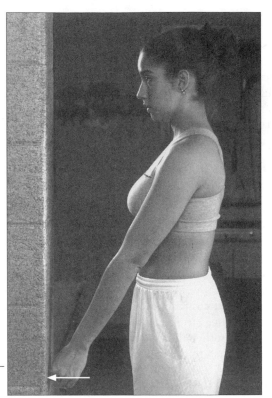

Figure 17.56
Isometric flexion.

Shoulder Flexion

This exercise strengthens the shoulder flexors. The patient stands facing a doorway or wall, with the involved arm slightly forward and the radial hand on the door frame or wall. The patient attempts to move the arm forward while pushing the hand against the door frame (figure 17.56).

Shoulder Abduction

This exercise strengthens the shoulder abductors. The patient stands with the involved side facing a wall or doorway. The arm is positioned in slight abduction with the dorsum of the hand against the wall. The patient keeps the elbow extended and pushes the arm against the wall, attempting to move the arm into abduction.

Figure 17.57
Isometric extension.

Shoulder Extension

This exercise strengthens the shoulder extensors. The patient stands with the back to the wall and positions the arm slightly behind the body, with the ulnar hand against the wall. The patient pushes the hand backward to the wall, keeping the elbow extended (figure 17.57).

Shoulder Medial rotation

This exercise strengthens the internal rotators. The patient stands facing a doorway with the elbow flexed to 90° and the anterior distal forearm placed against the surface of the door frame. With the elbow at his or her side, the patient attempts to roll the forearm inward toward the abdomen.

Figure 17.58 Isometric shoulder external rotation.

Shoulder Lateral rotation

This exercise strengthens the shoulder external rotators. The patient stands facing a doorway with the elbow flexed to 90° and the posterior distal surface of the forearm against the door frame. The elbow is kept in to the side as the patient attempts to roll the forearm outward (figure 17.58).

Isolated-Plane Isotonic Exercises

As mentioned previously, initial strengthening exercises should include primarily straight-plane activities. Once strength is sufficient to control the joint during motion, multiplane and diagonal exercises can begin. Here we look first at straight-plane exercises and then move to multiplane exercises. Keep in mind that although this section includes many of the commonly used exercises, the listing here is far from exhaustive.

Although shoulder motion includes muscle function of scapulothoracic and glenohumeral muscles, patients can and should perform isolated exercises of the muscles for each joint until the muscles have sufficient strength to control the joints during functional motions. To make it easier to identify specific exercise functions, the straight-plane exercises for the scapulothoracic and glenohumeral muscle groups are presented separately. Most are considered relative to the specific motion and muscles they address and are presented from easiest to more difficult.

Scapulothoracic Exercises

If the patient has pain with the shoulder in elevated positions, it is best to provide manual resistance with the shoulder in the lower planes of motion. An advantage of manual resistance is that it can be performed with the patient in any position. As the patient's strength increases, resistance can be offered in planes of motion that are more elevated.

Manual Resistance to Scapula

Patients can do this exercise early in the rehabilitation program for glenohumeral injuries, because it does not stress the glenohumeral joint and assists in minimizing atrophy of scapular rotators. The patient is sidelying with his or her hand on the table to isolate the scapular muscles (figure 17.59a). If glenohumeral joint adduction is uncomfortable, the hand need not be placed on the table, and the clinician can support the arm between his or her side and arm (figure 17.59b). The rehabilitation clinician faces the patient and places his or her hands on the medial scapular border to resist the combined movements of retraction and depression of the scapula; he or she places the other hand on the anterior shoulder to resist protraction and elevation of the scapula in the opposite direction. Manual resistance can also be offered to isolated scapular movements if there is weakness in specific muscles.

Figure 17.59 Manual resistance to scapula: *(a)* with hand on table, *(b)* with arm supported in non-weight-bearing position.

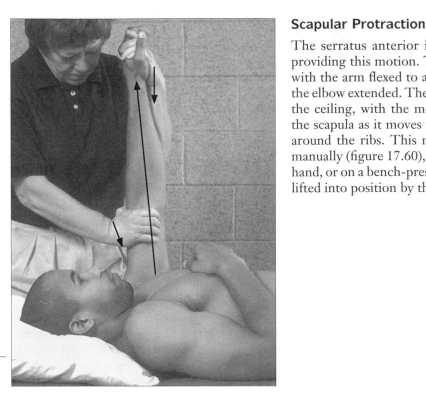

Figure 17.60 Serratus anterior.

Scapular Protraction

The serratus anterior is the primary muscle providing this motion. The patient lies supine with the arm flexed to about 110° to 120° and the elbow extended. The hand is pushed toward the ceiling, with the movement coming from the scapula as it moves forward and anteriorly around the ribs. This motion can be resisted manually (figure 17.60), with a dumbbell in the hand, or on a bench-press machine with the bar lifted into position by the clinician.

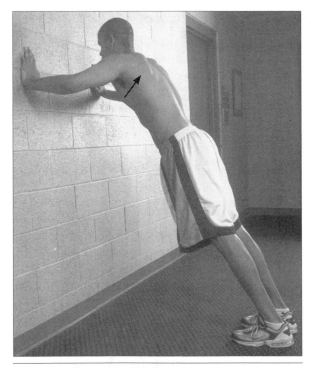

Figure 17.61 Push-up plus.

The serratus anterior can also be strengthened using a push-up plus. The patient performs a push-up with the emphasis on the additional push at the end to facilitate the serratus anterior; once the elbows are extended, the patient attempts to push the body away from the hands an additional distance, moving the scapulae forward around the rib cage. The lowest-level resistance for this exercise is with a wall push-up (figure 17.61); progression is to an incline push-up, then to a modified position on hands and knees, then to a regular push-up position, and finally to a decline push-up position with the feet higher than the hands. With the feet higher than the hands, the serratus anterior and the upper trapezius are particularly facilitated (Lear and Gross 1998). Patients with anterior instability or who have had recent shoulder surgery should avoid lowering the body so that the shoulders move in front of the plane of the elbows during push-ups so undue stress on the anterior shoulder is prevented.

The serratus anterior can also be strengthened using rubber tubing or pulleys. The tubing or pulleys are anchored just below shoulder level, and the patient stands or sits with his or her back to the anchor. With the elbow flexed, the patient pushes the band forward and slightly upward, reaching as far as possible with the elbow extended and the scapula punched forward (figure 17.62). A substitution to avoid in this exercise is using the trunk to rotate the arm forward rather than using the serratus anterior to punch the scapula forward.

An alternative exercise using rubber tubing can be performed with the patient supine and the tubing under the shoulders and back area. The patient grasps the ends of the tubing and starts with the elbows extended and the shoulders flexed to 90° so that the hands are toward the ceiling and the tubing is taut. The patient punches the hands toward the ceiling, protracting the scapulae.

Figure 17.62
Serratus anterior with rubber tubing: *(a)* start position, *(b)* end position.

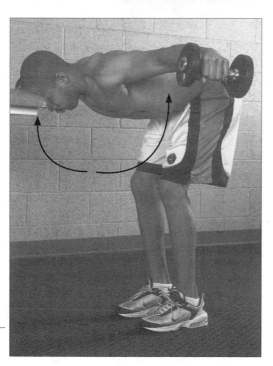

Figure 17.63
Reverse flys.

Scapular Retraction

Scapular retraction is produced by the rhomboids and middle trapezius. An early-phase exercise for strengthening these muscles is a scapular squeeze. The patient keeps his or her elbows at the sides and squeezes the shoulder blades together, holding for 5 to 10 s. This exercise can be performed frequently throughout the day.

The prone fly and rows strengthen these muscles. The prone fly, also called the reverse fly, can be performed with the patient prone and the arm hanging over the table. An alternative position is shown in figure 17.63, with the patient flexed at the hips and the head supported on the table so that the back is straight. The patient lifts a weight in horizontal extension as the scapulae are squeezed together. The elbows remain extended but not locked throughout the movement. Although the patient need perform the exercise with only the involved extremity, a greater facilitation of the muscles occurs if both arms perform the exercise simultaneously. A substitution seen in this exercise is shoulder horizontal extension without scapular retraction.

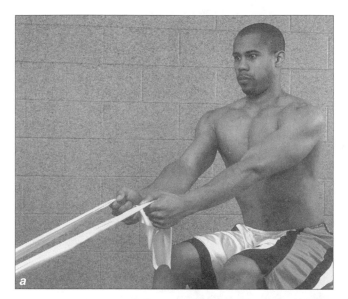

A row exercise can be performed in prone or sitting. In prone, the patient stands flexed at the waist or lies prone with the arm over the edge of the table. The patient lifts the weight toward the ceiling as high as possible; the elbow bends as the weight moves close to the anterior shoulder.

If performing the row in sitting, the patient faces rubber tubing or pulleys that are anchored to a door at or below shoulder level. The patient leans forward from the hip, keeping the back straight, with the scapulae in a protracted position and then moves to an erect position and simultaneously pulls to retract the scapulae, squeezing them together and keeping the elbows at the sides (figure 17.64). A substitution in this exercise is moving the pulley or tubing primarily with the trunk, hips, or shoulder extensors and not retracting the scapulae.

Figure 17.64
Row, seated: *(a)* start position, *(b)* end position.

Scapular Depression

This motion is performed by the lower trapezius and pectoralis minor. The patient performs the seated push-up or press-up while seated in a chair with the hands on the chair seat. The patient pushes down to lift the hips off the chair (figure 17.65a). These muscles can also be strengthened with the use of a pulley or rubber tubing. The pulley or tubing is positioned high overhead, and the patient grasps the handle with the elbow straight and the shoulder in flexion (figure 17.65b). Keeping the shoulder and elbow joints in their start positions throughout the exercise, the patient depresses the scapula downward toward the buttocks. A latissimus pull-down bar using both hands, the involved arm positioned at the end of the bar and the uninvolved arm positioned closer to the middle of the bar, can also be used for this exercise. Substitutions most common in this exercise are shoulder extension and elbow flexion. The patient should not alter positions of the shoulder and elbow throughout the exercise.

An alternative for this exercise can be performed with the resistance device anchored to the shoulder; in this position the shoulder is not placed in an elevated position (figure 17.65c). This exercise isolates the depressors and does not put stress on the glenohumeral joint.

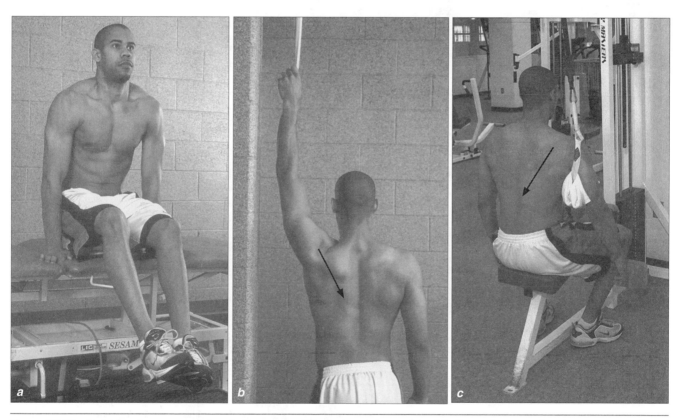

Figure 17.65 Scapular depressors: *(a)* seated press-up, *(b)* overhead depression, *(c)* alternative scapular depressor exercise position.

Bouhler Exercises

These three exercises strengthen the lower trapezius as it functions in upward rotation of the scapula. The patient stands with the back and heels near a wall. With the abdominals tightened to prevent the back from arching, the patient raises the arms overhead with the elbows straight and close to the ears. In the first exercise, the thumbs face the wall and are pushed to the wall (figure 17.66a). In the second exercise, the arms are in the same position as in the first exercise, but the thumbs face each other as the arms are moved to the wall (figure 17.66b). In the last exercise, the arms are positioned at a 45° angle from the body and are moved to the wall as the shoulder blades are squeezed together (figure 17.66c). In each exercise the patient holds the position for 5 to 10 s and repeats the exercise several times.

To perform these exercises at a more advanced level, the patient is prone, either on a table or on a Swiss ball. Weights can be added to the hands for additional resistance (figure 17.66d). Substitutions for this exercise in any position or difficulty level include arching the back, bending the elbows, abducting the arms, and standing away from the wall.

Figure 17.66 Bouhler exercises: *(a)* thumbs to the wall, *(b)* thumbs facing each other, *(c)* arms at 45° angle, *(d)* progression in an antigravity position with weights.

Scapular Elevation

This motion is performed by the upper trapezius and levator scapulae. These muscles are normally not weak and often overpower their synergists and their antagonists, resulting in a muscle imbalance. They are often used incorrectly during shoulder elevation as substitution for weak rotator cuff muscles, contributing to faulty mechanics, muscle imbalance, and prolonged injury recovery. In patients who have weakness of these muscles, initial strengthening can include shoulder shrugs and manual resistance to shrugs. A more advanced exercise uses weight during shrugs.

Once the patient is able to elevate the shoulder without pain, he or she can perform additional exercises such as an upright row; however, to reduce the risk of rotator cuff impingement, the patient should not elevate the elbows higher than the shoulders. An advanced exercise that can be used in the later stages of strengthening is the upright press with dumbbells or machines, also known as the overhead press or military press. Impingement can be a problem with this exercise, so the clinician must use caution in determining whether to include this exercise.

Scapular Rotation

Upward rotation is performed by the serratus anterior and trapezius muscles. Downward rotation is performed by the levator scapulae, rhomboids, and pectoralis minor. Full-range-of-motion exercise for scapular rotation also includes glenohumeral motion, so it is important for the rehabilitation clinician to be sure that glenohumeral joint stability is adequate before including these full-motion scapular activities in the rehabilitation program.

An upward scapular rotation exercise uses full shoulder elevation in either flexion or abduction. These exercises are performed with the elbow straight and the thumb facing upward to reduce rotator cuff impingement. The arm is elevated until the hand is overhead (figure 17.67).

Downward scapular rotation occurs during shoulder extension and adduction. In a prone position with the arm over the edge of the table, the patient lifts the hand toward the hip, leading with the ulnar aspect and maintaining elbow extension throughout the motion (figure 17.68).

Latissimus pull-downs are an advanced exercise for downward rotation. The hands are shoulder-width apart on the lat bar, and the elbows are kept straight throughout the exercise. Keeping the scapulae set, the patient brings the arms down to the front of the thighs.

In performing each of these exercises, the patient must maintain scapular control and correct glenohumeral positioning. The most frequent substitution in these exercises is shrugging the scapula and initiating the movement with the upper trapezius rather than allowing all scapular rotators to work correctly.

Figure 17.67   Scapular upward rotation.

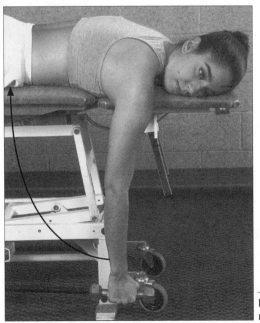

Figure 17.68   Scapular downward rotation.

Glenohumeral Exercises

Glenohumeral exercises performed in the lower levels of shoulder elevation emphasize the glenohumeral muscles. Once the shoulder is elevated, scapular muscles are also stressed with the exercise to maintain the shoulder position. Early strengthening of the shoulder may necessarily start in the lower levels of elevation until sufficient scapular muscle strength is present for stabilizing the shoulder in its correct position. Shoulder exercises should be divided into three levels: below 60°, 60° to 100°, and above 100°. Because scapular stabilization is a prerequisite to good shoulder motion, scapular muscle strength, first in the low and then in the middle ranges of shoulder motion, should be achieved before advancing to higher ranges of motion. As shoulder elevation increases, scapular muscles must work harder to simultaneously provide both scapular stabilization and scapular motion.

Lateral rotation

This motion is performed by the infraspinatus, teres minor, and posterior deltoid. The exercises should be performed in the scapular plane. In sidelying on the uninvolved side with a towel roll placed under the arm, the patient positions the elbow at 90° and lifts the weight upward toward the ceiling (figure 17.69a). Movement includes rolling of the forearm without moving the arm off the towel roll. Substitutions to watch and correct include shoulder extension, shoulder abduction, elbow extension, wrist extension, and rolling the trunk backward. Stabilization is important if the patient is to achieve the desired gains from the exercise. This exercise can also be performed in prone with the shoulder at 90° abduction (figure 17.69b), or in standing with rubber tubing or pulleys with the elbow at the side (figure 17.69c). Once scapular stability is achieved, this exercise can be performed with the arm abducted to 90°. Initially, it may be necessary to support the elbow (figure 17.69d); but as strength improves, elbow support becomes unnecessary (figure 17.69e). In the elevated position, the elbow remains elevated, and the shoulder is maintained at 90° abduction without horizontal adduction or abduction.

Figure 17.69 Lateral rotation: *(a)* sidelying, *(b)* prone, *(c)* standing, *(d)* in 90° of abduction with support, *(e)* without support.

Medial rotation

The subscapularis is the primary muscle responsible for medial rotation. It receives assistance from other muscles including the teres major, latissimus dorsi, anterior deltoid, and pectoralis major.

The patient can be sidelying on the involved side or supine. The elbow is flexed to 90°. If the patient is supine, the arm is abducted slightly. If the patient is sidelying, the elbow is next to the side. The elbow position is maintained throughout the exercise as the hand is moved toward the abdomen (figure 17.70).

This exercise can also be performed in standing using rubber tubing or pulleys and following the progression discussed for lateral rotation. A towel roll is placed between the trunk and arm, with the forearm kept parallel to the floor

Figure 17.70　Medial rotation.

similar to the position shown in figure 17.69c. From a starting position away from the body, the patient moves the forearm toward the abdomen. Common substitution patterns are rotation of the trunk, horizontal flexion of the shoulder, forward motion of the elbow, and elbow motion.

Once the scapular muscles are able to stabilize the scapula, the exercise is performed with the arm abducted to 90°. Initially, the elbow can be supported, but progression should be toward the more aggressive position for the exercise without elbow support.

Abduction

This motion is produced by force-couple activity of the deltoid with the supraspinatus. The other rotator cuff muscles also play an important role during shoulder abduction and flexion as they co-contract during abduction to depress the humeral head into the glenoid. Thus, the rotator cuff and deltoid collectively stabilize the glenohumeral joint during elevation activities. It is important that the scapular stabilizers also work to position the scapula during abduction. In the early strengthening stages it may be necessary to remind the patient to fix or 'set' the scapula before moving the humerus so that proper sequencing of shoulder motion occurs.

Abduction can be performed in the coronal plane, but the recommendation is to perform this exercise in the scapular plane, approximately 30° forward of the frontal plane. This position maximally facilitates the rotator cuff muscles. This position of the humerus in the plane of the scapula is called **scaption**, a term originally created and defined by Jacqueline Perry, M.D.

Abduction can be performed in sidelying with the elbow extended and the arm resting along the length of the trunk and thigh. The scapula is set and the arm is lifted into scaption.

The best position to strengthen the supraspinatus is prone with the shoulder elevated to 100° in the scapular plane and laterally rotated so the thumb faces the ceiling (Blackburn et al. 1990; Worrell et al. 1992). The elbow is maintained in an extended position as the arm is lifted in horizontal abduction to the ceiling.

Two alternative positions are both performed in sitting if a patient finds it too uncomfortable to lie prone. The patient sets the scapula and raises the arm with the elbow straight in a scapular plane. In one exercise, the thumb is pointed toward the floor so that the arm is in medial rotation (figure 17.71a). Although this position facilitates the greatest response from the supraspinatus, it may also aggravate the supraspinatus tendon by impinging it. If this occurs, the patient should limit elevation to within a pain-free range of motion. The second position is performed with the thumb pointed toward the ceiling (figure 17.71b). This position facilitates the scapular stabilizers. You should correct substitutions for these exercises, which include trunk lateral flexion, shoulder shrugging, moving the arm more into flexion and out of the scapular plane, and flexing the elbow.

Figure 17.71 Shoulder abduction in scapular plane (scaption): *(a)* thumbs down with medial rotation, *(b)* thumbs up with lateral rotation.

Horizontal Abduction (Extension)

Horizontal abduction, or horizontal extension, performed in the prone position with the arm in lateral rotation, demands output from the teres minor and infraspinatus muscles. This exercise also strengthens the posterior deltoid and scapular stabilizers. The patient lies prone with the arm over the edge of the table. The arm is elevated into horizontal extension (abduction) with the arm in lateral rotation. Common substitutions are rolling the trunk rather than lifting the arm, moving out of the plane of motion and placing the hand closer to the hip, and bending the elbow.

Key Shoulder Exercises

For several years many clinicians advocated specific exercises to strengthen the shoulder, but few offered concrete evidence that their exercises were beneficial. Although the results are arguably inconclusive, the findings presented by Bradley and Tibone (1991) shed some light on what many consider significant exercises that should be part of a general shoulder rehabilitation program (table 17.1). The authors defined a significant exercise as one that produced substantial effort in more than one muscle investigated. In their research, the four scapular rotator exercises that met this criterion were scaption with thumbs up, rowing, push-up plus, and the seated press-up. The glenohumeral exercises that met this criterion were scaption with medial rotation, horizontal abduction with lateral rotation, and the seated press-up. Other exercises beneficial to at least one muscle included medial rotation, lateral rotation, coronal plane abduction, fly (horizontal adduction), a regular push-up without the plus, a push-up with the hands apart, bench press, military press, and shoulder extension in prone.

Based on the information from Blackburn et al. (1990) and Worrell et al. (1992), there are two additional rotator cuff exercises that should be included, both performed in prone: the ones mentioned above for the supraspinatus and the infraspinatus and teres minor.

Table 17.1 Shoulder Rehabilitation Exercises

Exercises	Muscles significantly activated
Scaption with thumbs up	Scapular stabilizers
Rowing	Rhomboids, trapezius
Push-up plus	Serratus anterior, pectoralis minor
Seated press-up	Scapular rotators, pectoralis major, lattisimus dorsi
Scaption with thumbs down	Subscapularis, anterior deltoid, posterior deltoid, supraspinatus
Horizontal abduction in external rotation	Infraspinatus, teres minor, posterior deltoid

Based on Bradley and Tibone 1991.

STABILIZATION EXERCISES

▶ Several kinds of stabilization exercises help to restore the scapular stability crucial to shoulder motion. Advanced open chain exercises for shoulder stability include isokinetic exercises and open chain elastic-band exercises.

The importance of stability during shoulder motion cannot be overstated. As previously discussed, trunk or core stabilization must provide a firm base from which the scapula can operate. Scapular stabilization must provide a firm foundation for shoulder movement. Rotator cuff stabilization allows the humerus smooth, synchronous glenohumeral motion for functional upper-extremity activity.

Trunk stabilization exercises are discussed in chapter 16. A few will be mentioned later in this chapter, but only as they relate to shoulder exercises. Refer to chapter 16 for specific trunk stabilization exercises.

Shoulder stabilization exercises are important in that they aid strength development and also facilitate neuromuscular reeducation of the shoulder. They stimulate the afferent receptors to provide appropriate feedback into the central nervous system, to reeducate and reactivate the proprioceptive pathways that will eventually lead to proper functional performance.

Although some of these exercises are open kinetic chain activities, many are closed kinetic chain activities. One can argue that because most people involved in physical activity do not perform closed kinetic chain activities, use of closed kinetic chain exercises for the upper extremities is not germane in a rehabilitation program. Closed kinetic chain exercises are useful for the upper extremity for a couple of reasons. In a close-chain position, the shoulder has more stability through increased joint congruity; less stress is applied to the ligaments, and joint proprioceptors are stimulated. Closed kinetic chain exercise also facilitates cocontraction of muscles around the shoulder. This cocontraction during closed kinetic chain exercises permits stabilization activities to be initiated with less shear force applied to the static structures and also facilitates dynamic stabilization of the joints (Lephart and Henry 1996).

It is not necessary that every exercise mimic functional motions. In fact, in the early and middle stages of rehabilitation, it is important to improve muscle strength before functional movements can be safely executed. Neither straight-plane exercises nor pure closed kinetic chain exercises are necessarily functional; they do not mimic most of the shoulder's functional movements. They are crucial in a therapeutic exercise program, though, in that they facilitate, develop, and improve specific muscle activity that permits progression to functional shoulder movement.

Scapular Stabilization

Because scapular stability is vital to functional shoulder motions, scapular stabilization exercises should begin early in the rehabilitation program. Scapular stabilization exercises should be included in any shoulder rehabilitation program. A variety of scapular stabilization exercises are outlined here. The progression begins with isometric stabilization exercises and advances to stabilization during arm movement, first in simple planes and then in diagonal planes. The progression also begins with movements in the lower shoulder positions (30°-60° elevation) where the scapula has relatively little motion and its muscles work to primarily stabilize the scapular for glenohumeral motion and advances to middle-range positions of shoulder elevation (60°-100°) where the scapular muscles must work to stabilize and move the scapula simultaneously. Exercises in shoulder positions over 100° are initiated only after strength and control in the lower ranges are achieved; it is the higher ranges of motion that the scapular muscles are most stressed as they must continue to provide glenohumeral stability and also work to move the scapula in its final degrees of motion when the muscles are at their shortest and weakest positions. In the final phases of stabilization, movements include a combination of high (over 100° elevation) and low joint positions, use increased resistance, and are performed with greater speeds. These activities then become more functionally based.

Swiss-Ball Stabilization

Various exercises using Swiss balls can facilitate scapular stabilization. In a basic exercise that can begin early in the rehabilitation program, the ball is placed on a table or on the floor, and the patient bears weight through the shoulder as he or she moves the ball from side to side, forward and back, and in circles. The patient can also lie prone on the Swiss ball with the feet off the floor and the body anchored with the hands on the floor, shoulder-width apart. The patient then moves the body forward and back and from side to side on the ball while maintaining weight bearing through the arms (figure 17.72a).

If the patient does not have 90° of shoulder motion so the Swiss ball activity is not possible, the patient can begin in lower degrees by placing the ball on a table, floor, or wall. The patient bears weight on the arm and rolls the ball in varying patterns.

A more advanced weight-bearing exercise with the Swiss ball has the patient's lower body on a table and the hands placed on the ball while the upper body is over the edge of the table. The patient moves the ball out and away from the body as far as possible, then moves the ball closer (figure 17.72b).

Figure 17.72 Swiss ball weight-bearing exercises: *(a)* prone on a ball, *(b)* prone on a table.

Rhythmic Stabilization

These exercises assist in reeducating the proprioceptors and improve kinesthetic awareness. In the first exercise, the patient lies supine and places the arm in a scapular plane at approximately 100° elevation (figure 17.73a). The patient can hold a weight in this position, maintaining the angle with eyes closed, or the clinician can offer manual resistance in different directions while the patient provides an isometric resistance to the movements. You can repeat the exercise in different positions, each time requiring the patient to position and maintain the arm at the desired angle with the eyes closed.

Another rhythmic stabilization exercise can be performed with the patient in standing and bearing weight on the arms on a tabletop. The rehabilitation clinician offers resistance to the patient as the patient shifts weight from one arm to the other (figure 17.73b).

Additional weight-bearing exercises are performed with the patient in a quadruped position. The shoulders should be directly over the hands, and the hips should be forward of the knees so that the weight is primarily borne on the upper extremities. If the patient is unable to hold this position, the hips may be positioned directly over the knees to equalize weight distribution between the upper and lower extremities. The simplest exercise is to have the patient shift weight from the left to the right arm. You can offer manual resistance as the patient attempts to stabilize in the quadruped

(continued)

Figure 17.73 Rhythmic stabilization: *(a)* open kinetic chain, *(b)* weight bearing in standing, *(c)* quadruped weight bearing, *(d)* tripod weight bearing.

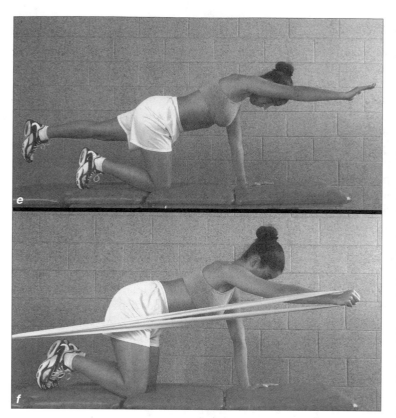

position as you attempt to move the patient off balance (figure 17.73c). Once the patient can do this without difficulty, he or she balances in a tripod position with the uninvolved arm off the table (figure 17.73d). From this exercise the patient can advance to a biped position with the involved arm and the opposite leg bearing the weight (figure 17.73e). Once again, the patient's hips should be ahead of the knees, and the shoulder should be directly over the hand so that the upper extremity is the primary weight-bearing extremity. In any of these positions, you can offer manual resistance as the patient attempts to maintain balance. For additional challenge, you can provide resistance to the uninvolved arm using a pulley or rubber tubing while the involved arm maintains balance (figure 17.73f) or you can apply proprioceptive neuromuscular facilitation (PNF) manual resistance to the uninvolved arm (figure 17.73g).

A more difficult exercise for rhythmic stabilization is with the patient in a unilateral weight-bearing position sideways on the involved arm, lower extremities extended at the knees as seen in figure 17.73h. The rehabilitation clinician provides manual resistance as the patient attempts to maintain balance.

Figure 17.73 *(continued)* Rhythmic stabilization: *(e)* bipod weight bearing, *(f)* with rubber-tubing resistance to involved extremity, *(g)* with PNF manual resistance to uninvolved extremity, *(h)* unilateral weight bearing.

Distal Movement Stabilization

These activities involve movement of the distal extremity, requiring movement control and strength as well as stabilization of the shoulder. You must be careful to have the patient maintain correct scapular position throughout each of these exercises. Verbal cueing may be necessary as a reminder to maintain proper scapular positioning. In one activity the patient lies prone with a roller stool under the hips or pelvis; feet are off the floor and hands are on the floor. The patient then moves across the floor, using only the arms to move the roller stool (figure 17.74a). Another distal movement activity is performed with a weighted ball in the hand. The patient stands or sits with the arm outstretched at from 60° to 110° elevation in the scapular plane. In this position the patient spells out the alphabet with the ball (figure 17.74b). Heavier balls provide additional resistance.

The Body Blade (Hymanson, Inc., Los Angeles, CA), B.O.I.N.G. (exclusively distributed by OPTP, Minneapolis, MN), and other commercially available rhythmic-wand equipment are useful in rhythmic stabilization exercises. They can be used in different positions, beginning in the scapular plane at 30° elevation (figure 17.74c) and advancing to overhead positions as strength improves.

Upper-body ergometers are another means of offering distal movement and proximal stabilization. These machines also provide cardiovascular exercise.

Figure 17.74 Distal movement stabilization exercises: *(a)* walk while prone on roller stool, *(b)* alphabet with distal weight, *(c)* rhythmic wand.

Proprioceptive Neuromuscular Facilitation

Proprioceptive neuromuscular facilitation (PNF) is useful in shoulder rehabilitation. There are a number of advantages to using PNF. There is no cost because this form of exercise uses the clinician's manual resistance; PNF is appropriate throughout most of the program. In the early rehabilitation stages, PNF can enhance neuromuscular control, and at later stages it can improve strength and coordination of muscle firing. Techniques include isometrics, concentrics, eccentrics, and rhythmic stabilization. Proprioceptive neuromuscular facilitation incorporates functional positions because it uses multiplane motions.

In the early rehabilitation stages, PNF is commonly used for rhythmic stabilization (figure 17.75). This assists in reeducating synchronous muscle firing and providing joint stability. Moving through functional patterns can stimulate neuromuscular control for stability and synchronous patterns of movement. The rehabilitation clinician provides isometric resistance at points in the range of motion that are weak.

In later rehabilitation stages, PNF can increase coordination through use of eccentric resistance in functional planes and through use of combinations of eccentric with concentric and isometric resistance as the arm moves through its motion patterns. In this activity the patient attempts to move the arm through either a D1 or D2 flexion-extension pattern at a constant rate of speed as the rehabilitation clinician provides various types of resistance—eccentric, concentric, and isometric.

Figure 17.75 Proprioceptive neuromuscular facilitation: rhythmic stabilization.

Advanced Open Chain Exercises

These exercises can incorporate various types of equipment. They are performed unsupported, first in straight-plane and then in diagonal positions. The unsupported position is the primary distinction between these and earlier exercises.

Isokinetic Exercises

Many rehabilitation facilities have isokinetic machines. These machines can be useful for monitoring and advancing shoulder strength. Unless the unit is used for range of motion or isometrics, isokinetic machines are generally not introduced into a rehabilitation program until the later stages after healing is to a level where injured structures will tolerate the stresses that these machines produce. Early exercises are performed in straight-plane motions, isolating specific muscles to perform the desired activity. As the patient's strength improves, diagonal patterns are used and the patient performs a more normal movement pattern using a summation of trunk and hip forces to produce normal shoulder motion (figure 17.76).

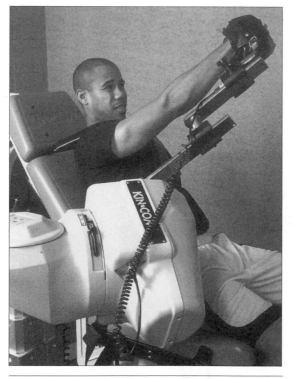

Figure 17.76 Isokinetic exercises for the shoulder.

Open Chain Elastic-Band Exercises

Once the patient achieves appropriate strength levels for shoulder stabilization during arm movement, elastic-band or rubber-tubing activities in an open kinetic chain can provide additional resistance and challenge. The challenge is to maintain stability during resisted arm movement. This is the next step once closed kinetic chain stabilization has been achieved. The patient is now required to execute resistive exercises without the feedback of the clinician in PNF and without the feedback of joint compression that closed kinetic chain activities provide. These exercises include a combination of concentric and eccentric resistance. The need for dynamic stabilization during these exercises more closely resembles functional activity demands; and these exercises are designed to prepare the shoulder for the next level of resistive exercises, plyometrics.

For shoulder-related fact sheets and patient information brochures and booklets, see the American Academy of Orthopaedic Surgeons Web site at: http://orthoinfo.aaos.org/category.cfm?topcategory= Shoulder.

Figure 17.77 Straight-plane external elastic-band exercises.

Straight-Plane Exercises

By now the patient should be able to maintain joint stability with the arm in at least 45-60° of elevation. Straight-plane exercises include medial and lateral rotation with the elbow at shoulder level and in the scapular plane. As control is achieved, the arm is elevated to 90° (figure 17.77). You must correct errors in execution. Common errors include dropping the elbow, horizontally extending the arm during lateral rotation and horizontally flexing it during medial rotation, and flexing the elbow during lateral rotation and extending it during medial rotation.

Diagonal-Plane Exercises

These exercises are performed once the patient demonstrates proper stabilization and control in straight-plane exercises. Proprioceptive neuromuscular facilitation movements in D1 and D2 flexion and extension patterns are used (figure 17.78). It is important for the patient to execute the motion correctly and to maintain appropriate joint stability throughout the motion. Joint stability is not maintained if the patient shrugs the shoulder during activity or initiates the activity with a shoulder shrug.

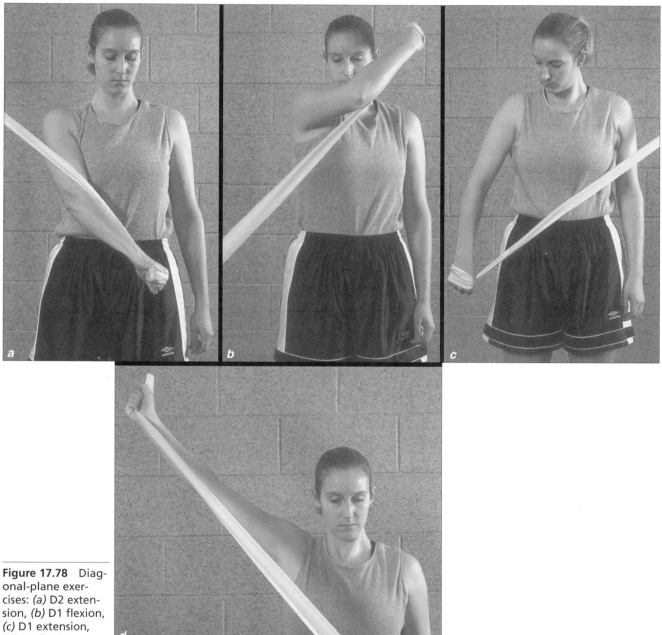

Figure 17.78 Diagonal-plane exercises: *(a)* D2 extension, *(b)* D1 flexion, *(c)* D1 extension, *(d)* D2 flexion.

PLYOMETRIC EXERCISES

▶ Patients who have achieved strength and stability of the shoulder can go on to perform plyometric exercises on unstable surfaces, plyometric push-ups, weight-bearing activities, and medicine-ball exercises.

Once the patient has achieved strength, and static and simple dynamic stabilization control, he or she progresses to plyometric exercises before performing functional activities. Plyometrics are the most demanding in the series outlined because they require maximum strength, optimal joint stabilization during high-level dynamic activities, and agility and coordination throughout the activity.

Unstable Surfaces

Exercises on unstable surfaces provide dynamic stabilization stress to the shoulder. Muscles must provide dynamic shoulder stability while simultaneously maintaining balance on a moving surface. A slide board can be used to stress joint stabilization in flexion-extension and horizontal abduction-adduction movements. In the progression, the patient is first on hands and knees and then on hands and feet. It is important that the weight be forward on the hands with the knees behind the hips. As the progression continues, the patient's feet are raised on a bench or stool, and finally the patient is positioned on a Swiss ball.

A Fitter (Fitter International, Calgary, AB, Canada) or simple device, such as a slide board or balance board, can be used as an unstable surface. The patient begins on hands and knees with the hands on the apparatus and moves the hands from side to side and forward and backward. Circular patterns can be used on the slide board (figure 17.79a). If on a balance board, the board can be maintained in a balance position or moved from side to side while the ends of the board are kept off the floor. Progression for this exercise includes advancing to a hands-and-feet position and finally to placing the legs on a Swiss ball while performing the upper extremity activity (figure 17.79b).

If available, more elaborate devices such as a computerized balance system or other commercially available balance system can be useful in providing an unstable base for dynamic stabilization exercises (figure 17.79c).

Figure 17.79 Unstable surface exercises: *(a)* Slide board while on knees, *(b)* balance board, *(c)* commercially available balance system.

Plyometric Push-Ups

The progression of plyometric push-ups begins with a wall push-up. The patient pushes him- or herself away from the wall with enough force to remove the hands from the wall. When the patient's hands come off the wall, the rehabilitation clinician pushes the patient back toward the wall and the patient stops his or her movement toward the wall by 'catching' him- or herself with both hands on the wall. The impact force is absorbed by bending the elbows as the body returns to the starting position. This exercise progresses to an incline push-up. The patient pushes off the incline support, such as a tabletop or counter, to lose hand contact and is pushed back to the starting position by the, as was done with the wall push-ups.

An additional progression involves having the patient perform a regular or modified push-up, first with the uninvolved hand on a medicine ball and the involved hand on the floor, then with both hands on the ball (figure 17.80, a and b).

Plyometric push-ups can also be performed on a trampoline. With the patient in a regular push-up position and the hands on the trampoline, the individual 'jumps' the hands off the trampoline and lands them out to the side, and then 'jumps' them back to the center on the next push-up movement.

The most difficult plyometric push-up is performed with boxes. Two boxes of the same height are placed on either side of the patient. The recommended starting height is 10 to 15 cm (3-6 in.). The patient begins with the hands on the floor in either a modified or regular push-up position and pushes up and away from the floor to position each hand on the box adjacent to each arm. The patient then drops the hands to the floor and repeats the push-up to the boxes (figure 17.80c).

Figure 17.80 Plyometric push-up variations: *(a)* push-up with hands on small medicine balls, *(b)* push-up with both hands on one large medicine ball, *(c)* box jump.

Resisted Movement in Weight Bearing

These exercises require good strength, control, and endurance. A stair machine, a step machine, or a treadmill can be used. The patient begins with hands on the machine and knees on the floor (figure 17.81). The patient 'walks' the hands as the treadmill's belt or stair machine's steps move. The speed of the machine depends on the patient's abilities. The recommendation is to use a manual setting initially, but a random setting may be appropriate as the patient progresses. Bouts of 30 s to 1 min provide the patient ample challenge, initially. As the patient improves, speed, time, and resistance may be increased. Wearing gloves during the exercise will protect the patient's hands.

Medicine-Ball Exercises

These exercises begin with a lightweight ball—approximately 0.9 kg (2 lb)—and can increase as the patient is able to maintain control and still execute the exercise correctly.

Figure 17.81 Resisted movement in weight bearing: *(a)* on stair machine on knees, *(b)* on treadmill on toes.

Rotation Progression

A beginning exercise is performed with the patient in supine and the shoulder at 90° abduction and laterally rotated with the entire arm supported on the table. The forearm should be supported on the table to prevent excessive lateral rotation during the initial phases of this progression. The medicine ball is dropped from the level of the rehabilitation clinician's shoulder to the patient's hand. Initially, the patient only catches the ball, but the patient should quickly advance to catching and tossing the ball back to the clinician (figure 17.82a). When the individual can perform this exercise without pain and through good motion, the clinician stands away from the patient toward the patient's feet and tosses the ball to the patient. The patient catches the ball and returns the toss, keeping the shoulder at 90° abduction and allowing it to laterally rotate as the ball is caught. The arm should move into medial rotation when the ball is thrown back to the rehabilitation clinician. If this is not difficult, the patient performs the exercise with the forearm unprotected by the table and then with the upper arm off the table as well. When the patient demonstrates good control, ease in allowing lateral rotation in the catch, and smooth medial rotation during the throw, he or she performs the

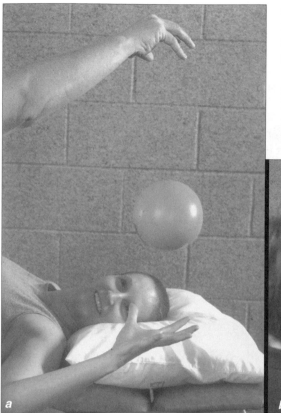

exercise in a standing or kneeling position (figure 17.82b). This exercise increases eccentric and concentric requirements of the medial rotators. The patient must maintain an elevated elbow at 90° of shoulder abduction and elbow flexion at 90°.

This exercise is also performed with the patient's back to the rehabilitation clinician (figure 17.82c). The patient tosses the ball backward as the arm is moved into lateral rotation. This position requires eccentric and concentric activity of the lateral rotators. The arm is maintained at 90° abduction throughout the exercise.

Figure 17.82 Medicine-ball progression: *(a)* drop-and-catch, *(b)* standing forward toss, *(c)* backward toss.

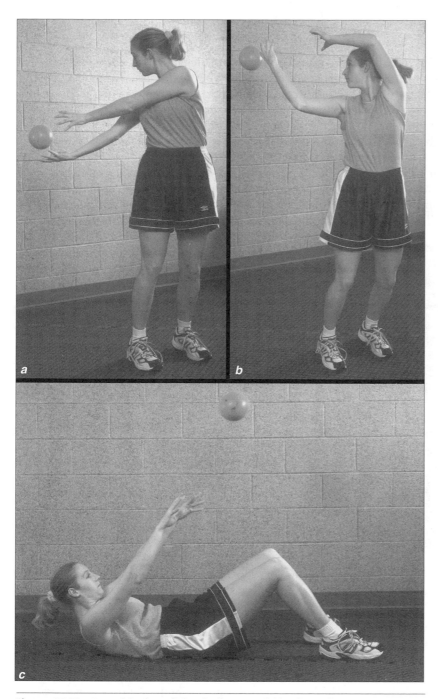

Rotational Tosses

Additional medicine-ball exercises include rotational tosses. The trunk is rotated from one side as the ball is thrown and continues to rotate during a full follow-through position. This exercise is performed to both sides and facing the wall or the clinician as well as with the patient's back to the wall or clinician (figure 17.83a). This activity is important in facilitating a functional motion, and it also assists in trunk strengthening.

In this exercise's progression, the arms are kept at a low level at first to produce less stress on scapular stabilizers and then placed in the more stressful elevated position, at shoulder level as strength and control improve. In the final position, the patient tosses the ball overhead (figure 17.83b). The overhead exercises can be performed in a standing or kneeling position or in the more difficult supine position (figure 17.83c). The supine position adds more resistance to the abdominals.

Figure 17.83 Rotational medicine-ball tosses: *(a)* backward with arms at low level; *(b)* backward overhead toss, standing; *(c)* overhead toss, supine.

FUNCTIONAL ACTIVITIES

▶ Functional exercises for patients with shoulder injuries progress gradually in time, resistance, and/or distance. For overhead activities, the progression is from lower to higher movements.

At this point, the specifics of the program are dictated by the patient's activity demands. If a patient participates in a throwing sport, during the plyometric exercise phase he or she can begin throwing a foam rubber ball or knotted sock toward a mirror, watching for form and motion pattern (figure 17.84). A tennis player can begin forehand and backhand strokes in the same manner in front of a mirror. This helps to promote proprioception and correct technique through the additional afferent feedback that comes from the visual system.

Chapter 10 covers progressive functional programs, outlining specific sequences of exercises as a guide for setting a patient on a course of functional return to full activity participation. The most important point to remember is that the program must present a gradual progression of time, resistance, and/or distance. If one element is increased, another may be decreased to allow the body to adjust to new stresses. For example, if a pitcher increases throwing speed from 50% to 75% of his or her normal speed, a reduction in throwing distance or repetitions may be necessary. An increase in the program is usually added only every third day of activity. This allows the body the time it needs for adjustment to new levels of stress before application of additional levels. For example, if a golfer is now able to perform a full swing with the long irons, it will be three days before he or she advances to using the woods.

In overhead events, the patient progresses through a program of low- and medium-height movements and attempts high movements last. For example, a tennis player begins functional activities with forehand and backhand groundstrokes. It is not until the individual accomplishes full-distance and full-force hits with these strokes that he or she progresses to overhead strokes. Because serves are the most strenuous activity, they are the last stroke the patient attempts. Partial force is used in the initial stages of serve activities, with progression to normal serves.

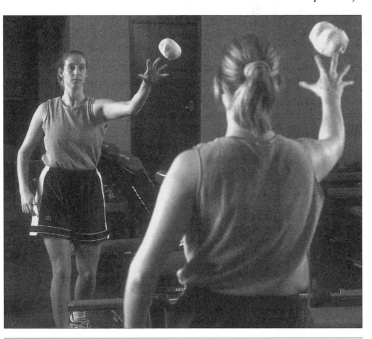

Figure 17.84 Mirror feedback.

SPECIAL REHABILITATION APPLICATIONS

▶ Among the types of shoulder injuries that raise special concerns and call for particular exercise approaches are instability, impingement, traumatic rotator cuff conditions, glenoid labral tears, adhesive capsulitis, acromioclavicular sprains, and biceps tendon injuries.

The combination and progression of exercises used in each rehabilitation program are determined individually according to the patient and the injury. Some injuries dictate special concerns for the rehabilitation clinician. Some of these injuries and the concerns unique to them are addressed here.

Shoulder Instability

The shoulder has two systems of stability, the **static restraints** and the **dynamic restraints**. The static restraints include the ligaments, capsule, and glenoid labrum. The dynamic restraints are the neuromuscular components. If the static restraint is damaged by joint sprains, subluxations, or dislocations, the neural input from the proprioceptors located within the injured static structures is compromised. Damage to static restraints also causes a deficiency in muscle function. Instability is the result. A secondary problem that can result from instability is rotator cuff tendinitis that can lead to rotator cuff tears with repetitive impingement and breakdown. If instability is not corrected either by surgery to reinforce static structures, or by rehabilitation to restore dynamic structures, or both, reinjury is perpetuated with continued activity until the joint becomes so unstable that it may sublux or dislocate or the impinged soft tissues break down and tear with relatively little stress.

Before you design a therapeutic exercise program for a patient with shoulder instability, you must consider several factors. The most common instability is anterior instability, which occurs when anterior structures become damaged. Inferior instability is the result of injury and laxity of the inferior capsule and support structures. Posterior instability, which is less common, occurs with damage to the posterior joint structures.

Two acronyms, AMBRI and TUBS, indicate the difference between nontraumatic and traumatic shoulder instability and present guidelines for treatment. The acronym **AMBRI** stands for 'Atraumatic, Multidirectional, Bilateral, Rehabilitation effective, Inferior capsular shift required.' Patients with this condition usually have bilateral shoulder laxity, as well as hypermobility in most joints. The instability is multi-directional but usually responds well to the conservative treatment of rehabilitation. If surgery is necessary, an inferior capsular shift is usually the procedure of choice. More recently, some surgeons have used an electrothermally assisted capsular shift to relieve multi-directional instability.

Anterior Instability

Shoulders with **TUBS** (**T**raumatic, **U**nilateral, **B**ankart lesion, **S**urgery required) are shoulders that have incurred a traumatic injury. A **Bankart lesion**, or tear of the anterior capsulolabral complex, is present and surgery is required to relieve the problem.

Patients in overhead-throwing sports commonly develop anterior instability because the throwing motion places repetitive stresses on the anterior joint structures. Often accompanying and encouraging this problem is a concomitant posterior capsule and rotator cuff tightness of the medial rotators. In these patients, the rehabilitation program for instability should include stretching of these structures.

The rehabilitation processes for surgically corrected anterior instability and nonrepaired instability are similar. The greatest differences may be their time lines, but the exercise sequence is essentially the same. A nonrepaired shoulder may require longer immobilization time and, thus, a delay in the total rehabilitation process. The arm is immobilized in a sling for approximately three weeks for the surgically repaired shoulder, but the time in a sling can be longer for the nonrepaired shoulder. Older patients are the exception. Generally, patients over 30 are started on early postoperative exercise intervention because a frozen shoulder is a common complication if motion is not initiated soon after any surgical shoulder procedure. The time required for a complete rehabilitation program varies from younger to older patients and from one sport to another. Patients in overhead sports such as baseball or volleyball may require a longer rehabilitation process than those whose shoulder demands are minimal, such as soccer players. An average program may take anywhere from 15 to 26 weeks.

After the first week following surgery or injury, the shoulder is taken out of the sling to permit active–assistive range of motion in straight-plane flexion. Gentle, passive motion to no more than 0° lateral rotation with the elbow at the side can also begin. Abduction to 30° is also permitted. Isometrics in nonstress positions are initiated after the first week. Care must be taken to avoid lateral rotation greater than 20° to 30° and abduction greater than 30° to 40°. The anterior shoulder joint should be minimally stressed during the first three weeks. Manual resistance to scapular stabilizers, avoiding stress to the glenohumeral (GH) joint, should begin early in the program. The most stressful position for the anterior joint is lateral rotation with abduction; this position should be avoided for the first several weeks.

During the first two weeks, grade I and II joint mobilization techniques to the GH joint in a resting position may provide pain relief. Simple, mild distraction with oscillation may be beneficial.

During the time the patient is wearing a sling, he or she may develop trigger points in the upper trapezius and levator scapulae as well as other neck and shoulder muscles. These trigger points should be treated during this time.

By the sixth week, passive shoulder flexion range of motion should be normal, and passive lateral rotation should be approximately 50° to 60° with the elbow at the side. By the 8th to

10th week, full passive range of motion should be present in all motions except lateral rotation, which should be at approximately 75°. Between weeks 10 and 12, full passive motion should be possible in all movements.

After the third week, gentle, active-resistive isotonic exercises for medial rotation, lateral rotation to about 20° to 30° with the elbow near the side, and abduction to 20° can begin in a scapular plane. Scapular exercises should advance as tolerated without the imposition of additional stress on the glenohumeral joint.

Joint mobilizations in the grade III range can begin in the third week. These should begin in the resting position. If a capsular pattern is present, the clinician should identify those portions of the capsule that are restricted and perform joint mobilizations to improve mobility in the appropriate ranges. Stress to the anterior capsule should be mild and start at III-.

By the end of the third or fourth week, the shoulder sling is removed. This can be an apprehensive time for the patient. The lack of support can also be initially fatiguing for the shoulder. The patient should be encouraged to support the arm throughout the day by placing it on top of a table or desk while sitting, and by putting the hand in a pocket when standing to permit some muscle rest. Trigger point treatment during this time may be effective if trigger points are found to be the source of the patient's discomfort.

By the 6th to 10th week, the rotator cuff exercises can go through increased ranges of motion as long as the anterior joint is not stressed. The program should continue with low weights and high repetitions. The elbow is kept near the side, but lateral rotation can progress to approximately 45°. Mild isokinetic exercises with the shoulder stabilized can begin during this time.

Joint mobilization by the 6th week can be any grade. By this time, repaired structures should be of sufficient strength to withstand joint mobilization forces. It is important for the clinician to emphasize attaining full range of motion in all planes by this time. If necessary, the clinician may apply joint mobilization in other loose-pack positions besides the resting position. Home exercises for range of motion gains can also be more aggressive at this time.

When the patient has full lateral rotation, eccentric exercises can begin. These start with the arm in the low position, less than 60°, and progress to the higher positions as tolerated. Once strength and control of the joints during motion are achieved, overhead activities, plyometrics, and finally functional activities can be added to the therapeutic exercise program.

Throughout the program, the clinician must receive feedback from the patient about the shoulder's response to activity. Pain should not be present with any activities. Scapular stability must be present before the patient advances to activities that place the arm above shoulder level. If this precept is not respected, rotator cuff tendinitis may occur and delay the patient's return to sport participation.

Posterior Instability

Traumatic posterior instability most often occurs from a fall on an outstretched, adducted and medially rotated shoulder. Impact forces are directed through the extremity, forcing the humeral head posteriorly. Swimmers, pitchers, and tennis players are more susceptible to posterior instability problems.

In posterior instability, positions to avoid initially are those that put stress on the posterior capsule: flexion with adduction and medial rotation. The rehabilitation process follows a similar routine presented above for anterior instability, but different motions are restricted. Excessive medial rotation and horizontal adduction should be performed carefully after the first three to four weeks, but active assisted lateral rotation and abduction can begin on post-op day 3 to 7, depending on surgeon preference. Isometric exercises for shoulder flexion, extension, abduction, adduction, and lateral rotation can begin after post-op day 7. Weight-bearing activities in a quadruped position should be avoided initially. These can put undue additional stress on the posterior capsule and cause additional damage. Other exercises that should be modified or avoided because of the posterior capsule stress they impose include chest fly, bench press, and push-ups. These activities should be added to the program carefully and not until the later stages of therapeutic exercise. In the early and middle phases, exercises should be performed with the shoulder in some lateral rotation and abduction. Scapular stabilization exercises should be performed in a supine position with glenohumeral lateral rotation and should advance to a sitting position, in which joint stability is more difficult to maintain than it is in supine. Seated, weight-bearing exercises that do not stress the posterior capsule can start earlier than quadruped weight-bearing exercises. Medial rotation exercises are performed from full lateral rotation to neutral in the early phases. Horizontal adduction exercises are avoided early in the program. When added later, they begin with horizontal adduction limitations to approximately 45° forward of the frontal plane. Gradually, full horizontal adduction is instituted in the later stages. Quadruped weight-bearing exercises for the shoulder begin in the later phase of rehabilitation after the patient has achieved stabilization and adequate strength and after adequate tissue-healing time has passed. When the bench press is initiated in the later phases, it should be performed with a wide grip so that the arms are in abduction and horizontal extension.

Initial positions to avoid with inferior instability injuries include placing the arm overhead and allowing it to hang at the side unsupported. The upright press and shrugs are exercises that the patient should avoid because of the stress they place on the inferior capsule.

Case Study

A 16-year-old basketball player was seen by the physician after experiencing a right shoulder subluxation. The injury occurred as he was going under the basket for a layup and his arm was caught by an opponent and pulled into horizontal extension with lateral rotation. He has no history of prior injury. The physician has placed the arm in a sling and instructed you to begin a rehabilitation program for this patient. It has been one week since the injury. The patient reports some difficulty sleeping at night; he cannot get comfortable as a result of the pain. He reports that he wears the sling all the time except for showers, as the physician has instructed. On examination, you find some discoloration in the upper arm, but the swelling of last week is gone. There is some muscle spasm and tenderness to palpation of the infraspinatus, supraspinatus, teres minor, rhomboids, upper trapezius, and levator scapula. You notice that atrophy of the supraspinatus is already evident after one week. Range of motion of the shoulder is 40° flexion, 20° abduction, and unable to achieve lateral rotation by 10° from neutral (remains in medial rotation).

Questions for Analysis

1. What will be your initial treatment?

2. Outline the exercises you will use for this patient during the first week of treatment.

3. What precautions must you take with his treatments?

4. Give a general outline of progression for his rehabilitation program, specifying what guidelines

Shoulder Impingement

Shoulder impingement is associated with unique factors that you must consider in developing and executing a therapeutic exercise program. These are discussed as program considerations before the case study is presented.

Program Considerations

The subacromial space is not a large area—a little wider than a pencil. Because the space is not large to begin with, even a slight alteration in its normal structure can have significant consequences, especially to a patient who places great stresses on the joint.

There are two types of impingement, primary and secondary. Primary impingement is the result of structures present within the subacromial space that narrow the normal size of the space to compromise the soft-tissue structures within it—the rotator cuff tendons (supraspinatus and infraspinatus), biceps tendon, and subacromial bursa. Among these structural factors are a congenital anomaly of the acromion structure, an osteophyte on the distal acromion, a narrower-than-normal subacromial space, and a larger-than-normal tendon. All these structural variations narrow an already small space and cause the soft-tissue structures to become impinged. Most often the cause of primary impingement is either a congenital anomaly in the distal acromion configuration or a bone spur.

Acquired or secondary impingement reduces the subacromial space because of alterations in the shoulder's function that lead to instability. These factors can include capsular laxity or tightness, postural deviations, rotator cuff weakness, and scapular rotator muscle imbalances. Cervical radiculopathy can also result in impingement if muscle weakness occurs and causes muscle imbalances during shoulder motion. If the capsule is loose, the humerus moves forward during follow-through of throwing motions. If the posterior capsule is tight, it tends to push the humerus upward into the anterior joint during shoulder motions, narrowing the subacromial space. Normal function of the rotator cuff is to depress the humeral head during shoulder elevation motions to provide for adequate subacromial space; but if the rotator cuff is weak, the humeral head will ride higher than it should in the glenoid and cause impingement. When the scapular rotator muscles are imbalanced, the upper trapezius and levator scapulae usually overpower the weaker lower trapezius. This causes poor scapulohumeral rhythm and narrows the subacromial space under the coracoacromial arch during shoulder motion because scapular elevation and upward rotation will not occur with shoulder elevation (Kamkar, Irrgang, and Whitney 1993). Poor posture causes the shoulders to round forward so that the greater tubercle is more directly under the acromial arch to cause impingement earlier in the range of motion. Each of these secondary problems can result in subacromial impingement. Uncorrected secondary impingement leads to a gradual, progressive shredding of the rotator cuff tendon and ultimately results in rotator cuff tears. Secondary impingement and rotator cuff tears are more common in athletes over the age of 30 than in those who are younger.

Secondary and primary impingement both result in inflammation of the soft-tissue structures in the subacromial space. This inflammation most commonly includes the supraspinatus tendon. The infraspinatus tendon can sometimes be affected as well. The subacromial bursa and biceps tendon can also be involved. Impingement, then, causes tendinitis or bursitis. Inflammation of the rotator cuff tendons weakens the tendon and can lead to tendon rupture if the condition is poorly managed or untreated.

Secondary impingement can be resolved through conservative efforts if the cause of the impingement is corrected. The cause must be determined before treatment can be successful. Secondary factors of muscle imbalance and asynchronous shoulder motion are commonly seen in primary impingement, leading to pain and rotator cuff tendinitis. Primary impingement is surgically corrected, but both primary and secondary problems should be treated with rehabilitation. The most common surgical correction is either removal of the osteophyte (if present) or an anterior acromioplasty.

Rehabilitation emphasizes control of the inflammation, correction of the secondary cause, and restoration of normal shoulder function. Initially, the focus is on pain and inflammation control and achievement of full range of motion. Placing the shoulder in a resting position with the arm slightly abducted and flexed helps to provide optimal circulation to the tendons. Gentle grade I and II mobilizations can be helpful in relieving pain. If inferior capsule tightness is present, inferior glenohumeral glide mobilizations should be used to increase capsule mobility, permitting the rotator cuff to position the humerus caudally during arm elevation. The rehabilitation clinician can massage the supraspinatus tendon by placing the patient's hand behind the hip to expose the anterior humerus and providing deep cross-friction to the tender area until the pain subsides (figure 17.23). Scapular stabilization strengthening exercises can take place, without stress applied to the rotator cuff tendons, and should be a part of the early program. Early on, the program should incorporate simple neuromuscular reeducation techniques for proprioception and improved kinesthetic awareness of the scapular rotators for correct scapular positioning during arm movement. Rotator cuff exercises in a pain-free range of motion are important at this time as well. Most rotator cuff exercises should be performed in the lower positions (below 60°), and the scapula should be in a 'set' position. Resistive exercises should begin with high repetitions and lower weights.

Progression of exercises is based on the patient's pain and strength. Exercises that produce pain should be avoided. In the early stages, these exercises include activities that place the arm above 60° to 90° or behind the back, as well as diagonal-plane motions. As the tendon's inflammation subsides and the patient achieves scapular stabilization strength, he or she can add higher shoulder positions and more stressful exercises to the rehabilitation program. Finally, the plyometric and functional exercises are incorporated into the program before the patient returns to full activity.

Case Study

A 40-year-old, competitive tennis player reports to you that she has had shoulder pain since the first half of the tennis season. She is now unable to serve without pain. She has pain in the beginning of her warm-ups but before a match begins, the pain goes away. About 2 h after a match, her pain is significant. She has pain in the deltoid insertion area. The doctor has ruled out primary impingement but feels that a course of rehabilitation is necessary before the patient returns to tennis. On examination this patient has full range of motion except that she is lacking about 10° in elevation. Pain occurs in the end ranges of movement and above 90° of elevation. She has a forward-head, round-shouldered posture. Her glenohumeral rotators and abductors are weak and painful. She has weakness in the lower trapezius and rhomboids.

Questions for Analysis

1. What is the cause of her secondary impingement?

2. What will you do to relieve the causes?

3. What will your first treatment include?

4. How will you help the patient progress in her rehabilitation program?

5. What guidelines will you use for her progression?

6. What functional program will you use to prepare her for her return to tennis?

Traumatic Rotator Cuff Conditions

Traumatic rotator cuff injuries are different from degenerative tears that occur in older patients. You must take into account several unique factors associated with traumatic rotator cuff injuries before developing a therapeutic exercise program for a patient with this type of injury.

Program Considerations

Traumatic rotator cuff conditions can include acute rotator cuff strain, a partial tear, a complete tear, and postsurgical conditions. Although rotator cuff tears are more commonly seen in older individuals, patients now begin sport participation at an earlier age and at a greater intensity level than earlier generations did, so rotator cuff tears are increasingly seen in younger patients as well. A sudden traumatic event such as a shoulder dislocation or a fall on the outstretched, laterally rotated arm can cause rotator cuff tears at almost any age, and may occur in a healthy rotator cuff or in one that has minor asymptomatic changes. Tears can also occur in rotator cuff muscles that have undergone repetitive stresses over time. These conditions are associated especially with overhead physical activities in which the musculotendinous unit has encountered chronic stress and fiber damage. An open repair is necessary for most rotator cuff tears in patients who wish to remain active. Following surgical repair, the starting point, duration, and progression of the rehabilitation process depends on the size of the tear, the extent of the surgical repair, the state of integrity of the deltoid (whether it was cut or preserved in surgery), and the age of the patient. A sling or abduction brace may be used immediately postoperatively and continued for about six weeks. After 7 to 10 days of immobilization, mild passive and active assistive range-of-motion exercises may be possible, but this depends on the surgeon's preference. Early exercises can include passive and active assistive elevation and lateral rotation, extension, and medial rotation. Pendulum exercises are also appropriate. Joint mobilization for pain relief (grades I and II) can be used. Active–lateral and medial rotation can be performed with the elbow at the side and extended. Manual resistance to scapular rotators in sidelying with the arm at the side can be useful. Trigger point treatments may be necessary if indicated. Distal joint movements such as elbow and wrist flexion and extension and ball squeezes should be performed to minimize atrophy of the muscles in the distal segments. At the end of the first three weeks, rubber tubing or manual-resistance medial and lateral rotation with the elbow at the side, and rhythmic stabilization with the arm at 100° to 120° flexion, can begin.

The time to start active exercises depends on the size of the tear and the type of repair, but an average time point is approximately six to eight weeks after the surgery. At this time, joint mobilization for increased mobility (grades III and IV) can begin. Active range of motion can be performed in the scapular plane and can be accompanied by isometric exercises in different arm positions as long as the motion is pain free. Resistive exercises such as those done with rubber tubing should continue for the rotator cuff if the arm is kept at the side. If scapular stabilization is adequate, gentle guided medial and lateral rotation with the arm at 90° abduction can begin. Biceps and triceps exercises can be performed against resistance. Antigravity shoulder extension, supine fly, and prone fly to no more than a horizontal neutral position, as well as weight-bearing scapular stabilization exercises, are suitable at this time. Exercises are kept in a straight plane.

At 10 to 12 weeks, the patient should have nearly full range of motion. More vigorous stretching exercises, such as overhead hangs, are permissible if full motion is not present. Exercises should remain in a pain-free range. Sidelying exercises for the lateral and medial rotators can begin; these should initially use low resistance and high repetitions. Isokinetic exercises in the scapular plane are appropriate once the patient has sufficient single-plane strength in the rotator cuff and scapular stabilizers. Proprioceptive neuromuscular facilitation patterns of resistance can be used.

After 12 weeks, the scapular stabilizers should have adequate strength to control the scapula in planes higher than 60° to 90° elevation. The shoulder should be able to tolerate an aggressive strengthening program. Resisted diagonal movements begin in the lower levels, progress to shoulder level, and then progress to above shoulder levels. Plyometrics such as medicine-ball exercises can be started.

At 15 to 18 weeks, resisted rotation exercises with the arm at 90° abduction can be performed, as can aggressive resistive exercises for all shoulder muscle groups. Toward the end of this time, a progression of functional activities can begin—when the patient has full pain-free motion, normal strength of all shoulder muscles, and normal scapulohumeral synchronized motion. By 21 to 26 weeks the patient should be able to return to full participation.

The difference in rehabilitation for a conservatively managed and postoperative rotator cuff injury lies primarily in the initial treatment and the progression rate. In conservative treatment, the inflammation following injury must be initially treated with modalities and activity modification. Isometric exercises can begin earlier for conservatively treated injuries, and active motion can be initiated early as long as the shoulder remains pain free and scapular strength is sufficient to maintain proper scapular stabilization during shoulder motion. Early shoulder medial and lateral rotation motions are performed with the elbow near the side in a scapular plane. Shoulder elevation can occur to 90° as long as the shoulder is pain free and scapular stabilization is maintained. Resistance exercises begin with high repetitions and low resistance and progress to higher resistance with increased scapular and glenohumeral control.

Case Study

An 18-year-old baseball pitcher with shoulder instability underwent a glenohumeral capsular shift reconstruction one week ago. The surgeon wants you to begin the rehabilitation process today. The patient's shoulder is supported on a bolster with the arm in partial abduction and medial rotation. Examination reveals a nicely healing surgical scar over the anterior-inferior aspect of the shoulder. Passive range of motion measures 80° flexion, 80° abduction, and lateral rotation stops at 10° from neutral (unable to achieve lateral rotation). There is tenderness over the supraspinatus muscle belly, and the upper trapezius and levator scapula muscles are tense and tender to palpation.

Questions for Analysis

1. What will your treatment session today include? What precautions must you consider?

2. Give this patient an outline of your rehabilitation program with an estimate of how long it will be before he begins a pitching program.

3. Outline his pitching progression program.

Arthroscopic Decompression

The advancement of arthroscopic procedures to improve subacromial arch space has permitted a relatively rapid recovery following surgery to relieve subacromial impingement.

Program Considerations

Debridement of rotator cuff tendons and decompression of the subacromial space via an **arthroscopy** permits early rehabilitation because there has been no disruption of the deltoid and the surgical insult is less than with open surgical repairs and techniques. A decompression is used to relieve primary impingement, and a debridement is used to relieve chronic tendinitis or synovitis.

Rehabilitation following arthroscopic decompression can begin immediately after surgery. The first week or two involves primarily pain and swelling modulation and range-of-motion exercises. Grade I and II joint mobilization can be used to achieve pain relief. Early motion exercises can include Codman's exercises and active assistive range-of-motion exercises with a wand, pulley, or the rehabilitation clinician. Medial and lateral rotation motion exercises start with the elbow near the side with a towel roll between the side and elbow and progress to positioning the shoulder at 45° and then 90° of abduction during rotation exercises. Motion activities can also include capsular stretches and joint mobilization. Submaximal isometric exercises can be initiated in the first two weeks postoperatively. Scapular stabilization exercises and biceps and triceps exercises are important in the early program as well. Early neuromuscular control exercises such as proprioception drills for glenohumeral positioning with eyes closed can be started early.

Once pain is under control and near-full motion is possible, straight-plane resistive exercises can be initiated, first below 60° in the scapular plane. As scapular stabilization improves, lateral and medial rotation are performed at 90° of abduction, first with the arm supported, and then with the arm unsupported during exercise. Isokinetics in the scapular plane can begin. Full range of motion and good capsular mobility should be present before the patient moves to the next step of the progression. Once scapular stabilization and straight-plane strength are good, diagonal-plane exercises using pulleys or rubber tubing can begin. These are followed by first low-level, then higher-level, and finally overhead medicine-ball activities. Plyometrics are followed by functional exercises before the patient finally returns to full sport participation. The entire rehabilitation process may average three to five months.

Case Study

A 19-year-old volleyball player underwent an arthroscopic decompression of her right-dominant shoulder after an eight-week course of rehabilitation did not alleviate her shoulder pain. The surgery was two days ago. The surgeon wants her to begin a rehabilitation program today. On examination she reports normal postoperative shoulder pain, but no more rotator cuff pain. There is minimal ecchymosis around the shoulder. The surgical portal sites are covered with adhesive suture strips. There is some spasm in the rotator cuff muscles and upper trapezius. Range of motion of the shoulder is 150° flexion, 100° abduction, 80° lateral rotation, and 90° medial rotation. Her strength has diminished from preoperative levels and is now 3/5 in the rotator cuff muscles, 3 – /5 in shoulder abduction, 3/5 in shoulder flexion, and 4 – /5 in the scapular rotators. The patient tends to shrug her shoulder when she elevates the arm.

Questions for Analysis

1. What will you include in your treatment today?

2. What instructions will you give the patient today?

3. What will the next three treatment sessions include?

4. Explain what you will use as guidelines to determine when she is ready to progress from straight-plane to diagonal-plane exercises, from diagonal plane to plyometrics, and from plyometrics to functional exercises.

5. List four exercises for each exercise level and indicate your justification for their inclusion.

6. Describe the functional program you will use before the patient's return to volleyball.

Glenoid Labral Tears

Glenoid labral tears are difficult to identify. Nevertheless, when they are diagnosed, and whether an anterior or posterior tear is present, special considerations are warranted in the development of a therapeutic exercise program. We look at these considerations first and then at a case study.

Program Considerations

Glenoid labrum tears are primarily the bane of throwing athletes. The large compression and shear forces generated during deceleration in throwing are mainly responsible for causing degenerative tears, abrupt tears, or detachments of the glenoid labrum. The labrum frequently tears superiorly either on the posterior or anterior glenoid in throwers. This type of lesion is referred to as a SLAP lesion—Superior Labrum tear Anterior and Posterior in location. The anterior-superior lesion occurs because of the tremendous throwing deceleration forces applied in this area where the long head of the biceps tendon attaches to the labrum. The posterior-superior lesions are thought to occur because of glenohumeral joint instability. If a glenoid labrum tear is present, instability is frequently an accompanying problem and should be examined and treated as part of the total rehabilitation process.

Labral tears often involve the long head of the biceps, especially during deceleration and follow-through throwing phases. When the biceps-labral complex is involved, the labrum can be torn from the superior aspect of the glenoid, and the biceps tendon can be either avulsed with the labrum or suffer a partial tear at its proximal insertion. One surgeon's group noted that 83% of labral tears also involved the biceps-labral complex (Andrews, Carson, & McLeod 1985). Based on this information, it may be presumed that the majority of glenoid labrum tears do not merely involve the labrum.

Whether or not instability is present, the usual treatment choice is to try a conservative approach with rehabilitation first. If this is unsuccessful, excision of the torn segment may be necessary. If instability is present, open reduction to remove the avulsed segment and stabilize the joint may be necessary. A variety of surgical repairs are used for this problem, including a Bankart repair and capsulolabral reconstruction.

If the patient undergoes an arthroscopic excision, the rehabilitation process follows the program used for arthroscopic debridement presented earlier with full recovery in approximately 3 to 5 months. If an open repair is necessary, the rehabilitation process will be delayed because of the required additional time of immobilization; the rehabilitation program proceeds more slowly and cautiously because the greater shoulder area involved and the risk of damaging the surgical repair if the rehabilitation is too aggressive. An open repair will damage the proprioceptors more than an arthroscopic procedure, so rehabilitation for these procedures should emphasize proprioceptive activities once active motion is possible. The open surgical cases will more closely follow the time line outlined for the rotator cuff repair program discussed previously; refer to that program for guidelines on procedures and timelines.

Case Study

A 17-year-old lacrosse player injured his right-dominant shoulder when another player ran into him while his arm was abducted. He suffered a torn glenoid and was in rehabilitation for three weeks following the injury. The following winter, he slipped on the ice and landed on an outstretched arm, causing his shoulder to sublux. He underwent an open debridement and anterior capsular reconstruction last week and is now ready for rehabilitation. The arm is in an abduction bolster harness, but the surgeon wants it removed during therapeutic exercises. Shoulder motion is 60° flexion, 60° abduction, and lateral rotation stops at 10° from neutral (unable to achieve lateral rotation). Rotator cuff strength in the middle of available range is 3+/5. The surgical scar is well healed, but there is ecchymosis surrounding the anterior shoulder area and into the upper arm. The upper trapezius and pectoralis major muscles are tender to palpation and in spasm.

Questions for Analysis

1. What will be your first treatment?

2. What will be included in your first two weeks of treatment?

3. When will you begin passive range of motion?

4. When will you begin resistive exercises, and what will they first include?

5. What precautions must you be aware of in this case?

Adhesive Capsulitis

Adhesive capsulitis is more commonly seen in patients over the age of 30 than in younger patients but does occur in younger age groups. Understanding the condition is essential to designing a therapeutic exercise program. Elements unique to this injury are discussed and a case study is then presented.

Program Considerations

Adhesive capsulitis is commonly referred to as a frozen shoulder. The generic term for adhesions in the capsule is arthrofibrosis. An idiopathic frozen shoulder occurs spontaneously with no known trauma or aggravating incident. Idiopathic frozen shoulder occurs predominantly in middle-aged patients—usually over 30, usually female—and typically in the nondominant shoulder. Although adhesive capsulitis is a malady of older patients, the shoulder can become restricted in its motion in younger patients because of a variety of predisposing factors. These factors can include surgery that changes the biomechanics of the shoulder; prolonged immobilization of the shoulder; scar-tissue adhesions in the capsule or ligaments surrounding the shoulder; and prolonged inflammation of the tendons, bursa, and other soft tissue around the shoulder. This condition is termed traumatic or secondary adhesive capsulitis when there is a sudden onset of injury or of immobilization resulting in loss of motion.

Immobilization causes adhesions in connective tissue that can reduce muscular tissue mobility. Reduced muscle tissue mobility decreases the number of sarcomeres present in the muscle (Akeson et al. 1973). The additional changes that occur with immobilization in muscle, joints, and supportive tissue were discussed in chapter 2. When the joint capsule is affected, loss of motion is most notable in lateral rotation, abduction, and flexion of the shoulder. A capsular pattern of motion loss becomes apparent, with lateral rotation more limited than abduction, abduction more limited than flexion, and flexion more limited than medial rotation (Cyriax 1975).

When adhesive capsulitis is in stage I, shoulder pain, pain at end ranges of movement, difficulty sleeping on the shoulder and progressive loss of motion are hallmark signs. It is during this time that the capsular scar tissue is forming and maturing. Lateral rotation will demonstrate loss of available motion, but other movements may or may not show evidence of lost motion. The most effective treatment at this time is active range-of-motion exercises. Joint mobilization should not be painful and should be oriented more toward pain relief than mobility gains. Stronger mobilization grades only aggravate the capsule and may promote an inflammatory response or cause a reactive muscle spasm that will increase pain. Active range-of-motion exercises maintain muscle length. Attempts at stretching the capsule at this time cause pain but little change in mobility.

In stage II, adhesive capsulitis has become mature, the glenohumeral joint has lost its normal mobility, and the shoulder is very stiff. Pain is present at the end of available motion. The patient may complain of pain in the elbow and is unable to lie on the shoulder. At this time more aggressive joint mobilization can be used as long as an inflammatory response is not created. Continued active stretches should also be used. Strengthening exercises in the available ranges should be a part of the program. Ultrasound before joint mobilization may permit more optimal results from the mobilization.

In the third stage, the patient's pain is evident before the end of capsular restriction is reached. The primary area of pain is distal on the arm, not in the shoulder. Pain is present at rest as well as during activity. Passive range-of-motion assessment demonstrates a hard, leathery end-feel with motion loss in a capsular pattern. Scapulohumeral rhythm is lost because glenohumeral capsular restrictions prevent normal motion between the scapulothoracic and glenohumeral joints. Because glenohumeral rhythm is lost, attempts at arm elevation include shoulder shrugging, and the scapula moves at the same time and rate as the humerus. Grades III and IV joint mobilizations can be used at this time. Continued range-of-motion exercises and active stretches are used throughout the day to promote mobility gains. Self-mobilization techniques are taught to the patient. Strength exercises for the scapular rotators, rotator cuff, and large glenohumeral muscles (deltoid, pectoralis major, teres major, and latissimus) should be provided in a progressive program.

If the patient is not seen until the third stage, treatment for 3 to 6 months may be necessary to resolve the condition. Without treatment, the adhesive capsulitis takes longer to resolve, perhaps between 18 and 24 months.

Case Study

A 45-year-old golfer had noticed a gradual loss of motion in his left nondominant shoulder over the past several months. He went to the physician when he was unable to retrieve his wallet out of his back pocket and was diagnosed with a frozen shoulder. He is unable to lie on the left side and has pain with sudden movements and when just sitting. He is concerned about getting his shoulder ready for golf season, which begins in three months. On examination, you find that he has 120° of flexion, 80° of abduction, 35° of lateral rotation, and 60° of medial rotation and that he is able to reach across in horizontal adduction to get his elbow even with his left ear. He has pain about 10° to 15° before the end range of all motions, and you observe a stiff end-feel at the end of each movement. Joint mobilization assessment indicates tightness throughout the capsule, especially the inferior and posterior capsule. Palpation reveals tenderness in all the rotator cuff muscles and some tension in the pectoralis major, upper trapezius, and levator scapulae. The patient's posture is good, but when he moves the arm there is no scapulohumeral rhythm, and he shrugs the shoulder toward his ear to initiate shoulder flexion motions.

Questions for Analysis

1. What stage of adhesive capsulitis is he in?

2. What will be your first treatment for him?

3. What home exercises will you give him on the first day?

4. Outline a progressive program for him including modalities, exercises, mobilization techniques, and functional progression for returning to golf.

Electrothermally Assisted Capsular shift

Electrothermally assisted capsular shift is a procedure for which long-term results have not been defined because of its newness to medicine. There remain many unanswered questions regarding the proper rehabilitation course. There is little research on postoperative treatment procedures. One study indicated that early range of motion and a slow but progressive strengthening program produce successful results over a 12-week therapeutic exercise treatment course (Ellenbecker and Mattalino 1999). This section presents the information currently available about the procedure and the postoperative course.

Program Considerations

The electrothermally assisted capsular shift procedure is a relatively new arthroscopic technique used to address glenohumeral instability. The long-term effects of the procedure are still being investigated and are at this point unknown because the technique has been used only since the late 1990s (Gerber and Warner 2002). The arthroscopic technique incorporates the use of a thermally assisted coagulator probe that is set at or above 65° C and is swept along the capsule between the glenoid and the humeral head to denature the capsule (Hayashi et al. 1997). The capsule immediately shrinks like a plastic shrink-wrap, reducing the joint's laxity.

It is thought that the heat causes the collagen to denature and fuse when fibroblasts invade the area. The fibroblasts are thought to use the denatured collagen as a scaffold in the new collagen matrix formation during the inflammatory healing phase (Hayashi et al. 1996). It is during this time that immobilization of the shoulder must occur so that the collagen matrix formation will result in appropriate capsular tightening.

The shoulder is kept immobilized for 7 to 14 days, although wrist and elbow motions are permitted. Active abduction is initiated about 10 to 14 days postoperatively. Lateral rotation is permitted to 45° with the elbow at the side and to 90° abduction after about two weeks.

Forward flexion is kept to 90°, and extension is limited to 20° hyperextension. Some physicians will allow active motion three days after the procedure with lateral rotation to 0° and scapular plane flexion to 90° for the first four weeks (Gerber and Warner 2002).

Since joint proprioceptors may have been damaged during the surgery, it is important to include exercises to restore proprioception. These can begin with early-stage activities within the allowed ranges of motion early in the program and advance as mobility and proprioception increase.

Submaximal isometric strengthening exercises can be performed after the first week or two as long as the patient stays within the range-of-motion restrictions and abduction is kept at 0°. Scapular stabilization exercises can be performed without placing undue stress on the glenohumeral joint. Resisted elbow and wrist motions should also be a part of the program. Joint mobilization to the AC, SC, and scapulothoracic joints are allowed.

At four to eight weeks, all motions should be within normal limits except lateral rotation, which is limited to 15° less than that on the contralateral side. Posterior capsular stretching is initiated at this time. Light resistive exercises with high repetitions and low resistance can begin as long as the patient remains pain free. Strenuous overhead activities should be avoided at this time, but controlled diagonal movements can be initiated. Proprioceptive exercises within the patient's motion and tolerance are started at this time.

After week 8, the patient should have full range of motion except in lateral rotation at 90° of abduction. More aggressive strength exercises are started as long as the patient remains pain free. Wall push-ups may be tolerated as the patient nears the 12-week mark.

After week 12, the patient should be able to tolerate plyometric exercises. The progression is the usual one previously discussed, starting with low-level movements and progressing to overhead movements once control is achieved at the lower elevation levels. The final step consists of functional activities and drills before return to full participation and normal activities.

Acromioclavicular Sprain

Although first-degree sprains are not usually difficult to manage, the treatment approach for more severe AC sprains is more complex. Considerations for the various degrees of AC sprains are presented, followed by a case study.

Case Study

A 21-year-old swimmer underwent an electrothermal capsular shift 10 days ago for anterior instability. The physician reports that the patient had no other joint damage and that no other surgical procedure was necessary. She is now to begin rehabilitation. She has some mild postoperative pain, but nothing unusual. She is to wear a sling for another four weeks but is permitted to remove the sling for rehabilitation. Her shoulder range of motion is 40° flexion, 30° abduction, and −5° lateral rotation (unable to achieve neutral rotation from medial rotation by 5°). The rotator cuff and scapular rotators are grossly 4 − /5 in strength, but there is more weakness in the scapular rotators than in the rotator cuff.

Questions for Analysis

1. What will be your first day's treatment?

2. What precautions will you provide this patient?

3. Outline your treatment progression for her.

4. What will you include in your functional program before her return to full sport participation?

Program Considerations

Most sprains, regardless of severity, are not surgically repaired and are treated conservatively. The speed with which conservative care is advanced depends on the severity of the injury. In mild sprains, the shoulder may be immobilized in a sling for a few days to relieve the traction discomfort caused by the weight of the arm pulling on the AC joint. Modalities are used to relieve pain, swelling, and muscle spasm. Active and active–assistive range of motion exercises are initiated on day 1 or 2 following the injury. Isometrics to tolerance can also begin immediately. Once full motion is restored, a progression of strengthening exercises is used until the patient has full function without pain and is able to return to full sport participation.

In type II and III sprains, the AC ligament is torn. In type II sprains the coracoclavicular ligament is intact, but in type III sprains it is not. Some deformity is present in both type II and type III sprains. Attempts at immobilization are made, but they are often unsuccessful because of the discomfort and restriction of the immobilizing device and the difficulty in stabilizing the AC joint. The benefits of surgical repair for type III sprains are disputable. Most often the treatment option selected is nonsurgical: A sling is used to relieve the distraction force of the weight of the arm on the AC joint. Some deformity usually persists, but this is a cosmetic issue and does not interfere with activity and shoulder function. The more severe injuries (types IV, V, and VI) are often surgically repaired, because significant damage to both static and dynamic structures around the joint has occurred.

In the type II and III injuries, the shoulder may be immobilized for one to three weeks. Active–assistive range of motion of the glenohumeral joint may begin early. If proprioception is deficient, basic exercises to restore it can begin early in the program and advance as pain subsides and motion and strength improve. Strengthening exercises (below 60°) follow a normal progression from stabilization, straight-plane, and low-level exercises to higher-level exercises and diagonal movements. Plyometric exercises are followed by functional exercises. Normal progression to heavy lifting occurs at about 8 to 12 weeks postinjury, and the patient returns to full participation after having performed functional exercises correctly.

Case Study

A 17-year-old wrestler incurred a type II sprain of his right AC joint in last week's match. He is to begin rehabilitation today. The shoulder has been in a sling for the past week. The patient is able to take the arm out of the sling for brief periods of time, but he reports that keeping the sling off for longer than 4 h causes an ache in the top of the shoulder. The muscles also feel tired. Examination reveals 150° of shoulder flexion, 120° of shoulder abduction, 60° of lateral rotation, and 75° of medial rotation. Strength tests reveal grades of 4 – /5 in the pectoralis major and rotator cuff; 3+/5 in the rhomboids, lower trapezius, and serratus anterior; and 4/5 in the deltoid and latissimus dorsi. You can palpate trigger points in the upper trapezius, pectoralis major, and supraspinatus muscles.

Questions for Analysis

1. What will your first treatment session include?

2. What are your goals for the first treatment session?

3. What instructions will you give the patient before he leaves today?

4. Outline the rehabilitation course, including a time line you anticipate for program changes and four examples of each type of exercise.

5. What will your functional exercise program include before return to sport participation?

Biceps Tendon Injuries

Although it might seem appropriate to deal with the biceps tendon in the chapter on the elbow, the biceps tendon plays an important role in shoulder stabilization. For this reason, injuries to the biceps tendon are discussed here.

Program Considerations

The most common injury seen in the biceps tendon is tendinitis. Tears, subluxations, and dislocations can also occur. Bicipital tendinitis occurs primarily in the long head and is usually secondary to shoulder instability, impingement, rotator cuff pathology, or other inflammations of the shoulder. The patient reports tenderness in the bicipital groove. Cervical pathology can refer into the biceps area and must be ruled out if no frank injury has occurred to cause the pain.

Biceps tendon ruptures are often associated with rotator cuff pathology, and most occur in middle-aged individuals. A sudden muscle contraction while the muscle is on stretch is a common mechanism of injury. Complete ruptures may display a 'Popeye' muscle, but partial ruptures are not as obvious. Pain, spasm, and swelling are immediate signs. If the long head of the biceps is ruptured in a young patient, surgery may be indicated. The same injury in an older patient may or may not require surgery. Because the long head of the biceps provides glenohumeral stability, its surgical repair can be important in the younger and more active population.

Rehabilitation treatment must include an examination of the rotator cuff, because its pathology is often related with biceps pathology. Control of pain, swelling, and inflammation is an initial goal of treatment. Use of modalities, anti-inflammatories, and rest initially may be beneficial. Rest is usually accompanied by active–assistive range-of-motion exercises. Therapeutic exercises progress as tolerated to include an exercise sequence similar to that listed for conditions discussed earlier. It should also obviously include supination and elbow flexion exercises.

Case Study

Three days ago a 21-year-old gymnast experienced a ruptured biceps injury while practicing on the rings. He is now ready to begin a rehabilitation program. There is ecchymosis in the distal arm and into the forearm. The area has swelling, and the biceps muscle feels tight from spasm. Elbow motion is lacking 15° of extension and has 120° of flexion. The patient has full passive supination but actively supinates to 45°. Elbow flexion is 3+/5 and painful. The patient admits to having had shoulder pain last season that kept him out of competition for one month. This season the pain has been present but tolerable. He indicates that he has never injured his neck but that sometimes it feels stiff.

Questions for Analysis

1. What will your first treatment include, and what are your goals for the first treatment?

2. What other areas should you investigate before deciding on your course of treatment?

3. When do you expect to achieve full range of motion in the elbow?

4. When will you begin strengthening exercises, and what will your first week of exercises include?

SUMMARY

1. Explain how knowledge of the mechanics of an activity impacts the establishment of a therapeutic exercise program.

   The shoulder is a complex structure composed of several joints and many muscles that must work synchronously to produce injury-free motion. When activity is not synchronous or when trauma occurs, the result is an injury that can affect the entire shoulder function. During specific motions such as pitching, swinging a golf club, swimming, or performing hits and serves in tennis, the shoulder and its joints and muscles must work in a specifically timed and synchronous manner to produce the desired effect with minimal risk of injury. The rehabilitation clinician must have an awareness and appreciation of these activities to properly rehabilitate the patient for return to full participation.

2. Discuss the importance of stability in shoulder rehabilitation.

   Stability of the glenohumeral and scapulothoracic joints is crucial to performance and to reduced injury risk for the shoulder. Studies have demonstrated the significance of good stabilization of these joints and the importance of good therapeutic exercise programs to permit restoration of stability of these areas.

3. Explain the role of scapular stabilization in shoulder function.

   Basic to shoulder function is scapular stabilization during shoulder activities. Scapular muscles serve as the foundation from which the shoulder moves; so when scapular muscles do not function properly, either because of weakness, loss of motion, or reduced endurance, the shoulder is at great risk of injury.

4. Describe two soft-tissue mobilization techniques for the shoulder.

   Cross-friction massage to the biceps tendon and anterior rotator cuff muscles is commonly performed with tendinitis injuries. Trigger point releases to rotator cuff muscles, such as the supraspinatus in the supraspinatus fossa or the teres minor at the lateral border of the scapula, are commonly performed to relieve pain and improve motion.

5. List three joint mobilizations for the shoulder.

   Shoulder joint mobilization techniques should include techniques for the specifically restricted joints. If the AC joint is restricted, PA, AP, and inferior glides can be used. If the scapula is restricted, scapular distraction is appropriate. If the glenohumeral joint is restricted, an arm pull is a gross technique, and an inferior glide is a more specific technique for improving joint mobility. Joint mobilization must be performed in grades III and IV to gain motion.

6. Identify three strengthening exercises for the scapulae and three for the glenohumeral muscles.

   Scapular muscle-strengthening exercises can include maneuvers such as push-up-plus, prone fly, and Bouhler exercises. Glenohumeral muscle strengthening exercises can include medial and lateral rotation exercises starting with isometric exercises and moving to rubber tubing and free-weight exercises, as well as abduction in the scapular plane.

7. Discuss the general progression of strengthening exercises for the shoulder.

   The specific progression depends on the specific injury and its severity. A general progression of strengthening exercises begins with scapular stabilization exercises and isometric rotator cuff exercises. Manual resistance to the scapular muscles can begin early in the program. From there the exercises include active resistive exercises in the lower third of shoulder motion until the scapular muscles are strong enough to provide scapular control in the middle ranges of motion and finally in motion over

100°, so overhead exercises can be performed without loss of control of scapular and glenohumeral positioning. Eccentric exercises for the rotator cuff using rubber tubing, medicine balls, and even manual resistance begin in straight planes and progress to diagonal planes. Exercises in both weight bearing and non-weight bearing are used for stabilization and strengthening. Plyometric activities begin slowly and progress as the patient gains proficiency. Functional exercises using sport equipment such as a tennis racket or golf club then begin, at first in low ranges of motion with reduced force until control and proficiency have been demonstrated. Exercises next progress to greater ranges of motion and begin to mimic the actual activity. Functional overhead activities are the last item to be added to the program. In addition to the shoulder, the biceps, triceps, and abdominal muscles must also be included in the program.

8. List precautions for a therapeutic exercise program following a rotator cuff repair.

    Care must be taken to allow tissue healing before exercises begin. Range of motion usually begins at 7 to 10 days. If immobilization continues for an extended period of time, there can be complications such as adhesive capsulitis, especially in patients over age 30. Range-of-motion exercises begin with activities such as Codman's and must progress on the basis of the status of the healing tissues. Strength exercises begin slowly with high endurance and low resistance, progressing as the patient gains control and strength. Scapular exercises can be initiated early, but rotator cuff exercises begin with submaximal isometrics. Range-of-motion gains in lateral rotation occur slowly and cautiously.

9. Outline key factors for a program for a biceps rupture.

    Active range of motion for shoulder, elbow, and forearm is followed by strengthening exercises for motions including elbow flexion, supination, and shoulder flexion and extension. Progression of exercises follows a pattern similar to that for other shoulder programs, according to considerations regarding pain, control, and tissue healing.

CRITICAL THINKING QUESTIONS

1. If you were Bob in the opening scenario for this chapter, what techniques would you have used to relieve P.G.'s posterior shoulder tightness and the scapular muscle weakness? What plyometric progression would you have used to advance him to functional activities? What criteria would you have used to begin his functional activities, and what would your throwing progression have been?

2. If an injured wrestler who experienced a shoulder dislocation two weeks ago comes to you to begin rehabilitation, what must be your greatest precaution with him? How much elevation can you safely place the shoulder in? What is your reasoning for this amount of motion? What exercises should you be able to do with him at two weeks postinjury?

3. If the rehabilitation process and the results for electrothermally assisted capsular shift procedures have not yet been fully documented, what guidelines can you use when a patient comes to you after this procedure has been performed on his or her shoulder? Based on your knowledge of healing and the shoulder, what precautions should be taken, and what exercises can you perform in the first three to six weeks postoperatively?

4. Recall the case of the 40-year-old tennis player presented in the section on impingement in this chapter. Have you figured out the cause of her problem? If posture is a primary contributing factor, what instructions will you give her to relieve the cause? What exercises will reinforce your efforts to change her posture? If her posture has been incorrect for some time, what soft-tissue changes would you expect will need to be treated?

5. If you have a patient whose diagnosis has been narrowed down to a rotator cuff tendinitis, shoulder instability, shoulder impingement, capsulitis, and cervical radiculopathy, how will you determine which diagnosis is correct? What tests will you use to differentiate between these diagnoses? Would the rehabilitation program change with different diagnoses? Why or why not?

LAB ACTIVITIES

1. With your lab partner as a patient, perform grades I, II, III, and IV joint mobilization on all shoulder complex joints. For the glenohumeral joint, apply an inferior glide to determine joint mobility. Identify how large the movement is for each of the grades as you go through the joint's total mobility range. Now repeat the examination on another person. How does the range of mobility of each joint compare between the individuals?

2. Apply the following joint mobilization techniques on your partner. While applying each technique, notice where the resistance to movement occurs and where movement stops. Why are these items important to assess for each motion and joint?

   a. Glenohumeral anterior glide

   b. Glenohumeral posterior glide

   c. Glenohumeral lateral glide

   d. Scapulothoracic glides

   e. Acromioclavicular inferior glide

   f. Acromioclavicular anterior-posterior glides

   g. Sternoclavicular AP glide

   h. Sternoclavicular PA glide

3. Locate the trigger points for the following muscles on your lab partner:

   a. Subscapularis

   b. Supraspinatus

   c. Infraspinatus

   d. Teres minor

   What muscles contained your lab partner's most sensitive trigger points? Perform an ice-and-stretch technique on the most sensitive areas after you have examined for active range of motion of the muscle. After the treatment, have your partner repeat the active ROM so you can determine the effectiveness of your treatment. How did the AROM change from before to after the treatment? Why?

4. If your partner has a tight anterior and inferior capsule, list the flexibility exercises you would give him. Have your partner go through them and tell you where the stretch is felt.

5. If your partner has a tight posterior capsule, list the flexibility exercises you would give her. Have your partner go through them and tell you where the stretch is felt.

6. Go through wand exercises to increase shoulder flexion, abduction, horizontal abduction, and lateral rotation with your partner. List all possible substitution patterns he performs and the verbal cues you use to correct these patterns.

7. Perform isolated scapular resistance exercises on your partner in all possible planes in sidelying and supine. How many repetitions for each exercise was she able to perform before fatigue occurred? How were you able to identify when she fatigued?

8. Have your partner perform a progression of push-up exercises beginning with wall push-ups and ending with box jumps on the floor (use footstools). List the progression you used and the number of repetitions your partner was able to do. What are you looking for in terms of his performance? How are you determining when he has performed enough repetitions to acquire adequate fatigue levels?

9. Have your partner perform one exercise each for the lower trapezius, middle trapezius, serratus anterior, and rhomboids. List the exercise and how many repetitions your partner was able to perform. What would be a progression for each exercise and when would you advance your partner to the next level?

10. Have your partner perform one exercise for the shoulder abductors, MR, and LR. Describe the exercise you have selected, why you have selected it, how many repetitions your partner was able to perform, possible substitution patterns to watch for, and your next progression for each exercise.

11. Have your partner perform any two of the scapular stabilization exercises in this chapter. What muscle did you partner feel the exercise working, and what possible substitution patterns could have been used?

12. Have your partner perform any two of the plyometric or functional exercises in this chapter. What purpose do they serve (goals for the exercise), and what substitution patterns could be used for each? How will you determine when she should advance to the next level of exercise (what are your criteria)? Can you think of another plyometric or functional exercise that is not in this chapter?

REFERENCES

Akeson, W.H., Woo, S.L-Y., Amiel, D., Coutts, R.D., and D. Daniel. 1973. The connective tissue response to immobility: Biochemical changes in periarticular connective tissue of the immobilized rabbit knee. *Clinical Orthopedics & Related Research* 93:356-362.

Andrews, J.R., Carson, W.G. Jr., and W.D. McLeod. 1985. Glenoid labrum tears related to the long head of the biceps. *American Journal of Sports Medicine*. 13:337-41.

Blackburn, T.A., McLeod, W.D., White, B., and L. Wofford. 1990. EMG analysis of posterior rotator cuff exercises. *Athletic Training*. 24:40, 42-45.

Bradley, J.P., and J.E. Tibone. 1991. Electromyographic analysis of muscle action about the shoulder. *Clinics in Sports Medicine* 10:789-805.

Cyriax, J.H. 1975. *Textbook of orthopaedic medicine. Vol. 1. Diagnosis of soft tissue lesions.* 6th ed. Baltimore: Williams & Wilkins.

Denegar, C.R., E. Saliba, and S. Saliba. 2005. *Therapeutic modalities for musculoskeletal injuries.* 2nd. ed. Champaign, IL: Human Kinetics.

Ellenbecker, T.S., and A.J. Mattalino. 1999. Glenohumeral joint range of motion and rotator cuff strength following arthroscopic anterior stabilization with thermal capsulorrhaphy. *Journal of Orthopaedic & Sports Physical Therapy* 29:160-167.

Gerber, A. and J.J. Warner. 2002. Thermal capsulorrhaphy to treat shoulder instability. *Clinical Orthopaedics & Related Research.* 400:105-116.

Hayashi, K., Thabit, G. III, Bogdanske, J.J., Mascio, L.N., and M.D. Markel. 1996. The effect of nonablative laser energy on the ultrastructure of joint capsular collagen. *Arthroscopy: The Journal of Arthroscopic and Related Surgery* 12:474-481.

Hayashi, K., Thabit, G. III, Massa, K.L., Bogdanske, J.J., Cooley, A.J., Orwin, J.F., and M.D. Markel. 1997. The effect of thermal heating on the length and histologic properties of the glenohumeral joint capsule. *American Journal of Sports Medicine* 25:107-112.

Host, H.H. 1995. Scapular taping in the treatment of anterior shoulder impingement. *Physical Therapy* 75:803-812.

Jobe, F.W., Moynes, D.R., and D.J. Antonelli. 1985. Rotator cuff function during a golf swing. *American Journal of Sports Medicine* 14:388-392.

Kamkar, A., Irrgang, J.J., and S.L. Whitney. 1993. Nonoperative management of secondary shoulder impingement syndrome. *Journal of Orthopaedic & Sports Physical Therapy* 17:212-224.

Kelley, M.J. 1995. Anatomic and biomechanical rationale for rehabilitation of the athlete's shoulder. *Journal of Sports Rehabilitation* 4:122-154.

Kibler, W.B. 1995. Biomechanical analysis of the shoulder during tennis activities. *Clinics in Sports Medicine* 14:79-85.

Lear, L.J., and M.T. Gross. 1998. An electromyographical analysis of the scapular stabilizing synergists during a push-up progression. *Journal of Orthopaedic & Sports Physical Therapy* 28:146-157.

Lephart, S.M., and T.J. Henry. 1996. The physiological basis for open and closed kinetic chain rehabilitation for the upper extremity. *Journal of Sport Rehabilitation* 5:71-87.

McQuade, K.J., Dawson, J., and G.L. Smidt. 1998. Scapulothoracic muscle fatigue associated with alterations in scapulohumeral rhythm kinematics during maximum resistive shoulder elevation. *Journal of Orthopaedics & Sports Physical Therapy* 28:74-80.

Morin, G.E., Tiberio, D., and G. Austin. 1997. The effect of upper trapezius taping on electromyographic activity in the upper and middle trapezius region. *Journal of Sports Rehabilitation* 6:309-318.

Moynes, D.R., Perry, J., Antonelli, D.J., and F.W. Jobe. 1986. Electromyography and motion analysis of the upper extremity in sports. *Physical Therapy* 66:1905-1911.

Nuber, G.W., Jobe, F.W., Perry, J., Moynes, D.R., and D. Antonelli. 1986. Fine wire electromyography analysis of muscles of the shoulder during swimming. *American Journal of Sports Medicine* 14:7-11.

Pappas, A.M., Zawacki, R.M., and T.J. Sullivan. 1985. Biomechanics of baseball pitching, a preliminary report. *American Journal of Sports Medicine* 13:216-222.

Perry, J. 1978. Normal upper extremity kinesiology. *Physical Therapy* 58:265-278.

Perry, J. 1983. Anatomy and biomechanics of the shoulder in throwing, swimming, gymnastics, and tennis. *Clinics in Sports Medicine* 2:247-270.

Pink, M., Perry, J., Browne, A., Scovazzo, M.L., and J. Kerrigan. 1991. The normal shoulder during freestyle swimming. *American Journal of Sports Medicine* 19:569-576.

Richardson, A.B., Jobe, F.W., and H.R. Collins. 1980. The shoulder in competitive swimming. *American Journal of Sports Medicine* 8:159-163.

Ryu, R.K.N., McCormick, J., Jobe, F.W., Moynes, D.R., and D.J. Antonelli. 1988. An electromyographic analysis of shoulder function in tennis players. *American Journal of Sports Medicine* 16:481-485.

Travell, J.G., and D.G. Simons. 1983. *Myofascial pain and dysfunction. The trigger point manual.* Vol. 1. Baltimore: Williams & Wilkins.

Worrell, T.W., Corey, B.J., York, S. L., and J. Santicstaban. 1992. An analysis of supraspinatus EMG activity and shoulder isometric force development. *Medicine and Science in Sport and Exercise.* 24: 744-748.

SUGGESTED READING

Allegrucci, M., Whitney, S.L., and J.J. Irrgang. 1994. Clinical implications of secondary impingement of the shoulder in freestyle swimmers. *Journal of Orthopaedic & Sports Physical Therapy* 20:312-318.

Andrews, J.R., and K.E. Wilk. 1994. *The athlete's shoulder.* New York: Churchill Livingstone.

Bonci, C.M., Sloane, B., and K. Middleton. 1992. Nonsurgical/surgical rehabilitation of the unstable shoulder. *Journal of Sport Rehabilitation* 1:146-171.

Braatz, J.H., and P.P. Gogia. 1987. The mechanics of pitching. *Journal of Orthopaedic & Sports Physical Therapy* 9:56-69.

Brewster, C., and D.R. Moynes Schwab. 1993. Rehabilitation of the shoulder following rotator cuff injury or surgery. *Journal of Orthopaedic & Sports Physical Therapy* 18:422-426.

Culham, E., and M. Peat. 1993. Functional anatomy of the shoulder complex. *Journal of Orthopaedic & Sports Physical Therapy* 18:342-350.

Davies, G.J., and S. Dickoff-Hoffman. 1993. Neuromuscular testing and rehabilitation of the shoulder complex. *Journal of Orthopaedic & Sports Physical Therapy* 18:449-458.

Dillman, C.J., Fleisig, G.S., and J.R. Andrews. 1993. Biomechanics of pitching with emphasis upon shoulder kinematics. *Journal of Orthopaedic & Sports Physical Therapy* 18:402-408.

Grubbs, N. 1993. Frozen shoulder syndrome: A review of literature. *Journal of Orthopaedic & Sports Physical Therapy* 18:479-487.

Jobe, F.W., and J.P. Bradley. 1989. The diagnosis and nonoperative treatment of shoulder injuries in athletes. *Clinics in Sports Medicine* 8:419-438.

Jobe, F.W., Moynes, D.R., and C.E. Brewster. 1987. Rehabilitation of shoulder joint instabilities. *Orthopedic Clinics of North America* 18:473-482.

Litchfield, R., Hawkins, R., Dillman, C.J., Atkins, J., and G. Hagerman. 1993. Rehabilitation for the overhead athlete. *Journal of Orthopaedic & Sports Physical Therapy* 18:433-442.

McQuade, K.J., and G.L. Smidt. 1998. Dynamic scapulohumeral rhythm: The effects of external resistance during elevation of the arm in the scapular plane. *Journal of Orthopaedic & Sports Physical Therapy* 27:125-133.

Meister, K., and J.R. Andrews. 1993. Classification and treatment of rotator cuff injuries in the overhand athlete. *Journal of Orthopaedic & Sports Physical Therapy* 18:413-421.

Moynes, D.R. 1983. Prevention of injury to the shoulder through exercises and therapy. *Clinics in Sports Medicine* 2:413-422.

Pappas, A.M., Zawacki, R.M., and C.F. McCarthy. 1985. Rehabilitation of the pitching shoulder. *American Journal of Sports Medicine* 13:223-235.

Payne, R.M., and M. Voight. 1993. The role of the scapula. *Journal of Orthopaedic & Sports Physical Therapy* 18:386-391.

Pezzullo, D.J., Karas, S., and J.J. Irrgang. 1995. Functional plyometric exercises for the throwing athlete. *Journal of Athletic Training* 30:22-26.

Plancher, K.D., Litchfield, R., and R.J. Hawkins. 1995. Rehabilitation of the shoulder in tennis players. *Clinics in Sports Medicine* 14:111-137.

Stone, J.A., Lueken, J.S., Partin, N.B., Timm, K.E., and E.J. Ryan. 1993. Closed kinetic chain rehabilitation for the glenohumeral joint. *Journal of Athletic Training* 28:34-37.

Wilk, K.E., and C. Arrigo. 1993. Current concepts in the rehabilitation of the athletic shoulder. *Journal of Orthopaedic & Sports Physical Therapy* 18:365-378.

Wilk, K.E., Voight, M.L., Keirns, M.A., Gambetta, V., Andrews, J.R., and C.J. Dillman. 1993. Stretch shortening drills for the upper extremities: Theory and clinical application. *Journal of Orthopaedic & Sports Physical Therapy* 17:225-239.

Zmierski, T., Kegerreis, S., and J. Scarpaci. 1995. Scapular muscle strengthening. *Journal of Sport Rehabilitation* 4:244-252.

18

Elbow and Forearm

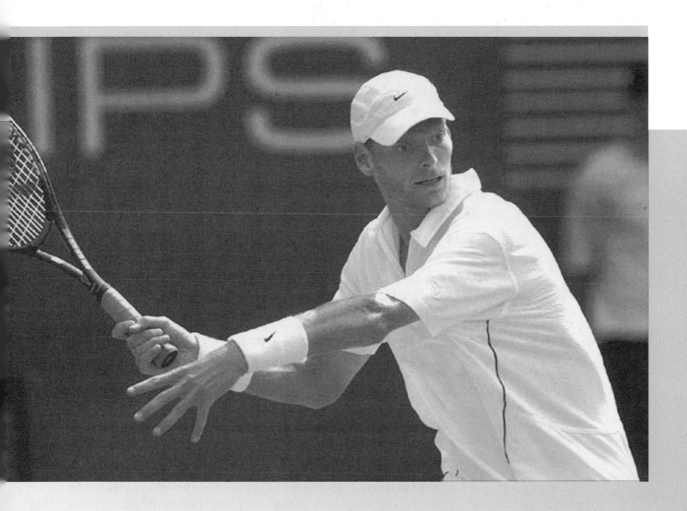

Objectives

After completing this chapter, you should be able to do the following:

1. Discuss why you should avoid overstretching the elbow, especially during the inflammation phase of healing.

2. Describe the convex-concave rules for the various elbow joints.

3. Identify the resting positions for the elbow joints.

4. Identify three soft-tissue mobilization techniques for the elbow.

5. List three joint mobilizations for the elbow.

6. Explain three strengthening exercises for the elbow, and their purpose.

7. Discuss the general progression of strengthening exercises for the elbow.

8. Outline a therapeutic exercise program for epicondylitis.

9. Indicate precautions to consider in a Little League elbow therapeutic exercise program.

10. List precautions, following an ulnar nerve transposition, for a therapeutic exercise program.

11. Explain the differences in rehabilitation programs for an arthroscopic debridement and a medial collateral reconstruction.

■ **The quality of a person's life is in direct proportion to their commitment to excellence, regardless of their chosen field of endeavor.**

Vince Lombardi, 1913-1970; Green Bay Packers Head Coach, 1959-1968

Like the spine and the shoulder, the elbow has special and distinct characteristics that must be considered in developing rehabilitation programs for elbow injuries. As the joint between two long lever arms, the elbow can experience large force applications from its proximal and distal arms. Open chain activities apply large velocities with sudden acceleration and deceleration forces from the proximal arm of the joint, while closed chain activities apply compressive stresses and torsional forces from the distal arm. The elbow muscles must work synchronously with adjacent structures, and the joint and muscles must have the flexibility necessary to withstand these forces.

Because the elbow lies between the shoulder and wrist, some muscles that traverse the elbow also affect the shoulder or wrist. It is difficult to separate these and thus was difficult to decide which chapter some of the techniques and exercises should be delegated to. It may seem that some of the techniques and exercises presented in this chapter would be better suited to the shoulder chapter or the wrist chapter. That may be the case, but how best to classify the exercise depends on the injury. For example, if a patient has a tennis-elbow injury, exercises and techniques for wrist extensor muscles are appropriately discussed in the context of the elbow. However, if a patient has a wrist sprain, those same techniques and exercises for wrist extensor muscles are best addressed in a discussion of wrist injuries. For this reason, some of the techniques and exercises you read about in this chapter are also referred to in the next chapter on the wrist and hand.

This chapter outlines basic considerations for elbow rehabilitation and then presents soft-tissue and joint mobilization techniques, flexibility and strength exercises, and plyometric and functional considerations. Distinctive considerations for some of the more commonly seen elbow injuries are discussed, and case studies for these injuries are presented so that you can problem solve and devise your own rehabilitation program.

GENERAL REHABILITATION CONSIDERATIONS

The elbow is unique in several ways, and the rehabilitation clinician needs to understand its distinctive characteristics to properly design and execute a therapeutic exercise program. The following sections focus on these characteristics.

▶ The design and execution of a therapeutic exercise program for the elbow must take into account the types of joint stresses incurred by the elbow, its unique structure, the mobility of its joints, and the amount of force application that is appropriate.

Joint Stresses

As mentioned in chapter 17, overhead motions are actually a total body movement that includes a summation of forces and properly timed execution of movement, started in the lower extremities and trunk and transferred to the shoulder, elbow, and hand. As the summation of forces accelerates the extremity in throwing sports, the elbow and forearm velocity must occur at high rates to successfully propel the hand or object at the desired speed. Researchers have reported different angular velocities for different sports. Baseball pitching produces the highest velocity at 2,300°/s (Feltner and Dapena 1986). Javelin athletes experience an angular velocity of 1,900°/s (Mero et al. 1994); the tennis serve has been recorded at 982°/s (Kibler 1995); and in fast-pitch softball, 680°/s velocities have been recorded (Ellenbecker and Mattalino 1997).

Most of these overhead motions place additional valgus or varus stress on the elbow joint. The greatest force applications occur during acceleration and deceleration phases of movement. High demands are placed on the biceps, brachioradialis, and brachialis during deceleration to slow forearm motion and prevent overextension and injury to the elbow. During acceleration the elbow experiences compressive forces laterally and distraction forces medially. The medial stresses can result in injuries such as neuritis, tendinitis, and medial joint sprains and muscle sprains. The lateral stresses can cause osteochondritis dissecans in young athletes, and bony osteophytes, articular damage, and degeneration in older athletes. It is common for athletes with an extended throwing career to develop flexion contractures because of articular and muscular changes. Proper mechanics, timing, and balanced joint and muscle function are crucial in the prevention of elbow injuries. If biomechanics are altered because of these deficiencies, the stresses are magnified. In pitching, the forces applied are a valgus distraction stress medially with a lateral compressive force. Tennis produces stress over the lateral epicondyle during the backhand stroke and medial epicondyle stresses during overhead serves and late-hit forehand strokes. Gymnastics, an upper-extremity weight-bearing sport, places excessive lateral stress on the joint because of the elbow's normal valgus position. Golfers with incorrect mechanics can place excessive medial force on the trailing elbow or excessive lateral force on the leading elbow. Pitchers with inflexibility of hips, trunk, or shoulder open up too soon and increase the elbow's medial joint stress. If tightness, weakness, or fatigue causes the elbow to drop, increased medial joint stresses are placed on the elbow during the cocking phase in pitching. In tennis, increased lateral stress is placed on the elbow when the player leads with the elbow on the backhand, and increased medial stress is applied on the forehand stroke when the ball is hit late.

It is important for the rehabilitation clinician to understand these concepts because the rehabilitation program should include an assessment of the patient's skill execution. Incorrect techniques may be the underlying cause of the problem, and the program must include correction of those techniques to prevent recurrence of the injury.

Unique Structure

The elbow has unique anatomical characteristics that can be advantageous or disadvantageous. The joint has a high degree of congruency within the ulnohumeral joint. That makes it stable. One of the more distinctive characteristics is that a muscle, not its tendon, traverses the joint. The brachialis muscle not only traverses the joint, but it also inserts onto the elbow's anterior superior capsule. This can cause problems when elbow immobilization is required following injury. Scarring and limitation of motion can easily occur in this area. Immobilization should be used cautiously, and extended periods of immobilization should be avoided. More than two weeks of immobilization can cause severe restrictions of the elbow's joint mobility. Complicating this reality that adhesions occur relatively easily in the elbow is the fact that the joint's anterior capsule is relatively thin and can easily incur damage with aggressive stretching, resulting in additional scarring. For this reason, it is important that aggressive, high-intensity stretching at the elbow be avoided. This is particularly crucial during the inflammation phase when the area is weaker and more easily aggravated than will be the case later. Soft-tissue tearing, scarring, and loss of joint motion can occur with passive overstretching. Early stretching techniques should include primarily active stretches. Passive range-of-motion exercises are permissible, but they should be pain free and should be performed in controlled and monitored situations.

Joint Mobility

The elbow has three joints that should be examined for joint mobility: the ulnohumeral, humeroradial, and radioulnar joints. Each joint has different resting and close-packed positions that you should recall when performing mobilization techniques. The ulnohumeral joint's resting position is at 70° elbow flexion with 10° supination, and its close-packed position is in full extension. The humeroradial joint's resting position is at full extension and full supination, and its close-packed position is at midflexion with midpronation. The radioulnar joint's resting position is at 70° elbow flexion with 35° supination, and its close-packed position is at full pronation or full supination. Joint mobilization should be performed initially in the resting position, where there is the greatest mobility and the least stress is applied to the joint. In later stages, it may be necessary to move the joint into other loose-packed positions to perform mobilizations. The close-packed position can also be used as an exercise position for unstable joints to provide increased stability during resistance activities.

Because the ulnohumeral and radiohumeral joints have the concave ulna and concave radius moving on the convex humerus, the concave-convex rule applies for mobilization techniques to these joints. The mobilization force application should be in the same direction as the restricted movement. Joint distraction applied in a resting position will stretch the anterior and posterior capsule. If the elbow is placed in flexion, and distraction is applied, the posterior capsule is stretched to increase elbow flexion; but if distraction is applied with the joint in extension, the anterior capsule is stretched to increase elbow extension.

The radius and ulna are connected by two joints, the proximal radioulnar joint at the elbow and the distal radioulnar joint at the wrist. Both joints must have normal movement to produce full supination and pronation. The proximal joint at the elbow is formed by the convex radial head in the concave ulnar notch. This joint abides by the convex-concave mobilization rule. The mobilization force application is in the opposite direction of restricted movement. To improve supination, the force is applied anterior to posterior; to improve pronation, the force is applied posterior to anterior.

Force Applications

Depending on the specific injury, the clinician may need to take special precautions with some strength exercises. Stresses applied to the elbow during strengthening can be excessive, depending on the arm position and the weight lifted. Lifting weights with the elbow extended places more stress on the anterior elbow, while lifting weights with the elbow flexed places more stress on the posterior elbow. Because of lever-arm lengths, a resultant force of up to three times body weight occurs when the elbow is flexed 30° (Ellenbecker and Mattalino 1997). Lighter weights or cuffs attached to the mid-forearm reduce these stresses.

An exercise such as a push-up delivers stress to the elbow, but the arm position determines the degree of stress. In a normal push-up position, the greatest compression force at the elbow is 45% of body weight, but the compression force is decreased if the hands are moved farther apart (Donkers et al 1993). In the superior position the compression force is decreased in the elbow, but the valgus torque is increased by 54% (Ellenbecker and Mattalino 1997).

Low-resistance, high-repetition strength exercises are commonly used in the early phases of elbow rehabilitation to reduce excessive stresses such as these on the joint. Once healing of tissue has occurred and neuromuscular control and strength gains are such that good joint control is possible, increased weights can be used.

REHABILITATION TECHNIQUES

Soft-Tissue Mobilization

▶ A therapeutic exercise program for the elbow includes trigger point release, ice-and-stretch, and cross-friction massage for the elbow movers and the wrist and finger movers, as well as cross-friction massage for elbow tendinitis.

The techniques addressed here are primarily trigger point release, ice-and-stretch, and cross-friction massage techniques. The trigger point referral patterns, trigger point releases, and ice-and-stretch procedures described here are based on the work of Travell and Simons (1983). The muscles mentioned here are also muscles that are addressed in chapter 19 on the wrist and hand, because most of the muscles originating at the elbow function at the wrist and hand.

It is important to note the locations of the patient's pain. Pain assessment necessitates investigation and elimination or confirmation of trigger points, neurological pathology, or localized injury as the source of the pain. If pain is not neurologically based, trigger points may often be the source, especially when the site of injury is different from the location of pain.

Elbow Movers

Along with pure elbow muscles, elbow movers also include muscles that cross the shoulder, biceps, and triceps but whose primary function is at the elbow.

Biceps Brachii

Trigger points of this muscle refer pain to the anterior deltoid and antecubital space, as well as into the suprascapular and distal biceps regions (figure 18.1, a and b). Trigger point release is performed with the patient supine or seated and the elbow slightly flexed and forearm supinated. The trigger points on the distal one third of the muscle are palpated first superficially, then more deeply for tender areas or taut bands. A strumming of the taut band, a deep pressure over the trigger point, or a pincher grasp on the muscle can be used (figure 18.1c).

Ice-and-stretch is performed with the patient sitting. The shoulder is abducted to 90°, laterally rotated, and horizontally abducted. The elbow is extended and the forearm pronated to put the biceps on stretch as ice sweeps are made from distal to the elbow proximally along the upper arm and to the shoulder (figure 18.1d).

Brachialis

The brachialis trigger points refer pain to the anterior carpometacarpal thumb joint and thumb's dorsal web space (figure 18.2a). They can also refer to the anterior arm and antecubital space (figure 18.2b). Trigger point release is performed with the patient supine or sitting and the elbow flexed about 45°. The biceps muscle is pushed medially to gain access to the brachialis (figure 18.2c). The distal trigger points most commonly refer to the thumb or antecubital space, and the more proximal points refer to the arm.

Ice-and-stretch is performed with the muscle on stretch and the patient in sitting or supine. The elbow is extended with support behind it as ice is stroked in the direction of pain referral from the elbow, either proximally along the arm or distally along the forearm to the thumb (figure 18.2d).

Triceps Brachii and Anconeus

The three heads of this muscle refer pain along the posterior arm to the shoulder and sometimes into the upper trapezius. They can refer pain into the lateral epicondyle, medial epicondyle, and olecranon process; along the lateral, posterior, or posterior forearm; along the posterior arm to the posterior shoulder; and to the fourth and fifth digits (figure 18.3, a–c). The anconeus muscle refers pain locally to the lateral epicondyle (figure 18.3d).

If the patient has good passive motion in a relaxed position but is unable to place the elbow next to the ear while the shoulder is in an end-flexion position and the elbow is fully extended, it is likely the patient has a triceps trigger point. Another position the patient will not achieve if a triceps trigger point is present is with the hand touching the scapula, fully flexing both the shoulder and elbow to achieve that position.

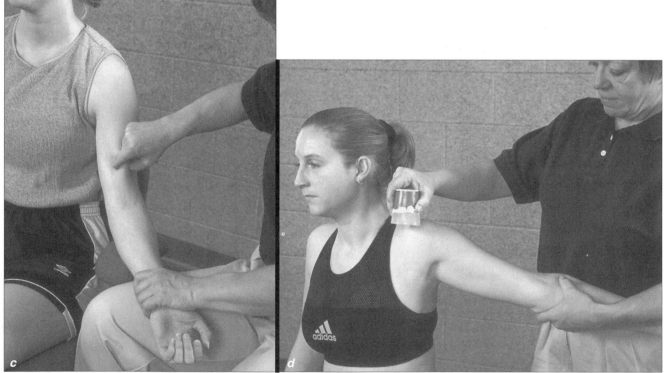

Figure 18.1 Biceps brachii: *(a-b)* pain-referral patterns, *(c)* trigger point release, *(d)* ice-and-stretch.

Figure 18.2 Brachialis: *(a-b)* pain-referral patterns, *(c)* trigger point release, *(d)* ice-and-stretch.

Trigger point release is performed with the muscle relaxed, the elbow in slight flexion, and the patient in supine. The taut band can be treated with a pincher grasp, or deep pressure over the trigger point sites can be used (figure 18.3e). Clusters of trigger points are often located in the medial and long triceps heads.

Ice-and-stretch is performed with the patient supine or sitting. The triceps is placed on stretch with the shoulder and elbow flexed as the ice is applied from the scapula along the posterior arm and forearm (figure 18.3f).

Figure 18.3
Triceps and anconeus: *(a-d)* pain-referral patterns, *(e)* trigger point release, *(f)* ice-and-stretch.

Supinator

The most common site of pain referral for this muscle is locally around the lateral epicondyle and lateral elbow region (figure 18.4a). The supinator can also refer to the dorsal thumb web space (figure 18.4b). A supinator trigger point is commonly seen with tennis elbow.

Trigger point release is performed with the elbow slightly flexed and fully supinated. The brachioradialis muscle is pushed laterally and deep pressure is applied to the supinator between the biceps tendon and brachioradialis muscle (figure 18.4c).

Ice-and-stretch is applied with the patient relaxed in supine or sitting. With the elbow in extension and the forearm in pronation, ice strokes are swept from the elbow in the direction of referred pain, either superiorly along the lateral arm or inferiorly along the radial aspect of the forearm to the thumb (figure 18.4d).

Figure 18.4 Supinator: *(a-b)* pain-referral patterns, *(c)* myofascial release, *(d)* ice-and-stretch.

Wrist and Finger Movers

It may seem odd to discuss wrist and finger muscles in the elbow chapter, but the long wrist and finger muscles also act on the elbow because they insert proximal to the elbow joint. Although their main function is in the distal upper extremity, the location of their proximal insertion necessitates attention to these muscles in the context of the elbow.

Wrist Extensors and Brachioradialis

Although the extensor carpi radialis rarely has active trigger points, the other muscles here are often activated with lateral epicondylitis. The radial extensors refer pain to the lateral epicondyle, to the hand's dorsum, and in the anatomical snuffbox area (figure 18.5, b and c). The ulnar extensors refer pain to the posterior ulnar wrist (figure 18.5a). The brachioradialis refers pain to the lateral epicondyle, to the thumb's web space, and less often along its muscle belly (figure 18.5d).

Trigger point release is performed with the patient in sitting and the relaxed forearm supported in partial flexion and full pronation. The wrist is hanging down in wrist flexion. The trigger points can be treated with either direct pressure (figure 18.5, e-g) or a pincher grasp (figure 18.5h).

Ice-and-stretch is performed with the patient supine or sitting and a support placed under the elbow. For the wrist extensors, the elbow is placed on stretch in an extended position, forearm pronated and wrist flexed as the ice strokes are swept from just above the elbow downward along the posterior forearm and past the wrist (figure 18.5i). For the brachioradialis, the stretch and ice sweeps are similar except that the wrist is placed in flexion with ulnar deviation and forearm pronation (figure 18.5j).

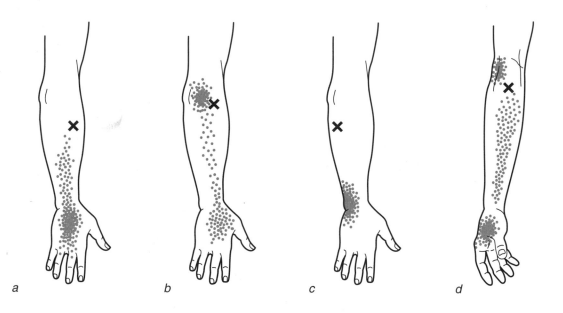

a　　　　b　　　　c　　　　d

Figure 18.5 Brachioradialis and wrist extensor myofascial release: *(a)* pain-referral patterns for extensor carpi radialis brevis, *(b)* extensor carpi radialis longus, *(c)* extensor carpi ulnaris, *(d)* brachioradialis. Trigger point release of *(e)* extensor carpi radialis longus, *(f)* extensor carpi radialis brevis, *(g)* extensor carpi ulnaris, *(h)* brachioradialis using pincher grasp. *(i)* Ice-and-stretch of wrist extensor, *(j)* brachioradialis.

Figure 18.5 *(continued)*

Finger Extensors

These muscles can refer pain during injuries such as lateral epicondylitis. They refer pain down the forearm along the back of the hand and to the fingers they move (figure 18.6, a–c). The lateral epicondyle is a common pain-referral site. Pain and stiffness of the fingers and hand can also be present even though the source of pain is more proximal.

Trigger point release is performed with the elbow in flexion, the forearm pronated, and the wrist flexed. The middle-finger extensor trigger point is located about 3 to 4 cm (1.2-1.6 in.) distally from the radial head and can be treated with direct pressure or a pincher grasp (figure 18.6d). The ring- and little-finger extensor trigger points are located deep and lateral to the extensor carpi ulnaris. The extensor indicis trigger point is distal on the forearm between the radius and ulna.

Ice-and-stretch is applied with the forearm supported, the elbow extended, and the wrist and fingers flexed as ice is swept distally from the muscle's proximal insertion on the lateral epicondyle toward the fingers (figure 18.6e).

Figure 18.6 Finger extensor myofascial release: *(a)* middle-finger extensor, *(b)* ring-finger extensor, *(c)* extensor indicis, *(d)* trigger point release, *(e)* ice-and-stretch.

Finger and Wrist Flexors, and Pronator Teres

The finger flexors refer into and beyond the end of the digits they move; patients commonly complain of an exploding, lightning-like pain that shoots out the end of the finger. The wrist flexors refer to the side of the wrist they flex, and the pronator teres refers to the radial wrist with overflow along the radial aspect of the anterior forearm and into the base of the thumb (figure 18.7, a–e).

Trigger point release is performed with the forearm supported and in supination. The wrist should be in a relaxed extension position. Deep pressure is applied to the trigger point areas (figure 18.7f).

Ice-and-stretch is applied with the patient sitting or supine. The forearm is supported in supination, and the elbow is extended. Ice strokes are swept from proximal to the medial epicondyle to distally along the anterior forearm to the wrist and into the digit being treated. an extension stretch is applied to the wrist and fingers while ice-and-stretch is performed (figure 18.7g).

Figure 18.7 Pain-referral patterns for: *(a)* flexor carpi radialis, *(b)* flexor carpi ulnaris, *(c)* flexor digitorum superficialis (dark 5 radial head, light 5 humeral head), *(d)* flexor pollicus longus, *(e)* pronator teres. *(f)* Pronator teres, and wrist and finger flexor trigger point release about 3 cm distal and slightly lateral to the medial epicondyle, *(g)* ice-and-stretch.

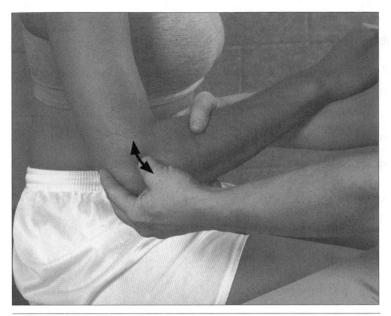

Cross-Friction Massage

This technique is usually performed over the lateral or medial epicondyle as part of the treatment for tendinitis. The area of tenderness is isolated with a finger or thumb pad. Pressure over the area is maintained while deep friction is applied to the area. The finger or thumb moves the overlying soft tissue against the underlying bone in a direction perpendicular to the fiber direction: Figure 18.8 shows application over the lateral epicondyle. Sometimes it may be necessary to pull the skin taut with the other hand while applying the cross-friction massage to maintain pressure over an isolated area. Mobile skin and subcutaneous tissue can easily cause the finger or thumb to move off the site.

Figure 18.8 Transverse friction massage.

JOINT MOBILIZATION

▶ Joint mobilization for the elbow addresses the ulnohumeral joint, the radiohumeral joint, and the proximal radioulnar joint.

The capsular pattern demonstrating capsular tightness in the elbow in flexion is more limited than in extension; supination and pronation are equally limited. A patient who presents with this type of motion loss should be treated with joint mobilization. Since three joints are enclosed in one capsule, capsular restriction can impact all the joints.

If the elbow is very inflamed, initial joint mobilization techniques are mild (grades I and II) for pain relief. Application of more aggressive grades (IIIs and IVs) should be postponed until the inflammation and elbow pain are under control. Aggressive techniques applied too soon may cause additional damage to the weak capsule.

Joint mobilization should be performed in the resting position when grades I and II are being applied, and in later stages during the initial applications of the more aggressive grades. This maximizes the effects of the mobilization techniques without aggravating the joint.

While applying joint mobilization, the clinician should always use good body mechanics. The hand applying the force should be positioned as close to the joint as possible. Keep in mind the principles of glide, roll, and spin so you apply forces properly to achieve the desired movement. Both the radial head and ulna are concave surfaces and move on a convex capitulum and convex trochlea, respectively, so force mobilization applications are in the same direction as the restricted movement. In the proximal radioulnar joint, however, the force is applied in the direction opposite the restricted movement because the convex-concave rule applies at this joint.

The joint mobilization techniques presented here are the most commonly used techniques for the elbow. As with any joint mobilization procedure, it is important to visualize the joint surfaces and apply the mobilization force parallel to the surface. You must respect precautions and contraindications, and you must consider the healing-tissue time line and strength of new tissue when deciding whether to apply joint mobilization and how much force to use. The elbow's anterior capsule relationship with the brachialis presents unique problems and must be approached cautiously. As always, application of joint mobilization to hypermobile joints is contraindicated. Improper technique, incorrect force application, excessive force, and inappropriate timing of application can all result in unnecessary injury or damage to the joint's structures. You must be aware of the appropriateness or inappropriateness of accessory and physiological joint mobilization application before you decide to use the techniques. If you are unsure, it is better to refrain from using joint mobilization.

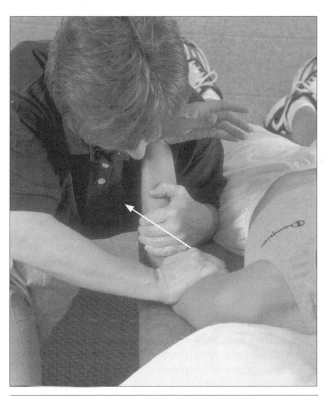

Figure 18.9   Ulnohumeral joint distraction mobilization.

Ulnohumeral Joint

This joint is also referred to as the humeroulnar joint. Although the elbow has three joints, the ulnohumeral joint is often considered the primary joint. Even though all three joints lie within the same capsule, joint mobilization for each joint can produce significant range-of-motion gains. The resting position for the ulnohumeral joint is 70° flexion with 10° supination.

Joint Distraction

This technique can be used with oscillation in grades I and II. Grade III most often uses sustained distraction. This technique is used for pain relief and relaxation in the lower grades (I and II) and to increase flexion and extension in the higher grades (III and IV). The patient lies supine with the elbow flexed to 70° and the forearm in slight supination. The patient's wrist rests against the clinician's shoulder. The humerus is fixated with a stabilization strap, with the help of an assistant or the rehabilitation clinician's hand. The rehabilitation clinician's hands are placed on top of each other around the proximal forearm near the elbow joint, or one hand is used if the other hand is stabilizing the patient's arm. The clinician applies a distraction force around the humeral axis by leaning backward (figure 18.9).

Medial Glide

This technique is used to improve elbow flexion or extension. The patient sits or stands, and the rehabilitation clinician faces and stands alongside the patient. The patient's forearm is positioned in the ulnohumeral joint's resting position and placed along the rehabilitation clinician's rib cage. The rehabilitation clinician's stabilizing hand's thenar eminence is placed against the patient's medial epicondyle while the mobilizing hand applies a sustained 10 s pressure against the radius to create a medial glide of the ulna with the humerus stabilized (figure 18.10). The pressure against the medial elbow may cause discomfort or injury to the ulnar nerve and must be applied with caution.

Figure 18.10   Medial ulnohumeral glide mobilization.

Lateral Glide

This technique can also be used to improve elbow flexion and extension. The patient and clinician positions are similar as for the medial glide except the clinician's hand placement is reversed so the stabilizing hand is on the patient's lateral epicondyle and the mobilizing hand applies a lateral pressure against the proximal ulna on the medial forearm.

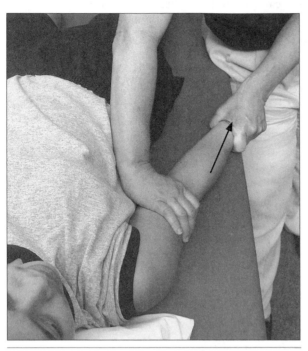

Figure 18.11   Radiohumeral distraction mobilization.

Radiohumeral Joint

This joint is also referred to as the humeroradial joint. The radiohumeral joint lies lateral to the ulnohumeral joint and should not be ignored when elbow capsular restriction is present. Mobilization of this specific joint can make significant differences in overall elbow mobility. The resting position for the radiohumeral joint is full extension with full supination.

Distraction

This technique is used to improve elbow extension and radial motion. The patient lies supine or sits in a chair with the arm slightly abducted and supported on the table. The joint is in its resting position. The rehabilitation clinician stabilizes the arm with a hand on the distal humerus and the index finger palpating the radiohumeral joint space. The mobilizing hand is placed around the distal radius but not on the distal ulna. The mobilization force is applied when the clinician laterally bends his or her trunk away from the patient's arm (figure 18.11). A traction force can be simultaneously applied to the joint.

Anterior and Posterior Glides

The anterior glide is also known as a posterior–anterior ventral glide and increases flexion. The posterior glide, also known as a dorsal anterior–posterior glide, increases extension. The patient lies supine with the arm supported on a towel roll on the table. The forearm is supinated, and the elbow is extended as far as possible. The rehabilitation clinician places the stabilizing hand on the medial distal humerus and the mobilizing hand on the proximal radius, with the fingers on the posterior aspect and the thenar eminence on the anterior aspect. To create a posterior glide, the thenar eminence moves the radial head posteriorly. To create an anterior glide, the fingers pull the radial head in a posterior-to-anterior direction (figure 18.12).

Figure 18.12 Radiohumeral anterior-posterior/posterior-anterior mobilization.

Figure 18.13 Radioulnar dorsal glide mobilization.

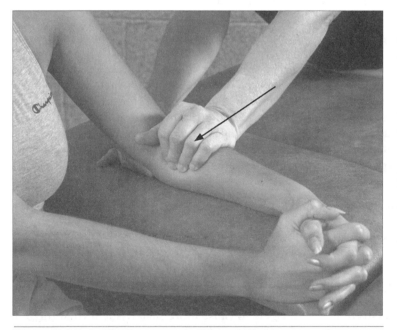

Figure 18.14 Radioulnar ventral glide mobilization.

Proximal Radioulnar Joint

Although this joint is not actually part of the elbow's flexion-extension joint, the fact that it lies within the same capsule with the other two elbow joints means that it should be considered part of the elbow. In fact, restriction of this joint can impact overall elbow movement and therefore should not be ignored. The resting position for the proximal radioulnar joint is 70° flexion with 35° supination.

Dorsal Glide

This technique is used to improve pronation. The patient is in sitting or supine with the arm supported on the table. The joint is placed in its resting position. The rehabilitation clinician faces the patient. The proximal ulna is stabilized by the medial hand, and the mobilizing hand is wrapped around the radial head with the thenar eminence on the anterior aspect. A downward pressure is exerted from the rehabilitation clinician's shoulder to move the radial head posteriorly (figure 18.13).

Ventral Glide

This technique is used to improve supination. The patient is sitting in a chair or supine with the forearm supported on the table. The elbow can be positioned either in the resting position in early treatments or closer to the closed-pack position for a more aggressive application in later treatments. The stabilizing hand is placed around the proximal ulna, and the mobilizing hand is placed around the head of the radius with the palm on the dorsal surface and the fingers anteriorly positioned. The radial head is moved with a posterior-to-anterior force, using primarily the heel of the hand (figure 18.14).

FLEXIBILITY EXERCISES

▶ Normal flexibility of the elbow is restored through use of prolonged stretches including equipment stretches, as well as active and assisted stretching.

The best way to achieve normal elbow flexibility is to prevent loss of motion. Methods of doing this include the use of continuous passive motion (CPM) machines, early mobilization following injury, and abbreviated periods of immobilization when appropriate. When loss of motion occurs, a variety of methods can be used to regain normal motion. The elbow heals as other areas of the body do, producing collagen that becomes scar tissue. As the collagen matures, stretching techniques and forces must change to affect the collagen arrangement and ultimately its strength. Short, active stretches can be used early to improve motion, but more prolonged stretches are necessary later when the collagen matures. These principles and guidelines are discussed in chapters 2 and 5.

Prolonged Stretches

Prolonged stretches to the elbow must be applied with caution. Light forces are applied so as not to disrupt the anterior capsule and still achieve greater joint motion. Prolonged stretches are used only after active stretches have not been successful in restoring elbow motion.

Night Splints

For patients whose motion gains are either difficult to achieve or are progressing slower than normal, a night splint can provide prolonged, low-level forces to effectively increase connective tissue lengthening. The patient wears the brace while sleeping but usually not during the day because the brace prevents the individual from using the arm. The force and angle of the brace can be adjusted to meet the individual patient's needs. It may take a couple of nights for the patient to adjust to the brace; however, continued wear, if tolerated, can significantly improve range of motion.

Equipment Stretches

Although they are not as long as the night-splint stretches, the stretches described in this section are considered prolonged stretches. The mere fact that they use equipment makes it more likely that application may be too aggressive. You must be careful to use less force than you think is needed, because a longer stretch duration has a significantly greater impact on tissues than a brief stretch using the same force. Rather than applying too much force and creating capsular damage, you should begin with a force lighter than you think necessary and increase it if the results and patient response indicate that this is appropriate.

Flexion-Extension Stretches

Often a variety of machines are readily available in the clinic to provide a prolonged stretch. These can be applied for at least 10 to 15 min and longer, if the patient is able to tolerate them. A few pounds of force are applied while the shoulder is stabilized. As discussed earlier, the elbow is unique in that a muscle belly crosses the joint and can complicate attempts to regain lost motion in the joint. You must be careful not to apply too much force and overstretch the soft tissue to cause more scar-tissue formation. The recommendation is to apply no more than 1.8 kg (4 lb) of force to a stretch to increase flexion range of motion. An isokinetic machine can be used to position the elbow on stretch in either flexion or extension with the speed set at zero to maintain the desired angle (figure 18.15a). An Iso-quad exercise unit can also be used to apply a prolonged stretch. If neither of these machines is available, the patient can use free weights in the supine position: a 4.5-kg (10-lb) weight at the shoulder to prevent the shoulder from elevating off the table, and a 1.8-kg (4-lb) weight attached to the wrist. The distal arm should have a towel roll under it to protect the elbow from excessive posterior pressure on the table (figure 18.15b).

Figure 18.15 Flexion-extension equipment stretches: *(a)* using an isometric machine set at zero speed to produce a prolonged stretch, *(b)* using a free-weight equipment stretch with 4.5 kg (10 lb) at the shoulder to stabilize it, and no more than 1.8 kg (4 lb) at the wrist to produce the stretch.

Pronation-Supination Stretches

A weighted bar can be used to increase either supination or pronation. The patient sits with the elbow supported on a table; the elbow is positioned directly under the shoulder. A bar, wand, or broom handle is held in the patient's hand with the forearm positioned at end range in either supination or pronation (figure 18.16). A more effective stretch is produced if the bar is secured in place with a strap wrapped around the hand and bar; this permits muscle relaxation to improve the stretch results. The position is maintained for at least 5 min.

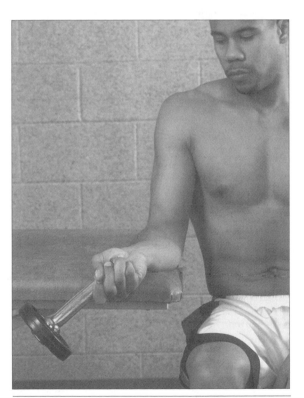

Figure 18.16 Supination equipment stretches.

Active Stretches

Active stretches are performed by the patient throughout the day. They do not require a great deal of equipment so are convenient and easy to apply. Active stretches can affect both muscle and joint structures.

Elbow Flexor Stretch

This exercise stretches the elbow flexors and anterior joint to increase extension. The patient sits or lies supine and places the uninvolved forearm across the abdomen to put the dorsum of the hand just above the involved posterior elbow. With the forearm supinated, the involved elbow is allowed to relax into extension and kept in this position for several minutes. This exercise can be easily performed throughout the day while the patient is sitting. Common substitutions for this stretch that patients should avoid include scapular protraction, forward trunk lean, and shoulder extension.

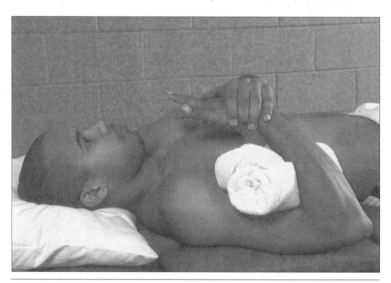

Figure 18.17 The elbow extensor stretch can be performed in supine or sitting.

Elbow Extensor Stretch

This exercise stretches the triceps and posterior joint to increase flexion. The patient grasps the involved forearm with the uninvolved hand. The elbow is stabilized next to the side or on a tabletop. The patient attempts to pull the involved forearm toward the shoulder with the uninvolved hand (figure 18.17). This stretch can be made more effective and more comfortable if a rolled-up towel or pad is placed in the antecubital fossa; the pad provides a distraction on the joint during the stretch. The stretch is held and repeated several times. The most common error for this exercise is shoulder extension and scapular retraction.

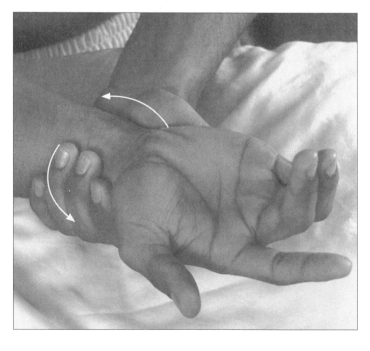

Pronator Stretch

This exercise increases supination and stretches the pronators. The patient sits with the elbow flexed to 90° and stabilized at the side. The forearm is positioned in as much supination as possible. The uninvolved hand is placed in an underhand grasp on the distal forearm so that the finger pads are on the volar aspect of the radius and the base of the hand is on the dorsal aspect of the ulna. The finger pads pull the radius downward as the base of the hand pushes the ulna upward (figure 18.18). The most common error in this stretch is movement inward by the elbow, and trunk lean toward the arm. The arm should be placed securely against the ribs to prevent movement during the stretch.

Figure 18.18 Pronator stretch.

Supinator Stretch

This stretch increases pronation by stretching the supinators. The patient sits with the elbow stabilized at the side and flexed to 90°. The forearm is actively positioned in as much pronation as possible. The patient grasps the distal forearm with the uninvolved hand in an overhand grasp by placing the finger pads around the ventral aspect of the ulna and the base of the hand on the dorsal aspect of the radius. The finger pads are pulled upward as the base of the hand is pushed downward (figure 18.19). A common error for this exercise is elbow movement away from the side as the shoulder abducts, and trunk lean away from the arm. The elbow must remain in contact with the lateral trunk.

Figure 18.19 Supinator stretch.

Assisted Stretches

The clinician should apply any stretch to the anterior joint cautiously. Overstretching this area can result in more adhesions or myositis ossificans. Contract-relax-stretch techniques with active contraction of the antagonists can be used in assistive stretches.

Elbow Flexion-Extension

These exercises are performed in sitting or supine, with the rehabilitation clinician supporting and stabilizing the elbow. The clinician's other hand is placed on the wrist. The stretch to increase flexion is applied by the rehabilitation clinician's hand at the patient's wrist, with the patient's hand moving toward his or her shoulder. Placing the clinician's other hand or a rolled-up towel in the antecubital fossa provides joint distraction to make the stretch more comfortable and more effective. This exercise should be performed in supination and pronation and can be controlled by the clinician's distal hand on the patient's wrist. If not properly stabilized, the shoulder can elevate to give a false impression of improved range of movement. The long head of the triceps can be stretched with the patient in sitting. The elbow is flexed by the clinician's hand on the distal forearm. The shoulder is then flexed overhead by the other hand on the patient's elbow (figure 18.20a).

To increase extension, the rehabilitation clinician applies the stretch by supporting the elbow and guiding the shoulder into hyperextension as the elbow is extended (figure 18.20b). This stretches the biceps and other anterior elbow structures. The shoulder should not protract during the stretch. The biceps is stretched when the forearm is in pronation, but the stretch should also be applied in supination.

Figure 18.20 Assisted elbow flexion-extension stretches: *(a)* stretch for long head of the triceps, *(b)* stretch for the biceps.

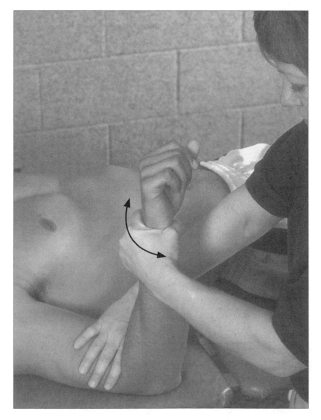

Supination-Pronation Stretches

These forearm stretches should be performed with the elbow flexed and extended. The patient can be sitting or supine. The rehabilitation clinician places the stabilizing hand on the distal arm, and the other hand grasps the wrist and supports the hand. The radius is rolled around the ulna, with overpressure applied at the end of each range in supination and pronation (figure 18.21). The arm must be stabilized so the shoulder is not allowed to abduct or adduct. The distal force application should be applied such that the stretch occurs at the radioulnar joints, avoiding a twisting of the hand.

Figure 18.21 Assisted supination-pronation stretches.

STRENGTHENING EXERCISES

▶ Strengthening exercises for the elbow use isometric resistance, manual resistance, straight-plane resistance, plyometrics, carryover shoulder exercises, and isokinetics in a careful progression.

As with other joints, the most basic elbow strengthening exercises include isometrics. Isotonic exercises in straight-plane motions advance to diagonal-plane motions before plyometric exercises become a part of the strength progression. The final part of the therapeutic exercise program includes the functional exercises before the patient's return to full participation.

Isometric Resistance Exercises

The patient can perform the following resistance exercises independently and frequently throughout the day. Each exercise is held for 6 s and repeated around 10 times each session. The patient should demonstrate correct execution of the exercises before performing them independently.

Elbow Flexion

The involved elbow is flexed, and the patient's other hand is placed on the distal forearm. The patient attempts to move the elbow into flexion while using the opposing hand to resist the movement (figure 18.22). This exercise should be performed in supination, pronation, and neutral, as well as at several different angles of elbow flexion.

Elbow Extension

For this exercise the resistance is applied to the distal forearm as the patient attempts to extend the elbow. This exercise should be performed at several different positions in the range of motion.

Manual-Resistance Exercises

Straight-plane manual resistance is provided by the rehabilitation clinician. It is important that the elbow moves through the full range of motion. The movement should be smooth, so the clinician needs to alter the resistance force according to changes in the patient's strength as the elbow moves through the range of motion. If an area of weakness is present, the rehabilitation clinician can offer an isometric resistance at that point in the motion before proceeding through the remaining motion; if an isometric is used, the patient should be informed prior to performing the exercise. You can begin manual resistance early and use it throughout the rehabilitation program, because you can easily alter the resistance to meet the resistance needs and still respect tissue-healing precautions.

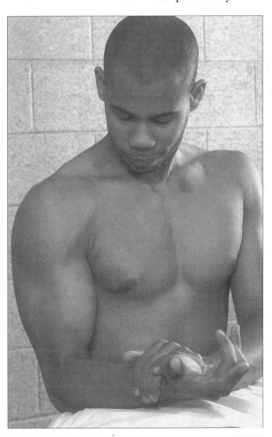

Figure 18.22 Isometric flexion.

Elbow Flexion-Extension

The best position for strengthening exercises is with the forearm in an antigravity position. This utilizes the weight of the forearm as additional resistance. For elbow flexion the patient is sitting or supine. Supine position is preferred because the elbow is more easily stabilized and able to go through a full range of motion. The rehabilitation clinician stabilizes the shoulder with one hand and resists elbow flexion with the other hand over the distal forearm (figure 18.23a). To resist primarily the biceps, the forearm is supinated. To eliminate the biceps and resist primarily the brachialis, the forearm is pronated. To add more resistance to the brachioradialis, the forearm is in neutral. Common substitutions in this exercise include shoulder flexion, shoulder shrugging, and scapular retraction.

Elbow extension is performed with the patient prone to maximize gravity's effect at end-range extension. The arm is abducted and supported on the table, with the forearm hanging over the side. A towel support is placed under the distal arm to increase patient comfort and elevate that arm to a level position on the table. The rehabilitation clinician stabilizes the arm with one hand and provides resistance to elbow extension at the distal forearm with the other (figure 18.23b). This exercise can also be performed with the patient in sitting with the shoulder fully elevated and the elbow overhead. This position provides maximal gravity resistance in the middle of the range of motion. A common substitution is scapular protraction.

Figure 18.23 Manual resistance: *(a)* resisted elbow flexion in supination, *(b)* resisted elbow extension.

Figure 18.24 Manual resistance to supination and pronation.

Supination-Pronation

This exercise can be performed with the patient sitting or supine. The elbow is flexed to 90°, and the rehabilitation clinician places both hands around the patient's distal forearm. As the patient supinates, the rehabilitation clinician provides resistance to the movement. Resistance is reversed for pronation (figure 18.24). The elbow should be held to the patient's side to prevent shoulder abduction with pronation and adduction with supination.

Straight-Plane Resisted Exercises

It is important for the patient to perform these exercises through a full range of motion in a slow and controlled manner.

Flexion

Depending on the forearm position, the biceps, brachialis, and/or brachioradialis are strengthened. Supination emphasizes the biceps, pronation emphasizes the brachialis, and neutral works the brachioradialis.

The patient stands with the uninvolved hand behind the involved distal arm just above the elbow. The weight is held in the hand in a supinated, pronated, or neutral position as the patient slowly flexes the elbow (figure 18.25a). In this position the maximum resistance occurs at midrange. The hand is held behind the elbow to stabilize the arm and prevent use of the shoulder to lift the weight, the most common substitution in this exercise. Another substitution is to heft the weight up with a sudden shrug movement of the shoulder or the use of momentum. If this occurs, lower the resistance.

An alternative position is with the shoulder flexed to 90° and the arm supported to maintain this position while the elbow is flexed against resistance (figure 18.25b). This position provides maximum resistance in the beginning of the exercise.

This exercise can also be performed with rubber tubing or pulleys. The pulley or tubing is anchored low, near the ground, if maximum resistance is to occur at midrange. Changing the anchor position changes the point in the motion where maximum resistance occurs. Refer to chapter 7 for additional information on joint positions and maximum resistance. It is important to stabilize the arm by placing the opposite hand behind the upper arm as seen in figure 18.25c.

Figure 18.25 Elbow flexion: *(a)* maximum resistance occurs at 90° elbow flexion, *(b)* maximum resistance occurs at the start of elbow flexion, *(c)* maximum resistance can change in the ROM, depending on where the rubber band or pulley is positioned relative to elbow motion.

Extension

This exercise strengthens the triceps and anconeus. To provide maximum resistance at mid-range, the exercise is performed with the shoulder elevated overhead so that the elbow is directly over the shoulder. The arm position is maintained with support from the opposite hand (figure 18.26a). If the long head of the triceps is to be emphasized less, the exercise can be performed with the patient supine (figure 18.26b).

To emphasize resistance at end range, the patient leans over at the waist in standing or lies prone on a table with the arm parallel to the floor and the elbow flexed. The elbow is extended alongside the body in either the trunk flexion or prone position (figure 18.26c). A common substitution is shoulder extension.

Equipment such as the latissimus pulldown bar can also be used to strengthen elbow extensors. The patient positions the bar so that the elbows are at the sides and flexed. Maintaining arm position, the patient lowers the bar by extending the elbows (figure 18.26d).

Figure 18.26 Elbow extension: *(a-b)* maximum resistance occurs at 90°, *(c)* maximum resistance occurs at end range, *(d)* using the latissimus pull-down bar to strengthen triceps.

Supination

This exercise is performed with the patient sitting and the forearm supported over the end of a table. A weighted bar is held at one end with the forearm in pronation. The patient rotates the bar upward until the bar is pointing toward the ceiling for a concentric exercise (18.27a). To perform an eccentric exercise the patient returns to the start position with palm turned down. Common errors with this exercise include letting the weight fall rather than controlling its movement and speed, shoulder adduction, and elbow extension.

Pronation

In this exercise, the patient is seated as for the supination exercise just described. The patient begins with the forearm in full supination and rotates the bar into pronation to the midposition for a concentric exercise, and then returning to full supination for an eccentric exercise (18.27b). Substitutions for this exercise include shoulder abduction and elbow flexion. The weight should be controlled throughout the range of motion.

It is incorrect to use a dumbbell to perform this exercise, because one end of the dumbbell will act as a counterbalance force for the other end, making the exercise ineffective.

Figure 18.27 *(a)* Supination, *(b)* pronation.

Plyometric Exercises

The patient progresses to diagonal-plane (multiplane) activities after good strength in straight-plane exercises is achieved. These exercises are more strenuous since they demand simultaneous muscle performance in multiple planes, continued control of the extremity, and accuracy of performance. These exercises serve as a transition phase and prepare the elbow and its surrounding structures for the next phase, functional activities.

Carryover Shoulder Exercises

Many of the closed kinetic chain exercises discussed in chapter 17 are appropriate for the elbow. Instead of repeating details here, I suggest that you refer to chapter 17 for a listing and for information about progression of these exercises. The push-up, seated push-up, Swiss-ball weight-bearing exercises, rhythmic stabilization activities, and distal movement stabilization exercises are all appropriate for the elbow.

Rubber tubing diagonal patterns in D1 and D2 flexion and extension can incorporate elbow movements or flexion or extension, or can maintain a stationary elbow position throughout the patterns. Which pattern to use depends on the patient's sport. For example, a pitcher or tennis player should use D2 flexion and extension patterns, because those patterns most closely mimic the motions in those sports. A breaststroke swimmer, on the other hand, should use D1 flexion and extension patterns.

Unstable-surface activities as discussed in chapter 17 are recommended for middle-phase elbow rehabilitation. Resisted movements using the treadmill or stair machine, and medicine-ball exercises and their progressions, are also applicable for elbow therapeutic exercise progressions.

Isokinetics

Isokinetic equipment is used initially in straight-plane exercises with stabilization and isolation of desired motions during middle-phase and late-phase rehabilitation. Elbow flexion-extension and forearm pronation-supination can all be performed on the equipment. As the patient progresses, diagonal patterns can be used as a progression into more-functional exercises.

FUNCTIONAL ACTIVITIES

▶ Functional activities for the elbow, progressing in distances, forces, and speeds, prepare the patient for return to sport participation.

Once the patient is able to meet the challenge of plyometric exercises, functional activities are the next logical step and the final preparation before one allows a full return to normal activities. Many of the functional programs discussed in chapters 10 and 17 can be used very appropriately for the elbow. Of course, specific applications depend on the patient's sport or activity.

Functional exercises should include warm-up and cool-down activities. Overhead activity progressions should begin with easy activities at diminished distances, forces, and speeds and should gradually increase only one component at a time until the patient performs all activities at normal performance levels. Increases should occur no more often than every third exercise session to permit adequate adaptation to increased stress levels. If a patient experiences pain with any increase, he or she should return to the previous level of exercises for an additional three days before attempting to try the next level again.

Rather than repeating programs that have already been described, I suggest that you refer to chapters 10 and 17 for details on programs, their progressions, and the precautions that guide those progressions.

SPECIAL REHABILITATION APPLICATIONS

▶ Common elbow injuries that warrant special considerations in therapeutic exercise program design are epicondylitis, Little League elbow, sprains, ulnar nerve injury, dislocation, and postarthroscopy conditions.

We will now look at rehabilitation programs for some of the more common elbow injuries. For each injury, specific aspects unique to that injury and the rehabilitation program for that injury are presented. These discussions are followed by a case study for you to solve that will enable you to apply your new knowledge of elbow rehabilitation.

Epicondylitis

Epicondylitis or tendinitis is commonly seen in the elbow. As discussed in chapter 15, among the most important aspects of treatment of these conditions are discovering and correcting the cause of the problem. If you do not correct the cause of the injury, the risk of its recurring is very high. Because the elbow sits on either side of two long lever arms, it can be susceptible to tendinitis, especially when the forces applied are exaggerated because of poor technique.

Program Considerations

Lateral epicondylitis is often referred to as tennis elbow, and medial epicondylitis is commonly known as golfer's elbow. These both come under the general heading of tendinitis and usually result from cumulative trauma. Lateral epicondylitis most commonly involves the extensor carpi radialis brevis. It is the result of various improper techniques on the tennis backhand, including hitting the ball too late or flipping the wrist into extension. Medial epicondylitis is seen in golfers who throw the club down with the back arm to hack at the ball rather than moving the club through with the trunk and front arm. Tennis players who hit a forearm stroke with the elbow ahead of the racket and gymnasts who bear weight on hyperextended elbows are also subject to medial epicondylitis.

In either tennis elbow or golfer's elbow, the patient experiences a gradual onset of epicondyle pain. It may begin with pain only after activity. Then it may progress to some pain at the start of activity that resolves as the activity continues but returns after activity. Eventually, pain occurs with daily activities and then at rest. Grasping objects and shaking hands are painful. Extending the wrist against resistance in lateral epicondylitis and flexing the wrist against resistance in medial epicondylitis are painful. The pain is localized to the epicondyle, but if left untreated can extend into the muscle bellies of the forearm. Pronation or supination activities can become painful. Grip strength weakens, as does wrist flexion or extension for medial or lateral epicondylitis, respectively. Pain can restrict full range of wrist motion, especially when it is combined with elbow extension.

As with other tendinitis treatments, the cause of the injury must be determined and corrected to diminish the risk of reinjury. The inflammation must be treated and deficiencies rehabilitated. Modalities such as ultrasound, phonophoresis, and iontophoresis are commonly used for these conditions. Cross-friction massage to the tender epicondylar areas is used to reduce tissue adhesions and increase local circulation. Weakness and loss of flexibility are often secondary occurrences with epicondylitis. Elbow, wrist, and finger flexion and extension and forearm supination and pronation should be returned to normal ranges of motion through a variety of flexibility exercises. If joint mobility is restricted, mobilization techniques are indicated. End-range stretches and mobilizations should not be aggressive, especially in the early rehabilitation phases when inflammation is significant. Patients who have been long-term participants in tennis or throwing sports may have developed flexion contractures and valgus deformities. These may result from repetitive microtears, scarring, and ossification of the flexor muscles and anterior capsule or hypertrophic bone changes (Ellenbecker and Mattalino 1997). In the presence of these ossification changes, attempts to stretch the elbow are frustrating and are not advised. During the early rehabilitation phase, stretching exercises should be active and within the patient's comfort range.

In the middle rehabilitation phase, if normal range of motion is still lacking, mobilization should be initiated. If a bony end-feel is palpated at less than normal extension, the patient may have structural changes that prohibit full extension. If the end-feel is capsular, however, joint mobilization techniques are indicated. Joint mobility of the wrist, forearm, and elbow is a consideration for epicondylitis treatment because muscles originating on the epicondyle affect wrist and forearm movement. If the muscles are not moved through their full range of motion, loss of mobility can occur. Specific wrist mobilizations and flexibility exercises are discussed in chapter 19. In addition to mobilization techniques, active assistive and passive stretching exercises can be used to improve wrist, forearm, and elbow motion in this phase.

Strengthening includes isometrics, eccentrics, concentrics, and plyometrics that are provided in a progression. Chapter 15 contains information on the rationale for and progression of exercises in the treatment of tendinitis. Isometrics should be used in the early rehabilitation phase if the tendons are very inflamed and other strength exercises are too painful. Effective strengthening exercises for tendinitis include an eccentric exercise program (Stanish et al. 2000. This starts with submaximal eccentric exercises using weights or rubber tubing and progresses to more aggressive use of heavier weights with increased speeds as tolerated by the injury. In the early rehabilitation phase, shoulder and trunk exercises should be included to maintain conditioning levels in these areas.

Middle-phase rehabilitation includes the use of diagonal motions, increased resistance, and more functional patterns of movement to prepare the injury for plyometric exercises. Many exercises in this phase are those listed in the shoulder rehabilitation program in chapter 17. Motions begin in a slow and controlled manner and progress to faster movements while the patient maintains control of the arm throughout the motion. Closed kinetic chain exercises and neuromuscular facilitation exercises are used in this phase. Isokinetic exercises, first in straight planes and then in diagonal planes, are suitable in this phase. Isokinetic exercises should be at higher speeds and should emphasize muscle endurance. In later stages of the middle phase, the patient can use the isokinetic equipment to perform full-body initiated and diagonal activities that mimic normal motions. All exercises should remain pain free with no associated post-exercise discomfort.

Plyometrics in the final phases of rehabilitation emphasize functional movements that prepare the patient for functional exercises before returning to full participation. These exercises are discussed in chapter 17. The progression is the same as that presented for the shoulder, beginning with easier plyometrics and advancing to higher-speed and/or more resistance as the injured segment adapts and the patient is able to tolerate increased stresses. It is during this phase that the isokinetic exercises are performed in functional patterns, using total-body performance positions. They should mimic normal activity patterns of movement as closely as possible.

Functional activities are individually determined and are based on the patient's sport and activity requirements. Guidelines for functional activity progressions are universal and are based on the patient's response to the exercises. As a rule, increases occur no more frequently than every third day. Only one parameter is increased at one time. In other words, if a pitcher increases throwing distance on a particular day, speed of the throw is not changed on the same day. In fact, it may be prudent to reduce the speed when increasing distance and to gradually build up the throwing speed to the levels that were being attained before the distance increase. If the patient experiences pain with any program increase, he or she returns to the immediately preceding program level for another three sessions before advancing.

Bracing can assist the patient in pain-free performance. A counter-force brace is approximately 5 cm (2 in.) wide or slightly larger and is made of nonelastic strapping, usually secured with Velcro (figure 18.28). Its purpose is to reduce wrist extensor activity and disperse the stresses applied to the extensor tendons (Groppel and Nirschl 1986). The brace should be worn during the treatment phase and also when the patient returns to normal participation.

Figure 18.28   Counterforce brace.

Before the racket-sport patient begins functional activities prior to returning to competition, his or her equipment should be examined for appropriateness. Racket weight, stiffness, and size should be evaluated. A heavy racket requires greater strength, energy expenditure, and muscle endurance. A stiff racket allows the patient to exert greater power on the ball, but it also absorbs less impact stress and transfers the unabsorbed stress to the patient's arm. A tightly strung racket also increases impact-stress transfer to the arm, so a patient returning to participation may be advised to reduce the string tension of the racket slightly. A combination of a less stiff racket and less string tension permits more force absorption in the racket because the ball is in contact with the racket longer (Newton's second law of motion). As the impact force is spread out over a longer period of time, it is reduced.

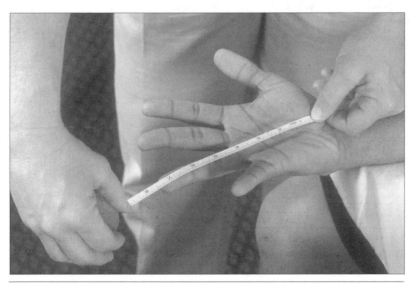

Figure 18.29   Racket-grip measurement.

Grip size is another factor that requires assessment before the patient uses a racket. A grip that is too small can increase the strength requirements, add stress to the epicondyles, and increase fatigue of the forearm muscles. Proper grip size is determined by measuring the distance from the tip of the ring finger to the proximal palmar crease (Nirschl 1977) (figure 18.29). To measure grip size, place the hand flat on a table top with the palm facing up and fingers extended. Extend a tape measure along the palm and to the end of the fingers between the third and fourth fingers. The distance to the nearest eighth of an inch between the middle palm crease and the height of the fourth finger tip is the person's grip size.

Occasionally, surgery is necessary to completely resolve more persistent cases of epicondylitis. In lateral epicondylitis, the extensor carpi radialis brevis tendon is detached from the lateral epicondyle, and debridement of the area is the common procedure. Medial surgical release commonly involves the pronator teres and flexor carpi ulnaris tendons.

Postoperative rehabilitation includes the use of an elbow immobilizer immediately after surgery and continuing for about one week. The brace may be continued for occasional support when the elbow gets fatigued, for up to three weeks postoperatively. Active range-of-motion exercises for the wrist and fingers can start after surgery, although the patient will probably not want to begin these until at least the second postoperative day. Gentle active and active assistive range of motion of the elbow can begin around day 5. By the third week the patient should have full range of motion.

At two weeks, active exercise against gravity without resistance can begin, as can squeezing a soft ball. Pronation and supination motion exercises for the elbow and wrist, as well as flexion and extension motion exercises, should continue.

By three weeks, low-resistance, low-repetition exercises can start with isometrics and straight-plane exercises. Full motion should be present by this time. The patient progresses as tolerated into higher-repetition exercises before moving into heavier weights.

Diagonal-plane exercises can begin at four to eight weeks, depending on the patient's pain tolerance and strength. Once the patient displays good strength and control without pain in diagonal motions, it is appropriate to begin plyometrics.

By three to four months, the patient can begin functional activities if there is no pain with plyometrics and if normal strength, muscle endurance, and flexibility are present. Patients undergoing medial epicondylar releases may not be able to return to full participation for five to six months, and those undergoing lateral epicondylar releases may return to function four to five months postoperatively.

Case Study

A 24-year-old, right-hand-dominant female tennis player has been playing with tennis elbow for the past six months. It started when she bought a new Kevlar tennis racket and began attempting to put topspin on her serve. The condition has advanced to a level such that she now has pain throughout her game; she is not playing well any more, has a difficult time opening doors and turning the key to start her car, and is unable to carry her gym bag in the right hand. The forearm feels stiff most of the time. Examination reveals tenderness over the lateral epicondyle extending into the proximal forearm along the radial wrist extensors. Resisted wrist extension is weak and painful. Grip strength measured with a grip dynamometer on the right is 15.8 kg (35 lb) and painful compared to the pain-free left grip strength of 34 kg (75 lb). Her wrist flexion range of motion is limited to 45° because of pain. There is no restriction of joint accessory movements. Passive elbow extension increases the wrist flexion pain.

Questions for Analysis

1. What will your first treatment session include?

2. What are your initial treatment goals?

3. What will be your instructions to the patient in the first treatment?

4. How do you plan to increase her range of motion?

5. Outline your program for strengthening the wrist and identify the guidelines you will use.

6. What suggestions regarding equipment will you make to the patient?

7. Describe a functional activity progression for the patient and identify the criteria you will use to determine when she is ready to return to full participation in tennis.

Little League Elbow

Little League elbow is another type of inflammation of the elbow, but it is unique because it occurs only in youngsters. Its name comes from the population it is most frequently seen in, pitchers of Little League baseball. It has been a common enough problem that youth league governing bodies have attempted to regulate pitching in this population, but the problem remains. Special issues surrounding this injury are presented before a case study is provided for you to solve.

Program Considerations

Little league elbow is unique to the preadolescent population. It involves a number of conditions that have the common thread of elbow pathology secondary to pitching. The most common site of pathology is the medial elbow because of the excessive traction forces applied to the medial epicondyle epiphyseal plate during acceleration. Curves and breaking pitches increase the demands on wrist flexion and pronation, increasing the medial epicondyle stresses. Injury to the inherently weak epiphyseal plate may begin as an inflammation and can progress to an avulsion of the plate with repetitive trauma. In severe cases, osteochondritis dissecans of the radioulnar joint can occur.

Less frequently, the lateral, anterior, or posterior elbow is affected by excessive stresses applied during throwing. The pronator teres increases stresses laterally during extreme pronation, and increased hyperextension forces on follow-through can increase anterior and posterior joint stresses.

In the more common medial Little League elbow, the athlete experiences progressive medial elbow pain with activity, pain with end-motion finger and wrist extension, tenderness to medial epicondyle palpation, and pain and weakness with resisted wrist and finger flexion. Swelling and, in more severe cases, ecchymosis, can be present over the medial epicondyle.

Common causes for little league elbow are improper warm-up or lack of warm-up, improper or insufficient conditioning, poor pitching mechanics, inadequate rest between games, pitching too many innings, and pitching curves and breaking-ball pitches. It is recommended that adequate conditioning programs and proper warm-up and cool-down procedures be included in a team's program, and that adherence to Little League baseball pitching rules be enforced for practices as well as games. Those rules include permitting an adolescent to pitch no more than six innings and mandating rest of three days between pitching rotations. Patients should avoid those activities that produce little league elbow. If an injury occurs, it becomes even more important for the patient to adhere to recommendations that minimize elbow stresses.

If growth plate damage is evident with the injury, the individual should be advised to stop pitching for the rest of the baseball season. Early-phase treatment for little league elbow includes rest, ice, and in advanced cases, immobilization. Active range-of-motion exercises to tolerance are encouraged. Passive stretches should be avoided. Because of the age of the patient, using heavy weights is not advisable because these could aggravate sensitive growth plates. Exercises are neither as aggressive nor as intensive as they are for adult patients, but the program should follow the same progression. This progression emphasizes range of motion and calming of the inflammation in the initial rehabilitation phase, with advancement to a progressive strengthening program before functional activities are initiated. Valgus stress should be avoided until it does not cause pain. A gradual throwing progression is included when the elbow is pain free and has full range of motion and normal muscle strength and muscle endurance.

Sprains

Sprains in the elbow most commonly occur as hyperextension injuries. Capsular injury of the elbow can be frustrating if not treated correctly at the very beginning. Special considerations relating to this type of injury are presented followed by a case study.

Program Considerations

The most common sprains in the elbow occur as a hyperextension injury or a medial collateral ligament sprain. A hyperextension sprain can occur when a football opponent runs into and past an outstretched blocking arm or when a gymnast does a handstand. Any sudden valgus force such as a sidearm throw by a shortstop, or a wrench of the elbow by a wrestling

---

Case Study

A nine-year-old baseball pitcher is in the middle of his season. For the past month he has experienced progressive medial elbow pain on his left throwing elbow. He is the team's top pitcher and usually pitches three days a week. An invitational tournament his team is competing in is planned for next weekend, and he wants to pitch. His parents are reluctant to allow him to do so, but they want your opinion. He has full range of motion of the elbow, but wrist extension is painful in the last 10°. Resisted pronation and wrist flexion are weak and painful. The medial epicondyle is tender to palpation and edematous.

Questions for Analysis

1. What will be your recommendation to the patient regarding the weekend invitational tournament?

2. What will be your recommendations on future pitching?

3. What treatment procedure will you recommend he follow to reduce the pain and inflammation?

4. What will be your instructions about exercises he should perform?

5. How much information will you give the patient's parents?

opponent, can also cause a sprain. In a hyperextension injury, the anterior capsule is injured; but in a medial collateral stress injury, the medial or ulnar collateral ligament (UCL), the primary stabilizing unit for the elbow, is injured.

Hyperextension injuries cause pain in the anterior joint and can also cause a bone contusion and pain of the olecranon or olecranon fossa. Ulnar collateral ligament sprains cause medial joint pain. A support brace may be used during the first couple of weeks following injury to support and protect the area. Initial rehabilitation includes treatment to relieve pain and swelling. Cross-friction massage to adherent scar tissue in the area can also relieve pain but should not be performed within the first 7 to 10 days following injury. Active and active assistive ranges of motion are used in the early phase, along with mild straight-plane strengthening exercises. Pain during activity should be avoided. Strengthening exercises should include the biceps and triceps, as well as wrist and finger flexors and extensors and forearm pronators and supinators. Following hyperextension injuries, the biceps, brachialis, brachioradialis, and supinator play an important role in providing dynamic stability anteriorly, and the triceps and biceps co-contract to provide weight-bearing stability. Following a UCL sprain, the supinators can assist in stability. Resistance to the flexor carpi ulnaris may aggravate the UCL in early rehabilitation and should be deferred until the middle rehabilitation phase. By the middle phase, full range of motion of the elbow should be present. Strengthening exercises for the flexor carpi ulnaris in wrist flexion and ulnar deviation should be instituted if they haven't yet been initiated. Straight-plane exercises continue, but resistance and repetition levels can increase. Eccentric and concentric exercises are used. By the end of the middle phase, diagonal-plane movements can begin with proprioceptive neuromuscular facilitation stabilization activities and closed kinetic chain exercises; rubber tubing can be added as long as the stresses do not cause pain either during or after the exercise. Isokinetics are appropriate, beginning with straight-plane movement and progressing to diagonal planes of movement.

In the late phase, plyometric exercises begin. These are the same exercises as those described for epicondylitis. Functional planes of movement are used during these exercises. The patient should be able to maintain good joint stability during all activities. The goal in this final phase is to prepare the injury site for functional activities.

Ulnar collateral ligament repair

Instability of the elbow occurs primarily in tears of the UCL. In these cases, surgical repair may be required if conservative care does not resolve the instability. Postoperative rehabilitation depends on the surgical technique used. Surgical reconstruction is performed using an autogenous graft with detachment of the flexor/pronator tendon group if the ligament lacks any viable tissue. This situation requires a longer postoperative rehabilitation process than when the ligament contains viable tissue and can be salvaged without detaching the flexor/pronator mass.

Following surgery, the elbow is locked at 90° in an adjustable elbow flexion splint for the first week. During this time, the patient can perform active wrist and finger motion exercises. Submaximal isometric exercises for the biceps and the shoulder can occur as long as the patient avoids shoulder lateral rotation, which would increase valgus elbow stress. The patient can also squeeze a ball.

By the end of the second week, the brace's motion stops are positioned 30° from extension and at 100° of flexion. Submaximal wrist and elbow isometrics can start after the second week. The patient should now start to actively move the elbow in the range of motion allowed by the brace. Each week the brace is adjusted to increase motion in both flexion and extension until it is set to full motion by the sixth week. With each change in brace positions, the patient's active motion is also improved through active exercises.

After three weeks, a gradual progression of strength exercises can be added to the program. These exercises include wrist and elbow flexion and extension and forearm pronation and supination, against mild resistance. Beginning proprioception exercises for joint-position sense with eyes closed is appropriate, but valgus stress to the elbow should be avoided. Proprioceptive exercises that avoid valgus stresses can advance as tolerated. Shoulder exercises with the exception of lateral-rotation motions are performed as well. Lateral rotation can start after the sixth week. Concentric, eccentric, and mild isokinetics can be used in straight-plane movements. Co-contraction exercises for the biceps and triceps can be started if valgus stress is avoided. Closed kinetic chain exercises and other stabilization exercises are permissible once the patient has strength and control of the elbow.

Full range of motion should be present by week 6 to 8. The muscles providing dynamic stability—the biceps, pronators, and wrist flexors—are important for assisting the UCL and should be well strengthened. After the sixth week, diagonal movements can begin if adequate strength and control without pain are present in the elbow. Work on proprioceptive neuro-muscular facilitation patterns, rubber tubing exercises, more aggressive stabilization exercises, and diagonal isokinetics at high speeds can all be started at this time.

In the final phase, plyometrics begin, after week 9. As with other plyometric activities, these begin with lower-stress activities at reduced speeds and resistance, and then increase to higher speeds and place additional stress on the elbow. Medicine ball tosses, push-up progressions, and functional isokinetic motions are included.

Functional exercises can begin in week 10 to 14. The timing depends on the patient's response to the exercises and the patient's sport. A pitcher may need to wait longer before beginning throwing activities because of the higher elbow stresses in pitching compared with those in a less intense sport, such as golf. The progression of functional activities and the precautions to observe are the same as for other injuries. Following UCL reconstruction surgery, it is common for a patient to return to full participation by week 22 to 26. These figures are based on averages, and you must always remember that time lines vary from one patient to another.

Ulnar Nerve Injury

Injury to the ulnar nerve can occur in any setting but seems most prevalent in throwing sports such as baseball (pitching). The most frequent cause in this population is incorrect mechanics. This injury is treated with both operative and nonoperative techniques. Considerations in therapeutic exercise for both treatments are presented here.

Case Study

A 30-year-old right-handed golfer injured his right elbow when he hit a divot and tore his ulnar collateral ligament. He attempted to continue playing through the season, but pain persisted. The elbow became unstable, and he underwent a medial collateral reconstruction. The surgery was 10 days ago, and he has been instructed by the surgeon to begin rehabilitation. The elbow is in a functional brace's motion blocks that are at 30° from extension and 100° flexion. Supination is possible to neutral. Your examination reveals mild discoloration still present in the forearm and distal upper arm medially. There is spasm in the upper trapezius and biceps. Active range of motion out of the brace is 60° from extension to 100° into flexion. Wrist extensors have 4/5 strength, the shoulder grossly has 4–/5 strength, the biceps and triceps are also 4–/5, and the wrist flexors are 3–/5. There are active trigger points in the forearm on the flexor and extensor surfaces.

Questions for Analysis

1. What will your first treatment session include?

2. What precautions will you give the patient?

3. When will you start pronation and supination motion activities?

4. What strengthening exercises will you include in the first week, and how will you advance them?

5. At what motion limits will you set the brace in week 5?

6. When will you start shoulder external-rotation exercises?

7. What functional-exercise program will you will establish for the patient, and when will you start it?

Program Considerations

Repetitive overhand throwing activities, especially in patients whose shoulder lateral rotation in the cocking phase is reduced, places excessive stress on the medial elbow structures. The ulnar nerve can become stretched, mechanically irritated, or even subluxed out of its sulcus. Adjacent soft-tissue structures can also compress the nerve. The patient commonly complains of fourth- and fifth-digit numbness or tingling and posteromedial elbow pain. Nonoperative treatment includes initial treatments to reduce the inflammation and pain. Exercises to improve range of motion and strength are similar to those for other elbow injuries. Mobilization can be performed if the joint is hypomobile. Strength exercises are initially low-resistance, high-repetition loads in straight-plane motions. Muscles for all shoulder, elbow, wrist, and forearm motions should be strengthened. If shoulder inflexibility, shoulder weakness, or poor athletic technique is contributing to the elbow injury, it must be corrected. Initial exercises should not place valgus stress on the elbow. As the strength increases, valgus stress is applied gradually. The final phases of the program include a progression from diagonal motions to plyometrics to functional activities before return to full sport participation.

When operative repair is necessary for a subluxating or dislocating ulnar nerve, the surgical technique most commonly used is the creation of fascial slings to support the ulnar nerve along with an anterior transposition of the nerve. Postoperatively, the elbow is placed in a hinged elbow brace that is positioned at 90° flexion for two weeks. After the first week, the brace motion stops are positioned at 30° to 15° from extension and at 100° to 120° flexion. The brace is discontinued by the third week. By about the sixth week, the patient should have full range of motion in all planes. Gentle gripping using a foam ball starts during the first week along with isometric exercises for the shoulder. Active range-of-motion exercises for pronation, supination, and wrist and finger flexion and extension are also included.

By week 2, isometrics for the elbow and wrist can begin. The splint can be removed for the patient to perform active and passive range-of-motion exercises. Early proprioceptive exercises for position sense are started. Mild manual-resistance exercises and light weights can be used for the wrist. By the third week, resistance exercises for the wrist, forearm, and elbow can include low-resistance, high-repetition exercises in all planes. Exercises are started in straight-plane motions and progress to diagonal planes as the strength and control improve.

By the eighth week, plyometrics can start with their normal progression from low-load, controlled movement to increased loads with higher speeds of movement. Functional activities can begin at week 10 to 12 with full return to full participation usually seen after week 12 to 16.

Case Study

A 19-year-old right-handed volleyball frontline player suffered a subluxed ulnar nerve at the end of the season. She underwent ulnar nerve transplantation two days ago. The surgeon wants her to begin her rehabilitation program today. She has a posterior splint set at 90°. She has some pain over the surgical site, but nothing significant. There is some tension in the upper trapezius muscle, and it is tender to palpation. Wrist extension and supination movements cause some medial elbow pain at the end range. Wrist flexion motion is lacking about 10°, and the patient reports that the wrist feels weak and sore from the surgery. Pronation is also weak. Shoulder flexion is lacking about 10°, lateral rotation is lacking about 20°, and there is some weakness in the rotator cuff.

Questions for Analysis

1. What will your first treatment session include?

2. What home exercises will you give the patient?

3. What exercises will the program include for the next three weeks?

4. Outline a functional-exercise program that the patient will use when she is ready for functional activities.

Dislocation

When an elbow dislocation occurs, there is no doubt about it because the deformity is obvious. If there has been no vascular compromise and surgery is not required, a therapeutic exercise program can follow the course described next. As is assumed with any therapeutic exercise program, modalities to relieve pain and swelling and to promote healing are applied before and even during the early stages of the therapeutic exercise program.

Program Considerations

Elbow dislocations occur primarily posteriorly and follow sudden hyperextension and abduction force applications. The injury produces an obvious deformity.

The elbow should be placed in a posterior immobilizing splint at 90° for about a week. Active wrist and shoulder motion in the splint is desirable. Isometric exercises to the elbow and mild resistive exercises to the wrist can be used initially. The patient can squeeze a ball throughout the day. After about five days, the splint can be removed for gentle active range of motion to tolerance in all elbow and forearm planes. Passive motion is avoided.

After the first week, the splint is removed but used as needed when fatigue occurs. After two weeks, the splint is discarded and active range-of-motion exercises are continued. Mild resistive exercises to the elbow with emphasis on high repetitions and low resistance begin. Straight-plane exercises are used initially and advance to diagonal-plane exercises when the patient demonstrates good control, strength, and coordination. By week 6 the patient should have full range of motion in all planes. Joint mobilization can be started by week 4 to 6 if needed.

Strength exercises progress in the same way as for other elbow injuries from isometric to isotonic to isokinetic. Emphasis is on strengthening the elbow flexors to provide dynamic stabilization against hyperextension. Resistive exercises begin in straight planes and progress to diagonal planes, to plyometrics, and finally to functional activities by week 8 to 10. A hyperextension brace may be necessary to offer the patient additional protection against hyperextension forces. It may take the patient 16 to 26 weeks to return to full participation.

Case Study

A 20-year-old right-handed gymnast fell off the balance beam and landed on her left hyperextended elbow, dislocating the elbow, five days ago. Surgery was not necessary, but the orthopedist has placed the elbow in a 90° splint and wants you to begin rehabilitation on it today. Elbow range of motion lacks 50° of extension and can flex to 100°. Supination is 10°, and pronation is 20°. Edema and ecchymosis surround the elbow and extend into the mid-forearm and mid-upper arm. Spasm is present in the biceps, triceps, and upper trapezius. Strength is difficult to test in the elbow because the patient complains of pain and offers minimal resistance to resisted elbow flexion and extension. Wrist movements demonstrate 4/5 strength, and grip strength is 75% compared to that on the right. Shoulder strength overall is 4+/5.

Questions for Analysis

1. What will your first treatment session include?

2. What instructions for home exercises will you give the patient?

3. What exercises will you include as part of the first week's treatment program?

4. What are your goals for the first week?

5. What will be your progression of flexibility and strength exercises?

6. What functional-exercise program will you include for rehabilitation?

Arthroscopy

Although arthroscopic surgery is less complicated than an open procedure and leads to less tissue damage, respect for tissue healing is still warranted. As the therapeutic exercise program begins, the rehabilitation clinician must not lose sight of the fact that the patient has had surgery and that tissue healing is ongoing.

Program Considerations

The most common arthroscopic procedure performed on the elbow is debridement of synovitis and removal of loose bodies. Postoperative rehabilitation following this procedure is more accelerated than with open procedures, because less damage and insult have occurred. The arm is often placed in a sling for one or two days (or three days if the pain warrants it) following the surgery. In addition to pain and edema control, initial treatment includes active and mild passive range of motion and joint mobilization for pain modulation. Shoulder and wrist range-of-motion exercises are also performed. Gripping exercises can also be used in the first two or three postoperative days.

Full range of motion should be possible by the third postoperative day. The sling can be discarded, and mild resistive exercises to the elbow can begin. If debridement has occurred in the posterior elbow, it may be uncomfortable for the patient to perform end-range flexion-extension exercises. These exercises should be performed in a straight plane within a pain-free range of motion, especially during the first three to four weeks. Shoulder strengthening and wrist and forearm strengthening are also performed within pain-free limits. Proprioception exercises begin within the first week.

By week 3 to 4, the patient begins the middle rehabilitation phase; isokinetic exercises can begin in straight planes, advancing as indicated to diagonal planes. Rubber tubing and other eccentric exercises can begin. Diagonal planes with resistive exercises can be used once good strength and control are seen in straight-plane exercises.

Plyometric exercises can begin once the patient shows good control and strength in diagonal-plane activities. This can be as early as the third week but may not be possible until the fifth or sixth week, depending on the patient's response to the surgery and exercises. Functional activities begin once plyometric exercises are completed and the patient is pain free and has full range of motion and normal strength. By around week 8, the patient may be ready to return to full sport participation once all functional-activity progressions have been completed.

Case Study

A 35-year-old, right-handed, recreational baseball pitcher underwent arthroscopic removal of loose bodies from the posterior elbow yesterday. The surgeon wants him to begin rehabilitation today. The patient reports mild postoperative pain, but nothing unusual. He is wearing an arm sling, but he has been told he can remove it throughout the day. There is swelling around the surgical site. The dressing does not indicate any unusual postoperative drainage. The elbow range of motion is lacking 30° in extension and flexes to 100°. Pronation is 70° and supination is 50°. Wrist flexion and extension are each 60°. There is some spasm in the triceps. Manual muscle testing reveals 4–/5 strength in the biceps and triceps with some tenderness to triceps resistance, 4–/5 wrist flexion and extension without pain, and 4/5 strength throughout the shoulder.

Questions for Analysis

1. What will your first treatment be?

2. What instructions will you give the patient before he leaves today?

3. Outline your expected progression of exercises for the next two weeks. What guidelines will you use to determine when the patient should begin a progressive throwing program?

4. What will you tell him when he asks you how soon he can get back to playing baseball?

SUMMARY

1. Discuss why overstretching the elbow should be avoided, especially during the inflammation phase of healing.

   The brachialis inserts onto the elbow's anterior superior capsule; adhesions occur relatively easily in the elbow; and the anterior capsule is relatively thin and can be easily damaged with aggressive stretching, resulting in additional scarring.

2. Describe the convex-concave rules for the various elbow joints.

   The radial head and ulna both are concave surfaces and move on a convex capitulum and convex trochlea, respectively, so force applications are in the same direction as the restricted movement. In the proximal radioulnar joint, the force is applied in the direction opposite the restricted movement because this joint is a convex surface moving on a concave surface.

3. Identify the resting positions for the elbow joints.

   As outlined in table 6.3, the resting position for the humeroulnar joint is 70° elbow flexion and 10° supination. The resting position for the humeroradial joint is full elbow extension with full supination. The radioulnar joint's resting position is 70° elbow flexion with 35° supination.

4. Identify three soft-tissue mobilization techniques for the elbow.

   Cross-friction is used for the biceps tendon; trigger point release is used for the brachialis; and trigger point release is used for the triceps.

5. List three joint mobilizations for the elbow.

   Distraction of the ulnohumeral joint is used for general relaxation and pain relief; posterior glide of the radiohumeral joint is used to increase extension; and ventral glide of the radioulnar joint is used for increasing supination.

6. Explain three strengthening exercises for the elbow and their purpose.

   Elbow flexion in a supinated position for primarily increasing strength of the biceps, elbow flexion in pronation for primarily strengthening brachialis, and elbow flexion in neutral for primarily strengthening brachioradialis.

7. Discuss the general progression of strengthening exercises for the elbow.

   Range of motion begins with cautious active motion and incorporates low-intensity long-term stretches only if active exercises cannot restore range of motion. Isometric strengthening exercises are followed by light-resistance exercises and then more-intense strengthening exercises as strength increases. Eccentric exercises are preceded by concentric exercises, using careful stabilization to isolate the correct muscles. Shoulder and wrist exercises are included in the program. Exercises are performed initially in straight plane and advanced to diagonal plane as strength and control improve. Plyometric exercises are added after strength and motion are adequate, and functional activities that prepare the patient for return to sport are the last exercises included.

8. Outline a therapeutic exercise program for epicondylitis.

   Basic to any tendinitis program is discovering the underlying cause and correcting it. Pain, edema, and inflammation relief with modalities is initiated before therapeutic exercises. Soft-tissue mobilizations such as friction massage and myofascial release are used for soft-tissue-related restrictions and pain, and joint mobilization is used with capsular pattern losses of motion. Active range-of-motion exercises can be performed during the soft-tissue and joint mobilization applications. Isometric and manual resistance in straight-plane exercises are followed by greater-resistance and diagonal-plane activities as strength progresses. Plyometric exercises with medicine balls and rubber resistance are followed by functional activities that begin at low resistance and low intensity and progress as the patient's control and execution improve.

9. Indicate precautions that should be considered in a Little League elbow therapeutic exercise program.

If growth-plate damage is evident when an injury occurs, the patient should be advised to stop pitching for the rest of the baseball season. Active range-of-motion exercises (only to tolerance) are encouraged. Passive stretches should be avoided. Use of heavy weights is not advisable, because this could aggravate sensitive growth plates. Exercises should be neither as aggressive nor as intensive as they are for older patients. Valgus stress should be avoided until it does not cause pain.

10. List precautions for a therapeutic exercise program following an ulnar nerve transposition.

Tissue healing must be respected. Exercises begin more slowly than they do with nonoperative treatment for nerve injuries. Straight-plane exercises precede diagonal-plane exercises. While the elbow is in a postoperative sling, handgrip exercises can be used to start early strengthening. Active exercises should be used for stretching. Gentle cross-friction massage should be used only after three weeks if a loss of range of motion persists.

11. Explain the differences in rehabilitation programs for an arthroscopic debridement and a medial collateral reconstruction.

Because the medial collateral reconstruction is an open procedure, rehabilitation is a much slower process than with some alternative procedures. The period of immobilization is longer, and exercises are less aggressive in the early stages of the program. Loss of motion is a more significant factor, so motion and mobility activities are more prominent in the early phases.

CRITICAL THINKING QUESTIONS

1. Joan is faced with a probable Little League elbow tendinitis in the opening scenario. What other possible diagnoses could Steve have? What tests should Joan perform to determine what the problem is? What recommendations should she make to Mr. Turner for care? What precautions should Joan take in making recommendations to him?

2. How does the rehabilitation program for an elbow differ for a dislocation as compared to a sprain? How are the precautions different? Is the progression of exercises different, and if so, how?

3. Can you identify the differences between a medial and a lateral epicondylitis? What structures are affected? How are the mechanisms of injury different? Would the rehabilitation programs be different? If so, how?

LAB ACTIVITIES

1. Locate the trigger points for the following muscles on your lab partner:
   a. Biceps
   b. Brachialis
   c. Triceps
   d. Brachioradialis

   Where were your partner's most sensitive trigger points? Perform an ice-and-stretch technique on each of them and provide your partner with a home exercise for each tender trigger point.

2. Locate the lateral epicondyle where the long finger extensors insert on the humerus. Can you palpate each extensor tendon as they come off the epicondyle? Can you identify the tendon that is most often the source of lateral epicondylitis? Explain why an individual with lateral epicondylitis has pain when grasping.

3. Examine your lab partner's joint mobilization for all three joints. How does the mobility of each one compare to the others? Which of the three joints has the greatest mobility; which one has the least amount of movement? Visualize in each joint's motion where the resistance to movement begins. Is it before or after half of the total joint mobility?

4. Perform the following joint mobilizations on your lab partner and identify what restriction would be best treated with each mobilization:
   a. Humeroulnar joint
   b. Distraction
   c. Medial glide
   d. Lateral glide
   e. Humeroradial joint
   f. Distraction
   g. Dorsal glide
   h. Ventral glide
   i. Proximal radioulnar joint
   j. Dorsal glide of radial head
   k. Ventral glide of radial head

5. Have your partner perform two stretches each for elbow flexion, elbow extension, pronation, and supination. Identify possible substitutions you must watch for with each exercise.

6. Apply manual resistance to your partner for each of the motions listed with your partner in supine. Have him or her go through 10 repetitions for each exercise. Be sure to apply a maximum resistance but produce a smooth concentric movement throughout the full range of motion. After that is completed, apply eccentric resistance to the same motions for 10 repetitions each. Which was more fatiguing for your partner? Which was more difficult for you to perform? Why?
   a. Elbow flexion
   b. Elbow extension
   c. Pronation
   d. Supination

7. Using a dumbbell or cuff weight, have your partner perform a triceps extension exercise in three different antigravity positions, 10 repetitions in each position. Repeat the activity for the elbow flexors. Which position was the most difficult to perform and why?

8. Have your partner use a free weight to perform a supination-pronation exercise while sitting. As your partner goes through the range of motion slowly, have him identify what muscles are being used at various portions of the range of motion. If you wanted to work only supinators in both concentric and eccentric motions, explain how you would have the patient perform the exercises.

9. If your partner has tennis elbow, what specific activities would you have her perform? You should concentrate on eccentric activities. What would they be, and how many repetitions and sets would you have her do today? Have your partner perform them as you state them. Have you changed your mind on the goals you set before the exercises were performed? What made you either keep them or change them from your original goals?

10. Develop a series of three plyometric exercises you would use for an elbow patient's rehabilitation program. Have your partner perform them and identify the easiest and most difficult exercise. What substitution patterns could he develop as fatigue occurred? What would you set as your criteria for progression from one exercise to the next? Justify why you have set these criteria.

11. List three sport-specific exercises you would have an elbow patient who is a softball left fielder perform before you allowed her to return to full play. Justify why you have selected these criteria.

REFERENCES

Donkers, M.J., An, K.N., Chao, E.Y., and B.F. Morrey. 1993. Hand position affects elbow joint load during push-up exercise. *Journal of Biomechanics* 26:625–632.

Ellenbecker, T.S., and E.G. Mattalino. 1997. *The elbow in sport.* Champaign, IL: Human Kinetics.

Feltner, M., and J. Dapena. 1986. Dynamics of the shoulder and elbow joints of the throwing arm during a baseball pitch. *International Journal of Sport Biomechanics* 2:235–259.

Groppel, J.L., and R.P. Nirschl. 1986. A mechanical and electromyographical analysis of the effects of various joint counterforce braces on the tennis player. *American Journal of Sports Medicine* 14: 195–200.

Kibler, W.B. 1995. Pathophysiology of overload injuries around the elbow. *Clinics in Sports Medicine* 14:447–457.

Mero, A., Komi, T.V., Korjus, T., Navarro, E., and R.J. Gregor. 1994. Body segment contributions to javelin throwing during final thrust phases. *Journal of Applied Biomechanics* 10:166–177.

Nirschl, R.P. 1977. Tennis elbow. *Primary Care* 4:367–382.

Stanish, W.D, Curwin, S. and S. Mandel. 2000. *Tendinitis: Its etiology and treatment.* New York: Oxford University Press.

Travell, J.G., and D.G. Simons. 1983. *Myofascial pain and dysfunction. The trigger point manual.* Vol. 1. Baltimore: Williams & Wilkins.

SUGGESTED READING

Adriani, E., Luziatelli, S., and P.P. Mariani. 1993. Medial instability of the elbow: Surgical management and rehabilitation. *Journal of Sports Traumatology and Related Research* 15:45–52.

Andrews, J.R., and J.A. Whiteside. 1993. Common elbow problems in the athlete. *Journal of Orthopaedic & Sports Physical Therapy* 17:289–295.

Barker, C. 1988. Evaluation, treatment, and rehabilitation involving a submuscular transposition of the ulnar nerve at the elbow. *Athletic Training* 23:10–12.

Ellenbecker, T.S. 1995. Rehabilitation of shoulder and elbow injuries in tennis players. *Clinics in Sports Medicine* 14:87–104.

Jobe, F.W., and G. Nuber. 1986. Throwing injuries of the elbow. *Clinics in Sports Medicine* 5:621–636.

Lee, D.G. 1986. "Tennis elbow": A manual therapist's perspective. *Journal of Orthopaedic & Sports Physical Therapy* 8:134–142.

Morris, M., Jobe, F.W., Perry, J., Pink, M., and B.S. Healy. 1989. Electromyographic analysis of elbow function in tennis players. *American Journal of Sports Medicine* 17:241–247.

Ollivierre, C.O., and R.P. Nirschl. 1996. Tennis elbow. Current concepts of treatment and rehabilitation. *Sports Medicine* 22:133–139.

Sisto, D.J., Jobe, F.W., Moynes, D.R., and D.J. Antonelli. 1987. An electromyographic analysis of the elbow in pitching. *American Journal of Sports Medicine* 15:260–263.

Stroyan, M., and K.E. Wilk. 1993. The functional anatomy of the elbow complex. *Journal of Orthopaedic & Sports Physical Therapy* 17:279–288.

Werner, S.L., Fleisig, G.S., Dillman, C.J., and J.R. Andrews. 1993. Biomechanics of the elbow during baseball pitching. *Journal of Orthopaedic & Sports Physical Therapy* 17:274–278.

Wilk, K.E., Arrigo, C., and J.R. Andrews. 1993. Rehabilitation of the elbow in the throwing athlete. *Journal of Orthopaedic & Sports Physical Therapy* 17:305–317.

Wrist and Hand

Objectives

After completing this chapter, you should be able to do the following:

1. Explain the pulley system of the fingers.
2. Explain why reducing edema in the hand is important.
3. Discuss the trimuscular system of the hand and explain its importance to hand function.
4. Identify the precision pinches and power grips of the hand.
5. Explain the difference between static and dynamic splints.
6. Identify what motion is increased with carpal radial glide joint mobilization.
7. Explain the force application sequence to improve long finger flexor and extensor motion.
8. Explain how the intrinsic stretches differ from the extrinsic stretches.
9. Discuss the difference in gliding exercises for the flexor profundus and superficialis tendons.
10. Present the differences between long flexor and long extensor tendons.
11. Explain what procedures should be used to eliminate an extensor lag of a distal phalanx.
12. Identify the early signs of RSD.

Three weeks ago Danny was playing soccer with his friends when he was tripped and fell, landing on his outstretched hands. His right hand was severely cut by a piece of broken glass hidden in the grass. The surgeon repaired his lacerated long finger flexor tendons and placed the hand in an extension-restricted splint, but now wants Deanna Murray, rehabilitation clinician, to begin the rehabilitation process on the hand.

Deanna has had experience with repaired tendons and appreciates the precautions she must consider, especially because the repair is only three weeks old. She is concerned about the adhesions that have begun to form between the long flexor superficialis and profundus tendons and other soft tissue in the anterior finger region, and the impact that might have on the finger's hood mechanism. If the hood mechanism is harmed, the intrinsic muscles can be affected, which will impair the hand's function; so Deanna understands she has to proceed cautiously with Danny's rehabilitation program.

■ **What lies behind us and what lies before us are tiny matters compared to what lies within us.**

Ralph Waldo Emerson, 1803–1882, American essayist and poet

We use our hands daily for hundreds of activities, not thinking of it as anything beyond the ordinary. However; if we reflect on the hand at all, we realize that it is an extremely complex structure and vital to our daily tasks. Many health care professionals have little regard for finger and hand injuries, but these can be among the most devastating injuries if not properly cared for, if only because the hand plays such an important role in everyday activities. It is my hope that by the end of this chapter you will gain an appreciation for hand and finger injuries to realize that a finger sprain is not *just* a sprain. The hand is much more complex than many think, and a seemingly minimal imbalance in the hand can cause profound effects on its abilities. Before we can discuss rehabilitation techniques for the wrist and hand, we must review their unique function and structure. It is important to gain an understanding of the wrist's and hand's structure and function, because they play a vital role in the techniques and applications of therapeutic exercises in a rehabilitation program.

Many texts have been written on the anatomy, biomechanics, and function of the wrist and hand. We will be only skimming the surface of this body of knowledge. A complete investigation of the hand's structure and function is beyond the scope of this chapter, but information vital to establishing a safe and appropriate rehabilitation program for the wrist and hand is presented. I refer you to the suggested readings at the end of this chapter for additional information.

This chapter includes structural and functional information that you will need in order to create an appropriate rehabilitation program for wrist and hand injuries. A presentation of soft-tissue and joint mobilization techniques includes information organized similarly to that in previous chapters. The exercises presented are limited to flexibility, strengthening, and coordination exercises for the wrist and hand. You should realize, however, that the wrist is intimately connected to the elbow and closely associated with the shoulder, so a therapeutic exercise program should also include activities for these areas. Specific injuries commonly seen in the wrist and hand are discussed, along with rehabilitation programs used to treat these injuries.

GENERAL REHABILITATION CONSIDERATIONS

▶ The hand's many special characteristics include its skeletal structure, its tendon sheaths and pulleys, its fascia and ligaments, and two categories of muscles. Edema is an important consideration in the hand, as are the tendon zones, tendon excursion, the various ways the hand is used, and splinting principles.

The wrist and hand is a complex unit composed of 29 bones, more than 30 tendinous insertions, and an involved neurological system that is vital to the unit's function. Twenty-five percent of the entire body's pacinian corpuscles' sensory endings are located in the hands. The hand's many compactly arranged muscles, including nine for the thumb and seven for the index finger alone, hint at the complexity of its function. The thumb and index finger are used primarily for fine activities requiring dexterity, whereas the middle, ring, and little fingers act primarily as a stabilizing vise for grasping activities. It is important that all of the structures within the hand work in a balanced, coordinated manner for the hand to function optimally.

Skeletal Structure

Three flexion arches, the proximal and distal transverse arches and a longitudinal arch, are formed by the bones of the wrist and hand. The proximal and distal transverse arches are formed by the carpals and metacarpals, respectively. The longitudinal arch runs from the carpals out to the ends of the fingers (figure 19.1). These arches form an equiangular spiral that provides for tremendous adaptation in grasping activities. If these equiangular structures are impaired because of joint restriction or muscle weakness, the hand loses its adaptability.

The concave radius joins with the convex proximal carpal row to form the wrist joint. This joint has motions of flexion, extension, abduction, and adduction. Adduction is commonly referred to as ulnar deviation or *ulnar flexion*, and abduction is referred to as radial deviation or *radial flexion*. These four motions combine to produce circumduction of the wrist. The distal ulna and radius are supported by the distal radioulnar ligament and the interosseous membrane, and allow forearm supination and pronation movement along with the proximal radioulnar joint. Restricted mobility at either joint prevents full supination-pronation motion.

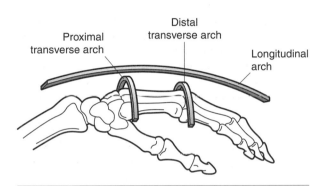

Figure 19.1 Hand arches.

Reprinted from Fess and Philips 1987.

The carpal bones also form several joints with each other, and the distal row forms the carpometacarpal joints with the metacarpals. The intercarpal joints are irregular in structure and are strongly held in place by ligaments, making it difficult to dislocate any carpal. The carpometacarpal joints are for the most part saddle joints that permit various degrees of flexion, extension, abduction, and adduction of the metacarpals. The thumb and fourth and fifth metacarpals also rotate to provide opposition of the thumb and little finger and grasping by the hand.

The metacarpophalangeal (MCP) joints are formed by the convex metacarpals and concave proximal phalanges. The interphalangeal (IP) joints are named as either proximal (PIP) or distal (DIP) interphalangeal joints. Collateral ligaments provide stability to these joints. When the fingers are relaxed they are in partial flexion of the IP and MCP joints. Their arrangement is such that it forms a cascade of progressive flexion from the second through the fifth digits; there is pathology present if this cascade is not seen.

Fascia and Ligaments

In addition to the ligaments connecting and supporting the joints throughout the wrist and hand, several other static structures add support to the area. The thick palmar fascia has two layers, superficial and deep. The superficial layer, an extension of the flexor retinaculum (transverse carpal ligament) and the palmaris longus tendon when it is present, expands over the volar hand and runs into each of the fingers. The deep layer covers the floor of the palm and runs between the thenar and hypothenar eminences. The fascia on the dorsum of the hand is in two layers as well but is not as thick as the palmar fascia. The palmar fascia serves to cushion and protect the hand's structures and to assist in maintaining the hand's concavity.

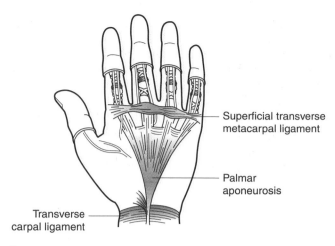

Superficial transverse metacarpal ligament

Palmar aponeurosis

Transverse carpal ligament

a

b

Figure 19.2 *(a)* Palmar soft-tissue elements *(b)* flexor tendon pulley system.

The flexor and extensor tendons are held in place by retinacula positioned throughout the wrist and hand. At the wrist, the flexor tendons are kept from bowstringing away from the wrist by the transverse carpal ligament. This ligament forms the roof of the carpal tunnel and maintains all of the finger flexor tendons except the palmaris longus and flexor carpi ulnaris, the nerves, and the arteries in the carpal tunnel. The extensor retinaculum on the dorsal wrist keeps the extensor tendons from bowstringing away from the wrist.

An extracapsular ligament, the transverse metacarpal ligament, connects the volar plate of one metatarsal head to the volar plate of its adjacent metatarsal heads (figure 19.2). This ligament is important in maintaining the distal transverse arch, and its normal flexibility is vital to hand functions such as prehensile grip and grasping activities. There are several fascial restraints in the digits that maintain alignment of the tendons in the fingers that also provide the pulley system for the tendons.

Tendon Sheaths and Pulleys

The flexor tendons are surrounded by a complex system of sheaths that serve to protect and nourish the tendons. The sheath system of the extensor tendons is not as elaborate; the extensor tendons are enclosed in sheaths at the wrist when they travel under the extensor retinaculum, but otherwise they are extrasynovial. The flexor sheaths begin proximal to the wrist and extend to the distal digits.

There is an elaborate pulley system on the flexor aspect of the fingers. This system is a series of fibrous tunnels that extends from the metacarpal head of each digit to the insertion of the distal finger flexor tendons. These pulleys are similar to the hoops along a fishing rod, positioned to keep the fishing line in place as it travels along the pole. There are five annular pulleys and three cruciate pulleys along the fingers (figure 19.2). Disruption of the key pulleys can cause bowstringing of the flexor tendons. The pulleys that are key to preventing bowstringing are A2 and A4 (Doyle and Blythe 1975). When the pulley system of any finger is disrupted, the mechanical advantage of the tendon is impaired and normal function is lost.

Muscles

Hand muscles are divided into two categories, extrinsic and intrinsic. Extrinsic muscles originate outside the hand whereas intrinsic muscles originate and terminate within the hand. There are 20 extrinsic muscles and 19 intrinsic muscles. The extrinsic muscles are attached to the long tendons. The thenar eminence contains the four intrinsic muscles of the thumb, and the hypothenar eminence contains the three intrinsic muscles of the fifth finger. If the hand is to operate well and avoid deformity following an injury, a balanced system must exist between the intrinsic and extrinsic muscles.

The long finger extensors run to the second through fifth fingers. At the distal metacarpal area they are connected by the juncturae tendinum, a fibrous band that limits independent motion of the extensor tendons. The extensor tendons are connected to the proximal phalanx by sagittal bands that attach on the volar plate to keep the extensor tendons from bowstringing and transmit the extensor tendons' extension force to the metacarpophalangeal joints. Distal to the MCP joints, the extensor tendons split into three segments: the central slip, which attaches to the base of the middle phalanx, and two lateral bands that insert when they rejoin at the distal phalanx (figure 19.3).

The long finger flexors include the flexor digitorum superficialis (FDS) and the flexor digitorum profundus (FDP). Both tendons pass deep in the hand. The FDS flexes the PIP joint. Each FDS tendon has its own separate muscle belly, so each can operate independently of the other. Each superficialis tendon splits before it attaches to the base of the middle phalanx and permits the deeper FDP tendon to emerge and attach to the distal phalanx (figure 19.4). The tendons of the FDP, unlike those of the FDS, do not possess separate muscle bellies, so distal phalanx flexion of the fingers cannot be isolated in their movements.

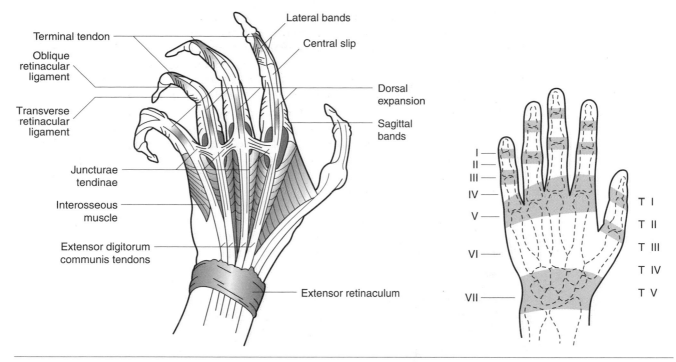

Figure 19.3 Dorsal soft-tissue elements and zones.

Extensor tendon zones from Kleinert, Schepel, and Gill 1981.

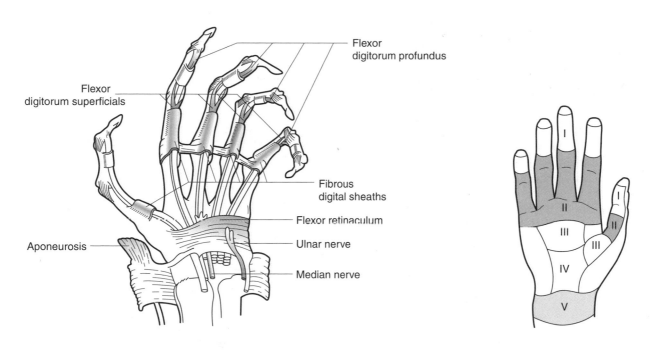

Figure 19.4 Palmar surface of the hand and zones.

Flexor tendon zones from American Society for Surgery of the Hand 1983.

Whereas the long finger muscles are used for gross-motor activity, the intrinsic muscles are used for fine-motor activities. They control the more intricate movements of the fingers. The lumbricals and interossei have unique attachments and arrangements with the long flexor and extensor tendons and the ligaments of the fingers. The lumbricals originate from the deep flexor tendons in the palm and insert on the extensor tendon expansion. This unique arrangement allows the lumbricals to function as MCP flexors and IP extensors because their line of force is anterior to the MCP joint, causing flexion at this joint and their line of force is posterior to the IP joint, resulting in IP extension. The dorsal and palmar interossei are responsible for finger abduction and adduction, respectively. Because they are more superficial than the lumbricals, they can be palpated.

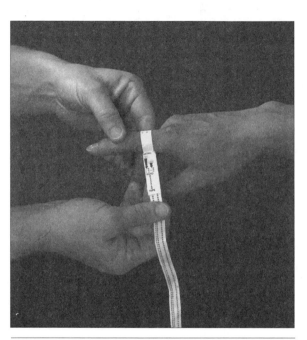

Figure 19.5   Circumferential gauge.

Edema

Skin covering the volar hand is thick, inelastic, and hairless and is attached to the palmar fascia to allow for grasping objects without their slipping out of the hand. The dorsal skin is elastic, mobile, and easily separated from the underlying fascia to permit skin mobility during grasping activities. Because the dorsal skin is loose and pliable compared to the volar skin, edema frequently accumulates in the dorsum of the hand. Pooled edema rich in proteins easily leads to contractures. Excessive swelling on the back of the hand can cause the hand arches to collapse anteriorly and adduct the thumb. Excessive swelling also requires a greater excursion of the skin to flex the hand. If the skin is already stretched because of the edema, the hand's ability to move the fingers through their full motion is impaired because the skin extensibility is already used by the edema. Fibrous tissue formation secondary to prolonged edema can cause reduced mobility and function of the hand.

Efforts by the rehabilitation clinician to reduce early edema are crucial. A circumferential gauge can be used to determine edema of the hand and fingers (figure 19.5). A string wrapped around the finger or hand and then measured for its length can also be used. Compressive dressings, elevation, ice, and compressive machines, as well as other modalities, can be used to reduce edema formation and reduce disability secondary to edema effects.

Tendon Zones

The flexor and extensor surfaces of the hand are divided into zones. Each zone has characteristics that are unique and impact both the physician's surgical approach and the clinician's rehabilitation approach. For this reason we consider them briefly here. There are five flexor and seven extensor zones of the wrist, hand, and four medial digits. The thumb has three flexor and five extensor zones.

Flexor Tendon Zones

Zone V begins in the forearm at the musculotendinous junction of the extrinsic muscles and goes to the wrist (figure 19.4). The tendons are surrounded by loose tendon sheaths. Injured tendons can become adherent to the sheath and surrounding soft-tissue structures. Following injury in this area, the rehabilitation clinician must prevent adhesions or restore normal gliding of tendons if they do occur.

Zone IV is at the wrist. This is the location of the carpal tunnel, the site of carpal tunnel syndrome. Because of the proximity of several tendons, nerves, and blood vessels, adhesions between tendons are a common problem following surgery or injury. The rehabilitation clinician must be aware of these problems and prevent them.

Zone III is in the palm after the flexor tendons leave the carpal tunnel. This is where the lumbricals attach to the FDP tendons. Because the extrinsic tendons have more room, they often heal without difficulty or complications. The intrinsic muscles, however, can have adhesions and contractures from prolonged flexor positioning of the palm. Gentle passive range-of-motion (ROM) exercises for the intrinsics can help prevent these complications.

Zone II is from the distal palmar crease, where the synovial sheaths begin, to the middle phalanx where the split slips of the FDS insert on the phalanx and near where the FDP traverses anteriorly from below the superficialis. This is the site of the flexor tendon sheaths. Injuries to the tendons in this region can result in adhesions of the tendons to their sheaths, or adhesions between the superficialis and profundus, and loss of motion. This is a particular concern if any of the pulleys are damaged, especially A2 and A4. These complications can seriously inhibit normal tendon gliding and prevent full restoration of function. This area has been called "no man's land" because of the inhibition of normal function after injury or surgery to this area, but more recent advances in surgical techniques permit improved function following surgery. This topic is discussed more thoroughly in the tendon injury section of this chapter.

Zone I is the area of the DIP joint. The only tendon involved here is the FDP as it inserts on the distal phalanx. Tendons are commonly ruptured from this location. These injuries require careful rehabilitation, because complications such as poor tendon gliding, contractures, and repair failures can occur.

The thumb zones include T I, T II, and T III. These zones are comparable to zones I, II, and III, respectively, of the fingers. Tendon injuries in these zones do not carry with them as strong a risk of adhesions, because the only tendon enclosed in a sheath is the flexor pollicis longus.

Extensor Tendon Zones

Zone VII is located at the wrist joints (figure 19.3). This area contains both wrist extensors and extrinsic finger extensors. The tendons in this area have synovial sheaths, are close together, and are covered by the dorsal retinaculum. This can be an area of adhesion formation after injury or immobilization. If an injury in this area involves only the wrist extensors, the wrist is the only joint in need of immobilization and should be positioned in approximately 45° of extension. However, if the long finger extensors are also involved, the wrist and MCP joints should both be positioned in extension. Because of the synovial sheaths in this area, the problems in rehabilitation of extensor zone VII are similar to those seen in flexor zone II (Evans 1989). The rehabilitation clinician must be cognizant of the risks of losing tendon gliding capabilities and should take steps to prevent and treat this complication. Tendon adhesions can cause loss of normal tendon gliding, can reduce wrist motion and strength, and can result in tendinitis. The treatment program, consisting of splinting and mobilization, is discussed later in this chapter.

Zones V and VI are from the hand distal to the extensor sheaths in the region of the CMC joints to distal of the MCP joints at the start of the extensor hood. Extensor tendons and sheaths can adhere to other surrounding soft-tissue structures, especially because they are close to the skin. Edema formation in the hand is usually seen in this area more predominantly than in the palmar aspect and should be controlled by the rehabilitation clinician. Control of edema will help reduce the risk of adhesion formation. Wrist immobilization for this area is approximately 45° extension at the wrist with the MCP and IP joints at 0° extension. Zones III and IV include the proximal phalanx and the PIP joints. When injuries occur to the extrinsic extensor tendon's central slip, what results is a boutonniere deformity where the PIP is positioned in flexion and the DIP in extension with the unbalanced pull of the intact lateral bands (see figure 19.60 on p. 735). Although stiffness of the PIP joint with loss of joint motion is a complication, immobilization of the digit is necessary, as discussed later in this chapter.

Zones I and II include the middle phalanx and the DIP joints. Ruptures of the distal tendon insertion resulting in mallet deformities occur commonly in this region. If untreated, a mallet deformity may lead to a swan-neck deformity, in which the PIP joint is hyperextended and the DIP joint is flexed. This occurs in the presence of a lax volar plate as the extensor mechanism slides proximally without its anchor at the distal phalanx. Splinting, and in some cases surgery, is necessary to correct this injury. Care must be taken during this time to guard against an extensor lag and local ischemia. Treatment of this injury is discussed in detail later. The thumb zones coincide with the zones of the finger, and injuries to those zones can be treated similarly to the corresponding finger zones. T I and T II coincide with zones I and II of the fingers. Zones T III and T IV coincide with zones V and VI of the fingers. Zone T V, like zone VII of the fingers, can suffer adhesions following injury. Web-space contracture, extensor pollicis longus adhesions, and reduced excursion of the thumb are common problems that the rehabilitation clinician must avoid.

Excursions

For the hand to close into a fist, a large excursion of the extensor tendons and dorsal surface of the hand and wrist must be possible. Adhesions can restrict this necessary mobility and reduce hand function. For this reason, early controlled passive motion of tendon injuries is vital to restoring full hand function. Care must be taken to maintain good tendon glide without risking tendon rupture.

As a tendon glides within its sheath, the adhesions are stretched. The normal excursion of a tendon is variable from one finger to another and is a matter of some dispute. The most commonly repeated values are based on the work of Bunnell reported by Boyes (1970) (table 19.1). The significance of these numbers for rehabilitation is twofold: They indicate how much excursion must be restored following injury or immobilization, and how much each healing tendon can move during immobilization without incurring damage. Based on Bunnell's work, it has been determined that a safe tendon-glide excursion of 5 mm would permit sufficient motion to minimize deleterious immobilization effects without endangering the extensor tendon (Duran and Houser 1975). Five millimeters of motion changes in terms of degrees from finger to finger, depending on the full arc of motion available (Evans and Burkhalter 1986). Table 19.2 lists the degrees of motion permitted with 5 mm (.2 in.) of movement for each digit at the MCP joint. These degrees, which become important in splint design when one is deciding the MCP angle of the splint for hand position after tendon repair, are discussed later. These excursions are also important for understanding the limitations of motion permitted in the early rehabilitation process to allow tendon gliding motion without causing tendon disruption.

Table 19.1
Extensor Tendon Excursions

	Extensor digitorum communis				
	Index	Long	Ring	Small	Extensor pollicus longus
Total	54 mm	55 mm	55 mm	35 mm	58 mm
Wrist	38 mm	41 mm	39 mm	20 mm	33 mm
MCP	15 mm	16 mm	11 mm	12 mm	7 mm
PIP	2 mm	3 mm	3 mm	2 mm	—
DIP	0	0	0	0	—
IP	—	—	—	—	8 mm

Adapted, by permission, from J.H. Boyes, 1970, *Bunnell's surgery of the hand* (Philadelphia: Lippincott). Copyright by Lippincott, Williams & Wilkins.

Table 19.2

Excursion of Extensor Digitorum Communis at the MCP Joint

Index finger	28.3°
Middle finger	27.5°
Ring finger	40.9°
Little finger	38.3°

Reprinted from Evans and Burkhalter 1986.

Use of the Hand

The hand is a trimuscular system that uses the three muscle groups, the extrinsic flexors, the extrinsic extensors, and the intrinsic muscles, to provide balanced, controlled function. If any of these muscle groups does not function normally because of either weakness or loss of mobility, balance is lost and the hand is not be able to work in its normal capacity.

Because of the hand's complex system of joints and muscles, uses of the hand as a tool are numerous. The hand can be used to transmit force or to provide movement to produce a desired effect. About 20% of its responsibility involves force transmission (Bowers and Tribuzi 1992). This force transmission occurs through power grips, also known as palmar grips, including the clenched fist, the cylinder grasp, the spherical grasp, and the hook (figure 19.6). In these grasps, the thumb is positioned in opposition to the other fingers to permit a firm grasp on an object. The majority of daily hand activities involve these palmar grips. Because palmar grasping is so vital to hand function, the hand is most commonly splinted in a palmar position with the thumb in slight opposition, facing the other fingers.

Figure 19.6 Power grips: *(a)* hook, *(b)* cylinder, *(c)* spherical, *(d)* fist.

The rest of the time, the hand provides movement to accomplish intricate tasks. These tasks include many activities, such as typing, sewing, or writing. They also include prehensile, or grip, activities in which the thumb and finger muscles co-contract to produce a desired activity. The three pinches are the digital prehension pinch (also known as 3-jaw chuck), the lateral prehension pinch (also known as key pinch), and the tip-to-tip prehension pinch (figure 19.7). The digital prehension pinch is used to handle and maneuver small tools in intricate activities. The lateral prehension pinch places the thumb tip against the side of the index finger and is used to grasp objects such as a key or book. The tip-to-tip prehension pinch uses thumb opposition to position the tip of the thumb facing the tip of another finger. It is used most often to pick up small objects.

In the precision pinches, the fingers are flexed and abducted at the MCP joints with some opposition present. The movements involved in precision activities vary in excursion and number of digits involved, but usually include the motions of flexion and rotation with some ulnar deviation. Unless the object being manipulated is heavy or large, primarily the radial digits are involved in precision activities. The power grips use the ulnar aspect of the hand to grasp the object and deliver the power and stability while the radial aspect of the hand provides the precision for the activity. Golf presents an example of this utilization of the power grip. In a power grip, the fingers flex and rotate and move into ulnar deviation so that the fingertips point toward the thenar eminence to hold the object in the hand and stabilize the thumb in abduction.

All these motions and grips must be restored to the injured hand. The clinician accomplishes this through awareness of the component motions these activities require, restoration of joint mobility, attainment of normal tendon glide, and balance of strength and flexibility.

Splinting

Braces and splints are orthotic devices commonly used in the treatment of hand injuries. They are either static or dynamic. Static splints are used to restrict motion to support and protect the hand, and dynamic splints are used to increase motion of the hand. The aim in using these devices is either to prevent damage and maintain balance or to improve balance. Splints are based on a three-point pressure system whereby two points of application are on one side of the hand, wrist, or forearm; and the fulcrum, or other point of application, is on the opposite side (figure 19.8). This system should be familiar because it was presented as a force system in chapter 3.

Figure 19.7   Prehension pinches: *(a)* digital, *(b)* lateral, *(c)* tip-to-tip.

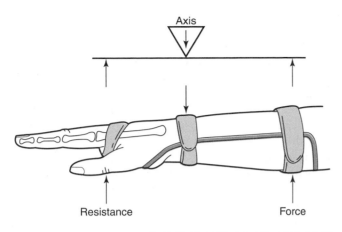

Figure 19.8 Three-point pressure system for splinting.

Splints are applied for varying amounts of time, depending on the structure injured, the repair, the adjacent structures and their influence on the injured tissue, and healing of the injured tissue. They may be applied during the day for periods of 3 to 8 weeks. Frequently, patients continue to use a night splint after they have reduced or discontinued splint use during the day. Use of night splints may continue for 10 to 12 weeks postinjury. Complex injuries commonly advance from an initial splint to a less restrictive splint during the day before removal of any day support is permitted.

Figure 19.9 Static tendon splint to restrict ROM.

Static Splints

Static splints do not have any moving parts (figure 19.9). They immobilize a joint to protect it from movement that would be deleterious. Periods of immobilization are frequently indicated following injury, and the static splint can prevent movement to allow scar-tissue formation to restore joint stability. If a joint has lost its mobility, a static splint places the joint on stretch by applying a low-level prolonged stretch and thus improving joint mobility. A static splint can also be designed to maintain ROM gains resulting from other rehabilitation techniques; this is called a static progressive splint.

Figure 19.10 Position of hand immobilization.

Although there are some exceptions, most often the hand is placed in a functional position with the wrist in slight extension, the fingers slightly flexed at the MCP and IP joints, and the thumb in slight opposition to the other fingers (figure 19.10). Only as many joints as necessary are immobilized so that mobility of the unaffected joints is optimized.

Dynamic Splints

Dynamic splints incorporate a system of movement through the use of springs, rubber bands, or other elastic elements. These devices are designed to produce passive or passive assistive motion in one line of pull and active resistive motion in the opposite direction. Dynamic splints can promote mobility by providing a continual, low-level stretch force to a joint. They are used when the patient lacks normal motion and is unable to achieve the desired mobility independently. The patient should be able to perceive the stretch force applied with the splint but should not find it painful. Because the device is worn for a prolonged period of time to influence scar-tissue remodeling, the force applied is low. These devices are usually worn at night so that they do not interfere with hand function during the day. The duration it is worn depends on the patient's tolerance, but the longer it is in place, the more successful the results are. As the joint's ROM increases, adjustments in the splint are necessary.

Dynamic splints are frequently used following tendon surgery to permit protected, guided movement of the tendon to maintain the tendon glide without risking tendon rupture. The device permits the appropriate degree of tendon motion based on the numbers presented in table 19.2. The tendon is held in its shortened position by rubber bands, and the splint keeps the opposing tendon from moving the digit beyond the designated degree of movement. The opposing tendon must work against the force of the rubber band to move the finger in the direction permitted, and the rubber band passively returns the finger to the resting position.

When splints are designed for the hand, fit, design, and purpose must be considerations. The purpose will determine what type of orthotic is used. The fit is individually determined based on the hand size and dimensions. The design is based on a combination of fit, purpose, and precautions.

Precautions in the design and construction are primarily two: friction and pressure. Whether the device is static or dynamic, friction can occur between the splint and the skin. When a splint does not fit correctly, it will move from its intended position and cause friction and irritation. The device should be held firmly, yet comfortably, in position by its straps and other structures; it may require periodic adjustments for maintenance of proper alignment and reduction of friction.

Pressure is particularly a problem when the splint is placed over bony prominences. The hand's most susceptible areas are the ulnar and radial styloid processes, pisiform, base of the fifth metacarpal, and metacarpal heads. Padding over these susceptible areas can be applied during splint construction and removed when the splint is worn to prevent pressure. If padding or relief is added after the splint is made, it may change the alignment and intended force application of the device.

The patient's skin should be routinely checked for redness and signs of pressure or friction. Adjustments may be necessary as the patient's condition changes. Wrist and hand splint construction can be complicated, depending on the injury. In complex cases, an occupational therapist, orthopedic technician, or other hand specialist typically constructs the orthotic. In these cases, the rehabilitation clinician plays an important role in reporting on the patient's tolerance of the device and can reinforce wear compliance.

SOFT-TISSUE MOBILIZATION

▶ Soft-tissue mobilization techniques used for the extrinsic and the intrinsic muscles of the hand include trigger point release and ice-and-stretch techniques.

Although soft-tissue treatment of many of the intrinsic muscles of the wrist and hand is discussed in chapter 18, other treatments have yet to be introduced. The soft-tissue mobilization techniques in this chapter are limited to trigger point release and ice-and-stretch techniques based on the work of Travell and Simons (1983). The pain-referral patterns and information presented here are also based on their work.

Extrinsic Muscles

Although there are several extrinsic muscles of the wrist and hand, they are grossly divided into two groups: flexors and extensors. The palmaris longus is described separately from the other flexors because its pain referral is different from theirs.

Palmaris Longus

The palmaris longus refers pain into the palm, but not the digits, and to a lesser extent along the distal anterior forearm. Because it inserts superficially, the pain is usually a prickly superficial sensation rather than the deep sensation of most muscle pain-referral patterns. The trigger point is a palpable band that is located in the medial aspect of the proximal anterior forearm as seen in figure 19.11a.

Trigger point release of this muscle is performed by placing direct pressure over the trigger point location or rolling across the band (figure 19.11b).

Ice-and-stretch is applied with the muscle on stretch. The elbow is supported on a padded surface while the fingers and wrist are extended. The ice is applied in parallel sweeps from the medial elbow along the medial forearm and into the palm as the elbow and fingers are passively moved into extension (figure 19.11c).

Figure 19.11 Palmaris longus: *(a)* pain-referral pattern, *(b)* trigger point release, *(c)* ice-and-stretch.

Pronator Teres, and Wrist and Long Finger Flexors

The wrist flexors and pronator teres refer pain into the wrist: the flexor carpi ulnaris to the ulnar aspect, the flexor carpi radialis to the radial aspect, and the pronator teres to the radial wrist. The long finger and thumb flexors refer pain into the digits they activate and extend the sensation of pain shooting out beyond the end of the digits (figure 19.12a). Pain patterns between the finger flexor superficialis and profundus have not been differentiated.

Trigger points are located within the forearm near the midbelly portion of each muscle. The exception is the flexor pollicis longus, whose trigger point is located on the distal forearm. Trigger point release is applied with the specific muscle in a relaxed position. Each muscle is treated with direct pressure over the tender trigger point until the discomfort subsides. Each trigger point elicits a local twitch response and produces a pain-referral pattern.

Ice-and-stretch is applied with the muscle on stretch and a support under the elbow (figure 19.12, b–c). The ice sweeps are made from the medial elbow downward to the specific digit being treated.

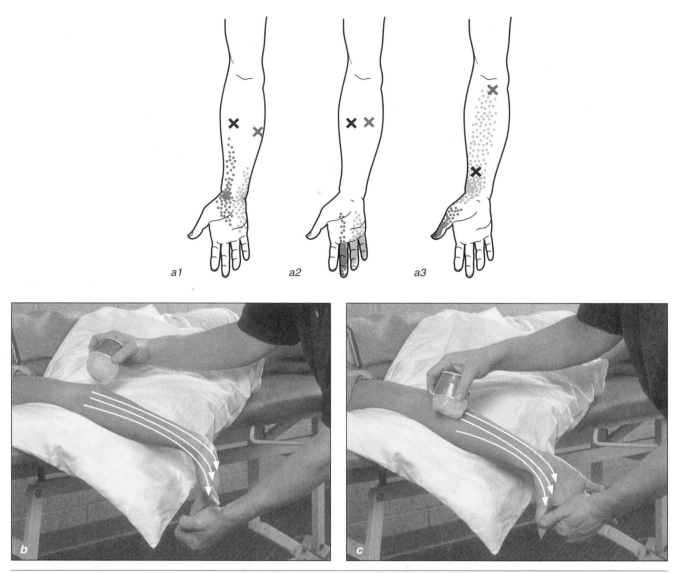

a1   *a2*   *a3*

b   *c*

Figure 19.12   Pronator teres, wrist and finger flexors: *(a)* pain-referral patterns, *(a1)* dark = flexor carpi radialis, light = flexor carpi ulnaris; *(a2)* dark = long finger flexors radial head, light = long finger flexors humeral head; *(a3)* dark = flexor pollicus longus, light = pronator teres, *(b)* ice-and-stretch to wrist and finger flexors, *(c)* ice-and-stretch to flexor pollicus longus and pronator teres.

Long Finger Extensors

In contrast with the long finger flexors, the long extensors refer pain into their digits short of the last phalanx. The pain is referred along the posterior forearm, with the primary pain occurring into the digit. The middle finger extensor can also refer to the lateral epicondyle. The extensor indicis refers to the ulnar wrist and into the dorsum of the hand but not the digit (figure 19.13,a–d). The trigger points are located in the belly of each muscle.

Extensor tendon trigger points are easily located as they produce a twitch response, especially the tendon to the long finger. It is located about 3 to 4 cm (about 7.5–10 in.) distal and dorsal to the radial head. Because the little- and ring-finger fibers are the deeper fibers of the muscle, they are more difficult to palpate but produce a twitch response when located. Deep pressure applied over these trigger points while the muscle is relaxed diminishes the discomfort (figure 19.13e).

Ice-and-stretch is performed with the forearm supported and the elbow extended. Ice sweeps, made from the elbow, move distally to the fingers with the wrist and fingers placed on stretch (figure 19.13f). If pain is referred to the lateral epicondyle, ice sweeps upward toward the epicondyle are also performed.

Figure 19.13   Long finger extensors: pain-referral patterns for *(a-b)* middle-finger extensor, *(c)* ring-finger extensor, *(d)* extensor incidis; *(e)* trigger point release; *(f)* ice-and-stretch.

Intrinsic Muscles

The intrinsic muscles are divided into three groups based on where they function: (1) at the thumb, (2) at the little finger, and (3) at the other finger muscles—the interossei and lumbricals. The thumb muscles lie within the thenar eminence, and the little finger muscles lie within the hypothenar eminence. Between these two prominences lie the interossei and lumbricals.

Thumb Muscles

The adductor pollicis refers pain to the base of the thumb, and the opponens pollicis refers pain to the radial volar wrist and along the palmar aspect of the thumb (figure 19.14, a-c). Each trigger point is near the middle aspect of the muscle belly.

Trigger point release of each muscle is applied with the muscle relaxed and pressure over the trigger point until a release is palpated or the discomfort diminishes (figure 19.14d).

Ice-and-stretch is applied with the muscle on stretch. The sweeps are applied across the thenar eminence and over the thumb (figure 19.14e).

Figure 19.14   Thumb intrinsics: pain-referral patterns for *(a-b)* adductor pollicis, *(c)* opponens pollicis; *(d)* trigger point release to adductor pollicus; *(e)* ice-and-stretch.

Interossei and Abductor Digiti Minimi

The dorsal interossei produce a strong pain referral along the radial side of the index finger, especially at the DIP joint. The other interossei refer pain along the side of the digit to which they attach (figure 19.15, a–d).

Trigger points can be palpated and treated using a pincher grip with the patient's fingers spread to move the metacarpals apart. While applying pressure on the dorsal surface, the rehabilitation clinician applies counterpressure on the palmar surface.

Ice-and-stretch is applied with the patient relaxed and the forearm supported. Only the first dorsal interossei can be reached with ice-and-stretch. With the thumb in abduction, the index finger is adducted toward the middle finger as an ice sweep is performed from proximal to the wrist and along the index finger (figure 19.15e).

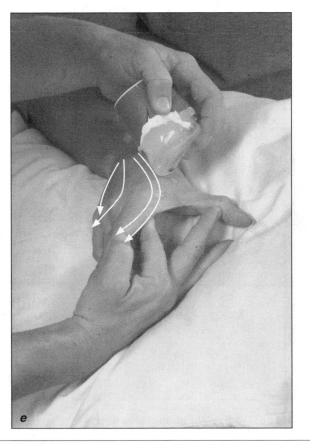

Figure 19.15 Interossei and abductor digiti minimi: pain-referral patterns for *(a-b)* first dorsal interosseus, *(c)* second dorsal interosseus, *(d)* abductor digiti minimi; *(e)* ice-and-stretch.

Figure 19.16   Palmar myofascial release.

Palmar Fascia

This myofascial technique is used to mobilize palmar fascia and the wrist retinaculum. The patient sits facing the rehabilitation clinician or lies supine with the forearm resting comfortably on the table. With the patient's hand in a palm-up position, the rehabilitation clinician grasps the patient's hand with the thumbs adjacent to each other over the base of the wrist and the fingers wrapped around the hand with the finger pads on the dorsum of the wrist. (figure 19.16). The rehabilitation clinician applies a lateral traction of the palmar soft tissue with his or her thumbs and their thenar eminences, as an upward force is applied by the finger pads on the wrist's dorsum.

JOINT MOBILIZATION

▶ Various joint mobilization techniques used to improve movement in the distal radioulnar joint, the wrist joint, and the carpometacarpal joints.

Most of the joint mobilization techniques discussed here are for joint accessory movements. They are based primarily on Maitland's (1991) work. There are certainly more movements available, but the movements discussed here are the techniques commonly used to improve joint mobility of the distal forearm, wrist, hand, and fingers.

Distal Radioulnar Joint

As with any elbow injury, both the proximal and distal radioulnar joints should be examined for restricted mobility. If any restriction is present, they should be mobilized according to restrictive findings.

Figure 19.17   Joint mobilization: radioulnar longitudinal distraction.

Longitudinal Traction

This is an accessory movement that is used to distract both the proximal and distal radioulnar joints. It can be performed in any position of elbow flexion or extension and any position of forearm supination or pronation. The greatest excursion occurs in a midposition of both flexion-extension and pronation-supination (Maitland 1991). This technique is often performed at the end range of the restricted movement.

The patient is positioned comfortably in either sitting or supine. The clinician faces the patient and places the stabilizing hand just proximal to the patient's elbow, with the web space wrapped around the patient's distal arm and the mobilizing hand wrapped around the anterior wrist (figure 19.17). The forearm of the mobilizing arm is in line with the patient's forearm. After the soft tissue's slack is taken up, either an oscillating longitudinal pull or a sustained traction is applied with the mobilizing arm.

Figure 19.18   Joint mobilization: distal radioulnar AP and PA glides.

Anteroposterior (AP) and Posteroanterior (PA) Glides

This mobilization technique is used to improve radioulnar mobility in supination and pronation. The rehabilitation clinician uses one hand to grasp the ulnar head and the other to grasp the radial head. The pad on one thenar eminence is used to apply the anteroposterior force on one bone; the fingers of the opposite hand, on the patient's posterior forearm, are used to apply the posteroanterior force on the other bone (figure 19.18). The vertical forces applied by the two hands should be equal in timing and degree. An AP force on the radius with a PA force on the ulna increases supination, and an AP force on the ulna with a PA force on the radius increases pronation.

Wrist Joint

Wrist mobilizations are performed with the patient in a comfortable position, either sitting or supine. The rehabilitation clinician is sitting or standing. A towel roll is placed under the patient's distal forearm with the wrist over the table edge.

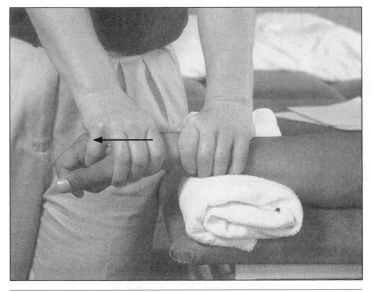

Figure 19.19   Joint mobilization: wrist traction.

Joint Traction

This maneuver is for general mobilization of the wrist. The forearm is in a comfortable position of pronation, and the wrist is in neutral. The rehabilitation clinician stabilizes the distal forearm with one hand around the radial and ulnar styloids and places the mobilizing hand over the distal carpal row. A traction force in a longitudinal direction is applied with the mobilizing hand (figure 19.19). The force can be either a sustained application or a traction oscillation.

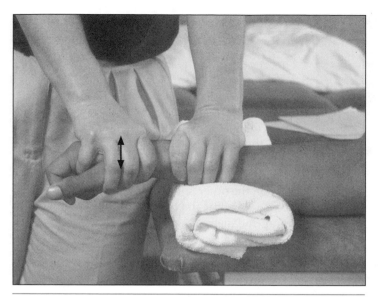

Figure 19.20 Joint mobilization: dorsal and volar glides of the wrist.

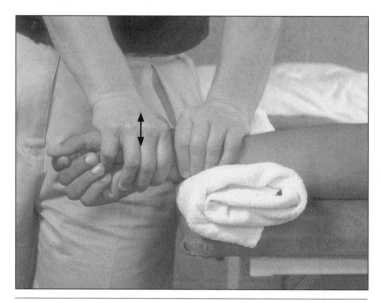

Figure 19.21 Joint mobilization: radial and ulnar glides of the wrist.

Dorsal Glide

This is a general maneuver used to increase wrist flexion. With the patient's forearm in pronation and the wrist in neutral, the rehabilitation clinician places the stabilizing hand over the radial and ulnar styloids and the mobilizing hand over the distal carpal row. An AP mobilizing force is applied by the distal, mobilizing hand (figure 19.20). The force should be applied at an angle parallel to the wrist joint.

Volar Glide

This is a general maneuver used to increase wrist extension. With the patient's forearm in pronation and the wrist in neutral, the rehabilitation clinician places the stabilizing hand over the radial and ulnar styloids and the mobilizing hand over the distal carpal row. Then a PA force is applied by the distal, mobilizing hand (figure 19.20). The force should be applied at an angle parallel to the wrist joint.

Radial Glide

This is a general technique used to increase ulnar deviation. The patient's forearm is positioned with the ulnar side upward and the wrist in neutral. The rehabilitation clinician places the stabilizing hand over the radial and ulnar styloids and the mobilizing hand over the distal carpal rows (figure 19.21). A vertically downward mobilizing force is applied by the mobilizing hand.

Ulnar Glide

This is a general technique used to increase radial deviation. The patient's forearm is positioned with the radial side upward and the wrist in neutral. The rehabilitation clinician places the stabilizing hand over the radial and ulnar styloids and the mobilizing hand over the distal carpal rows (figure 19.21). A vertically downward mobilizing force is applied by the mobilizing hand.

Specific Carpal Glides

Each of the carpals in the proximal and distal rows can be mobilized with each other and with the radius and ulna to improve flexion or extension motion in the wrist. Sometimes when individual carpal joints are restricted, individual joint mobilization techniques are necessary. The concave-convex rule applies to these joints, so it is important to know the joint's configuration before deciding whether a PA or an AP mobilization force is appropriate (figure 19.22).

The radius and ulna are concave surfaces, and the proximal carpal row provides the convex surfaces for the radiocarpal and ulnocarpal joints. To increase extension in the radiocarpal joints, the carpals are glided in a volar (anterior) direction. To increase flexion in the radiocarpal joints, the radius is glided in a volar direction. The ulnocarpal joint is mobilized by gliding the ulna in an anterior direction to unlock the articular disk that can obstruct wrist motion.

In the radial intercarpal joints, the convex scaphoid joins with the concave trapezium and trapezoid; this means that flexion is increased with a volar glide of the trapezium and

Key

1. Radius
2. Ulna
3. Scaphoid
4. Lunate
5. Triquetrum
6. Pisiform
7. Trapezium
8. Trapezoid
9. Capitate
10. Hamate

Figure 19.22   Convex-concave arrangement of carpal bones.

trapezoid on a fixed scaphoid, and extension is increased with a volar glide of the scaphoid on the distal carpal row. Because the capitate is the convex surface and the lunate is the concave surface of the capitate-lunate joint, flexion is increased by a volar glide of the lunate on the fixed capitate, and extension is increased by stabilizing the proximal lunate and performing a volar glide of the distal capitate.

The mobilization techniques for each of these joints are similar. The forearm is unsupported so that the weight of the arm can provide a slight traction force on the joints. In each case, mobilization is performed using a pinch grasp with both the stabilizing and mobilizing hands with the thumbs on the dorsum of the pronated wrist. The stabilizing finger and thumb grasp the bone that is to remain stationary, and the mobilizing finger and thumb grasp the bone to be mobilized (figure 19.23). Because the joints are small, the clinician's thumbs are nearly in contact with each other. The thumbs are used to apply a vertical downward force in a volar direction.

Figure 19.23   Joint mobilization: specific carpal glides.

Carpometacarpal Joints

For the finger and thumb carpometacarpal (CMC) joints, hand placements for stabilization and mobilization are similar. The stabilizing hand is placed in a thumb-and-index-finger pinch grasp over the carpal bone, and the mobilizing hand is placed in a similar grasp around the base of the metacarpal. Some distraction is applied to the joint while the mobilizing force is simultaneously applied. It is important to be careful not to squeeze the carpal but still grasp it firmly enough to provide adequate mobilization force. Because the CMC joints have a convex carpal and a concave metacarpal, flexion is increased with a volar (PA) glide of the distal segment, and extension is increased with a dorsal (AP) glide of the distal segment of the joint.

Finger Carpometacarpal Joints

Loss of mobility in these joints can restrict the individual's ability to make a fist and can reduce grip capabilities. Joint mobilization is often required to restore motion in these joints. Some of the most common techniques are presented here.

Joint Traction

This technique is used to relieve pain and provide a general increase in mobility. The carpal is stabilized, and the metacarpal is pulled in the direction of its long axis (figure 19.24).

Carpometacarpal Anteroposterior Glide

This technique is used to increase extension. The patient's hand is positioned in supination. The rehabilitation clinician stabilizes the patient's carpal with the thumb and index finger of one hand, and then places the thumb and index finger of the other hand over the metacarpal to be treated, with the thumb on the volar surface (figure 19.25). A downward force is applied by the thumb on the metacarpal in a direction vertical to the joint surface.

Figure 19.24 Joint mobilization: CMC distraction.

Figure 19.25 Joint mobilization: CMC AP glide joint mobilization.

Carpometacarpal Posteroanterior Glide

This technique is used to increase flexion. With the patient's hand in pronation, the rehabilitation clinician's grasps are similar to those described for AP glides except that the thumbs are placed on the dorsal surface and the fingers are placed on the volar surface (figure 19.26). A PA glide is applied to the metacarpal. If mobilizing the radial side, the clinician's fingers grasp around the first web space of the patient's hand. If mobilizing the ulnar hand, the rehabilitation clinician grasps the ulnar border of the hand.

Metacarpophalangeal Joint Rotation

Rotation of the MCP joints is an accessory movement that is necessary for full joint motion. If the finger is lacking the last few degrees of motion or the hand cannot make a complete fist, it may be that rotation of the MCP is limited. To perform the technique the MCP is positioned in 90° flexion. A distraction is applied to the joint as the distal segment of the joint is rotated medially and laterally (figure 19.27).

Figure 19.26 Joint mobilization: CMC PA (dorsal) glide.

Figure 19.27 Joint mobilization: MCP rotation.

Thumb Carpometacarpal Joint

As with carpometacarpal techniques for fingers 2 through 5, mobilization of the thumb is applied with the stabilizing hand using a thumb-and-index-finger pinch grasp over the carpal bone and the mobilizing hand placed around the metacarpal bone, close to the joint margin.

Carpometacarpal Traction

This technique is similar to the traction technique for the CMC joints of the fingers. The radial carpals are stabilized while a traction force is applied to the thumb metacarpal.

Figure 19.28 Joint mobilization: thumb CMC PA glide.

Carpometacarpal Posteroanterior Glide

This technique is used to increase extension. The rehabilitation clinician stabilizes the trapezium and trapezoid at the proximal aspect of the joint, using the thumb and index finger of one hand; the clinician holds the patient's first metacarpal with the opposite thumb along the posterior aspect, and the index finger around the anterior aspect. The rehabilitation clinician creates slight traction and applies a PA glide to the metacarpal using his or her thumb on its posterior surface (figure 19.28).

Carpometacarpal Anteroposterior Glide

This technique is used to increase flexion mobility. The rehabilitation clinician's hand placement is the same as for the PA glide, but the force is applied by the index finger on the volar surface of the metacarpal in an AP glide.

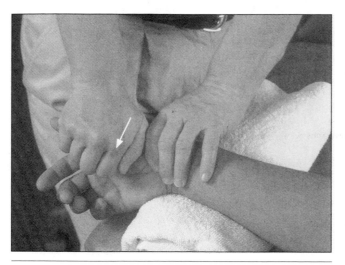

Figure 19.29   Joint mobilization: thumb CMC ulnar glide.

Carpometacarpal Ulnar Glide

Because the thumb's CMC joint is a saddle joint, it is convex at its proximal joint surface and concave at its distal joint surface for abduction-adduction movements. Mobilization for these movements is opposite to the direction of movement.

An ulnar glide increases abduction motion. With the forearm, wrist, and thumb positioned in neutral and the proximal aspect of the joint stabilized with the thumb and index finger of one hand, the rehabilitation clinician grasps the metacarpal with the other hand as shown in figure 19.29, and applies a downward force that is parallel to the joint surface.

Metacarpophalangeal and Interphalangeal Joints

The configuration of each of these joints is similar, so the mobilization techniques are similar. Each mobilization described can be used on any of these joints. Traction is applied during each mobilization technique to make the technique more comfortable and produce better results. The grasps should be firm enough to administer the mobilization force effectively but not tight enough to cause discomfort.

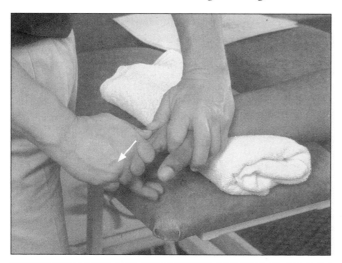

Figure 19.30   Joint mobilization: MCP distraction.

Traction

The proximal aspect of the joint is grasped with the stabilizing hand while the distal aspect of the joint is grasped by the index finger and thumb of the mobilizing hand (figure 19.30). The joint is positioned in slight flexion in a resting position. A traction force in line with the longitudinal axis is applied perpendicular to the joint surface.

Rotation

The proximal aspect of the joint is grasped with a lateral pinch of the thumb and index finger. The joint is in some flexion, and a mild traction force is applied by the mobilizing hand before medial and lateral rotation is applied.

Posteroanterior Glides and Anteroposterior Glides

Because the joints are a concave surface moving on a convex surface, the mobilization force is in the same direction of movement. To increase extension, an AP mobilization force is applied. Flexion is increased with a PA mobilization. The proximal aspect of the joint is stabilized while the distal aspect receives traction and a PA or AP force (figure 19.31).

Lateral Glides

Lateral glides are used to increase abduction and adduction of the MCP and IP joints. These are accessory movements that permit full joint motion. A radial or ulnar glide force is applied to the distal aspect of the joint, depending on the finger and movement desired (figure 19.32).

Figure 19.31 Joint mobilization: MCP AP and PA glides.

Figure 19.32 Joint mobilization: MCP lateral glides.

FLEXIBILITY EXERCISES

▶ Flexibility exercises for the hand are used to stretch the joints and ligaments, the extrinsic muscles, and the intrinsic muscles.

Range-of-motion exercises are divided into those for the intrinsic muscles and those for the extrinsic muscles. The two groups require different considerations for correct stretch application. Because extrinsic muscles cross multiple joints, the rehabilitation clinician must know these muscle insertion locations to apply appropriate stretches. Each joint the muscle crosses must be placed on stretch to produce optimal ROM changes, but the force should be applied precisely and in sequence from the most distal to the most proximal joint. When one joint is stretched, the other joints must be stabilized. If the proximal joint is not stabilized, the stretch force and surrounding tissue tension can cause the proximal joint to extend rather than flex. The force applied should be a slow, gentle, and sustained stretch to avoid incorrect stretch application or excessive force that can damage the small structures of the hand and fingers.

One finger should be stretched at a time. Joint mobilization is used before stretching so that the stretch of soft-tissue structures is more effective. If joint motion is restricted by extrinsic tightness, each joint is placed on stretch in the sequence just described to affect extrinsic structures but not intrinsic muscles. If joint motion is restricted by intrinsic tightness, the distal joint is stretched and the proximal joint is placed in the opposite direction in order to eliminate the stretch on extrinsic muscles and apply the intended stretch to the intrinsic muscles. For example, when the PIP joint is placed in flexion and the MCP joint is placed in extension, the intrinsic muscles are stretched and the extrinsic muscles are not; but when the PIP and MCP joints are placed in flexion, the extrinsic muscles are stretched but the intrinsics are not. If both structures have limited flexibility, stretching exercises in both positions are necessary.

Joints and Ligaments

As already mentioned, mobilization techniques—both accessory and physiological techniques—should be applied before joints are stretched. The accessory techniques are those already discussed, including motions that are not actively possible but that must take place for full motion to occur. These should be applied before the physiological motions. The physiological motions are those that can be actively produced, such as joint flexion and extension. Techniques used to produce the physiological motions are simply called stretching exercises.

Only one joint is stretched at a time. The other joints are positioned in neutral and kept relaxed to reduce soft-tissue tension on the joint being treated. When you are applying a stretch force, the distal portion of the joint's distal arm being stretched is the location of the stretch. You need to be careful, however, to apply the force on the joint's distal arm and not on the next distal joint. For example, when stretching a PIP joint, your force is on the distal portion of the middle phalanx, not on the DIP joint or the distal phalanx. Proper stabilization of the proximal phalanx must also occur for the stretch application to be correct (figure 19.33).

Figure 19.33 Stretch force application. *(a)* Incorrect: force is applied on the digit's distal segment. *(b)* Correct: force is applied at the distal joint first, then moves one joint at a time to the most proximal joint.

Figure 19.34
Thumb abduction
stretch.

Abduction movements are crucial to maintaining vital web space flexibility of the thumb and MCP extension movement of the fingers. Abduction of the fingers can assist in stretching the MCP collateral ligaments. Soft tissue of the web space is stretched with thumb abduction. These movements can be performed actively and passively. Passive movements can be performed by the clinician or the patient. The patient can stretch the finger MCPs by intertwining the fingers of the two hands together as in a praying position. The thumb's web space can be stretched by actively abducting the thumb or applying an abduction force at the CMC joint. Care must be taken not to apply the force on the MCP joint. The patient can also stretch the thumb's web space by placing the hand over the top of the knee, with the fingers separated from the thumb, and applying a downward force from the shoulder to push the hand on the knee (figure 19.34).

As mentioned earlier, the CMC and intermetacarpal joints form the palmar arches that are vital to hand formation and function. The second and third metacarpals, which have little mobility, form the peak of the palmar arches. The fourth, and especially the fifth, metacarpals move into flexion as the hand is formed into a fist; this motion is crucial to normal hand function and permits a firm grasp. The rehabilitation clinician can stretch these joints by placing his or her thumbs in the palm of the patient's hand and his or her fingers on the dorsum over the metacarpals. The thumbs are stabilizers as the fingers roll the metacarpals around the thumbs (figure 19.35). The palmar fascia can be stretched using the technique demonstrated in figure 19.16.

Wrist joint stretches are utilized with the fingers relaxed and the force applied proximal to the MCP joints. The patient can apply the stretches passively in all wrist motions (figure 19.36).

Figure 19.35 Range of motion of CMC and inter-metacarpal joints.

Figure 19.36 Wrist stretches.

The distal radioulnar joint stretches are the same as those for the proximal radio-ulnar joint. These are discussed in chapter 18 and are shown in figures 18.19 and 18.20. The stretch is applied at the distal radioulnar joint. The hand is not included in the stretch.

The oblique retinacular ligament acts on the IP joints similarly to the way the intrinsics act on the MCP and PIP joints. When the PIP joint is flexed, it extends the DIP joint. If passive DIP flexion is more with the PIP joint flexed than with the PIP extended, the oblique retinacular ligament is restricted. Tightness limits DIP flexion particularly during PIP extension. To stretch this ligament, the PIP joint is passively maintained in extension while the DIP joint is stretched into flexion.

Extrinsic Muscles

As mentioned previously, the stretch applied to extrinsics begins with the distal joint and proceeds in sequence distally to proximally. The force is applied slowly and deliberately without excessive stress to the structures. Contract-relax-stretch techniques can improve results of the stretch because of reflex inhibition. Application of a slight traction force on the joints makes the stretch more comfortable by reducing compressive forces on the joints.

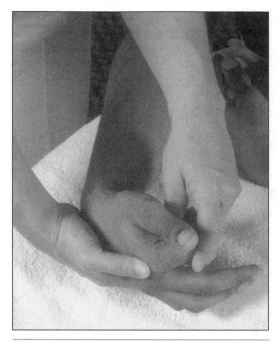

Figure 19.37   Extrinsic finger extensor stretch. In sequence: DIP, PIP, MCP, wrist elbow.

Because of the easy accessibility of the hand and wrist joints and the relatively small force required to stretch them, the patient can learn proper stretching techniques and can apply them frequently throughout the day.

Stretching for both the extrinsic extensors and extrinsic flexors starts distally and moves proximally. For example, improving flexion motion involves beginning at the DIP joint and stabilizing the PIP joint as the DIP is brought into flexion. Once the DIP joint is moved to its end position, the PIP joint is then moved into flexion. The MCP joint is then moved into flexion while the IP joints are held in their flexed positions. Finally, the wrist is brought into flexion to its end range with the finger maintained in its fully flexed position. Stretch to increase flexion is seen in figure 19.37. Stretches to increase flexion and extension of the extrinsic muscles are each applied in both elbow flexion and extension. The patient should feel a stretch on the forearm.

Wrist stretches should be applied with the fingers on stretch, because the long finger muscles can also influence wrist mobility. To increase wrist extension motion, the patient extends the fingers first and then moves the wrist into extension (figure 19.38a). As with stretches to the fingers, the wrist should be stretched with the elbow in flexion and in extension. The stretch should be felt on the anterior forearm.

A slow sustained stretch is applied to the finger and wrist extensors to increase wrist flexion. The stretch begins at the fingers and is applied last to the wrist (figure 19.38b). The stretch should be applied with the elbow flexed and extended until a stretch on the posterior forearm is felt.

Figure 19.38   Independent stretches to increase *(a)* wrist extension and *(b)* wrist flexion.

Intrinsic Muscles

Because the lumbricals and interossei flex the MCP joint and extend the IP joints, the stretch is applied in the opposite direction of their movement. The IP joints are maintained in a flexed position while a stretch to increase MCP extension is applied (figure 19.39). The wrist should be stabilized in neutral during this activity to prevent extrinsic muscle influences on the stretch.

Figure 19.39 Intrinsic stretch: IPs are flexed, MCP is extended, wrist is in neutral.

STRENGTHENING EXERCISES

▶ Strengthening exercises are used to restore normal glide of the hand's flexor and extensor tendons; and a large variety of resistive exercises promote strength of the wrist extensors, ulnar and radial extensors, and supinators and pronators.

During periods of immobilization, isometric exercises can be used for all wrist and hand muscles. Active exercises are good for maintaining motion and early strengthening. As the patient progresses, various equipment including weights, putty, and rubber bands can be used to further increase strength gains. In the early stages, the muscles may fatigue quickly, so the patient must be cautioned against overdoing it, causing undue stress. Since little functional hand activity is eccentric, concentric exercises, rather than eccentric exercises, for the fingers are the primary emphasis.

Tendon Glide Exercises

When restriction of normal tendon glide occurs because of adhesions of tendons or their sheaths, you must restore the normal tendon glide if full motion is to be achieved. When adhesions occur, they can occur anywhere along the tendon and can restrict tendon motion proximally and distally to the point of adhesion. Friction massage assists in reducing adhesions of superficial tendons, and exercises improve mobility of both superficial and deep tendons. Muscle activity aids in restoring proximal glide of the tendon. Active and passive exercises and splinting can restore distal glide of the tendon. Because active exercises can restore both proximal and distal tendon glide, it is advisable to use these whenever possible. The effectiveness of these exercises, however, is limited by the muscle's strength and endurance. Passive stretching and massage may be useful to improve tendon glide when these parameters are restricted.

Flexor Tendons

Gliding exercises for the long flexor tendons necessitate differentiating between the profundus and superficialis. You must isolate each tendon to facilitate gliding, because adhesions between the tendons restrict gliding. To show whether or not the tendons are gliding properly, the patient maintains extension of the MCP joint while flexing the PIP joints. With the fingers in this position, the clinician passively extends the DIP joint and should meet no resistance. If there is no resistance, it is normal and only the superficialis is being used. If the patient maintains this position with contraction of both muscles, normal tendon gliding is restricted. The MCP and PIP joints are stabilized in flexion while the patient attempts to flex and extend the DIP (figure 19.40a). To isolate the superficialis, the proximal phalanx is stabilized and the PIP joint is flexed and extended: Either one digit is stabilized at a time as shown in figure 19.40b, or all digits except the one being treated are stabilized. In this exercise the other IP joints are maintained in extension while the digit of interest is flexed. Because the profundus tendons all originate from the same muscle belly, it is easy to eliminate profundus activity by restricting movement of the other digits (figure 19.40c).

Figure 19.40   Isolation of tendons for gliding exercises: *(a)* flexor digitorum profundus, *(b)* flexor digitorum superficialis, *(c)* elimination of flexor digitorum profundus activity.

There are three functional flexor tendon gliding exercises that belong in a therapeutic exercise program when flexor tendon gliding is restricted. Keeping the MCP extended and flexing the IPs enhances gliding between the two longer finger flexor tendons (figure 19.41a). This is known as the hook position. The fist formation with the IP and MCP joints in flexion produces gliding of the profundus tendon within its sheath (figure 19.41b), and the position with the MCP and PIP joints flexed and the DIP joints extended (modified fist) provides optimal gliding of the superficialis tendons in their sheath (figure 19.41c). The start position for each of these flexor tendon gliding exercises is with all the fingers in full extension. As the patient performs each specific exercise, controlled digit movements are used throughout the entire motion.

Flexor pollicis longus gliding exercises are performed in a similar manner by moving the IP and MCP joints through a full range of flexion and extension. These exercises are initially performed with the wrist in neutral, but as the patient progresses, the wrist should be moved into flexion with finger flexion and into extension with finger extension.

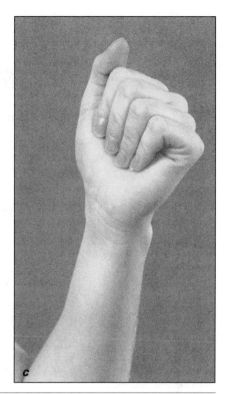

Figure 19.41 Flexor tendon gliding exercises: *(a)* Hook enhances gliding between FDS and FDP. *(b)* Fist enhances gliding of FDP. *(c)* Modified fist enhances gliding of FDS.

Extensor Tendons

Because the extensor tendons are flatter and wider than their flexor counterparts and because they have an intimate relationship with the intrinsic muscle system, they are more susceptible to adhesions. Adhesions can cause an extensor lag of the finger. If full extension occurs passively but not actively, adhesions may be the cause. This is particularly true if the digit's passive flexion is also limited, because the adhesion restricts full tendon excursion during a stretch. Care must be taken in stretching the extensor tendons following tendon repairs or fractures. The rehabilitation clinician must keep a close eye on increases in the extensor lag throughout the stretching process. If the extensor lag increases, it may be that the tendon is actually elongating (dehiscing) or tearing from its attachment. Emphasizing the use of active exercises for reducing extensor lag rather than passive forces to increase flexion motion helps to minimize this risk.

If an extensor lag is present at the MCP joint because of an adhesion, the adhesion is of the extensor digitorum communis (EDC) tendon. This tendon is the only extensor of the MCP joint. A gliding exercise for the EDC is performed by moving the hand from a hook to a fist formation as seen in figure 19.42. The MCP joint is moved from flexion to extension while the IP joints are kept in flexion to eliminate the intrinsic muscles. If the patient has difficulty maintaining flexion of the IP joints during this exercise, he or she can facilitate the activity by grasping a drinking straw or pencil in the fingers while moving the MCP joints. Wrist flexion and extension should also be added to the exercise when it is easy to perform with the wrist in neutral.

Figure 19.42 Extrinsic extensor gliding exercises: Keeping the IPs in flexion, the MCPs are moved into flexion and extension.

If the extensor lag occurs at either IP joint, it is the result of adhesions within the extensor mechanism and can include both intrinsic and extrinsic structures—the interossei, lumbricals, and EDC. To isolate the intrinsic muscles and facilitate their movement of IP extension, the MCP should be stabilized in flexion (figure 19.43a). As this exercise becomes easier, the MCP joint should be moved into extension. The most difficult position for this exercise is with the hand flat on a table and the proximal phalanx stabilized; in this position the patient attempts to lift the middle and distal phalanxes off the table (figure 19.43b).

Figure 19.43 Extensor gliding exercises. *(a)* Intrinsic: MCP flexion with IPs in extension. *(b)* Terminal extension: IP extension with MCP in extension.

Resistive Exercises

There are many variations for resistive exercises for the wrist and hand. Specific exercises are limited only by the rehabilitation clinician's imagination. A few of the more commonly used resistive exercises are outlined here. Common substitution patterns for the exercise are also listed. You should correct any errors in technique.

Wrist Extension

This exercise is used to increase the strength of the wrist extensors. The forearm rests on a tabletop in pronation with the hand over the end of the table. The patient lifts a dumbbell, moving through a full ROM from wrist flexion to wrist extension (figure 19.44). The forearm must stay in contact with the tabletop throughout the exercise; it may be necessary to stabilize the forearm with a hand across the proximal forearm. Substitutions seen in this exercise include flexing the elbow and moving the weight through a partial ROM.

Wrist Flexion

This exercise strengthens the wrist flexors. The patient sits next to a table with the forearm resting on the table in supination and the hand over the end of the table. He or she moves a dumbbell weight through a full ROM from wrist extension to flexion (figure 19.45). Substitutions for this exercise include flexing the elbow and moving the wrist through a partial ROM.

Figure 19.44 Wrist extension resistance exercise.

Ulnar and Radial Deviation

These exercises strengthen ulnar and radial flexors. To strengthen the ulnar flexors, a bar with a weighted end is placed in the hand, with the weight on the ulnar side. The patient stands with the elbow extended. The patient moves the wrist into ulnar deviation, lifting the weight as high as possible (figure 19.46a). He or she should maintain a firm grasp on the bar so that the wrist rather than the fingers is used to produce the motion. In addition to finger movement, shoulder extension is a common substitution.

To strengthen radial flexors, the patient's position remains the same, but the weighted bar is positioned with the weight on the radial aspect of the hand. The weight is lifted upward as high as possible toward the thumb (figure 19.46b). The patient must maintain a firm grasp to produce the motion from the wrist and not the fingers. Elbow flexion is a common substitution for this exercise.

Figure 19.45 Wrist flexion resistance exercise.

Figure 19.46 Ulnar (a) and radial (b) deviation resistance exercise.

Pronation and Supination

These exercises are demonstrated in chapter 18, figure 18.25. They can also be used to provide additional eccentric activity with rubber tubing. The rubber tubing is attached to a handle or weighted bar and anchored to the side of the table. To provide eccentric resistance to the supinators, the bar is positioned with the rubber tubing attached to the side of the table opposite the injured wrist. The bar is passively positioned with the forearm in supination. The patient then controls the bar as the rubber tubing pulls the forearm into pronation (figure 19.47a).

Eccentric resistance for the pronators is provided with the rubber tubing anchored to the table on the same side as the injured wrist. The bar is passively positioned with the forearm in pronation; and as the rubber tubing pulls the bar, the patient controls the supination motion of the forearm (figure 19.47b).

During each exercise, the forearm must remain stable on the tabletop, and no substitution by shoulder abduction or adduction is allowed.

Figure 19.47   Eccentric resistance exercises: *(a)* supination and *(b)* pronation.

Putty Exercises

A number of putty exercises can be incorporated into a program that the patient can perform at home or on road trips with the team. The putty comes in a variety of resistances, indicated by different colors, and can be changed for another color as the patient's strength improves. Some putty uses the addition of chips to increase resistance. Different colors can be used for different exercises to offer optimal resistance for each exercise. The patient can perform wrist flexion and extension by grasping the putty with the uninvolved hand and pulling on the putty with the involved hand (figure 19.48, a and b). The same precautions for substitutions apply as with the dumbbell exercises. Ulnar and radial deviation motions can also be resisted with putty. For ulnar deviation the patient places both hands with the lateral sides of the index fingers and thumbs adjacent to each other. With only wrist movement, he or she moves the hands laterally away from each other as the wrists move into ulnar deviation (figure 19.48c). For radial deviation, the patient positions the little finger of the involved hand on top of the thumb of the other hand. The putty is formed into a tube shape and is grasped by both hands. Stabilizing the uninvolved hand and the involved forearm and elbow, the patient moves the involved wrist into radial deviation. To perform pronation and supination, the patient uses the stabilizing hand to hold the putty while the involved forearm moves into supination and pronation as it grasps the putty (figure 19.48d). Supination-pronation motion should be limited to the forearm; no elbow motion is permitted.

Figure 19.48 Theraputty wrist exercises: *(a)* wrist flexion, *(b)* wrist extension, *(c)* ulnar deviation, *(d)* supination-pronation.

A number of finger exercises can be designed using putty of different strengths to provide a progressive resistive program. These are discussed next.

Grip Exercises

Grips using putty for resistance with the entire hand (spherical) (figure 19.49a), the thumb and index finger (hook) (figure 19.49b), and the thumb and fingers (cylinder) (figure 19.49c) address power-grip strengthening. The putty selected should provide enough resistance to make the exercise challenging but also be light enough to allow a full ROM. The hand is positioned as shown, and the putty is squeezed. It is then reshaped, and the exercise is repeated.

Patients can also perform precision grips using resistive putty (figure 19.50). The patient should do these exercises with each phalanx in slight flexion. The IP joints should not be extended. Precision-grip exercises can also be performed with clothespins. Wrapping rubber bands around the end of the clothespin provides additional resistance. As with the putty exercises, the patient should grasp the clothespins with the IP joints in slight flexion. Extension of any IP joint should not be permitted.

Flexion exercises can be performed against manual resistance, rubber bands, putty, or other objects. You can adjust these exercises according to the availability of your equipment.

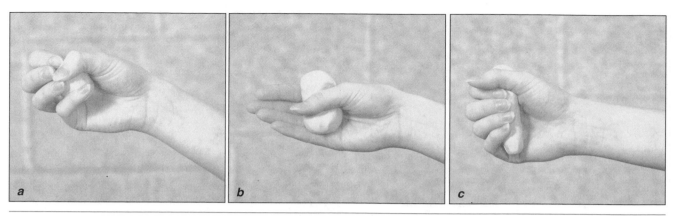

Figure 19.49 Theraputty power-grip exercises: *(a)* spherical, *(b)* hook, *(c)* cylinder.

Figure 19.50 Theraputty precision-grip exercises: *(a)* tip-to-tip, *(b)* digital prehension, *(c)* lateral prehension, *(d)* three-prong chuck.

Opposition Exercise

Gross finger-opposition strengthening exercise is shown in figure 19.51. The putty begins in a pancake on a tabletop (figure 19.51a). The patient places all the finger pads on the putty and pulls the finger pads together to pull the putty up into a cone shape (figure 19.51b). The intrinsic muscles are worked if the IP joints are kept in extension during the exercise. The extrinsics are worked if the IP joints are flexed during the exercise.

Figure 19.51 Gross opposition exercise for the intrinsic muscles: A cone should be formed in the middle as the patient repeats the exercise *(b)*.

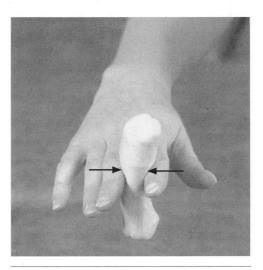

Figure 19.52 Finger adduction exercise.

Adduction

The patient can place the putty between any two fingers or between the index finger and the thumb; he or she then pulls the fingers together (figure 19.52). The IP and MCP joints should remain extended.

Finger Extension, and Thumb and Finger Abduction

Using putty or a rubber band, the patient places the item around the fingers and thumb and spreads these as far apart as possible (figure 19.53). Depending on the direction of movement, the abductors or extensors will be worked. This exercise can be used either on the entire group or on individual fingers.

Figure 19.53   *(a)* Multiple-finger and thumb extension with putty, *(b)* finger abduction with putty, *(c)* index-finger and thumb extension with putty, *(d)* two-finger abduction with rubber band, *(e)* multiple-finger abduction with rubber band, *(f)* thumb and fifth-finger abduction with rubber band.

Extensor Lag Exercises

To use the putty to strengthen the intrinsics, the patient places the putty on a tabletop. With the palm facing down and the MCP and IP joints flexed, the fingers push outward against the putty as the fingers move into extension (figure 19.54a).

A medicine ball, pushed while the MCP joints remain in flexion and the IP joints move from flexion into extension, will also provide resistance to the intrinsic muscles (figure 19.54b). This exercise becomes more challenging with the use of a heavier ball or with an increase in the surface friction.

Figure 19.54 Extensor lag exercises: *(a)* with putty, *(b)* with medicine ball.

Isokinetic Exercises

Wrist-strengthening exercises progress from straight plane to more functional diagonal planes, just as with other isokinetic protocols. Fast and slow speeds are used to enhance strength and muscle endurance. All exercises should remain pain free.

PLYOMETRIC EXERCISES

▶ In addition to plyometric exercises that are also used for the shoulder and elbow, plyometrics for the hand include activities using a medicine ball and isokinetic activities.

Many of the plyometric exercises for the shoulder and elbow are also used for the wrist and hand. A couple of additional exercises can be used for the hand. For specific information on the plyometric exercises for the shoulder and elbow, refer to chapters 17 and 18.

Ball Drop and Catch

This exercise uses a medicine ball small enough to be grasped in one hand. The patient stands with the arm outstretched in front and the hand positioned palm down. He or she grasps the medicine ball in the hand and allows it to drop, then immediately retrieves the ball before it reaches the floor by grasping with the hand in the palm-down position. As the exercise becomes easier, a heavier ball is selected. The patient should grasp the ball with all the fingers.

Other Plyometric Activities

Numerous other activities can be used as plyometric exercises for the hand. Some of these are bouncing a medicine ball against the wall or incline trampoline, boxing against a medicine bag, plyometric push-ups, and volleyball passes with a medicine ball.

FUNCTIONAL ACTIVITIES

▶ The great range of uses for the hand in sports means that the rehabilitation clinician working with a hand injury must understand the particular demands of each patient's sport and position.

Because the hand has wide variation of function, it is nearly impossible to define functional activities for the hand. Specific demands for functional activities are determined by the demands of the patient's sport or activity. A football quarterback's demands for hand function differ from those for the football lineman. The golfer's demands for hand function vary greatly from the basketball player's. The range of demands can include varying grips, varying positions, rapid or slow movements, sustained or changing grips, and forceful or light grasping. The rehabilitation clinician must understand the demands of each patient's activities and outline a functional exercise progression based on those requirements. Once a selection of exercises is made, a progression is designed using a planned program of increasing difficulty until the exercises mimic the stress levels the patient will encounter in full participation.

SPECIAL REHABILITATION APPLICATIONS

▶ Among the more common types of injuries to the hand are fractures, dislocations and sprains, overuse injuries including carpal tunnel syndrome, and tendon injuries. The rehabilitation clinician also encounters reflex sympathetic dystrophy of the hand.

Because the hand is so complex, with many structures in close contact with each other, an injury to one area or tissue can impact adjacent tissues and other segments within the wrist and hand. The rehabilitation clinician must be cognizant of this, must be keenly aware of the possibility of secondary involvement of other segments, and must do everything possible to attempt to prevent these complications.

Some of the more common injuries requiring rehabilitation are addressed here. Tendon rupture and repairs are not often seen in muscoloskeletal injuries, but the rehabilitation programs for them are outlined here since the clinician must take additional precautions when they do occur and necessitate a rehabilitation program.

Fractures

There are many bones in the wrist and hand. Which bone is fractured has a great impact on the rehabilitation process. This section presents some general concepts, applicable to all fractures, before addressing specific fractures. Although there are exceptions, a fracture is generally immobilized in a position so that the ligaments of the joints are placed on some stretch. This helps reduce the risk of contractures. Immobilization is often maintained for two to three weeks unless the fracture is unstable, displaced, or comminuted. Fractures that are unstable are often corrected with open reduction and internal fixation (ORIF), followed by immobilization. Open reduction and internal fixation is advantageous when the fracture is unstable, because it provides needed stability. However, because of the disruption of blood flow and increased soft-tissue damage that occurs with ORIF, healing time can be delayed.

Splints used to immobilize fractures should affect only as many joints as necessary to maintain good fracture alignment. Joints proximal and distal to the fracture site, and not included in the splint immobilization, should be moved through their ranges of motion regularly.

Distal Forearm and Wrist Fractures

The most common distal forearm fracture is the Colles fracture. The distal radius proximal to the wrist is fractured and is displaced dorsally. A Smith's fracture also involves the radius, but the distal radius fragment displaces volarly. Surgical repair is common with Smith's fractures but does not take place as often with a Colles fracture. A Barton's fracture occurs at the radial articular region and results in wrist subluxation as well as the fracture. While the Colles and Smith's fractures are most often the result of falling on an outstretched hand, the Barton's fracture occurs with a sudden violent wrist extension and pronation. The likelihood of its being unstable makes the need for ORIF highly probable.

As with all fractures, whether treated with open or closed reduction, management of pain and edema is the goal of early rehabilitation. Coban™ wrap is useful for controlling edema in the fingers and hand. Isotoner gloves are also used to reduce edema once the wrist cast is removed. Modalities are useful in controlling pain as well as edema. Early rehabilitation includes the use of active range-of-motion (AROM) exercises of the uninvolved joints. These exercises will encourage good tendon gliding, reduce edema, and relieve joint stiffness.

Immobilization casts or splints used for these fractures should permit full MCP flexion motion and full thumb opposition. Active range-of-motion exercises for the extrinsic finger muscles and the intrinsics should be permitted while the patient is in the splint or cast. The patient should be able to perform three exercises: MCP joint full flexion with IP extension, MCP joint extension with full IP flexion, MCP joint full flexion combined with IP joint full flexion.

It should be possible for AROM to approach passive range-of-motion (PROM) excursion. If full PROM is significantly greater than full AROM, the muscle may be atrophied and may lack sufficient strength, or the tendon is being restricted by adhesions, or both influences may be present. Active exercises, electrical stimulation, friction massage in regions where it is appropriate, proprioceptive neuromuscular facilitation, or biofeedback can be used to restore active motion while the wrist is immobilized.

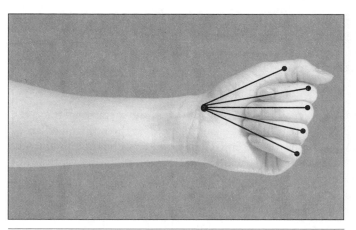

Figure 19.55 Finger alignment with MCP and PIP flexion.

It is common for distal radial fractures to be immobilized three to six weeks. Once immobilization is discontinued, the patient should attempt to regain full wrist motion and long tendon mobility. Joint mobilization with active stretches is used. Grades I and II joint mobilization can be used to relieve pain. Grades III and IV joint mobilizations are not incorporated into the program until the fracture is healed enough to withstand that stress. Range of motion in all planes should be emphasized. Many clinicians do not address radial and ulnar deviation, but these must be restored if the patient is to have full wrist function.

Isometric strengthening exercises can be used while the wrist is immobilized. Once the cast or splint is removed, the patient can begin low-resistance, low-repetition isotonic activities, progressing to higher repetitions and resistance as tolerated. If pain or swelling increases with exercises, the exercises are too aggressive and should be reduced in intensity or number of repetitions.

Once strength gains are substantial, the patient begins functional activities. Specific functional activities are determined by the patient's sport and position. Tennis has different requirements for the wrist than golf does, and golf and baseball differ in their demands. The rehabilitation clinician should be aware of the demands of the patient's sport and design a progressive functional program that will lead the patient to an appropriate return to that sport.

Carpal and Metacarpal Fractures

The carpal most frequently fractured is the scaphoid. Because of the bones' variability in blood supply, healing time is extremely varied, from 4 to 20 weeks, and depends primarily on the location and type of fracture. The area remains immobilized until radiography demonstrates signs of healing.

Edema control should be aggressive, and the patient should perform ROM of the uninvolved segments of the shoulder, elbow, and hand immediately and continually throughout the immobilization period. Pain should be avoided with these exercises.

Once the cast or splint is removed, ROM for the thumb should begin. These exercises should be active. If joint mobility is restricted in a capsular pattern, joint mobilization should be added to the program. The patient should perform active exercises with the proximal joint stabilized passively to ensure correct movement of the digit.

The hook of the hamate and the pisiform can incur fractures from impact with a baseball bat, golf club, or racket or from a fall on an outstretched arm. Because they are not often unstable, these fractures heal well most of the time with cast immobilization. As with other fractures in this area, ROM exercises for the shoulder, elbow, and other hand joints are routine while the splint is on, and restoration of full ROM for all joints should be the goal following cast removal. If pain occurs with hand and wrist activity following cast removal, a protective splint may be used at night and throughout the day to relieve the stress of motion and use. Progression of flexibility exercises should continue until full motion is achieved.

Joint mobilization of restricted metacarpal and carpal joints should be used to provide full physiological and accessory movements that are necessary for full hand and wrist function. Strengthening exercises are initiated when the cast is removed. Grip exercises are used early, because they help to mobilize the metacarpals and to restore the normal palmar arches. Wrist strengthening is also incorporated. The patient is weaned from the splint as pain and edema subside and motion and strength are restored.

Because the neck of the metacarpal is the weakest aspect of the bone, it is the most frequent site of metacarpal fractures. These fractures most commonly occur in the fourth and fifth metacarpals. Fractures here result primarily from compressive forces like those that occur when a fist is used to administer a direct blow. For this reason they are referred to as boxer's fractures. The alignment of the fingers determines whether the fracture can be treated with immobilization or whether it requires an ORIF. Normal oblique flexion of the digits with the MCP and PIP joints flexed causes an alignment of the digits such that they point toward the scaphoid tubercle (figure 19.55). If digit angulation is off by more than 20° to 30°, an ORIF may be necessary.

Two to four weeks of immobilization may be necessary for carpal and metacarpal fractures. Range-of-motion exercises while the cast is on are recommended for the uninvolved areas. Once the cast is removed, ROM exercises for the entire hand and wrist begin immediately. Active range-of-motion exercises are used for the metacarpal joints, and passive and active-motion exercises are used for the digits. This helps to reduce tendon adhesions. Intrinsic and extrinsic ROM exercises should be incorporated. Support for the metacarpals during finger ROM exercises should be provided either manually or with a splint. Once the fracture is well healed the patient progresses to PROM exercises to all areas, then to resistive exercises, and then to functional exercises. Joint mobilization can also be used to increase joint mobility in restricted segments. Resistive exercises begin with light weights and progress to heavier weights and more repetitions, using pain and edema as guidelines for advancing the patient.

A Bennett's fracture involves the first metacarpal. Because the thumb is responsible for at least 50% of hand function, appropriate management and treatment of thumb injuries are crucial. Proper angulation must be ensured with either closed or open reduction to ultimately permit good function of the thumb. The immobilization period is often four weeks. During that time, efforts to control edema and pain are important. The rehabilitation clinician should be aware that adhesions may occur in the first web space and should take steps to maintain appropriate web spacing during immobilization. If the web space is diminished, full thumb motion will be limited. Cast removal allows initiation of AROM exercises. Once union of the fracture site is observed on X-ray, usually about 6 to 8 weeks postinjury, PROM exercises can be used to regain motion. If PROM is significantly more than AROM, it is likely that tendon adhesions are present. Friction massage, electrical stimulation, and active and passive ROM exercises assist in restoring tendon glide. Dynamic splinting may be necessary when full ROM is not restored by 8 to 10 weeks. As with other fractures, resistive exercises begin after healing is apparent. Strengthening exercises should include both precision and power grasping activities and should also incorporate associated segments that have become weakened secondary to reduced use of the hand.

Phalangeal Fractures

Because of the long finger tendon forces, fractures of the proximal and middle phalanges often result in displacement and instability. Proximal phalanx fractures occur because of falls or direct blows to the phalanx, most often in the thumb and index finger. Middle phalanx fractures are not as common; these result from a crush injury such as occurs when a hand is stepped on. Distal phalanx fractures are common; these account for half of hand fractures. Proximal phalanx fractures typically result in flexion of the proximal bone segment from the pull of the interossei and extension of the distal segment because of the long extensor tendon's pull (figure 19.56). This fracture is reduced and immobilized with either open or closed reduction; the use of external wires is common. If the fracture is stable, buddy taping the fingers can immobilize the fracture and still permit tendon movement to reduce tendon gliding problems.

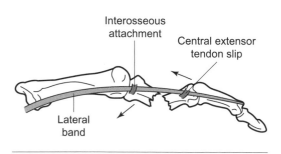

Figure 19.56 Forces affecting proximal phalanx fracture.

If the fracture is stable, motion exercises can begin as early as the first to second week. If the fracture is displaced, motion is usually started three to four weeks postinjury. Finger fractures are seldom immobilized for more than four weeks because of the deleterious effects of prolonged immobilization on surrounding soft-tissue structures.

One of the greatest complications of phalangeal immobilization is tendon adhesions, causing restriction of normal tendon gliding. Adhesions of the extensor tendon can result

Figure 19.57 Restraining exercise: The MCP and PIP joints are restrained while the DIP is moved.

Figure 19.58 Aggressive techniques to increase ROM: Tape is applied to increase IP joint flexion range of motion.

in an extensor lag and limited IP flexion. Adhesions of the long flexor tendons also prevent full extension. Scar massage can be used to limit adhesions and to treat them if they occur. Exercises that restrain specific motions to isolate tendon function can reduce tendon adhesions. For example, if the FDP is restricted, the MCP and PIP joints are positioned passively in flexion and blocked from moving while the DIP is moved into flexion and extension (figure 19.57).

Once the fracture is healed sufficiently to be stable, more aggressive PROM exercises and joint mobilization can be used to improve ROM. Dynamic splints can provide a continual low-level stress to tight structures. One can also apply tape to position digits into a stretch position (figure 19.58). These techniques should be used for 15- to 20-min periods throughout the day, as tolerated, to improve scar-tissue mobility and ROM. Caution is necessary in force application for prolonged stretching, especially with the extensor tendons, because it is relatively easy to overstretch the flat, broad extensor tendon. The end result is an extensor lag from overstretching the extensor tendon. If an extensor lag develops, an extension splint is required to correct it.

Stretching exercises should involve both intrinsic and extrinsic muscles. Intrinsic exercises are performed with the IP joints in flexion, and the MCP joints moving from flexion to extension, as seen in figure 19.39. Extrinsic muscles are stretched with the IP and MCP joints in various combinations of flexion and extension. Refer to figures 19.37 and 19.41 for these exercises.

Once the patient has achieved ROM, resistive exercises, including those using therapeutic putty and rubber bands and other exercises listed earlier, are necessary to restore full strength of the long finger flexors and extensors and the intrinsics. Wrist, elbow, and shoulder strength deficits should also be treated. Exercises begin with light resistance, increasing as the patient progresses. Exercises should emphasize full tendon and joint function that permit normal movement.

Dislocations and Sprains

Because dislocations are a severe form of sprain, these two injuries are addressed together. A dislocation, the most severe type of sprain, is immobilized for longer periods of time than a sprain. Dislocations and sprains occur primarily in the IP joints, and more commonly in the PIP than the DIP joints. A term commonly used for a finger sprain is "jammed finger." Sprains usually occur in ball-handling sports when the ball hits the end of the finger.

Program Considerations

When a dislocation occurs, the joint's supporting structures—the radial and ulnar collateral ligaments and the volar plate—have been damaged either individually or in any combination. Fractures can frequently accompany dislocations. If the dislocation is unstable, surgical repair using either a Kirschner wire or pin is often the standard course of treatment. This is accompanied by a postoperative cast or splint for three to five weeks. The wire or pin may be removed after three weeks, although use of the splint may continue. Removal of the splint to perform gentle active and passive PIP extension can be initiated with the surgeon's approval.

Case Study

A 21-year-old hockey forward suffered a fracture of the neck of the fourth MCP when he was involved in a fight during a game and hit an opponent. The hand was casted for two weeks and then placed in a splint that could be removed for his rehabilitation activities. The fracture is stable, so the physician wants to wean him from the splint over the next two weeks. The initial examination reveals some swelling in the hand and fingers. Wrist flexion is 50° and wrist extension is 65°. Ulnar deviation and radial deviation are 10°. Supination is 70° and pronation is 90°. MCP flexion is 45°, PIP flexion is 80°, and DIP flexion is 60°. The patient is unable to make a complete fist. The MCP and IP joints can extend passively to 0°. He is unable to simultaneously flex the MCP and extend the IP joints.

Questions for Analysis

1. What do you suspect this patient's primary problems are?

2. What will be included in your first three treatment sessions with him, assuming no regression with your treatments?

3. What will your initial goals during the first week be for him?

4. What precautions must you be aware of in treating him?

5. Describe three home exercises you will give this patient at the time of your first treatment.

6. List four strengthening exercises you will use with him.

7. What functional exercises will you incorporate into his rehabilitation program before he returns to hockey?

Exercises include activities that permit tendon gliding while protecting the injured joint. A gradually progressive program of strengthening exercises starts at six to eight weeks once the patient has achieved full motion.

If the dislocation is stable, the finger is immobilized similarly to the way it is for an unstable dislocation, with the PIP joint in 20° to 40° of flexion to permit maximal collateral ligament length and to control edema. Efforts should be made to control edema and pain even before motion exercises are started. In 7 to 10 days, AROM is initiated to prevent tendon gliding restrictions. These exercises are restricted by blocking individual joints. They should promote distal and proximal tendon gliding and emphasize both intrinsic and extrinsic muscles. Splinting is often discontinued after three weeks, with buddy taping applied to continue to protect the joint. Full active extension should be achieved within six to eight weeks. Resistive exercises can begin at around eight weeks.

If a finger is sprained, the immobilization and rehabilitation process will follow that outlined above for the stable dislocation, but the process may be accelerated. If the sprain is minor, less time will be necessary, but when the sprain is more severe, longer time will be required for a full recovery.

Overuse Injuries

The two most common overuse injuries of the wrist and hand are carpal tunnel syndrome and De Quervain's disease. Overuse is the term commonly used to describe these injuries, because trauma is produced over a period of time and applied at a greater rate than the structures can accommodate. Microscopic injury results and the structure is unable to rebuild before additional stress is applied. This creates an inflammatory response. If insult to the tissues continues, a chronic inflammatory response occurs and scar tissue develops, making the injury more difficult to manage. These injuries can be frustrating and challenging for

Case Study

A 16-year-old, right-handed volleyball setter suffered a dislocated dominant-hand middle finger three weeks ago. The finger has been in a partial flexion splint for the past three weeks. The physician has instructed the patient to tape the finger to her ring finger throughout the day except when in rehabilitation. She has been moving the wrist and MCP joint, but the finger has been immobilized since the injury. The edema is gone, but the finger is stiff in the IP joints. Passive DIP extension lacks 15° and flexion is to 30°, and PIP extension lacks 30° and flexion is to 50°,

Active DIP extension lacks 20° and flexion is to 25°, and PIP extension lacks 40° and flexion is to 50°. The patient is unable to make a complete fist because the middle finger does not flex into the palm. Her grip strength measurement is 13.6 kg (30 lb) on the right and 31.7 kg (70 lb) on the left. There is tenderness over the PIP collateral ligaments, especially on the radial side.

Questions for Analysis

1. What will your first treatment goals be for this patient today?

2. What will you attempt to accomplish in the next three treatments? How will you accomplish those goals?

3. What precautions should you consider in the treatments?

4. What are two exercises you will send home with the patient today?

5. What strengthening exercises will you use?

6. What functional activities will you eventually include in her therapeutic exercise program?

the rehabilitation clinician, especially when the patient has failed to seek treatment until the injury has become advanced. The key to successful treatment is early intervention and correction of the causes.

Carpal Tunnel Syndrome

This is also known as median nerve compression syndrome. The median nerve is compressed as it passes under the transverse carpal ligament and through the carpal tunnel. Compression of the median nerve results in loss of sensation over its distribution in the hand, as well as weakness and pain. Pain occurs primarily at night, when the wrist is placed in flexion while the patient sleeps. Prolonged flexion positioning of the wrist causes compression on the nerve and venous congestion, and thus pain. This problem often results from prolonged or repeated wrist extension positioning during daily activities. A gymnast with weak wrists who performs on the bars with the wrists in hyperextension can develop carpal tunnel syndrome.

If carpal tunnel syndrome occurs bilaterally, the cervical region should be investigated as the possible source of the problem. Cervical radiculopathy is a differential diagnosis that should be ruled out for any upper-extremity injury not specifically related to an incident. Obtaining an accurate history is important to correctly determining the cause of the patient's symptoms. If passively placing the neck in a quadrant position (extension with lateral flexion and rotation to the involved side) reproduces the patient's symptoms, cervical radiculopathy cannot be ruled out; further evaluation of the neck is necessary.

When treatment begins early, it can often succeed in relieving symptoms. Use of a splint to position the wrist in neutral, especially at night, is helpful in reducing median nerve compression and night pain. Modalities can be used to relieve the inflammation. Ice, contrast baths, phonophoresis, iontophoresis, or electrical stimulation can be helpful. Flexibility exercises for the wrist and long finger flexors, restriction of aggravating activities, and remedy of incorrect techniques all assist in relieving the pain. Strengthening exercises for all wrist, thumb, and finger movements—beginning with isometrics and advancing to isotonics, eccentric exercises, and concentric exercises—should progress when the inflammation is under control. Endurance, speed, and coordination all should be included in the progression of exercises.

If conservative treatment does not resolve the patient's carpal tunnel syndrome, surgical intervention for release of the transverse carpal ligament may be necessary. Gentle AROM may begin within three to seven days postoperatively. Once the sutures are removed, scar-tissue management and desensitization through massage and soft-tissue mobilization can begin. The patient can start doing progressive resistive exercises when tolerated. The progression of exercises follows a course similar to that discussed earlier for other wrist injuries.

De Quervain's Disease

De Quervain's tendinitis affects the first dorsal compartment and involves the abductor pollicis longus and the extensor pollicis brevis. These tendons travel together in the same synovial sheath in the first compartment and pass around the bony radial styloid process, a site of friction for the tendons. Repetitive stress and inflammation from friction of these tendons occur with activities such as weight training and rowing.

As with carpal tunnel syndrome, modalities can be useful conservative treatment for relief of the inflammation. A thumb spica splint is used to place the wrist in 15° of extension. The thumb is positioned in abduction, with the MCP joint in 10° flexion to put the affected tendons on slack. Although the splint is worn continually, it should be removed throughout the day for AROM exercises for the wrist and thumb. The patient should perform active range of motion of the fingers throughout the day.

Once pain and edema are reduced, mild strengthening and endurance activities can begin. The patient is gradually weaned from the splint during this stage. Gross- and fine-pinch activities, wrist and finger exercises, and endurance and coordination exercises should be a part of the strengthening program.

For surgical cases in which conservative treatment failed to resolve the injury, AROM exercises begin two to three days postoperatively to promote tendon gliding and prevent loss of motion. The wrist may be in a splint for about one week, but the patient removes it frequently during the day for ROM exercises. Pain and edema are controlled with various modalities, elevation, and active motion. The thumb should move in all its planes through full active motion. Thumb motion exercises should also include wrist motion.

Case Study

A 24-year-old crew team member underwent a surgical release of his right-nondominant first dorsal compartment three days ago. He has just seen the physician, who has removed the surgical dressing and instructed him to begin exercising the wrist and thumb. The physician has given the patient a splint to wear throughout the day except during treatments. Some swelling and tenderness are present over the scar. The wrist has good motion, but the thumb moves 10° at the MCP joint and 30° at the IP joint. There is some tenderness to radial deviation, but the patient has full motion.

Questions for Analysis

1. What will your treatment today include?

2. What instructions will you give the patient for home treatment?

3. What precautions must be considered?

4. What kind of ROM exercises will you give him?

5. When will you start working on strength, and what will the first strengthening exercises include?

6. What functional exercises will you advance the patient to before he returns to competition?

Once the sutures are removed and the scar is healed, scar-tissue desensitization and softening can begin with massage. Strengthening exercise progression, which can begin after 7 to 10 days, follows the same procedure as for other wrist injuries.

Tendon Injuries

Tendon gliding exercises have already been presented. These are important exercises to perform following any injury to the hand, because adhesions to either flexor or extensor tendons cause significant loss of motion and hand function. In addition, the rehabilitation clinician must have knowledge and understanding of the specific differences between flexor and extensor tendons to apply proper rehabilitation techniques to injuries affecting hand tendons.

Special Tendon Considerations

Although the biochemical structures of the hand's flexor and extensor tendons are similar, several differences govern variations in the rehabilitation of flexor and extensor tendon injuries. Some of the differences have already been mentioned. Among the more obvious differences is the presence of the strong pulley system for the flexor tendons versus the absence of any pulleys for the extensor tendons. The majority of the length of the flexor tendons is enclosed in sheaths, but the extensor tendons are primarily extrasynovial.

Normally, finger flexion strength is significantly greater than finger extension strength. The flexors require greater strength for activities such as grasping, propelling, and catching objects than the extensors require for opening the hand. When an injury occurs to an extensor tendon, care must be taken to prevent the stronger flexor muscles from overpowering and causing further damage to the weakened extensor tendon.

The extensor tendons are flatter and thinner than the flexor tendons; therefore overall they have less tensile strength than the larger-diameter, thicker flexor tendons. When the fingers flex into the hand, the extensor tendons undergo significant lengthening. These factors make the extensor tendon susceptible to stretch or rupture, especially when in a weakened condition following an injury.

Although the extensor tendons are not surrounded with tendon sheaths like the flexor tendons, both are at risk for adhesion formation with immobilization. Loss of extension motion can be more functionally debilitating than flexion motion loss (Stewart 1992). Because of the intricate relationship between the extensor tendons and the intrinsic muscles, loss of mobility of the extensor tendons can have a significant impact on the function of the interossei and lumbricals and can hamper the intrinsic and extrinsic muscle balance necessary for normal hand function.

Tendon ruptures and lacerations are the most common tendon injuries of the hand. The ruptures usually result from impact avulsions such as occur when a player's hand is hit with a baseball bat. Lacerations can result from cleats, contact with sharp objects hidden in the grass, and accidents in archery and many other activities. The timing of rehabilitation is crucial to rehabilitation success. Careful application of rehabilitative techniques is important to achieving desired end results. Recent advances in rehabilitation following tendon repair have improved surgical results and reduced the risk of tendon adhesions. New approaches to postoperative tendon repair include the use of early controlled motion during the first weeks after surgery rather than the more traditional three weeks or more of immobilization. Because of the relative fragility of extensor tendons, early controlled motion was first used primarily with flexor tendon injuries; but more recently, early controlled motion has proven successful with extensor tendon injuries as well. At present, most believe that early controlled motion is advantageous for both flexor and extensor hand tendons; however, there must remain a fine balance between the proper amount of motion for allowing tendon gliding, and too much motion, which causes elongation or rupture of fragile tendon tissue during the early healing phases. The rehabilitation clinician must feel free to coordinate a patient's rehabilitation program with a hand specialist if necessary.

Early controlled motion includes passive movement of the repaired tendon. The initial goal of early motion is to promote tendon gliding and good tendon healing simultaneously. The ultimate goal is to produce a good surgical and rehabilitative result. Areas of the hand, such as no man's land, that were previously approached with caution and misgiving because of poor surgical results can be successfully and effectively repaired using early controlled motion.

Early controlled motion is achieved using a splint that is applied approximately three days postoperatively. The splint is designed to limit flexion if an extensor tendon has been repaired and to limit extension if a flexor tendon has been repaired. The angles of the splints are based on the 5-mm rule discussed earlier in the context of excursion of tendons during finger motion. The splints include a passive elastic force that pulls the fingers passively in the direction of the repaired tendon's pull. For example, an extensor tendon repair splint is constructed to block MCP joint flexion at 30° for the index and middle fingers, MCP joint flexion at 38° for the ring and small fingers, and extension of the IP joints with the wrist at about 40°. An elastic system, attached to the fingers, passively extends the fingers so that active motion of the tendon is not required to pull the finger into a resting position after it has flexed.

Conversely, a flexor tendon repair is placed in a dorsal splint with the wrist in about 20° of flexion, the MPs in about 40° to 50° of flexion, and the IPs in extension. An elastic system is attached to the distal finger to pull the digit passively into flexion so as not to stress the newly repaired flexor tendon.

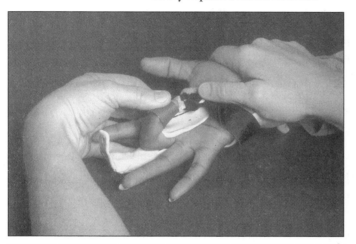

Figure 19.59 Passive range of motion in a splint.

It is necessary to take care with both these splints so that the tension of the rubber band is sufficient to permit passive flexion or extension of the digits, yet not strong enough to promote a contracture because the tension is too much for the opposing tendon to overcome.

While the repaired flexor tendon finger is in the splint, the IP joints are passively flexed frequently throughout the day (figure 19.59). The patient performs finger extension actively to return the finger to the splint surface. Also, so that a splinted tendon-repair finger moves frequently within the splint, have the patient extend the fingers against the rubber bands on the flexor surface and allow the bands to passively return the fingers to the resting position, throughout the day.

Tendon glide and careful avoidance of adhesions are the primary concerns during the early stages of postoperative rehabilitation. Extensor tendon repairs have the additional problem of possible extensor lag development. The rehabilitation clinician must be aware of these conditions and take steps to provide good care while protecting against these complications. Observation of joint mobility is necessary for assessing the presence of these potentially debilitating conditions. You must differentiate between capsular restriction and tendon adhesions when the patient's motion is less than normal. One way to do this is to examine the digit's ROM at the individual joints and the quantity of motion with all joints involved. For example, if the patient is able to fully extend the wrist and MCP, PIP, and DIP joints of a digit one at a time while the other digit's joints are positioned in flexion, but unable to fully extend them all at once, the joint capsules have good mobility, but the tendon is probably restricted.

Once sutures are removed, scar-tissue management and desensitization can begin with massage. The patient can be instructed to perform this technique frequently throughout the day. This will help reduce the risk of tendon adhesions, because the tendons lie so close to the surface in the hand and fingers.

When to begin strengthening exercises for repaired tendons is a point of controversy. If a tendon is adherent, strengthening exercises begin earlier than if it glides well. Strength exercises initially are light strengthening exercises, starting at four to five weeks postoperatively (Stewart 1992). Other determining factors include the type of tendon (extensor or flexor) and the zone in which the repair is located.

Flexor Tendons

Active range of motion begins at three to six weeks for flexor tendons. If there is good flexion movement, in terms of quality, not necessarily quantity, gentle active motion can begin. Blocking exercises that limit motion at the proximal joint while emphasizing the distal joint can be used during this phase. Placing the wrist in extension during finger flexion and in flexion during finger extension motions, permit the desired motion without placing undue stress on the tendons.

Tendon glide must be present before the patient can advance to resistive exercises. The patient's readiness is assessed using observation skills and the techniques already described to ascertain fluidity of movement and restriction of mobility. As a rule, if the patient is unable to passively simultaneously extend the wrist and MCP and IP joints, tendon gliding is restricted and needs to be treated before strengthening exercises begin.

Although some advocate the initiation of mild strengthening at four weeks postoperatively, the more typical time to begin strengthening is seven to eight weeks after surgery. To some extent, this time line depends on the location of the repair. Zone V repairs heal quickly because of their blood supply; patients with these repairs can begin isolated AROM exercises by the third week and mild strengthening by the fifth week. Flexor digitorum superficialis tendons can withstand resistive exercises sooner than the FDP tendon.

Mild strengthening exercises include isometrics with gradual buildup to maximum output, grasping exercises, prehension activities, and use of the hand in daily activities as long as the patient does not lift or hold any heavy objects. Repetitions should begin low and should increase over the next couple of weeks. Progression of resistance is slow, with careful attention to the deleterious effects of too rapid a progression: pain, swelling, and stiffness.

The therapeutic exercise program continues to progress, with increases in strength, muscle endurance, and coordination, as the patient tolerates. The normal progression to functional exercises and return to activities occurs within 12 weeks.

Extensor Tendons

The most common extensor avulsion tendon rupture is the mallet finger, in which the distal attachment of the extensor tendon is torn—usually when the digit is hit on the end and forced into sudden flexion. This rupture is frequently not surgically repaired but rather placed in a splint that maintains the DIP in 0° extension. Placing it in hyperextension risks local ischemia of the region. After six to eight weeks of continuous wear, the splint is removed and the digit is exercised with AROM, emphasizing full extension movement. Flexion exercises are active only and are gentle so that an extensor lag does not form as a result of overstretching the new connective tissue on the extensor tendon. If a lag develops, the digit must be placed in the splint once again for another couple of weeks before the patient resumes exercises. If the patient removes the finger splint during the initial six to eight weeks, the time count starts anew.

Extensor tendon injuries in zones III and IV cause what is known as a boutonniere deformity (figure 19.60). The cause, a disruption of the long extensor tendon's central slip, affects other structures within the extensor mechanism. The transverse retinacular ligament and the triangular ligament stretch with repeated motion of the digit without balance of the digit's forces. This causes an extensor lag at the PIP joint. When the lag occurs, the lateral bands of the extensor tendon move anteriorly to change the angle of pull of the intrinsics and create a hyperextension force at the DIP joint.

Treatment usually includes PIP joint immobilization in extension. Surgical repair of the central slip and lateral bands is occasionally required. The splint is commonly applied for six weeks, with isometric exercises

Figure 19.60   Boutonniere deformity.

beginning at three weeks while the digit is in the splint. The finger is taken out of the splint for gentle flexion AROM exercises at three to six weeks. To prevent tendon rupture, extension should be assisted. Early protective motion using a splint similar to the early protective extension splint, mentioned previously, can be used at three weeks.

When initiated, active exercises should stress active extension, isolating joint movement by blocking the proximal joints and advancing into combined joint extension movements. Passive stretching into flexion should be avoided for seven to eight weeks. Care must be taken throughout the therapeutic exercise process to avoid an extensor lag and flexor contractures. The rehabilitation clinician must monitor continuously for these problems.

Mild resistive extension exercises start at 8 to 10 weeks and progress as with flexor tendon injuries.

Extensor tendon injuries in zones V, VI, and VII vary from those in the other zones because they are not impacted by the extensor mechanism. Extraneous forces and deformity are less of a problem, so motion can begin earlier.

A splint is applied for three weeks immediately after injury or repair; the wearer is then weaned from it over the next two weeks. The wrist is maintained in about 30° to 45° extension with the MCPs and IPs in 0° extension. As with other tendon injuries, extensor lag and tendon adhesions must be prevented.

Gentle active motion can begin at three weeks with blocking exercises. Wrist extension and MCP flexion-extension with the IPs in extension, and hook exercises, are good tendon gliding exercises. At four weeks, full extension exercises for individual fingers begin; and at five or six weeks the hand exercises advance from a hook to a full fist. Resisted exercises and full stretch exercises begin after six weeks, progressing as with other hand therapeutic exercise programs.

Reflex Sympathetic Dystrophy

Reflex sympathetic dystrophy (RSD) more commonly involves the upper extremity than the lower extremity. It can occur as the result of an injury in any part of the extremity, but the

Case Study

A 16-year-old softball catcher suffered a mallet deformity of her dominant right-hand ring finger in a game three weeks ago. It has been in a splint for the past three weeks. The doctor wants the patient to begin active exercises today and wants her to continue to wear the splint but to remove it for her treatments. Your initial examination reveals the following ring-finger flexion/extension measurements: MCP 90°/0°, PIP 90°/0°, DIP 15°/10° from extension. When the patient simultaneously extends the wrist and finger, the DIP is lacks 20° extension. Grip strength measures 13.6 kg (30 lb) on the right and 34 kg (75 lb) on the left. Wrist extension is 4/5. Both ulnar and radial deviations have normal motion and strength. Wrist flexion is 4/5, finger flexion is 4/5, MCP extension is 4–/5, and finger abduction is 4–/5.

Questions for Analysis

1. What will your first treatment include?

2. What instructions will you give the patient for home exercises?

3. What precautions must you consider in her treatments?

4. What determining factors will you use to decide when she should begin her strengthening exercises?

5. List three strengthening exercises and explain why you have selected them.

6. Identify three functional exercises and indicate your guidelines for beginning them.

symptoms are most apparent in the hand. When it originates from a shoulder injury, it is sometimes referred to as shoulder-hand syndrome. It can be a difficult problem to treat.

Program Considerations

Reflex sympathetic dystrophy is believed to occur because of a reflex sympathetic response to an injury. Characteristic complaints include pain disproportionate to the degree of injury, stiffness that is exaggerated in relation to the expected response to the injury, edema in the hand, cyanotic discoloration with redness around the MCP and PIP joints, coldness, and excessive sweating in the hand. The edema is initially soft and pitting, but with time it becomes brawny and hard. X-rays can reveal bone demineralization. The skin appears tight and shiny because of immobilization and poor nutrition to the tissues. The patient tends to hold and protect the hand, moving the extremity minimally.

The most important aspect of treatment of RSD is early intervention. It is important to stop the sympathetic reflex cycle. The physician may attempt to select from a variety of medications or try a stellate ganglion block. The rehabilitation clinician can use a variety of techniques but must keep in mind that each patient with RSD may respond differently to these techniques.

Modalities can include a variety of methods such as various heat modalities to increase blood flow, reduce stiffness, and increase tissue extensibility for improved mobility. Heat, however, can sometimes cause increased edema. Electrical modalities, including high-voltage galvanic stimulation, transcutaneous electrical nerve stimulation, and functional electrical stimulation, can help reduce edema, decrease pain, and promote muscle activity, respectively. If tolerated, massage can be beneficial when pitting edema is present. It should be applied before exercise to maximize the effects of the exercise. Reduced edema can improve ROM and allow a greater excursion of muscle activity.

Splinting can be useful in preventing contractures. The wrist and hand are placed in a functional position with the wrist in slight extension, the MCP joints in midflexion, and the IP joints in extension. Continuous passive motion machines for the wrist and hand can also be useful in preventing contractures in the hand.

Exercises should be light and active. Exercise that is more than gentle often aggravates the patient's pain and increases stiffness. Low-repetition, active exercises are used to tolerance. These should include isolated joint motion and gross activities such as hook-grip, full-fist, and prehensile motions.

Case Study

An 18-year-old female gymnast was referred to you four weeks after incurring a hand injury. Your evaluation reveals pitting edema throughout the hand. The skin is red and shiny, with increased redness over the MCP and PIP joints. Active range-of-motion measurements of the fingers' extension/flexion were the following: Thumb MCP lacks 10°extension/25°, IP lacks 15°extension/20°; finger MCP lacks 25° extension/50°; index PIP lacks 20° extension/50° middle PIP lacks 30° extension/50°; ring –15°/60°; little –20°/50°; and all DIPs fixed at –20° extension. Wrist flexion is 30° and extension is 20°. The patient reports tenderness to light touch over the entire surface of the hand. The skin is cool and clammy to the touch.

Questions for Analysis

1. What are your initial goals for this patient?

2. What will your first treatment include?

3. What exercises will you initiate?

4. What instructions will you give the patient?

Passive motion and joint mobilization should not begin until the patient's pain is decreased. If pain intensifies, the exercises should return to previous levels of therapeutic activity. A gradual progression based on patient tolerance should include increased endurance exercises, strengthening, and functional activities.

SUMMARY

1. Explain the pulley system of the fingers.

   There is an elaborate pulley system on the flexor aspect of the fingers—a fibrous tunnel that extends from the metacarpal head of each digit to the insertion of the distal finger flexor tendons. These pulleys are similar to the hoops along a fishing rod, positioned to keep the fishing line in place as it travels along the pole. There are five annular pulleys and three cruciate pulleys along each finger. Disruption of the key pulleys can cause bowstringing of the flexor tendons. The key pulleys preventing bowstringing are A2 and A4. When the pulley system of any finger is disrupted, the mechanical advantage of the tendon is impaired and normal function is lost.

2. Explain why reducing edema in the hand is important.

   Because the dorsal skin is loose and pliable compared to the volar skin, edema frequently accumulates in the dorsum of the hand. Pooled edema rich in proteins easily leads to contractures. Excessive swelling on the back of the hand can cause the hand arches to collapse anteriorly and adduct the thumb. Excessive swelling also requires a greater excursion of the skin for the person to flex the hand. If the skin is already stretched because of the edema, the hand's ability to move the fingers through their full motion is impaired. Fibrous tissue formation secondary to the presence of prolonged edema can cause reduced mobility and function of the hand.

3. Discuss the trimuscular system of the hand and explain why it is important to hand function.

   Three muscle groups compose the trimuscular system of the hand—the extrinsic flexors, the extrinsic extensors, and the intrinsic muscles—and provide for balanced, controlled hand function. If any of these groups is not allowed to function normally, because of either weakness or loss of mobility, balance is lost and the hand is not able to work in its normal capacity.

4. Identify and explain the importance of the precision and power grips of the hand.

   The power grips, also known as palmar grips, include the clenched fist, the cylinder grasp, the spherical grasp, and the hook. In these grasps, the thumb is positioned in opposition to the other fingers to permit a firm grasp on an object. The majority of daily hand activities involve these palmar grips. Because palmar grasping is so vital to hand function, the hand is most commonly splinted in a palmar position with the thumb in slight opposition, facing the other fingers. The precision or prehensile grips include the digital prehension grip, the lateral prehension grip, and the tip-to-tip prehension grip. These movements include fine-tuned activities such as typing, sewing, or writing. These prehensile activities occur when the thumb and finger muscles co-contract to produce an activity requiring precision.

5. Explain the difference between static and dynamic splints.

   Overall, the aim of splints is either to prevent damage and maintain balance or to improve balance. Static splints restrict motion to support and protect the hand. Dynamic splints are used to increase motion of the hand. Splints are based on a three-point pressure system whereby two points of application are on one side of the hand, wrist, or forearm and the other point of application is on the opposite side.

6. Identify what motion is increased with carpal radial glide joint mobilization.

   A carpal radial glide is used to improve ulnar flexion of the wrist.

7. Explain the force application sequence for improving long finger flexor or extensor motion.

   The basic application sequence is the same for flexors and extensors. If the distal phalanx has limited flexion motion, the proximal joint is stabilized as the distal joint (DIP) is moved into flexion; then the PIP joint is moved into flexion as the MCP joint is stabilized while the DIP's flexed position is maintained. The MCP joint is then moved into flexion as the wrist is stabilized and the IP joints are kept in their flexion positions. Finally, the wrist is gradually moved into flexion. The stretch should be performed in both elbow flexion and elbow extension, and the forces applied gradually until the patient feels a stretch in the forearm.

8. Explain how the intrinsic stretches differ from the extrinsic stretches.

   Because the lumbricals and interossei flex the MCP joints and extend the IP joints, the stretch is applied in the opposite direction of their function or direction of motion. The IP joints are maintained in a flexed position while a stretch is applied to increase MCP extension. The wrist should be stabilized in neutral during this activity to prevent extrinsic muscle influences on the stretch.

9. Discuss the difference in gliding exercises for the flexor profundus and superficialis tendons.

   Three exercises for flexor tendon gliding include (1) keeping the MCP extended and flexing the IPs to enhance gliding between the two longer finger flexor tendons, (2) forming a fist with the IP and MCP joints in flexion to produce gliding of the profundus tendon within its sheath, and (3) positioning the MCP and PIP joints in flexion and extending the DIP joints. Flexor pollicis longus gliding exercises are performed in a similar manner by moving the IP and MCP joints through a full range of flexion and extension. These exercises are initially performed with the wrist in neutral; but as the patient progresses, the wrist should be moved into flexion with finger flexion and into extension with finger extension. A gliding exercise for the EDC is performed by moving the hand from a hook to a fist formation. The MCP joint is moved from flexion to extension while the IP joints are kept in flexion to eliminate the intrinsic muscles. If the patient has difficulty maintaining flexion of the IP joints during this activity, he or she can grasp a drinking straw or pencil in the fingers while moving the MCP joints. Wrist flexion and extension should also be added to the exercise when it is easy for the patient to perform the exercise with the wrist in neutral.

10. Present the differences between long flexor and long extensor tendons.

    Among the more obvious differences is the presence of the strong pulley system for the flexor tendons versus the absence of any pulleys for the extensor tendons. The majority of the length of the flexor tendons is enclosed in sheaths, but the extensor tendons are primarily extrasynovial. Finger flexion strength is significantly greater than finger extension strength. The extensor tendons are flatter and thinner than the flexor tendons; for this reason they have less overall tensile strength than the larger-diameter, thicker flexor tendons. When the fingers close into the hand, the extensor tendons undergo significant lengthening. The flexor tendons are surrounded with tendon sheaths and risk loss of tendon glide and formation of adhesions with immobilization. Loss of extensor motion can be more functionally debilitating than flexion motion loss.

11. Explain what procedures should be used to eliminate an extensor lag of a distal phalanx.

A gliding exercise for the EDC can be used to reduce adhesions that may be causing an extensor lag and is described in the answer to question 9. If the extensor lag occurs at either IP joint, it is the result of adhesions within the extensor mechanism and can include both intrinsic and extrinsic structures, the interossei, lumbricals, and EDC. To isolate the intrinsic muscles and facilitate their movement into IP extension, the MCP should be stabilized in flexion. As this exercise becomes easier, the MCP joint should be moved into extension. In the most difficult position for this exercise, the hand is flat on a table and the proximal phalanx stabilized, and the patient attempts to extend the distal phalanx off the table.

12. Identify the early signs of RSD.

Early complaints include pain disproportionate to the degree of injury, stiffness that is exaggerated in relation to the expected response to the injury, pitting edema in the hand, cyanotic discoloration with redness around the MCP and PIP joints, coldness, and excessive sweating in the hand.

CRITICAL THINKING QUESTIONS

1. Why do you suspect that tendinitis and overuse injuries are common in the hand and wrist? On the basis of the anatomy and the causes of overuse injuries, what sports would you suspect would have a higher-than-average incidence of overuse injuries of the hand and wrist, and why? Given this, what efforts can be made to prevent these injuries in these sports?

2. If a patient suffers a scaphoid fracture, how long would you expect him or her to complain of pain? If the wrist pain continues for several weeks beyond your expectations, what would you suspect is the reason? What would you do in this situation?

3. In the opening scenario, what test did Deanna use to determine that adhesions were forming between the flexor digitorum superficialis and profundus? What specific techniques would you use to reduce these adhesions? What exercises and home program would you give Danny to help create more mobility between the tissues? How would the adhesions interfere with hand function by affecting the intrinsic muscles?

4. If a mallet finger injury begins to lose active extension after having started rehabilitation exercises, what would you suspect is the cause? How would you remedy the situation to restore active extension?

LAB ACTIVITIES

1. Locate the trigger points for the following muscles on your lab partner:
   a. Wrist extensors
   b. Wrist flexors
   c. Long finger flexors
   d. Long finger extensors
   e. Pollicis adductor

   Where were your partner's most sensitive trigger points? Perform an ice-and-stretch technique on each of them and provide your partner with a home exercise for each tender trigger point.

2. Perform the following joint mobilizations on your lab partner and identify what restriction would be best treated with each mobilization:

   a. Distal radioulnar joint

   - Distraction

   - Dorsal glide of radius

   - Ventral glide of radius

   b. Radiocarpal joint

   - Distraction

   - AP glides

   - PA glides

   - Lateral glides

   c. MCP and IP joints

   - Distraction

   - Rotation

   - AP glides

   - PA glides

3. Examine your partner's finger motion using all of the tendon gliding exercises. Identify which structure each motion is assessing.

4. Instruct your partner in the flexor tendon gliding exercises and have him perform 10 of each. Instruct your partner in the extensor tendon gliding exercises and have him perform 10 of each. What are the differences in how each of the exercises feel as they are being performed?

5. Demonstrate how you would apply a stretch to the lumbricals. What are the key factors you need to consider in positioning for this stretch? Why?

6. List two exercises you would give a patient to strengthen the finger extensors. Identify the purpose of each exercise and when in the rehabilitation program they could be added.

7. List two strengthening exercises for the finger flexors and identify a progression for each of them. What would be your criteria for advancing a patient from one level of an exercise to another?

8. List three strengthening exercises for the intrinsic muscles of the hand and identify the substitution patterns you need to watch for during the patient's performance of each exercise.

9. List three sport-specific exercises you would have a softball left fielder perform before she returns to full participation. She is recovering from a second degree PIP sprain of the third finger. Explain why you have selected these criteria; what is your rationale?

REFERENCES

Bowers, W.H., and S.M. Tribuzi. 1992. Functional anatomy. In Concepts in hand rehabilitation, ed. B.G. Stanley and S.M. Tribuzi. Philadelphia: Davis.

Boyes, J.H. 1970. *Bunnell's surgery of the hand*. Philadelphia: Lippincott.

Doyle, J.R., and W.F. Blythe. 1975. The finger flexor tendon sheaths and pulleys. Anatomy and reconstruction. In A.A.O.S.: *Symposium on tendon surgery of the hand*. St. Louis: Mosby.

Duran, R.J., and R.G. Houser. 1975. Controlled passive motion following flexor tendon repair in zones 2 and 3. In *A.A.O.S. Symposium on tendon surgery of the hand*. St. Louis: Mosby.

Evans, R.B. 1989. Clinical application of controlled stress to the healing extensor tendon: A review of 112 cases. *Physical Therapy* 69:1041–1049.

Evans, R.B., and W.E. Burkhalter. 1986. A study of the dynamic anatomy of extensor tendons and implications for treatment. *Journal of Hand Surgery* (Am) 11:774–779.

Maitland, G.D. 1991. *Peripheral manipulation.* Boston; London: Butterworth-Heinemann.

Stewart, K.M. 1992. Tendon injuries. In *Concepts in hand rehabilitation*, ed. B.G. Stanley and S.M. Tribuzi. Philadelphia: Davis.

Travell, J.G., and D.G. Simons. 1983. Myofascial pain and dysfunction. *The trigger point manual.* Vol. 1. Baltimore: Williams and Wilkins.

SUGGESTED READING

Brunet, M.E., Haddad, R.J., Sanchez, J., and E. Leonard. 1984. How I manage sprained finger in athletes. *Physician and Sportmedicine* 12:99–108.

Burnett, W.R. 1992. Rehabilitation techniques for ligament injuries of the hand. *Hand Clinics* 8: 803–815.

Clemens, S., and B. Foss-Campbell. 1993. Rehabilitation following traumatic hand injury: Hand therapists' perspective. Part 1: Acute phase of hand rehabilitation. *Plastic Surgical Nursing* 13: 129–139.

Dovelle, S., and P.K. Heeter. 1985. Early controlled mobilization following extensor tendon repair in zone V-VI of the hand: Preliminary report. *Contemporary Orthopaedics* 11:41–44.

Evans, R.B., and D.E. Thompson. 1992. An analysis of factors that support early active short arc motion of the repaired central slip. *Journal of Hand Therapy* 5:187–201.

Halikis, M.N., and J. Taleisnik. 1996. Soft-tissue injuries of the wrist. *Clinics in Sports Medicine* 15: 235–259.

Hunter, J.M., Schneider, L.H., Mackin, E.J., and A.D. Callahan, eds. 1990. *Rehabilitation of the Hand. Surgery and Therapy.* St. Louis: Mosby.

Kleinert, H.E., and C. Verdan. 1983. Report of the committee on tendon injuries. *Journal of Hand Surgery* (Am) 7:794–798.

Levine, W.R. 1992. Rehabilitation techniques for ligament injuries of the wrist. *Hand Clinics* 8: 669–677.

May, E.J., Silfverskiold, K.L., and C.J. Sollerman. 1992. Controlled mobilization after flexor tendon repair in zone II: A prospective comparison of three methods. *Journal of Hand Surgery* 5:942–952.

Wadsworth, C.T. 1983. Clinical anatomy and mechanics of the wrist and hand. Journal of Orthopaedic and Sports Physical Therapy 4:206–216.

Wehbe, M.A. 1996. Early motion after hand and wrist reconstruction. *Hand Clinics* 12:25–29.

Zimmerman, G.R. 1994. Carpal tunnel syndrome. *Journal of Athletic Training* 29:22–30.

Foot, Ankle, and Leg

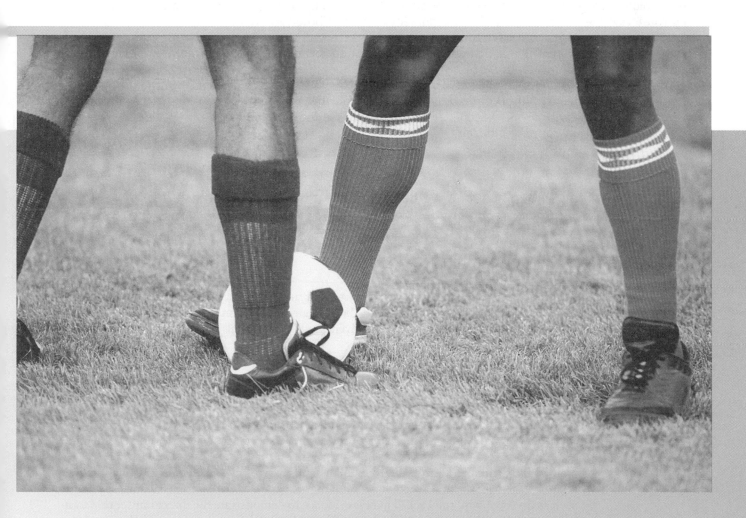

After two months of persistent heel pain, cross country runner Catie felt she could no longer hope the pain would go away on its own and decided to seek care for it. After Benjamin Charles had performed his evaluation, he informed Catie that the problem was plantar fasciitis.

Benjamin concluded from his examination that Catie had a few problems that were contributing to the plantar fasciitis. Her excessive pronation would have to be corrected with orthotics; the tight hip rotators were causing altered knee alignment that contributed to increased torsional stress on the plantar fascia and would have to be stretched and corrected, as would the tightness in the iliotibial band and Achilles. The muscle imbalance in Catie's quads and hamstrings was another possible contributing factor that would be resolved with strengthening activities. Benjamin also explained to Catie that not only were her shoes too worn to wear running; they also did not have the proper supports her foot needs. Although there were several problems, Benjamin was optimistic that they were all correctable with proper rehabilitation and changes in footwear so that Catie would be able to resume her normal running program.

■ **Growth begins when we begin to accept our own weakness.**

Jean Vanier, 1928–, founder of L'Arche community

The foot and ankle are complex structures that impact the entire extremity, because they form the base that moves the rest of the body from one location to another. Injuries in these areas can affect the efficiency and effectiveness of body propulsion, the primary function of the lower extremities.

Injuries to the foot and ankle are common. A key responsibility of the rehabilitation clinician is to use his or her skill and knowledge of the foot and ankle to provide the patient with an appropriate and efficient recovery program that will permit a full return to full participation.

The foot, ankle, and extremity, like the hand, wrist, and forearm, are complex structures composed of many bones, joints, and muscles. There are 26 bones and 33 joints in the foot, ankle, and extremity, along with several intrinsic and extrinsic muscles. These structures are divided into segments within the foot, ankle, and extremity; each segment forms integral relationships with the other segments within the area as well as with more proximal segments such as the knee, hip, and back. There is evidence to demonstrate the direct impact that foot position and mechanics have on the knee (Tiberio 1987; Klingman, Liaos, and Hardin 1997; Powers, Maffucci, and Hampton 1995) and other more distal segments (Massie and Spiker 1990). It is important, then, that you have knowledge of the structure and function of the distal lower extremity so that the rehabilitation program you establish will return the patient to full function without applying additional stresses to more proximal segments.

This chapter reviews the basic structure of the extremity, ankle, and foot as it pertains to the normal function of those segments as well as the more proximal segments. We will pay specific attention to concepts that directly relate to rehabilitation following injury. The second half of the chapter addresses specific injuries most commonly seen in the leg, ankle, and foot, along with case studies.

▶ Normal foot mechanics in ambulation depends on the correct timing and coordination of the motions of many joints and the extrinsic and intrinsic muscles of the lower leg and foot. Subtalar motion and position also influence movement of the lower extremity.

GENERAL REHABILITATION CONSIDERATIONS

Before discussing the foot and ankle, we need to define some of the more common terms used to describe these body segments. These terms are often misused, so establishing definitions helps to ensure common understanding.

Terminology

One possible reason for confusion about terms relating to the foot may be that the foot is not in the same plane as the rest of the body: the foot is at roughly a 90° angle to the extremity. Another possible reason is that the foot seldom moves in cardinal, or straight, planes; many of the joints are multiplanar. As a point of reference, ankle and foot motions in the cardinal planes (frontal, sagittal, and transverse) and multiplanes are defined here.

Pronation is a multiplanar rotational motion that occurs in the subtalar and transverse tarsal joints and is the combination of dorsiflexion, abduction, and eversion in non-weight bearing. This motion is sometimes incorrectly referred to as eversion. Dorsiflexion is the sagittal plane movement in which the ankle joint angle is decreased as the dorsal foot is moved upward toward the anterior surface of the extremity. Abduction is the transverse plane movement of the foot in which the lateral foot is moved away from the midline. Eversion is a frontal plane movement in which the plantar foot rotates outward so that the lateral border is lifted upward.

Supination is a multiplanar rotational motion that includes plantar flexion, adduction, and inversion in non-weight bearing. This combined motion is sometimes incorrectly referred to as inversion. Plantar flexion is the sagittal plane motion in which the foot moves downward and the dorsal foot moves away from the anterior surface of the extremity. Adduction is the transverse plane movement of the foot in which the medial foot is moved toward the midline. Inversion is a frontal plane movement in which the plantar foot rotates inward so that the medial border is lifted upward. These isolated, straight-plane motions of adduction-abduction, inversion-eversion, and dorsiflexion-plantar flexion do not occur in functional activities (figure 20.1). In open chain motion, pronation and supination occur as a result of the calcaneus moving on the talus. In closed chain activities, the calcaneus is anchored by body weight so pronation and supination occur more because the talus is moving on the calcaneus. Therefore, in weight bearing, pronation occurs as the talus moves medially (adducts) and plantarflexes on the calcaneus, and the calcaneus everts, pulling the cuboid and navicular into abduction and eversion, Likewiase, supination in weight bearing occurs when the talus abducts and dorsiflexes while the calcaneus inverts to pull the cuboid and navicular into adduction and inversion. Along with pronation and supination in the closed kinetic chain, associated motions take place further up the chain. With pronation, the tibia extremity medially rotates, the knee flexes, and the hip flexes and medially rotates. Conversely, with supination, the tibia laterally rotates; the knee extends; and the hip extends, abducts, and laterally rotates. Because supination and pronation occur in the subtalar joint, the subtalar joint is instrumental in foot motion and in control of the other joints. For example, if the subtalar joint in the closed kinetic chain is positioned in pronation, the tibia will medially rotate, the knee will flex, and the hip will medially rotate and flex. If the subtalar joint stays in pronation when it should be in supination during ambulation, injuries can result in either the foot or more proximal segments, especially if those segments are forced to be in an abnormal position during the gait cycle because of subtalar pronation. These injuries are discussed later in this chapter.

Extremity, Foot, and Ankle Joints

Specifics of gait analysis are discussed in chapter 12. Reviewing that chapter may help you understand some additional concepts presented here. The first structure to hit the ground in walking is the calcaneus. It, along with the talus, forms the subtalar joint; and the talus along with the tibia and fibula forms the talocrural joint. Normal function of these two joints permits us to land the foot on the ground and adapt to variations in ground topography while maintaining a steady gait. Although the talocrural joint is actually the ankle joint, both the talocrural and subtalar joints are often thought of as the ankle. The talocrural joint moves primarily in dorsiflexion and plantar flexion. The subtalar joint is responsible for inversion and eversion. Pronation and its component motions allow the foot to be a mobile adapter to accommodate for uneven surfaces. Supination allows the foot to become more rigid, provide for power transfer, and permit appropriate force application needed for propulsion in ambulation. As mentioned in chapter 12, these motions must occur at specific times for gait to be normal.

Figure 20.1   Foot planar motions: *(a)* adduction, *(b)* inversion, *(c)* dorsiflexion, *(d)* abduction, *(e)* eversion, *(f)* plantar flexion.

The talocrural joint is a mortise joint, with a convex talar dome in contact with a concave tibial mortise. The lateral malleolus is posterior and distal to the medial malleolus. This arrangement allows more inversion and eversion to occur in the subtalar joint, and also causes plantar flexion to occur more in a posterolateral direction and dorsiflexion to occur more in an anteromedial direction. As the ankle goes into plantar flexion, the talus moves anteriorly so that the posterior, narrower aspect of the talus sits in the mortise joint. This can contribute to instability of the ankle in plantar flexion and is one reason that women wearing high-heeled shoes, and individuals landing from a jump with the foot in plantar flexion, are especially susceptible to ankle sprains. Conversely, the most stable close-packed position for the talus is with the ankle in dorsiflexion when the wider anterior talus is wedged up into the mortise joint. During dorsiflexion, the fibula glides superiorly and rotates laterally; and in plantar flexion, it moves inferiorly and rotates medially. If these fibular motions are not present, full ankle dorsiflexion and plantar flexion cannot occur. Distal to the talocrural and subtalar joints are the midtarsal joints, a combination of the talonavicular and calcaneocuboid articulations. Their position is determined by the subtalar joint position; the midtarsal joints become locked during supination and unlocked during pronation. Movements of the midtarsal joints closely follow movements of the subtalar and talocrural joints. During supination, the navicular and cuboid bones move medially and inferiorly, and during pronation they move laterally and superiorly.

The tarsometatarsal joints are divided into five rays. The first ray is the joint between the first metatarsal and the medial cuneiform. Although the first ray has triplanar motion, its movements are generally referred to as plantar flexion and dorsiflexion. Movement of the first ray occurs equally in plantar flexion and dorsiflexion, with each movement equivalent to about a thumb's width of motion. The second ray includes the joint between the second metatarsal and the middle cuneiform, the third ray includes the third metatarsal and the lateral cuneiform, the fourth ray is the fourth metatarsal alone, and the fifth ray is the fifth metatarsal alone.

Metatarsophalangeal (MTP) joints permit flexion-extension, abduction-adduction, and accessory rotation and dorsal-plantar glides. The interphalangeal (IP) joints, which are hinge joints, permit flexion and extension with accessory rotation and dorsal-plantar glides. The first MTP joint must have about 65° of hyperextension for heel off and toe off during gait.

Muscle Function

There are 12 extrinsic muscles and 11 intrinsic muscles of the extremity and foot. The extrinsic muscles are divided into four compartments or groups: anterior, lateral, posterior superficial, and posterior deep (figure 20.2). The anterior compartment muscles cross the ankle joint anteriorly and provide for dorsiflexion, and lateral and posterior compartment muscles cross the ankle posteriorly and are plantar flexors (figure 20.3). The muscles that have the greatest mechanical advantage to produce inversion and eversion because of their positions are the anterior and posterior tibialis medially and the peroneals laterally.

The posterior extremity has a superficial and a deep compartment; the two compartments are separated by deep fascia, the intermuscular septum. The superficial group includes the large plantar flexors, the soleus, gastrocnemius, and plantaris. The deep posterior muscles originate from the same location as the anterior compartment muscles but traverse posteriorly.

The intrinsic foot muscles are contained within the foot itself. Their purpose is to provide stability to the toes, tarsometatarsal joints, and midfoot while extrinsic muscles move the joints. They attempt to keep the toes on the ground until toe-off during gait and convert the toes to rigid beams for propulsion in gait. These muscles are weakened with ankle injuries and must be rehabilitated along with the extrinsic muscles. In a foot that is unstable, such as a foot that is hypermobile or one that has excessive pronation, the intrinsics are required to work far beyond normal expectations. Excessive sweating of the foot and consequent foot odor are evidence of intrinsic muscle over activity.

Foot Arches

There are three arches of the foot, the medial and lateral longitudinal arches and the transverse arch. These arches are formed by the architecture of the tarsals and their arrangement with each other, the ligaments, and the supporting muscles. The primary tensile supporting structure for the longitudinal arches is the plantar fascia;

Figure 20.2   Cross section of the lower-leg muscle compartments.

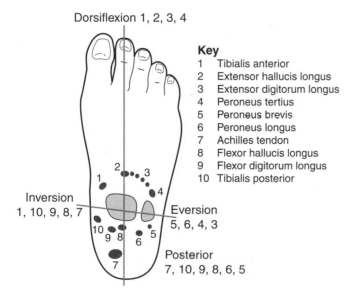

Figure 20.3   Ankle motions. The vertical axis divides muscles that provide inversion and eversion, whereas the horizontal axis divides dorsiflexors from plantar flexors. Muscles are listed in order of their mechanical advantage for motion.

the transverse arch is supported by the peroneus longus. These arches protect the underlying blood vessels and nerves and provide an efficient system of support for the body's weight. If the arches are unable to maintain a normal configuration, an imbalance is created, and abnormal stresses applied to the foot can cause injury. The normal alignment of the longitudinal arches is determined through use of the Feiss line test. In non-weight bearing, a line is drawn from tip of the medial malleolus to the first metatarsal head. This line should cross over the navicular tubercle. In weight bearing, the navicular tubercle should remain on the line or slightly below it.

Subtalar Neutral Position

Because the subtalar joint has a significant impact on the entire lower extremity, the rehabilitation clinician must know what normal subtalar motion and position are to be able to assess and treat an abnormal subtalar joint.

Subtalar neutral is the position in which the talus is equally palpable from its medial or its lateral aspect within the subtalar joint. It is at this point that the talus and navicular are most congruent and the alignment of the subtalar bones is optimal. Subtalar neutral should be assessed in both weight bearing and non-weight bearing (Lattanza, Gray, and Kantner 1988). In non-weight bearing, the patient lies prone with the opposite extremity flexed at the hip and knee and the hip in abduction and lateral rotation to stabilize the pelvis. With the patient's foot and distal extremity to be examined over the edge of the table, the clinician places a thumb and index finger on the medial and lateral aspects of the talus. Using his or her thumb, the clinician locates the medial aspect, in a depression slightly inferior and anterior to the medial malleolus and just proximal to the navicular. He or she locates the lateral aspect, anterior to the lateral malleolus, using the index finger (figure 20.4). As the talus is palpated with one hand, the other hand grasps the fourth and fifth metatarsal heads and moves the foot into dorsiflexion until resistance is felt. In this position, the forefoot is in pronated and supinated to invert and evert the rearfoot. When the forefoot is supinated, the talus is inverted so that the lateral border can be palpated; and when the forefoot is pronated, the talus is everted so that the medial border can be palpated. The foot is rocked back and forth in the two directions with progressively smaller arcs until the talus is centrally positioned and cannot be palpated on either the medial or the lateral aspect or is palpated equally on each side. If subtalar neutral is being palpated in weight bearing, the patient is asked to raise and lower the longitudinal arch to rotate the forefoot until subtalar neutral is determined.

Once subtalar neutral is determined, range of motion of the rearfoot based on calcaneal position can be assessed. Normal rearfoot motion is 30° with one-third in eversion and two-thirds in inversion. A perpendicular line bisecting the posterior calcaneus and a line bisecting the posterior tibia are used as reference points. The calcaneus is passively moved into eversion and inversion, and measurements are taken at the end range of each position (figure 20.5).

Figure 20.4   Subtalar neutral positioning.

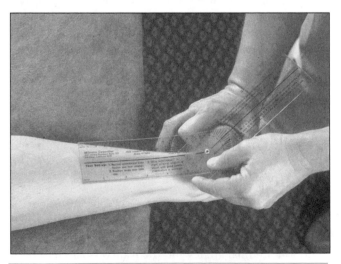

Figure 20.5   Measurement of subtalar range of motion. Lines bisecting the calcaneous and leg are used to define subtalar or rearfoot inversion and eversion range of motion.

COMMON STRUCTURAL DEFORMITIES

▶ Pes cavus and planus, hallux valgus, tibial torsion, tibial varum, and rearfoot and forefoot varus and valgus are among the common structural deformities of the foot and leg.

Although the deformities we will consider are not injuries but structural deviations, they can often lead to injuries. Athletic activity imposes greater-than-normal forces on the foot and thereby exaggerates the impact of a deformity. The rehabilitation clinician must be familiar with these deformities and their impact on the patient to provide appropriate treatment programs.

Pes Cavus

In pes cavus, the foot has an abnormally high longitudinal arch (figure 20.6). The navicular tubercle is above Feiss' line in both weight bearing and non-weight bearing. This is a rigid foot with limited stress-absorption abilities. The foot does not pronate as it should to absorb impact stresses, so the forces are transmitted up the extremity. Pes cavus feet can lead to fallen transverse arches, hammertoes or claw toes, corns, stress fractures, and other overuse injuries.

Figure 20.6   Pes cavus.

Figure 20.7   Pes planus.

Pes Planus

In pes planus, the foot has an abnormally low longitudinal arch (figure 20.7). A rigid pes planus has the navicular tubercle below Feiss' line in both weight bearing and non-weight bearing. A flexible pes planus foot has the navicular tubercle below Feiss' line in weight bearing but on Feiss' line during non-weight bearing.

Either rigid or flexible pes planus can lead to injuries. During weight bearing, the foot is unable to form a rigid lever for efficiency of propulsion and remains in a pronated position when it should be supinated. This imposes additional stresses on more proximal extremity segments. During heel-off and just before toe-off, the extremity and hip are laterally rotating, a motion in conflict with pronation, so torque forces become exaggerated. This is especially true at the knee, particularly at the patellofemoral joint. The condition also places torsion on the plantar fascia and Achilles tendon, because they should be supinating but are pronating. Common terms for the foot with pes planus are pronated foot, flatfoot, and pancake arch.

Figure 20.8   Hallux valgus.

Figure 20.9   Measuring tibial torsion: Tibial torsion is the angle formed between the line through the malleoli and the plane of the tabletop when the femoral condyles on the table and the patella are facing the ceiling.

Hallux Valgus

This condition is also known as a bunion. Hallux valgus is present when the first MTP joint is greater than 10° in valgus with the first toe pointed laterally toward the other toes (figure 20.8). The condition is most commonly seen in a pes planus foot. With the foot in pronation, the force at toe-off is transmitted though the medial aspect of the first ray. This increases medial joint stress. The first ray deviates medially, and the phalanx deviates laterally.

Tibial Torsion

Tibial torsion is present when the tibia is rotated on its long axis. Normally, the midline of the patella is in line with the first- and second-toe web space. In tibial torsion, the foot is rotated laterally to the patella's midline. One can quantify this with the patient supine and the medial and lateral femoral condyles in the transverse plane and the patella facing the ceiling. The rehabilitation clinician measures the angle between the plane of the table and the line between the medial and lateral malleolus (figure 20.9). Normal value is 15°, with a normal range of 2° to 3° in either direction.

Patients with tibial torsion experience increased stress to the knee. Because the tibia is laterally rotated relative to the patella, an increased torque is applied to the patellar tendon. Lateral rotation of the tibia can also be related to prolonged pronation, lateral thigh tightness, and altered patellofemoral alignment.

Figure 20.10 Measuring tibial varum: The line bisecting the leg should be vertical if normal tibial alignment is present.

Tibial Varum

Tibial varum is present when the distal tibia is closer to the midline than the proximal tibia. This can be measured with the patient in standing. With the patient's feet shoulder-width apart, the rehabilitation clinician places the goniometer's stationary arm on the floor and the movable arm along a posterior line bisecting the distal tibia (figure 20.10). The movable arm should be vertical.

Tibial varum is usually accompanied by genu varum and coxa valgus. This deformity places exaggerated stresses on the knee, Achilles, and hip.

Rearfoot Varus and Valgus

The rearfoot is composed of the talus and calcaneus, and its alignment is sometimes referred to as subtalar varus and valgus. Its alignment is determined by the position of the calcaneus relative to that of the posterior extremity. Rearfoot varus (figure 20.11b) is present when the calcaneus is inverted relative to the posterior bisection of the extremity. Rearfoot valgus is present when the calcaneus is everted relative to the tibia (figure 20.11c). The source of rearfoot varus is difficult to ascertain: it may be within the talus, the calcaneus, or both.

Rearfoot varus should be examined in both a relaxed standing position and a subtalar neutral position. Ideally, the results should be the same in the two positions. In a foot that has compensated for the deformity, the calcaneus is perpendicular to the floor in neutral and everted in resting standing. If a foot is uncompensated, the calcaneus remains in eversion in both positions, but the amount of eversion is less in neutral.

With rearfoot varus, the foot remains partially or fully pronated until heel-off during the weight-bearing phase of gait. More pronation than normal must occur to get the inverted heel to the ground. Once the foot is off the ground, the calcaneus rapidly supinates to catch up to the position it should be in at heel strike. This causes a medial heel whip immediately after toe-off, which you can see as you observe the patient posteriorly.

Because the rearfoot does not supinate adequately, hypermobility of the forefoot occurs, and the first ray is unable to get fully stabilized for propulsion. This causes transferal of increased shear and loading forces to the second metatarsal head, and sometimes to the third and fourth metatarsal heads. This in turn causes calluses predominantly over the second metatarsal head and secondarily over the third and fourth metatarsal heads (figure 20.11a). The rearfoot position is important to recognize because it is a key determining factor for the rest of the foot and has a significant impact on the knee and hip.

a   b   c

Figure 20.11 Varus and valgus rearfoot deformities: *(a)* callus pattern for compensated subtalar varus, *(b)* varus, *(c)* valgus.

Forefoot Varus and Valgus

A forefoot varus is an inversion deformity of the midtarsal joint. It is identified through comparison of the plane of the five metatarsal heads with the perpendicular line of the calcaneal bisection. For this examination, the patient lies prone and the rearfoot is placed and maintained in subtalar neutral. The forefoot is loaded on the fifth metatarsal head, and the foot is passively moved into dorsiflexion. In the normal forefoot, the line in the plane of the metatarsals and the line bisecting the calcaneus are perpendicular to each other (figure 20.12b). In forefoot varus, the medial forefoot is higher than the lateral side (inverted) (figure 20.12a). A related condition is first-ray dorsiflexion.

In compensated forefoot varus, the subtalar joint is pronated to allow the medial toes to get to the ground. This calcaneal pronation persists at a time when the joint should be starting to supinate. The rearfoot is unable to supinate in time for heel-off and toe-off because the forefoot is still in contact with the ground, forcing the rearfoot to remain pronated. A slight heel-whip may be seen at heel-off; but it usually is ineffective, because the deformity in the forefoot causing the compensation is still in contact with the ground.

With the rearfoot in pronation throughout propulsion, the body's weight is distributed more medially than normal, and the midtarsal joint becomes hypermobile. This causes the first ray to become unstable and incapable of carrying its propulsive load. The weight and force are then transferred to the second and third metatarsal heads, where callus formations appear as a result of this increased shear and force stress. Because the body's weight is more medially distributed than normal, the foot abducts and a callus forms on the medial hallux from shearing stresses as the body moves over this aspect of the hallux (figure 20.12d).

If the forefoot varus is uncompensated, the individual stays on the lateral aspect of the foot and is unable to pronate as much as he or she should normally. The forefoot varus does not permit the rearfoot to pronate in relaxed standing, so the calcaneus may appear either erect or slightly inverted. Callus formation in this case occurs over the lateral aspect of the foot and over the fifth metatarsal head, because rotation occurs off the fifth metatarsal head and weight bearing is primarily over the lateral foot (figure 20.12e). The rotation is secondary to the rearfoot's failure to go through a full excursion of supination, thereby limiting extremity lateral rotation; the body attempts to abduct the foot so the tibia can tilt to evert the foot to get the propulsive forces delivered from the medial foot, as close to the first metatarsal as possible.

Forefoot valgus is the opposite condition. The metatarsal line of the heads line is higher on the lateral side than on the medial side (everted) (figure 20.12c). A related condition is first-ray plantar flexion. If the first ray is rigid with little available mobility, during ambulation the first ray will hit the ground too early and the peroneus longus will assist by moving the weight more medially to transfer weight to the other foot. In a very rigid first ray, the fifth ray's ability to get to the ground is limited because the foot supinates too early in the mid-weight-bearing phase. With the forefoot in extreme valgus because of the rigid first ray, the forefoot inversion on the rearfoot is severely limited. The rearfoot then attempts to compensate by supinating during midstance. This causes the fifth ray to hit the ground suddenly and undergo increased loading before heel-off. This, in turn, causes the lateral foot to become unstable; and to compensate, the rearfoot moves into pronation at heel-off. The pronation imposes increased shearing forces on the forefoot. Because of the increased shearing forces and the increased time the first ray spends on the ground, there is usually a large callus buildup over the medial first metatarsal head. There is also a callus over the fifth metatarsal head because of the increased friction (figure 20.12f).

On the other hand, if the first ray is mobile, the rearfoot will pronate normally, and no problems should become evident because motion will occur fairly normally. A large callus forms over the first metatarsal head because of the prolonged contact of the first ray with the ground in its plantar-flexed position (figure 20.12g).

Figure 20.12 Forefoot alignment—varus and valgus deformities: *(a)* forefoot varus alignment relative to rearfoot, *(b)* normal forefoot and rearfoot alignment, *(c)* forefoot valgus, *(d)* callus pattern for compensated forefoot varus, *(e)* uncompensated forefoot varus, *(f)* callus pattern for compensated forefoot valgus with a rigid first ray, *(g)* compensated forefoot valgus and rearfoot varus with a flexible first ray.

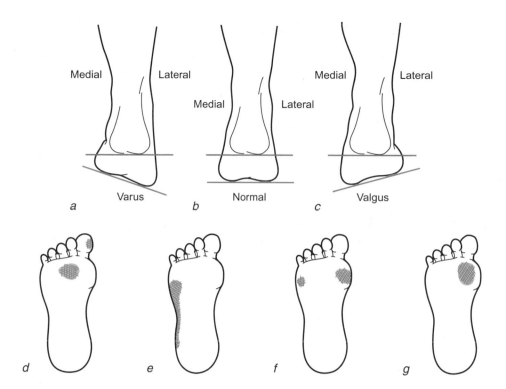

ORTHOTIC TREATMENT FOR FOOT DEFORMITIES

▶ Orthotic devices for the correction of foot deformities are either premade or custom made. The orthotist relies on a number of patient characteristics to design an orthotic device that fits that patient.

Normal foot mechanics during ambulation includes pronation immediately after heel strike and continuing through 25% of the stance phase. During midstance, the rearfoot moves to a neutral position with the calcaneus erect and all the metatarsal heads in contact with the ground. From that point until toe-off, the rearfoot continues its progression toward supination in preparation for converting the foot from a mobile adapter to a rigid lever for propulsion. If the patient's foot does not function in this manner, increased stresses are applied to segments within the foot or extremity. The purpose of foot orthotics is to make the abnormal foot's function closer to that of a normal foot, thereby reducing the abnormal stresses imposed on the foot and extremity. Although not all patients have correct foot alignment and function, many patients who have poor alignment do not have symptoms of pathology. For these asymptomatic patients, orthotics may not be indicated. Foot orthotics are used to correct or support symptomatic rearfoot and/or forefoot malalignments to reduce joint stresses and improve the patient's mechanical efficiency.

Premade Orthotics

Several types of orthotics are available. The type a patient uses depends on that person's specific needs. There are premade orthotics and custom-made orthotics. Premade orthotics, the off-the-shelf variety, are less expensive than custom orthotics and in some situations may meet the patient's needs. These include items such as heel cushions that assist in shock absorption at heel strike and that can also alter heel position if varus or valgus wedges are attached to them. A variety of pads and inserts can assist in reducing stress on specific areas of the foot. These items include metatarsal pads, arch cookies, heel pads, and other supportive devices. Premade arch supports can help support pes planus feet and feet with excessive pronation. Full-length insoles can replace the regular inner liners in shoes and further add to shock absorption.

Custom Orthotics

Custom orthotics are built to satisfy the individual's specific needs, either to absorb stress or to correct alignment. Some of the more common types of orthotics are briefly described next.

Three Types of Orthotics

Custom orthotics are either accommodating or functional and are of three basic types: rigid, semirigid, and soft. The more rigid the orthotic, the more exact the fit must be in order for the device to be effective. Soft orthotics, often made of soft polyethylene foam, are used for cavus or rigid feet to provide stress absorption. They are known as accommodative; they do not so much correct mechanics as accommodate and attempt to relieve symptoms by reducing stresses without altering the foot position.

Most athletic orthotics are of the semirigid variety. They contain a rigid shell, usually made of acrylic plastic or thermoplastic polymer, with a soft covering. These are functional orthotics but may also have accommodating aspects. Their purpose is to change the position of the rearfoot or forefoot (or both) to improve alignment, reduce shear stresses, reduce shock, and stabilize and support the foot joints. The shell has either intrinsic or extrinsic posts to correct the deformities. These posts are in the rearfoot or forefoot or both, depending on the correction needed. Extrinsic posts can be made from a variety of materials with varying densities, including ethyl vinyl acetate (EVA), polyethylene, crepe rubber, and polyplastic (figure 20.13).

Figure 20.13 Custom orthotics are made from a variety of substances and are rigid, semirigid, and soft.

Specialty orthotic devices can also be constructed for specific needs of the patient. Special orthotics can be designed to accommodate for the stresses applied in aerobics by providing more control for loading on the anterior foot. Cycling orthotics must be lightweight and must provide control for the anterior foot, which bears the weight during cycling. A low-profile orthotic can be designed to conform to special footwear such as ski boots, soccer shoes, track racing shoes, and dress shoes.

Three Impression Methods

The three most common methods of taking foot impressions are to use plaster casts, foam boxes, or wax. With the plaster cast method, the patient is prone as he or she would be if you were finding subtalar neutral. A traditional plaster cast using a double layer of plaster splint material is applied to the plantar foot. While the plaster dries, the foot is passively maintained in a subtalar neutral position. This method is the most useful when the orthotic is to be functional. Although the procedure can be messy, the molds are durable after they dry and can be taken or sent through the mail to an orthotics lab without being damaged.

With the foam-box method, the patient's foot is pushed into a box of foam material much like that used by florists. The foot is actively maintained as close to subtalar neutral as possible. This is not an accurate method to use for flexible feet because it can be difficult for a patient with a flexible foot to maintain subtalar neutral. A foam box impression is most commonly used for an accommodative orthotic device, or devices that do not require a precision fit.

The wax method uses warm wax sheets that are molded to the plantar surface of the foot. The rearfoot is maintained in subtalar neutral as the wax cools and hardens. This method is not used if the impressions are to be sent elsewhere, because it is not easy to transport them and the wax melts in heat and cracks in cold weather. The method can be used if the orthotics are constructed in-house.

Orthotic Evaluation

In addition to impression molds of the feet, assessment of various patient characteristics is necessary for an orthotic to be designed to fit accurately. Information that the orthotist needs includes the following items, with the examination presented in the process often followed, moving from non-weight bearing elements to weight bearing observations:

1. **The patient's height, weight, age, and gender.** Some materials have limited ability to withstand stresses beyond specific weights, so the patient's size determines the material used for the orthotic.
2. **The patient's shoe size and style.** Different orthotics are required for different shoe styles and sizes. For example, a sprinter's practice shoe will permit insertion of a different orthotic than the sprinter's race shoe.
3. **The patient's occupation and activity level.** Different orthotics are designed to withstand different stresses, so the orthotist will use information about the patient's activities and sport participation to decide on the specific construction of the orthotic. For example, a soccer player will use a low-profile device that fits in the shoe and absorbs shock during quick running starts and stops.
4. **Special problems.** Surgery, neuromuscular deficiencies, and other medical abnormalities can alter the body's ability to tolerate changes. For example, an open reduction and internal fixation (ORIF) of the ankle may cause soft-tissue adhesions that affect the patient's ability to tolerate a great deal of change rearfoot position.
5. **The patient's primary and other complaints.** These are what you are trying to relieve by providing the orthotic.
6. **Subtalar range of motion.** Subtalar mobility is determined using the method described earlier with the subtalar joint in neutral. Normal subtalar motion is 30° with a 2 to 1 ratio of inversion to eversion. On the form, this amount of motion is indicated as "average." If the total motion is less than 15°, limited rearfoot mobility that can cause forefoot accommodation or changes is present. If eversion motion is less than 5° with the rearfoot in a neutral position, the rearfoot has restricted mobility. If the rearfoot is restricted and there is no forefoot accommodation, a rigid foot may be present. Subtalar mobility of greater than 30° indicates an unstable foot that is in pronation more than it should be. The axis measurement needs to be indicated only if there is an extreme and obvious abnormality. Normal movement of the talus and calcaneus in the subtalar joint is a 1:1 ratio. The axis is considered high if there is more movement of the talus in its transverse plane than movement of the calcaneus in the frontal plane. If, however, there is more calcaneus movement than talus movement, the axis is low.
7. **Midtarsal (global) range of motion.** This is a subjective assessment of gross midfoot mobility. With the rearfoot locked in subtalar neutral, the forefoot is supinated and pronated. Normal mobility should allow full but not excessive motion. This is a difficult motion to assess until you have performed the maneuver many times to obtain an impression of what is loose, what is normal, and what is restricted.
8. **Midtarsal (integrity) range of motion.** In the non-weight bearing position, the foot is positioned first in subtalar neutral, and then the calcaneus is supinated against the cuboid to lock it in position. A normal position is stable with average motion of the forefoot. If the forefoot can be moved freely, the foot is unstable.
9. **First ray range of motion.** This is the amount of flexibility of the first ray. As mentioned previously, the first ray should move about one thumb's width each in plantar flexion and in dorsiflexion. If it moves well in one direction but not the other, it is semirigid. If it is limited in both directions, it is rigid.
10. **First metatarsal ray position.** With the rearfoot aligned in neutral, the forefoot toes should be on the same plane. If the first ray is sits above the forefoot plane, the first ray is dorsiflexed; if it sits below the plane, it is plantar flexed.
11. **Hallux dorsiflexion (open chain).** The hallux should have 60° to 65° of dorsiflexion for normal ambulation. In a rearfoot neutral position, the #1 MP joint should have the ability to be dorsiflexed passively to at least 65°. Patients with a lower value may have problems such as sesamoiditis, plantar fasciitis, or tendinitis. An adjustment in the orthotic may be necessary if the patient's motion is less than 60°.

(continued)

Orthotic Evaluation *(continued)*

12. Ankle dorsiflexion. This is measured in subtalar neutral with passive pressure applied to the ankle into dorsiflexion. Normal dorsiflexion needed for ambulation is 10°. If the ankle does not have this motion, pronation may occur to compensate and allow the patient the mobility needed. An adjustment in the orthotic to relieve stress on the Achilles and plantar fascia may be necessary if the patient lacks full ankle dorsiflexion.

13. Toe positions. These are good indicators of rearfoot deformities. For example, hallux valgus (HAV) may be an indication of excessive pronation, and hammertoes or claw toes (Contracted) are an indication of pes cavus. A Morton's toe may necessitate a change in the orthotic to redistribute weight from the second toe onto the great toe. Normal toes should be straight.

14. Location of corns and calluses. This is important in that corns and calluses are indicators of accommodating or non-accommodating forefoot and rearfoot deformities.

15. Foot appearance: semi-weight bearing arch. The arches are examined with the patient in a sitting position. The feet are resting on the ground. The determination of high, medium, or low arch is based on Feiss' line and the relative position of the navicular.

16. Foot appearance: weight bearing arch. The same examination of arches is made with the patient in full weight bearing. Changes in arch height from resting to weight bearing may indicate accommodations in the foot.

17. Hallux dorsiflexion (closed chain). With the patient in full weight bearing, the MP joint of the great toe is passively dorsiflexed. Care must be taken to have movement occur at the MP joint and not the IP joint.

18. Tibial varum. If this value is beyond 4°, it is abnormal. Tibial varum also adds to foot-deformity stresses and can increase pronation.

19. Knee positions. Knee positions can contribute significantly to foot deformities. For example, genu valgus can be associated with pronation.

20. Calcaneal stance position. In full weight bearing, the calcaneus position relative to the leg is observed in three different positions, subtalar neutral, relaxed standing, and in a half-squat position. These positions are useful in determining whether an accommodation is occurring.

21. Short leg. If leg length differences are greater than 0.5 inches, the differences between the two should be recorded. Differences greater than one-half inch can promote supination in the short leg and pronation in the long leg.

BIOMECHANICAL
S E R V I C E S

1050 Central Ave., Suite D. Brea, CA 92821

(714) 990-5932

Acct. No.:_____

Practitioner's Name: _____

Address: _____

Telephone: _____

Date: _____

Patient Name: _____ Gender: _____ (1) Age: _____ Weight: _____ Height: _____

Shoe Size: _____ Shoe Style: _____ Heel Height: _____

(2) Sport/Activity Level: _____ Previous Orthotic Therapy _____

(3) Medical History (Neuromotor, structural, surgical) _____

_____

_____

---

(4) Primary complaint: _____

_____

Other complaints: (Knee/hip/back)

_____

_____

_____

(5) Calcaneal stance position:

(Resting/relaxed)

Left	Inverted	Rectus	Everted
Right	Inverted	Rectus	Everted

(Neutral subtalar)

Left	Inverted	Rectus	Everted
Right	Inverted	Rectus	Everted

(6) Foot appearance:

(weight-bearing arch)

Left	High	Med	Low
Right	High	Med	Low

(non-weight-bearing arch)

Left	High	Med	Low
Right	High	Med	Low

(7) Toe positions:

Left	Straight	Contracted
	Subluxed	HAV
Right	Straight	Contracted
	Subluxed	HAV

(8) Knee positions:

Left	Genu Varum	Straight
	Genu Valgum	
Right	Genu Varum	Straight
	Genu Valgum	

(9) Tibial Varum (if any):

Degrees   Right _____   Left _____

Short leg (if any):

Left/right _____ MM/inches

(10) First metatarsal ray position:

Left	Normal	Plantar flexed
	Dorsiflexed	
Right	Normal	Plantar flexed
	Dorsiflexed	

(11) Range of motion:

Subtalar:

Left	Restricted	Loose
	Within normal limits	
Right	Restricted	Loose
	Within normal limits	

(12) Midtarsal:

Left	Restricted	Loose
	Within normal limits	
Right	Restricted	Loose
	Within normal limits	

(13) First metatarsal segment:

Left	Flexible	Semi-rigid
	Rigid	
Right	Flexible	Semi-rigid
	Rigid	

(14) Hallux dorsiflexion:

Left	65°	25°
	45°	None
Right	65°	25°
	45°	None

(15) Ankle dorsiflexion:

Left	10°	5–6°
	7–8°	3–4° or less
Right	10°	5–6°
	7–8°	3–4° or less

Area of pain:

(16) Corns/calluses:

R   L

Your diagnosis:

_____

_____

_____

_____

Courtesy of Biomechanical Services.

757

The firmer the orthotic, the less error is tolerated in the fit. Rigid orthotics require the most precision in creating the foot's impression. The softer orthotics tolerate a larger margin of error in the impressions from which they are made. If a semirigid orthotic is desired, an accurate impression should be used.

DETERMINING PROPER FOOTWEAR FOR PATIENTS

▶ To help a patient select a shoe, the rehabilitation clinician must understand shoe structure, not the wear pattern on the patient's current shoes, ascertain the patient's injury history, understand how a shoe should fit, and consider the purpose the shoe will be used for.

A frequently asked question regarding footwear is "What's the best shoe?" There is not a single best shoe. The best shoe is the one that meets an individual's needs. There are many athletic shoes to choose from and new models are released every six months; it is more important for the rehabilitation clinician to be aware of general functional concepts and purposes of shoe components than it is to have knowledge of specific models. He or she can select a shoe on the basis of this general information as it applies to specific models.

Shoes have many functions, including protecting the foot's skin and other soft-tissue structures, providing traction for improved propulsion, reducing shock impact during propulsion activities, increasing foot stability, and accommodating or correcting foot deformities. Companies emphasize style characteristics and fashion trends to increase the popularity of shoes. Ultimately, a shoe should be chosen on the basis of structure, function, and fit, not color, style, or name.

Shoe Structure

All shoes have the same basic structure consisting of an upper and a lower section. The upper section of an athletic shoe includes the vamp, toe box, saddle, collar, insole board, sock liner, and heel counter. The lower section includes the outsole, wedge, and midsole (figure 20.14).

Figure 20.14 Shoe anatomy: *(a)* upper section, *(b)* lower section.

The vamp, which covers the toes and forefoot, includes the toe box. Running shoes whose vamp is made of nylon or another fabric usually have a mudguard around the rim of the toe box. The toe box can vary in width and height from one style and company to another. The toe box functions to retain the shape of the shoe's forefoot and to provide room for the toes. The saddle, the midsection of the shoe along the longitudinal arch, is usually reinforced to provide support to the midfoot. The heel counter is an important stabilizer for the rearfoot. A foxing, an additional piece in many athletic shoes, further reinforces the rearfoot to assist in maintaining the counter's shape. The medial aspect of the counter is sometimes extended forward to resist pronation. The collar is the top rim of the shoe's heel, often padded to reduce friction on the Achilles. Sometimes it is angled inward slightly to provide a snugger fit around the ankle. The insole board lies between the upper and lower segments of the shoe and serves as the attachment for the two segments. A sock liner on top of the insole board is used for shock absorption and friction reduction. The sock liner may be either glued into the shoe or just inserted in it.

The outsole is the portion of the lower segment of the shoe that is in contact with the ground. This is composed of a durable material and has a variety of designs of ripples, waves, and nubs.

The midsole and wedge are made of a variety of substances including EVA, gas-filled or gel-filled chambers, and polyurethane. These sections provide shock attenuation, stability, and control. They can include wedges to provide stability, varying densities to reduce pronation, and special materials to reduce impact stresses.

Figure 20.15 Shoe last: *(a)* straight, *(b)* curved. Last determines the shoe's shape, size, style, and fit.

The last is an important component of a shoe. It is the insole board and is made of a firm substance and determines the shoe's shape, size, style, and fit. The most common types of last are the straight last and the curved last (figure 20.15). The straight last, which can be bisected lengthwise into two equal parts, offers the foot the most medial support and is recommended for pronators. Curved lasts are flared inward to varying degrees. These provide the least amount of medial support and should be avoided by persons who excessively pronate. A curve-lasted shoe is generally more flexible than a straight-lasted shoe. Construction of the shoe around the last involves attaching the outsole and midsole to the bottom of the last and attaching the heel counter, toe box, and upper section of the shoe to the top of the last.

A last is either a board last, a slip last, or a combination last. You can easily see the last by removing the sock liner. A board last is made of a cardboard or cardboard like material that provides for a stiff sole and thus adds to the stability to the foot. A slip-lasted shoe looks like a moccasin, with the upper section stitched along its bottom to the last. This shoe is appropriate for a more rigid foot and offers more flexibility than a board-lasted shoe. A combination last has a board-lasted rearfoot and a slip-lasted forefoot. This type of last is designed to offer rearfoot stability and forefoot flexibility, as well as ease of shoe bend to reduce stresses on the plantar fascia and Achilles during heel-off and toe-off.

Shoe Wear

An examination of the patient's worn shoes can give clues to foot deformities, helping the rehabilitation clinician guide the patient toward the most appropriate shoe. If the heel counter and medial heel are collapsed to the medial side of the shoe, the patient excessively pronates. A medial wedge, or increased density of the medial wedge or midsole, along with a strong heel counter will provide increased stability. This patient should use a board-lasted shoe.

If the lateral heel counter of the worn shoe is moved laterally, the patient has a rigid foot and needs a shoe with a slip last, a lot of cushion but no medial wedge, and a firm heel counter.

If the patient's hallux has a blackened toenail, the toe box may not be deep enough. If the hallux is wearing through the upper section of the shoe, the patient may have a rigid first ray and require increased shock absorption in the forefoot. The forefoot of the shoe for this type of foot needs to be rigid to protect the first ray.

Although shoe wear is a good indicator of deformities, a shoe that has noticeable wear is one that should be replaced. The life of a shoe depends on the patient, the frequency of participation, and the surfaces on which the patient plays the sport. Footwear varies greatly in longevity. It is important, however, that the shoe be replaced once a wear pattern is seen. A worn shoe changes the mechanics and stresses applied to the foot and can magnify any structural deformity.

Injury History

A profile of the patient's injury history also aids in determining the correct shoe for that person. For example, if the patient has a history of Achilles tendinitis, the cause may be either excessive pronation or tightness in the Achilles. This patient should find a shoe that has good heel-counter stability, a straight board or combination last, good forefoot flexibility, and a higher-than-normal elevation in the wedge to relieve Achilles stress.

If the patient has a history of knee pain, excessive pronation may be the cause. A board-lasted shoe with good rearfoot control and a firm heel counter is appropriate for this patient. Plantar fasciitis is also related to excessive pronation, so a similar shoe would be appropriate for a patient with a history of plantar fasciitis.

Proper Shoe Fit

Once the specific needs of the patient have been determined, the shoe must be fit properly. Shoe size is most easily determined using the Brannock measuring device found in shoe stores

Figure 20.16   Brannock measuring device.

(figure 20.16). This determines the width and length of the shoe. A good heel fit is critical for an athletic shoe. The shoe should fit snugly to provide adequate support for the rearfoot. There should be approximately one thumb's width between the end of the longest toe and the end of the shoe. The toe box should have adequate depth and width for the forefoot and toes. The bend in the vamp should coincide with the bend of the patient's forefoot. A good heel counter should feel firm and have little give when it is squeezed. The vamp should bend easily when you grasp the heel and try to bend the shoe by applying pressure with the index finger of your other hand. If a shoe is board lasted, it should be difficult to wring the shoe and produce much motion when stabilizing the heel and rotating the vamp.

Shoes should be evaluated to make sure that the heel counter is perpendicular to the sole, the sole is parallel to the floor, and the last is the same on the right as on the left shoe. It is also important to ascertain that there are no abnormalities in stitching, construction, or angle from one shoe to the other. Because there is no quality control in shoe manufacturing, errors in production are not uncommon. A construction error can cause an injury or aggravate any structural deformity.

Patients should try on shoes in the store, wearing socks of the same type and thickness as those they will use with the shoes. An individual should be able to give shoes a good trial in the store on a treadmill or track or be able to run outside before purchasing them. It is best to try shoes on in the later part of the day when foot volume is greater than in the morning. Because foot size may vary from right to left, it is advisable to try on both shoes, properly laced. It is a good idea to try on a variety of shoes and compare comfort and fit. The patient should be sure to ask about the store's return policy. The store should stand behind the product and permit exchanges if someone who has tried a shoe at home finds that it does not meet specific needs or is uncomfortable.

Shoe Types

Because different activities place different stresses on the foot, requirements for an athletic shoe differ among sports. There are as many types of shoes as there are sports. It is not advisable for a patient to wear a shoe intended for use in one sport for a second sport. The shoe is not designed to meet the demands of another sport.

Tennis Shoes

Tennis involves sudden stops and changes in direction and many lateral movements, so safe tennis participation requires good medial and lateral support to protect the lateral ligaments and peroneals. Because most tennis is played on a variety of outdoor surfaces, the outsole should be durable; the material should be able to adapt to differing playing surfaces and allow some sliding on the court. A toe guard or reinforcement over the medial toes will prolong the life of the shoe and protect it against toe drag on the serve. In a shoe appropriate for tennis, the heel and toe are at about the same level, whereas a running shoe has an elevated heel to reduce stress on the Achilles. Because placing the foot in a plantar-flexed position makes the ankle susceptible to inversion sprains and because tennis involves lateral movements, a tennis shoe is flat.

Running Shoes

In addition to the elevated heel, a running shoe should be flexible so that the foot does not have to work excessively to bend the shoe during heel-off. The shoe should have good cushion in the rear and forefoot yet provide stability to the heel.

Aerobics Shoes

Aerobics shoes should have good forefoot cushioning, and many have additional cushioning in the sock liner. A reinforced toe box supports the forefoot primarily during forefoot-impact activities. The forefoot should have good flexibility to allow the foot to bend easily during aerobic activities; in many shoes this flexibility comes from flex bars cut into the sole. There should be good rearfoot stability with a good heel counter for adequate ankle support during medial and lateral activities. Stability is necessary for the multidirectional movements in aerobics. Stability straps in the midfoot region can provide medial-lateral stability in the midsole and the upper section. In some shoes, a mid-height upper section provides added medial-lateral support without interfering with plantar flexion-dorsiflexion. Aerobic shoes come in leather and synthetic materials; synthetic material is usually lighter and does not absorb as much moisture as the leather.

Volleyball Shoes

Volleyball shoes must meet the demands of sudden stops, starts, jumps, and lateral moves. The shoe should not have an elevation to the heel but should have a durable outsole, good medial-lateral stability, and sufficient traction; it should be lightweight and flexible enough not to contribute to jumping fatigue. Stabilizing straps add medial-lateral support and forefoot stability. A gum-rubber sole increases traction and durability. Additional leather guards prolong the life of the shoe by protecting the toes from excessive wear during drag.

Basketball Shoes

Basketball shoes must provide cushion during jumps, stability during quick stops and starts and changes in direction, and ease of foot-bend during running. Mid- and high-top shoes provide medial-lateral support, as do the forefoot support straps and sole design. A good heel counter also provides stability. Flex joints in the sole of the forefoot facilitate bending, and the midsole is composed of a shock-absorbing substance such as EVA. Basketball court surfaces are rough on the outsole, so a basketball shoe should have a stitched rubber outsole with a reinforced toe region.

Soccer Shoes

A soccer shoe should have a flexible sole to permit ease in dorsiflexion-plantar flexion motion of the ankle. The cleats should be placed in areas that do not promote undue pressure on or irritation of the foot; rearfoot cleat placement should be around the perimeter to avoid heel irritation. Cleats vary according to the surface the patient plays on. Short cleats are appropriate for hard turf, whereas long cleats are suitable for softer surfaces such as wet grass.

Walking Shoes

Walking shoes have many of the same characteristics as running shoes. The heel is slightly raised, but not as much as in a running shoe, and a firm heel counter provides for rearfoot and impact stability. The forefoot is usually more flexible. The outer sole has a rocker bottom to provide efficiency and to lessen energy requirements during heel strike and rolling from heel-off to toe-off. The shank portion of the midsole is usually stiffer in a walking shoe to provide for better medial-lateral stability. Selection of a walking shoe should be based on the type of walking the patient performs. Olympic walkers require flexibility for economy of movement; off-trail walkers need stability and traction for uneven surfaces; and power and fitness walkers need stability and cushioning.

Mountaineering Shoes

Requirements for mountaineering shoes vary according to the specific activity involved. Hiking, climbing, and high-altitude climbing each place different demands on the feet and will require different shoes.

Hiking is one of the most popular mountaineering sports. A hiking shoe should provide stability and should have a good heel counter and midsole for medial-lateral support. Hiking shoes should be waterproof or water resistant and should have a very durable outsole. The outsole should have good traction for uneven and rough terrain. The upper section height should be mid to high for rough terrain and mid to low for easy terrain. A hiking shoe needs to be lightweight and comfortable; it should not have pressure points and should not need to be broken in.

Cross-Training Shoes

Cross-training shoes are designed to meet the needs of individuals involved in multiple activities. The goal is to meet all the needs of all the people all the time. The problem is that these shoes usually do not meet any specific need most of the time. There are various styles of shoes in this category. A person who wants a cross-training shoe should select the shoe that meets the demands of the activity he or she participates in most of the time.

Lacing Patterns

Some shoes, especially running shoes, have multiple eyelets that the wearer can select from when lacing the shoe. These allow the use of a variety of lacing patterns to meet specific needs. Alternative lacing patterns can add to the support the shoe provides or accommodate for some deformities. A person who has a narrow foot should use the eyelets farthest from the tongue of the shoe, which will pull the sides of the shoe more closely together (figure 20.17a). People with wide feet should use the eyelets closest to the tongue (figure 20.17b).

Women often have the problem of a wide forefoot and a narrower heel than is accounted for in the construction of a shoe. They can accommodate for this by using two laces, one for the lower eyelets and the other for the higher eyelets, and tying the upper lace more tightly to support the heel (figure 20.17c).

Patients with high arches should avoid lacing a shoe in the traditional crisscross pattern but instead should use a straight-across pattern (figure 20.17d).

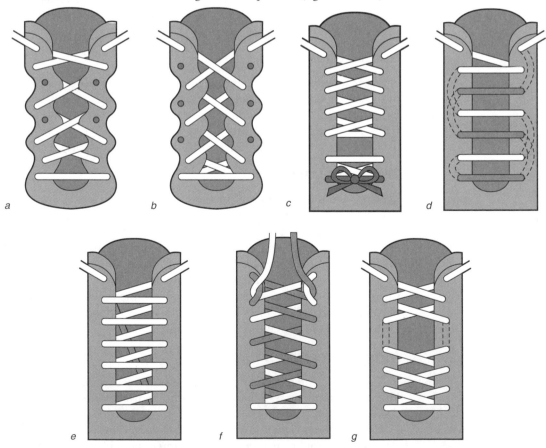

Figure 20.17 Shoe-lacing patterns for *(a)* narrow feet, *(b)* wide feet, *(c)* wide forefoot and narrow heel (using two laces), *(d)* high arches, *(e)* toe problems, *(f)* heel blisters, *(g)* dorsal foot bump.
Reprinted by permission from C. Frey 1998.

People with toe problems can obtain some relief by using the laces to lift up the forefoot of the shoe. As the shoe is tied, the lace that goes through the eyelet nearest the problem toe is brought directly to an eyelet at the top of the shoe. Pulling on this lace lifts up part of the forefoot (figure 20.17e).

Heel blisters are often caused by friction of the shoe over the heel. The wearer can decrease the friction by securing the heel more firmly in the shoe using a loop-through technique at the top of the shoe as seen in figure 20.17f. The lace should be pulled tighter at the top of the shoe than at the bottom.

A bump on the top of the foot can be painful with regular-lacing-pattern pressure. To relieve pressure on the top of the foot, don't cross the laces; instead, keep the laces on the same side of the shoe and skip the eyelet at the painful level (figure 20.17g).

SOFT-TISSUE MOBILIZATION

▶ Soft-tissue mobilization is used to treat common myofascial pain referred from the leg and foot. Treatment is applied to superficial intrinsic foot muscles, deep intrinsic foot muscles, and several muscles extrinsic to the foot.

As with the upper extremity, pain and referred pain in the lower extremity can come from several sources. Sciatica is a common pain-referral source in the lower extremity, with symptoms extending anywhere from the back to the toes. Before the rehabilitation clinician treats a pain locale, he or she must identify the source. If the pain is myofascially based, soft-tissue mobilization techniques can be effective in relieving the pain. The areas discussed here are common myofascial pain-referral patterns from the muscles of the extremity and foot. These pain-referral patterns and the treatments presented are based on the work of Travell and Simons (1992). The following sections deal with identification of trigger points and pain-referral patterns for the muscles and then present trigger point release and ice-and-stretch techniques. Remember that ice-and-stretch applications are repeated several times. The procedure is to apply the ice during the passive stretch and then to perform active shortening and repeated stretches. After the ice-and-stretch application, the patient should actively move the muscle through its full range of motion several times.

Superficial Intrinsic Foot Muscles

These muscles include the extensor digitorum brevis, extensor hallucis brevis, abductor hallucis, flexor digitorum brevis, and abductor digiti minimi. These muscles generally refer pain over the muscle site with a small degree of radiation that remains locally in the foot. The intrinsic toe extensors refer to the dorsum of the foot in the area of their muscle bellies (figure 20.18a). The abductor hallucis brevis refers to the medial heel with some radiation into the medial arch (figure 20.18c). The abductor digiti minimi refers pain along the fifth metatarsal's plantar aspect (figure 20.18b); the short toe flexors refer pain to the second through fourth metatarsal heads (figure 20.18d). Pain reports of these muscles include deep aching pain that has not responded to self-remedy attempts.

Deep pressure is applied to relieve the trigger point (figure 20.18, e-f). A local twitch is not commonly seen, but the patient may demonstrate a jump response to pressure over the trigger point. Ice-and-stretch is applied with the patient in a comfortable position. For application to the toe extensors, the foot is plantar flexed and the toes moved passively into flexion as the ice strokes are brought from the anterior extremity along the foot's dorsum to the toes (figure 20.18g). For ice-and-stretch to the abductors and intrinsic toe flexors, the ankle can remain in a neutral position. The abductor hallucis and intrinsic toe flexors are positioned in flexion while the ice is stroked from the plantar heel toward the toes (figure 20.18, h-j).

Figure 20.18 Superficial intrinsic muscle pain-referral patterns: *(a)* extensor digitorum brevis and extensor hallucis brevis, *(b)* abductor digiti minimi, *(c)* abductor hallucis, *(d)* flexor digitorum brevis. Trigger point release of *(e)* extensor digitorum brevis, *(f)* abductor hallucis. Ice-and-stretch for *(g)* extrinsic toe extensors, *(h)* flexor digitorum brevis, *(i)* abductor hallucis, *(j)* flexor digitorum brevis.

Figure 20.19 Self-application: massage to plantar foot.

The patient can perform self-massage techniques using a tennis or golf ball, a ridged vegetable can, or a rolling pin. In sitting, the patient places the plantar foot on top of the object being used and applies pressure downward on the knee while rolling the foot back and forth over the object (figure 20.19).

Deep Intrinsic Foot Muscles

These muscles include the quadratus plantae, lumbricals, flexor hallucis brevis, adductor hallucis, flexor digiti minimi brevis, and interossei. Like the pain-referral pattern of the superficial group, the pain-referral pattern of these muscles is primarily localized and over the region of their trigger points (figure 20.20, a-d). The pain is often described as a feeling of swelling and numbness that restricts walking. The quadratus plantae refers pain to the heel; the flexor hallucis brevis refers pain to the plantar and medial aspect of the head of the first metatarsal. The adductor hallucis refers pain to the ball of the foot; the interossei refer pain to the corresponding digit and along the dorsal and ventral aspects of the distal portion of the metatarsal to which they attach. The pain patterns of the lumbricals and flexor digiti minimi have not been determined.

Because these muscles lie deep to the plantar aponeurosis, long tendons, and superficial intrinsic muscles, deep palpation is required to affect them. Direct pressure over the trigger point is effective in releasing the painful trigger point (figure 20.20e).

The deep intrinsic muscles most amenable to ice-and-stretch techniques are the flexor hallucis brevis and the adductor hallucis. These muscles are treated with the ankle in neutral and the hallux hyperextended as sweeps are made from the heel toward the toe (figure 20.20f).

Extrinsic Muscles

As in the upper extremity, several extrinsic muscles function in the foot and ankle. They are presented here according to the extremity compartments they lie in, moving from anterior to lateral and posterior.

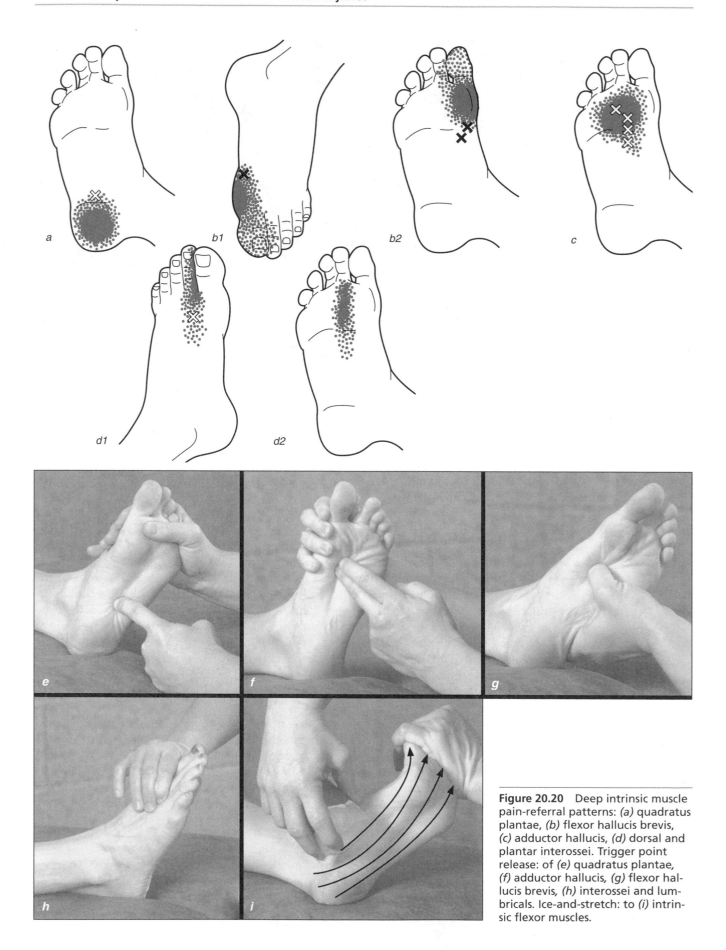

Figure 20.20 Deep intrinsic muscle pain-referral patterns: *(a)* quadratus plantae, *(b)* flexor hallucis brevis, *(c)* adductor hallucis, *(d)* dorsal and plantar interossei. Trigger point release: of *(e)* quadratus plantae, *(f)* adductor hallucis, *(g)* flexor hallucis brevis, *(h)* interossei and lumbricals. Ice-and-stretch: to *(i)* intrinsic flexor muscles.

Tibialis Anterior

The tibialis anterior refers pain to the anteromedial ankle and over the dorsal and medial big toe (figure 20.21a). It can occasionally refer pain along the anterior shin. This trigger point usually occurs in conjunction with trigger points of other muscles.

Trigger point release is performed with flat palpation of the trigger point located at the border of the proximal and middle third of the anterior extremity near the tibial ridge (figure 20.21b). The area is tender to palpation, and a taut band can be palpated. A local twitch response may be elicited with snapping palpation of the trigger point. Direct pressure to the patient's tolerance relaxes the band and relieves the pain.

Ice-and-stretch is applied as the foot is plantar flexed and pronated; ice sweeps are made from the knee distally toward the foot (figure 20.21c).

Figure 20.21   Tibialis anterior: (a) pain-referral pattern, (b) trigger point release, (c) ice-and-stretch in plantar flexion, (d) ice-and-stretch in plantar flexion with pronation added.

Peroneals

The peroneus longus and brevis refer pain to the lateral malleolus and proximally and distally to it (figure 20.22a). The longus pain may also spill over to the middle lateral extremity. The peroneus tertius refers pain to the anterolateral ankle and into the lateral heel. Individuals with a Morton's toe and excessive pronation are more prone to these complaints. Snapping palpation of the peroneus longus elicits a local twitch response that produces ankle plantar flexion and eversion. Its trigger point is located about 2 to 4 cm (0.8-1.6 in.) distal to the fibular head near the shaft of the fibula (figure 20.22b). The peroneus brevis trigger point is located at the juncture of the middle and distal thirds of the extremity. The peroneus tertius trigger points are just anterior and distal to those of the peroneus brevis.

Ice-and-stretch is applied to the peroneus longus and brevis with a passive stretch of the ankle into inversion and dorsiflexion while proximal-to-distal sweeps of ice are made along the lateral extremity. To treat the peroneus tertius, the rehabilitation clinician performs a plantar-flexion and inversion stretch and applies ice more anteriorly on the distal extremity (figure 20.22c).

Figure 20.22 Peroneal pain patterns *(a)*, trigger point release to peroneus longus *(b)*, and ice-and-stretch for peroneus tertius *(c)*.

Gastrocnemius

This muscle has four trigger points with different referral patterns. They can refer pain to the medial arch with spillover into the medial calf (figure 20.23a1), close to the medial border of the medial gastrocnemius head (figure 20.23a2), close to the lateral border of the lateral gastrocnemius head (figure 20.23a3), and slightly more distal on the lateral head of the gastrocnemius (figure 20.23a4). Nocturnal cramps are often associated with these trigger points.

Trigger point release using deep pressure can be performed with the patient either lying or kneeling (figure 20.23b). Either a flat thumb pressure or a pincher grasp can be used. If the muscle is taut, a flat pressure is easier and more comfortable to administer. Trigger point release is best performed with the ankle in slight plantar flexion to place the muscle on slack. A pincher grasp of the lateral head is easily used with the thumb on the lateral border and the fingers at the midline groove between the two gastrocnemius heads. Flat pressure should be used in the popliteal area.

Ice-and-stretch is applied with the patient in prone and the foot over the edge of the table. While the rehabilitation clinician uses his or her knee to dorsiflex the ankle with pressure over the ball of the patient's foot, he or she applies ice from above the knee in a distal direction toward the plantar foot (figure 20.23c).

Figure 20.23 Gastrocnemius trigger point: *(a)* pain-referral pattern, *(b)* trigger point release of lateral head, *(c)* ice-and-stretch.

Soleus

The most common site of pain referral of the soleus is into the posterior and plantar heel area and into the distal Achilles. The soleus occasionally refers pain into the upper calf and rarely into the ipsilateral sacroiliac joint (figure 20.24a). Heel pain during weight bearing and nocturnal deep heel pain may be primary complaints, and dorsiflexion is limited.

Trigger point release uses either a pincher or flat-pressure application. The patient can be either in prone with the knee flexed to keep the gastrocnemius slack (figure 20.24b) or in a kneeling position. The distal trigger points are located just distal to the medial and lateral gastrocnemius muscle belly bulges. Direct pressure to the patient's tolerance is applied until the muscle becomes relaxed and the pain subsides.

Ice-and-stretch is performed with the knee in flexion. The patient can be kneeling or prone (figure 20.24c). As the ankle is passively dorsiflexed, the ice is swept from proximal to distal across the posterior extremity and into the plantar foot.

Figure 20.24   Soleus: *(a)* pain-referral pattern, *(b)* trigger point release, *(c)* ice-and-stretch.

Tibialis Posterior

Trigger point activation of this muscle makes it painful for the patient to run or walk on uneven surfaces when the muscle's activity is increased for providing additional stabilization for the foot. The pain can refer into the Achilles tendon with spillover into the midcalf proximally and the heel, instep, and plantar foot and toes distally (figure 20.25a).

Because the tibialis posterior is the deepest muscle of the extremity, it is not possible to make direct contact with it through deep pressure. Deep pressure to more superficial muscles can be used to apply indirect pressure. The rehabilitation clinician presses deeply between the soleus and the medial border of the posterior tibia (figure 20.25b). Ice-and-stretch is applied with the patient prone and the foot over the edge of the table. The ankle is stretched into dorsiflexion and eversion as the ice sweeps begin at the posterior knee and extend distally into the plantar foot (figure 20.25c).

Figure 20.25 Tibialis posterior: *(a)* pain-referral pattern, *(b)* trigger point release (medial approach), *(c)* ice-and-stretch.

Long Toe Extensors

These muscles include the extensor digitorum longus and the extensor hallucis longus. Trigger points can cause night cramps in the toe extensors. The most common pain-referral pattern for these muscles is along the anterior ankle, along the dorsum of the foot over the metatarsals, and extending distally into the toes and proximally into the distal extremity (figure 20.26a).

Trigger point release is performed on the extensor digitorum longus through application of pressure over the muscle about 8 cm (3 in.) distal and slightly anterior of the fibular head (figure 20.26b). Trigger point release for the extensor hallucis longus is applied anterior of the fibula at the location of the juncture of the middle and distal thirds of the extremity (figure 20.26c).

Ice-and-stretch is applied with the patient supine. The ankle and toes are passively plantar flexed with pressure on the distal toes while ice sweeps are applied from the anterior and lateral proximal extremity distally over the ankle and foot to the toes (figure 20.26d).

Figure 20.26 Long toe extensors: *(a)* pain-referral patterns, *(b)* trigger point release of extensor digitorum longus, *(c)* trigger point release of extensor hallucis longus, *(d)* ice-and-stretch.

Long Toe Flexors

The most common symptom reported with active trigger points of the long toe flexors is pain in the feet during walking. The referral pain pattern for the flexor digitorum longus is into the sole of the forefoot with occasional spillover into the toes and medial calf (figure 20.27a1). The flexor hallucis longus refers pain to the plantar great toe and into the first metatarsal head (figure 20.27a2).

For trigger point release, the patient is in side-lying on the involved side with the knee flexed and the ankle in a relaxed plantar-flexed position. Using a flat-pressure technique, the rehabilitation clinician applies pressure on the medial proximal extremity between the tibia and gastrocnemius-soleus complex (figure 20.27b). Once the gastrocnemius is pushed posteriorly, pressure is applied downward and then laterally. The flexor hallucis longus is treated with the patient in prone; deep pressure is applied through the soleus lateral to the midline and at the juncture of the middle and lower thirds of the extremity (figure 20.27c).

Ice-and-stretch is performed with the patient prone and the knee passively flexed. As the ankle is passively dorsiflexed and everted and the toes are extended, ice sweeps are applied from the proximal calf along the medial ankle into the plantar foot to the toes (figure 20.27d).

Figure 20.27   Long toe flexors: *(a)* pain-referral pattern, *(b)* trigger point release of flexor digitorum longus, *(c)* trigger point release of flexor hallucis longus, *(d)* ice-and-stretch.

DEEP-TISSUE MASSAGE

▶ The rehabilitation clinician uses deep-tissue massage of the foot and ankle to promote tissue flexibility and improve range of motion. Patients can perform self-massage on foot intrinsic muscles.

Soft-tissue restriction often occurs after a patient has experienced excessive edema or immobilization of the ankle, foot, or extremity. Either the prolonged presence of edema or reduced tissue mobility can result in adhesions. Good tissue flexibility and restoration of normal range of motion can occur with release of adhesions. Deep-tissue massage techniques, discussed in chapter 6, can be useful in accomplishing these goals. Review the discussion of proper application of these massage techniques before using them. The patient can perform deep massage to foot intrinsic muscles that are in spasm or that have myofascial tightness. Sitting in a chair, the patient places the bare foot on the side of a ribbed fruit or vegetable can positioned on the floor. Applying some downward force on the knee with the hands, the patient rolls the foot back and forth over the can to provide a self-massage.

JOINT MOBILIZATION

▶ Joint mobilizations—glides or oscillations—are used to reduce pain and swelling or to improve mobility in many joints in the ankle.

Joint mobilization is often necessary in the ankle, especially after periods of immobilization. The techniques can be either repeated sustained glides or oscillations. In more restricted joints, sustained glides may be more effective than oscillations. Oscillation may be more comfortable for the patient and is frequently used in distractions to aid in reduction of swelling and pain (grades I and II). More aggressive grades (III and IV) are used to improve mobility.

To determine whether joint mobilization for mobility is indicated, the rehabilitation clinician assesses the joint's capsular pattern and motion loss and also compares the involved with the uninvolved segment. The normal capsular pattern for the talocrural joint is more limitation of plantar flexion than of dorsiflexion; in the subtalar joint, inversion is more limited than eversion. The great toe's MTP and all the toes' IP joints have capsular patterns of more limitation of extension than flexion. Refer to chapter 6 for this information and for details on close-packed and resting positions for these joints.

As with other joints, precautions and contraindications should be respected. Body mechanics, force direction application, and amount of force should be proper in all techniques. The hands should be as close to the joint as possible, with one hand acting as the stabilizing hand and the other applying the mobilization force. The convex-concave rule determines the direction of the mobilization force. That is, when a convex surface is moved on a concave surface, the force is applied in the direction opposite than that of the bone's movement; when a concave surface is moved on a convex surface, the force is applied in the same direction as the bone's movement. Many of the mobilization techniques in this chapter are based on Maitland's (1991) work.

Tibiofibular Joint

The tibia and fibula articulate with each other proximally in the distal knee region and distally at the ankle mortise joint. Both proximal and distal articulations must have restored mobility for ankle motion to be normal.

Superior Tibiofibular Joint

Mobilization of the superior tibiofibular joint should accompany any restricted movement of the distal tibiofibular joint. Normal mobility of this joint allows the fibular head to move anteriorly during knee flexion and posteriorly during knee extension. Mobilization glides for this joint include anterior-posterior (AP) and posterior-anterior (PA) movements of the fibular head. These can be performed either separately or in one continuous motion from full anterior to full posterior positions. Assessment of the joint's mobility, though, should be performed in one direction at a time.

The patient can be either in supine with the knee flexed and the foot flat on the table, or in sitting with the extremity over the table's edge and with the rehabilitation clinician stabilizing the distal extremity between his or her knees. The rehabilitation clinician's medial hand stabilizes the tibia, and the lateral hand grasps the fibular head with the thumb pad anteriorly and the index and middle fingers posteriorly (figure 20.28a). Compression of the peroneal nerve behind the fibula should be avoided. The lateral hand glides the fibular head anteriorly and posteriorly.

When each movement is performed individually, the patient is positioned to provide the clinician the best mechanical advantage and ease of force application. For an AP mobilization force, the patient is positioned supine with the knee in extension. The tibia is stabilized with the medial hand over the proximal tibia, and the lateral hand's fleshy aspect of the thenar eminence over the fibular head and proximal fibula to act as the mobilizing hand. A vertical downward force is applied by the mobilizing hand on the fibular head to produce a posterior glide of the fibula (figure 20.28b).

PA mobilization of the proximal tibiofibular joint is performed with the patient in side-lying. The weight of the extremity stabilizes the tibia while the rehabilitation clinician's distal hand stabilizes the middle extremity. The mobilizing hand applies an anterior glide with the pad of the wrist against the fibular head.

Figure 20.28 Proximal tibiofibular joint mobilization: *(a)* AP-PA mobilization, *(b)* posterior glide.

Figure 20.29 Distal tibiofibular joint mobilization, posterior glide.

Inferior Tibiofibular Joint

During dorsiflexion, the distal fibula moves superiorly from the tibia and rotates medially. During plantar flexion, the distal fibula moves in the opposite directions. Normal ankle motion depends on good fibular mobility. Restriction of joint play between the fibula and tibia may require fibular mobilization in both AP and PA directions to restore normal motion.

An AP glide is performed with the patient supine. The clinician places the medial hand over the medial malleolus to stabilize the tibia and places the thenar eminence of the lateral hand over the lateral malleolus and distal fibula. A posterior glide is performed using a downward movement of the lateral hand (figure 20.29).

A PA glide is performed with the patient prone and the distal extremity over the edge of the table. The base of the lateral hand is placed over the lateral malleolus while the medial hand stabilizes the distal tibia. The anterior force is applied perpendicular to the plane of the distal tibiofibular joint.

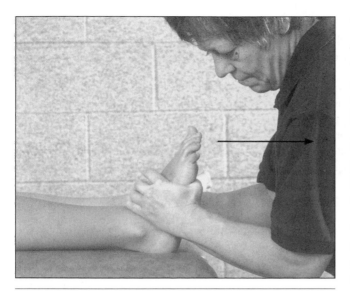

Figure 20.30 Talocrural distraction joint mobilization.

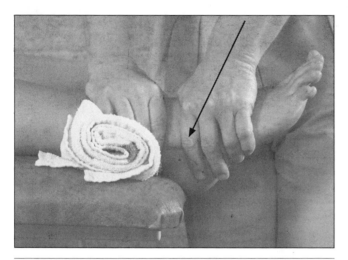

Figure 20.31 Talocrural posterior glide joint mobilization.

Figure 20.32 Alternative AP talocrural glide joint mobilization.

Talocrural Joint

There are several joints throughout the ankle and foot. The talocrural joint is the true ankle joint, allowing flexion and extension motion. The next sections present some of the most common joint mobilization techniques for this joint.

Distraction

Distraction movement is used to increase general joint play in the ankle joint and can also be used with lower grades of mobilization to relieve pain.

The patient is supine with the hip and knee extended. The rehabilitation clinician faces the foot and grasps the foot's dorsum with both hands, intertwining or overlapping the fingers of the two hands on top of the foot and placing the thumbs on the plantar aspect (figure 20.30). The clinician leans backward to apply a distraction force.

Anterior Glide

This technique is used to increase ankle plantar flexion. It is also known as a ventral glide or PA movement.

With the patient prone and his or her foot comfortably over the end of the table, the rehabilitation clinician places a pad or rolled towel for comfort under the distal extremity. The stabilizing hand is placed on the anterior extremity just above the malleoli, and the mobilizing hand cups the talus and calcaneus. The talus and calcaneus are glided anteriorly with downward force applied by the mobilizing hand.

Posterior Glide

This technique is used to increase dorsiflexion and is also known as a dorsal glide or AP glide.

The patient is supine with the knee extended; the clinician faces the foot. The stabilizing hand is placed anteriorly around the distal extremity, and the mobilizing hand is placed around the proximal foot with the thumb and index finger in contact with the malleoli. The talus is glided posteriorly in the plane of the joint (figure 20.31).

Alternative Technique for Dorsiflexion

An alternative technique for gaining dorsiflexion utilizes a mobilization strap. With the patient standing in a forward-backward stride position on a table, and a mobilization strap secured around the distal tibia and fibula and the clinician's hips, the rehabilitation clinician places the web of the thumb and index finger around the anterior ankle joint. The belt is used to stabilize the ankle. With the knee partially flexed the clinician uses the hips to pull the strap forward (figure 20.32).

Figure 20.33   Subtalar joint distraction joint mobilization.

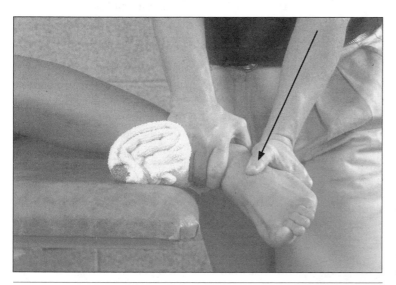

Figure 20.34   Subtalar joint medial glide joint mobilization.

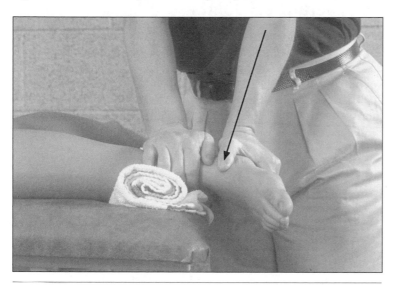

Figure 20.35   Subtalar joint lateral glide joint mobilization.

Subtalar Joint

The subtalar joint allows inversion and eversion movements to permit ambulation on uneven surfaces without injury. Some, but not all, mobilization techniques for the subtalar joint are presented here. Hand positions for some of these techniques, such as distraction, are subtly different from those for talocrural mobilization but nonetheless important.

Distraction

This technique is used to reduce pain and to improve general mobility. The patient is supine with the foot over the end of the table, and the rehabilitation clinician faces the foot. The stabilizing hand grasps the talus anteriorly, and the mobilizing hand cups the posterior calcaneus (figure 20.33). The calcaneus is pulled distally from the long axis of the extremity.

Medial Glide

This technique is used to increase eversion. With the patient sidelying on the uninvolved side and the involved ankle off the end of the table, a towel roll is placed under the distal extremity. The distal extremity is stabilized with the cephalic hand over the lateral extremity, and the caudal hand is positioned with its heel on the lateral calcaneus and the fingers on the plantar surface (figure 20.34). A downward medial glide is applied to the calcaneus.

Lateral Glide

This maneuver is used to increase subtalar inversion. With the patient in sidelying on the involved side, the foot over the end of the table, and the distal extremity supported with a towel, the rehabilitation clinician stabilizes the extremity with the cephalic hand over the medial distal extremity. The mobilizing hand is placed with the heel of the hand over the medial calcaneus and the fingers on the plantar aspect (figure 20.35). A lateral glide is applied, with the force directly downward and parallel to the joint surface.

Intertarsal Joints

These mobilizations can be performed on all midtarsal joints, including the talonavicular, calcaneocuboid, and naviculocuneiform.

Anterior Glide

This technique increases midfoot plantar flexion. With the patient prone, the rehabilitation clinician grasps the midfoot with one thumb, reinforced by the other thumb, over the bone to be mobilized. The forefoot is stabilized with the hands while the thumbs are used to provide a PA movement of the bone (figure 20.36).

Figure 20.36   Anterior glide intertarsal joint mobilization.

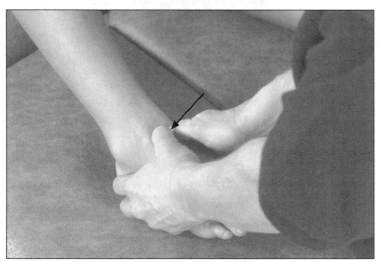

Posterior Glide

This technique is used to increase midfoot dorsiflexion. With the patient supine, the rehabilitation clinician stabilizes the rearfoot with one hand, and places the thumb of the other hand on the dorsum and the fingers on the plantar aspect of the bone to be mobilized. The mobilizing hand applies an AP movement in the plane of the joint surface (figure 20.37).

Figure 20.37   Intertarsal posterior glide joint mobilization.

Intermetatarsal Joints

Anterior and posterior glides can increase intermetatarsal mobility. The rehabilitation clinician stabilizes one metatarsal and grasps the adjacent one, with the thumb on the dorsum and the fingers on the plantar aspect. An AP-PA force is applied to the metatarsal (figure 20.38). A gross AP and PA glide can also be applied to the intertarsal joints: the proximal tarsal row is stabilized, and the distal row is mobilized in either an anterior or a posterior direction.

Figure 20.38   Intermetatarsal glide joint mobilization.

Figure 20.39 Metatarsophalangeal distraction joint mobilization.

Tarsometatarsal, Metatarsophalangeal, and Interphalangeal Joints

Many of the basic hand positions and force applications are the same for these joints, so they are grouped together. You must realize, however, that specific finger and hand positions vary according to the particular joint being mobilized.

Distraction

Distraction is a general technique that can enhance general joint mobility and relaxation. The phalanx is grasped with the thumb and fingers while the metatarsal is stabilized with the opposite hand (figure 20.39). A distraction force is applied to the phalanx.

Anterior and Posterior Glides

Anterior glides increase toe extension at the MTP and IP joints, and posterior glides increase toe flexion at the MTP and IP joints. For the MTP and tarsometatarsal joints, the metatarsal is stabilized with one hand while the mobilizing hand grasps the proximal phalanx and applies an AP-PA glide. Slight traction can be simultaneously applied to provide more comfort for the patient. For the IP joints, the proximal phalanx is stabilized while the mobilizing force is applied to the adjacent distal phalanx.

FLEXIBILITY EXERCISES

▶ There are many flexibility exercises for the ankle, foot, and lower leg. Among those often used are gastrocnemius, soleus, and Achilles stretches; ankle exercises the patient can do throughout the day; and BAPS board exercises.

The following sections present some of the more commonly used techniques for improving ankle, and foot flexibility. As with most exercises, the rehabilitation clinician must have knowledge of the body's mechanics, the muscle's function, and appropriate application of forces to design an effective flexibility exercise program.

Although there are some exceptions, the active flexibility exercises are held for 15 to 20 s and repeated four to five times. If the patient has less-than-normal flexibility, he or she should repeat the exercises frequently throughout the day.

Gastrocnemius Stretch

Because the gastrocnemius extends from above the knee to the calcaneus, both the knee and ankle joints must be placed on stretch to effectively stretch the muscle.

Standing Position

This stretch is performed with the patient in a straddle position with the extremity to be stretched behind the opposite extremity. The patient places his or her body weight on the arms, which are supported on the wall and on the front foot while the back extremity remains extended at the knee. The heel should remain in contact with the floor; the hip should be forward of the knee; and the foot should be in a straight line or the toes slightly turned inward (figure 20.40). Common substitutions are allowing the midfoot to collapse by rotating the foot outward, lifting the heel off the floor, bending the knee, or moving the hips posteriorly.

Sitting Position

If the patient is non-weight bearing, he or she can use this gastrocnemius stretch to increase flexibility until weight bearing is permissible.

With the patient in a long sitting position, a stretch strap or towel is hooked around the forefoot. Keeping the knee straight, the patient pulls on the strap to dorsiflex the ankle. Additional stretch can be applied with active contraction of the ankle dorsiflexors. Common substitutions in this exercise are hip rotation and foot pronation.

Soleus Stretch

Because the soleus does not cross the knee joint, to isolate this muscle the stretch should be applied with the knee flexed. This eliminates the stretch on the gastrocnemius and isolates the stretch to the soleus. As with the gastrocnemius stretch, this stretch can be performed in weight bearing or non-weight bearing.

Standing Position

In the standing position, the patient is in a position similar to that described for the gastrocnemius. With the involved extremity behind the uninvolved extremity, he or she keeps the foot flat on the floor with the foot turned slightly inward, and then slowly flexes the knee until a stretch is felt in the calf (figure 20.41). Common substitutions are outward rotation of the foot, knee valgus positioning, and posterior movement of the hip as the knee is flexed.

Figure 20.40   Gastrocnemious stretch in standing.   **Figure 20.41**   Soleus stretch in standing.

Sitting Position

A soleus stretch, if partial weight bearing is allowed, can be performed with the patient in sitting and the feet on the floor. The forefoot is on a 1/2 foam roller, and the heel is off (figure 20.42a). The patient attempts to push the heel to the floor, feeling the stretch in the distal calf.

Using a stretch strap in sitting, the patient positions the involved extremity with slight knee flexion. The strap is placed around the forefoot, and the patient pulls the strap to dorsiflex the foot while maintaining the knee in flexion (figure 20.42b). As with the gastrocnemius stretch in this position, additional stretch can be applied with the simultaneous activation of the ankle dorsiflexors. Common substitutions include increasing knee flexion rather than ankle dorsiflexion and placing the strap too proximal on the foot to apply an effective stretch force.

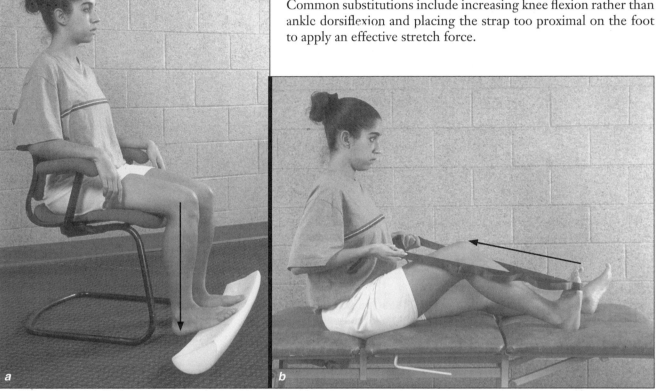

Figure 20.42 Soleus stretch in sitting: *(a)* with 1/2 foam roller, *(b)* with stretch strap.

Achilles Stretch

If the Achilles is the restricted structure, a prolonged stretch is most effective for increasing motion. Because of the connective tissue structure of the thick Achilles tendon, short-term stretches do not change its length. To perform a prolonged stretch, the patient stands with the back to a wall. The feet are positioned either on an incline (figure 20.43a) or on the edge of a book (figure 20.43b), with the heel no more than 2.5 cm (1 in.) from the wall. A towel roll is placed between the posterior knees and the wall to prevent knee hyperextension. The patient stands in this position for a prolonged period, at least 5 min and as much as 20 min if tolerable. It is useful to place a chair next to the patient so that he or she can place the hands on the back of the chair for stabilization and support. Once the stretch is released, the patient commonly feels stiffness in the posterior calf or ankle area, but this should subside quickly. Common substitutions are standing with the feet in pronation, standing too far away from the wall, and hyperextension of the knees.

Figure 20.43   Achilles prolonged stretch: *(a)* using an incline, *(b)* using a book. A towel roll should be placed behind the knees to prevent knee hyperextension.

Some people attempt to stretch the Achilles or gastrocnemius on the edge of a step. This is ineffective because the very muscle that is being stretched is simultaneously contracting to maintain balance.

Dorsiflexor Stretch

Ankles lacking full plantar flexion can be stretched with the patient sitting on the heels. With very tight ankles, full weight bearing onto the ankles in this position may be too uncomfortable. The recommendation is that the patient lean forward on the hands and pushes the hips back toward the heels as tolerated. Eventually, if there are no knee injuries, he or she should be able to sit fully on the ankles. In this position, the anterior ankles should be flat on the floor or mat (figure 20.44). A less aggressive stretch can be performed in standing, using a foam roller. The patient places the dorsum of the foot on the foam roller on the floor and pushes the ankle downward toward the floor.

Ankle Pumps, Alphabet, and Toe Exercises

General active exercises that the patient can perform independently throughout the day to increase ankle motion include ankle pumps and the alphabet. Leaving the heel on the floor for ankle pumps, the patient taps the foot up and down, going as high as possible each time he or she raises the foot. In another active-motion exercise, the patient spells the alphabet with the toes and foot while keeping the heel on the floor. These

Figure 20.44   Ankle dorsiflexor stretch, sitting. If the patient has a history of knee problems, this position should be avoided.

exercises can also be performed with the ankle elevated and can be useful in reducing edema. Patients can perform active toe motions, including curling, extending, abduction, and adduction, throughout the day.

BAPS Board

The BAPS board, or Biomechanical Ankle Proprioception System, is used to increase ankle flexibility and can also be used for strengthening. It consists of a board, or platform, and a variety of sizes of half-balls to which the platform is attached. The size of half-ball selected for an exercise depends on the patient's range of motion and the goal of the exercise. Patients may begin by sitting in a chair and placing the involved foot on the board to perform active range-of-motion exercises. They can advance to weight bearing on two extremities and then weight bearing on only the involved extremity to do full range-of-motion exercises for the ankle (figure 20.45). Once the patient has attained full range of motion and control on the BAPS board, you can add weights to the board to provide resistance to specific muscle groups. You can also use the board as a proprioception exercise device by having the patient single-extremity stand on the involved limb and slowly perform controlled isolated motions of inversion-eversion or plantar flexion-dorsiflexion.

Figure 20.45 BAPS board: *(a)* double-leg support, *(b)* single-leg support.

Additional Active-Motion Exercises

Cardiovascular exercises that can be used to improve ankle range of motion while simultaneously contributing to cardiovascular fitness include exercises on the stationary bike and the cross-country ski machine (figure 20.46). Both machines facilitate range of motion of the ankle, especially when the patient has received careful instruction in proper exercise execution. You should teach the patient ankling on the bike: dorsiflexing the ankle on extremity lift and plantar flexing the ankle on the downstroke. On the cross-country ski machine, the patient should attempt to push off from the posterior extremity by lifting the heel, and bearing weight on the ball of the foot before pulling the extremity and ankle forward and upward.

Figure 20.46   Other ankle range-of-motion exercises: *(a)* on stationary bike, *(b)* on cross-country skier.

STRENGTHENING EXERCISES

▶ Strengthening activities for the foot and ankle include isometrics, rubber tubing activities, exercises specifically for the toes, body-weight resistance for the ankle and foot, and resistance with equipment.

Strengthening exercises that can be used earliest in a rehabilitation program include isometrics. The patient can perform these even while the foot is in a cast or immobilizer. Normal progression is to isotonics and isokinetics. Isotonic exercises include those using rubber tubing, free weights, machine weights, and body resistance. Isokinetic exercises usually do not start until the patient's foot and ankle have sufficient strength to control isotonic activities.

Isometrics

Isometrics are held at the maximum contraction for 6 s, with a slow buildup and release of the force so that the total contraction is about 10 s long. No movement is produced.

Inversion

Sitting with the inside of the foot against a table extremity, the patient pushes the foot into the table extremity, attempting to invert the foot. The foot should not move, and the patient should feel the muscles working on the inside of the extremity. Common substitutions for this exercise are hip abduction, hip rotation, and tibial rotation.

Eversion

Sitting with the outside of the foot against a wall or table extremity, the patient pushes the foot into the wall or table extremity, attempting to evert the foot. The patient should feel the lateral extremity muscles working. Common substitutions include hip adduction, hip rotation, and tibial rotation.

Figure 20.47   Isometric exercise for dorsiflexion.

Dorsiflexion

Sitting with the uninvolved heel on top of the involved foot, the patient pushes the involved foot upward against the top foot, attempting to dorsiflex the ankle (figure 20.47). The patient should feel the anterior extremity muscles working. Common substitutions include hip flexion and foot eversion.

Rubber-Tubing Exercises

Because the various ankle muscle groups have different strengths, you must examine the patient's strength for each exercise before determining which rubber-tubing resistance is most appropriate for obtaining the desired results from the resistive exercise. Normally, ankle plantar flexors are the strongest, and ankle evertors are the weakest. Injured ankles have reduced levels of strength in all motions, but most of the time, the proportional strength remains close to normal. In other words, even though a patient's ankle has less-than-normal strength, the plantar flexors are still the strongest muscle group and the ankle evertors the weakest. These exercises can also be performed with either manual resistance or pulleys.

Eversion

This exercise strengthens ankle evertors. The patient sits in a chair, with the tubing around the forefoot and anchored to a table extremity near the uninvolved extremity. The ankle begins in inversion and is moved against the tubing into a full range of eversion (figure 20.48a). The most common substitutions for this exercise are hip abduction and rotation. To eliminate substitutions, you should instruct the patient in the proper technique and caution against moving the knee. Placing the hands on either side of the knee to stabilize the thigh also reduces substitutions. The patient can also perform this exercise in a long sitting position, but it is more difficult to stabilize the thigh and avoid hip substitutions in this position (figure 20.48b).

Inversion

This exercise is used to strengthen ankle inverters. The patient sits in a chair with the tubing around the forefoot and anchored to a table extremity near the involved side. He or she starts with the ankle in full eversion and moves it into a full range of motion to end-range inversion (figure 20.48c). Hip adduction and rotation are the most common substitutions in this exercise.

Dorsiflexion

This exercise strengthens the ankle dorsiflexors. The patient sits with the tubing around the forefoot and anchored to a table extremity, which the patient faces (figure 20.48d). The patient pulls the foot toward the shin, dorsiflexing the ankle. The most common substitution is knee flexion.

Plantar Flexion

This exercise can be used to strengthen plantar flexors if the patient is non-weight bearing. The patient is in a long sitting position with the tubing around the plantar foot and grasped in both hands (figure 20.48e). Maintaining a firm tension on the tubing and starting with the foot in full dorsiflexion, the patient pushes the foot against the tubing to move the ankle into full plantar flexion.

Figure 20.48   Tubing exercises: *(a)* eversion, *(b)* eversion in long sitting, *(c)* inversion, *(d)* dorsiflexion, *(e)* plantar flexion.

This exercise can also be performed with the knee in flexion and the patient sitting on a table with his or her extremity hanging off the table. In this position, plantar-flexion motion isolates and strengthens the soleus muscle.

If the patient has good strength in the early ranges of plantar flexion but is unable to stand in full plantar flexion, the tubing can be used to facilitate strength in the weak part of the motion. To do this, the patient places the foot in the weak range of motion and positions the tubing around the plantar foot. While the patient maintains the ankle position, he or she increases tension on the tubing by pulling on it with the arms to provide the resistance in the weak position. Maintaining good tension on the tubing, the patient slowly dorsiflexes the ankle to facilitate an eccentric contraction of the plantar flexors. This technique can be used to isolate weak positions in the other motions as well.

Figure 20.49   Toe exercises: *(a)* towel roll, *(b)* marble pickup.

Toe Exercises

Strengthening toe muscles helps to restore optimal foot function. Both intrinsic and extrinsic toe muscles are strengthened with these exercises. The long toe muscles can also add support to the ankle.

Towel Roll

This exercise strengthens primarily intrinsic muscles but also strengthens long toe flexors. The patient sits on a chair with a towel placed on the floor in front of the chair. Without shoes or socks, the patient uses the toes to curl the towel toward him- or herself (figure 20.49a). Resistance can be provided by placing a weight at the end of the towel, using a wet towel, or using newspaper. A common substitution is knee flexion motion. The thigh and extremity should not move during the exercise.

Marble Pickup

This exercise strengthens extrinsic and intrinsic toe flexors and can also help to facilitate ankle inverters or evertors. The patient uses the toes to pick up marbles that have been placed on the floor. The marbles are placed in the hand on the same side to facilitate eversion and in the hand on the opposite side to facilitate inversion (figure 20.49b). Objects such as a pencil, pieces of paper, or a towel can be used in place of the marbles.

Body-Weight Resistance Exercises

Exercises for both the gastrocnemius and soleus are necessary for complete restoration of strength. Exercises already mentioned for the long toe extensors also help to strengthen the posterior muscles. Body weight is an excellent form of resistance that strengthens many body segments, including the ankle and foot.

Heel Raises

This exercise strengthens the calf muscles. With feet about shoulder-width apart, the patient rises up on the toes as high as possible and then returns to feet flat on the floor. This exercise is more difficult when performed on an incline (figure 20.50) or on the edge of a stair, and also when it is performed on only the involved extremity. Common substitutions include using the hamstrings by flexing the knees during the heel raise, moving the body forward or rocking rather than moving straight upward, and placing most of the body weight on the uninvolved extremity rather than equally distributing the weight over both extremities.

Weigh-Scale Exercise

If the patient has difficulty bearing weight on the involved extremity, or is apprehensive about transferring weight onto that side, a weigh scale is an effective tool for teaching weight transfer and for helping the individual gain confidence in the involved extremity as well as improving strength.

This exercise uses a balance weight scale and a platform of height equal to that of the scale's foot plate. The platform is placed next to the scale. The patient stands with the uninvolved extremity on the platform and the involved extremity on the scale, and initially stands with most weight on the uninvolved extremity (figure 20.51). The scale balance is moved to a desired weight for the exercise. The patient is instructed to transfer enough weight to the involved side to move the balance arm to the top of the scale and then maintain the balance arm in the up position while performing a heel raise. As the patient's strength improves, the weight on the scale is increased until the patient is able to perform a single-extremity heel raise with full body weight.

This exercise is also good for weight-transfer instruction for gait training. The technique is similar, but the instruction is to move weight from the left to the right lower extremity. The scale weight is increased as the patient improves in ability to transfer weight properly.

Toe Raise

This exercise increases strength of the ankle dorsiflexors. The patient stands on an incline with the heel on the higher aspect of the incline. Keeping the heels in contact with the incline, he or she lifts the toes and forefoot upward and off the incline (figure 20.52). If this exercise is too difficult, the patient can start by performing the exercise on the floor. Use of the incline requires the muscle to work through a greater range of motion and increases the difficulty of the exercise. Common substitutions include hip flexion, forward trunk flexion, and body sway. For optimal results, correct improper execution.

Figure 20.50 Heel raise on an incline.

Figure 20.51 Weigh-scale exercises can be used to teach weight transfer and to increase strength of the involved extremity.

Figure 20.52 Toe raise on an incline.

Equipment Resistance

In addition to body weight, several kinds of equipment can be used to strengthen the ankle and foot. Presented here are a few of the possibilities.

Free Weights

Cuff weights can be used in strengthening exercises for ankle inversion, eversion, and dorsiflexion. The patient, placed in an antigravity position for the muscle being exercised with the cuff weight wrapped around the midfoot, moves the ankle through a full range of motion. For dorsiflexion, the position is sitting (figure 20.53a). For inversion and eversion, the position is sidelying on the involved side and on the uninvolved side, respectively (figure 20.53b).

Figure 20.53 Cuff-weight exercises: *(a)* dorsiflexion, *(b)* inversion. The weight should be lifted through a full range of motion.

Machine Weights

Calf raises in the standing and seated positions using machines strengthen the calf muscles. Standing calf raises can be performed on machines designed specifically for that exercise, or on machines such as an upright press or bench press that can be modified for use as a calf-raise machine. A seated heel-raise exercise to isolate the soleus muscle can be performed on a hamstring-curl machine.

The exercise difficulty can be increased by placing an incline under the foot in the seated heel raise or having the patient on a step in the standing heel raise. These modifications require the muscle to move through a greater range of motion, increasing the exercise difficulty.

PROPRIOCEPTION EXERCISES

▶ Proprioception is an important part of any ankle rehabilitation program. Proprioceptive exercises for posture and balance help improve ankle stability.

Proprioception is fundamental for kinesthesia and balance control. Research shows that deficits in these areas exist following ankle sprains, especially chronic ankle sprains (Forkin et al. 1996; Lofvenberg et al. 1995). Posture and balance, important factors in controlling ankle stability, can be improved with rehabilitation (Leanderson et al. 1996; Bernier and Perrin 1998). It is important, then, to include proprioception exercises in an ankle rehabilitation program. If a patient is non-weight bearing, early kinesthetic exercises can include mirroring activities with the two ankles, with the patient's eyes closed. The alphabet exercise mentioned earlier can also help improve kinesthetic awareness.

Once the patient is weight bearing, additional proprioception exercises can be incorporated into the program. One of the beginning weight-bearing exercises is a tandem stance with the involved foot directly behind the uninvolved foot so the front foot's heel touches the back foot's toes. This position should be held for 30 s with no loss of balance. Another beginning exercise is the stork stand. The patient stands on the involved extremity while attempting to maintain balance for 30 s (figure 20.54). Having accomplished this, the individual performs the exercise with eyes closed to eliminate the visual component of balance. The next level is to have the patient stork stand on an unstable surface, such as a trampoline, a foam roller, or a 1/2 roller (figure 20.55).

Figure 20.54 Stork stand.

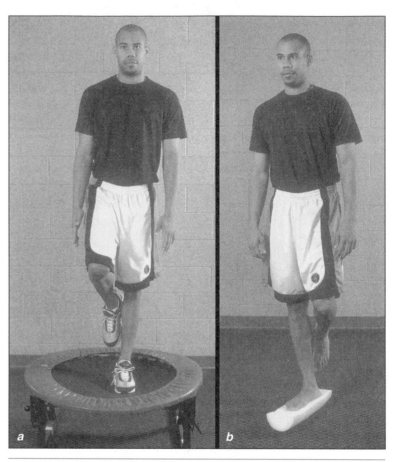

Figure 20.55 Advanced stork-stand exercises: *(a)* on trampoline, *(b)* on foam roller.

To progress to more advanced balance activities, the patient either attempts to maintain balance while performing another activity with another body part, so that concentration on balance is diverted, or performs additional activity with the lower extremity while maintaining balance. For example, a football receiver or softball or baseball player can catch a medicine ball while balancing on a foam roller or trampoline. The ball is thrown at different levels and to different sides of the body so that the patient must move to reach for it and still maintain balance. If the patient is a basketball player, bouncing a ball while maintaining balance on an unstable surface is a good activity (figure 20.56a). Setting a volleyball while stork standing on an uneven surface diverts the volleyball player's conscious effort from balance to enhance autonomic responses for balance.

Various kinds of balance boards can be either made or purchased. Wobble boards, circle boards, BAPS boards, and balance boards can all be used for balance work. A board placed on top of a PVC pipe is a simple balance board. In an exercise with this type of board the patient attempts to keep the ends of the board off the floor (figure 20.56b). This exercise becomes more difficult if the patient rolls the board side to side, still keeping the ends of the board off the floor, or if smaller pipes are used so that the ends of the board are closer to the floor.

Figure 20.56 Advanced balance exercises: *(a)* sports activity on unstable surface, *(b)* balance board.

Once the patient demonstrates good balance, he or she can advance to more complex exercises that require a combination of balance, agility, control, coordination, and strength. These exercises include activities with equipment such as the Fitter, tubing, slide board, and boxes. The Fitter and slide board are used to develop eccentric and concentric strength and proprioception of the intrinsic and extrinsic muscles (figure 20.57a). They can also assist in cardiovascular development. With tubing attached to the waist, the patient begins with left-to-right lateral or forward-backward jumps and progresses to single-extremity lateral and forward-backward jumps (figure 20.57b). Tubing exercises facilitate concentric strength, eccentric strength, power, control, coordination, and agility.

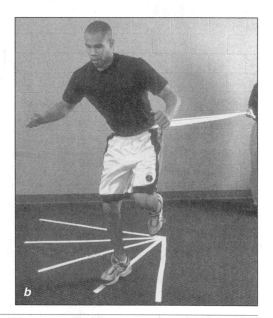

Figure 20.57 Agility exercises: *(a)* slide board, *(b)* tubing exercise—lateral, left-to-right activity.

Box activities are used as plyometric exercises to promote power and agility. Patients can perform various exercises created and designed by the rehabilitation clinician. Generic examples of these activities include rapid lateral jumping (figure 20.58a), rapid front-to-side agility step-ups (figure 20.58b), and multidirectional-change jumps (figure 20.58, c–d).

Plyometric jumps can advance to lateral high jumps (figure 20.58e) and box drop-jumps. For additional suggestions on plyometric exercises for the lower extremities, refer to chapter 9.

Figure 20.58   Plyometric box activities: *(a)* jump-over side-to-side, *(b)* alternate jumps side-to-front-to-side, *(c-d)* rapid sequencing from one box to another, *(e)* lateral high jumps.

Treadmill Activities

The treadmill can be used for more than gait analysis, walking, and running. It can be used to identify subtle differences between the involved and the uninvolved extremity during running. Besides using the treadmill to visually observe walking and running mechanics, you can use it as an auditory tool for defining running abnormalities. Listening to the foot hit the treadmill becomes a comparative tool; if the patient's feet do not sound the same at impact, it is likely that the individual has a different pattern between the involved and uninvolved extremity. Increasing the speed of the treadmill will also reveal differences in stride, gait, and weight transfer that you may not see at slower speeds.

The treadmill can also be used for facilitation, range-of-motion, strength, agility, and coordination exercises. Walking backward on a treadmill—retro walking (figure 20.59a)—has been shown to increase range of motion and muscle activity demands on the knee and ankle (Cipriani, Armstrong, and Gaul 1995). In retro walking, ankle dorsiflexion needs are increased, greater eccentric activity is required of the gastrocnemius, and the anterior tibialis also is more active. Many believe that these increased demands aid in facilitating the kinesthetic system and that they improve lower-extremity proprioception. Varying the speed of the treadmill alters demands on the muscles.

Agility and coordination exercises on the treadmill include activities such as side shuffles and cariocas going to both the left and the right (figure 20.59b). The patient may start with sets of 30 s bouts in each direction and then increase the time on each bout or increase the number of repetitions as improvement occurs. Requiring make more rapid changes from left side to right side increases the agility demands of the exercise. Placing the treadmill on an incline or increasing the speed also increases the difficulty.

Figure 20.59 Treadmill activites: *(a)* retro walking on an incline, *(b)* carioca on an incline.

Hopping Activities

Hopping exercises are often a necessary part of an ankle rehabilitation program because many athletic events include some type of hopping or jumping. These exercises can begin on a soft, force-absorbing surface such as a trampoline or mat and then advance to the patient's normal playing-field surface. Many different combinations of hopping activities are possible. Which specific patterns to select may depend on the patient's sport requirements, the injured ankle's deficiencies, and general conditioning demands. Some patterns are box hops, side-to-side hops, forward-backward hops, cross-pattern hops, high hops, long hops, zigzag hops, and circular hops. Some of these are presented as suggestions in figure 20.60. Patients may begin with two-legged hops and advance to one-legged hops. They may also alternate extremities or perform hops in combinations, such as two on the left and then two on the right, or two on the injured side and then one on the uninjured side.

Forward-backward hop: Hop forward and backward between two quadrants.

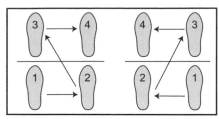

Cross-pattern hop: Hop in an X pattern.

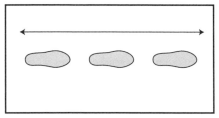

Straight-line hop: Hop forward and then backward along a 15- to 20-ft line.

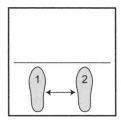

Side-to-side hop: Hop laterally between two quadrants.

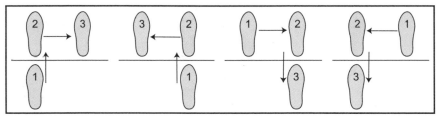

Triangular hop: Hop within three different quadrants. There are four triangles, each requiring a different diagonal hop.

Circular hop: Hop from square to square in a circular pattern. Sets are performed clockwise and counterclockwise.

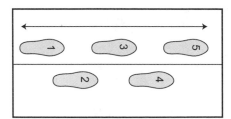

Zigzag hop: Hop from side to side across a 15- to 20-ft line while moving forward and then backward.

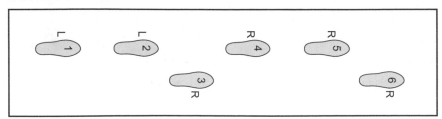

Mixed patterns: Various combination hop patterns can be used, such as two on the injured (i.e., left) side and one on the uninjured (i.e., right) side.

Figure 20.60 Suggestions for hopping patterns. You can design a number of hopping patterns, limited only by your imagination.

FUNCTIONAL EXERCISES

▶ By the end of the rehabilitation program, a patient with a foot or ankle injury must be able to perform functional activities—for example, zigzag runs and 90° cuts to the left and right—without hesitation, smoothly, and efficiently.

As the patient nears reentry into full participation, functional exercises must become a part of the complete rehabilitation program so that the patient's return is smooth and uneventful. As mentioned throughout this book, functional activities should mimic the patient's activity requirements. These functional activities are also a reliable means of final examination of the patient's ability to perform accurately and safely (Bolgla and Keskula 1997).

Functional activities for individuals will vary somewhat, but many running activities include many of the same functional activities. These include activities such as single, double, or triple hops; zigzag runs with rapid changes in direction; backward running; sprinting; running circles in clockwise, counterclockwise, backward, and forward directions; 90° cuts to the left and to the right; and running figure 8s. The patient should be able to perform the exercises without hesitation, smoothly in both directions and without favoring the involved extremity, and rapidly and efficiently.

Functional exercises should also encompass activity-specific drills and skill activities that are unique to the demands of each patient. You must have an appreciation and understanding of activities so that you can incorporate correct drills and exercises into the final phase of the patient's rehabilitation program.

SPECIAL REHABILITATION APPLICATIONS

▶ The rehabilitation clinician sees a number of common foot and ankle injuries that call for specific approaches within the therapeutic exercise program. Some of these injuries are sprains and dislocations, Achilles tendon injuries, shinsplints, compartment syndromes, a variety of foot injuries, and fractures.

This section deals with specific injuries to the foot and ankle. Injuries to the extremity, especially the ankle, are among the most common orthopedic injuries. Some—certainly not all—of the more frequently seen injuries are discussed in the following sections.

Ankle Sprain or Dislocation

An ankle dislocation is on the same continuum as an ankle sprain, so we will consider these two injuries together. As with other sprains, the severity determines the rate of rehabilitation progression and the time when various therapeutic exercises can begin. The more extensive the injury and the consequent tissue damage, the less aggressive the program can be, especially in the initial stages. It is important for the rehabilitation clinician to understand concepts and time lines and to assess the severity of the injury before proceeding with a rehabilitation program.

Discoloration is the result of bleeding in the area. It is generally a sign of the severity of the sprain as well. If no discoloration occurs, the sprain is likely to be mild or first degree, and the patient's other symptoms should be consistent with this assessment. If discoloration occurs, at least a second-degree sprain is present. Instability indicates a possible third-degree sprain of at least one ligament. Rehabilitation for second- and third-degree sprains proceeds more slowly than for first-degree sprains. A first-degree ankle sprain may restrict the patient from normal activities for no more than one week, with return to full participation in two to three weeks or less; but a second-degree sprain may restrict the patient from participation for three weeks and full participation for four to six weeks. Third-degree ankle sprains vary widely in recovery times, which may depend, at least, on the course of treatment provided (Konradsen, Holmer, and Sondergaard 1991). Third-degree sprains can take as little as six weeks or as much as three or more months to improve before the patient can return to full participation.

Third-degree sprains and dislocations can be treated either conservatively with rehabilitation or with surgery and rehabilitation. The choice is often made according to the patient's objective and subjective findings, age, level of sport participation, and surgeon's preference. Ankle instabilities may be surgically repaired. Studies show that early rehabilitation with controlled weight bearing in a boot, with early active-motion and therapeutic exercise, yields better results than the more conservative approach of prolonged casting with a slower initiation of rehabilitation (Konradsen, Holmer, and Sondergaard 1991; Glascoe et al. 1999).

The patient's ability to recover from an ankle sprain is dependent on the history of prior injuries. Multiple episodes of ankle sprains may result in an unstable ankle, making the rehabilitation process more complex and more difficult. The clinician must obtain an accurate history from the patient before instituting a therapeutic exercise program, because a prior history of ankle sprains can alter the program progression and anticipated results.

Chronic ankle sprains also affect other factors. One of these is additional scar tissue with probable adhesions that limits joint mobility and soft-tissue mobility. Repeated ankle sprains can result in chronic muscle weakness and reduced kinesthetic awareness, making the ankle susceptible to additional injury (Garn and Newton 1988). Chronic ankle sprains may also lead to compensatory changes with alterations in gait, strength, and flexibility, reducing the mechanical effectiveness of the ankle and foot. Because of these additional factors, chronic ankle sprains require more time to properly rehabilitate and achieve an appropriate recovery status (Seto and Brewster 1994).

Most ankle sprains are inversion sprains. The specific ankle ligaments and structures involved and the severity of the injury depend on the mechanical forces applied and the angle of stress application. Ankle sprains may also involve other structures; for example, there may be an avulsion fracture of the malleoli, peroneal strains or dislocations, or other tendon injuries. Of the ankle ligaments, the anterior talofibular is the most commonly injured ligament, and the calcaneofibular is the next most commonly injured ligament.

Occasionally, the tibiofibular ligament is injured. This ligament injury deserves careful consideration. The function of the tibiofibular ligament is to hold the tibia and fibula in alignment and formation of the ankle mortise joint. When weight is borne on the extremity, the force tends to spread the two bones apart. If the tibiofibular ligament is injured, repetitive stress with weight bearing can inhibit the healing process. If this ligament is injured, the patient should be instructed in non-weight bearing or partial weight bearing on crutches to ambulate pain free until full weight bearing does not cause pain. If this is not done, the ligament can develop chronic inflammation and can become difficult to treat successfully.

More typical ankle sprains permit weight bearing to tolerance. The rule of thumb is that if the patient is able to ambulate without limping, crutches are not required; however, if pain or dysfunction causes an abnormal gait, crutches with either partial or non-weight bearing are used. In most cases, weight bearing can be partial, to tolerance.

Control of edema and pain is the first priority, as with any injury. Common methods of reducing edema and pain include the use of ice and modalities along with strapping or bracing. Active range-of-motion exercises can be instituted early, usually within the first three days, to restore ankle range of motion. Joint mobilization and soft-tissue mobilization techniques are used as indicated and on the basis of the assessment before treatment. With chronic sprains, it is common to observe scar-tissue adhesions in the joints and surrounding tissue. Sometimes intertarsal and metatarsal joints become restricted, especially if the patient has been using an immobilizer boot or a cast.

Non-weight-bearing exercises can be used early in the therapeutic exercise program for strengthening. These include isometric exercises, aquatic exercises, and manual resistance. The BAPS board in a seated position can be used during partial weight-bearing periods.

Ankle inversion-eversion strength is important to ankle stability. Exercises for muscles controlling these movements must certainly be included among therapeutic exercises for a sprained ankle. Isometrics, manual resistance, pulleys, tubing, and aquatic exercises can all provide good strengthening activities for these groups. Closed kinetic chain exercises for inversion and eversion movements make strengthening of these motions more functional and enhance proprioceptive gains.

Once full weight bearing is pain free, gait training and closed kinetic chain exercises can be used to produce additional strength and coordination. Balance activities can progress from stork standing on the floor to stork standing on a 1/2 foam roller, trampoline, or other unstable surface. Initial closed chain strengthening exercises begin with low resistance, repetitions, and sets, and increase to more resistance, repetitions, and sets as the patient progresses. Early closed chain activities are performed slowly and in a controlled manner, but as the patient gains strength and control of the ankle, quicker movements requiring greater control and strength are added. This places demands on strength as well as the balance, coordination, and agility systems. When the patient has pain-free full motion and approximately 90% strength, plyometrics can be incorporated into the program. The final phase includes functional activities before return to full sport participation.

Throughout the progression, you must watch for signs of increased inflammatory response indicating that too much stress is being applied to the ankle. These signs include postexercise swelling, and pain either during or after the treatment session. If these signs are present, you should reduce the severity of the program for one to three days before advancing the patient to the next level of exercise difficulty.

It is advisable to have the patient refrain from wearing a protective brace during therapeutic exercises, but he or she may choose to use a supportive ankle device before returning to full sport participation. During therapeutic exercises the patient performs activities under controlled circumstances and in a restricted environment so risk of injury is reduced; but on returning to participation, he or she performs in an unpredictable environment, which creates an increased risk of injuring scar tissue that has less-than-maximum tensile strength. Because it may take a year or more for the tensile strength of injured tissue to achieve maximal levels, it is advisable for the patient to have the additional protection of ankle supports. A number of studies have demonstrated increased ankle stability with these devices (Sitler et al. 1994; Gross et al. 1987; Rovere et al. 1988; Kimura et al. 1987).

Case Study

A 16-year-old volleyball hitter jumped up for a hit and landed on another player's foot, causing an inversion sprain to the right ankle three days ago. She felt a pop and had immediate swelling. She was unable to bear weight on the ankle at the time. X-rays were negative, but the patient was placed on crutches, with weight bearing to tolerance. Ice, elevation, and taping have been applied periodically for the past three days, but the patient comes to you today to start her rehabilitation program. She denies any previous ankle injury. So far she has performed only alphabet exercises because it was too painful for her to do anything else. She can bear about 11 kg (25 lb) of weight on the foot in standing before she complains of pain in the lateral ankle and above the ankle joint. Her pain is located over the anterior talofibular, anterior tibiofibular, and calcaneofibular joints, with most of the pain over the first two ligaments. She has moderate swelling of the ankle, foot, and toes, with ecchymosis over the midfoot to the toes. She is able to wiggle her toes through about 50% normal motion. Her ankle range of motion is at 45° of plantar flexion, 10° of inversion with pain, 10° of eversion, and -10° dorsiflexion and is painful. Her ankle strength is restricted by pain on dorsiflexion and inversion. Since she is unable to bear weight on the foot, you cannot assess antigravity strength of the calf. You are easily able to overcome plantar flexion with manual resistance. Eversion is 4/5. Joint mobility is normal. Soft-tissue mobility is limited by the edema present, but you are unable to palpate any abnormal soft-tissue restriction.

Questions for Analysis

1. What are your goals for today's treatment?

2. What treatment will you provide for the patient today?

3. What home instructions will you give her?

4. What precautions will you give her?

5. What will be your guidelines for deciding when she can begin resistive weight-bearing exercises?

6. List three agility exercises that you will include in the patient's program when she is able to do them.

7. What will your functional testing include before her return to full sport participation?

Peroneal Tendon Dislocation

Peroneal tendon dislocations can often be overlooked, probably because they frequently occur in conjunction with other injuries. For this reason, they are also frustrating to resolve unless discovered through the use of good evaluation techniques.

Peroneal tendon dislocation occurs most commonly through two mechanisms, ankle dorsiflexion with active peroneal contraction, and an inversion sprain (Baumhauer, Shereff, and Gould 1997). In an inversion ankle sprain, the peroneal tendons are most susceptible to dislocation with the ankle in 15° to 25° of plantar flexion. This position places the tendons in a tenuous position along the distal fibula. If an inversion ankle sprain occurs with the ankle in less than 15° plantar flexion, the peroneal retinaculum can be stretched, leading to instability of the peroneal tendons. Skiers are commonly subjected to these injuries. If the ankle is in more than 25° of plantar flexion, the peroneal tendons move into a deep-seated position posterior to the fibular head and are stable in that position with little chance of dislocation.

Peroneal dislocations are usually self-reduced once the ankle is in a nonstressed position. The patient typically complains of a painful, snapping sensation in the posterolateral ankle with walking or ankle circumduction. Swelling along the tendon is sometimes observable. Treatment includes controlling the inflammation with modalities. Stabilization of the tendons with taping and pad support can sometimes help to relieve the subluxation episodes. If conservative treatment fails to prevent recurrent dislocations, surgical repair may be necessary.

Postoperative care includes soft-tissue massage around the surgical site to reduce soft-tissue adhesions in the area once the sutures have been removed. Joint mobilization techniques should be used in areas that demonstrate restricted joint mobility. Active range of motion is permitted anywhere from 10 to 21 days postoperatively. Ankle plantar flexion and eversion are motions that cause the least disruption of the tendons and can take place passively relatively early in the program.

Once weight bearing is permitted, the exercises and progression mentioned earlier for other ankle and extremity injuries can begin. A weigh-scale weight-bearing progression can be useful in helping the patient gain confidence in the injured extremity. Balance activities once the patient is fully weight bearing can begin with a stork stand and progress to more difficult exercises as strength and control are achieved. Strengthening exercises can begin with isometrics and progress to isotonics using techniques such as manual resistance, pulleys or tubing, and progressive standing heel raises. Other lower-extremity muscle groups in the hip and knee should be strengthened as well, because those areas have likely diminished in strength following the injury and surgery.

When the patient has achieved full range of motion and adequate strength for control, balance exercises during dynamic activities can begin, and the patient can then progress to agility exercises. Agility exercises on boxes, jumping with tubing resistance, and lateral movements are the final agility activities before functional activities.

Achilles Tendon Injuries

The most common injuries to the Achilles tendon are a rupture and tendinitis. Either injury can be debilitating and can restrict the patient from a rapid return to sport participation. The rehabilitation clinician's proper management of each injury is important to a safe and prompt return.

Tendinitis

If not treated correctly, tendinitis can be a frustrating and prolonged condition. Causes must be addressed and the inflammation brought under control before therapeutic exercises can be started.

Achilles tendinitis is usually a gradual-onset injury that originates secondary to overuse. Overuse of the Achilles tendon occurs when the tendon undergoes excessive stresses without sufficient time between stress applications to adjust to those stress levels. Excessive stress can be the result of cumulative forces caused by inherently poor foot mechanics, increased

Case Study

A 20-year-old tennis player was downhill skiing during winter break with his family. While he was on the slopes, maneuvering to the right, he fell forward and dislocated his left peroneus longus tendon. The injury was surgically repaired. The ankle was placed in an immobilizer boot, and the patient was non-weight bearing for two weeks. He is now able to partial weight bear to about 75% on the left and is to start rehabilitation. He presents to you today still non-weight bearing on the left. He admits that he is fearful of bearing weight on the extremity. His hip and knee strength is grossly 4/5. Ankle dorsiflexion and inversion are 3/5, and ankle eversion is 2+/5. His ankle range of motion is 0° inversion, 5° eversion, 40° plantar flexion, and -5° dorsiflexion. Joint mobility is moderately restricted in the subtalar and intertarsal joints. The calcaneocuboid and cuboid-metatarsal joints are also restricted. Soft-tissue mobility around the surgical scar, along the lateral foot, and into the posterior ankle is moderately limited. There is mild to moderate swelling around the ankle.

Questions for Analysis

1. What are your patient's primary deficiencies?

2. What will your first treatment today include?

3. What will your goals for today's treatment be?

4. What instructions will you give the patient today before he goes home?

5. What do you expect to accomplish in the next two weeks of treatment?

6. List precautions that you must respect at this point in the rehabilitation program.

7. List three strengthening exercises that you will use when the ankle is ready, and explain their progression.

8. What agility exercises will you eventually include in the therapeutic exercise program?

conditioning sessions, improper surfaces and playing fields, inadequate or improper footwear, weakness, or inflexibility. As with other tendinitis conditions, it is necessary to correct the fundamental causative factor or factors in order for there to be complete recovery with reduced risk of reinjury.

A foot with excessive pronation increases Achilles tendon stress. The Achilles tendon's normal configuration has a medial spiral rotation from its origin in the gastrocnemius-soleus complex, where it begins as a flat, fan-shaped tendon, to its insertion on the calcaneus where it ends as a rounded cord (figure 20.61). This spiral rotation begins about 12 to 15 cm (4.7–5.9 in.) above its insertion (Stanish & Curwin 2000). This twist of the tendon is an area of stress concentration, especially 2 to 5 cm (0.8–2.0 in.) above its calcaneal insertion where the rotation is at its greatest. This is coupled with the fact that this region is also an area of reduced circulation within the tendon. This site is the most common location for tendinitis in the Achilles.

With the calcaneus in eversion, the Achilles tendon suffers an additional torque force. Tightness in the Achilles causes even more pronation to occur. If pronation is prolonged into the phase of heel-off and beyond when the foot should be inverting, a wringing of the tendon occurs, increasing stress to the Achilles at its most vulnerable site. In cases of repetitive stress and prolonged tendinitis, a nodule of scar tissue from microscopic tears can often be palpated on the tendon 2 to 5 cm (0.8–2.0 in.) above its calcaneal insertion. The nodule is usually larger and more tender on the medial aspect, where the tendon incurs more stress.

Figure 20.61 Achilles tendon.

As with other cases of tendinitis, the patient's history typically includes a gradual progression of pain. The pain begins as tenderness that occurs during running but that goes away if the individual continues running. Gradually, pain persists longer and longer into the run until it continues after running and even during simple daily activities such as walking. Stiffness can occur after periods of inactivity or sitting. Eventually, pain is present with rest.

Common signs are reduced ankle dorsiflexion; tenderness along the Achilles, especially 2 to 5 cm (0.8–2.0 in.) above the calcaneal insertion where a nodule can be palpated; possible swelling; possible weakness; possible crepitus to palpation; and pain with unilateral hopping.

Treatment includes initially correcting the cause and reducing the inflammation. If the cause is excessive pronation, orthotics may be necessary. A low-dye strapping technique to stabilize the calcaneus and reduce pronation can be used either alone or in combination with heel cups or medial heel wedges to assess the effectiveness of orthotics. Use of commercially available arch supports can also determine whether custom orthotics may be necessary. Inflexibility, weakness, scar-tissue adhesions and joint immobility from previous injuries, and alterations in footwear should all be assessed and corrected as necessary. A good history must include inquiries regarding recent changes in conditioning or workout sessions that may have overstressed the tendon. Changes in surfaces, for example when an individual goes from flat surfaces to hills or from soft to hard surfaces, may also be a contributing factor that must be corrected.

In extreme cases it may be necessary to have the patient temporarily cease the aggravating activity until the inflammation is under control. Anti-inflammatory techniques include the use of various modalities, such as ultrasound, phonophoresis, iontophoresis, electrical stimulation, ice, and others presented in Denegar and colleagues (2005). Cross-friction massage over the nodule and other areas of soft-tissue restriction can help to mobilize the adherent scar tissue to reduce pain and improve soft-tissue mobility.

Therapeutic exercises must include stretching and flexibility activities for restricted areas. Hamstring and hip muscle tightness can influence Achilles flexibility and should be evaluated and corrected as needed. Gastrocnemius and soleus tightness should also be addressed with the flexibility exercises presented earlier.

You should initiate strengthening exercises cautiously because it is important to avoid exacerbation of the pain. Weight-bearing strengthening exercises can begin when the patient reports pain at around 5/10. Before that, rubber band exercises for ankle inversion, eversion, and dorsiflexion strength are appropriate. The patient can perform rubber band exercises for ankle plantar flexion through a full, pain-free range of motion. Weight-bearing Achilles exercises can include heel raises on a extremity press machine, standing heel raises beginning on a flat surface and progressing to an incline, and heel raises with weights. Once weight-bearing exercises have begun, the patient can perform eccentric heel raises beginning with a slow heel-drop on the floor and progressing from a medium speed on the floor, to a fast speed on the floor, to a slow speed on an incline, to a medium speed on an incline, and finally to a rapid heel-drop on an incline with three sets of 15 to 25. Other exercises for the lower extremity include squats, lunges, and knee flexion strengthening exercises as tolerated. When the patient's pain level is 2-3/10, agility exercises are suitable. Plyometrics start once the patient is pain free. At no time throughout the therapeutic exercise program should any exercise increase Achilles pain. If any progression results in Achilles pain, the patient should return to previous levels of activity for another one or two treatment sessions until he or she is able to progress to the next level without pain.

Once the patient is able to perform plyometric exercises well and without pain, functional activities are the last step before full return to sport participation. Throughout the program, the patient must communicate to the rehabilitation clinician any changes in Achilles pain and the response to treatment. You must respect the patient's pain and realize that each person will respond differently to an exercise progression. The key to the success of the program is correcting the underlying causes of the Achilles tendinitis and getting the inflammation under control before the patient advances in the program.

Retrocalcaneal bursitis is often mistaken for Achilles tendinitis. Bursitis occurs over the posterior aspect of the calcaneus where the bursa is located. This is an unusual location for Achilles tendinitis to occur, so a patient presenting with complaints of pain in this area should be examined for bursitis as well as tendinitis. A pump bump is frequently present because a heel-whip occurs as the calcaneus moves toward supination after being positioned in pronation longer than it should be during late stance and heel-off. The bursa becomes irritated with friction against the shoe's heel counter, especially with a heel whip. Treatment includes symptomatic relief of the inflammation along with correction of the cause of the bursitis. In addition to excessive pronation, other causative factors of bursitis include tight Achilles, tight plantar fascia, and poor shoes.

Case Study

A 24-year-old, male recreational runner reports to you with complaints of pain in the right extremity just above the ankle. He reports that about two months ago while he was running, he stepped off a curb and rolled his right ankle but continued running. The ankle swelled slightly but did not require him to cut back on his running program. He did not think much about it because it did not seem to cause any problems. This patient usually runs about 8 km (5 miles) once a day but has recently increased running to twice a day in preparation for an upcoming marathon. Because the marathon course is hilly, he has recently made it a point to run at least one steep hill during his workouts. When the pain began he would continue running, and the pain would go away; but it soon lingered longer into the run until it now is present throughout the run and has forced him to reduce his mileage. He has pain after prolonged sitting, while climbing stairs, and while walking barefoot. He reports that he feels a creaking in the back of his ankle when he walks. He does a few stretches but usually does not have time after his run to do any stretch more than once, holding each stretch for 20 s.

Your examination reveals that dorsiflexion in subtalar neutral −5°. The calcaneus inversion-eversion motion is a total of 35°, and the midfoot is loose when you lock the rearfoot and passively invert and evert the midfoot. Strength for heel raise in weight bearing is slightly less than normal, with pain occurring after about eight repetitions. There is a tender nodule about 3 cm (1.2 in.) above the base of the heel on the Achilles tendon. The nodule is significant in size, protruding about 2 mm medially and 1 mm laterally on the Achilles tendon. You can feel crepitus in the tendon as you passively dorsiflex and plantar flex the ankle.

Questions for Analysis

1. How do you think the ankle rollover incident has affected the Achilles tendon injury?

2. How will you describe for the patient the probable causes for his Achilles tendon injury?

3. What will your advice be regarding his workout program?

4. Describe what your first treatment session with the patient will include.

5. What home exercises will you give him?

6. What factors will you consider in deciding when to begin strengthening exercises?

7. What will you tell the patient when he asks you how long this will take to resolve?

Achilles Rupture

Treatment programs for Achilles ruptures have become less conservative in recent years, primarily because of the poor results seen with delayed rehabilitation. This section presents a program of treatment and then a case study for you to solve.

An Achilles rupture most commonly occurs in individuals in the fourth and fifth decades of life. In younger athletes, a rupture occurs when the foot is anchored and the patient is thrust forward to produce a sudden stretch on the tendon. A typical history for the older patient includes an incident in which the patient was running or cutting and felt as though he or she had been shot in the extremity. A younger athlete may be in a football pileup with one player on top of his foot and then be pushed forward by another player who comes into the pileup. A pop can be felt or heard. The pain is usually intense, and the patient is unable to walk on the extremity. Passively squeezing a normal calf muscle causes a plantar-flexion movement of the ankle, but this does not occur with a torn Achilles tendon (Thompson test).

Surgical repair, either open or subcutaneous, most recently has been the treatment of choice. Conservative care with immobilization often lends itself to poor results, especially in the athletic population. Following repair, the leg is placed either in a series of progressively reduced plantar-flexion casts or, more commonly, in a hinged ankle walking boot with ankle immobilization. The boot is initially positioned in plantar flexion and gradually positioned to neutral. The patient may be non-weight bearing initially and progress to partial weight bearing before weight bearing as tolerated is allowed.

Initial treatments include cardiovascular conditioning and exercises for the uninvolved lower-extremity segments and other body segments. Isometric exercises in the immobilization boot can be encouraged, but the patient should be instructed to perform a slow buildup to maximum with a maximal hold and a gradual release of muscle tension. Once the surgeon permits treatment to the involved segment, this should initially involve efforts to reduce edema and scar-tissue adhesions. Soft-tissue massage and mobilization, along with joint mobilization, often begin early to assist in restoring flexibility and range of motion. Active and passive range-of-motion exercises and strengthening exercises for ankle inverters, evertors, dorsiflexors, and plantar flexors begin in non-weight bearing and progress as tolerated to partial and then full weight bearing. Use of a rubber band for ankle motions once the patient is out of the boot assists in promoting strength. When the patient is permitted partial weight bearing, he or she can begin to use the BAPS board in sitting. Other activities can include exercise on a stationary bike, the towel-roll exercise, and marble pickups for extrinsic and intrinsic muscles. Plantar foot massage with a ribbed can, golf ball, or rolling pin is also appropriate during this time.

If the patient is on crutches, it is best to encourage a correct heel-toe gait. If the patient acquires bad habits on crutches, they may extend into full weight bearing and become difficult to correct. Gait training is a necessary part of the therapeutic exercise program once the patient is fully weight bearing.

Patients are typically reluctant to bear weight on the involved extremity once they are permitted full weight bearing without the boot. Weight transfer from the uninvolved to the involved extremity through the use of the weigh scale, with progressive increases in the weight placed on the scale, is a good way to help the patient develop confidence in weight bearing on the involved extremity. The scale can also be used to control and increase resistance in heel-raise exercises. This can be an especially significant exercise if the surgeon is permitting limited weight bearing on the extremity. The scale exercise can also be used in full-weight-bearing exercise, and can be used for monitoring and recording increases in the patient's ability to bear weight on the involved extremity through a full range of motion.

When the patient is able to bear full weight on the involved extremity, stork-standing exercises can improve balance and proprioception. Additional strength activities should include exercises for the entire lower extremity because it is likely that with inactivity, an antalgic gait, and surgery, the entire lower extremity is weaker than normal. These exercises can involve activities such as resisted hip exercises and knee exercises, as well as weight-bearing exercises such as squats and lunges. These exercises are discussed in chapters 21 and 22. Other activities include step exercises, balance and agility exercises, and eventually plyometric exercises as described earlier in this chapter. Functional exercises are part of the final phase of the rehabilitation program and are specific to the patient's sport.

During the early phase of the program, manual-resistance exercises for the hip and knee are feasible even when the extremity is immobilized. Trunk exercises can also be included in the early phase. Manual resistance to the ankle can begin once the immobilization brace or cast is off. Weight-bearing exercises are gradually increased in the program as the patient tolerates them. Initially, the resistance and repetitions are low, and emphasis should be on correct technique and proper execution. The patient may tolerate increased repetitions better than increased resistance in the early days of therapeutic exercise.

Resistance exercise beyond body weight is frequently added to the program around 8 to 12 weeks postoperatively. Once the patient has 10° to 15° of dorsiflexion, usually toward the end of the second month or the beginning of the third, jogging activities can begin. Straight jogging on a flat surface is permitted until the patient is up to 3.2 km (2 miles). After that, agility drills are appropriate.

Progression of the strengthening exercises is determined by tissue healing times, the patient's flexibility and mobility, and his or her tolerance. Pain and swelling are the primary signs to avoid with any exercise. It is desirable to achieve muscle fatigue without causing pain or swelling with strengthening exercises. Exercise stress is gradually increased, and the response to any increase in exercise stress—either increased difficulty in an exercise or the addition of new exercises—must be carefully monitored. You must rely on your own observational skills, as well as on the patient's reports of the Achilles response to changes in therapeutic exercises, to gauge the effectiveness of the program. These factors dictate alterations.

Case Study

Two weeks ago, a 45-year-old male tennis player was running to return a drop shot when he suddenly felt as though he had been shot in the left calf. He had intense pain and was unable to stand or walk. He was taken to the emergency room, placed on crutches, given ice, and instructed to follow up with an orthopedic surgeon. He underwent surgical repair for a ruptured Achilles tendon 10 days ago. His surgeon wants him to begin his rehabilitation program today. He has a walking boot fixed at 10° plantar flexion and is permitted partial weight bearing to 50%. He is apprehensive about putting weight on the left extremity and continues to walk non-weight bearing on the left. He does not have much pain in the Achilles because he is not moving it much. Although the surgical scar is well healed, there is moderate swelling throughout the foot and distal extremity. His active ankle movement is 30° plantar flexion and –15° dorsiflexion. Inversion-eversion is stiff and 20°. Joint mobility of the tarsals and metatarsals is restricted overall at about 50% normal mobility. Strength of the hip and knee is 4–/5; ankle dorsiflexion, inversion, and eversion are 3/5; and plantar flexion is 2/5. Palpation reveals myofascial tenderness with soft-tissue restriction throughout the calf muscles and the presence of adhesions in the dorsum of the foot and around the ankle. The surgical site has moderate adhesions of the scar to underlying soft tissue.

Questions for Analysis

1. How will you outline for the patient the general course of treatment progression?

2. What are your short-term goals with this patient, and when would you expect to achieve them?

3. What will your treatment include today?

4. What instructions will you give him today for a home program?

5. How aggressive will you be with your treatments during the next two weeks?

6. When will you begin strengthening exercises, and what will they initially include?

7. List three agility exercises you will give the patient when he is able to perform them, before he progresses to functional exercises.

Other Tendinitis

Although several tendons in the foot, ankle, and extremity can develop tendinitis, the most common sites are the tibialis posterior and the peroneal tendons. These tendons become inflamed most often because of overuse secondary to excessive pronation combined with increased mileage on hard surfaces.

The tibialis posterior works eccentrically to decelerate subtalar pronation and medial rotation of the tibia at heel strike, and concentrically as a supinator and inverter of the subtalar joint and lateral rotator of the tibia during stance. The peroneus longus and brevis work as pronators of the subtalar joint and as plantar flexors and evertors of the first ray during the non-weight-bearing phase of gait. During midstance and heel-off, they evert the foot to transfer weight from the lateral to the medial foot. These lateral and medial muscles both act as stabilizers of the foot during weight bearing. The tibialis posterior stabilizes the midtarsal joint, and the peroneus longus stabilizes the first ray to accept the load as it is transferred from the lateral to the medial foot at heel-off. When the foot is pronated longer than it should be in weight bearing, excessive loads are placed on these tendons. If the excessive load from changes in workouts, poor shoes, or ungiving surfaces causes breakdown that the tendon insufficiently recovers from before the next workout, tendinitis can occur.

Tibialis posterior tendinitis results in pain in the posteromedial ankle region and/or into the tendon's insertion site on the navicular and surrounding tarsals. Peroneal tendinitis pain, located in the posterolateral ankle region, can run along the tendon on the lateral foot.

As with Achilles tendinitis, it is crucial for the clinician to identify the causes if a treatment program is to have lasting effects. Once you have identified the causes, you can take steps to alleviate them. If the injury is not severe, it may be possible for the patient to continue sport participation once the causes have been corrected. In severe cases it may be necessary for the patient to refrain from full participation until the inflammation is alleviated.

Initial treatment includes the use of anti-inflammatory modalities that have been discussed previously. The patient should be instructed in proper stretching exercises for tight areas. These may often include structures adjacent to the injured area. For example, a tight iliotibial band or piriformis may impact the tibialis posterior tendinitis, making it necessary to include stretches for these structures in the therapeutic exercise program.

Strengthening activities once the inflammation is under control include those exercises discussed previously. The patient should do concentric and eccentric exercises for all ankle muscles, especially those deficient in strength or endurance, as well as the injured structures. Antigravity positioning using weights, rubber tubing, or manual resistance for inverters and evertors provides additional resistance to those muscles. Marble pickups with placement of the marbles in the ipsilateral or contralateral hand, lateral towel roll, and inversion-eversion on a BAPS board or wobble board are important exercises for peroneal and tibialis posterior tendons. Balance activities provide stress to lateral ankle tendons. The Fitter and rolling balance board can also be used for lateral ankle-stressing exercises. Resistive exercises for ankle dorsiflexors and plantar flexors should also be included.

Agility exercises and functional exercises are the same as for other injuries; you should add these to the program once the inflammation is gone and the patient is pain free with activity.

Case Study

A 16-year-old, female cross country runner presents to you with a two-month history of medial ankle pain. She does not remember injuring the ankle. The pain was tolerable, even though it has increased in duration during her workouts, until this past week, when she began increasing the intensity of her workouts in preparation for the start of the cross country competitive season. The pain is now present throughout her workouts and does not go away when she stops running as it had in the past. She has pain if she stands too long and when she walks. She reports that she has been meaning to buy new running shoes because the ones she wears now are worn out, but she thought she would wait until she saw you to ask your advice on what to buy.

Your examination reveals ankle dorsiflexion in subtalar neutral to 0°, plantar flexion to 55°, and inversion-eversion to 30°. The midfoot is loose with the rearfoot locked. In non-weight bearing, the patient has a normal arch, but in weight bearing the navicular is close to the floor and the calcaneus is everted. In walking, the calcaneus never inverts to a vertical position. The patient's shoes are collapsed medially in the heel. Palpation reveals tenderness under the navicular and running along the tibialis posterior tendon posterior and superior to the ankle.

Questions for Analysis

1. What will your first treatment today include?

2. What will you give the patient today for a home program?

3. Do you think she will need orthotics, and if so, why?

4. What will your recommendations be on shoe selection?

5. What are your short-term goals, and what is your best estimate on when to anticipate reaching them?

6. What are your criteria for when to begin strengthening exercises?

7. List three agility exercises you will include when appropriate.

8. What functional activities will you include in the patient's program?

9. What will your criteria be for her return to normal running activities?

Shin splints

Shin splints are also known as medial tibial stress syndrome. This is a stress-reaction inflammation of the periosteal and musculotendinous fascial junctions. The pain is located in the middle and distal third of the extremity. The pain may vary in intensity, from pain that resolves after running to pain that interferes with daily activities.

This condition is usually seen in distance runners and is commonly caused by training errors coupled with improper or poor shoes and a tight Achilles (Kohn 1997). Treatment includes correction of the causes along with reduced activity until symptoms are under control. In addition, modalities should be used to relieve the inflammation. Stretching of the Achilles and other tight structures should be performed throughout the day. Soft-tissue release through deep-tissue massage can be useful in relieving adhesions that occur and that add to the patient's pain.

If shin splints occur on the lateral extremity, the cause is usually an overuse inflammatory reaction of the tibialis anterior and extensor digitorum communis, compounded by excessive pronation, hill running, poor shoes, or training errors. This condition is usually relieved with changes in shoes, training methods, and orthotics.

Case Study

An 18-year-old, male sprinter presents to you with complaints of lateral and anterior extremity pain that began about one week ago. He has started training for the track season and is distance running to create a cardiovascular base. He reports that he had this pain last year but it went away after a couple of weeks, so he didn't think too much about it; however, this year, his first year as an intercollegiate athlete, the pain seems more intense. He likes the team's shoes, which he started wearing when he began training this year; he had never used the brand before.

Your examination reveals tightness in the Achilles with ankle dorsiflexion to 0°. Hamstring range of motion is 65° in a straight-extremity raise. His new shoes have a stiff sole. He is tender to palpation of the tibialis anterior.

Questions for Analysis

1. What will your first treatment today include?

2. What will you give the patient for a home program?

3. What will be your recommendations regarding his shoes?

4. What will be your recommendations regarding his workouts?

5. What are your short-term goals for him?

6. List three exercises you will include in his program.

Athletes may experience lateral extremity pain at the outset of preseason conditioning if they have not maintained an appropriate activity level up to that time. In these cases, the pain should resolve with time as the patient becomes conditioned. Ice-and-stretch can provide symptomatic relief in the short term. If symptoms continue beyond normal expectations, the patient should be referred to the physician to rule out anterior compartment syndrome.

Compartment Syndromes

There are various degrees of compartment syndromes, ranging from slight discomfort to emergency situations. Increased pressure within the extremity compartments can be an irritating problem at the least and possibly a dangerous situation.

The four compartments of the extremity are divided by thick, inelastic fascial coverings. The fascia creates unyielding walls that enclose the muscles in each compartment. If volume changes occur in a compartment, there is no room for expansion, and pressure builds up within the compartment. If pressure persists, a compromise of tissue, vascular, and neural structures can result. Although any of the compartments can experience compartment syndrome, the most commonly affected one is the anterior compartment.

An increase in compartment volume is commonly the result of edema from intense activity or the result of an injury, such as a crush injury or fracture, which causes bleeding and soft-tissue swelling. Activity-induced compartment syndrome is usually chronic, whereas injury-induced compartment syndrome is acute. The acute condition results from an increase in arterial flow from the injury, with a reduction in venous return because of pressure on the vessels, and leads to ischemic pain and tissue death if it persists.

The patient complains of intense pain that is not relieved by any treatment or positioning and of pain with passive plantar flexion. Palpation of the area reveals a hardness and tension of the soft tissues. As the condition advances, the distal pulses are diminished, and neurological changes can be observed.

Because tissue life is being threatened, this is considered a medical emergency and must be referred to the physician immediately. A surgical fasciotomy is usually performed to release the pressure.

In chronic compartment syndrome, the symptoms are different in some ways and similar in others. The patient has recurrent, usually bilateral, extremity pain and tightness in the compartment during activity, but the symptoms subside with rest. Edema and tenderness can be palpated, and some patients also experience paresthesia. This occurs because arterial flow from increased muscle activity is greater than the capillary perfusion rate. The local blood flow is restricted—much like cars in a rush-hour traffic jam. Many fast-moving cars are suddenly forced to slow down because the number of vehicles is beyond the capacity of the road to handle them all at one time. Once the number of vehicles on the road decreases, the traffic moves smoothly again.

In some chronic cases, fasciotomy for compartment release can be avoided with conservative treatment. Conservative treatment includes extremity-stretching exercises and strengthening exercises for balanced strength among all muscle groups. The patient should work out on softer surfaces and wear running shoes that absorb shock. Orthotics that reduce shock may also be helpful.

Patients who undergo fasciotomy may be placed on crutches, non-weight bearing, for 7 to 10 days. Isometric and active range-of-motion exercises can begin within a week of surgery. Once the wound is healed, aquatic exercises are useful for gaining range of motion and strength. Myofascial release and massage for soft-tissue mobility, joint mobilization if indicated following immobilization, and gait training may all be necessary if the patient shows deficiencies on the initial examination. Once the patient is fully weight bearing, closed

Case Study

A 16-year-old, female cross country runner fractured her right tibia in a motor-vehicle accident 5 years ago. The extremity was in a cast for two months before the patient underwent a rehabilitation program. One month ago she was competing in a cross country race and began experiencing right shin and foot numbness and burning. After that she continued to experience the same symptoms during her workouts. She underwent an anterior and a posterior compartment release and removal of extensive scar tissue two weeks ago. The surgeon wants her to begin rehabilitation today.

She is partially weight bearing on crutches, but the surgeon has instructed her to ambulate without the crutches within the next couple of days. She admits that she lacks the confidence to get rid of the crutches. Your examination reveals well-healed surgical scars anteriorly and posteriorly on the extremity. You note the presence of mild edema and stiffness to passive range of motion, but the patient has no pain. Dorsiflexion is –5°; plantar flexion is 35°. Inversion-eversion is 30°. Palpation reveals mild soft-tissue restriction around the surgical scars and moderate tissue restriction in the calf and anterior extremity.

Questions for Analysis

1. What are your goals for the patient's first treatment with you today?

2. What modalities will you use, if any, and why?

3. What exercises will you initiate today?

4. What home program and instructions will you give the patient before she leaves today?

5. What are your goals for her for the next two weeks, and how will you attempt to accomplish them?

6. What specific activities will you have the patient perform the first day she is on a treadmill?

7. Outline a progressive running program that you will give the patient when she is ready to begin running.

kinetic chain exercises can begin with a progression of the resistive exercises discussed previously. Rubber tubing exercises can be used before full-weight-bearing activities. At four to six weeks, treadmill and stair-climber exercises can begin if the patient has shown strength and flexibility gains.

Return to running activities is commonly slower in posterior compartment releases than in anterior compartment releases. Return to running activities proceeds slowly on the basis of the patient's symptoms and the healing progression. Jogging is the initial speed, which progresses to slow running, then to fast running before return to normal speeds. Initial jogging distances may be no more than 0.8 km (0.5) miles with a gradual progression to 3.2 to 4.8 km (2–3 miles) before the patient has a medical release to return to former running distances. Running should be on soft, flat surfaces before the patient progresses to hill running.

Foot Injuries

A number of common and some unusual foot problems can also arise. Some of the more commonly seen conditions are presented here.

Plantar Fasciitis

Of all foot injuries, plantar fasciitis is among the most common. Its cause can be any number of factors, and you must recognize and correct the cause to correct the problem and reduce the risk of reinjury.

The thick aponeurosis that covers the plantar foot from the calcaneus to the MTP joints is the plantar fascia. It is a thick connective tissue structure that protects the structures in the plantar foot, provides flexibility for shock absorption, and creates a windlass mechanism that transforms the foot into a rigid lever for transferring propulsion forces during push-off. It can become irritated when subjected to abnormal stress, usually during running activities. Patients in any sport involving these activities can be susceptible to plantar fasciitis. High arches and excessive pronation can both be culprits that increase normal stress loads and lead to plantar fasciitis. These inherent structural stresses are usually combined with other factors such as increased workout levels, poor shoes, restricted dorsiflexion from tight Achilles or calf muscles, restricted great-toe dorsiflexion, and workouts on hard surfaces.

The most classic symptom of plantar fasciitis is heel pain with weight bearing when the person arises in the morning, as well as after prolonged sitting, that decreases with continued walking. In more severe cases, pain can occur at rest and extend into the midarch region. The pain is usually unilateral. X rays often reveal a heel spur; however, the source of pain is not the heel spur but the soft tissue that is inflamed because of the irritation and stress it is experiencing. Repetitive stresses applied to the plantar fascia at its origin on the calcaneus commonly result in the development of exostosis at the location where the fascia attaches.

Treatment must include correction of the underlying causes. This frequently involves flexibility exercises for tight structures, proper shoe selection, orthotics if needed to correct abnormal foot structure, changes in conditioning, and changes in workout surfaces. Treatment must also include modalities to relieve the inflammation. Occasionally, the physician may opt for a cortisone injection into the inflamed area. Alternative methods that may provide relief to the inflamed tissues include using a heel cup with strapping techniques, applying a low-dye strapping technique to the arch to reduce the stress on the plantar fascia, putting heel lifts in the shoes to reduce the stress from a tight Achilles tendon, and providing a heel cup to increase calcaneal stability and provide a cushion to the plantar calcaneus. Stretching of the Achilles and calf must be performed soon in the program so that the heel lift can be discarded as soon as possible; prolonged use of the heel lift can encourage tightness and prevent restoration of full motion. Calf stretching must be performed with the ankle in subtalar neutral so that the foot does not collapse and give a false impression of stretching the calf. Stretching of the plantar fascia and great toe can be performed with the ankle in dorsiflexion and the great toe in hyperextension. Massage with golf balls, a rolling pin, or a ribbed can may provide additional relief.

If orthotics seem necessary, before they are provided the rehabilitation clinician should attempt temporary orthotic relief to assess whether an orthotic can achieve the desired result. If either a temporary orthotic or a low-dye strapping technique provides significant relief, this is a good indication that a permanent orthotic is needed.

Once the inflammation is under control and flexibility exercises have been provided, the patient should begin strengthening exercises for the ankle inverters and the intrinsic and extrinsic toe flexors. These muscles can assist in supporting the arch and plantar fascia. Marble pickups with deposit into the opposite hand and towel-roll, heel raise, and resisted inversion exercises are all appropriate for plantar fasciitis.

Only in extreme cases will the patient have to refrain from normal activities. Pain is normally the limiting factor; but because the fascia is inflamed, it is susceptible to tears, especially during sudden acceleration or push-off movements. If a rupture of the plantar fascia occurs, pain and swelling will prevent the patient from ambulating normally. A stiff-soled shoe or partial weight bearing on crutches for three to seven days may be necessary. Treatment for a plantar fascia rupture follows a course similar to that for plantar fasciitis. Inflammation control, flexibility exercises, and the usual progression to strengthening, coordination, agility, and functional activities are normal program components.

Case Study

A 19-year-old basketball player has developed right plantar fasciitis over the past month. The pain is present when he gets up in the morning and when he stands after sitting in class for an hour. He is able to perform his workouts without any difficulty, but he has noticed that the pain is worse the morning after a particularly hard workout. Your examination reveals higher-than-normal arches of both feet. Ankle dorsiflexion in subtalar neutral is −5°. Great-toe hyperextension is 50°. There is tenderness to pressure over the plantar medial calcaneus where the plantar fascia inserts. Shoe wear is excessive on the lateral aspect of the shoe.

Questions for Analysis

1. What will your first treatment include?

2. What home exercises will you give the patient before he leaves today?

3. What accommodations will you place in his shoes or on his feet?

4. What strengthening exercises will you give him, and when will you give them?

5. If you decide that the patient needs orthotics, what specifications will you want in them?

Tarsal Tunnel Syndrome

The tarsal tunnel is formed by the medial malleolus, calcaneus, talus, and deltoid ligament's posterior aspect. Tarsal tunnel syndrome is an entrapment of the posterior tibial nerve as it passes under the flexor retinaculum posterior to the medial malleolus along with the tendons of the tibialis posterior, flexor digitorum longus, and flexor hallucis longus (figure 20.62). Excessive pronation, especially with improper shoes, can cause increased tension on the flexor retinaculum to increase compression on the nerve. Dancers, especially tap dancers who wear rigid shoes and sustain high-impact forces, are susceptible to tarsal tunnel syndrome. Swelling from trauma or tendinitis can also cause tarsal tunnel syndrome. Symptoms during weight bearing include a burning pain, tingling, and numbness in the medial and plantar foot. Tinel's sign is often positive. Toe flexor and abductor hallucis weakness and decreased ability to plantar flex and invert the foot can be noted in more advanced cases.

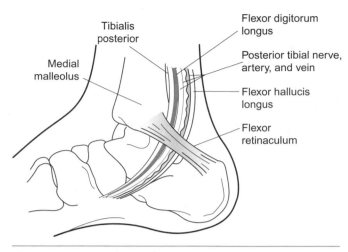

Figure 20.62 Tarsal tunnel.

Only severe cases require cessation of activities or surgery. Most cases can be treated conservatively. Treatment includes orthotics to reduce pronation and reduce posterior tibial nerve irritation, modalities such as phonophoresis or iontophoresis to diminish inflammation, and therapeutic exercises to resolve weakness. Properly fitted shoes and anti-inflammatory medications are also useful. Flexibility exercises and soft-tissue mobilization for release of adhesions can also be beneficial for pain relief. If shoe compression on the medial foot contributes to the problem, use of padding for nerve relief can reduce symptoms.

Cases requiring surgical release of the retinaculum may necessitate either a walking boot or a non-weight-bearing posterior splint for about 2 weeks postoperatively. A normal therapeutic exercise progression is followed by jogging at around 6 to 8 weeks and return to full participation at around 10 to 12 weeks following surgery.

Sesamoiditis

The two sesamoids under the first metatarsal head function to enhance the windlass mechanism of the foot for increased propulsion and to disperse the weight-bearing forces. A sesamoiditis does not actually involve the sesamoids but rather the soft tissue surrounding the bones. Restriction of soft tissue around the sesamoids, a tight Achilles tendon, plantar-flexed first ray, reduced great-toe hyperextension motion, and a restricted midfoot can all be underlying causes of sesamoiditis. Occasionally, cleat misplacement on shoes can increase pressure on the sesamoids and cause soft-tissue inflammation. Hyperextension of 65° is required for walking and running activities. Less hyperextension than that can increase forces imposed on the sesamoid region during propulsion.

The patient complains of pain with running, especially during push-off. The pain is located over the first metatarsal head. Standing heel raises with pressure over the first metatarsal head are painful, as is passive dorsiflexion of the great toe. Palpation reveals tenderness of the sesamoids.

Treatment includes relieving the inflammation and correcting the underlying cause. Flexibility exercises to correct tight structures are vital. Soft-tissue mobilization is usually necessary, because the soft tissue becomes adherent around the sesamoids and further restricts great-toe hyperextension motion. A pad or orthotic with a cutout for the first ray and with an extension pad to the second metatarsal head and toe can help to reduce stress on the sesamoids. Placing the foot in a rigid-soled shoe also limits the stress applied to the sesamoids.

This injury is self-limiting and does not usually require cessation of activity. Modification of shoe wear, correction of the causes, and modifications in activity usually will allow the patient to continue some level of participation.

Turf Toe

Turf toe is a hyperextension injury to the first MTP joint that occurs when the phalanx is jammed into the metatarsal. Improperly fitting shoes and high acceleration forces are common accompanying factors.

Symptoms include tenderness, swelling, and reduced range of motion of the great toe. Rehabilitation includes modalities to reduce the swelling and pain, scar-tissue mobilization, and active range-of-motion exercises. Ankle dorsiflexion with toe flexion-extension can be performed in a whirlpool initially and then in weight bearing as tolerated. Joint mobilizations, initially in grades I and II for pain relief but later in grades III and IV for joint mobility, are included. Strengthening exercises including closed kinetic chain activities and progressing to jumping and plyometric exercises are added as the patient tolerates them.

Case Study

An 18-year-old, male collegiate freshman sprinter had a plantar wart removed from the medial aspect of the ball of his left foot five years ago. Recently the ball of the foot has become progressively painful during running. He does not remember any injury to the foot recently. Your examination reveals an area of swelling with hard scar tissue around the first metatarsal head. His great-toe hyperextension is 45°. He complains of pain when you attempt to hyperextend the toe beyond that point. He is unable to stand on his toes without pain. His ankle dorsiflexion in subtalar neutral is –5°. Mobilization of the sesamoids is difficult, with mobility about 50% compared to that of the right foot. The patient reports pain when you attempt to mobilize the sesamoids with medial-lateral and superior-inferior glides.

Questions for Analysis

1. What is your determination of the cause of the patient's pain?

2. What will your treatment for him today include?

3. What modifications will you place on his foot or in his shoe that will permit him to continue his workout program?

4. What instructions will you give the patient for his workout tomorrow and for his home program?

5. How will your treatment program change as he improves over the next few weeks?

Shoe fit should be appropriate before the patient is allowed to return to participation. A rigid toe box and plantar-flexion positioning of the first ray with strapping or padding can be useful in reducing pain when the patient returns to the sport.

Fractures

The primary concern with a fracture in a young patient is that it may include the growth plates. If this occurs, further development and bone growth can be severely impaired. Stress fractures and acute fractures are more common than one might think. Each is treated differently; programs and considerations related to these fractures are outlined here.

Fractures can occur in any of the extremity, ankle, or foot bones. Stress fractures result from repetitive stress to the tibia and metatarsal bones, whereas acute fractures result from sudden application of excessive forces. In younger patients, epiphyseal plate fractures can occur, especially in the distal fibula and tibia. Acute fractures vary greatly in their presentation and according to how the forces are applied. Lateral stresses to the ankle can result in malleolar fractures; compression forces from jumping can cause talus, tibia, and metatarsal fractures; crush injuries from having the foot stepped on can cause metatarsal and phalangeal fractures; other phalangeal fractures can occur as a result of stubbing a toe; and torsional stresses can cause fractures of the tibia and foot.

Phalangeal fractures are painful but seldom casted. The fractured phalanx is commonly buddy taped to an adjacent toe. Metatarsal fractures of the second, third, and fourth metatarsals are commonly placed in a CAM boot to restrict movement during ambulation. Crutches are sometimes needed if the patient is unable to ambulate normally. Fractures of the first metatarsal require special attention because this is a major weight-bearing bone. Fifth metatarsal fractures also deserve special attention because they can cause problems that linger, depending on the fracture's location. Tarsal fractures can be interarticular and involve interarticular ligamentous damage. If the fracture is displaced, surgery is usually indicated. Ankle fractures are often surgically repaired, because even minimal displacement of fragments produces better results than conservative management (Thigpen 1983). Fractures in young patients should be referred to an orthopedic surgeon because epiphyseal injuries can impair normal bone growth.

Because the tibia, talus, calcaneus, and first ray are the primary weight-bearing structures of the foot and extremity, fractures to these bones require immobilization and non-weight bearing. The fibula is a non-weight-bearing bone, so walking boots or walking casts are usually used for fractures of this bone. Displaced fractures are surgically repaired whereas nondisplaced fractures may be immobilized with or without surgery.

Immobilization for fractures of the extremity, ankle, or foot must include immobilization of the ankle. Following immobilization, limited joint mobility is most often the greatest debilitating factor. The greater the damage, the more extensive the scar-tissue formation. The risk of increased formation of scar tissue is greater with a greater and more prolonged presence of edema. Immobilization and soft-tissue edema with subsequent scar-tissue adhesions combine to produce restricted joint mobility of the ankle and surrounding joints. Normal mobility of these joints must be restored to make full balance of function possible. If one joint is restricted, an adjacent joint suffers additional stress as it attempts to compensate for the lost mobility of the restricted joint. Over time, the increased stress can lead to tissue breakdown and injury.

In addition, the immobilization time required for fracture healing leads to capsular restriction, muscle weakness, balance and proprioception loss, and muscle endurance deficits. Joint motion and soft-tissue mobility must be emphasized in early rehabilitation, because the window of opportunity for regaining these elements is narrower than for the other factors. As scar tissue matures, the opportunity to impact changes in its length diminishes. If prolonged immobilization and extensive scar-tissue formation have occurred, prolonged stretches to affect more mature scar tissue may be necessary to increase mobility of shortened tissue or adherent collagen.

The typical duration of immobilization is three to six weeks. This may vary for stress fractures and surgically repaired fractures. Stress fractures are not frequently casted, but activity is reduced to relieve the stress and permit healing to occur. Fractures that undergo ORIF can usually advance to weight bearing sooner than conservatively treated fractures. Patients with fractures that involve the primary weight-bearing bones generally advance to weight bearing with more caution, and full weight bearing is delayed.

Joint mobilization and soft-tissue mobilization techniques are initiated as soon as safely possible. Modalities, such as heat or ultrasound, applied before mobilization techniques can be useful in preparing soft tissue and achieving better treatment results. Massage is useful in relieving edema. Deep-tissue massage, friction massage, and myofascial techniques are used to improve soft-tissue mobility.

Joint mobilization techniques for pain relief and joint mobility are often used in combination, beginning and ending with grade II mobilizations for pain relief. If a joint is very tender, grade III and IV techniques may not be possible until pain is under control. Active stretches, passive stretches, and contract-relax-stretch techniques are useful in increasing motion of both joint and soft-tissue structures.

Immobilization and periods of altered weight bearing necessitate gait-training instructions once the patient is able to resume full weight bearing. During partial weight bearing it is important to instruct the patient in a normal heel-toe gait to encourage proper gait patterning in preparation for full weight bearing. Once the patient is permitted to bear full weight on the extremity, pregait instruction, including weight-transfer activities and normal stride reeducation, is usually needed.

Closed kinetic chain exercises for strengthening, as well as static balance activities such as stork standing, can begin when full weight bearing is permitted. Therapeutic exercises proceed in the manner discussed earlier in this chapter. Advancement follows a logical progression from light to heavier weights, reduced to increased repetitions, static to dynamic balance and agility exercises, and simple to complex activities until the patient advances to plyometric exercises and finally to functional activities before returning to full activity.

The rate of progression is determined by the tissue-healing time line, the tissue's response to stresses, and the individual's ability to tolerate the therapeutic exercise progression. Functional testing before return to full participation must mimic demands that the patient will encounter during his or her ability to perform. Once all the parameters are improved and

Case Study

A 16-year-old wrestler sustained a left ankle lateral malleolar fracture during a wrestling match. He underwent an ORIF the following day and was placed on crutches, non-weight bearing for two weeks before advancing to partial weight bearing. It is now four weeks after the surgery and the patient is not yet full weight bearing, although the surgeon has instructed him to begin weight bearing to tolerance and to advance to weight bearing without the crutches. The patient admits to you that he is apprehensive about putting weight on the extremity for fear of breaking it again. The extremity had been placed in a cast following surgery until yesterday, when it was removed.

On examination, the patient's ankle moves to 10° plantar flexion for maximum dorsiflexion. Other measures include 30° of plantar flexion, 0° of eversion, and 5° of inversion. Ankle strength in these directions is 2+/5 in the available ranges of motion. His hip and knee ranges of motion are normal, but strength is 4–/5 for all of the muscle groups. The surgical scar is well healed, but sloughing skin is present around the ankle and there are dry scabs over the wound. Palpation reveals stiffness of soft tissue around the ankle and into the foot. The foot is mildly enlarged, but there is no pitting edema. Joint mobility of the ankle joints is restricted to no more than 30% of normal, and the intertarsal and metatarsal joints are restricted to 50% normal mobility.

Questions for Analysis

1. What are your goals for today's treatment session?

2. What home program will you send with the patient today?

3. The patient wants to attend a wrestling camp in 10 weeks; what will you tell him when he asks whether he will be able to attend the camp?

4. List your long- and short-term goals for the patient for the next six weeks.

5. What will be your criteria for advancing him to closed kinetic chain exercises?

6. List three closed kinetic exercises that you will give the patient the first day these types of exercises are in his program.

7. List three non-weight-bearing exercises that you will give him in the next week.

8. List three agility exercises you will use in the patient's program and the criteria he must meet before they are used.

the patient passes all the functional tests, without any difference in performance from left to right lower extremity, he or she may resume full participation. Depending on the extent of the injury, the time of immobilization, the age of the patient, and initial joint and soft-tissue restriction following immobilization, three to six months is considered a reasonable amount of time before the patient is able to resume participation.

SUMMARY

1. Discuss normal foot mechanics in ambulation.

The first structure to hit the ground during ambulation is the calcaneus. It, along with the talus, forms the subtalar joint; and the talus, along with the tibia and fibula, forms the talocrural joint. Normal function of these two joints permits us to land the foot on the ground and adapt to variations in ground topography and stresses while maintaining a steady gait. The talocrural joint moves primarily in dorsiflexion and plantar flexion. The subtalar joint is responsible for pronation and supination. Pronation and its component motions cause the foot to convert to a mobile adapter for accommodation to uneven surfaces. Supination causes the foot articulations to become more rigid and provide for power transfer to permit appropriate force distribution needed for propulsion in ambulation. As the ankle goes into plantar flexion, the talus moves anteriorly so that the posterior, narrower aspect of the talus sits in the mortise joint. During dorsiflexion, the fibula glides superiorly and rotates laterally; and in plantar flexion, it moves inferiorly and rotates medially. In addition to the talocrural and subtalar joints, the more distal tarsal bones of the foot form the midtarsal joint. This joint's movements closely follow the subtalar and talocrural joint movements. During supination, the navicular and cuboid bones move medially and inferiorly; during pronation they move laterally and superiorly. The first-ray movement occurs in plantar flexion and dorsiflexion and is equal in each direction, with each equal to about a thumb's width of motion. The second ray includes the joint between the second metatarsal and middle cuneiform; the third ray includes the third metatarsal and the lateral cuneiform; the fourth ray is the fourth metatarsal alone; and the fifth ray is the fifth metatarsal alone. Metatarsophalangeal joints permit flexion-extension, abduction-adduction, and accessory rotation and dorsal-plantar glides. The IP joints, which are hinge joints, permit flexion and extension with accessory rotation and dorsal-plantar glides. The first MTP joint must have about 60° to 65° of hyperextension for toe roll-off during gait.

2. Identify two foot deformities and discuss their impact on athletic injury.

   Pes cavus, a rigid foot, makes force absorption of the foot more limited, causing forces to be absorbed farther up the closed chain and thus risking injury to other structures. Pes planus, or flatfoot, causes the foot to move inefficiently, requiring more effort from, and subsequently applying more stress to, other structures. It also changes the mechanics of the extremity, increasing stresses applied to structures such as the Achilles, patella, and hip.

3. Describe the primary structures of a shoe.

   A shoe's main components include an upper and a lower section. The upper section includes the vamp, toe box, saddle, collar, insole board, sock liner, and heel counter. The lower section includes the outsole, wedge, and midsole. The vamp covers the toes and forefoot and includes the toe box. The toe box varies in width and height and functions to retain the shape of the shoe's forefoot and provide room for the toes. The saddle is the midsection of the shoe along the longitudinal arch, which is usually reinforced to assist in supporting the midfoot. The heel counter is an important stabilizer for the rearfoot. A foxing is an additional piece often seen in athletic shoes that further reinforces the rearfoot to assist in maintaining the counter's shape. The medial aspect of the counter is sometimes extended forward to resist pronation. The collar, the top rim of the shoe, is often padded to reduce friction on the Achilles. The insole board lies between the upper and lower segments and serves as the attachment for the two segments. A sock liner on top of the insole board is used for shock absorption and friction reduction for the foot.

4. List the important factors in shoe considerations for a pes cavus foot.

   Because a pes cavus foot is rigid and has limited stress-absorption capabilities, a shoe for someone with this deformity should have as much force absorption as possible. Factors such as a soft midsole, a curved last, and flexibility should be standards in a shoe for a rigid foot.

5. Outline key factors in an orthotic evaluation.

   (1) The patient's height and weight; (2) type of sport and activity level of the patient; (3) medical history; (4) the patient's primary and secondary complaints; (5) the calcaneal position in relaxed standing and in subtalar neutral standing; (6) the appearance of the arches in weight bearing and non-weight bearing; (7) toe positions; (8) knee positions; (9) tibial varum; (10) first-ray positions; (11) subtalar mobility; (12)

midtarsal mobility; (13) first-metatarsal mobility; (14) hallux dorsiflexion; (15) ankle dorsiflexion; and (16) location of corns and calluses. This last factor is important because corns and calluses are indicators of accommodating or nonaccommodating forefoot and rearfoot deformities.

6. Explain one joint mobilization technique for improving ankle dorsiflexion.

    A dorsal glide can be used: The stabilizing hand is placed anteriorly around the distal extremity, and the mobilizing hand is placed around the proximal foot with the thumb and index finger in contact with the malleoli. The talus is glided posteriorly in the plane of the joint.

7. List three stretching exercises for the ankle and extremity, including one that is not mentioned in the text.

    Some stretches for these structures are the standing gastrocnemius stretch, the seated soleus stretch with a strap, and standing sideways on an incline board with the ankle positioned in inversion.

8. Identify three strengthening exercises for the ankle and extremity.

    Exercises for strengthening the ankle and extremity include calf raises, toe raises, and eversion in sidelying with a weight attached to the ankle.

9. Explain three agility exercises.

    For agility the patient can do lateral jumps, zigzag runs, and rapid change-of-direction maneuvers performed on command.

10. Describe three functional exercises for the lower extremity.

    Some functional exercises for the lower extremity are side-to-side sprints; run, stop and jump exercises; and running and stopping while bouncing a basketball.

11. Provide an example of a therapeutic exercise program progression for an ankle sprain.

    Initial treatment includes modalities for edema and pain relief and reduction of inflammation. Joint mobilization and soft-tissue mobilization may be necessary if those structures are impaired in their normal movement. Active and passive range-of-motion exercises are accompanied by mild strengthening exercises, such as isometrics, manual resistance, and rubber band exercises. If the patient has been non-weight bearing, it may be necessary to use exercises with a weight scale to reintroduce the concept of weight bearing on the extremity as a prelude to gait training. Body-weight resistance exercises and machine-weight resistance exercises are then included. Balance and proprioception exercises begin with simple stork standing and progress to standing on unstable surfaces, then moving on one extremity. Once strength, flexibility, and balance are restored, plyometric and then functional activities are used before return to participation.

CRITICAL THINKING QUESTIONS

1. Explain how Benjamin concluded that Catie's plantar fasciitis was being caused by her pronation, hip tightness, and knee and tibial malalignments. Why would he suspect that Catie's thigh muscle imbalance was also contributing to the plantar fasciitis? What shoe characteristics should Catie look for when she buys her next running shoes?

2. If a patient had a leg-length discrepancy but no other major structural problems, would you expect to see an abnormal wear pattern on the bottom of his or her shoes? If so, what?

3. Using the repaired-Achilles case study presented earlier, what would you include in an aquatic exercise program for this patient for range of motion, strength, and cardiovascular conditioning? When could you begin his aquatic program?

LAB ACTIVITIES

1. Perform a deep-tissue massage to your lab partner's leg. Are you able to locate any areas of restriction? Is that same area also tender when you apply a deep massage to it? Why would this be?

2. Instruct your partner in a home treatment to release adhesions on the plantar foot. Give precise instructions in terms of what to use, how long to apply it, how much pressure to use, and what the expected outcome should be.

3. Locate the trigger points for the following muscles on your lab partner:

   a. Peroneus longus

   b. Gastrocnemius

   c. Soleus

   d. Abductor hallucis

   e. Flexor digitorum brevis

   f. Quadratus plantae

   g. Flexor hallucis brevis

   Where were your partner's most sensitive trigger points? Perform an ice-and-stretch technique on each of them and provide your partner with a home exercise for each tender trigger point

4. Perform grades II and IV joint mobilizations on your lab partner and identify what restriction would be best treated with each mobilization for the following joints:

   a. Tibiofibular joints

      - Superior: AP, PA glides

      - Inferior: AP, PA glides

   b. Talocrural joint

      - Distraction

      - Anterior glide

      - Posterior glide

   c. Subtalar joint

      - Distraction

      -Anterior glide

      -Posterior glide

   d. TMT, MTP, IP joints

      - Distraction

      - Anterior glide

      - Posterior glide

5. Have your partner perform a gastrocnemius and soleus stretch. What are the substitution patterns and where does s/he feel the stretch for each of the exercises? What verbal cues could you use to correct the errors in performance?

6. Have your partner perform a prolonged Achilles stretch for 3 minutes. How could she perform the exercise incorrectly so the stretch would not be optimally effective? When she steps out of the stretch, what does she feel?

7. Provide your partner with manual resistance to dorsiflexion, inversion, and eversion, 10 repetitions each. Be sure to provide enough resistance to make the motion smooth, accommodating your resistance to match his and still obtain a maximal output from him or her for each exercise. What position did you place him or her in to allow you to provide resistance most efficiently?

8. Now have him perform the same exercises as in question 7 with a Thera-band. First, how will you determine what color of theraband she should use for each exercise? Have her perform the exercise and then describe the differences in how the manual resistance and theraband resistance felt throughout the range of motion for each exercise. How do these results influence the factors you would use to decide what kind of exercise to include in a rehabilitation program?

9. Have your partner perform balance exercises that progress from static balance to dynamic balance to balance while performing distracting activities. Evaluate how your partner was able to perform the activities as you would for a chart note. Be sure to include the activity, repetitions, and your assessment on quality of performance.

10. Have your partner perform one agility drill that you design using tape marks on the floor. Diagram the exercise on paper. Have her perform it first without resistance then with resistance. Did your partner's ability to perform the activity change with the addition of resistance? If so, how did it change? What performance factors did you watch and correct for and what were your cues for correction? What sport athletes would benefit most from these activities as part of their rehabilitation program?

11. Design one plyometric or hopping activity. Describe it and identify why this is the one you selected. Have your partner perform it. What performance factors did you watch and correct for, and what were your cues for correction? What would be the criteria for your partner to advance to the next level of exercise? Which patients benefit most from these activities as part of their rehabilitation program?

REFERENCES

Baumhauer, J., Shereff, M., and J. Gould. 1997. Ankle pain in runners. In *Running injuries*, ed. G.N. Guten. Philadelphia: Saunders.

Bernier, J.N., and D.H. Perrin. 1998. Effect of coordination training on proprioception of the functionally unstable ankle. *Journal of Orthopaedic & Sports Physical Therapy* 27:264–275.

Bolgla, L.A., and D.R. Keskula. 1997. Reliability of lower extremity functional performance tests. *Journal of Orthopaedic & Sports Physical Therapy* 26:138–142.

Cipriani, D.J., Armstrong, C.W., and S. Gaul. 1995. Backward walking at three levels of treadmill inclination: An electromyographic and kinematic analysis. *Journal of Orthopaedic & Sports Physical Therapy* 22:95–102.

Denegar, C., E. Saliba, and S. Saliba. 2005. *Therapeutic modalities for musculoskeletal injuries*. 2nd ed. Champaign, IL: Human Kinetics.

Forkin, D.M., Koczur, C., Battle, R., and R.A. Newton. 1996. Evaluation of kinesthetic deficits indicative of balance control in gymnasts with unilateral chronic ankle sprains. *Journal of Orthopaedic & Sports Physical Therapy* 23:245–250.

Garn, S.N., and R.A. Newton. 1988. Kinesthetic awareness in subjects with multiple ankle sprains. *Physical Therapy* 68:1667–1671.

Glascoe, W.M., Allen, M.K., Awtry, B.F., and H.J. Yack. 1999. Weight-bearing immobilization and early exercise treatment following a grade II lateral ankle sprain. *Journal of Orthopaedic & Sports Physical Therapy* 29:394–399.

Gross, M.T., Bradshaw, M.K., Ventry, L.C., and K.H. Weller. 1987. Comparison of support provided by ankle taping and semirigid orthosis. *Journal of Orthopaedic & Sports Physical Therapy* 9:33–39.

Kimura, I.F., Nawoczenski, D.A., Epler, M., and M.G. Owen. 1987. Effect of the AirStirrup in controlling ankle inversion stress. *Journal of Orthopaedic & Sports Physical Therapy* 9:190–193.

Klingman, R.E., Liaos, S.M., and K.M. Hardin. 1997. The effect of subtalar joint posting on patellar glide position in subjects with excessive rearfoot pronation. *Journal of Orthopaedic & Sports Physical Therapy* 25:185–191.

Kohn, H.S. 1997. Shin pain and compartment syndromes in running. In *Running injuries*, ed. G.N. Guten. Philadelphia: Saunders.

Konradsen, L., Holmer, P., and Sondergaard, L. 1991. Early mobilizing treatment for grade III ankle ligament injuries. *Foot & Ankle* 12:69–73.

Lattanza, L., Gray, G.W., and R.M. Kantner. 1988. Closed versus open kinetic chain measurements of subtalar joint eversion: Implications for clinical practice. *Journal of Orthopaedic & Sports Physical Therapy* 9:310–314.

Leanderson, J., Eriksson, E., Nilsson, C., and A. Wykman. 1996. Proprioception in classical ballet dancers. *American Journal of Sports Medicine* 24:370–374.

Lofvenberg, R., Karrholm, J., Sundelin, G., and O. Ahlgren. 1995. Prolonged reaction time in patients with chronic lateral instability of the ankle. *American Journal of Sports Medicine* 23:414–417.

Maitland, G.D. 1991. *Peripheral manipulation*. Boston; London: Butterworth-Heinemann.

Massie, D.L., and J.C. Spiker. 1990. *Foot biomechanics and the relationship to rehabilitation of lower extremity injuries*. Berryville, VA: Forum Medicum.

Powers, C.M., Maffucci, R., and S. Hampton. 1995. Rearfoot posture in subjects with patellofemoral pain. *Journal of Orthopaedic & Sports Physical Therapy* 22:155–160.

Rovere, G.D., Clarke, T.J., Yates, C.S., and K. Burley. 1988. Retrospective comparison of taping and ankle stabilizers in preventing ankle injuries. *American Journal of Sports Medicine* 16:228–233.

Seto, J.L., and C.E. Brewster. 1994. Treatment approaches following foot and ankle injury. *Clinics in Sports Medicine* 13:695–719.

Sitler, M., Ryan, J., Wheeler, B., McBride, J., Arciero, R., Anderson, J., and M.B. Horodyski. 1994. The efficacy of a semirigid ankle stabilizer to reduce acute ankle injuries in basketball. *American Journal of Sports Medicine* 22:454–461.

Stanish, W.D, Curwin, S. and S. Mandel. 2000. *Tendinitis: Its etiology and treatment*. New York: Oxford University Press.

Thigpen, C.M. 1983. Early management of fractures of the foot and ankle. *Current concepts in trauma care* 6:4–8.

Tiberio, D. 1987. The effect of excessive subtalar joint pronation on patellofemoral mechanics: A theoretical model. *Journal of Orthopaedic & Sports Physical Therapy* 9:160–165.

Travell, J.G., and D.G. Simons. 1992. *Myofascial pain and dysfunction. The trigger point manual*. Vol. 2. Baltimore: Williams & Wilkins.

SUGGESTED READING

Batt, M.E. 1995. Shin splints—a review of terminology. *Clinical Journal of Sports Medicine* 5:53–57.

Janisse, D.J. 1994. Indications and prescriptions for orthoses in sports. *Orthopedic Clinics of North America* 25:95–107.

Loudin, J.K., and S.L. Bell. 1996. The foot and ankle: An overview of arthrokinematics and selected joint techniques. *Journal of Athletic Training* 31:173–178.

Mascaro, T.B., and L.E. Swanson. 1994. Rehabilitation of the foot and ankle. *Orthopedic Clinics of North America* 25:147–160.

McPoil, T.G. 1988. Footwear. *Physical Therapy* 68:1857–1865.

Reynolds, N.L., and T.W. Worrell. 1991. Chronic Achilles peritendinitis: Etiology, pathophysiology, and treatment. *Journal of Orthopaedic & Sports Physical Therapy* 13:171–176.

CHAPTER 21

Knee and Thigh

Objectives

After completing this chapter, you should be able to do the following:

1. Discuss the relationship and alignment between the patella and femur.

2. Identify postinjury factors that influence strength output.

3. Define quadriceps extensor lag and explain its significance.

4. Outline a general progression of rehabilitation for a knee.

5. Identify three soft-tissue mobilization techniques for the knee.

6. Identify three joint mobilization techniques for the knee, and their purpose.

7. Explain three flexibility exercises for the knee, and identify the structures they affect.

8. Explain three proprioception/balance exercises for the knee.

9. Identify three functional activities.

10. Identify three factors that influence PFD.

Three mornings a week Lewis King and his friends play a game of basketball at the university gym before going to work. It was their way of having fun and getting exercise at the same time. They have been following this routine since they were in their mid-30s, about 10 years ago.

About two weeks ago their routine was suddenly disrupted. Lewis jumped to retrieve a rebound and landed in severe pain. He felt as if someone had shot him in the thigh. Several hours later he underwent a quadriceps tendon repair and was placed on crutches. Today he had his first rehabilitation appointment with Donette Soo.

After Donette completed her examination, she explained to Lewis what she saw as primary problems and discussed how she thought they could best resolve those problems. Lewis agreed with her and realized that this was not going to be an easy or short process, but he was willing to work with her to get back onto the basketball court. He liked Donette's approach and appreciated the way she was able to explain things better than the doctor did, so he could understand them. He knew she would work him hard; but he also knew that if he wanted to play basketball again, he would have to work hard, and he was eager to start.

Although Donette explained to Lewis that it would not be an easy process and would require him to be committed and consistent in his rehabilitation, she also knew that the tissue's healing process had to be respected. Because it was only two weeks since his surgery, stress to the newly formed tissue was important, but too much stress could be detrimental. The proper amount of stress to the patellar tendon was important, but she could also start Lewis on more aggressive exercises on the hip and ankle and not stress the patellar tendon. She sensed that Lewis was the type of person who was eager and willing to work hard but would also understand precautions if he knew about them. As she does with all her patients, Donette would keep him well informed throughout his program about what he should and should not be doing and why.

■ **Character is what you are willing to do when the spotlight has been turned off, the applause has died down and no one is around to give you credit.**

Unknown Author

Passion and a quest for understanding drive the accumulation of knowledge that makes us all better rehabilitation clinicians. Perhaps one of the most passionately pursued orthopedic topics is the knee. A tremendous amount of research has provided us with a wealth of knowledge on the knee. There is still a plethora of information to be gleaned about the knee; but in the past several years, investigators have given us new insights and information regarding knee biomechanics, improved surgical procedures, and optimal rehabilitation techniques.

This chapter deals with thigh and knee injuries. Thigh injuries could just as easily have been considered along with the hip in the next chapter. Indeed, I will refer you from one chapter to the other, because there is an intimate relationship between the thigh and knee and the thigh and hip. I have placed most thigh injuries in this chapter only because the knee comes before the hip in the text. Thigh injuries that impact primarily the hip are presented in chapter 22.

As with the other chapters in part IV, this one begins with general information that impacts therapeutic exercise programs for knee and thigh injuries. This information is vital if the rehabilitation clinician is to design and establish an appropriate therapeutic exercise program for the various injuries of the knee and thigh. This chapter presents specific therapeutic exercise techniques, including soft-tissue and joint mobilization and exercises for flexibility, strength, and coordination. Recommendations for functional activities before the patient's return to full sport participation are also included. The final section of the chapter discusses rehabilitation programs for specific injuries commonly seen in the knee and thigh.

Controversy continues on the best surgical repair technique and the most appropriate postoperative and postinjury methods of rehabilitation for the knee. Over the past several years, treatments of knee injuries and postoperative care have changed dramatically. The trend has shifted from conservative care, including cast immobilization and non-weight bearing for six weeks following surgery or serious injury, to weight bearing to tolerance with hinged-splint immobilization. Although cast immobilization is rare today, many surgeons choose to remain conservative while others prefer a more accelerated approach. It is important for the rehabilitation clinician to work with the physician to provide a successful rehabilitation outcome for the patient. Both the physician's and the rehabilitation clinician's protocols for rehabilitation of knee and thigh injuries should be based on the severity of the injury, the structure injured, and the tissue healing time line. If there is to be an error, as with any rehabilitation program, it should be on the side of caution.

GENERAL REHABILITATION CONSIDERATIONS

▶ The knee encompasses two major joints, the tibiofemoral joint and the patellofemoral joint. The knee also contains a joint capsule, ligaments, menisci, and muscles. A therapeutic exercise program must take into account the knee's unique structure, as well as a number of biomechanical and physiological characteristics specific to the knee.

The knee is one of the most frequently injured joints. The forces applied to it during running, twisting, and lifting activities are complicated by the fact that there are two long lever arms on either end of the joint, making it a joint susceptible to stresses. For as shallow a joint as the knee is, complete dislocation is surprisingly rare. This may be so because of the strong static and dynamic structures that surround the joint. The ligaments and muscles of the knee give the joint a sound structure so tremendous forces are required to produce an injury. The more common knee injuries are discussed later in this chapter. This section deals with unique knee structures which serve to support and protect the joint but are impacted when injury occurs.

Knee Structure

Although at first glance the knee appears to be a relatively simple joint, it is actually a complex structure involving several factors that influence its function. When balance is lacking in structure or function, the knee becomes susceptible to injury. An understanding of the knee's structures and the ways they influence one another is basic to the ability to develop a therapeutic exercise program for any injury of the knee.

Tibiofemoral Joint

The knee joint is actually two joints, the tibiofemoral joint and the patellofemoral joint. The tibiofemoral joint has a concave tibia platform attached to a convex humerus. This means that during joint mobilization, the concave tibia moves on the convex femur in the same direction as the physiological movement of the joint. In other words, a posterior glide produces flexion and an anterior glide produces extension.

Capsule

The knee joint is the largest joint of the body and is surrounded by a capsule that aids in joint stability by merging with the collateral ligaments. The capsule also distributes the synovial fluid around the joint during movement and merges with many of the knee's bursae. If the joint capsule is restricted, a capsular pattern becomes apparent. The knee's capsular pattern is restriction of flexion more than of extension. The joint is in a resting position when it is in about 20° to 25° of flexion and in a fully close-packed position in full extension with lateral tibial rotation.

Ligaments

The collateral ligaments provide for protection and stability of medial and lateral or valgus and varus stress. The medial collateral ligament (MCL) is attached to the medial meniscus. This arrangement may be one reason the medial meniscus is often injured with MCL sprains. In addition to providing protection against valgus stresses, it helps to restrict lateral rotation of the tibia on the femur. The lateral collateral ligament (LCL) is not attached to the lateral meniscus and is taut during medial rotation of the tibia on the femur and when the knee incurs varus stress. Because valgus stress from lateral forces is more frequently applied to the knee than varus stresses, the MCL is the more frequently injured of these two ligaments.

The anterior and posterior cruciate ligaments (ACL and PCL, respectively) are structures unique to the knee. Their position within the knee joint allows them to provide distinctive anterior-posterior stability to the knee. The ligaments also provide the knee with rotational stability. Fibers of each ligament are taut throughout the knee's range of motion. Injury to either ligament can cause instability within the knee that can be disabling.

The ACL and PCL are enclosed within a synovial membrane that provides the ligaments with their primary blood supply. If a partial tear of either ligament occurs, the synovial membrane can become disrupted as well, compromising the ligament's vascular supply. If this happens, dehiscence or erosion of the ligament can eventually result.

The ACL is the most commonly injured knee ligament. It protects the knee from anterior translation of the tibia on the femur. The PCL is not as frequently injured because it is much stronger. It serves primarily to restrict knee hyperextension and posterior tibial displacement of the tibia on the femur.

Rotational stresses at the knee are restrained by all the ligaments. The cruciate ligaments twist and become taut during medial rotation. The collateral ligaments become taut to provide stability during lateral rotation. Rotation is a primary motion of the knee in both weight bearing and non-weight bearing. In weight bearing the femur rotates on the tibia, and in non-weight bearing the tibia rotates on the femur. Injury mechanisms that produce excessive rotational forces can cause damage to more than one ligament and can result in joint instability.

The knee's joint capsule and intra-articular structures, including the ACL, contain various neuroreceptors that provide the neural system with position-afferent information from the knee. We know that the ACL contains afferent mechanoreceptors that impact the knee's stability. The joint capsule has mechanoreceptors (Ruffini endings) that are sensitive to pressure and deformation (Freeman and Wyke 1967). Injury to the knee's ligamentous structures can damage these receptors, impairing proprioception. Therapeutic exercise programs must include proprioception facilitative techniques to restore the deficiencies resulting from interarticular knee injuries.

Although each ligament has its own responsibility in supporting and protecting the knee, ligaments also provide assistive support to other ligaments. These protective designs are referred to as primary and secondary restraint. As an example, the ACL is the primary restraint protecting the knee against anterior tibial translation; but if it is injured, other structures such as the capsule, other ligaments, and dynamic structures act as secondary restraints to continue to protect the joint. Sometimes the secondary structures are able to assume the responsibilities of providing normal stability to the joint and sometimes they fall short. Instability caused by ACL or PCL insufficiencies is often minimally supported by secondary structures (Butler, Noyes, and Grood 1980).

Meniscus

The medial and lateral meniscus serve to cushion the joint, deepen the socket, increase joint congruity to better distribute weight-bearing forces, assist in joint lubrication, and provide stability. These structures are commonly referred to as cartilage, although this is a misnomer. These structures are primarily fibrocartilage (hence the name), but this is certainly not their only component. The knee joint also has articular cartilage, so the term "cartilage" is not only erroneous but sometimes confusing, especially to the patient who has injured articular cartilage, not meniscus. Of the two menisci, the medial meniscus is the more frequently injured. It is attached to the MCL, the ACL, and the semimembranosus. This arrangement is believed to be one cause for the greater frequency of injury to the medial meniscus. Even though the lateral meniscus is not attached to the LCL but does connect to the popliteus and PCL, it has more freedom of movement and is not impacted by collateral ligament positioning and stresses.

When the knee moves sagittally in flexion and extension, the menisci follow the tibial movements. During flexion the menisci are pulled posteriorly via the semimembranosus and popliteus, and during extension they are pulled anteriorly by the meniscopatellar ligaments. During rotation the menisci follow the movements of the femur. During movement from extension into flexion, the femur slides posteriorly on the tibia so that in a squat or flexed position, the weight is borne primarily by the posterior aspect of the menisci, whereas in extension the femur is primarily on the anterior menisci. Compressive forces absorbed by the menisci are up to 50% to 60% of the knee's loads. When the knee is at 90° flexion and the primary force is applied at the posterior aspect of the joint, the meniscal load increases to 85% of the total knee joint compressive forces (Ahmed and Burke 1983). Meniscal posterior horn tears seem to be primarily degenerative tears, whereas anterior horn and lateral tears are often traumatic events. Posterior degenerative tears may be related to the increased forces absorbed by the menisci in flexion, as well as to the repetitive activity imposed on the menisci during squatting and other positional activities. On the other hand, acute tears occur most often during a running or cutting maneuver, when the knee is near extension.

The menisci are avascular except for roughly their peripheral 25%. This has a significant impact on conservative and surgical intervention following injury of the meniscus. This topic is discussed later in the chapter.

Screw Home Mechanism

The knee joint is a modified hinge joint. This means that although it is similar to a hinge joint, permitting movement in one plane, the bony segments are not entirely and purely congruent throughout. Because the medial aspect of the joint is larger and extends slightly more distally than the lateral side, when the knee moves into extension during weight bearing the tibia rotates laterally as the medial femoral condyle rotates on the medial tibial plateau. This mechanism, called the screw home mechanism, occurs in the last 30° of extension. It affords the joint greater stability than a pure hinge-joint arrangement would because it provides a kind of locking. The popliteus is responsible for unlocking the knee during movement from full extension into flexion. It does this by laterally rotating the femoral condyles with its medial tibial insertion anchored in weight bearing. In non-weight bearing, the popliteus unlocks the knee as it medially rotates the tibia with its proximal insertion stabilized.

Patellofemoral Joint

The patella, the largest sesamoid bone in the body, sits within the femoral groove. Its resting position is knee extension, and its close-packed position is knee flexion. The patella serves to increase the lever-arm length of the quadriceps tendon, adds to the cosmesis of the knee joint, and protects the knee from anterior blows. It is a site of common knee pain and dysfunction.

The quadriceps tendon and its medial and lateral expansions surround the patella. The tendon attachment from the patella to the tibial tubercle is sometimes referred to as the patellar ligament because it travels from bone to bone. This structure is also called the patellar tendon.

Patellar stability is the result of static and dynamic structures. The greatest bony contributor to patellar stability is the femoral sulcus formed by the medial and higher-ridged lateral epicondyles within which the patella sits. Ligamentous stability from the patellofemoral and patellotibial joints assists in providing static restraints. Active restraints from the quadriceps provide the greatest dynamic stability. The pes anserine group and the biceps femoris with their control of tibial rotation provide indirect secondary dynamic support. Tibial rotation changes the tibial tubercle position and can alter stability provided by the patellar tendon.

Patellar alignment is examined in static and dynamic positions. The patella is examined in long sitting for abnormalities in resting. Position of the patella during contraction of the quadriceps in long sitting and in weight bearing is also examined, because patellar movement in open and closed kinetic chain conditions may be different. A closed kinetic chain position can change the patellar alignment because other factors, such as hip rotation and foot pronation, alter the way the patella moves when the quadriceps contract.

Superior Tibiofibular Joint

This joint is not actually a joint of the knee because it is distal to the knee joint, but it can impact the ankle and knee joints. There are no physiological movements in this joint, but it must have full accessory motion for full ankle range of motion to occur. Reduced tibiofibular joint mobility can cause lateral knee pain by restricting soft-tissue mobility in the region.

Muscles

The quadriceps and hamstrings have been the most widely addressed muscles because of their prominence in knee control. Both groups also impact the hip, and because they do, positioning of the hip must always be a consideration when one is exercising the muscles at the knee.

The quadriceps provide the most dynamic restraint for the knee. The rectus femoris is the quadriceps component that also assists in hip flexion. Hip positioning determines where in the motion the rectus femoris is most contributory at the knee. In a supine straight-leg raise, it works throughout the motion; but in sitting, the rectus femoris works only in terminal extension (Close 1964).

Because of the angle of their pull and tendon insertions, the hamstrings also produce tibial rotation. The biceps femoris produces tibial lateral rotation, and the semimembranosus and semitendinosus produce tibial medial rotation. They provide dynamic secondary restraints to assist the ACL, and in ACL-deficient knees they must be trained to become more prominent stabilizers.

Rehabilitation of isolated hamstring muscles should include the additional movements of rotation along with hip extension and knee flexion. Eccentric and concentric activities for all their motions would most appropriately strengthen the hamstrings throughout all their functions.

Biomechanical and Physiological Concepts

An appreciation of biomechanical and physiological concepts helps the clinician understand the significance of specific therapeutic exercise applications for various knee injuries, as well as the indications and precautions.

Patellofemoral and Tibiofemoral Relationship

When the knee extends, the patella glides superiorly and inferiorly during knee flexion for a total excursion of 5 to 7 cm (2.0-2.8 in.). The patella must glide freely for full knee motion to be possible.

In a normal knee, the patella's inferior pole is at the knee joint's margin and rests on the supratrochlear fat pad. A patella that lies superior to this position is called **patella alta,** and one that is inferior to the normal position is called **patella baja.** Either position restricts full range of motion of the knee. Injuries of the patellar tendon, including ACL reconstructions utilizing the quadriceps tendon, may develop patella baja. Injuries such as repaired quadriceps ruptures are susceptible to developing patella alta. Patella baja or alta requires aggressive patellar mobilization and soft-tissue-stretching techniques. These techniques are discussed in detail later.

The patella glides in the femoral groove and makes contact with the femoral groove. When contact between the two segments is made, compressive forces are applied to the posterior patella. These compressive loads can reach up to 10 times body weight during daily activities (Brownstein et al. 1988). In full extension, the patella rests on the fat pad and is not in contact with the sulcus. The area of contact between the posterior patella and femoral groove migrates from the inferior pole to the superior aspect as the knee moves from about 10° to 20° of flexion to 90°. The area of contact is fairly uniform across the breadth of the patella. Once the knee approaches the end of flexion, however, the contact is on the odd facet medi-

Figure 21.1 Patellofemoral contact patterns.

Adapted by permission from Goodfellow, Hungerford, and Zindel 1976.

ally and the lateral-superior aspect of the patella until the patella rests on the top of the lateral condyle in full flexion (figure 21.1).

Of significance with this change in points of contact between the patella and femur is the fact that as the knee moves into flexion, the amount of contact pressure and area of contact both increase. **Contact pressure** is a ratio between the patellofemoral joint reaction force and the contact area. **Joint reaction force** is a compressive force equivalent to the resultant vector force (of the patellofemoral quadriceps and patellar tendon forces) that is perpendicular to the patellar contact surface. Stress to the patellofemoral joint is the force per area of contact. In a closed kinetic chain activity, the joint reaction forces and the area of contact both increase as the knee moves from extension to 90°; but the force applied is greater than the area of contact, so joint stress increases as the knee moves into flexion to 90°. As the knee moves from 90° toward 120°, the force decreases and the surface area of contact remains the same, so the stress decreases. The greatest compressive forces occur in the 60° to 90° positions (Huberti and Hayes 1984; Steinkamp et al. 1993). If a patella is not in good alignment within the femoral groove, the congruency between the two bones is altered, so compressive forces are distributed over a smaller area. This may be one reason why malalignment of the patella results in increased pain and irritation of the patellofemoral joint.

In an open kinetic chain activity, the joint stress is lowest at 90° and greatest at 0°. Although there may be some individual variations, open kinetic chain exercises are least irritating when performed from 60° to 90°, while closed kinetic chain exercises cause the least patellofemoral joint irritation in the ranges of 0° to 30° and greater than 90° (Grelsamer and Klein 1998).

During closed kinetic chain activities such as walking, patellofemoral compressive forces of about one half of body weight are produced, while stair climbing produces about three times body weight and squatting produces compressive forces of over seven times body weight (Reilly and Martens 1972). During open kinetic chain activities the amount of compressive force changes with the type of activity and the angle at which it occurs. If knee extension is performed with a weight attached to the end of the extremity, compressive forces reach their peak at 35° to 40°; but if the force is applied by a machine arm at right angles to the ankle such as in an N-K table or isokinetic machine, the peak compressive forces occur at 90° and decrease as the knee extends (Reilly and Martens 1972). On the basis of mathematical formulas, it has been estimated that isokinetic exercises reach a peak patellofemoral compressive force of about five times body weight (Kaufman et al. 1991).

Many functional activities are performed in the 0° to 40° range of motion. It is important when you are treating patients with patellofemoral pain to avoid painful arcs of motion. As a general rule, closed kinetic chain exercises from 0° to 40° of flexion provide less lateral patellar motion and less patellofemoral stress than open kinetic chain exercises, and open chain exercises in positions greater than 50° flexion are less stressful (Doucette and Child 1996; Steinkamp et al. 1993).

These numbers may seem confusing, but you need to understand their significance when treating patients with patellofemoral stress injuries. Several points are important to remember. The most patellofemoral stress in open chain exercises occurs in the first 30° of motion, and the least amount of stress occurs in the range of 60° to 90°. The least patellofemoral stress in closed chain activities occurs in the first 30° of motion, and the greatest amount of stress occurs in the range of 60° to 90°. Because there is no contact between the femur and patella in 0° to 10°, it should be safe to strengthen in this range with any exercise (Steinkamp 1993). The more inflamed the patellofemoral joint is, the more limited are the ranges of motion the patient is able to exercise within to strengthen the quadriceps without pain. Because the patella does not make contact with the femur until about 20° of flexion, very irritated patellofemoral joints may tolerate motion only in the first 20° of flexion. Full squat exercises and full range-of-motion exercises with weight boots or cuff weights attached to the ankle should be avoided until later in the treatment program when the inflammation is reduced and strength is improved enough for the patellofemoral joint to tolerate the greater stresses of these activities. It is logical to include a slow progression in range of motion as symptoms decrease and strength increases. If you use isokinetic exercises, avoid going into the 90° range of motion where peak patellar compressive forces are produced. Shortening the lever-arm length on weight machines can reduce the compressive forces.

Q-Angle

Q-angle is the angle that is formed by a line from the anterior superior iliac spine to the middle patella and a line from the middle patella to the tibial tubercle (figure 21.2). Lower normal Q-angle measurement is 10°. Upper normal values may vary for men and women because of the differences in pelvic structure and range from 12° to 15°. The Q-angle can change from non-weight bearing to weight bearing, because tibial rotation changes the Q-angle. If the patient has pronation in weight bearing, the tibia is medially rotated and increases the Q-angle. If the leg laterally rotates, the Q-angle decreases. A weak vastus medialis oblique (VMO) can also increase the Q-angle.

In the past, many thought the Q-angle key to patellofemoral alignment and symptoms. Because it can change with functional activities, unless it is profoundly excessive its significance with patellofemoral pain is not considered as great as in the past (Livingston 1998). The Q-angle should be assessed for gross abnormalities in non-weight bearing and for changes in standing. It may not be a primary cause of patellofemoral pain syndrome, as was once believed, but it may contribute to the syndrome when other conditions are present.

Lower-extremity Alignment

As mentioned earlier, excessive rearfoot pronation influences the patella's alignment because it increases tibial rotation and changes the quadriceps tendon pull on the patella. You should evaluate other lower-extremity alignments during a knee examination because alterations from normal can increase stress levels of various knee structures. For example, increased hip medial rotation, squinting patellae, genu recurvatum, patella alta, tibial varum, medial tibial rotation, and compensatory pronation are malalignments that can contribute to patellofemoral pain. Because the lower extremity is a closed kinetic chain during most of its functions, malalignment in one segment results in compensatory changes in another segment. Changes at the hip or at the foot cause compensatory alterations and increased stress in the knee. Compensatory pronation and hip medial rotation with resulting medial tibial rotation are two malalignment problems that should be investigated in patients with patellofemoral pain.

Figure 21.2 Measuring Q-angle.

Factors Influencing Postinjury Strength

Obviously, injury and surgery weaken the knee muscles. Other factors, however, influence knee strength and function. Some are not often considered, but all impact knee function and are important for that reason.

These factors—edema, pain, and abnormal ambulation—lead to impaired muscle function. Reduced function leads to atrophy and weakness of the muscle. Muscle weakness leads to reduced function and control of the body segment. The rehabilitation clinician must pay attention to these factors when examining a patient before initiating a therapeutic exercise program.

Edema

One of the important goals of first-aid treatment of musculoskeletal injuries is minimization of edema. Once edema forms, efforts should be made to relieve it as quickly as possible. One reason this is a priority is that edema causes an inhibition of quadriceps function. Studies have demonstrated that swelling in the knee joint causes a reflex shutdown of the quadriceps (McDonough and Weir 1996, Fahrer et al 1988, Spencer, Hayes, and Alexander 1984). Other researchers have injected plasma or saline in small quantities (20-30 ml) into normal knees and found a profound inhibition of quadriceps activity to levels 60% below normal (Young, Stokes, and Iles 1987; Spencer, Hayes, and Alexander 1984). As fluid quantity increases, quadriceps activity decreases.

(continued)

Pain

It is commonly understood that pain causes a reflex inhibition of muscle activity. Pain affects both the autonomic and the conscious pathways. The reflex response in the presence of pain is to withdraw. The conscious response is to refrain from activity that produces pain. If pain persists following an injury, the patient's ability to perform active muscle contraction is impaired. Use of electrical stimulation and other modalities to control pain before therapeutic exercise may result in improved strength-output levels during exercises. This can ultimately reduce the patient's rehabilitation time by enhancing strength gains.

Ambulation

Normal ambulation utilizes the right and left lower extremity equally, applying weight-bearing and propulsive forces equally on the two extremities. Weakness results when a patient sustains a lower-extremity injury that causes him or her to favor the extremity. An unequal gait produces less-than-normal stresses on the extremity as the patient spends less weight-bearing time on the extremity and applies less stress to it. An antalgic gait produces weakness not only in the injured segment but also throughout the entire lower extremity. Therefore, it is important to examine the total lower extremity following an injury and to correct secondary weaknesses that develop in the extremity's noninjured segments.

Rehabilitation Concepts

In addition to the routine rehabilitation concepts guiding development of a therapeutic exercise program, special factors enter into knee rehabilitation. The rehabilitation clinician must address them all if a rehabilitation program is to be successful. The following sections deal with the special factors that have the most influence.

Extensor Lag

Questions that have elicited particular interest are what types of resistive knee exercises optimally strengthen the quadriceps and which quadriceps muscle works at what time within the knee's range of motion. The condition in which full passive motion is present but active extension is incomplete is an extensor lag. Two deficiencies are typically present after a knee injury: VMO atrophy and an extensor lag. Because the two problems frequently appear concurrently, a clinical presumption has been that the extensor lag is the result of VMO insufficiency. The VMO's oblique fiber insertion has tended to support this presumption. Research has shown, however, that the VMO does not exert any more effort than any of the other quadriceps muscles during terminal extension (Lieb and Perry 1971). Muscle fiber atrophy is more prominent in the VMO, but the reason is unclear. The atrophy may be apparent not because it is greater in the VMO than in the other quadriceps muscles, but because the fascial covering of the muscle is thinner over the oblique fibers of the vastus medialis than in the rest of the quadriceps group. On the other hand, it may be true that VMO atrophy occurs more readily because the VMO is unable to perform its function as a patellar medial stabilizer as effectively as the other quadriceps muscles perform their task as knee extensor. Research evidence to confirm either suspicion is lacking.

Terminal extension is difficult for a weakened quadriceps to achieve. Some researchers hold that because of its fiber alignment, the function of the VMO is to maintain medial patellar alignment, providing dynamic restraint for the patella (Witvrouw et al. 1996). If this is the case, an extensor lag may occur not because the VMO is deficient, but because the force required of the quadriceps to produce the last 15° of extension is twice as great as for the other ranges of knee motion (Grood et al. 1984). The quadriceps muscles' loss of mechanical advantage (decreased lever-arm length) as the knee approaches its end range means that a much greater muscular effort is needed to complete the movement.

Some of the frequently used open kinetic chain exercises for strength gains are the quad set, the straight-leg raise, and the short-arc quad. Among these, the quad set is the most effective in producing total quadriceps activity (Gough and Ladley 1971). The rectus femoris works more during the straight-leg raise and the short-arc quad. Vastus medialis activity is most apparent during a quad set. As would be expected, quadriceps muscles work more during a knee extension exercise than during a straight-leg raise (Knight, Martin, and Londeree 1979). Open kinetic chain exercises are an important tool in restoring isolated quadriceps strength, so these exercises are key elements in a therapeutic exercise program for a patient with isolated quadriceps weakness.

Open and Closed Kinetic Chain Exercises

Open and closed kinetic chain exercises have been the subject of debate in knee rehabilitation, especially ACL rehabilitation, for the past several years. Most recently, the type of exercise most widely advocated for ACL injuries has been closed kinetic chain exercise. This is because research demonstrates a reduction in anterior shear stress and ACL strain in weight-bearing activities that are performed in 0° to 60°. The least amount of anterior displacement in an anterior cruciate-deficient knee during a closed chain exercise occurs at 60°, while the greatest displacement in an open chain exercise occurs at 30° (Jenkins et al. 1997). It has been assumed that closed kinetic chain exercises recruit a cocontraction of hamstrings and quadriceps to provide stability; this assumption has yet to be substantiated through research, and recent studies have indicated that it may not always be the case. For example, investigators have demonstrated that the lateral step-up exercise, thought to recruit cocontraction of hamstrings and quadriceps, recruits the vastus lateralis and vastus medialis components of the quadriceps significantly but does little to recruit the hamstrings (Worrell, Crisp, and LaRosa 1998). Joint compressive forces in closed kinetic chain exercises may be responsible for reducing the shearing forces and anterior translation that occur in open kinetic chain activities (Isear, Erikson, and Worrell 1997). Additional investigations are needed before judgment on this topic can be final.

In an open kinetic chain exercise as indicated in figure 21.3, less anterior shear stress is applied to the ACL in knee extension resistive exercises from 60° to 90° flexion, and more is applied in terminal-extension ranges of motion (Beynnon et al. 1995). The greatest shear stress to the ACL occurs from 0° to 40° flexion. The quandary for the clinician is that 30° is the best position for quadriceps strengthening but puts the greatest strain on the ACL. Less strain is applied to the ACL in closed kinetic chain, but increased stress is applied to the patellofemoral joint in closed kinetic chain activities beyond about 50° flexion (figure 21.4) This can create a dilemma regarding patients who have undergone ACL reconstructions and have patellofemoral pain. Closed kinetic chain activities are less stressful for an ACL injury, but many patients with patellofemoral pain have difficulty performing closed kinetic chain exercises because of the pain.

Figure 21.3 ACL strain with open kinetic chain activities.
Adapted by permission from Beynnon et al. 1995.

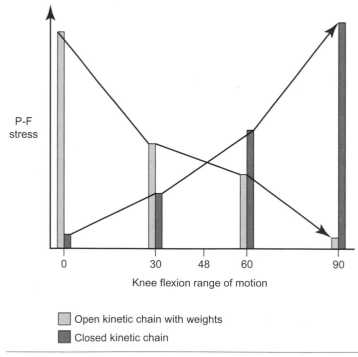

Figure 21.4 Patellofemoral joint stress at different angles.
Adapted by permission from Steinkamp et al. 1993.

Shear Stress

Aside from open kinetic chain activities, factors that also influence tibiofemoral shear stress include joint angle, location of the applied resistance, and the speed of the exercise. Peak shear stress occurs in the joint at around 28° to 14° of flexion. This may be one reason open chain exercises create their greatest shear force in 15° to 30°. Outside force that is applied more distally on the leg produces greater shear force than more proximally applied force. Manual resistance, especially in the early phases of therapeutic exercise, should be applied just distal to the knee joint to reduce shear-force applications. This is also true for exercise-machine arms used in open chain exercises.

Isokinetic exercise is not used until the later phases of rehabilitation because it is open chain; its lever arm can be shortened but still applies significant shear stresses. When isokinetic exercise is first used, the slower speeds should be avoided because slower speeds produce a greater torque to increase anterior tibial displacement and ACL strain.

Bracing

Perhaps more than any other joint, the knee is a frequent site for braces. There are three types of braces: prophylactic, rehabilitative, and functional. The prophylactic brace is used to prevent or reduce the severity of an injury, the rehabilitative brace restricts motion of an injured joint, and a functional brace improves stability of an unstable joint. A functional brace can also be a prophylactic brace.

There are custom-made braces and off-the-shelf braces. Custom-made braces, which are more expensive, can cost several hundred dollars or more. Off-the-shelf braces are similar in construction to the custom-made braces but come in generic sizes, usually ranging from extra small to extra large.

Braces are most often used for ACL injuries. Braces provide anterior stability during low-stress loads but have not shown adequate stability during more functional athletic load applications. Subjective reports often indicate a sense of security and improved performance when exercising with a brace as compared to exercising without one. Braces do seem to provide some proprioceptive feedback, and may be of value for this reason.

Patients who have patellofemoral pain often use knee sleeves. Once again, the proprioceptive benefit as reflected in subjective reports of decreased pain may be the primary advantage. The sleeves do not alter patellar glide or protect the knee from external stress. But one cannot dismiss the psychological benefits of increased confidence and assurance that using a sleeve may give the patient.

Program Progression

Tissue healing and the injury's response to exercise are primary factors that dictate rate of progression of a knee therapeutic exercise program. Parameters of range of motion, strength and endurance, balance and agility, and functional performance are advanced as with therapeutic exercise programs for other body segments. Careful observation by the rehabilitation clinician, as well as reliance on the patient for accurate communication regarding responses to exercise, is essential for a steady progression within a therapeutic exercise program.

Flexibility exercises, joint mobilization, and soft-tissue mobilization are all techniques that improve range of motion and flexibility. Strength and endurance exercises encompass a variety of activities that advance from static to dynamic and from isometric to isotonic to isokinetic. The method of advancing strength depends on the timing of the program, the patient's response, availability of equipment, and the rehabilitation clinician's preference. Isometric exercises are used more often when rehabilitation is in its early phases, when the knee is immobilized, when range-of-motion exercises are too painful for the patient, and when the aim is to isolate weak ranges of motion. In most cases a combination of open and closed kinetic chain exercises is beneficial.

Balance and agility exercises begin with double-support weight-bearing activities and progress to single-limb static balancing on a stable surface. Initial double-support activities might be as simple as gait training with correct weight transfer from the right to the left extremity. From there the activities advance to single-limb stance on a stable surface then on an unstable surface. Balance activities can begin at a low level when the patient is able to bear weight on the extremity. Once the patient is able to place total body weight on the injured extremity, single-limb stance activities can begin. For these the patient must be able to correctly shift weight without trunk lean onto the involved extremity. A trunk lean not only does not permit accurate body-weight transfer onto the extremity, but it also promotes bad weight-bearing habits that can become difficult to overcome.

Agility activities advance from balance and coordination exercises. Prerequisites to a patient's progressing to agility exercises are an intact neuromuscular response system, and strength and motion sufficient to return the body's center of gravity to within its base of support when balance is disturbed (Wegener, Kisner, and Nichols 1997). Agility exercises also demand appropriate coordination and muscle power, so they are the next logical step in the rehabilitation progression before functional activities. Agility exercises are dynamic; they may begin with no-impact activities and progress to high-impact activities. The lower-level agility exercises are unidirectional, and more advanced agility exercises are multidirectional. Agility activities begin at reduced speeds and advance to full speed as the patient progresses.

When adding a new agility exercise to a program, it is beneficial to include it early in the exercise session before the patient becomes fatigued. There is evidence to demonstrate that fatigue reduces the knee's proprioceptive function (Lattanzio et al. 1997). An agility activity requires proprioceptive feedback for proper execution. If fatigue reduces proprioceptive function, the execution will not be as good as it should be, and the application is undesirable because of the risk of engramming an incorrect execution.

Once the patient has mastered the agility exercises, the final step—functional activities—prepares the individual physically and psychologically for return to full participation. The program can advance to this phase when there is no evidence of pain or edema postexercise and when the injured knee has full range of motion, near-normal strength, and good balance. As with other therapeutic exercise programs, functional activities include specific activity-related drills that mimic the patient's normal activities. They are designed to come as close to normal participation demands as possible. They may begin at reduced stress levels, but as the patient's skills and confidence return, the stress of the activity is akin to the stress he or she will experience on returning to full participation.

The functional examination to determine the patient's readiness for return to full participation should mimic the patient's activities. The rehabilitation clinician should examine the patient for accurate execution, ability to use both lower extremities equally, without hesitation to use the involved extremity or inclination to favor it, and confidence in performance.

SOFT-TISSUE MOBILIZATION

▶ Soft-tissue mobilization for knee injuries addresses pain referred from the quadriceps, the hip adductors, the hamstrings, the popliteus, and the tensor fascia lata. Deep-tissue massage is typically for the quadriceps tendon and the iliotibial band.

Pain in the soft tissue surrounding the knee can result from injury to the local tissue or to distant tissue. The foot and hip can refer pain into the knee. Sciatica can also occur as knee pain without leg or back pain. You should examine these areas as possible sources of knee pain if there has been no frank injury. With injuries that might have involved other segments, assessment of these segments is also indicated. You must make a differential diagnosis to eliminate other sources of pain to provide appropriate rehabilitative care for the patient.

Muscles surrounding the knee have specific pain-referral patterns. They can refer pain if they are injured, if they have associated soft-tissue adhesions with restrictions of normal tissue mobility, or if they suffer loss of flexibility and are subjected to increased stress during activity. Trigger points become active with abnormal or excessive stress application. These issues are discussed in chapter 6.

Soft-tissue mobilization techniques discussed in this chapter include the common pain-referral patterns and trigger point release techniques identified and advanced by Travell and Simons (1992), deep-tissue massage for relief of scar-tissue adhesions, and cross-friction massage for tendinitis treatment. You should review chapter 6 for information on other soft-tissue mobilization techniques, such as effleurage for edema.

Hip muscles that cross the knee joint or impact knee movement are discussed here. Other hip muscles are addressed in chapter 22.

Quadriceps

For the most part, soft-tissue referral pain in the anterior aspect of the knee and thigh originates from the anterior thigh and hip muscles.

The pain-referral pattern for the quadriceps covers the anterior thigh and knee. The rectus femoris and vastus medialis are the only quadriceps muscles referring into the anterior knee. The vastus lateralis refers to the posterolateral knee. The vastus lateralis also refers pain anywhere along the lateral thigh to the knee and sometimes into the posterior knee. Proximal thigh pain caused by the vastus lateralis can make sleeping on that side uncomfortable. Rectus femoris pain is usually described as a deep thigh ache, especially at night. Referred pain from the vastus medialis can sometimes cause buckling of the knee. The vastus intermedius refers into the midthigh and the upper thigh (figure 21.5a).

You can provide trigger point release either by using finger-pad pressure or by grasping the taut band. The vastus medialis is usually treated with a finger pad technique. The hip and knee are in partial flexion and hip lateral rotation, supported for comfort. The distal trigger points are more often tender than the proximal trigger points. The distal trigger points are at the muscle's medial distal border, whereas the proximal trigger points are in the midthigh region of the muscle's medial border. The rectus femoris trigger point is inferior to the ASIS, just distal to the inguinal ligament. The vastus intermedius cannot be palpated directly but can be located lateral and deep to the rectus femoris on the proximal thigh distal and slightly lateral to the rectus femoris trigger point site. The vastus lateralis has multiple trigger points located in taut bands along the muscle and can be treated with finger-pad pressure (figure 21.5b).

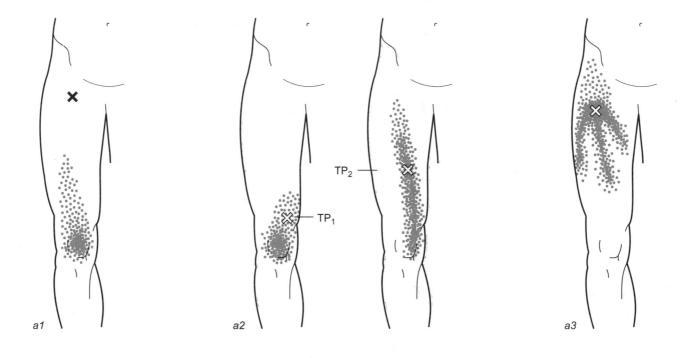

(continued)

Figure 21.5 Quadriceps: pain-referral patterns for the *(a1)* rectus femoris, *(a2)* the vastus medialis, *(a3)* the vastus intermedius , and *(a4)* the vastus lateralis.

Figure 21.5 *(continued)* Quadriceps: trigger point release for *(b1)* vastus medialis, *(b2)* vastus intermedius, and *(b3)* vastus lateralis.

Ice-and-stretch treatment is performed with the patient side-lying or supine for the rectus femoris and supine for the other quadriceps muscles. The hip is extended and the knee flexed for treatment to the rectus femoris with ice sweeps from proximal to distal along the muscle. For treatment to the vastus medialis, the hip is laterally rotated and flexed and the knee is flexed as the ice is swept from the medial superior thigh to below the knee. Ice-and-stretch for the vastus intermedius and vastus lateralis is performed with a stretch moving the knee into flexion as the ice is swept from the hip to below the knee.

Hip Adductors

The adductor longus and brevis refer pain deep into the groin, the anteromedial upper thigh, and the upper medial knee. The adductor magnus refers deep pain into the groin and distally over the anteromedial thigh. The gracilis referral pain is a superficial, hot, stinging pain along the inside of the thigh (figure 21.6a). The trigger points are located along each muscle belly.

Trigger point release is performed with the patient supine with the hip and knee flexed and the hip laterally rotated and abducted. A pillow placed beneath the thigh provides comfort. A pincher grasp or flat pressure with the finger pads can be used (figure 21.6b). The adductor longus proximal trigger points are in the muscle's upper third and best treated with a pincer grasp. Trigger points on the muscle's distal two-thirds are best treated with a flat pressure. Adductor brevis trigger points are located under the adductor longus and approached with indirect flat pressure. The adductor magnus trigger point can be located in the proximal third of the posteromedial thigh in a triangle formed by the ischial tuberosity and pubis proximally, the medial hamstrings posteriorly, and the gracilis anteriorly. Gracilis trigger points can be found in the upper third of the muscle, but may be difficult to locate. The adductor magnus trigger points can also be located beneath the gracilis and hamstrings posteriorly, just distal to the ischial tuberosity.

Ice-and-stretch is applied with the patient supine and the thigh abducted and laterally rotated and the knee flexed. Ice sweeps for the adductor magnus are applied from the knee proceeding proximally along the length of the muscle to the groin (figure 21.6c). The stretch is applied, moving the hip into abduction and flexion. Ice-and-stretch for the adductor magnus and brevis is performed with the patient's hip abducted and laterally rotated and the knee flexed with the foot against the opposite thigh. As the ice sweeps are moved from the knee and along the inner thigh to the groin, the muscle is stretched, moving the hip into as much flexion and abduction as tolerated (figure 21.7c). The gracilis muscle technique is similar to the hamstring technique with the knee straight.

TrP₁

b1

(continued)

Figure 21.6 Hip adductors: *(a)* pain-referral patterns, dark = adductor longus and brevis, medium = gracilis, light = adductor magnus; trigger point release for *(b1)* adductor magnus.

Figure 21.6 *(continued)* Hip adductors: trigger point release for *(b2)* anterior longus and brevis, *(b3)* adductor longus. Ice-and-stretch for *(c1)* adductor longus and brevis, *(c2)* adductor magnus.

Hamstrings

Pain referred from the hamstrings occurs in the gluteal fold and posterior knee with overflow along the muscle and into the distal medial calf (figure 21.7a). Semimembranosus and semitendinosus pain is often described as a sharp pain, whereas referred pain from the biceps femoris is more often a deep ache.

Trigger point release can be performed with the patient supine (for medial hamstrings only), sidelying, or prone, with the knee partially flexed to relax the hamstrings. Either a pincher grasp or flat pressure can be used for the medial hamstrings, but the lateral hamstrings are best approached with a flat pressure (figure 21.7b). A twitch response is usually seen with trigger point contact on the medial hamstrings. The trigger points are located in the middle third of the muscles.

Ice-and-stretch of the hamstrings is performed with the patient supine and the opposite extremity in extension. The involved extremity is supported at the ankle by the rehabilitation clinician. The initial distal-to-proximal ice sweeps are performed with the extremity abducted to passively lengthen the adductor magnus. Once the extremity is abducted as far as possible (the thigh should be almost parallel with the table top), the sweeps move in a proximal to distal direction while the hip is moved into adduction while maintaining hip flexion; the knee is maintained in extension throughout the motion (figure 21.7c). Once the extremity reaches a vertical position, the clinician stops the movement and dorsiflexes the ankle and extends the cold application to the calf. Passive adduction is then resumed to the end of adduction motion while in full flexion.

Figure 21.7 Hamstrings: pain-referral patterns. Dark = medial hamstrings, light = lateral hamstrings. Trigger point release *(b1)* lateral hamstrings, *(b2)* medial hamstrings, *(c)* ice-and-stretch.

Popliteus

The pain-referral pattern of the popliteus muscle (figure 21.8a) is commonly reported as posterior knee pain during activities such as running, walking down stairs and hills, and squatting. The patient may complain of knee pain when fully extending the knee.

Trigger point release is performed with the patient sidelying on the affected side with the knee partially flexed, the leg laterally rotated slightly, and the ankle in moderate plantar flexion. A flat pressure is applied in a downward and anterior direction medial to the medial head of the gastrocnemius between it and the semitendinosus (figure 21.8b).

Ice-and-stretch is performed with the patient prone. Ice sweeps begin distally and move along the muscle's path in a proximal direction as the leg is laterally rotated and the knee extended but not locked (figure 21.8c).

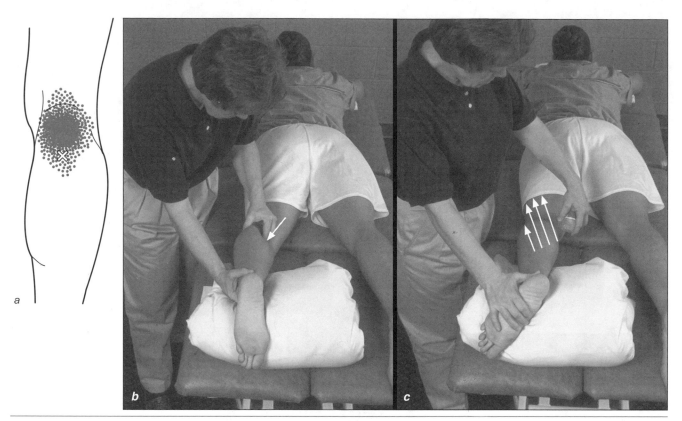

Figure 21.8   Popliteus: *(a)* pain-referral pattern, *(b)* trigger point release, *(c)* ice-and-stretch.

Tensor Fascia Lata

The tensor fascia lata refers a deep pain in the anterolateral hip from the greater trochanter and can extend as far as the knee (figure 21.9a). The pain can sometimes mimic trochanteric bursitis, making it painful to lie on the side or to run.

Trigger point release is performed with the patient supine and the knee supported in slight flexion to relax the muscle. A flat palpation of the muscle is performed distal to the anterior superior iliac spine and medial and proximal to the greater trochanter (figure 21.9b).

Ice-and-stretch is performed with the patient sidelying, the involved extremity on top. The rehabilitation clinician supports the extremity under the distal thigh and applies the ice sweeps from the anterolateral thigh distally and laterally to above the knee. The stretch is applied by stabilizing the pelvis with a hand on the lateral hip and lowering the thigh with the other hand as the thigh is moved into lateral rotation (figure 21.9c).

Deep-Tissue Massage

Two areas of the knee and thigh typically require deep-tissue massage, the quadriceps tendon and the iliotibial band (ITB). When the quadriceps tendon becomes inflamed, cross-friction massage is frequently used to relieve scar-tissue adhesions that can occur secondarily to the inflammation. The tendon fibers are cross-frictioned in the manner described in chapter 6. Because the tendon fibers run vertically from the patella to the tibial tuberosity, the cross-friction technique is applied horizontally across the fibers.

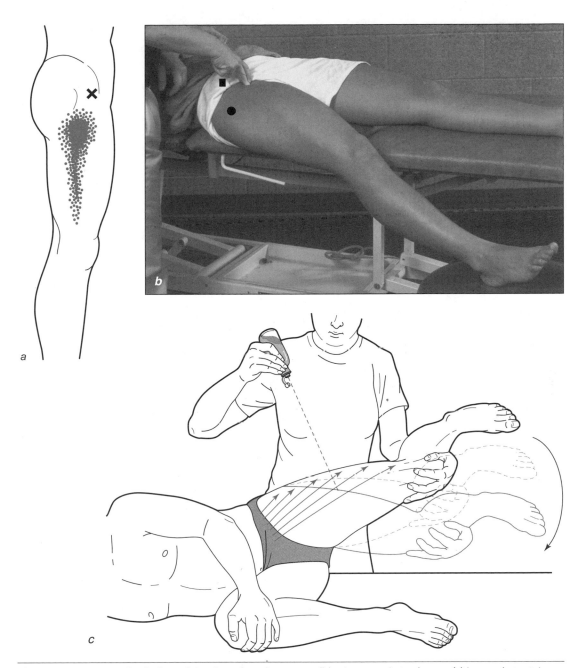

Figure 21.9 Tensor fascia lata: *(a)* pain-referral pattern, *(b)* trigger point release, *(c)* ice-and-stretch. ● = greater trochanter, ■ = ASIS.

Cross-friction massage can be used on surgical scars to prevent adhesions of skin to underlying structures. Even the portal sites of arthroscopy should be examined and treated as needed to prevent adhesions and promote good tissue mobility following surgery.

The tensor fascia lata is a frequent site of adhesions, especially following injury or the use of prolonged poor biomechanics such as seen with genu valgus. These areas along the ITB are relieved by deep-tissue massage. The rehabilitation clinician flexes the metacarpophalangeal and proximal interphalangeal joints and extends the distal interphalangeal joints so the finger pads rest in the palm. With the hand in this position, the clinician uses posterior surfaces of the middle and distal phalanx to apply pressure while guiding the hand along the patient's lateral thigh from the knee moving toward the hip. Soft-tissue restrictions can be palpated as "sticking points" as the hand moves along the lateral thigh. The clinician repeats the massage

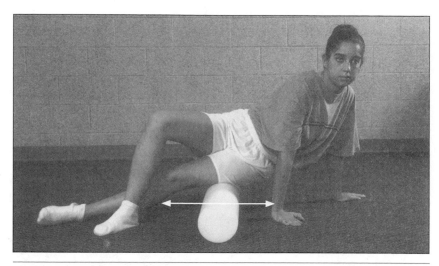

Figure 21.10   Iliotibial band foam-roller self-massage.

strokes several times, spending additional time on the more-restricted regions. As the restriction releases, tissue mobility is less inhibited and the patient reports less tenderness with the massage.

In an alternative technique, the patient can apply self-massage using a foam roller. The patient lies on the involved side, with the weight on both hands and the thigh on the foam roller (figure 21.10). He or she rolls from knee to thigh on the foam roller, spending more time on the areas that are tender and restricted. Normally, this should not produce tenderness, but tenderness will occur in areas of soft-tissue restriction.

The foam roller can also be used to massage the quadriceps muscle if it becomes restricted from immobilization or injury (figure 21.11). The patient lies prone with weight on both forearms and with the anterior thighs on the foam roller. He or she uses the arms to move the roller from the hips to the knees, spending more time over the tender sites.

Figure 21.11   Quadriceps foam-roller massage.

JOINT MOBILIZATION

▶ Joint mobilization techniques for the knee include anterior glides for extension, posterior glides for flexion, and rotational glides for terminal flexion and extension.

Injury, surgery, edema, and immobilization can lead to reduced joint mobility involving the patellofemoral joint, tibiofemoral joint, and proximal tibiofibular joint. Although the tibiofibular joint is not actually part of the knee, if it develops reduced mobility it can refer pain to the knee and affect ankle mobility. For this reason, you should assess the tibiofibular joint for mobility along with the knee joints before establishing a therapeutic exercise program.

Superior Tibiofibular Joint

Anterior and posterior glides are the mobilization techniques used for this joint. With the patient's knee and hip flexed and the foot resting on the tabletop, the rehabilitation clinician grasps the head of the fibula with the pads of the thumb anteriorly and the index and middle fingers posteriorly. The fibular head is moved anteriorly and then posteriorly (figure 21.12). The weight of the leg stabilizes the leg.

Figure 21.12 Joint mobilization: superior tibiofibular anterior and posterior glides.

Patellofemoral Mobilizations

Patellar mobility is necessary for full knee flexion-extension motion and tibial rotation.

Lateral Glide

The patient lies supine, and a rolled towel is placed under the knee for knee support. The rehabilitation clinician places both thumb pads on the medial surface of the patella. The thumbs move the patella laterally (figure 21.13a). Care must be taken to apply a lateral force, not a compressive force, on the patella.

Medial Glide

With the patient and the knee in the same position as just described, depending on which side of the treatment table the rehabilitation clinician is standing on, the clinician places the thumbs or fingertips on the lateral side of the patella and moves the patella in a medial direction (figure 21.13b). Compression of the patella into the femur should be avoided.

Inferior Glide

The patient and knee are in the position described for lateral glides. The rehabilitation clinician places a thumb and index finger around the superior rim of the patella. Being careful not to compress the patella on the femur, the clinician glides the patella distally in an inferior direction (figure 21.13c).

Superior Glide

With the patient in the position described for lateral glides, the rehabilitation clinician places a thumb and index finger around the inferior rim of the patella. A cephalic force is exerted on the patella (figure 21.13d). Compression of the patella on the femur should be avoided.

Figure 21.13   Patellofemoral joint mobilization: *(a)* lateral glide, *(b)* medial glide, *(c)* inferior glide, *(d)* superior glide.

Tibiofemoral Mobilizations

This is the joint most often mobilized to improve range of motion in the knee. Although the patellofemoral joint also can affect total range of motion, this joint has the greatest impact. For this reason, tibiofemoral mobilization techniques are outlined here.

Distraction

Distraction is a mobilization technique used for general restriction. The patient is supine with the knee supported by the rehabilitation clinician. The knee is partially flexed. The femur is stabilized with one hand proximal to the knee, and the mobilizing hand is placed above the ankle joint. The tibia is pulled distally by the mobilizing hand while the stabilizing hand secures the thigh (figure 21.14).

Figure 21.14   Joint mobilization: tibiofemoral distraction.

Anterior Glide

An anterior glide of the tibia is used to increase knee extension. This technique is performed with the patient prone. The knee is flexed with the thigh supported on the table and the patient's leg resting on the rehabilitation clinician's shoulder. A pad under the thigh will make the position more comfortable for the patient and align the thigh more appropriately for the glide. The patient's distal leg is supported on the rehabilitation clinician's shoulder. The clinician clasps his or her hands around the proximal leg near the knee and glides the tibia anteriorly on the femur (figure 21.15). The glide force must be parallel to the plane of the joint surface, so as the knee bends, the angle of the glide force changes. Before applying the mobilization force, the clinician must take note of how the joint is positioned and must apply the force accordingly. The hamstrings should remain relaxed to produce the most effective results.

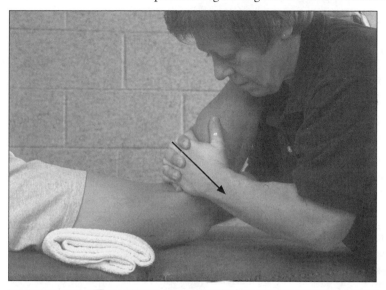

Figure 21.15   Joint mobilization: tibiofemoral anterior glide.

An alternative posterior-to-anterior mobilization technique is performed with the patient prone and the rehabilitation clinician supporting the tibia with the knee at 30° flexion. An anterior force is applied by the mobilizing hand just distal to the knee joint.

An anterior glide can also be performed with the patient sitting with the thighs on the table and the legs freely hanging over the side. The clinician secures the patient's leg between his or her knees to place the knee in a resting position and places both hands over the posterior proximal leg just below the knee.

Posterior Glide

A posterior glide of the tibia is used to increase knee flexion motion. The thigh is stabilized with the patient supine and a pad under the knee to position it in slight flexion. The rehabilitation clinician places the heels of his or her hands on the anterior proximal tibia and applies a posterior glide parallel to the joint surface (figure 21.16). In an alternative position, the patient is in sitting with the knee over the edge of the table and the thigh supported on the table with a towel roll under the distal thigh. The clinician secures the patient's leg between his or her knees to position the knee in a resting position The rehabilitation clinician applies a posterior glide at the tibial condyles.

Figure 21.16   Joint mobilization: tibiofemoral posterior glide.

Rotational Glides

If the patient is lacking the last few degrees of flexion or extension, it may be that the femur and tibia are not rotating properly. To gain those last few degrees of motion, you can mobilize the tibial condyles unilaterally.

Anterior Glide, Medial Condyle

This maneuver is used to gain lateral tibial rotation and knee extension. The patient is prone with a pad placed under the anterior thigh. The knee is flexed and supported by the rehabilitation clinician's stabilizing hand. The heel of the mobilizing hand is placed over the medial tibial plateau, and a posterior-anterior (PA) glide is applied to the medial plateau (figure 21.17).

Posterior Glide, Medial Condyle

This technique is used to gain medial tibial rotation and knee flexion. The patient is supine with a pad under the distal femur. The rehabilitation clinician applies an anterior-posterior (AP) glide with the heel of the hand on the medial tibial plateau (figure 21.18).

If the rehabilitation clinician applies the mobilizing force to the femur rather than to the tibia in AP glides or to the opposite side of the tibia in rotational glides, the opposite motions are influenced. For example, on an anterior glide of the tibia, the motion affected is knee extension. However, if the femur receives the anterior glide, knee flexion is the motion affected. So, too, if a posterior glide is applied to the lateral tibial condyle rather than to the medial tibial condyle, gains are seen in lateral rotation and extension; and if an anterior glide is applied to the lateral rather than to the medial tibial condyle, medial rotation and knee flexion are affected. If the mobilizing force is applied to the femur, the tibia must be anchored.

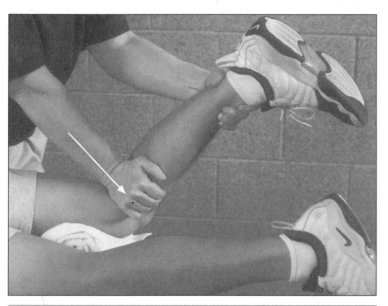

Figure 21.17   Joint mobilization: medial tibial condyle anterior glide.

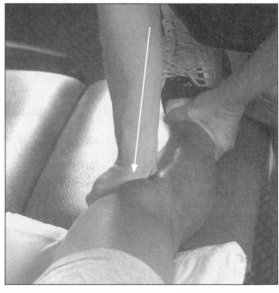

Figure 21.18   Joint mobilization: medial tibial condyle posterior glide.

FLEXIBILITY EXERCISES

▶ Flexibility exercises for the knee include prolonged extension and flexion stretches, as well as active stretches for the quadriceps and hamstrings.

Flexibility exercises for the knee can be active or passive. The specific techniques used depend on the type of tissue being stretched. If scar tissue is being stretched, the technique also depends on the age of the scar tissue. Recent scar tissue may be effectively stretched with active and short-term stretches. Scar tissue that is very adherent and is well into the remodeling phase of healing requires a combination of scar-tissue massage to loosen adhesions and long-term stretches to affect the tissue's plastic element.

Following surgical repair of the knee, orthopedic surgeons frequently have the patient's knee placed in a continuous passive motion (CPM) machine or begin early active motion. Although not used as frequently as they were a few years ago, CPMs are beneficial in reducing pain and edema and encouraging restoration of range of motion. One should not assume, however, that the CPM will restore full knee motion. You must assess the patient's knee motion at the time of the initial examination and frequently throughout the rehabilitation process.

The exercises presented here are divided into prolonged and active stretches. The active stretches include some exercises that use assistive equipment and some that require only the patient's active motion. During active stretches it is important for the patient to contract the opposing muscle whenever possible to enhance relaxation of the muscle being stretched and achieve a more effective stretch.

Prolonged Stretches

These stretches are used when scar tissue that is limiting motion is mature or is becoming mature, and a short-term stretch would be ineffective.

When using prolonged stretches, the rehabilitation clinician must inform the patient that the knee will feel stiff once the stretch is removed but that the stiffness sensation should resolve within a few minutes. It may be difficult for the patient to take the first few steps after a prolonged stretch. A prolonged stretch is more effective the longer it is applied. At first the patient may not feel that a stretch is being applied, but as time passes he or she will feel the stretch. A patient may not be able to tolerate a stretch for more than 5 or 10 min initially. If this is the case, and a weight is being used, the stretch weight should be decreased or removed to make a longer stretch tolerable. As the patient adjusts to the stretch, either the weight can be increased or the time can be lengthened; but the time should not be reduced. If an increased weight necessitates less time on the stretch, it is better to reduce the weight and permit a longer time on the stretch.

Prolonged Extension Stretch

These exercises are used to increase knee extension. They can be performed in two positions, prone or long sitting. The prone stretch can also increase rectus femoris length. The patient lies prone with the foot over the end of the table. A pad is placed under the thigh for patella comfort (figure 21.19). The patient relaxes the leg and maintains this position for 10 to 15 min. A weight on the ankle will increase the stretch force, but the weight should start light and increase only as the patient tolerates. If the hip flexes during the stretch, a stabilization strap across the hip and thigh may be necessary. You can increase the rectus femoris stretch by having the patient lie on the elbows to increase hip extension.

The other prolonged extension stretch is in the long sitting position. The knee is extended. A towel roll can be placed under the heel to lift the calf off the tabletop. A weight is applied to the thigh (figure 21.20). The patient can easily perform this stretch independently at home by placing the foot on

Figure 21.19 Prolonged extension stretch in prone.

Figure 21.20 Prolonged extension stretch in long sitting.

Figure 21.21   Prolonged knee flexion with rope system.

top of another chair or a coffee table and applying a weight on the thigh for a specified amount of time. The rehabilitation clinician must instruct the patient not to laterally rotate the leg. Applying hot packs before and during the stretch may permit a greater tolerance for the stretch.

Prolonged Flexion Stretch

The position used for this stretch depends on how much restriction of knee flexion movement is present. If restriction is severe, the patient is instructed to lie supine on a bed with a chair back against the bed. A pad is placed on the top of the chair back, and the posterior knee is positioned on top of the pad. The patient is instructed to relax the thigh and allow the leg to drop down, relaxing in this position for 10 to 15 min, if tolerable. Placing a weight around the ankle will increase the stretch force.

Using a rope-and-pulley system, the patient can perform a prolonged flexion stretch in sitting (figure 21.21). The rope is anchored to the back chair leg. The rope is attached around the patient's ankle and controlled by the patient's pulling on the rope. The patient is instructed to pull the leg back to a point that feels tight but not painful. He or she holds this position for several minutes before attempting to increase flexion farther. The exercise is repeated several times for a total of 10 to 15 min.

Active Stretches

A number of exercises are used to gain knee flexibility. The important point to remember for each stretch is to position the muscle so it is not working during the stretch. A hamstring stretch that many athletes use, standing and bending over to touch the floor, is a good example of what not to do. The hamstrings are used to hold the body upright; therefore, attempting to stretch the muscle in this position is futile because the muscle has to contract to maintain balance.

Active stretches can be repeated several times throughout the day. As discussed previously, a 20 s hold for about four repetitions is advocated. When possible, the opposing muscle should contract to produce a more effective stretch on the intended muscle.

Quadriceps Stretches

The quadriceps can be stretched using several different methods. Factors such as weight-bearing status, tolerance, agility, and balance ability determine which exercise is used. Listed here are a few examples.

Wall Slides

This exercise is used very early in the therapeutic exercise program when the patient does not have good muscular control of the joint, when the joint is painful, and when motion is significantly restricted because of pain, swelling, or recent immobilization.

The patient lies supine with the buttocks about 60 cm (2 ft) from the wall. A towel is placed between the foot and the wall, with the foot on the wall. The patient slides the foot down the wall, bending the knee as far as possible (figure 21.22). The foot, knee, and hip should remain in alignment with each other throughout the motion. The uninvolved extremity assists in returning the foot to the starting position. As motion

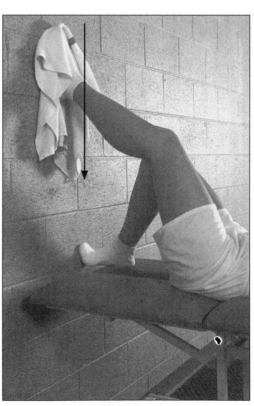

Figure 21.22   Wall slides.

improves, the buttocks are moved closer to the wall. If the patient is able to tolerate more movement, he or she can encourage more flexion by using the uninvolved extremity to push on the top of the involved extremity at the ankle.

Seated Knee Flexion

Once the patient has about 50° of flexion, he or she can perform stretches in sitting using the uninvolved extremity to move the involved knee into greater flexion. With the foot flat on the floor and the uninvolved foot across the involved ankle, the patient uses the uninvolved extremity to flex the involved knee as far as possible (figure 21.23). The knee must remain aligned with the foot and hip. This exercise can be performed throughout the day during sitting.

Standing Knee Flexion

Patients can perform this exercise once they have achieved near-normal flexibility. Standing near a table or wall to use as support, the patient grasps the foot behind the back and pulls it toward the buttocks. The body should remain in an upright position with the hips forward to include the rectus femoris in the stretch (figure 21.24).

If the patient is unable to reach the foot because of insufficient flexibility, he or she can use a stretch strap in standing. The strap is wrapped around the ankle and grasped behind the back. The strap is pulled to move the foot toward the buttock. An erect posture must be maintained for this exercise.

Figure 21.23   Seated knee flexion.

Figure 21.24   Knee flexion in standing.

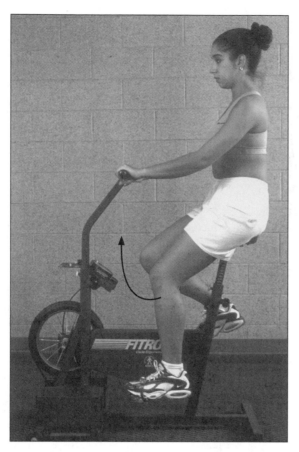

Figure 21.25
Range of motion
on stationary
bike.

Stationary Bike

Once the patient has about 90° of flexion and is allowed at least partial weight bearing, a stationary bike can be used to facilitate greater motion. With the feet secured on the foot pedals, the patient uses the uninvolved extremity to guide and control the involved extremity during pedaling. It is best to begin with a backward motion, because it is easier to achieve a full circle going backward than it is forward. Once the patient is moving the pedals smoothly in reverse, he or she can do forward cycling. The height of the seat should be such that at the bottom of the crank position, the knee is near full extension (figure 21.25). The patient may tend to shift from side to side at the hips as he or she attempts to move the crank through its full cycle, but this should be discouraged.

Hamstring Stretches

Hamstring stretches can be performed in a variety of positions. The important consideration in positioning the patient is that the muscle remains relaxed throughout the exercise. If the muscle works to maintain the position, the stretch will be ineffective.

Supine Stretches

Supine stretches ensure relaxation of the hamstrings, because the quadriceps are used to extend the knee during these exercises.

The patient lies supine with the uninvolved extremity extended. The involved knee is brought toward the chest, and the hands are clasped behind the thigh. The knee is then actively extended as far as possible so that a stretch is felt behind the knee or in the thigh (figure 21.26). The opposite extremity is kept in extension to stabilize the pelvis so that the ischial tuberosity does not roll upward and reduce the effectiveness of the stretch on the hamstrings.

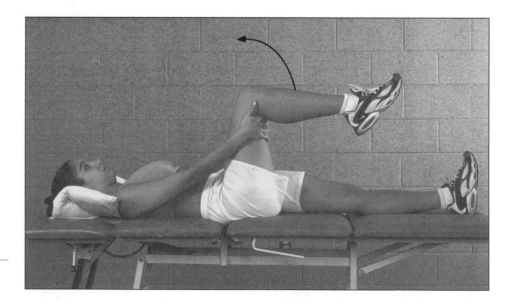

Figure 21.26 Hamstring
stretch, supine.

A stretch strap can be used around the foot if it is too difficult for the patient to reach the thigh. Another alternative is to have the patient lie supine in a doorway with the uninvolved extremity extended into the doorway and the involved foot on the wall (figure 21.27). The stretch is released by bending the knee. As the patient's flexibility increases, the buttocks are moved closer to the doorframe.

Figure 21.27 Hamstring stretch in doorway.

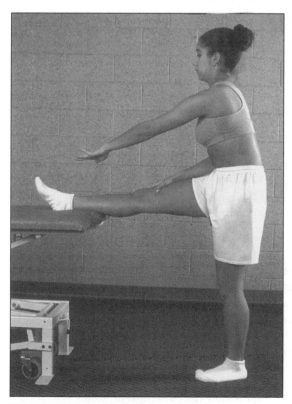

Figure 21.28 Hamstring stretch in standing.

Standing Stretch

Standing hamstring stretches assure stabilization of the pelvis because the supporting extremity remains in extension during the stretch. The height of the surface that the involved extremity is placed on depends on the patient's flexibility. With very tight hamstrings, it may be best to begin the stretch with the foot on a footstool or chair seat. The standing leg is positioned with the foot facing forward. The involved knee is kept extended during the stretch, with the foot facing the ceiling. The patient bends forward from the hips, not the back, and attempts to reach toward the toes with the opposite hand (figure 21.28). Reaching forward with the same hand allows trunk rotation. The back should remain straight during the stretch.

As the patient's flexibility improves, the height of the supporting object can be raised. If flexibility is normal, an individual should be able to touch the toes of the foot elevated to hip height with the opposite hand. The patient should not bounce during this exercise. Contraction of the quadriceps improves the flexibility during the stretch.

STRENGTHENING EXERCISES

▶ Patients with knee injuries perform many kinds of strengthening exercises, including isometrics, non-weight-bearing isotonics, weight-bearing resistive exercises, machine exercises, and isokinetic exercises.

Strengthening exercises can begin early in a therapeutic exercise program even if the knee is immobilized and weight bearing is not permitted. Isometrics can be used to retard muscle atrophy. Once active motion is permitted, isotonic activities against gravity can progress to exercises against resistance in the form of free weights, manual resistance, machine resistance, body weight when weight bearing is permitted, and isokinetic exercises.

The rehabilitation clinician must bear in mind that both hip and ankle muscles cross the knee joint and must be strengthened if they show weakness. The hip and lateral thigh muscles act as stabilizers for the knee and are important for knee control. Trunk muscles also are important for knee stability and must not be neglected. Although exercises for the trunk, hip, and ankle are not discussed here, they should be part of a total therapeutic exercise program for a patient with a knee injury.

Strengthening exercises should not cause pain or swelling either during or after the exercise. The clinician must solicit reliable feedback from the patient about the knee's response to exercises in the therapeutic exercise program, especially during the initial treatment phase and whenever there are increases in the program. Increased pain and swelling are indications that the exercises are too severe for the knee to tolerate. In the presence of these signs, the exercises should be reduced in intensity or severity. It is important not to provide too many new exercises that stress the same tissue at one time, because if the patient returns for the next treatment session with increased edema and/or pain, it is too difficult to assess which exercise caused the inflammatory response. In the early stages of a therapeutic exercise program when the rehabilitation clinician wants to move the rehabilitation process along but not overstress tissue, it is better to provide a balance of exercises that include perhaps only one or two strengthening exercises for various deficient areas rather than emphasizing only the quadriceps or only the hamstrings. For example, the first treatment session's strengthening exercises may include short-arc quads; manual resistance to hip abduction, adduction, and extension; and hamstring curls. In this case, if the patient returns with increased anterior knee pain, it is likely that the short-arc quads caused the irritation. If the patient had received short-arc quad exercises along with full-arc quad and standing squat exercises, it would be difficult to determine the cause of the new pain. Once the knee's reaction to stress has been established, it is easier to decide what exercises are likely to be tolerated; but in the beginning it is safer to add exercises cautiously.

Isometrics

Instructions of isometric exercises should emphasize a gradual buildup of the muscle contraction to a maximum level, a hold at the maximum level for 5 to 6 s, and then a gradual decline to full relaxation before the next repetition. A sudden contraction to maximal levels can cause discomfort and yields a less-than-optimal result. You should also instruct the patient to repeat the exercise in at least sets of 10 several times throughout the day.

Quad Set

This exercise strengthens the quadriceps. Perhaps the earliest exercise used to strengthen the quads, it can begin in the recovery room following surgery. With the patient supine, the uninvolved knee flexed with the foot flat on the tabletop, and the involved knee straight with the patella facing the ceiling, the patient pushes the back of the knee down onto the tabletop. Placing the hand on the quad to feel for muscle tightening helps facilitate a contraction. If the patient is unable to feel a contraction, have the individual perform the exercise with the uninvolved quadriceps to feel a normal contraction before performing the isometric with the involved knee.

If the patient is still unable to facilitate a quad contraction, you can lift the heel of the involved leg off the table about 15 cm (6 in.) and instruct the patient to hold this position as you reduce hand support. You should not completely remove your hand, though, because the patient will probably not be able to hold the position independently.

Figure 21.29 Quad set, prone.

Figure 21.30 Straight-leg raise.

If the patient has difficulty producing a quad set in supine, he or she can use an alternative position. The patient lies prone with a rolled towel under the ankle (figure 21.29). The patient then attempts to push the ankle into the towel roll, facilitating quadriceps activation. The clinician should palpate the quadriceps to monitor active contractions. Electrical stimulation can also be useful for quadriceps facilitation if the patient is unable to produce a good quad contraction with an active exercise.

Straight-Leg Raise

The straight-leg raise is a hip exercise; but because it requires the quadriceps to hold the knee in extension it is essentially an isometric exercise for the quadriceps, with the exception of the rectus femoris, which also acts at the hip.

The patient is supine with the uninvolved knee flexed and the involved knee extended. The patient first contracts the quadriceps muscle, then raises the involved extremity off the table about 20 cm (8 in.) and holds the leg at that level for about 5 s (figure 21.30). The extremity is then slowly lowered, and the quadriceps muscle is not relaxed until the extremity is on the table.

The exercise becomes more difficult if the patient is in a long sitting position rather than supine. It also is more difficult if the hip is laterally rotated during the lift rather than in a neutral position. Weights can also be used to increase the difficulty of the exercise.

Hamstring Sets

This isometric exercise assists in maintaining hamstring strength. With the patient supine, the uninvolved extremity extended, and the involved knee partially flexed, the patient pushes the heel into the table. No movement is produced. This exercise can be repeated at different knee joint angles.

Non-Weight-Bearing Isotonic Exercises

Strengthening can begin early in the therapeutic exercise program even though the patient is non-weight bearing or partial weight bearing. Open kinetic chain exercises can be useful at this stage of the program.

Short-Arc Quad Exercise

This exercise is a terminal-extension exercise to strengthen the quadriceps in the final degrees of knee extension. This exercise applies a significant stress to the ACL; therefore, this exercise should not be used early in an ACL injury or reconstruction.

A towel roll is placed under the knee to position the knee in partial flexion. The patient is supine to utilize the rectus femoris or sitting to increase the difficulty of the exercise. With the uninvolved knee flexed, the involved knee is straightened, held in full extension, and

Figure 21.31 Short-arc quad exercise.

Figure 21.32 Full-arc quad exercise.

then returned to the starting position (figure 21.31). The patient can be instructed to hold the position in full extension for about 5 s. A weight or manual resistance can be applied to the ankle to increase the difficulty of the exercise. The size of the towel roll can vary, depending on how much of an arc you want the patient to go through.

Full-Arc Quad Exercise

This exercise strengthens the quadriceps muscle, but it should be used with caution. The patellofemoral joint may be painful during this exercise; this is especially the case during the range of motion from 0° to 60° of flexion, because this range places more joint reaction force on the patellofemoral joint. The ACL is also stressed during the 0° to 60° arc of motion, so this exercise is inappropriate for recent ACL injuries.

The patient sits in a chair or on the edge of a table with the knees over the edge. The foot is lifted slowly upward to straighten the knee (figure 21.32). Manual resistance, ankle weights, or rubber-band resistance can be used to increase the exercise's difficulty.

This exercise can be used in partial ranges of motion. If necessary, the rehabilitation clinician can restrict motion manually to limit the patient's ability to extend or flex beyond a desired range; or an object such as a chair or bench can be used to block motion. Pain should not result either during or after this or any strength exercise.

Hamstring Curls

These exercises are used to increase hamstring strength. The patient lies prone with the foot over the edge of the table and the knee in full extension. The knee is flexed against gravity, manual resistance, a cuff weight, or rubber tubing. In standing, the patient is supported by the noninvolved extremity and the hands. The involved knee is flexed as far as possible. Gravity, cuff weights, manual resistance, or rubber tubing can be used to provide resistance (figure 21.33).

These two positions for the hamstring provide maximum resistance curl in different parts of the range of motion, so both positions can be used in a program. Maximal resistance in the prone exercise occurs in the beginning of the motion, in which the muscle is strongest, but the standing exercise provides maximum resistance at the end of the motion, wherein the muscle is at its physiologically weakest position.

Figure 21.33 Hamstring curl: *(a)* with cuff weight, *(b)* with rubber-band resistance.

Weight-Bearing Resistive Exercises

Once the patient is able to bear weight on the injured knee, weight-transfer activities and gait training may be necessary if the individual has been on crutches, has been non-weight bearing or partial weight bearing, or demonstrates a poor gait pattern. These activities, discussed in chapter 20, include weight-transfer exercises on a scale, gait-training activities, and use of a mirror for facilitation of weight transfer and proper gait.

Reciprocal Training

Machines such as a stationary bike, a treadmill for gait training, a step machine, or a ski machine can be useful once weight bearing is permitted. The stationary bike produces less tibiofemoral force stress than walking; it can also be used for strengthening and cardiovascular conditioning. Step machines used with controlled degrees of knee motion, and the ski machine, facilitate strength, motion, reciprocal motion between the right and lower extremities, and cardiovascular conditioning.

Platform Leg Press

Platform leg-press machines come in a variety of models and can be used in a variety of ways to exercise the quads. They are all closed kinetic chain units on which the feet remain stationary and the platform on which the body rests is moved by leg force. The most traditional method of machine use is with the patient supine and the involved foot on the platform. The patient pushes against the platform to move the sled away from the foot. The patient may initially use two legs and progress to a single-leg press (figure 21.34). Preselected and

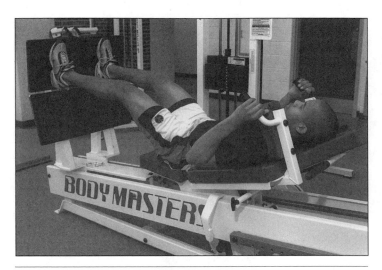

Figure 21.34   Platform leg press.

adjusted rubber bands or weights are used to vary the resistance. Ankle plantar flexion at the end of the motion can be added to provide ankle resistance. To reduce patellofemoral stress, the foot should be positioned on the platform so that the knee is flexed no more than 90° in the starting position. The knee should remain in alignment with the hip and ankle throughout the movement.

In the supine position, you can add resistive concentric and increased eccentric activity by having the patient push off the platform and catch himself or herself as the feet return to the platform. The speed of this exercise depends on the force with which the patient pushes off the platform and the amount of resistance used.

If the patient is in a tripod position on elbows and knees with the involved foot on the platform, the foot should be placed high on the platform to facilitate the quads and hip extensors. In this position, the patient can perform a slow and controlled motion as well as a rapid push-off and eccentric catch; however, the faster speed is more difficult and should be used only after the patient has demonstrated proficiency with the slower exercise.

Wall Squats

This exercise strengthens the quads. The patient stands with the back to the wall and the feet out in front. He or she squats to bend at the hips and knees, but the knees should remain over the ankles so that the leg does not go beyond a perpendicular line to the floor. If the knee is flexed more than 90°, patellofemoral stress increases and pain may result. The deeper the squat, the farther away from the wall the feet should start so that from the wall the knee is never flexed more than 90° in the squat position. Placing a ball between the knees is thought to increase response from the vastus medialis, but this theory has recently been challenged (Mirzabelgi et al. 1999).

The patient can hold this position in an isometric for several seconds or move up and down without pausing in the low position. A Swiss ball can be placed between the wall and the patient if repetitions without an isometric hold are used.

Common errors with this exercise include positioning the feet too close to the wall so that flexion goes beyond 90°, placing more weight on the uninvolved extremity, and hiking the hip so that the knee does not flex as much. If the patient is reluctant to bear weight equally on left and right extremities, a small platform placed under the uninvolved foot can facilitate increased weight bearing on the involved extremity.

You can advance this exercise by increasing the repetitions or sets, increasing the depth of the squat (as long as the knee does not move in front of the ankle in the end-squat position), or having the patient perform the exercise with one extremity only (figure 21.35).

Plié

This exercise strengthens the quads, especially the VMO. The patient stands with the feet in a wide stance with the hips and feet turned outward about 45°. The buttocks are squeezed as the patient slowly bends the knees, keeping the knees in line with the second toe (figure 21.36). The back should remain straight, so as the patient flexes the knees and hips, the trunk leans forward; the pelvis should not be allowed to move into a posterior tilt.

Common errors with this exercise include not aligning the knees over the second toes, causing the knees to move into a valgus position, not keeping the weight evenly distributed over right and left legs, and not keeping the back straight.

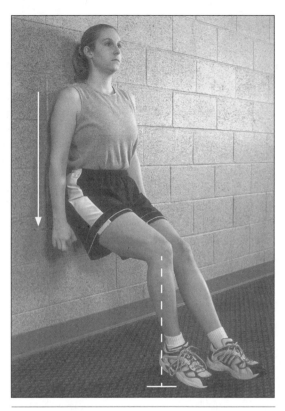

Figure 21.35 Wall squat using only right leg.

Figure 21.36 Plié.

Figure 21.37 Lunge.

Lunge

This exercise strengthens the hip extensors and quads. The patient stands with the feet in a forward-backward stance with the involved extremity in front. The quadriceps and buttocks are tightened, and the weight is shifted to the front extremity as the patient bends the knee (figure 21.37). The knee should remain in line with the second toe, and the arch should be lifted as weight is placed on the extremity. This position can be held for several seconds and then repeated.

Common errors are to allow the arch to fall and the knee to move into a valgus position. The knee should not move forward ahead of the foot. The leg should remain at an angle no more than perpendicular to the floor.

Figure 21.38   Minisquat on one leg.

Minisquats

This exercise strengthens the quads and buttock muscles. The patient stands with feet shoulder-width apart and toes turned slightly outward. Keeping the weight equally distributed, the patient squats to a comfortable position, maintaining the knees in alignment with the second toes. In a progression of this exercise, the patient grasps tubing that is anchored under the feet to increase resistance for home exercises. Holding weights in the hands increases eccentric and concentric resistance. Performing the exercise on only one extremity increases the difficulty (figure 21.38).

The back remains straight as the patient squats, so the hips flex and move posteriorly and the pelvis remains in neutral throughout the exercise. Common errors are valgus movement of the knees, trunk flexion, and hip hiking on the involved side to reduce knee flexion. If genu valgus is noted, the patient should be instructed to keep the knees over the second toe and to arch the foot; trunk flexion is corrected with verbal cueing for a straight back and instructions to push the hips back and to keep the chest up; hip hiking is corrected with instructions to bend the knee more and keep the hips level.

Step Exercises

The patient should not attempt these exercises until he or she is able to bear weight on the involved extremity in a single-leg stance position. Proper weight transfer is also a prerequisite for these exercises. The step height may begin at a low level, around 10 cm (4 in.) and increase to 20 cm (8 in.) as the patient gains strength and knee control. The rehabilitation clinician should observe the patient's exercise execution and correct errors as needed. The patient should perform the exercise in a slow and controlled manner. As with other weight-bearing resistive exercises, the knee should remain in line with the second toe throughout the motion. The knee should achieve extension at the top of the exercise, but it should not lock. During initial performance of these exercises, patients often demonstrate poor knee control evidenced by wobbling of the knee as the individual raises and lowers body weight. With gains in strength, the knee movement becomes steady with no lateral knee movement.

Common errors for these exercises include flexion at the hip and trunk to reduce the amount of quadriceps activity required, locking the knee in the extension position to reduce the need for muscular control, hip hiking to reduce the amount of knee flexion motion in the lowered position, jerking up and dropping down rather than maintaining a smooth and controlled motion throughout the motion, moving the knee into a valgus position and flattening the foot arch, and pushing off with the uninvolved leg. Usually, corrections for these errors require verbal cueing and placing the patient in front of a mirror for visual feedback during the exercise. If pushing off with the uninvolved leg, dropping down and jerking up, and trunk and hip flexion are not corrected with these cues, the height of the step may be preventing the patient from correcting the errors and it may be necessary to use a lower step.

You can advance these exercises by increasing the numbers of repetitions and sets, increasing the depth of the step, and adding weights to the hands.

Step-Up

This exercise strengthens the quads. The patient stands facing a step with the involved extremity on the step. The patient shifts the weight to the involved extremity and moves the uninvolved extremity up onto the step, straightening the knee to lift the body up. The patient should not push off with the uninvolved leg (figure 21.39). He or she then returns to the starting position.

Step-Down

This exercise strengthens the quads and gluteal muscles. It stresses the knee more than the step-up exercise does because the patient is moving forward on the extremity and the knee must move in front of the foot. If the exercise causes knee pain, it can be performed on a lower step; but if pain occurs on the lower step, the exercise should be deferred until knee control and strength increase. The patient stands on a step and slowly lowers the uninvolved extremity to the floor so that the heel touches the floor first (figure 21.40). The patient then returns to the start position, lifting the body backward. The patient should not push off with the uninvolved extremity.

Lateral Step-Up

This exercise strengthens the quads and isolates the quads more than the other step exercises do. The patient stands sideways on a step, with the involved extremity on the step and the uninvolved extremity on the ground. Only the heel of the uninvolved extremity is in contact with the ground; the toes remain off the ground throughout the exercise. The patient lifts the body weight up to the step by tightening the quads and gluteals (figure 21.41). The patient then slowly lowers the heel of the uninvolved extremity to the floor. If the patient flexes at the trunk, the hamstrings are working rather than the quadriceps.

You can provide additional overload by requiring the patient to land the heel of the uninvolved extremity out from the step to abduct the uninvolved extremity when it is lowered.

Figure 21.39 Step-up.

Figure 21.40 Step-down.

Figure 21.41 Lateral step-up.

Figure 21.42   Terminal extension.

Sit-to-Stand

This exercise strengthens the quadriceps and can increase strength in the mid-ranges of motion. The patient sits in a chair with both feet on the floor under the knees. Without using arms for assistance, the patient moves in a slow and controlled manner from the sit position to standing and then returns to the chair. The knees should remain in line with the second toes; weight should be equally distributed over right and left extremities; and the back should remain straight with the pelvis in neutral. Once the patient performs this exercise easily, he or she can advance to a single-leg exercise.

Common errors in this exercise include shifting the weight to the uninvolved side, bending the trunk, jerking up, and dropping down into the chair. Correction techniques are verbal cueing, using a mirror for visual feedback, or using a higher chair and later advancing to a lower chair as strength improves.

Terminal Extension

This exercise is used to increase weight-bearing strength in the terminal-extension range. A rubber band is anchored around a stable object such as an upright bar, door jamb, or table leg. It is placed around the knee. A pad or towel roll between the posterior knee and band will enhance comfort. The patient stands facing the door jamb or table with the knee slightly flexed to 30° to 45°, weight on the involved extremity, and the band taut. The quadriceps muscle is tightened to straighten but not lock the knee (figure 21.42). The position is held for up to 5 s and then slowly released and repeated several times.

Common substitutions for this exercise include rotating the hips, bending the trunk, and flexing the hips.

Machine Exercises

A number of machine and weight exercises are available for strengthening the knee. Some units vary in features or style from one brand to another but have underlying similarities and exercise the same muscles or muscle groups. Available equipment varies from one facility to another according to budget, space, and staff preferences. Whatever equipment is used, it is imperative for the rehabilitation clinician to be familiar with the machine, with the instructions for use and the indications, and with the precautions and dangers before using it with patients. The following sections describe exercises with a few of the more commonly used machines.

Knee Extension

This machine should be used with caution. I do not often use it because of its potential for injury to the patellofemoral joint and ACL. It provides an open kinetic chain exercise that produces patellofemoral compression in the early portion of motion and places shear stress on the ACL in the later portion of the motion. It is essential that you use this machine cautiously, if at all, and in limited degrees of motion.

I mention the knee extension unit here not because I advocate its use, but because many facilities have such a unit and therefore it is important for the rehabilitation clinician to be aware of it, how to use it, and its dangers.

The patient sits with the feet anchored around a weighted bar. To facilitate the rectus femoris, the patient should incline backward with the weight on the hands behind the hips. The individual then extends the knees (figure 21.43). If pain is produced with the machine, it should not be used.

Figure 21.43   Machine knee extension.

Figure 21.44 Machine leg press.

Machine Leg Press

The machine leg press unit strengthens the quads and calf and gluteal muscles. The patient sits (or lies supine) with the feet on a platform. The patient pushes the platform with the feet either to move the foot platform or to move the body away from the platform, depending on the machine (figure 21.44). The patient can perform the exercise with either both legs or one leg. The exercise should be performed slowly and in a controlled manner through a full range of motion.

Figure 21.45 Squat.

Squat

This exercise strengthens the quads and hip extensors. It is an advanced exercise that is not performed until a patient has demonstrated good strength and knee control with the step exercises and other closed chain activities previously outlined.

With the feet about shoulder-width apart, the weight is placed on the patient's shoulders. Keeping the back straight, the patient squats to no more than a 90° angle at the hips and knees (figure 21.45). The knees should remain in line with the second toe. The illustration demonstrates the exercise with a barbell, but the exercise can also be performed with adaptable machines such as a bench-press or heel-raise unit.

Figure 21.46 Machine hamstring curl.

Hamstring Curl

This exercise strengthens the hamstrings. Depending on the machine, the patient may lay prone, stand, or sit on the unit with the machine secured around the posterior ankle. The knee begins in an extended position, and the patient flexes the knee (figure 21.46).

Isokinetic Exercises

Isokinetic exercises for the quads and hamstrings usually begin after the patient has demonstrated control in isotonic exercises. Hamstrings and quadriceps can be exercised isokinetically, isometrically, or eccentrically on isokinetic machines. If facilitation of the rectus femoris is desired, the seat back should be reclined to extend the hip (figure 21.47). The hamstrings can be exercised in a seated position to maximize output at the knee or in prone.

Figure 21.47   Isokinetic exercises.

PROPRIOCEPTION EXERCISES

▶ A rehabilitation program for a patient with a knee injury includes a progression of proprioception exercises aimed at restoring balance, agility, and coordination.

Just as with other injured areas, balance, agility, and coordination must be restored following knee injury or surgery. Proprioception is the element basic to these parameters. Early proprioception exercises before weight bearing can include a variety of activities. For example, with eyes closed the patient can move the involved knee to mimic the uninvolved knee's position, or with eyes closed can position the knee at a designated angle. With the latter activity, the clinician measures the angle to determine the patient's ability to produce the desired angle.

Weight-bearing proprioception exercises are similar to those for the ankle as discussed in chapter 20. The patient performs stork standing on the floor with eyes open (figure 21.48a) and then eyes closed before advancing to stork standing on unstable surfaces such as the BAPS board (figure 21.48b), trampoline (figure 21.48c), or foam rollers.

Figure 21.48   Stork-standing balance progression: *(a)* on ground, *(b)* on BAPS, *(c)* on trampoline.

The next progression is to make the balance activity more challenging and to facilitate change in the activity from a conscious to a subconscious activity. To accomplish this you can have the patient perform a distracting activity while maintaining balance on an unstable surface. For example, the patient can stand on a foam roller while using an upper-extremity device such as a B.O.I.N.G., Body Blade, or other device (figure 21.49). Another example is shown in figure 20.56a.

Other balance and proprioception exercises include activities on balance boards, the Fitter, and slide boards. Activities that develop agility, coordination, and balance include jumping activities against rubber tubing with both legs and then with just the involved extremity; treadmill activities such as retro walking, side shuffle, and cariocas; and bilateral and unilateral hopping and jumping activities. Plyometric exercises with boxes develop agility and power in preparation for functional exercises. These advanced proprioception exercises are discussed in chapter 20 and shown in figure 20.58.

Figure 21.49   Advanced- and beginning-level distracting balance activities: *(a)* on ½ foam roller, *(b)* on foam roller.

FUNCTIONAL EXERCISES

▶ Functional exercises for the knee, which are similar to those for the ankle, use hopping, running, and cutting as well as sport-specific drill and skill activities.

Many of the functional exercises used for the knee are similar to those discussed in chapter 20 for the ankle. The exercises vary more according to the patient's activity demands than according to the lower-extremity segment injured, because a safe return to full participation depends on the entire lower extremity's ability to withstand stresses and perform properly regardless of the segment injured.

Functional activities include single, double, and triple hops; zigzag runs with sudden changes in direction; backward running with sudden changes to forward running; sprinting; running circles in clockwise and counterclockwise directions; 90° cuts to the left and to the right; and sport-specific drill and skill activities. Activity-specific drill and skill activities are dictated by the patient's specific sport or activity requirements. Because running, rapid changes of direction, and reliance on both lower extremities are vital to most sport participation, the running and hopping activities are universal and should be a part of most therapeutic exercise programs. These are discussed in detail in chapters 10 and 20.

Before returning to full participation, the patient must undergo an examination of functional activity performance. This examination uses many of the functional exercise activities the patient has been performing, and quality of performance is a crucial element. The patient should be able to perform all functional activities without psychological or physical impediment and should demonstrate equal use and performance with both lower extremities.

SPECIAL REHABILITATION APPLICATIONS

▶ Specific injuries to the knee and thigh that require particular types of therapeutic exercise approaches include ligament sprains, collateral ligament sprains, meniscus injuries, patellofemoral injuries, strains and contusions, and bone injuries.

This section deals with specific injuries to the knee and thigh. The more common injuries are discussed.

Ligament Sprains

Any ligament in the knee can become injured if the stresses applied are sufficient to overstress the ligament. Depending on the magnitude and direction of the forces applied, a single ligament or multiple structures can incur injury simultaneously. For the sake of simplicity, this discussion focuses primarily on injuries to individual ligaments.

Anterior Cruciate Ligament Sprain

The ACL is the knee ligament that is most frequently sprained. Considerations unique to this ligament are discussed here, and then a case study is presented.

Although daily activities apply around 454 N of stress to the ligament, it is able to tolerate up to 1,730 N before it ruptures (Dye and Cannon 1988; Markolf et al. 1990). It is in a position of maximum stress when the knee is either at full extension or at 90° flexion. The ACL is most typically injured when the knee suffers a valgus stress with lateral rotation in a foot-planted position as the athlete decelerates. The individual is often in a cutting maneuver, and the injury can occur with or without contact with another person. Sudden knee hyperextension with rotation is another mechanism of ACL injury.

When contact with another player occurs, the ACL is frequently only one of the structures injured. The MCL or medial meniscus, or both, can be involved along with the ACL when outside contact force is added to the internal stresses of cutting or hyperextension. When more than one structure is injured, the rehabilitation process becomes more complicated because it must address considerations other than those related to the ACL.

The individual may hear or feel a pop and then experience a giving way of the knee. Swelling occurs within the next 2 to 24 h, but is not apparent immediately.

Once an individual sustains an ACL injury, the decision about surgery must be made. Factors determining an individual's candidacy for ACL reconstructive surgery include age, activity level, desire to return to full participation, and knee instability. Long-term differences between ACL injuries that have been surgically treated and those that have not include arthritic changes, progressive instability, and an alteration in activity level; these changes are more prominent in ACL injuries that have not undergone reconstruction.

If a patient elects to have reconstructive surgery, motion recovery and return to participation results are best when surgery is delayed. Studies have demonstrated that surgical repair produces the best results when performed after the inflammation has subsided and full range of motion has been restored (Irrgang et al. 1997).

Over the years, many types of reconstructive surgeries for the ACL have been attempted. Surgical techniques continue to evolve, but currently the two most commonly accepted reconstructive procedures utilize either the patellar tendon or the medial hamstring tendon. The jury remains out on which technique is more effective and beneficial. The patellar tendon graft technique, which uses the central third of the patellar tendon with bone-plug ends from the patella and tibial tuberosity, is performed partially arthroscopically and also involves either one or two surgical incisions. Patellar tendon graft proponents point out that such a graft uses bone blocks, so less healing time is needed before return to full participation. The patellar tendon graft reconstruction allows immediate weight-bearing and allows therapeutic exercises two to three days following surgery. The rehabilitation time is three to six months. Advocates are also quick to point out that hamstring tendon graft reconstructions do not permit running for six months. In addition, because the fixation is not bone to bone, it has a more tenuous attachment site with greater risk of failure. Because of the weaker fixation, the rehabilitation program for the hamstring tendon graft begins later and the therapeutic exercise progression must be more conservative.

The semitendinosus and gracilis are used for the hamstring tendon procedure, which is a combined open and arthroscopic procedure. Advocates of the hamstring tendon graft procedure present the case that subjects who receive hamstring tendon grafts have fewer donor-site complications and regain quadriceps strength faster (Brown, Steiner, and Carson 1993). Donor-site problems seen with quadriceps tendon autografts include common complaints of patellofemoral pain or patellar tendinitis and, more rarely, problems of patellar tendon rupture and patellar fracture. There are pros and cons to both procedures. The physician's choice may depend on the patient's history and the physician's personal preference. The central-third patella tendon graft has high tensile strength, stiffness, and fixation strength, while the hamstring tendon graft has lower surgical morbidity during the harvesting (Brown, Steiner, and Carson 1993). If the ACL-deficient knee is chronic, a patellar tendon graft may be more successful because of its greater stiffness and the probable laxity that has developed in the knee's secondary restraining structures. If the patient has a history of patellar tendinitis, patellofemoral pain, or patellar dislocations or has a failed patellar tendon ACL reconstruction, he or she is a likely candidate for the hamstring tendon graft.

Rehabilitation following ACL reconstruction follows two schools of thought, one for delay and the other for acceleration. Some advocate using the accelerated program with competitive and serious recreational athletes and the more conservative program with less serious recreational athletes (Wilk et al. 1999). The primary differences between the two programs relate to the timing of weight-bearing and therapeutic exercises. Those in the delayed-program camp are concerned about the vulnerability of new tissue and feel that stressing the tissue too soon will risk detachment at the graft site, compromise the graft, and render the joint unstable. A delayed protocol includes touchdown weight bearing for the first four weeks postoperatively, knee extension motion limited by a locked brace to around 15° and full motion not permitted until week 4, and refraining from closed kinetic chain exercises for the first six to eight weeks. Running is restricted until about the fifth month, with full return to activities occurring six to nine months following surgery.

Those advocating the accelerated program for ACL reconstructions believe that there are few complications from the surgery with early weight-bearing and therapeutic exercise applications and that stability is not threatened with the accelerated protocol. Weight bearing is to tolerance immediately postoperatively. The patient may wear a brace, and it may or may not restrict knee range of motion, depending on physician preference. Within a week postoperatively, closed kinetic chain exercises are started, with return to full participation in five to six months.

Histologically, the ACL graft undergoes necrosis and remodeling once it is transplanted. Initially it is avascular, but revascularization occurs at 8 to 10 weeks and is completed around 16 weeks postoperatively. It is around 4 to 8 weeks that cellular proliferation into the graft site takes place. Because of proliferation and remodeling, it takes about 8 weeks for a graft to firmly attach to bone. Before this time, the graft is at risk of rupture. Once the graft is secure, it is safer to apply strain to the reconstructed site. A gradual progression of tissue remodeling occurs especially during the first 26 weeks, maturing the graft site and allowing it to manage progressively greater applied stresses. It may take at least a year for the graft to appear histologically normal, but it does not ever regain normal tensile strength. Although it is known that the graft strength is reduced, especially during the first few months following surgery, precise load-tolerance levels have not been determined. This means that the rehabilitation clinician must proceed with common sense, rely on available knowledge and on the patient's reports of the knee's response to treatment, and observe carefully to determine therapeutic exercise applications.

When you are designing a specific ACL rehabilitation program for a patient who has undergone reconstructive surgery, key considerations must include the type of graft and fixation used, the type of surgery performed, the surgeon's rehabilitation preferences, and other injuries present. Although the timing is different for exercises in delayed and accelerated programs, the exercises and the progression are essentially the same.

Two program timing progressions are provided here as examples of a delayed and an accelerated ACL program. In actuality, a patient's program may be accelerated or delayed or may be a combination of the two programs. Communication with the physician regarding the patient's progression is crucial to a safe and successful rehabilitation program.

Accelerated Postop Program

In an accelerated program, the patient ambulates with crutches, weight bearing to tolerance with full knee extension, immediately following surgery. Two days postoperatively, passive knee extension to 0°, active hip exercises including straight-leg raises, and ankle range-of-motion exercises begin. The patient may wear a knee brace, but it is set at 0° extension. Although CPMs are used infrequently, one may be used in conjunction with electrical stimulation to the quadriceps. By the end of the first week, the patient should have 90° range of motion with full extension.

During the second week, active range-of-motion exercises for the knee begin, as do patellar mobilization and soft-tissue mobilization. By the end of the second week, the patient should be ambulating without crutches, but he or she continues to use the brace. Gait training may be necessary. Some physicians discontinue the brace during the third week, whereas others continue it for about six weeks, with removal only for showers and passive exercises. Closed kinetic activities such as mini-squats and stationary-bike exercises with minimal tension are used during the second week. Hamstring curls, toe raises, and range of motion to 105° are included at this time.

By the third week, the patient can exercise in the pool, can add other exercise equipment, such as the ski machine and the stepper with no more than a 10-cm (4-in.) step, and can leg press through a 60° range of motion. The patient can do stork standing if weight transfer during ambulation is correct. By the end of the first month, the patient should have flexion to about 115° and full extension. Tibiofemoral joint mobilizations should be used if capsular tightness is evident. None of the exercises should increase pain or edema or give the patient the sensation of increased knee laxity.

During weeks 6 to 8, if there has been no increase in swelling and the patient has full active extension and flexion to 115° to 120° and good isometric quadriceps strength, he or she can begin ambulation without the brace. Step-up exercises on a 15-cm (6-in.) step, active knee extensions in 100° to 60° ranges of motion, and a treadmill walking program are implemented during this time. Research has demonstrated that a treadmill set at an incline slightly greater than 12% reduces ACL strain and patellofemoral strain but recruits greater quadriceps activity, and thus may be beneficial for ACL and patellofemoral rehabilitation programs (Lange et al. 1996).

During the weeks leading up to the third month, the exercises that the patient has done so far continue, progressing as tolerated and without pain and edema. By the third to fourth month, the patient can begin jogging and then progress to running and sprinting. During this time the patient advances to agility drills, plyometrics, and activity-specific drills, provided that full range of motion is present, strength is about 80% that of the uninvolved knee, and proprioception is good in static and dynamic balance activities.

During the fifth to sixth month, the program continues with strengthening and flexibility exercises and advances to more functional activities as the patient prepares to return to full sport participation. Because the physician often relies on the rehabilitation clinician for the information needed to determine readiness to return to full participation, an appropriate assessment is necessary. Before returning, the patient must pass all aspects of the functional examination; have full motion, strength, and normal proprioception; and be pain free without edema postexercise.

Conservative Postop Program

A delayed program has the same progression, but at a slower rate. Weight bearing progresses from non-weight bearing during the first two weeks, and then to toe-touch weight bearing during the third through sixth weeks. By the sixth to eighth week, the patient is full weight bearing. Patellar mobilization is started during week 2, and electrical stimulation and modalities for pain and edema modulation can begin during the first week. During the first week, stretching exercises for the hamstrings, gastrocnemius, ITB, and quads can begin along with straight-leg raises and quad sets. Cardiovascular activities are limited to an upper-body ergometer or unilateral stationary cycling with the uninvolved extremity.

Other exercises are not added until week 5 to 6, when the patient begins hamstring curls, hip exercises, and stationary-bike exercise. Extremity-press-machine exercise with restrictions in motion of 10° extension to around 60° to 70° of flexion can also start. Pregait activities that include weight shifting and proprioception exercises begin at this time.

Once the patient is full weight bearing, mini-squats, toe raises, wall sits, BAPS activities, and an aquatic program can be added. Active knee extensions from 90° to 30° are added as well. These exercises continue to progress as the patient is able to tolerate them, without increases in swelling or pain, throughout the program. At week 9 to 10, treadmill walking, stepper-machine exercises, and ski-machine activities can begin.

Jogging progressing to straight running is not permitted until about six months postoperatively. Cutting and lateral movements are permitted after the sixth month. A progression of plyometrics, agility exercises, and functional activities is gradually incorporated into the program.

During the 8th through 12th month, once the patient has passed the same examination tests as in the accelerated program, return to full sport participation is permitted.

Non-Operative Program

Patients who sustain partial ACL tears or who opt not to have surgery must undergo a therapeutic exercise program to rehabilitate the injured knee. The emphasis for these patients is on hamstring strengthening and use of the hamstrings to act as a secondary stabilizer for the ACL-deficient knee. A brace is usually used for three to six weeks, with partial weight bearing advancing to full weight bearing over the first three weeks. The brace may be restricted to 15° extension and 90° flexion and advance to 0° extension by week 3 to 5. During the first two to four weeks, the exercises include quad sets, hip exercises including straight-leg raises, knee flexion range-of-motion exercises, and hamstring curls. Patellar mobilization is performed. Electrical stimulation for quadriceps facilitation and pain- and edema-modulating modalities are also used.

During weeks 3 to 4 the brace is removed for range-of-motion exercises, cocontraction activities for the hamstrings and quadriceps, resisted hamstring curls, stationary-bike exercise, and other closed chain exercises such as minisquats and stork standing to begin. The patient can perform pool exercises and exercises emphasizing hamstring function.

By week 6, active extension to 0° is started, and step-up exercises and other previously mentioned strengthening exercises are used. A walking treadmill program also begins. A derotational brace is used during weight-bearing activities.

By week 8 to 10, jogging begins, progressing to running and sprinting. Once the patient is able to sprint, he or she can perform lateral activities. Agility exercises, plyometrics, and functional activities then progress as previously outlined.

Recovery from ACL reconstruction can be a slow process. In a prospective study, patients who underwent ACL reconstruction took anywhere from one to two years to regain full muscle function and pain relief (Risberg et al. 1999). The clinician must be careful always to consider the tissue healing time line and to coordinate intensity levels of therapeutic exercises with the time line. Optimal results are most likely to occur if these factors are respected.

Case Study

A 16-year-old, male soccer forward suffered a right ACL injury that was repaired last week. His physician instructed him in straight-leg-raise exercises and quad sets before discharging him from the hospital, but now the physician wants the patient to begin rehabilitation using an accelerated program. The patient is using crutches and bearing about 50% of his weight on the right lower extremity. He has a rehabilitative brace on the knee, with the knee joint set at 0° extension and 90° flexion. He is allowed to remove the brace for passive activities only. The knee has minor edema and some ecchymosis around the knee and into the proximal leg. The surgical repair was a patellar tendon transfer; the patient has two scars, one over the patellar tendon and one over the distal lateral thigh, in addition to portal scars from the arthroscopy. The surgical scars are healing well but still have sutures that will be removed next week. There are some soft-tissue adhesions around the knee, especially surrounding the surgical sites and the patellar pouch areas. The patient reports only minor postoperative pain. Patellar mobility is about 50% normal in all planes, but the patient does not report pain with movement. Alignment of the patella is normal, without the presence of patella alta or baja. The patient is able to perform a straight-leg raise but is unable to tolerate any resistance to the motion. Hip adduction is 3+/5, hip abduction is 4–/5, and hip extension is 4–/5. He reports some pain with attempts at full weight bearing but admits that he is very apprehensive about putting full weight on the extremity.

Questions for Analysis

1. What will your first treatment for this patient include today?

2. What will your goals for this first treatment today be?

3. What pregait activities will you use to encourage the patient to put more weight on the right lower extremity?

4. What instructions will you give him before he leaves today?

5. What exercises will you include in his program over the next two weeks?

6. Over the next six weeks, what exercises will you assign, and what will be your criteria for advancing the exercises during that time?

7. How long do you expect the patient's program to take, assuming that he follows a program without complications or problems?

8. When will you have him start on a treadmill, and what will be your first exercise on it?

9. Outline a progression from the treadmill to a full running program.

10. List four exercises you will include in the patient's functional activities program.

11. Describe the functional tests you will use before the patient is allowed back to full sport participation.

Posterior Cruciate Ligament Sprain

PCL injuries are not as frequently surgically repaired as ACL injuries. Necessary special considerations for this ligament are discussed here, and then case study is presented.

PCL injuries occur less often than ACL injuries. The common mechanisms of injury are either hyperextension of the knee or falling onto a flexed knee. Although reconstructions using the semitendinosus, middle third of the patellar tendon, or the medial gastrocnemius are occasionally performed, most often injury management is non-operative with emphasis on rehabilitation. Surgical repair is performed if the knee is unstable or if other ligaments have been injured as well as the PCL.

Stresses to the PCL are different from those applied to the ACL. The PCL experiences a progressive increase in shear stress in a resisted open kinetic chain flexion exercise as the knee moves from extension to flexion. The amount of PCL shear stress during resisted knee extension is a bit more controversial. Some investigations have found high PCL shear stresses in the 85° to 100° ranges of motion with less posterior shear as the knee reaches full extension when anterior shear stress increases (Wilk et al. 1999). In closed kinetic chain exercises, the posterior shear stress becomes progressively greater going from extension to flexion with the greatest stresses occurring in the 70 to 100° ranges of knee flexion. It is advisable, then to keep OKC extension exercises to no more than 60° of flexion, avoid OKC resisted flexion exercises until the PCL is adequately heeled to withstand those stresses, and keep CKC exercises in a similar range as the OKC extension exercises, 0° to 60° (Wilk et al. 1999).

PCL-deficient knees do not generally feel unstable unless the person is walking down an incline, because the PCL protects the tibia from posterior displacement on the femur (or anterior femoral displacement on the tibia). Most patients are able to return to full participation following an appropriate rehabilitation program without surgical reconstruction.

The initial goals of rehabilitation are to resolve the inflammation and restore range of motion. Once the inflammation is under control, important goals are restoration of strength, control, and normal function. Modalities for modulation of pain and edema along with electrical stimulation for muscular facilitation are used initially. Range-of-motion exercises include active knee extension and passive flexion. Active hamstring exercises should be avoided because they produce posterior translation of the tibia on the femur. Strong gastrocnemius contractions should also be avoided beyond 30° of knee flexion because of the translational stress applied to the joint and stress added to the PCL (Durselen, Claes, and Kiefer 1995).

Open kinetic chain exercises within a safe range of motion can provide good isolated strengthening for the quadriceps as long as patellofemoral pain is avoided. If patellofemoral pain occurs, the exercises should be modified to avoid the pain. Modifications can include changing the degrees of motion and angles of the exercise, reducing the resistance, reducing the lever arm of the applied resistance, and using low weights with higher repetitions. These exercises include quad sets, straight-leg raises, and quad range-of-motion exercises. Crutches are used in weight bearing to tolerance with gradual progression to weight bearing without assistive devices. A closed kinetic chain exercise in terminal extension with rubber tubing can be used to strengthen the hamstrings and produce minimal posterior tibial translation (see figure 21.42). The hamstrings can also be strengthened in an open kinetic chain exercise for the hip extensors if the patient keeps the knee extended to reduce the posterior tibial shear stress.

Once the patient has progressed to full weight bearing, other closed kinetic chain exercises can begin. Gait training may be necessary if the patient is unable to assume a normal gait. Weight transfer activities may be indicated if the patient is reluctant to bear weight on the extremity. Proprioception exercises should emphasize recruiting the quadriceps for posterior translation control, first in static positions and advancing through dynamic activities. By the third week, exercises such as wall squats progressing to standing squats, step-ups, and other CKC exercises can be added to the program. By about the sixth week, the program can progress from treadmill walking to jogging, running, increased weights, agility exercises, plyometrics (stressing deceleration activities, pivoting, lateral movements, and jumping), and functional activities. Knee control for posterior tibial translation should be emphasized throughout the program. By the 9th to 12th week, the patient should be able to begin functional and specific activities and return to full participation.

PCL injuries that are surgically reconstructed are immobilized with a brace that is locked in 0° extension for four weeks and is worn for a total of six to eight weeks, with free range of motion permitted in the last two weeks of wear. The brace is removed after the first week for passive exercises only. The patient is able to ambulate with PWB on the leg for the first three weeks with a progressive increase in weight bearing to full weight bearing by the end of the 3rd week. In the early phase, the leg should be supported when the patient is in long sitting to prevent posterior sag of the tibia on the femur. During the first week, quad sets, straight-leg raises, and short-arc quad (SAQ) exercises are started. Patellar mobilization is performed. Hip extension and knee flexion activities are avoided during the first three weeks, but hip adduction and abduction exercises can be used with resistance applied proximally on the leg. Once the patient is full weight bearing, weight transfer activities, wall squats, weight bearing proprioception and balance activities, and a stationary bike can be initiated and progressed as the patient tolerates it.

After about six weeks, the patient should have full passive range of motion and normal gait. Hip extension with the knee in extension, exercise on the stationary bike with toe clips to reduce hamstring activity, and progressive balance activities are also included.

By 6 to 10 weeks, mild resistive hamstring curls can be initiated along with treadmill walking, step machine, ski machine, and pool running activities. Resistive exercises continue to be progressive for the quads and other lower extremity muscle groups.

The progression for a surgically reconstructed PCL is the same as for the ACL program, with advancement to agility, plyometrics, and functional activities. The patient is able to return to full sport participation after 6 to 12 months, depending on the individual patient's response to the program.

Case Study

Last week an 18-year-old, female volleyball player injured the left posterior cruciate when landing hyperflexed after hitting a ball. The physician will not perform surgery because the knee is stable. He wants you to begin the rehabilitation process with the patient today.

Your examination reveals moderate edema around the knee. The patient has a brace and is able to bear partial weight on the left extremity. Her range of motion out of the brace is 30° to 60°. Her patellar mobility is limited by about 75%, but her knee is too flexed for you to decide whether the restriction is attributable to the knee position or to reduced patellar mobility. She has pain at 6/10. Although there is edema around the knee with some discoloration, the soft tissue feels tight from the edema pressure. Her strength is 4–/5 in hip flexors and abductors and 3+/5 in hip extensors, adductors, and quads. You have deferred hamstring testing because of the PCL injury.

Questions for Analysis

1. What will your first treatment with the patient today include?

2. What instructions will you give her to do at home?

3. What exercises will you include in today's session?

4. Outline your expected time line for beginning hamstring exercises, walking on a treadmill, and stationary cycling. Will you use pool exercises with the patient? If you will use the pool, list three exercises.

5. List four agility exercises and functional skill activities you will include in the last phases of her therapeutic exercise program.

6. List the functional tests you will use to determine when the patient is ready to return to full sport participation.

Collateral Ligament Sprains

The MCL can be injured by itself or in combination with other knee structures. Collateral ligament injury treatment is different from cruciate ligament treatment.

Medial collateral ligaments are more frequently injured than LCLs. An MCL injury occurs as the result of a valgus stress, and an LCL injury results from a varus stress to the knee. Medial collateral ligament injuries are rarely surgically repaired except when instability results from a combination of ACL and MCL tears. In those situations, the MCL may or may not be repaired even if the ACL is repaired.

The rehabilitation programs are similar for MCL and LCL injuries. Initial treatment includes modalities for pain and swelling modulation. The current philosophy in treating isolated collateral ligament injuries is to use a brace in conjunction with an early therapeutic exercise program (Reider 1996). The patient's injured knee is placed in a functional or rehabilitative brace with limits set at 0° extension and 90° flexion to control ligament stress yet still allow motion. The brace is worn for three to six weeks; and crutches, with either non-weight bearing or weight bearing to tolerance, are used for two to four weeks. During this time, active range-of-motion exercises, isometric exercises to retard quad and hamstring atrophy, and hip and ankle exercises are used. Patellar mobilization may be necessary if the joint becomes stiff. Cross-friction massage to soft tissues can be helpful in promoting healing and preventing adhesions. In 7 to 10 days, pool exercises are useful for range of motion and strength. After about two weeks, the stationary bike can be used if the knee has about 105° of flexion. Before that time, the patient can use the bike as a means of increasing range of motion.

A combination of open and closed kinetic chain exercises is used to increase hamstring and quadriceps strength. These exercises follow the progression outlined for cruciate ligament injuries and must not produce patellofemoral pain or increase collateral ligament pain. Once the patient is ambulating in full weight bearing, stork standing and other balance activities can begin. Walking on the treadmill with progression to jogging occurs once a normal walking gait has been achieved. Jogging then progresses to running and sprinting as long as pain and edema are avoided.

If full motion is not achieved by around week 5 or 6, joint mobilization techniques and prolonged stretches may be required. The patient progresses in strength and agility exercises as long as there are no deleterious signs. The program advances from agility and plyometrics to functional activities. A functional knee brace is often used before and after return to sport. The collateral ligament brace does not require the rotational stability that an ACL brace does, but it should have medial and lateral upright supports to control valgus and varus stress.

An individual's tolerance and the severity of the injury will determine the patient's rate of progression. Return to normal function can occur in as few as three to four weeks or can take as long as two to three months.

Meniscus Injuries

Among all the rehabilitation programs for knee injuries, the rehabilitation program for meniscal injuries has seen the greatest changes over the past several years. Current trends in treatment allow for a more rapid return to participation than in the past, with reduced deleterious effects.

Surgical treatment of meniscal injuries has evolved over the past several years. Arthrotomies for complete removal of damaged meniscus have been replaced by arthroscopic procedures for partial removal of torn segments, repair, and allograft replacements.

Isolated injury to the medial meniscus does not result in instability to the knee, but if a meniscal tear is combined with an ACL rupture, the knee becomes unstable. Isolated meniscal tears tend to be degenerative tears, whereas meniscal tears that accompany ACL injuries are more likely to be acute (Shelbourne et al. 1996). A stable knee with a meniscal injury may not be a candidate for a meniscal repair, but an unstable knee will become more unstable if

Case Study

A 17-year-old, male gymnast suffered a grade II sprain of his right MCL during a rings dismount three days ago. The physician wants him started on a rehabilitation program. For the past three days he has received ice, elevation, compression, and electrical stimulation for edema control. He is on crutches with a hinged brace set at 0° and 90°. He is bearing about 75% of his body weight on the right extremity when he ambulates. There is moderate swelling with tenderness to palpation along the MCL. His hip and hamstring strength is grossly 4/5. He has an extensor lag of 15°. He reports mild pain unless he attempts to bend the knee past 60°; then the pain level becomes moderate. Patellar mobility is normal.

Questions for Analysis

1. What will your first treatment for this patient today include?

2. What home program will you give him before he leaves your facility today?

3. Outline the exercise program you will have the patient perform for the next week. How will you determine his progression?

4. List three open kinetic chain and three closed kinetic chain exercises you will have him perform within the next two weeks, and list them in the order that you will assign them.

5. What agility exercises will you include in his program?

6. What plyometric exercises will you use?

7. Describe the functional activities you will use in your assessment to determine when the patient is ready to return to full sport participation.

---

the meniscus is removed or partially removed. Knees that undergo a meniscal repair with an ACL repair do better than with an isolated meniscal repair (Tenuta and Arciero 1994).

Lateral meniscal repairs and lateral meniscectomies have a greater success rate than medial meniscal repairs. One may presume that the higher success rate of lateral meniscectomies and their lower impact on ACL-deficient knees is attributable to the lower amount of movement on the lateral knee and the smaller attachment the lateral meniscus has to the knee.

Meniscal repairs must have a viable blood supply to be successful. The peripheral rim of the menisci has a blood supply, but the majority of its inner substance is avascular. Meniscal blood supply can reach inward as far as 6 mm (about 0.25 in). Tears that occur over the outer third of the meniscus have the best healing capabilities. Tears that extend inward farther than the blood supply do not do well with meniscal repair procedures. Surgeon's preferences regarding the width of the meniscal tears that do well with repairs are variable, and range from 2 mm to 6 mm (Scott, Jolly, and Henning 1986; Stone, Frewin, and Gonzales 1990). Up to 20% of all meniscal tears are reparable. Meniscal repair is advantageous over meniscectomy because the meniscus remains, and there is consistent evidence that even partial meniscectomy leads to osteoarthritic changes in the joint. The rehabilitation process, however, is significantly longer for a meniscal repair than for a meniscectomy. Whereas a rehabilitation program for a meniscectomy generally requires four to six weeks, a patient is often restricted from sport participation after a meniscal repair for four to six months.

The patient who has a medial meniscus and ACL injury that both require surgical repair is a difficult case for the surgeon and rehabilitation clinician. Meniscal repairs do better if performed as soon after the injury as possible. Following the meniscal repair, the postoperative care is conservative, with non-weight bearing and limited motion for up to six to eight weeks. On the other hand, the ACL repair is most successful when delayed until after the inflammation is resolved and with immediate postoperative partial to full weight bearing and motion.

Traditionally, the postoperative care for meniscal repairs has been conservative, but accelerated programs have been used more recently (Barber 1994). There is much controversy about use of an accelerated program for meniscal repairs. The conservative protocol guards the repair by using limited motion and weight bearing to reduce the shearing forces applied to the repair. The accelerated program limits the time on crutches and uses partial weight bearing and active motion in the early stage to apply appropriate stresses to healing tissue and prevent unwanted loss of motion and patellofemoral pain problems. The rehabilitation clinician must communicate with the physician to create a feasible rehabilitation program for the patient who has received a meniscal repair.

Conservative Postop Repair Program

A conservative postoperative meniscal repair program includes placing the patient on crutches, non-weight bearing on the involved extremity for six to eight weeks. Toe-touch weight bearing is sometimes allowed after two weeks, with slowly progressive increases in weight bearing to full weight bearing at six to eight weeks. A rehabilitative brace is used to keep the knee in a flexed position for about six weeks after surgery. During this time of immobilization, the patient can perform trunk, hip and ankle exercises. Manual resistance to the hip should be applied above the knee to prevent stress on the knee joint. Once the brace is removed, patellar mobilization, and after six to eight weeks tibiofemoral joint mobilizations, can be used. Active range of motion and a progressive strengthening program begin after the brace is removed. Crutches are discarded when the patient is able to walk normally and has adequate quadriceps strength to control the knee. Pivoting and acceleration-deceleration activities are not allowed for four to six months after surgery. From then on, the patient progresses to functional activities before returning to sport.

Accelerated Postop Repair Program

In an accelerated program, weight bearing is allowed as the patient tolerates it, but the patient uses crutches until he or she is able to walk normally. Range-of-motion exercises are used during the first postoperative week. Quad sets and straight-leg raises also begin during the first two weeks. The goal during the first few weeks is to achieve full range of motion without increased edema in the knee. By the end of week 2 to 3, the patient should be able to ambulate normally without crutches.

In week 2 to 4, the patient can use pool exercises, closed kinetic chain exercises including those on a stationary bike, mini-squats, and a walking treadmill program. By week 6 to 8, isokinetic exercises are suitable. Jogging progressing to running is added before lateral and pivoting movements are allowed. By that time the patient should have about 80% quad strength. The progression then follows that outlined for the ACL programs, with return to participation at 10 to 12 weeks postoperatively.

Meniscectomy Program

If the meniscus is not reparable, an arthroscopic partial meniscectomy is often the surgery of choice if the patient continues to experience knee locking or giving way following the injury. The patient may be placed on crutches immediately postoperatively because of reflex inhibition of muscle activity subsequent to surgery and edema. Weight bearing is to tolerance with the expectation that the patient will be able to walk without assistance in the next few postoperative days as the pain and edema subside and knee control improves. Quad sets and straight-leg-raise exercises can begin immediately postoperatively, but often the patient has difficulty with these exercises on the first day because of reflex inhibition. Electrical stimulation can aid the quadriceps in regaining function. A combination of open and closed kinetic chain exercises is used within the first two to three days after surgery. Gait-training and weight-transfer activities may be necessary if the patient demonstrates an abnormal gait. Wall slides for range of motion, ankle pumps, hip exercises, and hamstring stretches can begin on the first or second day. Minisquats, wall squats, step-ups and step-downs on a small step, standing terminal extensions, stationary-bike exercise, tubing exercises, and use of free weights can all start at this time as the patient tolerates. Once the patient is able to transfer weight appropriately onto the involved extremity, static balance activities are used to increase proprioception, advancing to dynamic balance activities.

By the second week, step-up exercises can usually be tolerated. Lunges can be added at this time. The slide board, ski machine, and stepper can also be used. A jogging program is started by week 3 to 5, progressing to running as the patient responds to the stresses appropriately without increased swelling or pain.

Isokinetic, agility, plyometric, and functional activities are the last progressions before the patient's return to full sport participation. These are added to the program once the patient has good control with adequate strength and coordination. Although the timing varies from one patient to another, these activities are usually added around week 5 to 6, with full return to participation within six to eight weeks postoperatively.

Postop Autograft Transplant Program

Rarely, the surgeon may opt to perform an autograft meniscus transplant. Transplantations can be performed arthroscopically or with an open procedure. Sutures with bone plugs at either end of the meniscus are used as the anchors for the graft (figure 21.50). Postoperative care guidelines have been primarily reported as case studies (Fritz, Irrgang, and Harner 1996). Program progression, as with other conditions, is based on a combination of tissue healing and knowledge of stresses and loads applied to the menisci.

Rehabilitation for meniscal transplants involves non-weight bearing or partial weight bearing on the involved extremity for six weeks. Continuous passive-motion and range-of-motion exercises are used immediately postoperatively, with flexion limited to 90°. The patient wears a brace to maintain the knee in extension when not exercising in order to reduce the shear stress on the graft for about six weeks. Patellar mobilization techniques can be used to maintain good patellar mobility while the patient is in the brace. Treatment goals in the first six weeks are to control the inflammation, maintain full knee extension, minimize quadriceps atrophy, and protect the graft.

Figure 21.50   Meniscal transplant.

After six weeks, gait training without the brace begins, as do closed kinetic chain exercises from full extension up to 60° flexion. As mentioned earlier, compressive loads on the menisci increase to 85% of those for the entire knee at 90° flexion; so flexion greater than 60° is avoided in the closed kinetic chain, but motion to 90° is permissible in an open kinetic chain motion. Continued protection of the graft with normal gait and increased motion and strength becomes a goal as the program progresses for the next six weeks. Closed chain exercises include toe raises, minisquats, wall sits, leg presses, and step-ups. Open chain exercises include range-of-motion exercises, hip exercises, and pool activities. Standing balance activities begin at this time. Progression continues as the patient tolerates and as he or she shows no signs of unwanted stress.

Rehabilitation progression for a meniscal transplant procedure follows that for most other programs but at a slower rate. Once the patient has adequate strength, range of motion, and coordination to control the knee, agility, plyometric, and functional activities proceed. Full return to normal participation may take around 8 to 10 months or longer.

Case Study

A 20-year-old male ice hockey forward experienced a left knee meniscal tear. He underwent an arthroscopic partial meniscectomy yesterday and comes to you today to begin his rehabilitation program. He is walking without crutches, but he has an antalgic gait on the left extremity. He reports mild pain and a sensation of tightness around the knee. Your examination reveals swelling of 2.5 cm (1 in.) around the knee. The patient's active range of motion is –15° extension and 90° flexion. Passive range of motion is 0° extension and 100° flexion. He is able to perform a straight-leg raise but cannot tolerate resistance in the motion. Other hip motions are 4/5. Hamstring strength is 4–/5. The patella is slightly restricted in mobility.

Questions for Analysis

1. What will your first treatment with the patient include today?

2. What will you give him as home exercises and instructions before he leaves today?

3. What are your goals with him for the first week of treatment?

4. Preseason hockey practice begins in two months. What will you tell the patient when he asks you whether he will be ready by then?

5. When do you expect him to be able to begin squats with weights?

6. What will you say when the patient asks you why he cannot straighten the knee when he could before the surgery?

7. Present a progression of proprioceptive exercises that you will have in this program. Discuss the progression of agility exercises you will use. List the functional activities you will include in the final phase of the patient's program.

Patellofemoral Injuries

Patellofemoral injuries can be complex injuries and frustratingly slow to respond to treatment. Several factors may contribute to patellofemoral injuries, especially those that are nontraumatic. This section deals with the most frequently seen injuries.

Patellar Dislocations and Subluxation

Patellar instability is more frequently seen in women than in men. This is thought to be the result of an increased Q-angle secondary to a wider pelvis, which increases the lateral vector force on the patella. Other predisposing factors include a shallow lateral femoral condyle or posterior patella, an improper position of the patella, and a weak VMO, especially if it is combined with tight or strong lateral structures.

The mechanism for injury is lateral rotation of the thigh with knee flexion on a planted foot. If the patella is subluxed, it often relocates independently. A frank dislocation may or may not relocate on its own. First-time dislocations may not relocate, but recurrent ones often do without assistance. Pain and edema are severe.

Treatment includes use of crutches with weight bearing to tolerance. An immobilizer brace may be initially used with progression to a functional brace to stabilize the patella. Therapeutic exercise progresses to the patient's tolerance. Electrical stimulation to the quadriceps and modalities for pain and edema control are applied in the early phase of a rehabilitation program, usually in the first two weeks. Increases in pain and edema are avoided throughout the program. Patellofemoral pain can be produced at any time, but especially in the early phases of rehabilitation when the area is still inflamed from the initial insult. All exercises should be pain free. If an exercise produces pain, it should be delayed until the patient is able to perform it without pain.

Initial exercises include straight leg raises and pain free short-arc exercises with progression into a greater arc of motion as strength gains and pain permit. Exercises are a combination of open and closed kinetic chain. Program emphasis should be on VMO strength and patellar control during activities. As strength and knee control improve, exercises progress to more rapid activities until functional speeds are possible with good patellar control.

Lower-extremity alignment should be examined in standing and walking, because pronation can increase the risk of patellar instability and can be corrected with orthotics.

The duration of a rehabilitation program depends on whether the dislocation or subluxation is a first-time event or a recurring injury. Recovery from an acute subluxation/dislocation can take more time than from a recurring injury. An average expected recovery period is 4 to 10 weeks; recurrent injuries are on the shorter side and first-time injuries require the longer recovery time.

Patella Plica Syndrome

Plicae are residual synovial folds that persist into adult life and can become symptomatic secondary to a persistent synovitis and resulting loss of normal elasticity (Galloway and Jokl 1990). A secondary synovitis can result from the presence of loose bodies, meniscal tears, instability, or chondromalacia. The plica as an extension of the synovium becomes inflamed. In persistent cases, the plica becomes fibrotic and can be palpated as a firm, inelastic band, usually on the medial aspect of the knee.

Conservative treatment includes modalities and medication to relieve the inflammation, hamstring stretching, and quadriceps strengthening. If conservative measures do not relieve the patient's pain, arthroscopic excision of the plicae may be necessary.

Rehabilitation following surgical excision follows a course similar to that for an arthroscopic partial meniscectomy. Therapeutic exercises can begin on the day of surgery and progress according to the patient's tolerance. The patient should be able to return to sport participation within three to six weeks after surgery if the postoperative course is normal.

Osgood-Schlatter Disease

In spite of its name, Osgood-Schlatter disease is not a disease but a mechanical disruption of the patellar tendon insertion site on the tibial tuberosity. It is an avulsion, an avascular necrosis, or an epiphysitis of the tibial tuberosity. It is most commonly seen in active adolescents, often after a recent growth spurt. A direct impact such as a fall on the tibial tuberosity can also cause the injury. The signs and symptoms are similar to those of a patellar tendinitis, with pain during activities such as running or jumping. Stiffness and edema can also be present.

Treatment for this condition has changed over the years. Cast immobilization used to be the preferred treatment method, but current treatment focuses on activity modification. An enlargement of the tibial tuberosity occurs, and only in extreme cases is this surgically excised. Patients can derive benefits from modalities for modulation of inflammation, pain and edema; stretching exercises for the hamstrings, ITB, and gastrocnemius; strengthening exercises to the quadriceps; and cross-friction massage to the patellar tendon. The injury is self-limiting in that the patient's activities are constrained by pain. Activity to tolerance is generally allowed once the inflammation has subsided.

Patellofemoral Syndrome

Syndromes of the patellofemoral joint can be caused by many different factors, individually or in combination. The term for this frustrating injury, "syndrome," demonstrates that the medical community has been unable to identify one specific etiology.

Mechanism

Patellofemoral pain is a common complaint among athletes as well as among those who do not participate in athletics. Anterior knee pain has been classified under various headings including chondromalacia patellae, patellofemoral stress syndrome, patellofemoral pain syndrome, extensor mechanism malalignment syndrome, runner's knee, and patellofemoral malalignment syndrome. Chondromalacia is a term that was used in the past to describe anterior knee pain. Chondromalacia refers to a specific injury that involves softening and degeneration of the patella's posterior articular cartilage and it is not an accurate diagnosis for most anterior knee pain conditions. The most commonly used terms today to describe anterior knee pain include patellofemoral pain syndrome (PFPS) or patellofemoral stress syndrome (PFSS).

Signs and Symptoms

Typical signs and symptoms of PFPS include stiffness after prolonged sitting, pain with activities such as stair climbing and running, and pain after activity. Crepitus is usually present. The patient may experience a giving way of the knee because of reflex inhibition secondary to pain, especially on stairs or ramps. Swelling is usually mild, but the posterior surface of the patella is tender to palpation.

Underlying Factors

PFPS is anterior knee pain and inflammation caused by abnormal stresses applied to the knee's extensor mechanism. Several underlying conditions can lead to PFPS. Patellofemoral pain syndrome can result from direct trauma to the patella, but is more often the result of cumulative stresses in the presence of additional contributing factors, both extrinsic and intrinsic to the joint itself. These factors are thought to include tightness in the ITB, hamstrings, and gastrocnemius; weakness in the VMO or imbalance of strength between the VMO and vastus lateralis; excessive pronation; increased Q-angle; knee hyperextension; and patellar alignment. It is likely that a patient has more than one of these factors to develop PFPS. Each elements should be evaluated when examining the patient with PFPS, because correction of or compensation for these malalignments must occur if the PFPS is to be resolved.

Normal function of all body segments relies on a balance of the surrounding structures. This balance includes adequate flexibility and proper strength so that forces are adequately and appropriately directed to produce the desired motion and force applications. If hamstring, gastrocnemius, ITB, or lateral connective tissue structures are tight, they apply an imbalance of forces on the knee. Tight hamstrings prevent full extension so the knee is in flexion during activities when it should be extended, increasing compressive forces on the patella anteriorly. If knee flexion is less than 60°, the need for increased knee flexion during ambulation is compensated by increased dorsiflexion to clear the toe. Normally 10° of dorsiflexion is necessary for ambulation; but if the gastrocnemius does not permit this motion or if the hamstrings increase the need for additional dorsiflexion but it is not available, the foot pronates in an attempt to increase flexibility. Excessive pronation necessitates tibial medial rotation, which increases the knee's valgus stress. A tight ITB pulls the patella laterally as the ITB moves posteriorly during knee flexion. In cases of severe distal tightness of the ITB, the patella is in a lateral tilt position because of the ITB's lateral pull on it.

If either the VMO is weak or an imbalance is present between the VMO and the vastus lateralis, the patella moves laterally during quadriceps contractions. This permits the patella's lateral rim to ride more on the lateral femoral condyle than in the intercondylar groove, where it normally glides during knee motion. If the vastus lateralis is tight, the lateral pull during quadriceps contractions is exaggerated. Repetitive gliding against the condyle leads to inflammation of the patella's articular surface.

If the knee is in hyperextension, the inferior pole of the patella is frequently tilted inward. This causes the patella to push into the fat pad in full extension, and to glide with an inferior tilt during knee motion, altering the relationship between the patella and femoral groove. The patella has increased contact inferiorly as it glides in the groove, increasing stresses at the inferior pole.

Patellar Orientation

Patellar orientation and alignment should be examined in a relaxed long sitting or supine position, and in closed chain positions in both static and dynamic conditions. Patellar alignment varies from one patient to another; it can also be different from left to right knee in the same individual. In a relaxed open chain position with the knee resting in slight flexion on a rolled towel and the femur in parallel alignment with the examination tabletop, the rehabilitation clinician should assess the patellar alignment in various planes. He or she should examine for the presence of a lateral glide, lateral tilt, inferior tilt, and rotation. In the examination position, the patella should rest slightly lateral to the center of the knee with the inferior pole at the knee's joint margin. If the patella's position is more than a few millimeters to the lateral aspect, it has a lateral glide. A medial glide is rare. When a finger is placed on the medial and lateral poles of the patella, they should be in the same plane; if the lateral finger is lower than the medial finger, the patella has a lateral tilt. A medial tilt is rare. When a finger is placed on the mid-superior patella surface and another is placed on the inferior patellar pole, they should be in the same plane; if the distal finger sits deeper than the proximal finger, the patella has an inferior tilt or posterior tilt. This is also referred to as an AP tilt. The superior medial and lateral poles should be in the same plane; if the lateral pole lies more superiorly on the knee and the medial pole lies more inferiorly, the patella is laterally rotated. If the medial pole lies more superiorly, the patella is medially rotated. A lateral rotation is more common than a medial rotation. These patellar positions are demonstrated in figure 21.51.

The patella's tracking pattern should be examined in non-weight bearing. With the patient contracting the quadriceps in full knee extension, the clinician observes the patella for its movement. Normal movement is 8 to 10 mm inferiorly on the femur, with some lateral motion. If lateral structures are tight or the VMO is weak, the patella will move more laterally with the lateral component occurring sooner in the motion. During knee movement into flexion, the patella migrates medially as the Q-angle decreases and the patella becomes centered in the trochlea.

Alignment should also be observed in standing, and movement of the patella should be observed while the patient performs an activity such as a lunge or step-down. Changes in patellar alignment and glide during weight bearing can indicate various influential factors that should be corrected, such as pronation, weakness, incorrect firing patterns, and tightness.

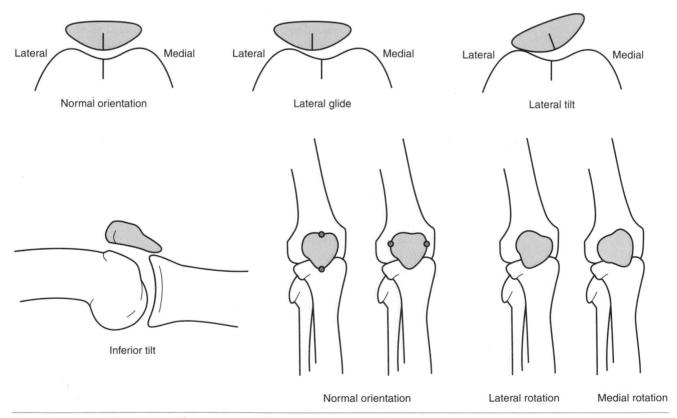

Figure 21.51 Patellar orientation.

Corrections

Common surgical procedures to treat patellofemoral pain and patellofemoral malalignment in the past included a lateral release in which the lateral retinaculum was cut, or an advancement of the tibial tubercle to allow a better patella alignment. It has been demonstrated, however, that patients with PFPS have better results with nonsurgical management that consists primarily of exercise (Karlsson, Thomee, and Sward 1996).

Determination of the underlying causes dictates what is included in the treatment program. Orthotics may be needed if pronation is present; flexibility exercises and soft-tissue mobilization techniques are necessary if tightness and adhesions exist; muscle reeducation for timing of contractions is necessary for imbalance in timing of activity or strength between the VMO and vastus lateralis; and strengthening exercises, especially for the VMO, are needed with all patellofemoral pain regardless of cause, because pain causes an inhibition reflex and weakens the quadriceps.

Patellar Taping Technique

A technique developed by Jenny McConnell, an Australian physiotherapist, uses a combination of taping to the patella and exercises. Her initial theory stated that the tape corrected patellar alignment to relieve pain and allow the patient to exercise to regain strength. Recent studies, however have shown conflicting results on the efficacy of patellar taping. Some have demonstrated that no change in patellar position occurs (Kowall et al. 1996) whereas others have demonstrated that a reduction in pain or minimal short-term changes in alignment do occur with the tape (Somes et al. 1997; Worrell et al. 1998); these studies, however, consistently point out that the effects of taping on patellar position were limited. Patellar position changed only at 10° of knee flexion (Worrell et al. 1998), and no change occurred in the open chain position (Somes et al. 1997). Changes that did occur lasted less than 15 minutes after activity was initiated. Empirical evidence persists to support the theory that McConnell taping reduces pain in spite of the now accepted fact that the tape does not change functional patellar alignment. It has been speculated that the tape may provide neural inhibition through neurosensory afferent stimulation of the large A fibers (Bockrath et al. 1993).

Research has shown that patellar taping facilitates a quicker response of the VMO during step-up activities and delays the onset of vastus lateralis response while increasing the onset of VMO response during a step-down exercise (Gilleard, McConnell, and Parsons 1998). It has yet to be determined whether this change in muscle response results from improved muscle response secondary to pain reduction or neurosensory facilitation.

Patellar Tape Applications

Although it has been demonstrated that patellar taping does not change the position of the patella, tape applications advocated by McConnell are presented here. The reason these techniques are presented is that the tape has shown to consistently reduce pain in spite of the reason for this remaining elusive. When more than one malalignment is present and one of them is a posterior tilt, the posterior tilt is corrected first; otherwise, the greatest malalignment is corrected first. The tapes used for patellar taping are Cover-Roll, used as a hypoallergenic cloth undertape to protect the skin, and Leukotape™, used to guide patellar alignment. The tape should reduce the patient's pain symptoms immediately. To evaluate its effectiveness, the patient should perform an activity that reproduces the pain such as a step-down and assess the pain level. After the tape is applied, the patient repeats the activity to reassess the pain level. Although the pain may or may not completely resolve, it will be significantly reduced with the tape application in 50% of the cases (Bockrath et al. 1993). If no change in pain is perceived, the correction tape should be reapplied in a different sequence. The tape can be worn for extended periods of time to effect a low-load, long-term stretch on soft tissues. It is worn 23 h a day with an hour off, usually after a shower, to relieve skin stress. With a reduction in pain, an increase in VMO facilitation and quadriceps strengthening can occur. The tape can get wet without any effect on its adhesion, but over time it loses its effectiveness. The top tape strip can be readjusted if it loosens. If taping proves effective, the patient can be instructed in tape application, removal, and skin care so that he or she can reapply the tape daily until symptoms subside. As quadriceps strength improves and pain decreases, the patient is weaned from the tape.

The cloth undertape is applied smoothly to the skin over the patella, and the correction tape is applied with force to correct patellar position. The tape is usually applied with the knee in extension and a rolled towel under the knee for comfort. If pain occurs during the middle range of a squat, the tape can be applied with the knee positioned in the painful range of flexion. The quadriceps must remain relaxed during any McConnell tape application.

For a lateral glide, the correction tape is applied from lateral to the lateral border of the patella with a medial pull on the tape over the medial femoral condyle (figure 21.52). The soft tissue over the medial femoral condyle is lifted toward the patella manually to create a fold in the skin on the medial side and provide a better pull of the tape. A couple of strips of correction tape may be necessary. Each strip should create a larger soft-tissue crease.

For a lateral tilt, a strip of tape is firmly anchored at the middle of the patella and pulled firmly toward the medial femoral condyle so that the lateral patellar border is lifted to move the patella level with the anterior femoral plane (figure 21.53). The soft tissue is lifted on the medial aspect to provide a better result.

Figure 21.52 Lateral glide correction.

Figure 21.53 Lateral tilt correction.

For a lateral rotation alignment, the tape is anchored on the inferior patellar pole. The patella is manually rotated in correct alignment while the tape is pulled upward and medially (figure 21.54).

If present, a posterior or inferior tilt is taped first to reduce infrapatellar fat-pad irritation with other tape applications. A posterior tilt is usually taped in combination with a lateral tilt or lateral glide. The tape is applied over the superior half of the patella to lift the inferior pole up and away from the fat pad (figure 21.55).

Skin irritation can occur with the use of tape. To minimize this risk, the tape should be removed carefully; an adhesive remover should be used after the tape has been taken off, and the skin should be carefully cleansed and conditioned with a moisturizer when the tape is not in use. If a small area of skin breakdown occurs, it should be covered with a protective dressing or, if possible, the tape should be averted from the area. If the breakdown area is too large, use of the tape should be discontinued until the skin heals. If an allergic reaction occurs, the tape should be discontinued.

Figure 21.54 Lateral rotation correction.

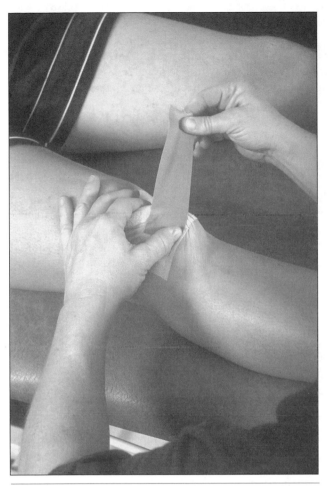

Figure 21.55 Inferior tilt correction.

Figure 21.56 Iliotibial band massage.

Soft-Tissue Mobility

Soft-tissue adhesions and tightness along the distal ITB and into the lateral retinaculum often play a role in patellar malalignment. These structures should be treated with deep-tissue massage and stretching. Deep-tissue massage can be applied by the rehabilitation clinician with the dorsal side of a flat fist (flexed MPs and PIPs, extended DIPs), with pressure delivered over the posterior middle and distal phalanges, as was discussed earlier in this chapter in the section "Deep-Tissue Massage." The patient can also be instructed to use a foam roller to perform self-massage techniques (figure 21.10). The patient can perform manual massage techniques over the distal lateral thigh throughout the day while sitting (figure 21.56).

The patient should receive instructions for stretching exercises for all tight muscle groups and should perform them throughout the day. The muscle groups commonly included are the hamstrings, gastrocnemius, and tensor fascia lata.

Additional Therapeutic Exercises

Therapeutic exercise is a vital part of the total rehabilitation program for patellofemoral pain. Stretching and strengthening exercises can alter patellar tracking to establish a more correct alignment (Doucette and Goble 1992). Because muscle imbalance can play a role in PFPS, it is logical to assume that improvement in muscle balances can impact improvement in this condition.

As for all extremity programs, exercises for core and pelvic stabilization should be included in the therapeutic exercise program. These exercises were presented in chapter 16 and include strengthening exercises for the abdominal obliques, lower abdominals, and spine extensors. In addition, lateral and posterior hip muscles should be strengthened to provide hip stability during knee activities.

Lower-limb alignment and mechanics have a direct impact on the patellofemoral joint. Muscles in distal and proximal segments must be corrected for imbalances along with the knee muscles if patellofemoral pain is to be resolved. Muscles controlling foot pronation, including the posterior tibialis, anterior tibialis, and peroneals, should be strengthened and reeducated for pronation control and foot stability during closed chain activities.

Pelvis stability is important in knee control. Hip muscles and abdominals, especially lower abdominals, play a key role in providing adequate knee control during closed chain activities. Pelvic stability and hip control deficits are often seen in PFPS. Stabilization and strengthening exercises for these groups should be included when deficiencies exist.

Quadriceps strength is primary to a successful rehabilitation program. Electrical stimulation and biofeedback can be used to facilitate quadriceps activation. These electrical modalities are used in open chain exercises such as straight-leg raise and SAQ and in closed chain exercises for concentric and eccentric activity such as walking, step-downs, and lunges. A combination of open and closed chain activities within a pain-free range of motion is part of a total therapeutic exercise program. Patellofemoral taping might be required, especially in the early phases of therapeutic exercise when patellofemoral pain prevents adequate quadriceps activation.

When the patient is able to perform closed chain activities in a slow and controlled manner and without pain, the speed of the activities is increased to challenge muscle recruitment patterns and prepare the patient for agility and functional activities. As the patient gains strength, control, and flexibility, he or she follows a progression of exercises similar to that for other knee injuries, advancing to increased stress and forces, more challenging coordination and agility activities, and finally functional activities. Return to full participation is possible once the patient is pain free; has normal flexibility, strength, agility, and power; and is able to demonstrate normal performance of activity-specific activities.

Patellar Tendinitis

Patellar tendinitis can be related to patellofemoral alignment, so the same factors discussed in PFPS should be assessed for patellar tendinitis. Patellar tendinitis is often called jumper's knee because jumping activities are the primary precipitating factor. With the energy absorption that occurs during landing from a jump, jumping on hard surfaces and excessive jump repetitions can overload the tendon beyond its stress-absorbing capabilities. Tissue breakdown then occurs. This stress is exaggerated with muscle imbalances of weakness or tightness or mechanical malalignments such as foot pronation.

Pain occurs in the patellar tendon between the patella and tibial tuberosity. Classic activities cause patellar tendon pain: Pressure over the tendon, quadriceps tightening (especially eccentric activity), and stair climbing (especially going down). There may be slight edema in the area.

Initial rehabilitation goals are to reduce the inflammation and pain. This is accomplished with modalities such as phonophoresis, iontophoresis, ice, and electrical stimulation. Cross-friction massage across the tendon can be useful in promoting healing and reducing soft-tissue adhesions. The rehabilitation clinician applies cross-friction to one tender location on the tendon until the pain is reduced or relieved; he or she then moves to another site on the tendon and repeats the procedure until all tender sites have been treated.

Therapeutic exercises should include a combination of flexibility and strength. Stretching exercises for the hamstrings, quadriceps, lateral thigh, and calf muscles are taught to the patient. Strengthening exercises include open chain exercises to isolate the quadriceps and closed chain exercises for functional stresses. They may begin with isometric exercises for the quadriceps and active exercises for the hamstrings, hip, and ankle; but this depends on the patient's tolerance. In some cases the patient tolerates concentric closed chain activity but the eccentric portion of the closed chain exercise is too painful to perform. If this is the case, the exercise should be either postponed until the patient can perform it pain free or modified to eliminate the eccentric phase.

The rate of the program's progression is purely dependent on the patient's response to the exercises. The exercises should be performed pain free. During eccentric exercises, mild pain may occur during the last of three sets, but it should resolve when the exercise is completed. The program for eccentric exercises for tendinitis is outlined in chapter 15.

When the patient is able to perform sport-specific activities without pain or hesitation, return to full sport participation is possible.

Tendon Rupture

Tendon ruptures occur most commonly in people 30 to 50 years old as a result of a sudden quadriceps contraction; the cause is probably a gradual degeneration, although prior complaints of tendinitis are not usual. Tendon ruptures occur more often in males than in females. As with Achilles tendon ruptures, the patient feels as though he has been shot or kicked in the knee. The patient is unable to bear weight on the extremity. The rupture can occur from either the tendon attachment between the patella and tibial tuberosity (patellar tendon rupture) or the tendon between the patella and quadriceps (quadriceps tendon rupture). Complete

Case Study

A 16-year-old, female cross country runner has had left knee pain for the past month. The pain has progressed so that it now interferes with her workouts and occurs even during walking. The physician has diagnosed PFPS and wants her to begin rehabilitation. Your examination reveals genu valgus and recurvatum with foot pronation in standing. The patient's running shoes have excessive wear on the lateral posterior heel so that the midsole is evident. The shoes have a sewn curved last. The patient's rearfoot and forefoot have excessive mobility. Straight-leg raise is to 70°; ankle dorsiflexion in rearfoot neutral is 0°. She has a positive Ober's test, and deep palpation reveals tenderness along the distal ITB. Her quadriceps strength is 4–/5, lower abdominal strength is 3/5, and hip extension strength is 4/5. Patellar alignment assessment reveals a posterior and lateral tilt. Patellar tracking in long sitting is lateral. In standing, lateral patellar tracking is less. When the patient performs a step-down exercise, pain is produced, and the knee wobbles. Palpation of the posterior patellar surface reveals tenderness medially and laterally, especially over the inferior aspect.

Questions for Analysis

1. What will your treatment for the patient include today?

2. What instructions will you send her home with today?

3. What will you tell her when she asks what she should do about her workouts?

4. Given her signs, what part of the range of motion would you expect the patient to have the most pain in?

5. List two elements you will use to strengthen the VMO during the first week.

6. What are your short-term and long-term goals for the patient, and when do you expect her to achieve them?

ruptures are surgically repaired, with the knee kept either locked in extension with a brace or on a CPM. Straight-leg raises, quad sets, and hip exercises are used during the first 10 days to two weeks. Patellar mobilizations are used to maintain patellar mobility. Weight bearing is restricted initially and then advanced to weight bearing as tolerated in the brace. After about three weeks, exercises begin out of the brace and follow a progression similar to that for other surgical repair programs. The period until return to full activity is four to nine months.

Strains and Contusions

The severity of a strain determines the length of recovery. Ecchymosis indicates at least a grade II strain and necessitates a longer recovery time than a strain that does not produce discoloration. Ecchymosis is often distal to the site of muscle tear, because gravity pulls the blood caudally.

Lack of normal flexibility, fatigue, incoordination, and a sudden violent contraction or stretch of a contracting muscle can all be frequent precipitating factors for muscle strains.

Initial treatment goals include relieving inflammation, pain, and spasm. Pulsed ultrasound is effective in promoting the absorption of ecchymosis. Electrical stimulation is useful in relieving pain and spasm. Stretches with activation of the antagonists assist in relieving muscle spasm and regaining range of motion.

If the patient is unable to ambulate normally, assistive devices are used with weight-bearing to tolerance. Strength exercises are incorporated into the program as the patient tolerates them. Active range of motion against gravity may be all that is tolerated initially, but progression to resisted open and closed chain exercises occurs within a few days. A variety of activities including proprioceptive neuromuscular facilitation, manual resistance, pool exercises, stationary-bike exercise, co-contraction exercises, and unilateral weight bearing can begin within one to three days once spasm and pain have subsided.

The program is quickly advanced to eccentric and isokinetic exercises. Eccentric exercises are important for muscle strains, because athletic activity places high eccentric demands on lower-extremity muscle groups (Stanton and Purdam 1995). Agility activities requiring more rapid muscle responses are introduced into the program as the patient gains strength, coordination, and balance control. After the patient is able to perform functional and sport-specific activities, he or she is ready to be tested functionally for return to full sport participation.

Hamstrings

Hamstring strains most commonly occur at the musculotendinous junction, either near the ischial tuberosity or more toward the mid-lateral aspect of the muscle where the biceps femoris tendon inserts more distally. Hamstring strains often occur during high-speed activities such as sprinting or during sudden changes in muscle activity.

Stretching exercises should begin within two to four days after an injury. Hamstring tightness is often a predisposing factor in strains. After an injury, additional flexibility loss occurs. Appropriately timed deep massage and cross-friction to the injury site promote healing and reduce scar-tissue adhesions that can further restrict hamstring mobility.

Strength exercises start as isometrics and progress to concentrics, and then eccentrics, before transitioning to isokinetics and faster-speed activities.

Quadriceps

The quadriceps are subject to strains, contusions, and other injuries, some severe and others not. The injuries requiring rehabilitation have unique characteristics that are outlined here, and then a case study is presented.

Strains

Jumping or sudden changes in direction are activities that often produce quadriceps strains. The treatment course follows the same routine as for hamstring strains. Stretching activities are started on day 2 to 4 and are accompanied initially with isometric exercises. Pool exercises, proprioceptive neuromuscular facilitation, passive stretching, and stationary-bike exercise are used early in the program. Isometric exercises are replaced with isotonic and open and closed chain activities and advance to eccentric activities as tolerated. Isokinetic, agility, plyometric, and functional activities progress as previously mentioned for other knee rehabilitation programs.

Contusions

Contusions occur more commonly in the quadriceps than strains do. Pain and spasm are the most debilitating symptoms, so initial treatment goals are to resolve these conditions and maintain flexibility. Electrical stimulation, pulsed ultrasound, and ice help to relieve spasm and pain. Mild active and passive stretches with contraction of the contralateral muscle are recommended after spasm is relaxed, usually on the second or third day postinjury. A stationary bike can be used to improve range of motion. Pool exercises can also relax the muscle. Pain reflexively inhibits the muscle, so quadriceps strengthening is necessary and can begin when muscle spasm has been relieved. The progression is the same as outlined for other injuries, with the rate of progression based on the patient's response to specific exercises. Recovery with full return to sport participation usually can occur in two to three weeks for moderate and severe contusions.

Myositis ossificans is a condition that results from either a severe direct blow or repetitive blows to the quadriceps that affects the periosteum of the femur and cause non-neoplastic bone formation in the muscle. A painful, rigid mass can be felt through deep palpation of the anterior thigh in the muscle belly. Loss of range of motion accompanies myositis ossificans.

Surgical treatment is indicated for unresolved conditions but is usually not performed until the growth has stabilized, about one year postinjury. Surgical excision before that time can exacerbate the problem. Conservative treatment involves the treatment course outlined for contusions.

Case Study

A 30-year-old male tennis player sprinted to return a ball at the net when he felt a tear in his right hamstring one week ago. He was unable to walk and sought medical attention. The physician has diagnosed a grade II hamstring strain and wants the patient to begin rehabilitation. The patient ambulates with a slight antalgic gait. His knee motion is 15° to 115°. Left straight-leg raise is 60°, but the patient states that he has always been tight in his hamstrings. His hamstring strength is 3/5 and painful with resistance. His quadriceps strength, ankle strength, and hip strength are each 4/5. A large area of ecchymosis is present posteriorly from the proximal thigh below the gluteal fold to about 10 cm (3.9 in.) distal to the knee. The ecchymotic region is most tender in the darkest area of discoloration along the mid-posterolateral thigh. There is a small indentation with tenderness to palpation about 10 cm distal and 5 cm lateral to the ischial tuberosity.

Questions for Analysis

1. What will you include in today's treatment for the patient?

2. What home program will you give him before he leaves today?

3. What are your short-term goals for him and when do you expect him to achieve them?

4. Outline the course of exercises for this patient for the next two weeks. What functional activities will you include in his program?

5. What will your criteria be for permitting the patient to return to full sport participation?

Iliotibial Band Syndrome

Iliotibial band syndrome is an overuse syndrome that results from friction between the ITB and the lateral femoral epicondyle. It is seen most often in middle- and long-distance runners. Friction is thought to take place at 30° of knee flexion when the ITB is pulled over the lateral femoral epicondyle and occurs during running when the tensor fascia lata and gluteus maximus, the muscles attaching to the ITB, are active and are pulling on the band during the initial stance phase (Orchard et al. 1996). During downhill running, more time is spent in flexion, increasing ITB stress.

Predisposing factors may include leg-length discrepancy, increased Q-angle, genu valgus, and foot pronation. Running hills and increased running distances can also lead to ITB syndrome.

The patient complains of pain along the ITB (especially over the lateral femoral epicondyle), increased pain with walking or running (especially down hills), edema, and crepitus. Snapping over the lateral femoral epicondyle can sometimes be felt.

Treatment must involve correction of predisposing factors, stretching, and strengthening. Modalities to relieve the inflammation and a workout modification are useful. Running at a faster speed may reduce ITB pain, because during faster running the knee is at more than 30° flexion in the early weight-bearing phase. When pain is relieved, strengthening exercises for deficiencies should proceed with the inclusion of open and closed kinetic chain exercises, concentric and eccentric closed chain activities, and a progression as previously presented for return to full sport participation.

Osseous Injuries

Fractures of the knee bones can be traumatic or stress related. Femur fractures are not common occurrences, fortunately, but tibial fractures are seen more frequently.

Fractures

Fractures of the knee result from direct blows and impact forces, torsional stresses, or compression loads. A patellar fracture usually occurs as the result of a direct blow, but a tibial fracture occurs most often because of torsional or compression forces. Epiphyseal plate injuries of the proximal tibia or distal femur occur in adolescent patients whose growth plates have not yet matured. Damage to these sites can alter bone growth. Tibial plateau fractures require non-weight bearing for six to eight weeks because of the tibia's major role in weight bearing. Displaced fractures require open reduction and internal fixation (ORIF).

Fractures repaired with ORIF procedures become more stable more quickly and can sometimes undergo a more accelerated therapeutic exercise program.

Chondral fractures and articular cartilage defects occur as a result of trauma to the articular surface, often a direct impact. These lesions occur most often in young adults. The lesions frequently develop into localized joint degeneration. Several treatment options are available for these isolated degenerative changes in the knee. Surgical options involve resurfacing of the chondral defect and commonly include arthroscopic debridement of the chondral surface. This is often accompanied by an abrasion arthroplasty, subchondral drilling, or creation of microfractures to stimulate bleeding to produce scarring that ultimately produces cartilage. Cartilage formation using these techniques is fibrocartilage, not hyaline cartilage, the normal articular cartilage. Fibrocartilage, unlike hyaline cartilage, has poor tolerance for weight-bearing activities.

Autologous-Chondrocyte Implantation

The most recent advances in cartilage transplant were developed by Swedish physicians (Brittberg et al. 1994). Chondral tissue is harvested from a non-weight-bearing surface of the patient's knee. The harvested cells regenerate chondrocytes in a laboratory until sufficient quantities are available to transplant into the chondral defect. The recent reports indicate that the cartilage graft is hyaline, not fibrocartilage. This technique offers patients with a rather narrow diagnosis of focal articular defects an opportunity to avoid osteoarthritis at the most or delaying arthritic symptoms to prolong physical activity at the least. This procedure is still under study, but cases that have been reported demonstrate favorable results.

Osseous/Chondral Post-op Rehabilitation

Rehabilitation following chondral-resurfacing techniques is similar to fracture rehabilitation in that weight bearing is either non-weight bearing or toe-touch weight bearing for six weeks. A brace locked in extension is used during ambulation to reduce shear stress on the lesion site. If debridement is the only procedure performed, weight bearing immediately postoperatively is to tolerance. If autologous-chondrocyte implantation is the surgical technique, the patient is initially NWB but progresses to toe-touch and full weight bearing within 4 to 6 weeks. Exercises with the knee positioned to minimize stress of the surgical site are permitted during the non-weight bearing phase: Electrical stimulation, isometric exercises, and other non-resistive open chain exercises Biofeedback for muscle reeducation is useful for quadriceps facilitation and control. Early range of motion may be achieved using either CPM machine or passive ROM activities or a combination of both. The goal during this period is to stimulate chondral formation without applying excessive loads to the lesion site. It is appropriate to add pool exercises in deep water for range of motion after the operative wounds are well healed. Patellar mobilization and soft-tissue mobilization can be used by the second post-op week. A stationary bike without resistance can be used after the third week. Active assistive range-of-motion exercises advancing to active range-of-motion exercises can also be used then. By week 3 or 4, the patient should be able to demonstrate good quad control without an extensor lag and should have near-normal range of motion. After the third week, mild resistive pool exercises in deep water are suitable.

After the sixth week, full weight bearing with crutches can begin. Crutches are not removed until the patient is able to ambulate normally, has no extensor lag, and has full motion in extension. The brace can be discontinued by this time. Pool exercises can progress from the deep to the shallow end with progressive weight bearing. Progressive resistive exercises in the open and closed kinetic chain, using small arcs of motion initially and advancing to larger arcs of motion, start after six weeks. Exercises should remain pain free in all arcs of motion. A ski machine or stepper can also be used. Once the patient is able to ambulate without crutches, treadmill activities can begin. Static balance exercises progress to dynamic balance exercises as tolerated.

A gradual progression from balance to coordination to agility exercises takes place as the patient gains strength and proprioception. Jogging then running is allowed at 6 to 8 months postoperatively. Full return to sport participation occurs at 7 to 12 months.

Bone-fracture rehabilitation programs follow the same basic progression, but the timing for return to full sport participation is more rapid. A general range of time for return to sport following a fracture is 4 to 8 months. The range varies according to whether the fracture is treated surgically or immobilized, the location and type of fracture, the age of the patient, and the physician's preference.

Osteochondritis Dissecans

Osteochondritis dissecans (OD) is a disease of unknown etiology without related trauma that affects the femoral epiphysis in juvenile OD and the femoral condyle in adult OD. A bone flake in juvenile OD or a bone fragment in adult OD occurs at various sites of the femoral condyle. Juvenile OD occurs in youths under age 15, and adult OD is seen in people over age 15. Symptoms include nonspecific knee pain, point tenderness over the site, and quadriceps atrophy. There is minimal effusion, and the patient may experience catching, locking, or giving way during ambulation.

Treatment for adult OD includes arthroscopic debridement of loose bodies. If the lesion is small, an abrasion arthroplasty or autogenous grafting can also be performed. Treatment for juvenile OD is more conservative, with prolonged rest, three months or more, occasionally with immobilization.

Rehabilitation for juvenile OD must attempt to reverse the deleterious effects of prolonged immobilization and inactivity. Cardiovascular exercise using the upper extremities, and lower-extremity exercises for the uninvolved segments help to maintain conditioning levels. Quad sets, straight-leg raises, and electrical stimulation can assist in retarding atrophy during immobilization.

Range-of-motion exercise, joint and soft-tissue mobilization, and active exercises are used once immobilization is removed. Weight-bearing exercises include weight-transfer activities and gait training. Pool exercises with progressive weight bearing can be used, and activities to restore proprioception using a BAPS board and a balance board, as well as stork standing, are helpful.

Rehabilitation following surgical treatment includes immediate weight bearing unless the lesion is large; in this case, weight bearing may be restricted. A gradual progression of exercises that do not produce pain takes place as with other knee lesions. An expected recovery to full sport participation usually takes about four to six months.

SUMMARY

1. Discuss the relationship and alignment between the patella and femur.

   Patellar stability is the result of static and dynamic structures. The bony configuration, with the patella seated within the femoral sulcus formed by the medial and higher-ridged lateral epicondyles, is the greatest bony contributor to patellar stability. Ligamentous stability from the patellofemoral and patellotibial joints assists in providing static restraints. Active restraints occur primarily from the quadriceps. The patella is in various degrees of contact within its groove in the femur during any specific point within the knee's range of motion. A combination of compressive forces and the amount of area of contact determines the patellofemoral joint stress.

2. Identify postinjury factors that influence strength output.

   Edema and pain both cause automatic withdrawal of quadriceps activity. An abnormal gait, using the injured extremity less than normal, also results in reduced muscle activity. These factors in combination contribute to further reduction of strength in the injured extremity.

3. Define quadriceps extensor lag and explain its significance.

   An extensor lag occurs when full passive motion of knee extension is present but the patient is unable to actively achieve full extension. It is an indication of quadriceps weakness.

4. Outline a general progression of rehabilitation for a knee.

   As with other body segments, specific applications depend on specific deficiencies. Modalities are used to relieve pain and edema and to encourage the healing process. Soft-tissue and joint mobilization techniques may be necessary. Range of motion, active and passive, is used to increase motion. Strengthening exercises can be started early in a pain-free range of motion or with isometric exercises. Manual resistance can progress to machine and body-weight resistances, rubber tubing, and isokinetics. Proprioception and balance activities begin with something simple like a stork stand and progress to balance activities on unstable surfaces. Once flexibility, balance, and strength have reached appropriate levels, plyometric exercises, such as target jumping, lateral jumps, box activities, and depth jumps, can be used. Functional activities that mimic the patient's specific sport are the final aspect of the therapeutic exercise program before full participation in the sport is permitted.

5. Identify three soft-tissue mobilization techniques for the knee.

   Three such techniques are foam roller myofascial release to the ITB, trigger point release to the quadriceps, and cross-friction massage to the patellar tendon.

6. Identify three joint mobilization techniques for the knee, and their purpose.

Lateral glides of the patella are used for full flexion-extension range of motion of the knee, posterior glide of the tibia on the femur is used to increase flexion, and rotational glides are used to increase terminal flexion and extension of the knee.

7. Explain three flexibility exercises for the knee and identify the structure they affect.

Flexibility exercises include standing knee flexion stretch for the quadriceps with the heel behind the buttocks, standing hamstring stretch with the involved extremity on an elevated surface, and the gastrocnemius stretch with the knee straight.

8. Explain three proprioceptive/balance exercises for the knee.

Exercises for proprioception/balance include stork standing with eyes open and then closed, stork standing on a 1/2 foam roller, and standing on a foam roller while catching a ball.

9. Identify three functional activities.

Three functional activities are running and cutting while dribbling a basketball, sprinting forward and then backward with rapid changes in direction, and lateral glides with pivots to left and right.

10. Identify three factors that influence PFPS.

Three such factors are weak quadriceps, weak hip and trunk control, and tight hamstrings.

CRITICAL THINKING QUESTIONS

1. In this chapter's opening scenario, how much knee flexion motion would you expect Lewis to have after two weeks of immobilization? What kind of motion exercise would he be able to start on his first day of rehabilitation? What strengthening exercises would you give him for his hip and ankle on his first day of rehabilitation? When you would expect him to have full knee motion? When would you start him on passive stretching exercises for his quads? Give your justification for this timetable.

2. When would you begin patellar mobilization on Lewis? When would you begin soft-tissue mobilization to the quadriceps repair site? Give your rationale for these timetables.

3. If you had two patients with knee injuries, one with an ACL sprain and the other with an MCL sprain, which one (if either) would you be more cautious with and why? How would their rehabilitation programs differ?

4. If a patient complains of patellar tendinitis, what structures would you investigate for possible causes? What key items would you include in your history questions? Would you use primarily open or closed chain exercises initially, and why?

5. A teenaged patient you have been rehabilitating for weakness following an anterior medial knee contusion continues to complain of pain in the knee even though his strength is improving. How would you approach the problem and what would you suspect?

LAB ACTIVITIES

1. Perform soft tissue mobilization on your lab partner's ITB. First examine the area for any restrictions, and then apply mobilization to relieve the main restrictive areas. Examine the area after your treatment. What changes do you and your partner (objectively and subjectively) observe? What do you think as occurred with the treatment? Use a foam roller to perform a soft tissue mobilization technique on the same area.

Compare the sensory changes between the two techniques. Based on the differences, what would be the advantages and disadvantages of each technique?

2. Locate the trigger points on your lab partner for the muscles listed. As you perform each one, indicate what the pain pattern would be if the trigger point was active.

    a. Rectus femoris

    b. Vastus lateralis

    c. Vastus medialis

    d. Popliteus

    e. Medial hamstrings

Where were your partner's most sensitive trigger points? Perform an ice-and-stretch technique on each of them and provide your partner with a home exercise for each tender trigger point.

3. Perform grades II and IV joint mobilizations on your lab partner and identify what restriction would be best treated with each mobilization for the following joints:

    a. Patellofemoral glides

      - Medial glide

      - Lateral glide

      - Superior glide

      - Inferior glide

    b. Tibiofemoral glides

      - Distraction

      - Anterior

      - Posterior

      - Anterior glide of the medial condyle

      - Posterior glide of the medial condyle

Are the medial and lateral patellofemoral glide excursions the same? Perform the tibiofemoral glides first in the resting position, and then in other open-packed positions. How does the amount of motion change with the different positions? What implications does this outcome have on treatment?

4. Have your partner perform two different prolonged stretch exercises to increase knee flexion. Is there an advantage of one over the other?

5. Identify short-term stretches you would give a patient to perform at home. Identify stretches that would be used to stretch a knee with extension limited to 15° of flexion and another stretch that could be used on a knee with extension limited to 90° of flexion. What factors do you have to consider that are unique to each condition when coming up with an exercise for each situation?

6. Have your partner perform two different exercises (same level of difficulty) to strengthen the quadriceps. How are they different? Why might you use one over the other? Explain your rationale.

7. Have your partner perform a lateral step-up exercise for 20 repetitions. What substitution patterns must you watch for and how would you correct them?

8. Have your partner perform a wall squat using three alternative ways of doing it so each exercise is a progression of the previous one. Have your partner perform 20 repetitions of each exercise. Does your partner confirm that the progression you created is a progression, or is a later exercise easier than a previous one? What are the substitution patterns you should watch for and what verbal cues would you give to correct them?

9. Have your partner perform three proprioceptive exercises, each one a progression of the previous exercise. What have you used to determine when your partner is able to progress to the next exercise (what is your criteria for progression)?

10. Evaluate your partner's patella alignment for lateral tilt, lateral shift or glide, inferior tilt, and rotation. What malalignments do you see? Is it bilateral? If there are malalignments, what might be possible reasons for them in your partner? What exercises might correct the alignment deficiencies?

11. Have your partner perform a quad set in straight leg sitting and a lunge in standing. What differences in patellar tracking do you see between the two positions? How would you correct any deficiencies you noted?

12. If a new patient (basketball forward) you are seeing for the first time today is diagnosed with an ACL reconstruction (patellar tendon graft), list in proper sequence all the exercises you would include in the rehabilitation program. You do not need to identify timing, only sequence in which you would add the exercise. Also indicate when you might consider discontinuing an exercise in the program and your rationale.

REFERENCES

Ahmed, A.M., and D.L. Burke. 1983. In vitro measurement of static pressure distribution in synovial joints: I. Tibial surface of the knee. *Journal of Biomedical Engineering* 105;216–225.

Barber, F.A. 1994. Accelerated rehabilitation for meniscus repairs. *Arthroscopy* 10:206–210.

Beynnon, B.D., Fleming, B.C., Johnson, R.J., Nichols, C.E., Renstom, P.A., and M.H. Pope. 1995. Anterior cruciate ligament strain behavior during rehabilitation exercises in vivo. *American Journal of Sports Medicine* 23:24–34.

Bockrath, K., Wooden, C., Worrell, T., Ingersoll, C.D., and T. Farr. 1993. Effects of patellar taping on patella position and perceived pain. *Medicine and Science in Sports and Exercise* 25:989–992.

Brittberg, M., Lindahl, A., Nilsson, A., Ohlsson, C., Isaksson, O., and L. Peterson. 1994. Treatment of deep cartilage defects in the knee with autologous chondrocyte transplantation. *New England Journal of Medicine* 331:889–895.

Brown, C.H., Steiner, M.E., and E.W. Carson. 1993. The use of hamstring tendons for anterior cruciate ligament reconstruction. Technique and results. *Clinics in Sports Medicine* 12:723–756.

Brownstein, B., Mangiene, R.E., Noyes, F.R., and S. Kryer. 1988. Anatomy and biomechanics. In *Physical therapy of the knee*, ed. R.E. Mangiene. New York: Churchill Livingstone.

Butler, D.L., Noyes, F.R., and E.S. Grood. 1980. Ligamentous restraints to anterior-posterior drawer in the human knee. *Journal of Bone and Joint Surgery* 62-A:259–270.

Close, J.R. 1964. *Motor function in the lower extremity. Analysis by electronic instrumentation.* Springfield, IL: Charles C Thomas.

Doucette, S.A., and D.D. Child. 1996. The effect of open and closed chain exercise and knee joint position on patellar tracking in lateral patellar compression syndrome. *Journal of Orthopaedic and Sports Physical Therapy* 23:104–110.

Doucette, S.A., and E.M. Goble. 1992. The effect of exercise on patellar tracking in lateral patellar compression syndrome. *American Journal of Sports Medicine* 20:434–440.

Durselen, L., Claes, L., and H. Kiefer. 1995. The influence of muscle forces and external loads on cruciate ligament strain. *American Journal of Sports Medicine* 23:129–136.

Dye, S.F., and W.D. Cannon. 1988. Anatomy and biomechanics of the anterior cruciate ligament. *Clinics in Sports Medicine* 7:715–725.

Fahrer, H. Rentsch, H.U., Gerber, N.J., Beyeler, C., Hess, C.W., and B. Grünig. 1988. Knee effusion and reflex inhibition of the quadriceps. A bar to effective training. *Journal of Bone & Joint Surgery* 70B:635-638.

Freeman, M.A., and B. Wyke. 1967. The innervation of the knee joint. An anatomical and histological study in the cat. *Journal of Anatomy* 101:505–532.

Fritz, J.M., Irrgang, J.J., and C.D. Harner. 1996. Rehabilitation following allograft meniscal transplantation: A review of the literature and case study. *Journal of Orthopaedic and Sports Physical Therapy* 24:98–106.

Galloway, M.T., and P. Jokl. 1990. Patella plica syndrome. *Annals of Sports Medicine* 5:34–41.

Gilleard, W., McConnell, J., and D. Parsons. 1998. The effect of patellar taping on the onset of vastus medialis obliquus and vastus lateralis muscle activity in persons with patellofemoral pain. *Physical Therapy* 78:25–32.

Gough, J.V., and G. Ladley. 1971. An investigation into the effectiveness of various forms of quadriceps exercises. *Physiotherapy* 57:356–361.

Grelsamer, R.P, and J.R. Klein. 1998. The biomechanics of the patellofemoral joint. *Journal of Orthopaedic and Sports Physical Therapy* 28:286–298.

Grood, E.S., Suntay, W.J., Noyes, F.R., and D.L. Butler. 1984. Biomechanics of the knee-extension exercise. Effect of cutting the anterior cruciate ligament. *Journal of Bone and Joint Surgery* 66-A: 725–734.

Huberti, H.H., and W.C. Hayes. 1984. Patellofemoral contact pressures. The influence of Q-angle and tendofemoral contact. *Journal of Bone and Joint Surgery* 66-A:715–724.

Irrgang, J.J., Harner, C.D., Fu, F.H., Silbey, M.B., and R. DiGiacomo. 1997. Loss of motion following ACL reconstruction: A second look. *Journal of Sport Rehabilitation* 6:213–225.

Isear, J.A. Jr., Erickson, J.C., and T.W. Worrell. 1997. EMG analysis of lower extremity muscle recruitment patterns during an unloaded squat. *Medicine and Science in Sports and Exercise* 29: 532–539.

Jenkins, W.L., Munns, S.W., Jayaraman, G., Wertzberger, K.L., and K. Neely. 1997. A measurement of anterior tibial displacement in the closed and open kinetic chain. *Journal of Orthopaedic and Sports Physical Therapy* 25:49–56.

Karlsson, J., Thomee, R., and L. Sward. 1996. Eleven year follow-up of patello-femoral pain syndrome. *Clinical Journal of Sport Medicine* 6:22–26.

Kaufman, K.R., An, K-N., Litchy, W.J., Morrey, B.F., and E.Y.S. Chao. 1991. Dynamic joint forces during knee isokinetic exercise. *American Journal of Sports Medicine* 19:305–316.

Knight, K.L., Martin, J.A., and B.R. Londeree. 1979. EMG comparison of quadriceps femoris activity during knee extension and straight leg raises. *American Journal of Physical Medicine and Rehabilitation* 58:57–67.

Kowall, M.G., Kolk, G., Nuber, G.W., Cassisi, J.E., and S.H. Stern. 1996. Patellar taping in the treatment of patellofemoral pain. A prospective randomized study. *American Journal of Sports Medicine* 24:61–66.

Lange, G.W., Hintermeister, R.A., Schlegel, T., Dillman, C.J., and J.R. Steadman. 1996. Electromyographic and kinematic analysis of graded treadmill walking and the implications for knee rehabilitation. *Journal of Orthopaedic and Sports Physical Therapy* 23:294–301.

Lattanzio, P.J., Petrella, R.J., Sproule, J.R., and P.J. Fowler. 1997. Effects of fatigue on knee proprioception. *Clinical Journal of Sport Medicine* 7:22–27.

Lieb, F.J., and J. Perry. 1971. Quadriceps function. An electromyographic study under isometric conditions. *Journal of Bone and Joint Surgery* 53-A:749–758.

Livingston, L.A. 1998. The quadriceps angle; a review of the literature. *Journal of Orthopaedic & Sports Physical Therapy*. 28: 105-109.

Markolf, K.L., Gorek, J.F., Kabo, J.M., and M.S. Shapiro. 1990. Direct measurement of resultant forces in the anterior cruciate ligament. An in vitro study performed with a new experimental technique. *Journal of Bone and Joint Surgery* 72-A:557–567.

McDonough, A.L. and J.P. Weir. 1996. The effect of postsurgical edema of the knee joint on reflex inhibition of the quadriceps femoris. *Journal of Sport Rehabilitation* 5:172-182.

Mirzabeigi, E., Jordan, C., Gronley, J.K., Rockowitz, N.L., and J. Perry. 1999. Isolation of the vastus medialis oblique muscle during exercise. American Journal of Sports Medicine 27: 50–53.

Orchard, J.W., Fricker, P.A., Abud, A.T., and B.R. Mason. 1996. Biomechanics of iliotibial band friction syndrome in runners. *American Journal of Sports Medicine* 24:375–379.

Reider, B. 1996. Medial collateral ligament injuries in athletes. *Sports Medicine* 21:147–156.

Reilly, D.T., and M. Martens. 1972. Experimental analysis of the quadriceps muscle force and patello-femoral joint reaction force for various activities. *Acta Orthopaedica Scandinavica* 43:126–137.

Risberg, M.A., Holm, I., Tjomsland, O., Ljunggren, E., and A. Ekeland. 1999. Prospective study of changes in impairments and disabilities after anterior cruciate ligament reconstruction. *Journal of Orthopaedic and Sports Physical Therapy* 29:400–412.

Scott, G.A., Jolly, B.L., and C.E. Henning. 1986. Combined posterior incision and arthroscopic intra-articular repair of the meniscus. *Journal of Bone and Joint Surgery* 68-A:847–861.

Shelbourne, K.D., Patel, D.V., Adsit, W.S., and D.A. Porter. 1996. Rehabilitation after meniscal repair. *Clinics in Sports Medicine* 15:595–612.

Somes, S., Worrell, T.W., Corey, B., and C.D. Ingersoll. 1997. Effects of patellar taping on patellar position in the open and closed kinetic chain: A preliminary study. *Journal of Sport Rehabilitation* 6: 299–308.

Spencer, J.D., Hayes, K.C., and I.J. Alexander. 1984. Knee joint effusion and quadriceps reflex inhibition in man. *Archives of Physical Medicine and Rehabilitation* 65:171–177.

Stanton, P., and C. Purdam. 1995. Hamstring injuries in sprinting—the role of eccentric exercise. *Physiotherapy in Sport.* 18:6-11.

Steinkamp, L.A., Dillingham, M.F., Markel, M.D., Hill, J.A., and K.R. Kaufman. 1993. Biomechanical considerations in patellofemoral joint rehabilitation. *American Journal of Sports Medicine* 21:438–444.

Stone, R.G., Frewin, P.R., and S. Gonzales. 1990. Long-term assessment of arthroscopic meniscus repair: A two- to six-year follow-up study. *Arthroscopy* 6:73–78.

Tenuta, J.J., and R.A. Arciero. 1994. Arthroscopic evaluation of meniscal repairs. Factors that effect healing. *American Journal of Sports Medicine* 22:797–802.

Travell, J.G., and D.G. Simons. 1992. *Myofascial pain and dysfunction. The trigger point manual.* Vol. 2. Baltimore: Williams & Wilkins.

Wegener, L., Kisner, C., and D. Nichols. 1997. Static and dynamic balance responses in persons with bilateral knee osteoarthritis. *Journal of Orthopaedic and Sports Physical Therapy* 25:13–18.

Wilk, K.E., Arrigo, C., Andrews, J.R., and W.G. Clancy Jr., 1999. Rehabilitation after anterior cruciate ligament reconstruction in the female athlete. *Journal of Athletic Training* 34:177–193.

Wilk, K.E., Andrews, J.R., Clancy, Jr., W.G., Crockett, H.C., and J.W. O'Mara. 1999. Rehabilitation programs for the PCL-injured and reconstructed knee. *Journal of Sport Rehabilitation.* 8:333-362.

Witvrouw, E., Sneyers, C., Lysens, L., Victor, J., and J. Bellemans. 1996. Reflex response times of vastus medialis oblique and vastus lateralis in normal subjects and in subjects with patellofemoral pain syndrome. *Journal of Orthopaedic and Sports Physical Therapy* 24:160–165.

Worrell, T.W., Crisp, E., and C. LaRosa. 1998. Electromyographic reliability and analysis of selected lower extremity muscles during lateral step-up conditions. *Journal of Athletic Training* 33:156–162.

Worrell, T.W., Ingersoll, C.D., Bockrath-Pugliese, K., and P. Minis. 1998. Effect of patellar taping and bracing on patellar position as determined by MRI in patients with patellofemoral pain. *Journal of Athletic Training.* 33:16–20.

Young, A., Stokes, M., and J.F. Iles. 1987. Effects of joint pathology on muscle. *Clinical Orthopaedics & Related Research.* 219:21–27.

SUGGESTED READING

Bailey, A. Goodstone, N., Roberts, S., Hughes, J. Roberts, S., van Niekerk, L., Richardson, J., and D. Rees. 2003. Rehabilitation after Oswestry autologous-chondrocyte implantation: the OsCell protocol. *Journal of Sport Rehabilitation.* 12:104-118.

Borsa, P.A., Sauers, E.L., and S.M.Lephart. 1999. Functional training for the restoration of dynamic stability in the PCL-injured knee. *Journal of Sport Rehabilitation.* 8:362-378.

Gillogly, S.D., Voight, M. and T. Blackburn. 1998. Treatment of articular cartilage defects of the knee with autologous chondrocyte implantation. *Journal of Orthopaedic & Sports Physical Therapy.* 28: 241-251.

Hip

Objectives

After completing this chapter, you should be able to do the following:

1. Discuss how anteversion and retroversion change lower-extremity mechanics.

2. Explain the mechanical factors involved in gait with hip abductor weakness and explain how a cane assists in normal gait.

3. Identify a joint mobilization technique for the hip and explain its benefit.

4. Identify a flexibility and a strengthening exercise for the hip.

5. Identify a proprioception exercise for the hip and indicate its progression.

6. List precautions for a hip-dislocation rehabilitation program.

tevie T. has worked with dancers for several years. Having responsibility for the city ballet company's rehabilitation programs, he is quite busy. Over the years he has come to realize that the novice dancers' injuries tend to be acute whereas the experienced dancers' injuries are more often chronic. Although he is able to resolve the acute injuries more quickly, Stevie sees the chronic injuries as a challenge—one that he is usually able to meet and resolve, much to his patients' delight.

Stevie's current patient, however, has been his greatest challenge yet. Joan Dean, the lead female dancer in the company, had been bothered with a groin strain for several months before she reported it. It occurred early in the season during rehearsal, and Joan had dismissed it as minor, not worth treating. But the problem has not gone away, and now that the company is at the peak of the performance season, the injury is aggravated with each performance. Still, Joan refuses to take any time off to allow the strain to heal.

■ **God gave us two ends—one to sit on and one to think with. Success depends on which one you use. Head you win, tail you lose.**

Author Unknown

At the conclusion of this final chapter you will have acquired the tools you need to work as a rehabilitation clinician, planning and providing sound therapeutic exercise programs to patients. Use your head with all the knowledge and experience it has gathered to be an exceptional clinician. To ascend to new levels of knowledge is a professional goal and a responsibility shared by those who have a desire to excel within their profession; individual professional greatness is measured not by what we know but by how we share what we know.

The actions of the rehabilitation clinician in hip rehabilitation must be carefully planned if the patient is to return to full participation promptly and in accordance with the clinician and patient's mutually established goals.

The hip joint is secured by a deep socket and is supported by strong muscles. It is an area that experiences repetitive, microtraumatic injuries more often than acute, macrotraumatic injuries. Like other segments, this area relies on a balance of muscle flexibility and strength, along with coordination of movement, to maintain a balance for function and health. By now you realize that if normal length, strength, or function of any element is lost or changed, other elements are impacted and the hip becomes prone to injury.

The hip is a common site for pain referral from other sources, so pain complaints of this area warrant a differential diagnosis before treatment can begin. Because of the various structures that can produce pain into the hip and groin, establishing the source of pain is not always easy. Hip or groin pain can be secondary to referral from sources such as lumbar disk disruption, spondylolysis, organ disease, myofascial pain, sacroiliac dysfunction, and the knee. The rehabilitation clinician must eliminate these possibilities of pain source before he or she can accurately treat the patient. During the initial examination, if the patient's pain is not reproduced by stress applied to peripheral structures but is reproduced when stress is applied to the hip, it is likely that the hip is the source of the pain. If there is no change in the patient's condition after four to six sessions or two weeks of treatment, reexamination for other sources of pain is indicated.

This chapter introduces basic concepts the rehabilitation clinician must consider for hip-injury rehabilitation, focusing on topics relevant to treatment and therapeutic exercise program progression. As with the other chapters in this part, specific techniques for soft-tissue and joint mobilization and exercises for flexibility, strength, and proprioception are presented. Once the foundations of a therapeutic exercise program have been established, specific injuries commonly seen in the hip are discussed along with program progression for these injuries. Cases are presented in connection with some injury programs to help you conceptualize how a program is put together and advanced for a specific patient.

GENERAL REHABILITATION CONSIDERATIONS

▶ A rehabilitation program for the hip must be based on knowledge of the hip's osseous structures, neural structures, and joint mobility and joint mechanics. The rehabilitation clinician must also be familiar with methods of reducing stress in an injured hip.

The hip is a stable joint with extensive range of motion in several planes. The socket is deep and is reinforced with strong ligaments for stability. Strength and motion are important for the hip because it serves as a force transmitter for both lower- and upper-limb activities and provides motion and strength for propulsion in walking and running.

Osseous Structures

The **acetabulum,** the hip socket, is in an inferior and anterolateral position. The femoral neck forms a 125° angle with the shaft of the femur, as shown in figure 22.1a (Kapandji 1986). An angle greater than 125°, called coxa valga, increases pressure into the joint (figure 22.1b); an angle less than 125°, called coxa vara, increases stress on the femoral neck (figure 22.1c). The femoral neck is rotated relative to the line of the femur's long axis. Normal alignment places the neck in a line that is 15° anterior to the line of the femur in the adult (figure 22.2). If the angle is greater than 15°, the leg is positioned in medial rotation; this condition is called **anteversion.** If it is less than 15°, **retroversion** occurs to position the leg in lateral rotation. Anteversion and retroversion alter knee alignment and change the forces acting throughout the entire lower extremity. Anteversion leads to medial hip rotation, squinting patellae, and/or foot adduction, causing the individual to ambulate with a toe-in gait. Retroversion results in lateral hip rotation, frog-eyed patellae, and/or foot abduction, and causes the person to ambulate with a toe-out gait. Anteversion and coxa valga each make the hip susceptible to dislocation.

Figure 22.1 Femoral neck angles: *(a)* normal; *(b)* coxa valga—increased angle with increased joint stress; *(c)* coxa vara—decreased angle with increased femoral neck load.

Figure 22.2 Femoral neck alignment with long axis of femur: *(a)* normal, *(b)* retroversion, *(c)* anteversion.

Anteversion is measured with the patient lying prone and the knee flexed to 90°. The rehabilitation clinician moves the patient's leg into medial rotation until palpation of the greater trochanter reveals that it is parallel to the tabletop (figure 22.3). A goniometer is then used to measure the difference between the tibial position and a line vertical to the tabletop. This value is the degree of anteversion.

Figure 22.3 Craig's test for femoral anteversion: greater trochanter is positioned parallel to the tabletop (a), and the angle between the lower leg's position in 90° flexion at this point and in a vertical position is measured (b).

Neural Structures

Nerves entering the lower extremity must pass through the hip region. Nerve irritations can occur when structures around the hip impinge on a nerve. The sciatic nerve passes beneath, occasionally through, the piriformis muscle and through the sciatic notch before it travels along the posterior thigh. Entrapment of the nerve in the piriformis region can occur and can cause neural irritation distally.

A sensory branch of the femoral nerve, the lateral femoral cutaneous nerve, travels through the psoas major muscle and then passes under the inguinal ligament near the anterior superior iliac spine (ASIS). Compression of this nerve by the inguinal ligament can cause aching and burning over the tensor fascia lata in the anterolateral thigh where it provides sensory innervation.

The obturator nerve enters the pelvis from the upper lumbar nerve roots and provides sensory and motor innervation to the medial thigh. Entrapment of this nerve can cause medial thigh sensory changes and adductor weakness.

Stablization

Chapter 16 mentioned pelvic or trunk stabilization and its importance in reduced injury risk and improved upper and lower extremity performance. As you recall, a portion of trunk stabilization depends upon the hip muscles. Specifically, the hip extensors and abductors play a very important role in pelvic stability. When you think about it, this makes intuitive sense. Since the gluteal muscles attach to the pelvis, and athletic performance and reduced injury risk are dependent upon a stable trunk or pelvis, then hip stability is also important for these same performance and injury-prevention elements. The hip muscles also serve as a means by which the power of the legs is transferred up the chain to other body segments during upper extremity activities such as pitching, golf, and tennis. As was mentioned in chapter 17, assuming the patient performs with good sequential motion, the legs and trunk provide 51% to 55% of the total kinetic energy and total force for overhead activities (Kibler 1995). This means that if the hips are weak, not only will there be less force applied where and when it is needed, but there will be increase stress applied to other segments to take up the slack of weak hip muscles. The hips must be the platform from which the pelvis functions just as the pelvis is the platform from which the scapula functions, and the scapula is the platform from which the shoulder joint functions. It is important, then, for the clinician to examine hip stability, especially strength of the hip extensors and abductors, for not only hip injury rehabilitation but also any extremity joint just as the clinician examines trunk stability for upper-and-lower extremity rehabilitation programs.

Joint Mobility

The joint configuration is a convex femoral head on a concave acetabulum, so glide of the femur on the pelvis occurs in the direction opposite to movement during open chain motion. The hip's capsular pattern has its most significant restriction of motion in medial rotation. Flexion and abduction are less limited, and extension is less limited than flexion or abduction. Lateral rotation is normal (Cyriax 1975).

The hip joint's close-packed position is full extension, abduction, and medial rotation. The resting position is 30° flexion and 30° abduction with slight lateral rotation.

Joint Mechanics

Pelvis movement has a direct influence on hip movement because the hip joint socket lies within the pelvic bones. Pelvic motion alters hip positioning, and hip abnormalities affect pelvic posture. An anterior pelvic tilt moves the anterior pelvis closer to the anterior femur, and a posterior pelvic tilt moves the posterior pelvis closer to the posterior femur. This change in position relationships alters the hip so that an anterior pelvic tilt increases hip flexion and a posterior pelvic tilt increases hip extension.

When a person moves from a two-leg to a one-leg stance, the center of gravity must be transferred toward the supporting leg. This places rotatory stress on the weight-bearing hip because gravity's pull on the non-weight bearing leg drops the pelvis on that side. To prevent pelvic drop and rotatory forces, the abductors on the weight-bearing leg must work to keep the hips level with each other. The force required of the abductors is significantly greater than the weight of the body, because their lever-arm length is less than that of the center of gravity (figure 22.4). If the abductors are not strong enough to counter the force of gravity that is pulling the non-weight-bearing hip downward and laterally rotating the pelvis, a normal gait is not possible. The patient either drops the non-weight-bearing hip and downwardly rotates the pelvis to the non-weight-bearing side, or tilts the trunk to lean over the weak weight-bearing hip during stance on the leg so that the center of gravity is closer to the fulcrum, the femoral head. If the center of gravity is moved far enough laterally to be placed on top of or lateral to the fulcrum, the abductors do not have to work.

If a cane is used on the side opposite the weakness, an upward force is transmitted through the cane to counterbalance the downward gravitational force on the same side (figure 22.5). Because the lever arm from the cane to the fulcrum at the weak hip is longer than the lever arm of the body's center of gravity, the necessary counterbalance force transmitted through the cane is relatively small. Patients who use a cane or a single crutch for ambulation need only apply light pressure on the handle to offset the gravitational pull and produce adequate substitution for the weak abductors.

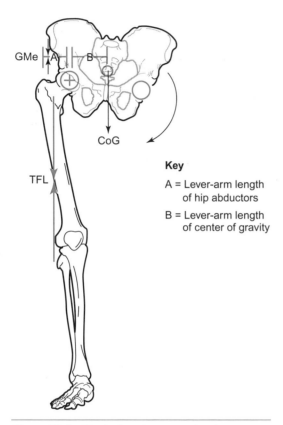

Key

A = Lever-arm length of hip abductors

B = Lever-arm length of center of gravity

Figure 22.4   Single-leg stance mechanics.

Key

1 = Femoral head

2 = Center of gravity (CoG)

3 = Cane

A = Lever-arm length for CoG

B = Lever-arm length for cane

Figure 22.5   Force application with cane use in ambulation.

Leg-length discrepancies can result from actual differences in length or from other unilateral differences such as genu valgus, coxa vara, rotated sacrum, or foot pronation, as well as from soft-tissue differences such as hip flexor tightness, abductor tightness, and muscle imbalances. When one leg is shorter than the other, the pelvis drops on the shorter side; and the trunk bends away from the short leg when weight bearing on the short leg. The greater the discrepancy, the more notable are these compensations. If a leg-length discrepancy is suspected, shoe wear is the most obvious indication that one is present. When a leg-length discrepancy is present, the clinician should assess all possible causes; correction or adaptation of the discrepancy may be necessary to alleviate the patient's pain.

Leg-length differences can eventually lead to osteoarthritis of the hip in the longer leg. This occurs because the longer leg is in a position of adducted angulation when weight bearing. This produces increased joint incongruence in which greater weight is borne on the superior lateral aspect of the acetabulum. The weight shift to the shorter leg is caused the leg-length difference; consequently, increased compressive forces are applied to the hip joint as the abductors on the longer leg increase their exertion to keep the pelvis level.

Stress-Reduction Concepts

One rule of thumb is that if a patient ambulates with an antalgic gait, he or she should use assistive devices until normal ambulation is possible. An abnormal gait may result from pain, inadequate muscle control, or apprehension; and if it continues, additional injury to the hip, back, or other lower-extremity segments can result. When weight bearing is permitted, an assistive device is used only as much as necessary to create a normal gait. As the precipitating factor is resolved, the patient is weaned from the crutches or cane until a normal gait without assistive devices is possible.

Stress can be reduced in the hip by shortening the stride length during walking or running. A smaller stride reduces the force and motion demands on the muscles, tendons, and ligaments. Application of a hip spica wrap can help diminish stride length.

General Rehabilitation Procedures

Hip-pain complaints without a specific injury can sometimes be difficult to interpret because of the various possible sources. Hip joint pain commonly refers to the groin, the anterior or medial proximal thigh, or the knee. Spinal-based pain can refer to the anterior hip, buttock, or thigh. Sacral pain can refer to the buttock or posterior or lateral thigh. Internal organs and the abdomen can refer pain to the groin. When a patient complains of pain in these areas without a specific history of injury, a differential diagnosis is necessary to eliminate these locations as sources of hip pain. The examination tests should reproduce the patient's pain complaints for a differential diagnosis.

Pain and inflammation control are the primary goals for initial treatment programs for hip injuries; the means of pain control include anti-inflammatory medication, reduced activity, and modalities. Some hip injuries are self-limiting in that pain is the determining factor with respect to participation. The patient may wish to continue normal participation in this case, because continued activity will not make the condition worse; but the recovery time may need to be longer because irritation is being introduced on a regular basis.

Therapeutic exercises include a progression of stretching or flexibility exercises, strengthening exercises, proprioception activities, and functional activities. When injuries result from predisposing factors rather than acute insult, those factors must be corrected to reduce the risk of recurrence. Since many hip muscles cross more than one joint, flexibility exercises require adequate stabilization of adjacent segments and proper application of the stretch force. Because the hip is so closely aligned with the pelvis, strengthening exercises must include pelvic and core stabilization exercises. Because the hip depends on the back, pelvis, knee, and ankle for its balance and quality of motion, exercises for deficiencies in these segments must be a part of the therapeutic exercise program for the hip.

Return to sport participation is possible when the patient is pain free with muscle balances intact and when performance of activity-specific activities is normal.

SOFT-TISSUE MOBILIZATION

▶ Soft-tissue mobilization techniques for the hip, including massage, scar-tissue mobilization, and cross-friction mobilization, are directed at the iliopsoas; the gluteus maximus, medius, and minimus; the piriformis; and the pectineus.

Because of the neurological, myofascial, orthopedic, and organ systems that can refer pain into the hip region, it is prudent for the rehabilitation clinician to identify any differential diagnosis that may be contributing to hip or groin pain. If myofascia is the expected source of pain, treatment can proceed. If changes in the patient's complaints do not occur with soft-tissue mobilization techniques, it is necessary to reassess for other probable causes.

Soft-tissue mobilization techniques for the hip include deep-tissue massage, scar-tissue mobilization, cross-friction massage, and myofascial release, including trigger point treatments and ice-and-stretch techniques. The myofascial release techniques and pain-referral information presented here are based on the work of Travell and Simons (1992). The quadratus lumborum muscle is discussed in chapter 16; the rectus femoris, hamstrings, adductors, and tensor fascia lata are addressed in chapter 21.

Myofascial techniques include direct pressure with the flat finger or thumb pad or with a pincher grasp of the muscle that is held until the muscle relaxes. If soft-tissue resistance is palpated after the initial application, the technique can be repeated. Cold-and-stretch techniques incorporate ice massage or cold spray applied in parallel sweeps, usually proximally to distally, with a simultaneous application of manual stretching. The rehabilitation clinician repeats this process three to five times, attempting to increase mobility with each application. He or she assists the patient in actively moving the leg to the starting position between bouts of ice-and-stretch. The patient performs several bouts of active motion following ice-and-stretch. Heat can be applied after the ice-and-stretch. Pain should not be produced during the application.

Iliopsoas

Pain from the iliopsoas trigger points is noticed particularly during weight bearing but is relieved with non-weight bearing. Pain is referred either throughout the lumbar paraspinal region on the same side as the lesion or into the anterior thigh and groin (figure 22.6a).

Myofascial release to the trigger points is performed using the finger or thumb pads. The patient is supine, with the abdominal muscles relaxed and the hip slightly flexed, abducted, and supported for relaxation. The distal trigger point is located on the lateral wall of the femoral triangle (figure 22.6b). It is important to avoid pressure on the medial side of the muscle, because the femoral nerve is located in this region. Just behind the ASIS and inside the rim of the iliac crest, the middle trigger point can be treated with finger-pad pressure pushing the muscle against the inside rim of the ilium. The third trigger point is more difficult to access because the patient must keep the abdominal muscles relaxed, and this is sometimes difficult to do. The region is lateral and just inferior to the umbilicus on the lateral rim of the rectus abdominis. Direct downward pressure is exerted slowly. Once past the rectus abdominis, the pressure continues downward and medially toward the spine. Depending on the patient's size, the psoas may or may not be directly palpated; but indirect pressure is effective if direct palpation is not possible.

Ice-and-stretch techniques are applied with the patient sidelying on the unaffected side and the top leg supported by the rehabilitation clinician in hip extension (figure 22.6c). Ice or cold spray sweeps are made from the abdomen downward past the thigh and to the knee, with stretch force applied to increase hip extension and medial rotation. Ice or cold spray sweeps are finally applied to the low back and posterior hip.

Figure 22.6 Iliopsoas trigger points: *(a)* pain-referral patterns, *(b)* trigger point release on distal trigger point, *(c)* ice-and-stretch. ● = ASIS.

Gluteus Maximus

The gluteus maximus refers pain locally in the buttock region around the sacrum or the gluteal fold above the ischial tuberosity (figure 22.7a). Pain related to this muscle is commonly reported after prolonged sitting, walking uphill, and swimming the freestyle stroke.

Trigger point myofascial release is performed with the patient in sidelying with the involved hip on top and a pad under the bottom hip for comfort. The top thigh is flexed comfortably. Pressure is applied with either a pincher grasp (to the inferior trigger points) or a finger or thumb pad (to the superior trigger points). A taut band can be palpated in the muscle's middle and distal fibers in the direction of fiber arrangement (figure 22.7b).

Cold-and-stretch is applied with the patient in sidelying and the top hip flexed and adducted with the knee resting on the table in front of the bottom extremity. The ice or cold spray sweeps start at the posterior iliac crest; they move along the muscle fiber direction to the mid-posterior thigh as stretch is applied, moving the hip into flexion (figure 22.7c).

Figure 22.7   Gluteus maximus trigger points: *(a)* pain-referral patterns, *(b)* trigger point release to superior trigger point, *(c)* ice-and-stretch. O = greater trochanter, □ = ischial tuberosity.

Gluteus Medius

Pain from the gluteus medius is aggravated with walking, lying supine, sidelying on the affected side, or sitting in a slouched position. The location of pain is along the posterior iliac crest, down the sacrum, and into the lateral posterior gluteal area; and the trigger points are along the iliac crest (figure 22.8a). Patients with Morton's toe are more susceptible to trigger points here. Ambulating with the hip medially rotated, unilateral standing, falling on the hip, prolonged tennis matches, walking on soft sand, and aerobics are all activities that can contribute to activation of these trigger points.

Trigger point release is performed with the patient sidelying; the affected hip is superior, and the hip is flexed and supported with a pillow between the knees and under the bottom hip for comfort (figure 22.8b). Thumb or finger pad pressure of the trigger points against the ilium is used along the iliac crest at the tender sites until their relaxation is palpated.

Ice-and-stretch is applied with the patient sidelying. The hip is in adduction behind the uninvolved extremity for stretch to the anterior fibers and in front of the uninvolved extremity for stretch to the posterior fibers. Parallel ice or cold spray sweeps are made from the iliac crest, over the lateral thigh to the knee (figure 22.8c).

Figure 22.8   Gluteus medius trigger points: *(a)* pain-referral patterns, *(b)* trigger point release to the posterior trigger point *(a1)*, *(c)* ice-and-stretch. ● = greater trochanter.

Gluteus Minimus

Pain from the gluteus minimus occurs with getting out of a chair and with walking. The pain-referral pattern is 1) over the lower lateral buttock, down the lateral thigh and into the lateral leg to the ankle for anterior trigger points or 2) over the lower posterior buttock, posterior thigh and into the proximal posterior calf for posterior trigger points (figure 22.9a). This can sometimes mimic a sciatic pain pattern, so sciatica should be ruled out.

Trigger point treatment is performed with the patient supine for anterior trigger point release, or sidelying on the unaffected side for posterior trigger point release (figure 22.9b). Because the gluteus minimus lies deep to the medius and maximus muscles, deep pressure is required for treatment. The gluteus medius and maximus should be relaxed, using supportive pillows for optimal effectiveness. The anterior fibers are palpated just distal to the ASIS on either side of the tensor fascia lata (TFL), deep to the TFL. The TFL is located by palpating for the muscle and simultaneously providing light resistance to hip medial rotation. The posterior trigger points are treated with the hip slightly flexed and adducted. They are located just above the piriformis toward the middle and lateral aspects of the piriformis.

Ice-and-stretch is applied with the patient in sidelying with the buttock close to the end of the table (figure 22.9c). With the

Figure 22.9   luteus minimus trigger points: *(a)* pain-referral patterns, *(b)* trigger point release, *(c)* ice-and-stretch.
● = greater trochanter, ■ = ASIS.

hip in adduction and supported by the rehabilitation clinician, ice or cold spray is applied in sweeping strokes from the iliac crest, down the lateral thigh to the lateral lower leg and ankle for the anterior trigger points and along the posterior hip, thigh, and calf for the posterior trigger points. The stretch force is applied with the hip in extension and adduction for the anterior fibers and in 30° flexion and medial rotation for the posterior fibers.

Piriformis

Activities such as sitting, standing, running and walking aggravate myofascial pain of the piriformis. Individuals who slip but catch themselves to stop a fall may aggravate piriformis trigger points. The piriformis refers pain into the sacroiliac area and the posterior hip (figure 22.10a). The pain can also extend into the upper two thirds of the posterior thigh.

Trigger point release can be performed with the patient prone or sidelying on the uninvolved side (figure 22.10b). A line from the greater trochanter to the superior border of the sciatic foramen is the course of the muscle. Two trigger points are found on this line; one is at the junction of the medial and middle third of the line and the other is at the junction of the middle and lateral third of the line.

Ice-and-stretch is performed with the patient sidelying and the hip in about 90° flexion and adducted in front of the bottom thigh. The sidelying patient keeps the flexed and adducted thigh anchored with his or her hand at the knee. The rehabilitation clinician then applies ice or cold spray sweeps from the sacrum to the lateral hip and down the posterior thigh (figure 22.10c). The stretch is applied at the pelvis with the clinician's hand on the patient's anterior pelvis to pull the pelvis posteriorly while the patient holds the thigh stable.

Figure 22.10 Piriformis trigger points: *(a)* pain-referral patterns, *(b)* trigger point release to lateral trigger point, *(c)* ice-and-stretch. ● = greater trochanter.

Pectineus

The pectineus muscle refers pain deep into the groin just below the inguinal ligament (figure 22.11a).

The trigger point is treated with the patient supine and the hip abducted, slightly flexed, and supported (figure 22.11b). Medial to the femoral artery, lateral to the adductor longus, and inferior to the inguinal ligament, finger-pad pressure is applied to the muscle's trigger point.

Ice-and-stretch is performed with the patient supine, the hip abducted and the knee and leg over the edge of the table (figure 22.11c). The stretch force is applied so that the hip becomes progressively more abducted and moves into extension.

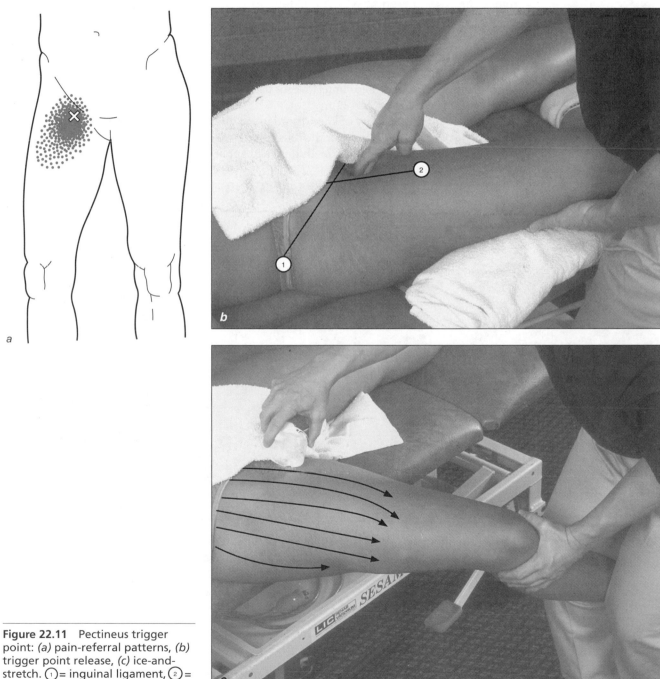

Figure 22.11 Pectineus trigger point: *(a)* pain-referral patterns, *(b)* trigger point release, *(c)* ice-and-stretch. ①= inguinal ligament, ②= femoral artery.

JOINT MOBILIZATION

▶ The rehabilitation clinician used joint mobilization of the hip to improve joint play and general hip mobility, as well as hip flexion, extension, abduction, and rotation. Patients can also apply self-mobilization techniques.

Whereas painful hip joints can benefit from grades I and II mobilization techniques, hip joints that display a capsular pattern of restricted movement can benefit from grades III and IV mobilization techniques. Although not always, oscillating techniques are often used for grades I and II and a sustained force for grades III and IV.

Because the proximal aspect of the hip joint is the pelvis, which is firmly attached to the trunk, there is little need to stabilize the hip joint of mobilization. The weight of the pelvis acts as an anchor.

Inferior Glide

This technique, also referred to as hip distraction or traction, helps the patient regain joint play, which is essential for all hip motions. Distraction is also useful in pain control. A history of knee disorders necessitates using an alternative technique. The patient lies supine while the rehabilitation clinician grasps the distal tibia and fibula of the affected leg and places the leg in a resting position. The patient is instructed to relax the hip and thigh muscles while the technique is applied. The clinician leans backward, using his or her body weight to supply the traction force (figure 22.12a).

If the patient has a history of knee disorders, an alternative position for an inferior glide is to have the patient's lower leg over the rehabilitation clinician's shoulder. The clinician clasps his or her hands around the proximal thigh and applies the inferior glide (figure 22.12b).

Figure 22.12 Joint mobilization—inferior glide: *(a)* with force applied in knee extension, *(b)* with force applied in knee flexion.

Lateral Glide

Lateral glides are used to promote gains in hip adduction and general mobility. The patient lies supine with the rehabilitation clinician standing at the side of the affected leg. A strap is secured around the proximal thigh and the clinician's hips (figure 22.13a). The rehabilitation clinician places his or her cephalic hand on the lateral pelvis to stabilize it and the caudal hand on the distal thigh. With the patient's thigh in slight flexion, the clinician transfers his or her weight from the front leg to the back leg, pushing his or her body against the strap to apply the traction force through the strap. The patient's hip can be placed in various positions of flexion and rotation for application of superior or inferior distractions with the lateral glide (figure 22.13, b and c).

Figure 22.13   Joint mobilization—lateral glide: *(a)* with hip in extension, *(b)* with leg in hip flexion and pelvis stabilized at opposite ASIS, *(c)* with hip in flexion and lateral rotation and pelvis stabilized at opposite ASIS.

Posterior Glide

The posterior (or dorsal) glide is useful for increasing hip flexion and medial rotation. The patient lies supine with the hip and knee flexed. The degree of hip flexion depends on the technique used. When a belt is used, partial flexion of the joints is necessary, with the belt placed around the distal thigh and secured to the rehabilitation clinician's shoulder. The clinician places the stabilizing hand under the belt and the mobilizing hand over the anterior proximal thigh. With the elbow kept extended, the rehabilitation clinician applies a downward force on the proximal thigh, using his or her legs, while the patient's thigh is kept stable with the belt (figure 22.14a).

An alternative position is with the hip in 90° flexion and about 10° adduction and the knee in full flexion. The rehabilitation clinician applies the posterior glide force through the long axis of the femur by leaning his or her body weight into the femur (figure 22.14b). Care must be taken not to apply the mobilizing force through the patella.

Figure 22.14   Joint mobilization—posterior glide: *(a)* with strap, *(b)* large axis.

Medial Glide

This mobilization technique is used to increase hip abduction and flexion. The patient is sidelying on the unaffected side while the rehabilitation clinician supports the leg at the distal thigh and knee and positions it in slight abduction and flexion (figure 22.15). The clinician's mobilizing hand is placed on the proximal thigh, and the mobilizing force is applied downward, parallel to the joint's plane.

Figure 22.15   Joint mobilization: medial glide.

Anterior Glide

This technique is also called a ventral or PA glide and is used to increase hip extension and lateral rotation. With the patient prone and the knee flexed, the rehabilitation clinician supports the distal thigh using the stabilizing hand; the mobilizing hand is at the proximal posterior thigh (figure 22.16a). The stabilizing hand keeps the hip positioned in slight extension or neutral while the mobilizing hand applies a downward force through an extended elbow; body weight exerts the force. The hip can be placed in various rotation positions for additional techniques.

Figure 22.16   Joint mobilization—anterior glide: *(a)* prone on table, without strap, *(b)* prone off table, with strap.

In an alternative position, the patient is prone, with the hips on the edge of the table and the noninvolved lower extremity supporting the body weight with its foot on the floor. The clinician can either support the patient's distal thigh in one hand or can have a stabilizing strap over the shoulder and wrapped around the distal thigh (figure 22.16b).

Self-Mobilization

The patient can perform self-distraction using a stretch strap. The patient is supine with the strap anchored around the foot and the anterior hip; the knee and hip are placed in flexed positions, about 90° each (figure 22.17). A pad is placed on the anterior thigh for comfort. Keeping the opposite hip flexed with hands supporting the thigh, the patient pushes the involved foot against the strap, attempting to extend the hip and knee.

In an alternative position, the patient places a weight cuff around the ankle and stands with the foot off a step, allowing gravity to create a distraction force on the hip. The position is maintained for several minutes, as tolerated.

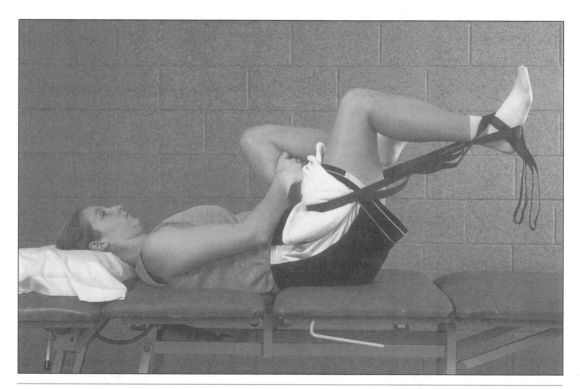

Figure 22.17   Joint mobilization: self-mobilization distraction.

FLEXIBILITY EXERCISES

▶ Active stretches and prolonged stretches are used to improve flexibility in the hip's lateral, anterior, medial, and posterior muscles.

Several muscles cross the hip joint, acting not only on the hip but also on the knee, back, or pelvis. For effective stretching at the hip, these segments must be positioned appropriately.

Active stretches are held for 15 to 20 s and are repeated about four times each. They should be repeated at least three to four times throughout the day. Active contraction of opposing muscles leads to improved results in flexibility exercises by enhancing relaxation of stretched muscle. Enough force is applied to move the muscle to a point at which the patient perceives a stretch without pain. Prolonged stretches are most effective in altering tissue length in scar tissue and connective tissue.

Lateral Muscles

Lateral hip muscles are frequently tight, and impact not only the hip but also the knee. Improper mechanics results, placing additional stress on the hip and knee joints and their structures.

Lower Lumbar Rotation

The lower lumbar muscles are stretched with the patient lying supine. The patient flexes the involved hip and knee and rotates the thigh across the body, keeping the ipsilateral shoulder on the ground. The contralateral hand can be used to apply additional stretch (figure 22.18). The stretch should be felt in the lower back and lateral hip. The more the hip is flexed, the lower the stretch is felt.

The ipsilateral shoulder must be kept on the ground. If necessary, the arm can be extended outward from the side to prevent the shoulder from rising up.

Figure 22.18   Lumbar rotation stretch.

Tensor Fascia Lata Stretch

The TFL, in addition to the other hip abductors, can be stretched in standing, sitting, or sidelying. In standing, the patient places the affected side closest to a wall about an arm's-length distance from the wall. The feet are crossed, with the affected extremity behind the uninvolved extremity. Placing the hand on the wall, the patient pushes the hips toward the wall, keeping both feet on the ground as the hand on the wall provides a push force (figure 22.19a). The patient should not rotate the body or bend the elbow. The stretch should be felt on the outside of the thigh.

In sitting, the patient has the uninvolved extremity out straight and the involved extremity flexed at the knee and hip; the foot of the involved extremity is placed flat on the ground on the outside of the uninvolved knee. The patient uses the hands to pull the involved knee across the body toward the opposite shoulder (figure 22.19b).

In sidelying, the patient lies on the uninvolved extremity with the top hip extended and the knee flexed. The top extremity is allowed to drop down behind the bottom extremity (figure 22.19c). The patient must not rotate the trunk to place the top hip behind the bottom hip. A pad under the bottom hip makes the position more comfortable. This position can be used for a prolonged stretch.

Figure 22.19 Tensor fascia lata stretch: *(a)* standing stretch, *(b)* seated stretch, *(c)* sidelying position for prolonged stretch.

Anterior Muscles

Hip flexors include the iliopsoas and rectus femoris. To include the rectus femoris in a stretch, the knee must be flexed. If the knee is extended, the iliopsoas will be the only hip flexor stretched. Positions for stretching these muscles are standing, kneeling, supine, and prone. In standing, the patient grasps the foot from behind to bring the heel to the buttock while keeping the knee pointing to the floor (figure 22.20a). The back must remain erect in order to prevent iliopsoas shortening, and the knee must be kept pointing to the floor to prevent shortening of the rectus femoris.

In kneeling, the involved extremity is the kneeling leg, and the opposite extremity bears weight on the foot in front. The patient transfers weight from the back knee to the front foot so that the weight moves in front of the back knee (figure 22.20b). The back should remain erect. The patient can apply additional stretch by attempting to flex the knee, although this can be a difficult maneuver. A pad can be placed under the knee for comfort.

In prone, the patient lies on the edge of a table with the uninvolved foot on the floor and the hip and knee slightly flexed to stabilize the pelvis. A pillow or wedge is placed under the thigh on the table. The patient rests with weight on the elbows. Additional stretch is applied with greater pillow height or flexing the knee. This position can be used for a prolonged stretch (figure 22.20c).

In supine, the stretch position is the Thomas hip flexor stretch. The patient lies with the buttocks on the end of the table. The uninvolved extremity is flexed at the hip and knee and can be supported by the patient's hands. The involved extremity is placed over the edge of the table so that the mid to upper thigh is at the edge (figure 22.20d). Substitutions during this stretch include hip abduction and lateral rotation. The extremity position can be aligned passively by the clinician or with use of stabilization straps. This position can be used for a prolonged stretch. Weights can be applied to the ankle for additional stretch force during a prolonged stretch.

(continued)

Figure 22.20 Anterior muscle stretch: (a) standing hip flexor stretch, (b) kneeling hip flexor stretch.

Figure 22.20 *(continued)* Anterior muscle stretch: *(c)* prone hip flexor stretch, *(d)* supine hip flexor stretch.

Medial Muscles

The adductors can be stretched in sitting, standing, or kneeling. The long adductors pass below the knee joint, so they are stretched when the knee is extended; the shorter adductors can be stretched with the knee flexed or extended.

In sitting, the patient flexes and abducts the hips and knees to place the bottom of the feet together. He or she pulls the feet toward the buttocks. In this position, the hands are placed on the ankles, and the forearms are placed along the inner lower legs. A stretch force is applied along the forearms to lower the knees (figure 22.21a). The stretch is felt in the groin. The back should be kept straight, with forward bending originating from hip flexion.

An alternative position is in long sitting with the hips abducted and the knees extended. The patient flexes forward from the hips, keeping the back straight, while placing the weight on the hands to keep the groin muscles relaxed (figure 22.21b). Additional stretch can be provided to the long adductors by rotating to the affected extremity and reaching for the toes.

In kneeling, the patient is on the uninvolved knee and places the involved extremity in abduction with the knee straight (figure 22.21c). The uninvolved hip is pushed laterally away from the involved extremity as the involved extremity is pushed downward. A pillow can be placed under the supporting knee for comfort, and the patient can use hand support if needed. The inside border of the involved foot should remain in contact with the floor so the hip does not rotate.

In standing, the patient stands sideways to a supporting object that is about hip height and places the involved extremity's foot on top of the object (figure 22.21d). Keeping the medial border of the foot facing downward, the patient squats on the supporting extremity while pushing on the involved lateral thigh. The patient should be cautioned regarding substitutions of hip or pelvis rotation.

Posterior Muscles

The hip extensors and lateral rotators are the posterior muscle groups. The hip extensors include the hamstrings and gluteals; the lateral rotator of primary concern is the piriformis.

Figure 22.21 Medial hip muscle stretch: *(a)* sitting position for short adductors, *(b)* long-sitting position for long adductors, *(c)* kneeling position, *(d)* standing position.

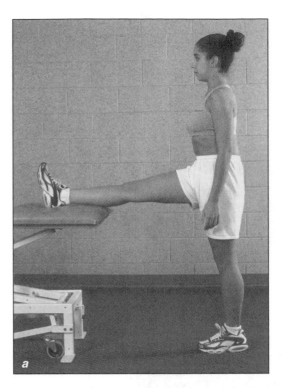

Hip Extensors

The hamstrings are frequently stretched with the patient standing or supine. In standing, the patient places the involved extremity on a supporting surface (figure 22.22a). The height is determined by the tightness of the hamstrings: The tighter the hamstrings, the lower the surface. The standing extremity should be positioned with the foot facing forward. Keeping the back straight, the patient leans forward from the hips toward the elevated foot. The involved extremity should be maintained with the foot facing the ceiling and in good body alignment, not in abduction. Reaching with the opposite hand prevents the pelvis from rotating and lessening the effectiveness of the stretch.

The hamstrings can be stretched in supine with the uninvolved extremity in full hip and knee extension. With the involved knee in extension, the patient places his or her hands around the posterior thigh and pulls the leg toward the chest (figure 22.22b). The back should not arch, and the uninvolved extremity's knee should not come off the supporting surface. The knee is extended until a stretch is felt.

The gluteals are stretched in a position similar to that for the supine hamstring stretch, with the difference being that the involved extremity's knee is flexed and the force pulls the knee toward the chest. The pelvis should not roll posteriorly, and the opposite thigh should not lift off the table (figure 22.22c).

Figure 22.22 Hip extensor muscle stretches: *(a)* standing hamstring stretch, *(b)* supine hamstring stretch, *(c)* supine gluteal stretch.

Piriformis

The piriformis can be effectively stretched in a supine, standing, or quadruped position. In supine, the patient lies with the knees crossed, the involved extremity on top of the uninvolved extremity. The knees are brought to the chest, and the patient pulls them, with the involved extremity's knee directed toward the opposite shoulder (figure 22.23a).

In a quadruped position, the patient crosses the involved extremity under the uninvolved extremity and leans the hips backward, keeping the uninvolvedextremity's knee off the floor and allowing it to move back (figure 22.23b). This permits the involved hip to adduct, flex, and medially rotate. In standing, the patient rests the involved extremity's leg on a tabletop with the hip in lateral rotation and flexion. He or she leans forward toward the tabletop to feel the stretch in the hip.

Figure 22.23   Piriformis stretches: *(a)* supine stretch, *(b)* quadruped stretch.

STRENGTHENING EXERCISES

▶ Strengthening exercises for the hip, which are analogous in their progression to those for other body segments, include isometric, body-weight resistance, rubber tubing, machine, free-weight, and Swiss-ball activities.

As with other body segments, hip exercises begin with isometrics and can be performed in various joint positions for optimal results. Isotonic exercises include concentric and eccentric exercises; these use gravity as resistance for the least difficult exercise and advance to various other forms of resistance including manual resistance, weight cuffs, rubber tubing, pulleys, and machines. Increased manual resistance and weight-cuff resistance are applied at the ankle. If less resistance is necessary, the same amount of resistance can be placed more proximally on the extremity.

The exercises should be performed in a smooth, controlled motion of the hip through a full range of motion. Substitutions of other muscles occur easily in the hip and must be carefully observed and corrected as needed by the rehabilitation clinician. Low intensity, high repetition resistance can be replaced with higher loads and fewer repetitions as strength and control improve.

Because the trunk, knee, and ankle are so intimately connected to the hip, strength, motion control and stabilization within all of these segments are vital to hip stability and quality of performance. Exercises to satisfy deficiencies in these areas must be part of a total hip rehabilitation program. As exercises for these segments have been presented in previous chapters, they are not repeated here.

Isometric Exercises

The patient can perform isometrics independently against his or her hand or a stationary object. To perform hip adduction in long or short sitting, the patient places either the hands or a rolled towel between the knees and attempts to push the knees together (figure 22.24a).

Hip abduction isometrics are performed in sitting. The patient moves the thigh outward as he or she resists the motion at the knee on the lateral distal thigh (figure 22.24b).

Figure 22.24   Isometric hip exercises: *(a)* hip adduction, *(b)* hip abduction.

Hip flexion is best performed while sitting in a chair. The patient places a hand on the distal thigh and resists attempts to lift the knee up. The patient should refrain from using the foot to push off the floor.

Hip extension is performed best in supine. The patient squeezes the buttocks to set the gluteals.

All isometric exercises are performed using a buildup to maximal tension. The tension is held for 5 or 6 s and then gradually released to full relaxation before the exercise is repeated. Isometrics are performed several times throughout the day in sets of at least 10 repetitions. They are used early in the rehabilitation program when the muscle is very weak or when range of motion is limited either by immobilization or by restricted mobility.

Body-Weight Resistance Exercises

In a 68-kg (150-lb) patient, the lower extremity weighs about 11 kg (25 lb). This can be substantial resistance for a very weak hip muscle. Weight should not be added to the extremity until the patient is able to control movement against gravity through a full range of motion.

If the patient is unable to lift the extremity against gravity, flexing the knee to perform the exercise can shorten the resistance lever-arm length. If antigravity exercises are too difficult for the patient, he or she can perform the same activity in standing; gravity is less in this position, but the muscle is still required to contract and move the hip.

Hip Abduction

With the patient in sidelying on the uninvolved extremity, the bottom extremity is flexed at the hip and knee for stability. The patient keeps the knee and hip extended and lifts the extremity against gravity (figure 22.25). Common substitutions in this exercise include rotating the hip, lying more toward the back, and moving the hip into flexion and out of the abduction plane. These substitution patterns should be corrected to prevent either the rotators or the hip flexors from performing the exercise.

Figure 22.25   Isotonic hip abduction exercises.

Hip Adduction

The patient lies on the involved side with the top extremity flexed at the hip and knee and the foot placed in front of the bottom knee. Keeping the involved extremity's knee and hip extended, the patient lifts the extremity against gravity (figure 22.26a). Common substitutions are rolling toward the back or flexing the hip to permit the hip flexors to perform the exercise. The exercise is more difficult because greater trunk stabilization is required if the patient lifts the top extremity into abduction and maintains that position while lifting the bottom extremity to meet the top extremity (figure 22.26b). An alternative position is with the top extremity placed on a supporting object such as the seat of a chair (figure 22.26c).

Figure 22.26 Isotonic hip adduction exercises: (a) without top leg support, (b) with additional requirements for trunk stabilization, (c) with top leg supported.

Hip Extension

The patient lies in prone with the extremity either supported in extension or positioned in flexion. Hip hyperextension is limited to about 15°, so when the patient begins in a fully extended position, the amount of motion the muscles produce is relatively small (figure 22.27a). If the patient lies prone with the extremity over the edge of a table, the hip begins in flexion and must travel through a greater range of motion (figure 22.27b). In either position, the patient should squeeze the gluteal muscles while lifting the extremity and should keep the knee extended to facilitate all hip extensor muscles. If the patient is to isolate the gluteals, the knee should be flexed; but remember that with a shorter lever-arm length, the resistance of the extremity is less. Common substitutions for this exercise are hip rotation and trunk rotation.

The patient can also strengthen hip extensors with a bridge exercise. The patient lies supine with the hips and knees flexed and with the feet flat on the floor. The hips are raised so that the hips and trunk form a straight line. The patient is then instructed to hold this position for several seconds. This exercise can be advanced to one-extremity support (figure 22.27c). A common substitution is dropping the hips, moving them into flexion.

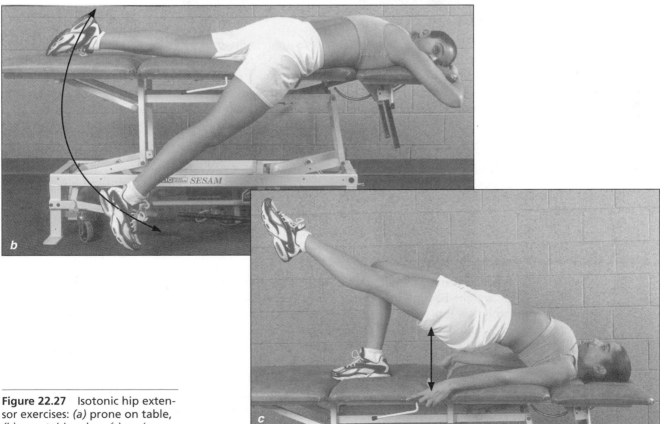

Figure 22.27 Isotonic hip extensor exercises: *(a)* prone on table, *(b)* over table edge, *(c)* supine.

A figure-4 exercise serves the dual purpose of strengthening hip extensors and lateral rotators. The patient lies prone; the involved extremity is flexed at the hip and knee, and the ankle is under the uninvolved thigh. If the patient lacks enough flexibility for the position, he or she should place the involved extremity's ankle on top of the uninvolved extremity as proximal along the extremity as possible. In a figure-4 position, the patient lifts the flexed knee as high as possible (figure 22.28). If the right knee is being lifted, the face should be turned to the left, and vice versa. Typical substitutions for this exercise are hip rotation and trunk rotation.

Figure 22.28 Figure-4 lift.

Hip Flexion

A straight-leg raise performed in supine strengthens the hip flexors. The uninvolved extremity is flexed at the hip and knee, with the foot flat on the supporting surface. The patient tightens the abdominals to prevent the back from arching, tightens the quadriceps to maintain knee extension, and lifts the involved extremity upward toward the ceiling. Rotation and hip abduction should be corrected if the patient attempts substitutions with these motions.

Rubber-Tubing Resistance Exercises

Rubber tubing or bands or weighted pulleys can be used progressively once the patient is able to perform antigravity exercises through a full range of motion. In the following descriptions of the exercises, the involved extremity is used as the exercising extremity, so it is advisable to use upper-body support devices for balance in order to promote better execution.

Rubber-tubing exercises can also be performed with the resistance attached to the uninvolved extremity so the involved extremity must work to support and stabilize the body during uninvolved extremity activities. When exercises are used with that goal, the use of upper-extremity support should be limited or eliminated to facilitate a greater effort from the weight-bearing hip. When the exercises are used for balance and proprioception, they can be executed either as explained here—in straight planes of movement—or in the more challenging diagonal proprioceptive neuromuscular facilitation planes.

If the patient performs the exercise using a substitution pattern, correct the execution by providing verbal and/or tactile cueing or by providing visual feedback with a mirror. If substitution continues with these corrections, the resistance may be too much for the patient to control properly, and he or she should use the next-lightest resistance band instead. The motion should be full and controlled by the patient throughout the exercise.

Figure 22.29   Rubber-tubing hip abduction.

Hip Abduction

With the tubing attached to a doorway or table leg, the patient places the tubing around the involved extremity's ankle. The patient stands sideways with the uninvolved side closest to the anchor site, takes the slack out of the tubing, tightens the quadriceps and gluteals, and abducts the extremity out to the side (figure 22.29). Common substitutions for this exercise include hip flexion, trunk forward lean, side lean to the opposite side, and hip hiking. If verbal and visual cueing do not correct the substitution patterns, a less-resistive band may be necessary. A full range of motion should be possible.

Hip Adduction

With the tubing anchored around a table leg or secured low in a closed doorway, the patient places the tubing around the involved extremity's ankle and stands sideways from the anchor site with the involved side closest to the anchor site. With the laxity taken out of the tubing, the patient moves the extremity with the knee straight across and in front of the uninvolved extremity. Common substitutions are rotating the trunk as the extremity moves across the body, flexing the hip too far forward, hip flexion, and trunk lean toward the tubing anchor.

Gluteus Medius

For this exercise, short-length tubing is wrapped around both ankles. In standing, the patient tightens the quadriceps and gluteals and extends the involved hip backward and outward to about a 45° angle (figure 22.30a). Placing both hands on a wall keeps the patient from substituting trunk forward bend and side-bend away from the involved extremity.

An alternative gluteus medius exercise is performed with the patient standing sideways with the uninvolved side about 5 to 10 cm (2–4 in.) from the wall. The uninvolved extremity's knee is flexed to 90° and is pressed sideways into the wall. The involved extremity is flexed slightly at the knee and should be in line with the ipsilateral shoulder and the second toe (figure 22.30b).

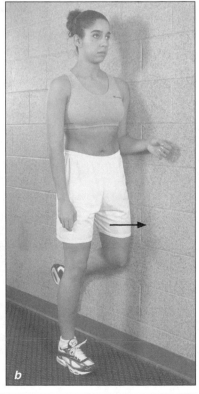

Figure 22.30   Gluteus medius strengthening: (a) with short-length thera-band, (b) the standing leg is the involved leg.

Figure 22.31   Rubber-tubing hip extension.

Hip Extension

With the tubing anchored around a table leg or low in a closed doorway, the patient places the tubing around the involved extremity's ankle and faces the anchor site. Taking the slack out of the tubing, the patient tightens the quadriceps and gluteals and extends the hip (figure 22.31). Common substitutions that should be corrected include trunk forward lean, hip abduction, and knee flexion.

Hip Flexion

With the tubing anchored around a table leg or low in a closed doorway, the patient stands with the tubing around the involved ankle and his or her back to the anchor site. After having removed the slack from the tubing, the patient tightens the quadriceps to keep the knee extended and flexes the hip. Common substitutions include backward trunk lean and knee flexion.

Hip Medial rotation

The tubing is anchored to between a closed door and doorframe about 30 to 45 cm (12–18 in.) from the floor. With the uninvolved side closest to the tubing anchor, the patient lies prone on the floor with the tubing around the involved ankle. The involved extremity's knee is flexed to 90°, and the slack is taken out of the tubing. The patient uses the involved hip to rotate the tubing away from the anchor site (figure 22.32). Common substitutions to avoid include pelvis rotation and hip extension.

Figure 22.32   Rubber-tubing internal rotation.

Hip Lateral rotation

With the tubing anchored as for hip medial rotation, the patient lies prone on the floor with the involved extremity closest to the anchor site and the tubing around the extremity's involved ankle. With the knee flexed to 90° and the slack taken out of the tubing, the patient pulls the involved extremity's foot toward the uninvolved extremity. Substitutions include extending the knee and rotating the hips or pelvis.

Machine and Equipment Exercises

Many resistive exercises for the hip are the same as those used for the knee as discussed in chapter 21. Some additional exercises are mentioned here, but you should revisit chapter 21 for additional hip exercises. Some of these are step exercises, wall squats, mini-squats, the plié, lunges, sit-to-stand, and leg press machine exercises.

Reciprocal-Exercise Equipment

Reciprocal-exercise equipment can be useful for range-of-motion gains, strengthening, and coordination. These can be used early in strengthening work when the patient may not have antigravity strength but is able to tolerate resistance in an upright posture that does not require full antigravity strength. These exercises include activities on machines such as the step machine, ski machine, or stationary bike (figure 22.33).

Figure 22.33 Reciprocal machines, such as the step machine *(a)* or stationary bike *(b)*, can be used to increase strength, ROM, and coordination.

Resistance Machines

Machines have a variety of resistance mechanisms, including weights pans, hydraulics, rubber, and asymmetrical cam systems. They all provide progressive resistance for a variety of exercises. Resistive increments vary from one type machine to another.

Figure 22.34   Isolated hip-motion exercises.

Hip Abduction, Adduction, Extension, and Flexion

Some machines offer progressive resistance only in single planes of motion while others provide resistance selections in multiple planes of hip motion. In each case the machine isolates a hip motion and does not utilize motion from other joints or other hip motions (figure 22.34). It is essential to provide instruction in the proper use of these machines. The patient should receive instruction on correct alignment, proper weight selection that can be controlled throughout the motion, and precise execution without improper substitution.

Recliner Leg Press

There are different models of leg presses on the market. The machines are closed kinetic chain devices that utilizes hip, knee, and ankle motions. The hip can be exercised in supine with the involved extremity placed on the platform so the knee and hip start the exercise at 90°. The patient pushes the extremity into extension so that the body moves away from the platform (figure 22.35).

The patient can take an alternative position to further increase hip-extension activity. With the patient in a quadruped position on the machine, the involved extremity is placed high on the platform and the patient bears weight on the uninvolved extremity's knee and elbows. The patient pushes on the platform to extend the involved extremity.

Figure 22.35   Recliner leg press exercises: *(a)* supine position, *(b)* prone position.

Figure 22.36 Squat exercise with free weights. Correct body alignment should be maintained.

Free-Weight Squats and Split Squats

Barbells and dumbbells can provide resistance to squat and split-squat exercises. The patient should be cautioned to keep good alignment of the knee and back in executing these exercises (figure 22.36). Weights should begin light and progress as the patient demonstrates control and adequate strength. These exercises can be advanced to have the patient stand with the involved extremity in the regular squat position and the uninvolved extremity on a box or step to place more resistance on the involved limb.

Swiss-Ball Exercises

Swiss-ball exercises can involve activities such as bridging with leg curls, first with both legs and then with the involved extremity only. This exercise facilitates the hip extensors. Hip flexor exercises on the Swiss ball are performed with the patient prone with hands on the floor and tibias on the ball. The patient pulls the knees toward the chest while maintaining balance on the ball (figure 22.37).

Both of these exercises become more difficult when manual resistance is applied to the movement of the ball: The clinician's hands provides friction against ball motion during the exercise.

Figure 22.37 Swiss-ball hip-flexion exercise: With legs on the ball, the knees and hips begin in an extended position. The patient pulls the knees toward the chest to end in the position shown.

PROPRIOCEPTION EXERCISES

▶ Proprioception exercises for the hip progress from static balance activities to distracting balance activities, then to agility exercises such as rapid box exercises, and finally to plyometrics.

Balance exercises can begin early in the therapeutic exercise program when the patient is able to bear weight on the extremity. As with other lower-extremity injuries, progression is from weight-transfer activities and gait training to stork standing with eyes open and then eyes closed. Balance begins with static activities and advances to distracting activities in which static balance is challenged while the patient performs other functions and dynamic activities. These can include the tubing exercises performed with the uninvolved extremity while the patient balances on the involved extremity on the ground or on a 1/2 foam roller; stork standing on a trampoline or BAPS board while catching or bouncing a ball; and using a balance board or other machine such as a Fitter or slide board.

As balance, proprioception, strength, and coordination improve, the patient progresses to agility exercises that demand higher proprioceptive responses and control. These include resistive weight-transfer activities, exercises using increased speed of movement, and finally explosive exercises using jumping and plyometrics.

Agility exercises were introduced in chapters 20 and 21. Some of these are rapid box exercises such as rapid step-up-and-step-down activities, changes in direction from left to center to right box steps, and hopping over boxes.

Rubber tubing can be used to increase resistance of rapid-direction-change exercises. With tubing attached to the waist, the patient can be required to jump to different targets on the floor, change directions of movement, and alternate patterns of jumps. Some of these exercises are detailed in chapter 20.

Plyometric exercises maximize use of the patient's agility, strength, power, and coordination; these begin when the patient has demonstrated good control in rapid agility exercises and has good strength and adequate flexibility to perform the exercises safely.

Plyometric exercises such as drop-and-jump activities, lateral jumps, and cone jumps can all be used for all lower-extremity injuries, including hip injuries. These activities are discussed in chapters 9 and 20.

FUNCTIONAL EXERCISES

▶ The rehabilitation clinician selects functional exercises for the hip, when the patient is ready for them, according to the patient's specific sport and position.

A wide variety of functional exercises can be included in hip rehabilitation. The primary factor in determining which ones to use in a hip program is the patient's sport and position within the sport. If the sport includes primarily running activities, then those types of activities are included in the functional program. If the patient's activity includes rapid changes of direction, acceleration, and deceleration, then the functional portion of the program includes those activities. If the patient's activity demands include jumping, pivoting, and backward motions, then those are added to the functional program.

Speed, distance, repetitions, and difficulty of the exercises are at a low level at first and are increased progressively as the patient is able to tolerate the added stress. A continuous progression to activities that precisely mimic the demands of the patient's activity is provided, as long as pain and other deleterious signs are avoided.

The patient may return to full activity participation once he or she is pain free; has normal strength, flexibility, and agility; can perform equally on the left and right lower extremities without hesitating or favoring the involved extremity; and uses both lower extremities normally.

SPECIAL REHABILITATION APPLICATIONS

Although hip injuries do not occur as often as injuries of the ankle and knee, they can be just as disabling and need proper rehabilitation if the patient is to have a successful return to sport participation. Younger patients whose bones have not matured sustain more growth plate injuries in the hip than they do ligamentous or musculotendinous injuries (Mellman et al. 1996). Some of the more common injuries and dysfunctions of the hip and their rehabilitation programs are discussed next.

> ► Among common hip injuries that the rehabilitation clinician encounters are muscle-imbalance syndromes, acute soft-tissue injuries, various inflammation conditions, and fractures and dislocation.

Muscle-Imbalance Syndromes

Many of the soft-tissue injuries around the pelvis, hip, and thigh result from muscle imbalances (Geraci 1994). These syndromes are characterized by tightness of a muscle group and weakness of its antagonist and compensatory muscle firing patterns in adjacent areas. The resulting symptoms typically include pain and reduced function and can cause structural changes. Changes in myofascial tissue are also commonly seen.

Hip Flexor Tightness Syndrome

This problem is common in gymnasts and dancers. Hip flexors are tight, and their antagonists, the hip and lumbar extensors, are weak and inhibited. This imbalance is characterized by an exaggerated anterior pelvic tilt and lumbar lordosis in standing. Lower lumbar spine dysfunctions including disk degeneration, spondylosis, spondylolysis, or spondylolisthesis can develop. Myofascial restriction is common in the lumbar paraspinals, quadratus lumborum, and latissimus dorsi.

Objective assessment findings demonstrate a positive Thomas test for hip tightness. In prone, assessment of muscle firing in hip extension reveals an asynchronous pattern. Normal firing sequence in prone hip extension is initiated by the hamstrings; next, the gluteus maximus fires, the firing sequential order is then the contralateral lumbosacral paraspinals, followed by the ipsilateral lumbosacral paraspinals, followed by the contralateral thoracolumbar paraspinals, and finally the ipsilateral thoracolumbar paraspinals fire (Geraci 1994). Excessive scapular muscle firing is seen as a compensation for weak, inhibited extensor muscles.

Treatment of this syndrome requires correction of shortened muscles, myofascial release of restricted soft tissue, correction of posture, strengthening of the weak muscles, and muscle reeducation to facilitate correct muscle firing patterns. When the antagonistic muscles are weak secondary to tightening of agonists, lengthening of the tight muscles often has a significant impact on positive strength changes in the antagonists. Pelvic stabilization activities and strengthening lower abdominals for pelvic support provide a base for posture correction. The use of electrical stimulation and instruction in muscle firing sequence patterns, beginning with slow sequences and progressing to more rapid firing sequences and finally to functional activities, can be helpful in muscle reeducation.

The patient can usually continue with some activities during the rehabilitation process, but he or she should be cautioned that performance may change as muscle firing patterns change. This can be frustrating for a patient who has adapted specific sport skills to compensate for imbalances.

Piriformis Syndrome

Buttock pain is the most distinguishing symptom of piriformis syndrome. Pain can also radiate distally into the thigh and lower leg, mimicking an S1 nerve root syndrome. Running, standing, or prolonged sitting can aggravate the piriformis. Clinical examination reveals tightness of the piriformis that is often accompanied by weakness. When the patient is relaxed in supine, the involved extremity is more laterally rotated than the contralateral leg. Palpation reveals tenderness, tightness, and soft-tissue restriction in the piriformis muscle. Active trigger points are often the source of pain referral into the lower extremity. Sciatic nerve irritation that occurs as the tight piriformis presses on the nerve can also refer pain into the lower extremity. The 15% of the population whose sciatic nerves pass through the piriformis muscle are more susceptible to this condition as the source of referred leg pain from the piriformis.

Common causes of piriformis syndrome include sacroiliac dysfunction; leg-length discrepancies; running on canted surfaces, creating a false leg-length difference; and muscle imbalances including tightness of the piriformis, hamstrings, and lateral thigh muscles.

Treatment includes correction of underlying causes, myofascial release and trigger point release techniques, stretching exercises, and strengthening exercises. The patient can usually continue sport participation during treatment. It is a self-limiting condition in that pain dictates the patient's ability to perform.

Case Study

A 25-year-old distance runner presents with complaints of right buttock and posterior thigh pain that has become progressively worse over the past three weeks. He has recently increased his distance from 6.4 to 9.7 km (4–6 miles). The pain occurs about 4.8 km (3 miles) into his run and remains. The patient reports that when he gets up from his desk after sitting for about 45 min, his right buttock is painful until he walks around for a few minutes. He had a back injury about five years ago that was treated, and he has not had any back problems since then. Standing trunk motions do not elicit pain in any direction. When he lies supine on the treatment table, his right leg is laterally rotated about 20° more than his left. Placing the hip in 60° flexion, adduction, and medial rotation elicits pain in the right buttock. Straight-leg raise is to 70° and negative for sciatic pain. Palpation of the right buttock reveals tenderness in the mid-buttock region to deep pressure. You can feel tightness in the piriformis. Resisted hip lateral rotation in this position is painful. Hip rotation is weak.

Questions for Analysis

1. What other tests should you perform to eliminate any other possible cause of the patient's problem?

2. What do you suspect is his problem?

3. What will be your first treatment for him today?

4. What instructions for home treatments will you give him before he leaves today?

5. What will your goals for the first week of treatment include?

6. What will you tell the patient when he asks you if he can continue running?

Acute Soft-Tissue Injuries

Injuries in this category include sprains, strains, and contusions. Traumatic bursitis can also come under this heading, but bursitis will be discussed in connection with repetitive stress injuries.

Contusions

Hip contusions are very common, especially in athletics. When they occur along the crest of the ilium, they are called a hip pointer. A hip pointer usually does not require rehabilitation unless it is severe and disabling. In these cases the patient experiences a rapid progressive onset of pain within 24 h following the injury; this pain increase is the result of edema and spasm of the muscles that attach to the iliac crest. These injuries involve hip and abdominal muscles that attach or cross the contusion site, so activities that elicit complaints of pain include hip motions of flexion and abduction and trunk motions, especially resisted motions. Ambulation is painful, especially long striding and faster speeds. Ecchymosis becomes evident within a day or two.

Treatment includes anti-inflammatory medication and modalities to absorb the ecchymosis, relieve muscle spasm, and encourage healing. The injury is self-limiting, primarily because of the muscle spasm and tenderness from the ecchymosis. Range of motion with the aid of electrical stimulation can be useful in restoring early active mobility and should be encouraged within the first or second day of the injury. Ultrasound is helpful for ecchymotic absorption. Light resistive strengthening exercises should be possible by day 2 or 3, depending on the severity of the injury. Resistive exercises progress in repetitions and resistance as the patient tolerates them.

Recovery depends on the severity of the injury; the quality of initial treatment in controlling the swelling, bleeding, and muscle spasm; and the timing of rehabilitation. With a moderate injury and appropriate care, the patient may return to full participation in less than one week, but more severe injuries with delayed care can disable the patient for at least a couple of weeks.

Groin Strain

Groin strains are defined as strains not only to the hip adductors but also to the hip flexors. The iliopsoas, rectus femoris, adductor longus, brevis, magnus, or sartorius may be involved. Most often, an adductor or the iliopsoas is the muscle injured. The muscle is injured when it is either brought beyond its normal limits of motion or produces a rapid forceful contraction. Premorbid contributing factors include muscle tightness, weakness, or imbalances. The injury is usually at the site of the musculotendinous junction and can be disabling in moderate or severe cases.

The patient has an antalgic gait favoring the injured leg, with an uneven stride cadence, shortened stride length, and reduced knee and hip motion. Muscle spasm, swelling, and tenderness to palpation of the injury site can also be present. Ecchymosis occurs in second- and third-degree strains.

Examination of the injured muscle includes resisted muscle activity tests to determine which motion produces the greatest pain response. Hip flexion with knee extension tests the iliopsoas; hip flexion with knee flexion tests the rectus femoris; hip flexion, lateral rotation, and abduction with resisted knee flexion tests the sartorius; and hip adduction tests the adductors.

Treatment includes modalities for pain control and spasm reduction. Electrical stimulation for muscle spasm reduction, along with assistive active range of motion and active range of motion, is used to regain lost range of motion as soon as possible. If the patient displays an antalgic gait, crutches are necessary until he or she demonstrates a normal gait. A hip spica wrap supports the muscle and reduces range of motion during ambulation to make walking more comfortable. Pool exercises and reciprocal-motion machines can be helpful after day 2 or 3. The patient begins with isometric exercises on day 2 or 3, and a gradual, progressive, resistive exercise program starts when the patient is able to move the limb in antigravity positions. Once the patient is able to weight transfer from one extremity to the other correctly, stork standing and progressive proprioception exercises are used to develop balance and, later, agility. Treadmill activities can begin when the patient walks normally without crutches; these entail first walking, then jogging, and finally running. Agility activities on the treadmill can be used when the patient demonstrates good muscle control and range of motion with closed kinetic chain exercises. Soft-tissue massage is helpful in reducing scar-tissue adhesions and stimulating blood flow to encourage healing after day 5 to 10, depending on the injury's severity and the extent of tissue damage.

Resistive tubing jumping, box drills, and lateral movements begin when good dynamic balance and muscle control are present. The patient advances to plyometrics then functional activities prior to his or her return to full activity.

Depending on the severity of the injury, the patient's program may span from less than a week to several weeks.

Sprains

Ligament sprains in the hip are relatively rare. The joint is stable because of its deep socket and strong ligamentous support and does not succumb easily to outside forces. Hip ligaments can incur sprains when a violent injury involving severe forces occurs. The hip is placed in a position of combined extreme flexion, abduction, and lateral rotation or combined extreme flexion, adduction, and medial rotation during these events.

Grades I and II joint mobilizations can relieve joint pain following a sprain. The patient can do pool exercises in small arcs of motion initially, with progression in the size of the arc of motion as the joint responds. Therapeutic exercises for flexibility and strength progress as in other hip rehabilitation programs.

Case Study

A 16-year-old sprinter injured her left hip when she was practicing three days ago. She has continued pain in the proximal inner thigh with some discoloration along the middle aspect of the inner thigh. She is unable to walk normally because of the pain. Your examination reveals hip abduction to 20°, limited by pain. The patient is unable to adduct the leg against gravity. Hip flexion is 4/5 but is not as tender as adduction. The inner thigh area feels tight and is tender to palpation from the middle thigh to the groin.

Questions for Analysis

1. What do you suspect is the patient's injury?

2. What other differential tests will you do?

3. What will her treatment today include?

4. What instructions for home care will you give her today?

5. Outline the progression of therapeutic exercises you will provide for this patient. What modalities will you use with her and why?

Inflammation Conditions

These injuries are overuse based and are the result of repetitive stresses applied at a rate greater than the body's ability to recover. Among the number of conditions that fall into this category are bursitis, tendinitis, and osteitis.

Bursitis

The most common bursitis in the hip is greater trochanteric bursitis; but other hip bursae, including the ischiogluteal and iliopectineal bursae, are also subject to inflammation.

If the patient's symptoms persist in spite of treatment efforts, other diagnoses must be considered. Additional diagnoses that should be ruled out include lumbar disk injury, facet syndrome, fracture, nerve entrapment, inguinal hernia, abdominal visceral diseases, hip joint disease, and bone tumor. Additional diagnoses for males are testicular torsion and chronic prostatitis.

Greater Trochanteric Bursitis

The greater trochanteric bursa is susceptible to bursitis when the patient's running mechanics increases stress to the bursa because the person has a greater-than-normal adduction angle or is running on a canted surface. Muscle imbalance between adductors and abductors, an increased Q-angle, leg-length discrepancy, and a wider pelvis are also precipitating causes for trochanteric bursitis. Falling on the lateral hip can cause a traumatic bursitis. Pain in the lateral hip can radiate distally down the thigh or proximally into the lateral buttock. There is pain with lying on the involved side and crossing the legs, as well as during running or walking.

The examination reveals tenderness to palpation over the greater trochanter, pain with hip rotation, and tightness of the ITB as demonstrated with a positive Ober's test. Resisted abduction is tender because of the pressure placed on the bursa by the contracting muscles. Passive hip flexion with adduction and medial rotation press the bursa against the greater trochanter and cause irritation. The patient may stand with the involved extremity more abducted or may place more weight on the contralateral leg.

Iliopectineal Bursitis

Dancers and skaters are the athletes who most commonly experience iliopectineal bursitis, although it can occur in most sports. The iliopectineal bursa lies superficially to the anterior acetabulum and deep to the iliopsoas tendon. Sudden flexion-extension activities, especially resisted motions, can aggravate the bursa. The bursa lies adjacent to the femoral nerve and can often irritate the nerve if it becomes inflamed and swollen. Pain occurs with either stretch or contraction of the iliopsoas muscle. The pain is located at the site of the bursa in the inguinal area, but it can also radiate into the hip, anterior thigh, or knee if the femoral nerve is also affected.

Ischiogluteal Bursitis

The ischiogluteal bursa lies between the ischial tuberosity and gluteus maximus. A traumatic bursitis can develop if the patient falls and lands on the buttocks, or it can develop over time consequent to prolonged sitting on hard surfaces or sitting with the legs crossed. Pain is present with hip or trunk flexion, stair climbing, and walking or running. Palpation of the ischial tuberosity with the patient in sidelying reveals localized tenderness with occasional radiation into the hamstrings or hip.

Treatment

Ultrasound and thermal techniques are the modalities most commonly employed for hip bursitis. Anti-inflammatory medications are provided either orally or by injection. Cross-friction massage reduces adhesions and promotes circulation. Therapeutic exercises should include stretching exercises to increase flexibility of tight muscles and strengthening to correct muscle imbalances. Correction of underlying causes such as running mechanics and running surfaces is necessary to reduce the risk of recurrence. The bursitis injury is self-limiting; and although a modification of activity level may be advantageous, total cessation of sport participation is left to the discretion of the rehabilitation clinician and/or physician. The amount of activity restriction depends on factors such as severity of the injury, type of sport, intensity of participation, and correction of mechanics.

Tendinitis

The adductor longus, iliopsoas, and rectus femoris tendons are the most common sites of tendinitis at the hip (Micheli and Coady 1997). Mechanisms of injury relate to overuse and can involve additional factors such as tightness, muscle imbalances, leg-length discrepancy, running on canted surfaces, increasing workloads too quickly, and incorrect mechanics. A gradual onset of pain in the groin (adductor longus) or inguinal area (rectus femoris or iliopsoas) is the primary complaint. The course of tendinitis in the hip follows that of tendinitis in other body segments, with a progression of pain into the patient's workout until daily activities such as walking and stair climbing are painful.

Examination reveals tenderness to palpation of the tendon. Crepitus may be felt. Stretching or resisted contraction can be painful. Flexibility is often reduced. Reduced stride length and diminished hip motion may be present in an antalgic gait.

Treatment follows the same course as for other tendinitis conditions. Anti-inflammatory medications and modalities for pain and inflammation control accompany therapeutic exercises. Stretching exercises and a graduated program of strengthening exercises including eccentrics are used as tolerated. Correction of the underlying causes is necessary. Cross-friction massage on the tendon reduces adhesion formation and promotes circulation. The patient's sport participation may have to be altered during treatment, depending on the severity of the injury.

Osteitis Pubis

Distance runners, race walkers, fencers, and soccer players are susceptible to osteitis pubis. This is an inflammatory condition of shear stresses caused by either repeated trauma or strain on the symphysis pubis joint. Pain onset is gradual and localized, with occasional radiation to the abdomen or groin. Aggravating activities include pivoting, jumping, sprinting, kicking, and sudden direction changes. Daily activities such as stair climbing can become painful. Stretching the legs into full abduction is painful, as is resisted adduction.

Treatment includes anti-inflammatory medication, modalities for pain relief, and therapeutic exercises for flexibility and strength as tolerated. The treatment progression follows that of a tendinitis program. This injury is self-limiting, but an initial reduction in normal activity helps to improve the response to treatment efforts and reduce recovery time.

Rice Krispie Syndromes

Snap, crackle, and pop sounds in the hip, resulting from a variety of factors, occur most commonly in dancers and gymnasts; but they can also occur in athletes in other sports such as skating and running.

The ITB can be the source of snapping in the hip. The snapping occurs when a tight ITB moves across the trochanteric bursa during hip flexion-extension. The condition becomes more noticeable with medial rotation when the band is moved across the bursa. It can cause pain and result in irritation of the trochanteric bursa or the proximal ITB.

Another malady found in dancers is the iliopsoas snap syndrome, which occurs when the hip is in about 45° flexion and moving into extension (Mellman et al. 1996). In this position the iliopsoas snaps against the iliopectineal bursa and anterior ridge of the acetabulum. Tightness of the iliopsoas or an anterior pelvic tilt can be the source of this syndrome, which can cause either bursitis or tendinitis in the area if it persists.

A clicking sound that accompanies pivoting movements may result from a torn acetabular labrum. The pivoting motion of the femur catches the labrum when the hip is in extension. A torn acetabular labrum presents with a sharp pain into the groin or anterior thigh.

Patients with the acetabular click syndrome should be referred to the physician for orthopedic examination. Patients with either iliopsoas or ITB syndrome should learn proper stretching exercises to lengthen shortened structures, should use stabilization techniques for proper pelvic and hip alignment, and should strengthen muscles if imbalances exist. Deep-tissue massage can be used to reduce adhesions, stimulate circulation, and reduce pain.

Case Study

A 16-year-old, male, competitive figure skater has been diagnosed with right iliopectineal bursitis. His physician has referred him to you for treatment. The patient presents with tenderness in the inguinal area for the past four weeks. Over that time the pain has increased to the point that it interferes with his practices. He is unable to lift his partner during their practices without intense pain. He also experiences pain throughout the practice, especially when he pivots, jumps, or lands on the right leg. During the past week he has noticed pain extending down the front of the thigh. Your examination reveals pain with resisted hip flexion and stretch into hip extension. The patient has pain and weakness to resisted hip flexion. He has a moderate lumbar lordosis and weakness in the lumbar extensors, and his hip-extension firing-pattern test reveals increased scapular activity with mild to moderate gluteal firing last in the sequence.

Questions for Analysis

1. List other tests for a differential diagnosis that you should perform today.

2. What treatment will you give the patient today?

3. What home instructions will you discuss with him?

4. What will you tell the patient when he asks if he can continue his workouts?

5. Outline your program for the patient for the next two weeks. What functional activities will you include in his program before full return to sport participation?

Fractures and Dislocation

Fractures fall into three main categories: traumatic, stress, and growth plate fractures. Traumatic fractures are not commonly seen in athletics because of the great forces required. Stress fractures, however, are more common. Growth plate fractures occur in younger athletes whose epiphyseal plates remain immature.

Traumatic Fractures

The traumatic fractures include avulsion fractures involving an apophysis that a muscle is attached to and nonapophyseal fractures that can include the pelvis or femur. Both types occur as the result of a high-energy violent trauma—the apophyseal fractures because of an internal force, and the non-apophyseal fractures because of an external force.

Avulsion Fractures

Avulsion fractures occur because of a sudden, forceful contraction of a muscle that pulls the apophysis away from the bone. The sites of avulsion fractures are at the origins of the hip's strong muscles. These locations include the ischium, ASIS, anterior inferior iliac spine, lesser trochanter, inferior pubic ramus, and iliac crest—the origin sites for the hamstrings, sartorius, rectus femoris, iliopsoas, adductors, and abdominals, respectively. The greater trochanter rarely is a site of avulsion fractures.

The patient has pain with active movement and attempts to shorten the muscle's motion during ambulation. For example, if the ischium is fractured, the patient ambulates with a shortened stride length and keeps the leg from moving very far in front of the body to reduce pull on the ischium by the hamstrings. Resistance against the muscle is more painful than stretching the muscle, but both elicit significant pain responses. The site is very tender to palpation, and edema and discoloration are present.

Treatment depends on the size of avulsion and its location. An open reduction and internal fixation may be necessary but often is not. Crutches with partial weight bearing to tolerance are used for the first three to six weeks until the patient is able to walk normally. Isometric exercises and active range-of-motion exercises, pain free, are used early in the therapeutic exercise program. Modalities for modulation of pain, edema, and muscle spasm are used initially. Strength exercises progress from isometric to isotonic. Pool exercises can be used after the first or second week. Isotonic exercises progress as the patient tolerates them pain free, moving to antigravity resistance and weight-resistance activities as tolerated. When the patient is able to bear total body weight on the extremity, he or she can perform stork standing and other static balance activities and then advance to dynamic balance activities and agility exercises. From this point the typical progression is to plyometrics and then to functional exercises before return to full sport participation.

Rehabilitation may take up to three months following an avulsion fracture. The time required for full recovery depends on the site of the fracture, type of treatment (surgical or nonsurgical), and the individual patient's ability to progress.

Non-Avulsion Fractures

Common sites of these fractures include the pelvis, acetabulum, femoral neck, and intertrochanteric femur. Fractures of this type, which are rare in athletics, cause significant pain. Most often they require hospitalization and surgical treatment, especially if the fracture is displaced. The rehabilitation process is prolonged, a minimum of three months. During immobilization or after surgery, isometric exercises are used to reduce muscle atrophy. Other exercises and weight bearing may be delayed in comparison to the timing for avulsion fractures, but the program progression is similar.

Stress Fractures

Stress fractures occur most commonly in patients who suddenly increase their training intensity. This type of fracture is most often seen in distance runners and soccer players. The common sites of stress fractures are the pubic ramus, femoral neck, and subtrochanteric region of the femur. In patients with coxa vara, stress loads placed on the femoral neck may be increased, predisposing these individuals to femoral neck stress fractures.

The patient reports a sharp, deep, localized pain that is aggravated with jumping and running. In the early stages, rest relieves the pain; but as the injury progresses, the pain continues during rest.

Treatment includes correction of the causative factors. Non-weight bearing or partial weight bearing on crutches is used for up to three weeks. Exercises on reciprocal machines such as the stationary bike or upper-body ergometer, pool exercises including deep-water running, and pain-free open kinetic chain exercises can take place early in the program. Hip, knee, ankle, and trunk exercises should be part of the program. As the patient progresses to full weight bearing with a normal gait and without pain, he or she performs progressive closed kinetic chain and proprioception exercises to make additional strength, balance, coordination, and agility gains.

Growth Plate Fractures

Slipped capital femoral epiphysis is a displacement of the femoral head from the femoral neck because of a weakness in the epiphyseal plate. It occurs in boys, ages 10 to 17, and in girls, ages 8 to 15. It is seen in youths, who have predisposing factors such as a recent growth spurt, an imbalance of sex hormones and growth hormones, and is overweight or has a lanky build. The patient reports an insidious, gradual onset of pain in the groin that can refer to the thigh and knee in chronic slips. Less often, the patient experiences an acute slipped capital femoral epiphysis that presents with a sudden onset of pain and disability following a traumatic event. Pain produces an antalgic gait.

Examination reveals restriction of hip medial rotation, abduction, and flexion, with the greatest restriction in medial rotation. During active hip flexion, the hip also moves into lateral rotation. In a relaxed position, the leg is in greater lateral rotation than the contralateral limb. Hip abductors are weak.

Possible differential diagnoses with groin, anterior thigh, and knee pain must be investigated. Other possible diagnoses are fracture, tumor, hernias, strains, and contusions. An evaluation of the patient's history, hip motion, motion patterns, pain level, and strength helps the rehabilitation clinician determine other possible sources of the patient's pain.

Treatment includes open reduction and internal fixation followed by partial weight bearing for two to six weeks. Isometric exercises immediately postoperatively, followed by open kinetic chain exercises, are used early in the rehabilitation process. Pool exercises after the surgical incision has healed and the patient is still partial weight bearing are used to achieve range-of-motion and strength gains. Once full weight bearing is permitted, the patient continues to use the crutches until normal gait and hip control are evident. Stork standing and other proprioception exercises progress as tolerated when unilateral weight-bearing activities are permissible. The therapeutic exercise progression follows that for other fractures once the patient is full weight bearing.

Dislocation

Because the hip socket is deep and the ligaments surrounding it are strong, the hip is rarely dislocated in sports: a large, violent force is required to disrupt the joint. One may see dislocations in high-energy sports with large external force applications such as downhill skiing, soccer, football, and rugby. Rarely are orthopedic injuries considered medical emergencies, but hip dislocations are emergencies because of the risk of arterial damage.

Rehabilitation of hip dislocations follows up to three weeks of bed immobilization. During this time, isometric hip exercises and isotonic exercises for the knee and ankle are used to retard atrophy. Theraband exercises for the ankle and knee can be performed in bed throughout the day. Manual resistance exercises can also be used. Activities that put the hip at risk for redislocation include hip adduction, hip flexion, and trunk forward bending. For this reason, the patient should not cross the legs, sit in a chair with the hip at 90° to the trunk, or bend over from the waist for 12 to 16 weeks postinjury.

Once the patient is permitted crutch ambulation, usually partial weight bearing to tolerance, active range-of-motion exercises can begin. All exercises should be pain free and should not include motion beyond active abilities. The patient uses crutches for about 6 to 8 weeks postinjury, until he or she is able to ambulate normally and demonstrates good hip control. Closed kinetic chain exercises begin when the patient begins weight bearing, but hip flexion beyond 90° is avoided for up to 12 to 16 weeks post-injury. Machine squats, leg press, and other resistive machines for the hip are appropriate after week 12. Pool exercises can be started around week 8; however, swimming should be avoided until week 12 when the hip strength is sufficient to provide hip stability against the water's resistance; the breaststroke should be avoided until week 16. The stationary bike can begin at week 12 to 16; treadmill walking begins during week 10 and is performed without an incline until week 12. When the patient demonstrates good hip control, walking can progress to jogging after week 14 to 16. The patient transitions to running, then to agility and sport-specific activities as he or she makes further gains in strength, control, and coordination, usually anywhere from week 20 to week 30.

Acetabular Labral Tears

A child or young athlete with complaints of hip pain that has not responded to treatment may have a labral tear. This sharp anterior hip, thigh, or groin pain may be accompanied by popping, clicking, or catching. The most common location of acetabular labral tear is seen in the anterior labrum (Farjo, Glick, and Sampson 1999). If the anterior labrum is torn, pain will increase with hip extension. If the patient reports a previous hip injury and complains of persistent vague, recurrent groin or thigh pain, the clinician should rule out a labrum tear (Binningsley 2003). The preferred method of treatment of labral tears is arthroscopic debridement (O'Kane 1999).

Immediately postoperatively, these patients may ambulate either NWB or PWB with crutches for the first several days. Within the first week, range of motion exercises can begin along with isometric exercises for hip muscles. Active ROM exercises can be started early. Once the portal wounds are healed, pool exercises can be initiated. When the patient is able to bear full weight on the extremity, proprioception and balance activities as well as strengthening exercises can be started. Jogging and running activities can begin around post-op week five.

Case Study

A 17-year-old, female, forward soccer player reports that she has had progressive anterior hip pain for the past four weeks. The pain has increased to the point that it bothers her on stairs and during walking and standing. She ambulates with an antalgic gait, using a shortened stride length and keeping the hip flexed and in a forward trunk lean. Your examination reveals tenderness to resisted hip flexion that increases with resisted knee extension applied simultaneously. Hip flexion is weak. Passive stretch of prone hip extension with knee flexion is more uncomfortable than hip extension with the knee extended. There is tenderness to palpation of the anterior inferior iliac spine, and pressure on this area reproduces the patient's pain.

Questions for Analysis

1. What do you suspect is the patient's problem?

2. What other differential diagnoses should you eliminate, and how would you accomplish this?

3. Explain what your treatment for her today will include.

4. What home instructions will you give the patient before she leaves today?

5. Outline the rehabilitation program you will place the patient on over the next two weeks. How will you decide when she is ready to resume full sport participation?

If the patient has no complications, he or she may begin agility activities by week six, move into functional, and then into sport specific activities by week eight to ten.

SUMMARY

1. Discuss how anteversion and retroversion change lower-extremity mechanics.

   Normal alignment places the neck in a line that is 15° anterior to the line of the femur in the adult. If the angle is greater than 15°, the hip is in anteversion. If it is less than 15°, the hip is in retroversion. Retroversion and anteversion alter knee alignment and change the forces acting throughout the entire lower extremity. Retroversion results in frog-eyed patellae, or calcaneal inversion, and causes the individual to ambulate with a toe-out gait. Anteversion causes squinting patellae, or foot pronation, and causes the individual to ambulate with a toe-in gait. Anteversion makes the hip susceptible to dislocation.

2. Explain the mechanical factors involved in gait with hip abductor weakness and explain how a cane assists in normal gait.

   When the person stands on the involved extremity, the abductors are not strong enough to counter the force of gravity pulling the non-weight-bearing hip downward and laterally rotating the pelvis, so a normal gait is not possible. The patient either drops the non-weight-bearing hip and downwardly rotates the pelvis to that side, or tilts the trunk to lurch over the weak hip during stance on the leg so that the center of gravity is closer to the fulcrum, the femoral head. If the center of gravity is moved far enough laterally to put it lateral to the fulcrum, the abductors do not have to work and the pelvis does not drop. If a cane is used on the side opposite the weakness, an upward force is transmitted through the cane to counterbalance the downward gravitational force on the same side. Because the lever-arm from the cane to the fulcrum is longer than the center of gravity's lever arm, the force that must be transmitted through the cane is relatively small.

3. Identify a joint mobilization technique for the hip and explain its benefit.

   Medial glide is used to increase hip extension and lateral rotation.

4. Identify a flexibility and a strengthening exercise for the hip.

   Thomas stretch is used to gain hip extension. A rubber tubing exercise moving into extension is used to increase hip extensor strength.

5. Identify a proprioceptive exercise for the hip and indicate its progression.

   In a proprioceptive exercise progression for the hip, the patient stork stands with eyes open, then with eyes closed, then on an unstable surface, then on an unstable surface while performing a distracting activity, and finally on the involved extremity while performing a resisted exercise with the uninvolved extremity.

6. List precautions for a hip-dislocation rehabilitation program.

   Activities that put the hip at risk for redislocation include hip adduction, hip flexion, and trunk forward bending. Therefore, the patient should not cross the legs, sit in a chair with the leg at 90° to the trunk, or bend over from the waist for 12 to 16 weeks postinjury.

CRITICAL THINKING QUESTIONS

1. If you were Stevie in the opening scenario, how would you manage Joan's injury? Would you insist that she take time off from her performances; would you rehabilitate the injury as if Joan were not performing daily; would you treat the injury to keep it from getting worse until the season was over and fully rehabilitate it then; would you

refuse to treat her unless she complied with your recommendations; or would you use some other approach? Give justifications for your decision and explain your treatment program.

2. If a patient complains of anterior hip pain, what possible diagnoses will you need to differentiate before beginning a rehabilitation program? (Hint: Do a mental review of all the structures from superficial to deep.) What differences would there be in the rehabilitation programs for those diagnoses?

3. If a gymnast sustained an anterior hip contusion on the bars, what possible secondary problems would cause her to require rehabilitation? What would be your rehabilitation approach to these problems?

LAB ACTIVITIES

1. Locate the trigger points on your lab partner for the muscles listed below. As you perform each one, indicate what the pain pattern would be if the trigger point was active.

   a. Piriformis

   b. Iliopsoas

   c. Gluteus medius

   d. Gluteus minimus

   Where were your partner's most sensitive trigger points? Perform an ice-and-stretch technique on each of them and provide your partner with a home exercise for each tender trigger point.

2. Perform grades I, II, III, and IV of joint mobilizations on your lab partner's hip joint. Examine the joint's total range of mobility. Where does the joint's resistance occur relative to the entire joint's mobility? Is it the same for the other hip joint? How does your partner's joint excursion and point of resistance compare with two other people in your class? Of what relevance is this to your thoughts on hip joint mobilization?

3. Perform grades II and IV joint mobilizations on your lab partner's hip and identify what motion restriction would be best treated with each mobilization:

   a. Anterior glide

   b. Posterior glide

   c. Inferior glide

   d. Medial glide

   Which one was the easiest to perform? Which one allowed you to feel the greatest motion within the joint? Given the size of the leg, what accommodations did you have to make in order to manage the leg during joint mobilization treatment?

4. Check your partner's sequential firing pattern during prone hip extension. Looking at when these muscles fire, what is his sequence? What is the normal sequence? Compare your partner's sequential firing pattern with the opposite leg. Are they the same? What would you do to correct the sequence-firing pattern if it was abnormal? Why should an abnormal sequence-firing pattern be corrected?

5. Examine your partner's hip ROM for flexion, extension, abduction, lateral rotation, and medial rotation. What are the ranges of motion for each movement? What is normal for each motion? Measure medial and lateral rotation with your partner in seated and prone positions. Do you get differences between the two positions? Why?

6. Have your partner perform the TFL stretch in standing, sitting, and sidelying as demonstrated earlier in the chapter. Hold each stretch for 30 to 60 seconds. Observe and correct for substitutions. Which one did she feel the greatest stretch? What do you think is the reason for this?

7. Have your partner perform the hip flexor stretches demonstrated earlier in this chapter. Hold each stretch for 30 to 60 seconds. Observe and correct for substitutions. Which position created the greatest stretch for him? What do you think is the reason for this?

8. Instruct your partner in a piriformis stretch. Notice if she performs it correctly and give verbal cueing to correct for any errors. Reverse positions so you are now the patient and have your partner instruct you in a different piriformis stretch, correcting with verbal cues any errors in your performance. What kind of substitutions could each of you use in these exercises?

9. Have your partner perform each of the hip extension exercises in figures 22.27 and 22.28 for 20 repetitions. Which exercise was the most difficult? Why?

10. Using rubber tubing or bands that provide sufficient resistance, have your partner perform resisted hip extension and abduction, each for 15 repetitions. What are the substitutions he could use for each exercise? What verbal cues should you use to correct these errors?

11. Have your partner perform two different exercises for proprioception. Which one was the easier one and which one was more difficult? How could you make them each more difficult?

12. Have your partner perform two plyometric exercises and identify how you would determine when she has progressed in one to go to the next. What substitutions would you be looking for and how would you correct them with verbal cues?

13. A cross-country runner strained his piriformis three weeks ago when he slipped on wet grass running up a hill. He has noticed that he is limping and does not have the stride length he usually has when he runs. He reports that he has pain with sitting, walking, and running. Why do you think he continues to have pain three weeks after the injury? What do you think will need to be resolved before he is able to resume racing without pain? Describe a progressive rehabilitation program, including all types of exercises you would incorporate into the program. What would be your guidelines for progression throughout the program?

REFERENCES

Binningsley, D. 2003. Tear of the acetabular labrum in an elite athlete. *British Journal of Sports Medicine* 37:84-88.

Cyriax, J.H. 1975. *Textbook of orthopaedic medicine. Vol. 1. Diagnosis of soft tissue lesions.* Baltimore: Williams & Wilkins.

Farjo, L.A., Glick, J.M. and T.G. Sampson. 1999. Hip arthroscopy for acetabular labral tears. *Arthroscopy* 15:132-137.

Geraci, M.C. 1994. Rehabilitation of pelvis, hip, and thigh injuries in sports. *Physical Medicine & Rehabilitation Clinics of North America* 5:157–174.

Kapandji, I.A. 1986. *The physiology of the joints. Vol. 2. Lower limb.* 5th ed. New York: Churchill Livingstone.

Kibler, W.B. 1995. Biomechanical analysis of the shoulder during tennis activities. *Clinics in Sports Medicine* 14:79-85.

Mellman, M.F., McPherson, E.J., Dorr, L.D., and P. Kwong. 1996. Differential diagnosis of back and lower extremity problems. In *The spine in sports*, ed. R.G. Watkins. St. Louis: Mosby.

Micheli, L.J., and C.M. Coady. 1997. Approaching hip, pelvis, and groin injuries in athletes. *Biomechanics* 4:22–26.

O'Kane, J.W. 1999. Anterior hip pain. *American Family Physician.* 60:1687-1696.

Travell, J.G., and D.G. Simons. 1992. *Myofascial pain and dysfunction. The trigger point manual.* Vol. 2. Baltimore: Williams & Wilkins.

Glossary

A band—The portion of the sarcomere where the thick filaments inter-digitate with the thin filaments.

ABCs of proprioception—Agility, balance, and coordination.

abduction—Lateral movement of a limb or segment away from the midline of the body or part.

absolute refractory period—The time immediately following a stimulus when depolarization prevents another response of the muscle cell from occurring.

acceleration—Rate at which velocity increases.

acceleration phase—That portion of swing in which momentum is increased and the non-weight-bearing limb has propulsion forward.

accessory joint motion—Necessary mobility for normal joint motion that cannot be voluntarily performed or controlled.

accommodating resistance—An activity where the resistance provided a muscle changes as the muscle moves through its range of motion. Isokinetic activity.

acetylcholine—A neurotransmitter at the myoneural junction of striated muscles. Causes vasodilation.

actin—One of two primary proteins of the thin filament of the sarcomere.

action peak—The second ground reaction force peak. The peak occurs during the last half of support and is usually less than impact peak.

action potential—A brief nerve impulse created from a rapid change in the membrane potential to cause a muscle contraction.

active assistive range of motion (AAROM)—Range of motion that is performed with a combination of voluntary activity of the muscles and passive assistance from an outside source.

active range of motion (AROM)—The amount of movement produced at a joint by the patient without assistance.

active stretch—A stretch that uses the patient's active muscle force to control and provide the force for the stretch.

active trigger point—A trigger point that is always tender and that can produce referred pain whether the muscle is active or inactive.

adduction—Lateral movement of a limb or segment toward the midline of the body or part.

adenosine diphosphate (ADP)—A phosphate compound that, when combined with a phosphate, forms adenosine triphosphate (ATP) for energy production. It is also the product of the breakdown of ATP during energy production.

adenosine triphosphate (ATP)—A phosphate compound that provides energy for muscle activity.

adrenaline—See epinephrine.

afferent muscle nerve fiber—A sensory nerve fiber from the muscle spindle and Golgi tendon organ. There are two primary types, A and C fibers. C fibers are pain receptors; A fibers are tension and length receptors. Group III delta are A receptors that responds to pressure pain. Group I are A receptors: Group Ia form muscle spindle primary endings and Group Ib form Golgi tendon organs. Group II are A receptors and form muscle spindle secondary endings.

afferent receptors—Sensory receptors that transmit information from the periphery to the central nervous system.

agility—The ability to control the direction of a body or its parts during rapid movement.

agonist(ic)—A muscle acting as a prime mover to produce a motion.

all-or-none principle—A motor unit does not respond until the stimulus is sufficient to produce an action potential. The action potential produces a reaction from the entire motor unit.

alpha motor neuron—An efferent nerve from the ventral horn of the spinal cord to the muscle.

amortization phase—The second phase of a plyometric activity that is the rapid transition from eccentric to concentric motion.

angiogenesis—Formation of new blood vessels.

angle of pull of a muscle—Angle formed by the muscle's line of pull and the line of the bone. Maximal isometric force occurs at a 90° angle of pull.

angular motion—Rotational movement on an axis through an arc.

antagonist(ic)—A muscle that opposes the motion of another muscle.

anteversion—Excessive anterior angulation of the femoral head, resulting in a toe-in gait.

arachidonic acid—An unsaturated essential fatty acid. Works as a precursor in the production of substances, including leukotrienes, prostaglandins, and thromboxanes.

Archimedes' principle of buoyancy—Principle stating that a body partially or fully immersed in a fluid will experience an upward thrust of that fluid that is equal to the weight of the fluid the body displaces.

areolar connective tissue—Loose connective tissue with unorganized structure and relatively long distances between cross-links.

arthrokinematics—The motions between the bones that make up a joint, including roll, slide, spin, compression, and distraction.

arthroscopy—Use of an endoscope to examine or surgically treat the interior aspect of a joint.

assessment—A conclusion based on the gathering of information through an evaluation.

ATPase (adenosine triphosphatase)—Myosin enzyme that is a catalyst the body uses to break down ATP into ADP and phosphate for energy production.

atrophy—Wasting away of tissue with a decrease in size and strength, especially from lack of use.

autogenic inhibition—A protective mechanism provided by the Golgi tendon organ, in which a Golgi tendon organ stimulus facilitated by a sudden stretch causes a reflex activation of the antagonist and relaxation of the agonist.

balance—The body's ability to maintain an equilibrium by controlling the body's center of gravity over its base of support.

ballistic stretching—A rapid stretch or bouncing technique used primarily in sport activities but seldom used in rehabilitation because of the increased risk of injury.

Bankart lesion—Tear of the capsulolabral complex from the glenoid rim.

barrier—A resistance that is felt when a part is moved through its passive range of motion in muscle energy techniques.

Barton's fracture—A fracture of the wrist that occurs with a sudden, violent wrist extension and pronation.

base of support—Two-dimensional area that lies within the points of contact between an object and the supporting surface.

basophil—See granular leukocyte.

Bennett's fracture—A fracture of the first metacarpal.

boutonniere deformity—Deformity characterized by flexion of the PIP joint and hyperextension of the DIP joint.

boxer's fracture—Fracture of the metacarpals secondary to a compressive force.

bradykinin—A local tissue hormone that is activated by the interaction of proteases upon the Hageman factor. A very potent local vasodilator. It increases vascular permeability and stimulates local pain receptors.

brain stem—Includes the midbrain, pons, medulla oblongata, and diencephalon to form the stem of the brain between the spinal cord and cerebrum.

Brannock measuring device—Used to determine shoe size (length and width).

bursa—Synovial-filled membrane that lies between adjacent structures to limit friction and ease movement.

bursitis—Inflammation or swelling of a bursa.

callus—Fibrous matrix formed at a bone's fractured sites. Immobilizes the bone fragments and serves as the foundation for eventual bone replacement.

capsular pattern—A characteristic pattern of motion unique to each joint when a loss of motion is caused by capsular tightness.

carpal tunnel syndrome—A condition of the wrist and hand characterized by compression of the median nerve as it passes through the carpal tunnel.

center of buoyancy—The center of gravity of the fluid displaced by a body in water and the point at which the buoyant force acts on the body.

center of gravity—The point on an object around which its weight is balanced.

central nervous system—The brain and spinal cord comprise the central nervous system.

cerebellum—That section of the brain that lies below the posterior cerebrum and behind the brain stem and is connected to the brain stem by paired peduncles.

cerebral cortex—The surface of the brain that contains primarily gray matter and nerve cell bodies.

cerebrum—The largest portion of the brain encompassing most of the skull.

chemoattractant—See chemotactic factor.

chemotactic factor—A chemical gradient. Also referred to as a chemotactin or chemoattractant. Occurs after an injury. Cells either become oriented along a chemical concentration gradient or move in the direction of that gradient. Example: Chemicals attract platelets, red blood cells, and polymorphonuclear leukocytes into an injured area.

chemotactin—See chemotactic factor.

chemotaxis—Movement of cells or chemicals in response to a chemical stimulus. Vital activities in wound healing that occur through complex and not totally understood processes.

claw toes—Toes that are extended at the metatarsophalangeal joints and flexed at the proximal and distal interphalangeal joints.

closed kinetic chain—Characterizing a motion in which the distal segment of an extremity is weight bearing and the body moves over the hand or foot.

close-packed position—The joint position in which the joint surfaces are most congruent with each other.

Codman's exercises—Low-level passive flexibility exercises for the shoulder that are performed by the patient. Also known as pendulum exercises.

cogwheel resistance—An abnormal response during muscle testing that is observed as a series of catch-and-release tensions rather than a smooth resistance, indicative of the individual's providing a less than maximal effort.

collagen—Major structure of the body's protein. There are five types in the body: type I, the most abundant type, is high in tensile strength and is found in dermis, fascia, and bone; type II is found in cartilage; type III is found in embryonic connective tissue; types IV and V are found in basement membranes. Forms inelastic bundles to provide structure, integrity, and tensile strength to tissues.

collagenase—An enzyme produced by newly formed epithelial cells and fibroblasts. Involved in the degradation of collagen during tissue repair. It is important in controlling the collagen content in a wound.

collar—The top rim of the shoe that is often padded to reduce friction on the Achilles.

Colles fracture—A fracture in which the distal radius proximal to the wrist is fractured and is displaced dorsally.

comparable sign—A sign produced by an active or passive movement or test that reproduces a patient's symptom, such as pain or protective muscle spasm.

compartment syndrome—A significant rise in intracompartmental pressure caused by severe bleeding within a muscular compartment that can compromise neurovascular structures.

complement system—Various proteins found in serum. Act as chemotactic factors for neutrophils and phagocytosis.

concave-convex rule—Roll and slide occur in the same direction when a concave surface moves on a convex surface.

concentric motion—Dynamic activity in which the muscle shortens.

concentric phase—The third phase of a plyometric activity, resulting from the combined eccentric and amortization phases. The concentric phase is the outcome phase. If the eccentric activity has been quickly performed and the amortization has occurred rapidly, the concentric phase will produce the desired powerful outcome.

contact pressure—Pressure that occurs between two objects in contact with each other.

contractility—The ability of a muscle fiber to contract.

contraction phase—That part of the mechanical response of a muscle twitch that follows the latency period during which the sarcomere's actin and myosin cross-bridge activity occurs.

contracture—Failure of a muscle to relax. Can occur after fatigue.

convex-concave rule—Roll and slide occur in opposite directions when a convex surface moves on a concave surface.

coordination—The ability of muscles and muscle groups to perform complicated movements.

coxa valga—Femoral neck angulation greater than 135°.

coxa vara—Femoral neck angulation less than 120°

creep—Permanent tissue elongation caused by low-level stress applied over an extended period.

crepitus—A cracking or grating sound or sensation caused by inflammation or degenerative changes.

cross-bridges—The "head" projections from the myosin filaments that link the thick filaments to the thin filaments through a complex process.

De Quervain's disease—Tenosynovitis of the abductor pollicis longus and extensor pollicis brevis tendons and their sheaths on the radial side of the thumb.

deceleration—Negative acceleration.

deceleration phase—That portion of swing in which the limb slows down in preparation for making initial contact with the ground. Also known as terminal swing.

dense connective tissue—Connective tissue with highly organized, parallel collagen fibers and more cross-links than loose connective tissue.

depression—A downward movement of the scapula.

dislocation—Complete disassociation or displacement of one joint surface on another.

dorsiflexion—The sagittal plane movement in which the ankle joint angle is decreased as the dorsal foot is moved upward toward the anterior surface of the lower leg.

double-crush syndrome—A condition in which an injury at one site produces signs and symptoms at another site.

double float—The nonsupport phase in a running stride.

double-limb support—The point of the gait cycle that occurs at the beginning of the stance phase during heel strike for one leg and the end of the stance phase just before toe-off for the other.

downward rotation—A movement of the scapula that causes the glenoid to face downward and backward. The inferior angle of the scapula moves medially, and the scapula slides backward.

drag—The water's resistance to a body moving through it. There are three types of drag: form drag, wave drag, and frictional drag.

drug interaction—A reaction in which one drug either enhances or reduces the effectiveness of other drugs that are also being taken.

duration of drug action—Amount of time the blood level of a drug is at or above the level needed to obtain a minimum therapeutic effect. Determined by the drug's half-life.

dynamic activity—Activity in which movement occurs.

dynamic restraint—One of two systems a joint has for its stability. Dynamic restraints are the neuromuscular components that provide movement.

dynamic splint—Splint used to increase motion or limit unwanted activity. It incorporates springs, rubber bands, or other elastic elements to provide a continual low-grade passive stretch, passive assistive motion, or active assistive motion to an area.

dynamometer—A device used to measure strength.

eccentric motion—A dynamic activity in which the muscle lengthens.

eccentric phase—The first phase of a plyometric activity during which the muscle is pre-stretched as it actively lengthens in preparation for performing the activity. The slack is taken out of the muscle, and its elastic components are put on stretch.

eddy—Circular motion of water layers pulling against a moving object.

elasticity—An object's ability to return to normal shape or size after a deforming force is applied.

elastin—An essential protein of connective-tissue elastic structures. Arranged in a wavy orientation. The wavy arrangement allows tissue to change with stress and to resume normal conditions after stress removal. It plays an as yet unknown role in the remodeling phase.

electrothermally assisted capsular shift—A relatively recently developed arthroscopic procedure used in the shoulder to reduce joint laxity.

elevation—An upward movement of the scapula.

end-feel—The nature of resistance that is felt at the end of joint movement.

endomysium—Connective-tissue layer covering a muscle fiber and continuous with the muscle fiber's membrane.

endothelial cells—Large flat cells that line blood and lymphatic vessels.

endothelial leukocyte—A large white blood cell that circulates in the bloodstream and tissues. Acts as a phagocyte to remove debris from an injured area.

endurance limit—See fatigue failure.

energy—The capacity to do work.

engram—A memory trace of an activity accomplished through repetitive application of stimuli.

eosinophil—See granular leukocyte.

epicondylitis—An overuse injury to the tendinous attachments of the flexor/pronator group at the medial epicondyle or the extensor/supinator group at the lateral epicondyle. Also referred to as tennis elbow.

epimysium—Connective-tissue layer covering an entire muscle.

epinephrine—A hormone. Also called adrenaline. A potent stimulator of the sympathetic nervous system. It is also a powerful vasopressor, increasing blood pressure, stimulating the heart muscle, accelerating the heart rate, and increasing cardiac output. It also increases such metabolic activities as glycogenolysis and glucose release.

erythrocyte—An element of blood. Also known as a red blood cell or corpuscle. Used by the body for oxygen transport.

eversion—Outward-turning motion of the foot that causes the bottom of the foot to face laterally.

examination—Includes subjective and objective components by which a clinician determines the severity, irritability, nature, and stage of a patient's injury. It serves as the basis upon which a rehabilitation program is based.

excursion—Amount of movement from one point to another.

extension—Straightening of a joint so that the two body segments move apart and increase the joint angle.

extensible—Able to lengthen. When muscle temperature increases, the muscle fibers and its connective tissue become more easily stretched.

extensor lag—Inability to fully extend the knee during active motion, but full passive motion is present.

extracellular matrix—The basic material from which tissue develops. Produced by fibroblasts in wounds. Composed of fibers and ground substance. Serves as a foundation on which anything is cast.

extrafusal fiber—A regular muscle fiber. Also known as a myofibril.

extrinsic foot muscles—Muscles that provide function of the toes, foot, and ankle but originate in the lower leg and terminate in the foot.

extrinsic muscles—Muscles that originate proximally from the hand or foot and terminate within the hand or foot.

exudate—Material that escapes from blood vessels following an injury. It contains high concentrations of protein, cells, and other materials from injured cells. As polymorphonuclear leukocytes die and decompose, the exudate may resemble pus although no infection is present.

factor XII—See Hageman factor.

fast-twitch fiber—A muscle fiber, also called a type II fiber or fast oxidative fiber, that is lighter in color than a slow-twitch fiber and that reaches its maximum tension approximately 50 ms after being stimulated.

fatigue—An inability to continue an activity.

fatigue failure—The point at which the cumulative stress of a repetitive submaximal load results in tissue failure. Also called endurance limit.

Feiss line—A line from the tip of the medial malleolus to the first metatarsal head. It is used as a point of reference to determine relative position of the navicular tubercle.

fibrin—Insoluble fibrous protein. Formed by fibrinogen. Important in clotting.

fibrinogen—A globulin present in plasma. Converts to fibrin to form a fibrin plug at the injury site.

fibrinolysin—An enzyme in plasma that is released in later healing. Converts fibrin into a soluble substance to unplug lymphatics.

fibroblast—A connective-tissue cell. Fibroblasts differentiate into chondroblasts, osteoblasts, and collagenoblasts. They form the fibrous tissues to support and bind a variety of the body's tissues.

fibrocyte—An inactive fibroblast. See fibroblast.

fibronectin—An adhesive glycoprotein found in most body tissues and serum. Fibronectin is plentiful in early granulation tissue formation but gradually disappears during the remodeling phase. Fibronectins cross-link to collagen in connective tissue, thereby playing a role in the adhesion of fibroblasts to fibrin. They are also involved in the collection of platelets in an injured area, and enhance myofibroblast activity.

first-class lever—A lever in which the fulcrum is between the resistance and the force.

first ray—The joint between the first metatarsal and the medial cuneiform. This is the primary weight-bearing ray of the foot and has triplanar motion.

flexibility—Mobility of a body segment, dependent on soft-tissue tolerance to movement and the ability of soft tissue to move with forces applied to it. Flexibility can involve soft-tissue mobility alone or in combination with joint motion. Used interchangeably with range of motion.

flexion—Bending of a joint so that the two body segments approach each other and decrease the joint angle.

fixation—A state of stabilization in which motion is restricted or prevented.

foam roller—Cylindrical therapeutic tool made of Ethafoam or polyurethane and used in rehabilitation in neurological, orthopedic, and sports medicine facilities.

foot abduction—The transverse plane movement of the foot in which the lateral foot is moved away from the midline.

foot adduction—The transverse plane movement of the foot in which the medial foot is moved toward the midline.

foot eversion—The frontal-plane movement in which the plantar foot rotates inward so that the medial border is lifted upward.

foot flat—That portion of the stance phase of the gait cycle in which the foot is flat on the floor. Also known as loading response.

foot inversion—The frontal-plane movement in which the plantar foot rotates outward so that the lateral border is lifted upward.

foot strike—Initial foot contact with the ground in running. The term replaces initial contact or heel strike.

force—A strength or energy that causes movement and has direction and magnitude.

force couple—Two equal forces acting in opposite but parallel directions to create a rotatory motion.

force deformation—The amount of force applied to maintain a change of length or deformation of tissue.

forefoot valgus—An eversion deformity of the midtarsal joint causing the medial forefoot to be lower than the lateral forefoot in non-weight bearing when viewed in the same plane as a perpendicular line bisecting the calcaneus.

forefoot varus—An inversion deformity of the midtarsal joint causing the medial forefoot to be higher than the lateral forefoot in non-weight bearing when viewed in the same plane as a perpendicular line bisecting the calcaneus.

form drag—The resistance an object encounters in a fluid, as determined by the object's size and shape.

foxing—An additional piece of the heel counter that is often seen in athletic shoes to further reinforce the rearfoot in order to help maintain the heel counter's shape.

free nerve endings—Small-diameter, unmyelinated afferent nerve endings located throughout soft-tissue and articular structures that perceive pain and temperature. They are nociceptors that are stimulated by pain and inflammation. Although they do not play a role in proprioception, they respond to any extreme joint position.

friction—Resistance to movement between two surfaces.

frictional drag—The result of water's surface tension. This is not a factor in therapeutic exercise.

frog's eye—Condition in which the patellae face outward in relation to each other rather than forward.

frontal (coronal) plane—Any vertical plane that divides the body into front and back parts.

functional evaluation—An assessment of the patient's ability to perform accurately and safely an exercise or skill drill before that patient is allowed to advance to the next level.

functional exercise—Activities that mimic the stresses, demands, and skills of the sport and advance a patient toward a safe and prompt return to sport participation.

gait cycle—The time from the point at which the heel of one foot touches the ground to the point at which it touches the ground again.

genu recurvatum—Excessive knee hyperextension.

genu valgus—Knee alignment in which the knees are angled toward each other. Also called genu valgum.

genu varum—Knee alignment in which the knees are bowed outward. Also called genu varus.

glycoprotein—One of a number of protein–carbohydrate compounds that are elements of ground substance. Includes fibronectin. Probably cross-links with collagen so that tissue is able to withstand pressure without harming tissue integrity.

glycosaminoglycan (GAG)—One of a number of compounds occur-ring mostly in proteoglycans. Glycosaminoglycans are non-fibrous elements of ground substance in the extracellular matrix. Examples: hyaluronic acid, proteoglycans. Different glycosaminoglycans have different functions—for example, stimulating fibroblast proliferation, promoting collagen synthesis and maturation, contributing to tissue resilience, and regulating cell function.

Golgi-Mazzoni corpuscles—These afferent receptors are located in joint capsules. They are stimulated by joint compression but not by joint motion. Any weight-bearing activity stimulates these slowly adapting receptors. They are not believed to play a role in proprioception except in identification of joint compression.

Golgi tendon organ (GTO)—A stretch receptor found in series within the musculotendinous structure. It responds to muscle contraction more than to muscle stretch to signal force.

goniometer—A tool used to measure joint range of motion. The device uses either a 180° or a 360° system.

goniometric terms—See abduction, adduction, depression, dorsiflexion, downward rotation, elevation, eversion, extension, external rotation, flexion, frontal (coronal) plane, horizontal extension, horizontal flexion, internal rotation, inversion, opposition, plantar flexion, pronation, protraction, radial deviation, retraction, sagittal plane, supination, transverse (horizontal) plane, ulnar deviation, upward rotation.

granular leukocyte—White blood cells, divided into three groups: neutrophils, eosinophils, and basophils. Among their functions are chemotaxis and phagocytosis, as well as release of histamine and serotonin to produce vasoactive reactions following injury.

granulation tissue—Newly formed vascular tissue that is produced during wound healing. Consists of fibroblasts, macrophages, and neovascular structure within a base of connective-tissue matrix of collagen, hyaluronic acid, and fibronectin. It has the velvety appearance of small, red, nodular masses seen in new tissue. It eventually forms the cicatrix of the wound.

granuloma—Hard mass of fibrous tissue. Occurs in chronic inflammatory conditions when the body produces collagen around a foreign substance to protect itself from that substance.

grasshopper eye—See frog's eye.

ground substance—Gel-like material in which connective-tissue cells and fibers are embedded. Part of the connective tissue or extracellular matrix. Reduces friction between the connective-tissue fibers when forces are applied to the structure. Adds to the area's density.

growth factor—A factor released by platelets and macrophages. Growth factors perform complex and numerous roles, including the stimulation of re-epithelialization, and are chemotactic for macrophages, monocytes, and neutrophils. The role of growth factors is not thoroughly understood but is believed to be important throughout tissue repair. Also referred to as growth hormone factor.

H band—That portion of the sarcomere that contains only thick filaments.

Hageman factor—An enzyme present in the blood. It initiates the blood coagulation process by converting prothrombin to thrombin following trauma to an area.

half-life—Amount of time it takes for the level of a drug in the bloodstream to diminish by one half. Determines the frequency with which a medication is taken.

hallux valgus—A condition also known as a bunion. Present when the first metatarsophalangeal joint is greater than 10° in valgus, so that the first toe points laterally toward the other toes.

hammertoe—Condition in which the toe is extended at the metatarso-phalangeal joint, flexed at the proximal interphalangeal joint, and extended at the distal interphalangeal joint.

heel counter—The portion of a shoe that circles the calcaneus and serves as an important rearfoot stabilizer.

heel-off—The portion of the stance phase of the gait cycle in which the weight begins to transfer to the front of the foot and the heel is lifted off the floor. Also known as terminal stance.

heel strike—The portion of the stance phase of the gait cycle in which the heel first comes in contact with the floor. Also known as initial contact.

hip pointer—a contusion along the iliac crest.

histamine—A local tissue hormone released by mast cells and granulo-cytes. Increases vascular permeability to proteins and fibronectin.

Hooke's law—Law stating that the stress applied to a body to deform it is proportional to the strain as long as the body's elasticity limit is not exceeded.

horizontal extension—A motion of the upper extremity in a transverse plane away from the midline of the body. Also called horizontal abduction.

horizontal flexion—A motion of the upper extremity in a transverse plane toward the midline of the body. Also called horizontal adduction.

hyaluronic acid—See glycosaminoglycan. A major component of early granulation tissue. Greatest amounts are seen in a wound during the first four to five days. Promotes cell movement and migration during repair. Stimulates fibroblast proliferation. Produces edema by absorbing large amounts of water to increase fibroblast migration.

hypertrophy—An increase in muscle bulk from an increase in size of the muscle fibers, not the number of muscle fibers. Hyper-trophy occurs with strength gains.

hysteresis—The process of tissue lengthening that results when the tissue is unable to withstand forces that are progressively applied to it.

I band—The portion of the sarcomere that contains only thin filaments.

impact peak—The ground reaction force that is a rapid peak occurring very quickly with impact at the foot's initial contact with the ground.

inertia—The tendency of an object at rest or in uniform motion to remain in that state until an external force is applied. See also Newton's first law of motion.

inflare—A pelvic girdle dysfunction in which the iliosacral joint is medially rotated.

inhibition—Transmission of an impulse that results in the cessation or decrease of an activity.

initial contact—See heel strike.

initial swing—The portion of the swing phase that includes early swing and acceleration.

insole board—The part of a shoe that lies between the upper and lower segments and that serves as the attachment for the two segments. Also called last.

internuncial transmission—Transmission of a message by a neuron that is interposed between two other neurons. The transmission rate is slower than that for monosynaptic transmission.

intrafusal muscle fiber—Modified muscle fiber that lies within a muscle spindle. The two types of muscle fibers are nuclear bag fibers and nuclear-chain fibers.

intrinsic foot muscles—Muscles that control the foot and toes and originate and terminate within the foot.

intrinsic muscles—Muscles that originate and terminate within the hand or foot.

inversion—An inward-turning motion of the foot that causes the bottom of the foot to face medially.

irritability—The amount of stimulation that is required to initiate a response, such as pain.

isokinetic—Characterizing a dynamic activity in which the velocity of movement remains the same and the resistance varies.

isometric—Characterizing an activity produced when muscle tension is created without a change in the muscle's length. An isometric activity is a static activity.

isotonic—Characterizing an activity during which a muscle's length changes.

joint reaction force—Forces that are transmitted from one segment to another through the connecting joint.

jump sign—A reflex response to a trigger point palpation that includes a wincing or withdrawal reaction by the patient.

juncturae tendinum—A fibrous band that limits independent motion of the extensor tendons of the hand.

kallikrein—A proteolytic enzyme found in blood plasma, lymph, and other exocrine secretions. Activated by the Hageman factor. Forms kinins and activates plasminogen, a precursor of plasmin. Increases vascular permeability and vasodilation.

kinetic energy—Energy that a body has because of its motion.

kinin—A generic term for polypeptides related to bradykinin. Kinins are potent local tissue hormones and are found in injured-tissue, released from plasma proteins. Examples: bradykinin, kallidin. Kinins mediate the classic signs of inflammation. Their action in the microvascular system is similar to that of histamine and serotonin in the early inflammation phase to cause increased microvascular permeability.

lactic acid—A by-product of muscle activity that leads to fatigue by reducing the muscle's calcium-binding capacity and impairing glycogen breakdown.

last—An important component of a shoe that determines the shoe's shape, size, style, and fit. It can be straight or curved. A shoe is constructed around a last that can be formed as a board last, slip last, or combination last.

latent trigger point—A trigger point that is painful only when it is palpated.

lateral rotation (LR)—Rotation of a joint around its axis away from the body's midline. Also inaccurately referred to as external rotation.

leukocyte—White blood cell or corpuscle. Types include polymorphonuclear leukocytes and mononuclear cells. These cells have notable phagocytic properties for removal of debris from an injury site.

leukotriene—A compound formed from arachidonic acid. Leukotrienes regulate inflammatory reactions. Some stimulate the movement of leukocytes into the area.

lever—A simple machine with a rigid bar and a fulcrum.

linear motion—Movement in a straight line.

line of gravity—Imaginary line through an object's center of gravity to the center of the earth.

line of pull of a muscle—The long axis of the muscle along which it exerts force.

lipid—A heterogeneous group of fats and fatlike substances, including fatty acids and steroids. Lipids serve as a source of fuel and are important to the structure and makeup of cells.

Little League elbow—A valgus traction force injury of the medial elbow that may start out as an inflammatory response or apophysitis and progress to an avulsion of the apophysis if the repetitive stress continues.

loading response—See foot flat.

local twitch response—An involuntary contraction of the muscle fibers in response to the snapping palpation.

loose-packed position—A joint position in which there is not complete congruency of joint surfaces with each other. Also called open-packed position. A joint demonstrates its greatest laxity in a loose-packed position.

lordosis—Excessive anterior convexity of the cervical and lumbar spine.

lymphocyte—A non-phagocytic leukocyte found in blood and lymph. These cells serve as important structures in the body's immune system by producing antibodies.

M band—The center of the A band where the thick filaments are attached.

macrophages—Mononuclear phagocytes that arise from stem cells in bone marrow. Considered one of the regulators of the repair process. They serve to phagocytize injury areas of debris, kill microorganisms, and secrete substances into an injury site, including enzymes, fibronectin, and coagulation factors. They play a role in keeping the inflammatory process localized and enhance collagen deposition and fibroblast proliferation.

mallet deformity—Avulsion of the extensor digitorum longus from the distal phalanx. Also known as baseball finger.

manipulation—Passive joint movement used to increase joint mobility. It incorporates a sudden, forceful thrust that is beyond the patient's control.

manual muscle test—An evaluation technique that uses manual resistance against a muscle or muscle group to provide a grade for that muscle or muscle group. Muscle grades range from 0 (zero) to 5 (normal).

manual therapy—The use of hands-on techniques for evaluating, treating, and improving the status of neuromusculoskeletal conditions.

massage—Manual manipulation of soft tissue to effect changes in the neuromuscular, lymph, cardiovascular, and connective-tissue systems.

mast cells—Connective-tissue cells. Also referred to as mastocytes and labrocytes. Store and produce various mediators of inflammation. Through their release of histamine, enzymes, and other mediators, mast cells cause increased local blood flow, attract immune cells, stimulate cell production of fibroblasts and endothelial cells, and promote and control remodeling of extracellular matrix.

matrix—Substance of a tissue. Can refer to intracellular or extra-cellular structure. Forms the basis from which a structure develops.

medial rotation (MR)—Rotation of a joint around its axis toward the midline of the body. Also incorrectly referred to as internal rotation.

Meissner's corpuscles—Sensory nerve endings that transmit light-touch sensation.

midsole—The middle portion of a shoe's outer sole that can be composed of a variety of substances. It can also include a wedge. The midsole provides shock attenuation, stability, and control.

midstance—The portion of the stance phase of the gait cycle in which the foot is directly under the body's weight and the entire foot is in contact with the floor. Also known as single-leg support.

midswing—Also known as swing-through.

mitochondria—Organelles of a cell that are the primary energy source for the cell and that contain the enzyme used to metabolize lactic acid for energy to form adenosine triphosphate.

mobilization—Passive joint movement for increasing joint mobility or reducing pain. The applied force is light enough that the patient can stop the movement at any time.

modality—A physical agent used to relieve pain, improve circulation, reduce spasm, and promote healing.

momentum—Amount of motion that a moving object has.

monocyte—Mononuclear phagocytic leukocyte. Monocytes are formed in the bone marrow and transported to tissues to become macrophages. They debride an injury site.

mononuclear phagocyte—Any cell capable of ingesting particulate matter. The term usually refers to macrophages (polymorphonuclear leukocytes) and monocytes (mononuclear phagocytes). These ingest microorganisms and debride an injury site.

monosynaptic response—A reflex response involving only one synapse that is between the afferent and efferent nerves.

monosynaptic transmission—The direct connection between a sensory nerve and a motor neuron. Also called a monosynaptic reflex.

motor unit—A neuromuscular unit composed of the nerve, or motor neuron, and the muscle fibers that it innervates.

mucopolysaccharide—Polysaccharide. Also called GAG. See glycosaminoglycan.

muscle endurance—Ability of a muscle or muscle group to perform repeated contractions against a less-than-maximal load.

muscle energy—A manual therapy technique using precisely applied active muscle contraction against a counterforce to correct alignment and improve function.

muscle energy technique—The use of muscle contraction to precipitate a correction of a joint's malalignment.

muscle spasm—Prolonged reflex muscle contraction.

muscle spindle—A neuromuscular spindle, composed of intrafusal muscle fibers, that lies between regular muscle fibers. With its complex afferent and efferent supply, it provides the body with sensory stimulation and motor responses. The muscle spindle is sensitive to stretch, and signals muscle length and rate of change in the muscle's length.

muscle stiffness—The change in a muscle's tension that occurs as the muscle's length changes; related to the strength of the muscle's cross-bridge connections and the amount of muscle hypertrophy. The more stiffness a muscle has, the more resistant it is to stretching. Muscle stiffness is related to muscle tone.

muscular endurance—A muscle or muscle group's ability to sustain a submaximal force during either static or dynamic activity over time.

muscular strength—The amount of force a muscle or muscle group exerts. The ability to resist or produce a force.

myoblast—A cell formed from myogenic cells in muscle. Myoblasts form myotubes that eventually evolve into muscle fiber.

myofibroblasts—Fibroblasts that have the ultrastructural features of a fibroblast as well as the qualities of a smooth muscle cell. They are responsible for wound contraction.

myogenic cells—Cells that arise from muscle and later become myoblasts. See myoblast.

myosin—The chief protein structure of the thick filament of the sarcomere.

myotatic reflex—See stretch reflex.

neural mobilization—A manual therapy technique that stretches neural and connective tissue structures to affect neural symptoms, restore tissue balance, and improve function.

neurotransmitters—Hormones such as norepinephrine, epinephrine, and acetylcholine that are found in capillary, arteriole, and artery walls. They are released at the injury site to enhance platelet and leukocyte adherence to the vessel surface.

neutral spine—See pelvic neutral.

neutrophil—See polymorphonuclear leukocyte.

Newton's first law of motion—Law stating that a body remains at rest or in uniform motion until an outside force acts on it.

Newton's second law of motion—Law stating that acceleration of an object is directly proportional to the force causing the motion and inversely proportional to the mass of the object being moved.

Newton's third law of motion—Law stating that for every action there is an equal and opposite reaction.

nociceptors—Afferent nerve endings that transmit pain stimuli.

norepinephrine—A hormone that acts as a powerful vasoconstrictor at the immediate onset of injury. It may last from a few seconds to a few minutes.

nuclear bag fiber—One of two intrafusal muscle fibers within a muscle spindle, named for its nuclei arrangement. The nuclei are bunched together in the middle of the fiber's central region.

nuclear chain fiber—One of two intrafusal muscle fibers within a muscle spindle. Its nuclei are arranged in a chain or row. It is the smaller of the intrafusal muscle fibers.

nystagmus—A reflexive attempt to keep the eyes steady during body motion.

objective evaluation—The portion of an examination by which the clinician discovers the observable signs and effects of an injury: The portion of observation, testing for quality and quantity of movement, strength, neurological and other special testing, and palpation.

oculomotor system—An afferent system for balance that uses the eyes to provide the central nervous system with information regarding the body's relative position in space.

open kinetic chain—Characterizing a motion in which the distal segment of an extremity moves freely in space.

open reduction internal fixation (ORIF)—Surgical reduction of a fracture with application of a fixation device, such as a pin or screw, to stabilize the fracture site.

opposition—A diagonal movement of the thumb across the palm of the hand to permit the thumb to make contact with one of the other fingers.

orthotic—In reference to the foot, an appliance designed to correct body-segment or foot alignment or function, absorb stress, or reduce pressure or symptoms. Orthotics can be custom made or preformed and can vary in composition, degree of control, and type of correction.

Osgood-Schlatter disease—An inflammation or avulsion of the tibial apophysis, occurring in active, prepubescent children.

osteitis pubis—An inflammatory condition of shear stresses caused by either repeated trauma or strain on the symphysis pubis joint.

osteoblasts—Osteogenic cells from periosteum. Lay down the callus of fractured bone. Convert later to chondrocytes.

osteochondritis dissecans—Avascular necrosis of a joint's articular surface.

osteoclasts—Large multinuclear cells. Resorb dead, necrotic bone tissue.

osteocyte—A cell characteristic of adult bone. Maintains new bone mineralization.

outsole—The portion of a shoe that includes the lower segment and is in contact with the ground.

overflow—Also known as irradiation. With increased voluntary effort or prolonged effort, motor activity spreads to additional motor units of the same muscle and to motor untis of other muscles.

overload principle—To gain strength, a muscle must be overloaded beyond its accustomed level.

overpressure—Movement of a joint beyond its normal mobility to assess and feel or produce a comparable sign.

pacinian corpuscles—Afferent nerve endings that lie throughout the joint capsule and periarticular structures. They are rapidly adapting receptors thought to be compression sensitive, especially during high-velocity changes when the joint accelerates or decelerates as it moves into its limits of motion.

paratendinitis—An inflammation and thickening of the paratenon sheath of tendons that do not have synovial sheaths.

Pascal's law—Law stating that pressure from a fluid is exerted equally on all surfaces of an immersed object at any given depth (i.e., the deeper the object is immersed, the greater the pressure it encounters).

passive physiological range of motion—The amount of range of motion achieved without the assistance of the patient.

passive range of motion (PROM)—See passive physiological range of motion.

passive stretch—A stretch for which application relies on an outside force. The patient remains relaxed throughout the stretch.

patella alta—Position of the patella higher than normal in the patellofemoral groove.

patella baja—Position of the patella lower than normal in the patellofemoral groove.

pathoneurodynamics—A term coined by David Butler to describe pathological conditions that produce referral patterns proximally and distally from the site of pathology.

pelvic neutral—The position in which the spine and sacrolumbar junction incur the least stress. This is usually a mid-position between the extremes of anterior and posterior pelvic tilt. Because of its impact on spine position, the position is also referred to as neutral spine or straight spine.

pelvic stabilization—Activities or exercises that are used to position and maintain the body in a pelvic neutral position. Also referred to as core stabilization or spinal stabilization activities.

periarticular connective tissue—Soft tissue surrounding a joint, such as ligaments, the joint capsule, fascia, tendons, and synovial membranes.

perimysium—Connective-tissue layer covering a group of muscle fibers (fascicle).

pes cavus—An abnormal condition in which the foot has an abnormally high longitudinal arch. Associated with a rigid foot.

pes planus—An abnormal condition in which the foot has a low longitudinal arch. Associated with a hypomobile foot. Also known as a pancake arch, flatfoot, or excessive pronation. Associated with a flexible foot.

phagocyte—Any cell that ingests particulate matter. Commonly referred to as polymorphonuclear leukocyte and mononuclear phagocyte, otherwise known as macrophage and monocyte. These cells ingest microorganisms and other particulate antigens to debride an area.

phospholipids—Lipids that contain phosphoric acid. Found in all cells and in layers of plasma membranes. Stimulate the clotting mechanism.

physically active—Characterizing an individual who engages in occupational, recreational, or athletic activities that require physical skills and utilize strength, power, endurance, speed, flexibility, range of motion, or agility. (Based on the National Athletic Trainers' Association definition.)

physiological advantage—A muscle's ability to shorten. A muscle has its greatest physiological advantage when at its resting length.

physiological joint motion—Joint motion that can be performed voluntarily, such as shoulder flexion and ankle inversion.

plan of treatment program—The components, frequency, and duration of a treatment program. Includes the establishment of short-term and long-term goals.

plantar flexion—An extension of the ankle that causes the dorsum (top) of the foot to move away from the lower leg so that the angle of the ankle increases.

plasmin—An enzyme that occurs in plasma as plasminogen. It is activated by kallikrein and other activators. It converts fibrin to soluble substances.

plasminogen activator—An enzyme. See fibrinolysin. Converts fibrin to a soluble substance.

plasticity—In muscle physiology, a permanent change in length that occurs after an elongation force is applied.

platelet-derived growth factor (PDGF)—Substance found in platelets. It is essential for the growth of connective-tissue cells and stimulates the migration of polymorphonuclear leukocytes.

platelets—Irregular cell fragments found in blood. The first cells seen at an injury site, platelets are classified as regulatory cells of healing. Release growth factors. Form a plug at the injury to stop bleeding.

plica—A redundant fold in the knee's synovial lining, palpated as a band extending medially from the patella.

plumb line—A string with a weight (formerly a lead weight, but any weight object will do) at the end. When suspended, the string forms a vertical line.

plyometric exercise—A lengthening of a muscle followed by a sudden shortening to produce increased power. Also called stretch-shortening exercise.

polymorphonuclear leukocytes—One of the granular leukocytes. Also referred to as PMNs or neutrophils. These cells are chemotactic and phagocytic in the healing process.

posture—The relative alignment of the various body segments with one another.

potential energy—Energy that is stored in a body.

power—Work produced over time.

preswing—See toe-off.

primary intention—Healing that occurs with minor or surgical wounds. Reepithelialization closes the wound within 48 h. Scarring is minimal when healing by primary intention occurs.

procedure (vs. modality)—A treatment technique that involves the clinician's active participation or supervision.

pronation—Movement of the palm backward or downward so that the palm faces in a posterior direction, opposite the anatomical position. Also, a multiplanar rotation of the subtalar and transverse tarsal joints that is the combination of dorsiflexion, abduction, and eversion.

proprioception—The body's ability to transmit afferent information regarding position sense, to interpret the information, and to respond consciously or unconsciously to stimulation through appropriate execution of posture and movement.

proprioceptive neuromuscular facilitation (PNF)—A combined movement pattern that uses neural stimulation to facilitate a proper muscle response.

prostaglandins (PGs)—Components stemming primarily from arachidonic acid. Release of these substances requires the presence of the complement system and follows kinin formation. Specific PG compound compositions are designated by adding a letter, "A" through "I," and a subscript number, 1 through 3, to designate the number of hydrocarbon bonds. Examples: PGE_1 and PGE_2. Prostaglandins mediate cell migration during inflammation and modulate serotonin and histamine. Some PGs increase pain sensitivity, induce fever, and suppress lymphocyte transformation, thereby inhibiting the inflammatory reaction. Mediate myofibroblasts. Prostaglandins initiate early phases of injury repair as well as playing a role in the later stages of inflammation.

protease—An enzyme that acts as a catalyst to split interior peptide bonds in protein. Activates kallikrein to release bradykinin, ultimately causing increased vascular permeability to result in an increase in concentration of proteins and cells in the wound spaces.

proteoglycan—Substances found in tissues, including synovial fluid and connective-tissue matrix. Proteoglycan solutions are very viscous lubricants and are sulfated glycosaminoglycans. See glycosaminoglycan. A proteoglycan provides a resilient matrix for inhibiting cell migration. Regulates cell function and proliferation and regulates collagen fibrillogenesis.

protraction—A forward movement of the scapula. Also called scapular abduction.

pump bump—Increased prominence of the posterior calcaneal tuberosity. Also know as a calcaneal exostosis.

Q-angle—The angle formed by a line from the anterior superior iliac spine to the middle patella and a line from the middle patella to the tibial tubercle.

radial deviation—A movement of the wrist toward the thumb side of the forearm. Also called radial flexion.

range of motion—Amount of movement within a joint. Range of motion is affected by soft-tissue mobility and can be influenced by strength when performed actively. Used interchangeably with flexibility.

rearfoot valgus—An abnormal condition in which the calcaneus is everted relative to the tibia.

rearfoot varus– An abnormal condition in which the calcaneus is inverted relative to the posterior bisection of the lower leg.

refraction—When a light ray moves from air through water, it bends as it moves from the air, which has a lower density than the water does, into the water with its higher density. This makes the pool bottom appear closer than it actually is and makes objects within the water appear distorted.

refractory period—The time immediately following a stimulation, when the muscle fiber is unable to respond to additional stimuli. It is divided into an absolute refractory period and a relative refractory period.

rehabilitation clinician—The medical professional responsible for the design, progression, supervision, and administration of a rehabilitation program for individuals involved in physical activity. Medical professionals who most often assume these responsibilities include certified athletic trainers and physical therapists.

relative density—See specific gravity.

relative refractory period—A period that follows depolarization after a membrane has become partially repolarized. During this period the membrane is able to respond again if the stimulus is stronger than the normal threshold level.

resisted range of motion (RROM)—Motion that occurs with resistance applied to the movement. Also referred to as strengthening exercises or progressive resistive exercises.

resting membrane potential—The electrical potential difference across an inactive cell's membrane.

reticulin—A collagen-like fiber. Some consider reticulin a type III collagen fiber. Forms the early framework for collagen deposition in a wound.

retraction—A backward movement of the scapula. Also called scapular adduction.

retroversion—Decreased anterior angulation of the femoral neck, resulting in a toe-out gait.

Romberg test—A test for balance in which a patient stands with feet together and eyes closed. Increased postural sway compared to when eyes are open is a positive sign.

Ruffini nerve endings—These afferent receptors are in the joint capsule on the flexion side of the joint. They are slowly adapting and respond more to loads on the connective tissue in which they are contained than to displacement of that connective tissue. These receptors are stimulated by extreme joint motion when the capsule is stressed in extension with rotation.

saddle—The portion of a shoe that includes the midsection along the longitudinal arch, usually reinforced to assist in supporting the midfoot.

sagittal plane—The anterior-posterior vertical plane through which the longitudinal axis passes and which divides the body into right and left halves.

SAID principle—specific adaptation to imposed demands. Tissue will adapt to the specific stresses applied to it. This is a principle upon which a therapeutic exercise program is designed.

sarcomere—The smallest contractile element of a muscle fiber.

sarcoplasmic reticulum—A highly specialized intracellular membrane system that stores and transports calcium.

satellite cells—Cells present in muscle. Regenerate new muscle tissue.

scaption—Elevation of the shoulder in the scapular plane 30° forward of the frontal plane. This alignment of the glenohumeral joint with the scapula on the rib cage places the rotator cuff in the least stressful position for exercise.

scoliosis—A lateral or S curvature of the spinal column.

secondary intention—Healing that occurs in large wounds associated with soft-tissue loss. The wound heals with granulation tissue from the bottom and sides of the wound. Epithelial tissue does not form until granulation tissue has filled the wound. Larger scar formation occurs with healing by secondary intention. Wound contraction is evident with this healing.

second-class lever—A lever in which the resistance is between the fulcrum and the force.

serotonin—A hormone released by mast cells and platelets. Produces vasoconstriction in small vessels after norepinephrine activity is completed; occurs only when blood vessel endothelial walls are damaged. In later phases, it is responsible for initiating reactions leading to collagen cross-linking. It also is involved in granuloma formation.

shin splints—A general term used to describe pain and inflammation of the musculotendinous unit and/or periosteum along the anteromedial border of the tibia. Also know as medial tibial stress syndrome.

single-leg support—The portion of the gait cycle in which the body weight is transferred entirely to the one supporting leg and the other leg is in the middle of its swing phase. Also known as midstance.

slow-twitch fiber—A muscle fiber that is a type I fiber or slow oxidative fiber, is darker in color than the fast-twitch fiber, and takes about 110 ms to reach its peak tension when stimulated.

Smith's fracture—A type of fracture in which the distal radius is fractured and the fragment is displaced palmarly.

sock liner—The portion of a shoe that lies on top of the insole board, used for shock absorption and friction reduction for the foot.

somatosensory system—Another term for the body's proprioceptive system.

specific gravity—The ratio of an object's weight to the weight of an equal volume of water. The term refers to the density of an object relative to that of water. This ratio is also called relative density. The specific gravity of water is 1.

spinal cord—Part of the central nervous system that extends from the brain to the second lumbar vertebra and contains a cervical and a lumbar enlargement where the dorsal and ventral roots leading to the extremities are contained.

spinal reflex—When an impulse goes from a dorsal root afferent nerve either to an internuncial connecting nerve or directly to an efferent nerve in the spinal cord, and then immediately out the ventral root to the muscle.

sprain—Stretching or tearing of a ligament or capsular structure.

squinting patellae—Patellae that are angled toward each other rather than facing forward.

stance phase—The portion of the gait cycle during which the foot is in contact with the floor and the extremity is bearing partial or total body weight.

static activity—An isometric activity in which no movement occurs.

static progressive splint—Change of static splints as motion of a segment changes so the desired goals, usually including increased motion, are achieved.

static restraint—One of two systems a joint has for its stability. Static restraints include ligaments, capsule, and other inert structures such as the glenoid labrum in the shoulder and the meniscus in the knee.

static splint— Splint used to support, protect, or restrict motion. It does not have any moving parts.

steady state of a drug—The state in which the average level of a drug remains constant in the blood: The amount of drug leaving the body is equal to the amount being absorbed. On average, a steady state occurs after five doses equal to the drug's half-life are administered.

step length—The distance from heel strike of one foot to heel strike of the other foot in one gait cycle.

strain—Amount of change in size or shape of an object caused by stress.

strength—A muscle's relative ability to resist or produce a force.

stress—Force required to change the shape or form of a body.

stretch reflex—The most basic sensorimotor response. Does not involve an internuncial neuron, but instead goes directly from the afferent sensory nerve (muscle spindle) to the spinal cord, where it makes contact with the motor nerve to permit a rapid muscle response.

stride length—The distance from heel strike of one foot to heel strike of the same foot in one gait cycle.

stride width—The body's side-to-side movement as weight is shifted from one lower extremity to the other.

structural fatigue—The point at which stress exceeds the tissue's ability to resist it and breakdown occurs.

subjective evaluation—The portion of an examination that includes the history of an injury, including the mechanism of injury, the patient's experience of pain and other symptoms, prior injuries, medical conditions, medications, and other pertinent social and medical factors. This information is provided by the patient or other individual.

subtalar joint—The joint formed by the talus and calcaneus. This joint allows inversion and eversion motion of the rearfoot.

subtalar neutral—The position in which the talus is palpable from its medial or its lateral aspect within the subtalar joint. The point at which the talus and navicular are most congruent and the alignment of the subtalar bones is optimal.

summation of forces—Sequential movement of body segments to increase force production for a desired motion.

supination—Movement of the palm forward or upward into the anatomical position. Also, the multiplanar rotation of the subtalar and transverse tarsal joints that includes plantar flexion, adduction, and inversion.

swan-neck deformity—A deformity caused by hyperextension at the PIP joint and hyperflexion at the DIP joint due to disruption of the volar plate and tensioning of the flexor tendons.

swing phase—The time during which the foot is not in contact with the floor and no weight is borne on the extremity.

swing-through—The middle of the swing phase, also called midswing.

Swiss ball—A large, vinyl ball developed by an Italian toy manufacturer that is used in physical therapy and therapeutic exercise programs.

synergist(ic)—A muscle that assists an agonist muscle.

talocrural joint—The true ankle joint that is formed by the talus and tibia with the fibula. The joint allows dorsiflexion and plantar flexion motions.

tarsal tunnel—Formed by the medial malleolus, calcaneus, talus, and deltoid ligament's posterior aspect.

tendinitis—The global term used to identify an inflammation of a tendon. Also spelled tendonitis.

tendinosis—A condition that involves microscopic tears of the tendon caused by repeated trauma.

tenocyte—Tendon cell. Converts to fibroblasts during healing of tendons.

tenosynovitis—An inflammation of the synovial sheath that surrounds a tendon.

tensile strength—Maximal amount of stress or force that a structure is able to withstand before tissue failure occurs. Tensile strength varies as tissue healing proceeds. One must take tensile strength of an injured structure into account when determining appropriate stress application in rehabilitation.

terminal stance—See heel-off.

terminal swing—The portion of the swing phase that includes late swing, or deceleration.

tetanus—An intermittent contraction of a muscle that is demonstrated as a fibrillation of the muscle.

tetany—A sustained maximal contraction of a muscle.

third-class lever—A lever in which the force is between the fulcrum and the resistance.

thoracic kyphosis—Excess posterior convexity of the thoracic spine.

thoracic outlet syndrome (TOS)—A clinical term that describes compression of the neurovascular structures as they exit through the thoracic outlet at the base of the neck.

threshold stimulation—The minimal stimulation required to initiate a muscular response.

thrombin—An enzyme that converts fibrinogen to fibrin to form a fibrin plug early in the inflammation phase. In later inflammation, it stimulates fibronectin production and fibroblast proliferation.

thromboxane—A compound that is produced by platelets and is unstable. Its half-life is 30 s. Related to prostaglandins. Acts as a vasoconstrictor and is a potent inducer of platelet aggregation.

tibial torsion—An abnormal structural condition in which the tibia is rotated along its longitudinal axis so that the foot is rotated laterally beyond the normal 15° in relation to the patella's midline.

tibial varum—An abnormal condition in which the distal tibia is closer to the midline than the proximal tibia.

toe box—The upper portion of the shoe that covers the toes. It varies in width and height, and functions to retain the shape of the shoe's forefoot and provide room for the toes.

toe-off—The portion of the gait cycle during which the foot comes off the floor and the swing phase begins. Also called push-off or preswing.

torque—The ability of a force to produce rotational movement.

transverse (horizontal) plane—A plane that divides the body or a body part into upper and lower parts. It is parallel to the horizon.

Trendelenburg gait—An abnormal gait secondary to gluteus medius weakness. The gait is also known as a gluteus medius gait and is seen as a drop of the pelvis on the uninvolved side during weight bearing on the involved side.

trigger point—According to Travell and Simons (1983, p. 3), a "focus of hyperirritability in a tissue that, when compressed, is locally tender and, if sufficiently hypersensitive, gives rise to referred pain and tenderness, and sometimes to referred autonomic phenomena and distortion of proprioception." A myofascial trigger point includes a taut band of muscle with its surrounding fascia.

tropomyosin—One of two primary proteins of the thin filament of the sarcomere.

troponin—A protein on the actin filament to which calcium ions bind during a sarcomere's cross-bridging process.

ulnar deviation—A movement of the wrist toward the little-finger side of the forearm. Also called ulnar flexion.

ultimate strength—The greatest load a tissue can tolerate before it reaches failure.

upward rotation—A movement of the scapula that causes the glenoid to face forward and upward. The inferior angle of the scapula moves laterally away from the spine, and the scapula slides forward.

Valsalva maneuver—When the breath is held, intrathoracic pressure is increased. This can lead to impeded venous return to the right atrium, causing increased peripheral venous pressure, increasing blood pressure and reducing cardiac output because of diminished cardiac volume.

vamp—The upper portion of a shoe that covers the toes and forefoot and includes the toe box.

velocity—Rate of change of position.

vestibular system—An afferent system within the inner ear that is responsible for sending messages to the central nervous system regarding vertical and horizontal position and motion.

viscoelasticity—The property of being both viscous and elastic.

viscosity—The resistance to movement within a fluid or fluid-like substance that is caused by the friction of the fluid's molecules. Viscosity limits the rate of muscle contraction: The faster the contraction, the greater the internal resistance and the less the force that can be generated.

volitional—The conscious performance or an activity.

wave drag—The water's resistance as a result of turbulence.

weight—The force of gravity. Commonly measured in kilograms (grams) or pounds (ounces).

work—Product of a force and the distance through which it is applied.

Z disk—The end of the sarcomere element where the thin filaments attach. Also known as the Z-line or Z-band.

Bibliography

Ahmed, A.M., and D.L. Burke. 1983. In vitro measurement of static pressure distribution in synovial joints: I. Tibial surface of the knee. Journal of Biomedical Engineering 105:216–225.

Akeson, W.H., Woo, S.L.-Y., Amiel, D., Coutts, R.D., and D. Daniel. 1973. The connective tissue response to immobility: Biochemical changes in periarticular connective tissue of the immobilized rabbit knee. Clinical Orthopedics & Related Research 93:356-362.

Allerheiligen, B., and R. Rogers. 1995. Plyometrics program design. Strength and Conditioning 17: 26–31.

Almekinders, L.C., and J.A. Gilbert. 1986. Healing of experimental muscle strains and the effects of non-steroidal antiinflammatory medication. American Journal of Sports Medicine 14:303–308.

Alon, R. 1990. Mindful spontaneity: Moving in tune with nature: Lessons in the Feldenkrais method. New York: Harper & Row.

American Academy of Orthopaedic Surgeons. 1965. Joint motion: Method of measuring and recording. New York: Churchill Livingstone.

Andrews, J.R., Carson, W.G. Jr., and W.D. McLeod. 1985. Glenoid labrum tears related to the long head of the biceps. American Journal of Sports Medicine 13:337-41.

Andriacchi, T.P., Sabiston, K., DeHaven, K., Dahners, L., Woo, S., Frank, C., Oakes, B., Brand, R., and J. Lewis. 1988. Ligament: Injury and repair. In Injury and repair of the musculoskeletal soft tissues, ed. S.L.-Y. Woo and J.A. Buckwalter. Park Ridge, IL: American Academy of Orthopaedic Surgeons.

Appell, H.-J. 1990. Muscular atrophy following immobilization: A review. Sports Medicine 10: 42–58.

Archambault, J.M., Wiley, J.P., and R.C. Bray. 1995. Exercise loading of tendons and the development of overuse injuries. Sports Medicine 20:77–89.

Barber, F.A. 1994. Accelerated rehabilitation for meniscus repairs. Arthroscopy 10:206–210.

Barlow, W. 1977. The Alexander Technique. New York: Knopf.

Barrack, R.L., Lund, P.J., and H.B. Skinner. 1994. Knee joint proprioception revisited. Journal of Sport Rehabilitation 3:18–42.

Baumhauer, J., Shereff, M., and J. Gould. 1997. Ankle pain in runners. In Running injuries, ed. G.N. Guten. Philadelphia: Saunders.

Beard, G., and E.C. Wood. 1969. Massage principles and techniques. Philadelphia: Saunders.

Berger, R.A. 1962. Optimal repetitions for the development of strength. Research Quarterly 33: 334–338.

Bernier, J.N., and D.H. Perrin. 1998. Effect of coordination training on proprioception of the functionally unstable ankle. Journal of Orthopaedic and Sports Physical Therapy 27:264–275.

Betz, P., Norlich, A., Wilske, J., Tubel, J., Penning, R., and W. Eisenmenger. 1992. Time-dependent appearance of myofibroblasts in granulation tissue of human skin wounds. International Journal of Legal Medicine 150:99–103.

Beynnon, B.D., Fleming, B.C., Johnson, R.J., Nichols, C.E., Renstrom, P.A., and M.H. Pope. 1995. Anterior cruciate ligament strain behavior during rehabilitation exercises in vivo. American Journal of Sports Medicine 23:24–34.

Billeter, H., and H. Hoppeler. 1992. Muscular basis of strength. In Strength and power in sport, ed. P.V. Komi. Boston: Blackwell Scientific.

Binningsley, D. 2003 Tear of the acetabular labrum in an elite athlete. British Journal of Sports Medicine. 37:84-88.

Blackburn, T.A., McLeod, W.D., White, B., and L. Wofford. 1990. EMG analysis of posterior rotator cuff exercises. Athletic Training. 24:40, 42-45.

Bockrath, K., Wooden, C., Worrell, T., Ingersoll, C.D., and T. Farr. 1993. Effects of patellar taping on patella position and perceived pain. Medicine and Science in Sports and Exercise 25:989–992.

Bogduk, N., and L.T. Twomey. 1987. Clinical anatomy of the lumbar spine. New York: Churchill Livingstone.

Bolgla, L.A., and D.R. Keskula. 1997. Reliability of lower extremity functional performance tests. Journal of Orthopaedic and Sports Physical Therapy 26:138–142.

Borcherding, S. 2000. Documentation manual for writing SOAP notes in occupational therapy. Thorofar, NJ: Slack.

Bowers, W.H., and S.M. Tribuzi. 1992. Functional anatomy. In Concepts in hand rehabilitation, ed. B.G. Stanley and S.M. Tribuzi. Philadelphia: Davis.

Boyes, J.H. 1970. Bunnell's surgery of the hand. Philadelphia: Lippincott.

Braatz, J.H., and P. P. Gogia. 1987. The mechanics of pitching. Journal of Orthopaedic and Sports Physical Therapy 9:56–69.

Bradley, J.P., and J.E. Tibone. 1991. Electromyographic analysis of muscle action about the shoulder. Clinics in Sports Medicine 10:789–805.

Brittberg, M., Lindahl, A., Nilsson, A., Ohlsson, C., Isaksson, O., and L. Peterson. 1994. Treatment of deep cartilage defects in the knee with autologous chondrocyte transplantation. New England Journal of Medicine 331:889–895.

Brown, C.H., Steiner, M.E., and E.W. Carson. 1993. The use of hamstring tendons for anterior cruciate ligament reconstruction. Technique and results. Clinics in Sports Medicine 12:723–756.

Brown, D.R. 1980. Neurosciences for allied health therapies. St. Louis: Mosby.

Brownstein, B., Mangiene, R.E., Noyes, F.R., and S. Kryer. 1988. Anatomy and biomechanics. In Physical therapy of the knee, ed. R.E. Mangiene. New York: Churchill Livingstone.

Buckwalter, J.A. 1996. Effects of early motion on healing of musculoskeletal tissues. Hand Clinics 12: 13–24.

Buckwalter, J.A., Rosenberg, L., Coutts, R., Hunziker, E., Reddi, A.H., and V. Mow. 1988. Articular cartilage: Injury and repair. In Injury and repair of the musculoskeletal soft tissues, ed. S.L.-Y. Woo and J.A. Buckwalter. Park Ridge, IL: American Academy of Orthopaedic Surgeons.

Butler, D.L., Grood, E.S., Noyes, F.R., and R.F. Zernicke. 1978. Biomechanics of ligaments and tendons. Exercise and Sport Sciences Reviews 6:125–281.

Butler, D.L., Noyes, F.R., and E.S. Grood. 1980. Ligamentous restraints to anterior-posterior drawer in the human knee. Journal of Bone and Joint Surgery 62-A:259–270.

Butler, D.S. 1991. Mobilization of the nervous system. New York: Churchill Livingstone.

Butler, D.S. 1994. Mobilization of the nervous system. Level II. 1996/97 course handbook. Marina Del Rey, CA: Neuro Orthopedic Insitute.

Cappaert, T.A. 2000. The sacroiliac joint as a factor in low back pain: a review. Journal of Sport Rehabilitation. 9:169-183.

Callagan, M.J., Selfe, J., Bagley, P.J., and J.A. Oldham. 2002. The effects of patellar taping on knee joint proprioception. Journal of Athletic Training 37:19-24.

Caplan, A.B., Carlson, J., Faulkner, J., Fischman, D., and W. Garrett, Jr. 1988. Skeletal muscle. In Injury and repair of the musculoskeletal soft tissues, ed. S.L.-Y. Woo and J.A. Buckwalter. Park Ridge, IL: American Academy of Orthopaedic Surgeons.

Chambers, H.G. and D.H. Sutherland. 2002. A practical guide to gait analysis. Journal of the American Academy of Orthopaedic Surgeons 10:222-273.

Christie, A.L. 1991. The tissue injury cycle and new advances toward its management in open wounds. Athletic Training 26:274–277.

Chu, D. 1989. Plyometric exercises with medicine balls. Livermore, CA: Bittersweet.

Chu, D. 1992. Jumping into plyometrics. Champaign, IL: Leisure Press.

Church, J.B., Wiggins, M.S., Moode, F.M., and R. Crist. 2001. Effect of warm-up and flexibility treatments on vertical jump performance. Journal of Strength & Conditioning Research 15:332-336.

Cipriani, D.J., Armstrong, C.W., and S. Gaul. 1995. Backward walking at three levels of treadmill inclination: An electromyographic and kinematic analysis. Journal of Orthopaedic and Sports Physical Therapy 22:95–102.

Clarke, D.H. 1971. The influence on muscular fatigue patterns of the intercontraction rest interval. Medicine and Science in Sports 3:83–88.

Clarke, D.H. 1975. Exercise physiology. Englewood Cliffs, NJ: Prentice-Hall.

Close, J.R. 1964. Motor function in the lower extremity: Analysis by electronic instrumentation. Springfield, IL: Charles C Thomas.

Connolly, J.F. 1988. Fracture complications, recognition, prevention, and management. Chicago: Year Book Medical.

Corrigan, B., and G.D. Maitland. 1989. Practical orthopedic medicine. London: Butterworth.

Cyriax, J.H. 1975. Textbook of orthopaedic medicine. Vol. 1. Diagnosis of soft tissue lesions. 6th ed. Baltimore: Williams & Wilkins.

Cyriax, J.H. 1977. Textbook of orthopaedic medicine. Vol. 2. Treatment by manipulation, massage and injection. Baltimore: Williams & Wilkins.

Davis, B.C., and R.A. Harrison. 1988. Hydrotherapy in practice. New York: Churchill Livingstone.

deAndrade, J.R., Grant, C., and A.S.-J. Dixon. 1965. Joint distension and reflex muscle inhibition in the knee. Journal of Bone and Joint Surgery 47A:313–322.

DeLorme, T.L., and A.L. Watkins. 1948. Technics of progressive resistance exercise. Archives of Physical Medicine 29:263–273.

Denegar, C., E. Saliba, and S. Saliba. 2005. Therapeutic modalities for musculoskeletal injuries. 2nd. ed. Champaign, IL: Human Kinetics.

Dillman, C.J. 1975. Kinematic analyses of running. Exercise and Sport Sciences Reviews. 3:193–218.

DiPietro, L.A. 1995. Wound healing: The role of the macrophage and other immune cells. Shock 4: 233–240.

Dommissee, G.F. 1975. Morphological aspects of the lumbar spine and lumbosacral region. Orthopedic Clinics of North America 6:163–175.

Donatelli, R., and A. Owens-Burkhart. 1981. Effects of immobilization on the extensibility of periarticular connective tissue. Journal of Orthopaedic and Sports Physical Therapy 9:67–72.

Donkers, M.J., An, K.N., Chao, E.Y., and B.F. Morrey. 1993. Hand position affects elbow joint load during push-up exercise. Journal of Biomechanics 26:625–632.

Doucette, S.A., and D.D. Child. 1996. The effect of open and closed chain exercise and knee joint position on patellar tracking in lateral patellar compression syndrome. Journal of Orthopaedic and Sports Physical Therapy 23:104–110.

Doucette, S.A., and E.M. Goble. 1992. The effect of exercise on patellar tracking in lateral patellar compression syndrome. American Journal of Sports Medicine 20:434–440.

Doyle, J.R., and W.F. Blythe. 1975. The finger flexor tendon sheaths and pulleys. Anatomy and reconstruction. In A.A.O.S. Symposium on Tendon Surgery of the Hand. St. Louis: Mosby.

Duran, R.J., and R.G. Houser. 1975. Controlled passive motion following flexor tendon repair in zones 2 and 3. In A.A.O.S. Symposium on Tendon Surgery of the Hand. St. Louis: Mosby.

Durselen, L., Claes, L., and H. Kiefer. 1995. The influence of muscle forces and external loads on cruciate ligament strain. American Journal of Sports Medicine 23:129–136.

Dye, S.F., and W.D. Cannon. 1988. Anatomy and biomechanics of the anterior cruciate ligament. Clinics in Sports Medicine 7:715–725.

Edlich, R.F., Towler, M.A., Goitz, R.J., Wilder, R.P., Buschbacher, L.P., Morgan, R.F., and J.G. Thacker. 1987. Bioengineering principles of hydrotherapy. Journal of Burn Care and Rehabilitation 8:580–584.

Eldred, E. 1967. Peripheral receptors: Their excitation and relation to reflex patterns. American Journal of Physical Medicine 46:69–87.

Ellenbecker, T.S., and A.J. Mattalino. 1997. The elbow in sport. Champaign, IL: Human Kinetics.

Ellenbecker, T.S., and A.J. Mattalino. 1999. Glenohumeral joint range of motion and rotator cuff strength following arthroscopic anterior stabilization with thermal capsulorraphy. Journal of Orthopaedic and Sports Physical Therapy 29:160–167.

Elliot, D.H. 1965. Structure and function of mammalian tendon. Biology Review 40:392–421.

Enwemeka, C.S. 1989. Inflammation, cellularity, and fibrillogenesis in regenerating tendon: Implications for tendon rehabilitation. Physical Therapy 69:816–825.

Esch, D., and M. Lepley. 1974. Evaluation of joint motion: Methods of measurement and recording. Minneapolis: University of Minnesota Press.

Evans, R.B. 1989. Clinical application of controlled stress to the healing extensor tendon: A review of 112 cases. Physical Therapy 69:1041–1049.

Evans, R.B., and W.E. Burkhalter. 1986. A study of the dynamic anatomy of extensor tendons and implications for treatment. Journal of Hand Surgery (Am) 11:774–779.

Evans, R.B., Eggers, G.W.N., Butler, J.K., and J. Blumel. 1960. Experimental immobilization and remobilization of rat knee joints. Journal of Bone and Joint Surgery 42A:737–758.

Fahrer, H. Rentsch, H.U., Gerber, N.J., Beyeler, C., Hess, C.W., and B. Grünig. 1988. Knee effusion and reflex inhibition of the quadriceps. A bar to effective training. Journal of Bone & Joint Surgery 70B:635-638.

Farjo, L.A., Glick, J.M. and T.G. Sampson. 1999. Hip arthroscopy for acetabular labral tears. Arthroscopy 15:132-137.

Feigenbaum, M.S., and M.L. Pollock. 1999. Prescription of resistance training for health and disease. Medicine & Science in Sport & Exercise 31:38-45.

Feltner, M., and J. Dapena. 1986. Dynamics of the shoulder and elbow joints of the throwing arm during a baseball pitch. International Journal of Sport Biomechanics 2:235–259.

Finsterbush, A., and B. Friedman. 1975. Reversibility of joint changes produced by immobilization in rabbits. Clinics in Orthopaedics and Related Research 111:290–298.

Fisher, A.C., Mullins, S.A., and P.A. Frey. 1993. Athletic trainers' attitudes and judgments of injured athletes' rehabilitation adherence. Journal of Athletic Training 28:43–47.

Forkin, D.M., Koczur, C., Battle, R., and R.A. Newton. 1996. Evaluation of kinesthetic deficits indicative of balance control in gymnasts with unilateral chronic ankle sprains. Journal of Orthopaedic and Sports Physical Therapy 23:245–250.

Freeman, M.A., and B. Wyke. 1967. The innervation of the knee joint. An anatomical and histological study in the cat. Journal of Anatomy 101:505–532.

Fritz, J.M., Irrgang, J.J., and C.D. Harner. 1996. Rehabilitation following allograft meniscal transplantation: A review of the literature and case study. Journal of Orthopaedic and Sports Physical Therapy 24:98–106.

Galloway, M.T., and P. Jokl. 1990. Patella plica syndrome. Annals of Sports Medicine 5:34–41.

Gambetta, V. 1986. In roundtable discussion: Blelik, E., Chu, D.A., Costello, F., Gambetta, V., Lundin, P., Rogers, R., Santos, J., and F. Wilt. 1986. Practical considerations for utilizing plyometrics. Part 1. National Strength Coaches Association Journal 8:14–22.

Garn, S.N., and R.A. Newton. 1988. Kinesthetic awareness in subjects with multiple ankle sprains. Physical Therapy 68:1667–1671.

Garrett, W.E., Jr. 1990. Muscle strain injuries: Clinical and basic aspects. Medicine and Science in Sport and Exercise 22:436–443.

Gelberman, R., An, K.-A., Banes, A., and V. Goldberg. 1988. Tendon. In Injury and repair of the musculoskeletal soft tissues, ed. S.L.-Y. Woo and J.A. Buckwalter. Park Ridge, IL: American Academy of Orthopaedic Surgeons.

Gelberman, R.H., Woo, S.L.-Y., Lothringer, K., Akeson, W.H., and D. Amiel. 1982. Effects of early intermittent passive mobilization on healing canine flexor tendons. Journal of Hand Surgery 7: 170–175.

Geraci, M.C. 1994. Rehabilitation of pelvis, hip, and thigh injuries in sports. Physical Medicine and Rehabilitation Clinics of North America 5:157–174.

Gerber, A. and J.J. Warner. 2002. Thermal capsulorrhaphy to treat shoulder instability. Clinical Orthopaedics & Related Research 400:105-116.

Gerhardt, J.J., and O.A. Russe. 1975. International SFTR method of measuring and recording joint motion. Bern: Huber.

Gilleard, W., McConnell, J., and D. Parsons. 1998. The effect of patellar taping on the onset of vastus medialis obliquus and vastus lateralis muscle activity in persons with patellofemoral pain. Physical Therapy 78:25–32.

Glascoe, W.M., Allen, M.K., Awtry, B.F., and H.J. Yack. 1999. Weight-bearing immobilization and early exercise treatment following a grade II lateral ankle sprain. Journal of Orthopaedic and Sports Physical Therapy 29:394–399.

Gough, J.V., and G. Ladley. 1971. An investigation into the effectiveness of various forms of quadriceps exercises. Physiotherapy 57:356–361.

Greenman, P.E. 1996. Principles of manual medicine. Baltimore: Williams & Wilkins.

Grelsamer, R.P., and J.R. Klein. 1998. The biomechanics of the patellofemoral joint. Journal of Orthopaedic and Sports Physical Therapy 28:286–298.

Grigg, P. 1994. Peripheral neural mechanisms in proprioception. Journal of Sport Rehabilitation 3: 2–17.

Grood, E.S., Suntay, W.J., Noyes, F.R., and D.L. Butler. 1984. Biomechanics of the knee-extension exercise. Effect of cutting the anterior cruciate ligament. Journal of Bone and Joint Surgery 66A: 725–734.

Groppel, J.L., and R.P. Nirschl. 1986. A mechanical and electromyographical analysis of the effects of various joint counterforce braces on the tennis player. American Journal of Sports Medicine 14: 195–200.

Gross, M.T. 1992. Chronic tendinitis: Pathomechanics of injury, factors affecting the healing response, and treatment. Journal of Orthopaedic & Sports Physical Therapy 16:248-261.

Gross, M.T., Bradshaw, M.K., Ventry, L.C., and K.H. Weller. 1987. Comparison of support provided by ankle taping and semirigid orthosis. Journal of Orthopaedic and Sports Physical Therapy 9: 33–39.

Harrison, R.A., Hillman, M., and S. Bulstrode. 1992. Loading of the lower limb when walking partially immersed: Implications for clinical practice. Physiotherapy 78 (3):164-167.

Hay, J. 1993. The biomechanics of sports techniques. 4th ed. Englewood Cliffs, NJ: Prentice-Hall.

Hayashi, K., Thabit, G., III, Bogdanske, J.J., Mascio, L.N., and M.D. Markel. 1996. The effect of nonablative laser energy on the ultrastructure of joint capsular collagen. Arthroscopy: The Journal of Arthroscopic and Related Surgery 12:474–481.

Hayashi, K., Thabit, G., III, Massa, K.L., Bogdanske, J.J., Cooley, A.J., Orwin, J.F., and M.D. Markel. 1997. The effect of thermal heating on the length and histologic properties of the glenohumeral joint capsule. American Journal of Sports Medicine 25:107–112.

Heppenstall, R.B. 1980. Fracture healing. In Fracture treatment and healing, ed. R.B. Heppenstall. Philadelphia: Saunders.

Hertling, D., and R.M. Kessler. 1990. Management of common musculoskeletal disorders. 2nd ed. Philadelphia: Lippincott.

Hettinger, T., and E. Müller. 1953. Muscle strength and muscle training. Arbeitsphysiologie 15: 111–126.

Hillman, S. 2005. Introduction to athletic training. 2nd. ed. Champaign, IL: Human Kinetics.

Hislop, H.J. and J. Montgomery. 2002. Daniels and Worthingham's muscle testing. Techniques of manual examination. Philadelphia: WB Saunders.

Hom, D.B. 1995. Growth factors in wound healing. Otolaryngologic Clinics of North America 28: 933–953.

Hoppenfeld, S. 1976. Physical examination of the spine and extremities. New York: Appleton-Century-Crofts.

Hortobagy, T., and F.I. Katch. 1990. Eccentric and concentric torque–velocity relationships during arm flexion and extension. European Journal of Applied Physiology 60:395–401.

Host, H.H. 1995. Scapular taping in the treatment of anterior shoulder impingement. Journal of Orthopaedic and Sports Physical Therapy 75:803–812.

Houglum, J.E. 1998. Pharmocologic considerations in the treatment of injured athletes with non-steroidal anti-inflammatory drugs. Journal of Athletic Training 33:259–263.

Houglum, J.E., Harrelson, G.L., and D. Leaver-Dunn. 2005. Principles of pharmacology for athletic trainers. Thorofare, NJ: Slack, Inc.

Houglum, P.A. 1992. Soft tissue healing and its impact on rehabilitation. Journal of Sport Rehabilitation 1:19–39.

Huberti, H.H., and W.C. Hayes. 1984. Patellofemoral contact pressures. The influence of Q-angle and tendofemoral contact. Journal of Bone and Joint Surgery 66A:715–724.

Hunter, G.R. 1994. Muscle physiology. In Essentials of strength training and conditioning, ed. T.R. Baechle. Champaign, IL: Human Kinetics.

Iqbal, S., Schwellnus, M.P., Noakes, T., and C. Lombard. 1994. A fivefold reduction in the incidence of recurrent ankle sprains in soccer players using the Sport-Stirrup orthosis. 1994. American Journal of Sports Medicine 22:601–606.

Irrgang, J.J., Harner, C.D., Fu, F.H., Silbey, M.B., and R. DiGiacomo. 1997. Loss of motion following ACL reconstruction: A second look. Journal of Sport Rehabilitation 6:213–225.

Isear, J.A., Jr., Erickson, J.C., and T.W. Worrell. 1997. EMG analysis of lower extremity muscle recruitment patterns during an unloaded squat. Medicine and Science in Sports and Exercise 29: 532–539.

Jenkins, W.L., Munns, S.W., Jayaraman, G., Wertzberger, K.L., and K. Neely. 1997. A measurement of anterior tibial displacement in the closed and open kinetic chain. Journal of Orthopaedic and Sports Physical Therapy 25:49–56.

Jobe, F.W., Moynes, D.R., and D.J. Antonelli. 1985. Rotator cuff function during a golf swing. American Journal of Sports Medicine 14:388-392.

Kaltenborn, F.M. 2002. Mobilization of the extremity joints Vol 1. The extremities. 5th ed. Minneapolis: OTPT.

Kamkar, A., Irrgang, J.J., and S.L. Whitney. 1993. Nonoperative management of secondary shoulder impingement syndrome. Journal of Orthopaedic & Sports Physical Therapy 17:212-224.

Kapandji, I.A. 1986. The physiology of the joints. Vol. 2. Lower limb. 5th ed. New York: Churchill Livingstone.

Karlsson, J., Thomee, R., and L. Sward. 1996. Eleven year follow-up of patello-femoral pain syndrome. Clinical Journal of Sport Medicine 6:22–26.

Karpovich, P.V., Herden, E.L., Jr., Asa, M.M., and G.P. Karpovich. 1959. Electrogoniometer: A new device for study of joints in action. Federation Proceedings 18:79.

Kaufman, K.R., An, K.-N., Litchy, W.J., Morrey, B.F., and Chao, E.Y.S. 1991. Dynamic joint forces during knee isokinetic exercise. American Journal of Sports Medicine 19:305–316.

Keith, R.H., Granter, C.V., Hamilton, B.B., and F.S. Sherwin. 1987. The functional independence measure: A new tool for rehabilitation. In Advances in clinical rehabilitation, ed. M.G. Eisenberg and R.C. Grzesink. New York: Springer.

Kelley, M.J. 1995. Anatomic and biomechanical rationale for rehabilitation of the athlete's shoulder. Journal of Sports Rehabilitation 4:122–154.

Kendall, F.P., McCreary, E.K., and P.G. Provance. 1993. Muscles: Testing and function. 4th ed. Baltimore: Williams & Wilkins.

Kessler, R.M., and D. Hertling. 1983. Management of common musculoskeletal disorders. Philadelphia: Harper & Row.

Kibler, W.B. 1990. Concepts in exercise rehabilitation of athletic injury. In Sports-induced inflammation, ed. W.B. Leadbetter, J.A. Buckwalter, and S.L. Gordon. Park Ridge, IL: American Academy of Orthopaedic Surgeons.

Kibler, W.B. 1995a. Biomechanical analysis of the shoulder during tennis activities. Clinics in Sports Medicine 14:79–85.

Kibler, W.B. 1995b. Pathophysiology of overload injuries around the elbow. Clinics in Sports Medicine 14:447–457.

Kimura, I.F., Nawoczenski, D.A., Epler, M., and M.G. Owen. 1987. Effect of the AirStirrup in controlling ankle inversion stress. Journal of Orthopaedic and Sports Physical Therapy 9:190–193.

Kirsner, R.S., and W.H. Eaglstein. 1993. The wound healing process. Dermatological Clinics 11:629–638.

Klein, L., Heiple, K.G., Torzilli, P.A., Goldberg, V.M., and A.H. Burstein. 1989. Prevention of ligament and meniscus atrophy by active joint motion in a non–weight bearing model. Journal of Orthopaedic Research 7:80–85.

Klingman, R.F., Liaos, S.M., and K.M. Hardin. 1997. The effect of subtalar joint posting on patellar glide position in subjects with excessive rearfoot pronation. Journal of Orthopaedic and Sports Physical Therapy 25:185–191.

Knight, K.L. 1985. Guidelines for rehabilitation of sports injuries. Clinics in Sports Medicine 4:405–416.

Knight, K.L., Martin, J.A., and B.R. Londeree. 1979. EMG comparison of quadriceps femoris activity during knee extension and straight leg raises. American Journal of Physical Medicine and Rehabilitation 58:57–67.

Knott, M., and D.E. Voss. 1968. Proprioceptive neuromuscular facilitation. New York: Harper & Row.

Kohn, H.S. 1997. Shin pain and compartment syndromes in running. In Running injuries, ed. G.N. Guten. Philadelphia: Saunders.

Konradsen, L., Holmer, P., and Sondergaard, L. 1991. Early mobilizing treatment for grade III ankle ligament injuries. Foot & Ankle 12:69–73.

Koopman, C.F. 1995. Cutaneous wound healing: An overview. Otolaryngologic Clinics of North America 28:835–845.

Kottke, F.J. 1990. Therapeutic exercise to develop neuromuscular coordination. In Krusen's handbook of physical medicine and rehabilitation, ed. F.J. Kottke and J.F. Lehmann. Philadelphia: Saunders.

Kottke, F.J., Pauley, D.L., and R.A. Ptak. 1966. The rationale for prolonged stretching for correction of shortening of connective tissue. Archives of Physical Medicine and Rehabilitation 47:345–352.

Koury, J.M. 1996. Aquatic therapy programming. Champaign, IL: Human Kinetics.

Koutedakis, Y. 1989. Muscle elasticity—plyometrics: Some physiological and practical considerations. Journal of Applied Research in Coaching and Athletics 4:35–49.

Kowall, M.G., Kolk, G., Nuber, G.W., Cassisi, J.E., and S.H. Stern. 1996. Patellar taping in the treatment of patellofemoral pain. A prospective randomized study. American Journal of Sports Medicine 24:61–66.

Kubler-Ross, E. 1969. On death and dying. New York: Macmillan.

Lane, J.M., and J.R. Werntz. 1987. Biology of fracture healing. In Fracture healing, ed. J.M. Lane. New York: Churchill Livingstone.

Lange, G.W., Hintermeister, R.A., Schlegel, T., Dillman, C.J., and J.R. Steadman. 1996. Electromyographic and kinematic analysis of graded treadmill walking and the implications for knee rehabilitation. Journal of Orthopaedic and Sports Physical Therapy 23:294–301.

Lattanza, L., Gray, G.W., and R.M. Kantner. 1988. Closed versus open kinetic chain measurements of subtalar joint eversion: Implications for clinical practice. Journal of Orthopaedic and Sports Physical Therapy 9:310–314.

Lattanzio, P.J., Petrella, R.J., Sproule, J.R., and P.J. Fowler. 1997. Effects of fatigue on knee proprioception. Clinical Journal of Sport Medicine 7:22–27.

Leadbetter, W.B. 1994. Soft tissue athletic injury. In Sports injuries: Mechanisms, prevention, treatment, ed. F.H. Fu and D.A. Stone. Baltimore: Williams & Wilkins.

Leanderson, J., Eriksson, E., Nilsson, C., and A. Wykman. 1996. Proprioception in classical ballet dancers. American Journal of Sports Medicine 24:370–374.

Lear, L.J., and M.T. Gross. 1998. An electromyographical analysis of the scapular stabilizing synergists during a push-up progression. Journal of Orthopaedic and Sports Physical Therapy 28:146–157.

Lehmann, J.F. and B.J. DeLateur. 1990. Gait analysis: Diagnosis and management. In Krusen's handbook of physical medicine and rehabilitation, ed. F.J. Kottke and J.F. Lehmann. Philadelphia: Saunders.

Leib, F.J., and J. Perry. 1971. Quadriceps function. An electromyographic study under isometric conditions. Journal of Bone and Joint Surgery 53A:749–758.

Lephart, S.M., and T.J. Henry. 1996. The physiological basis for open and closed kinetic chain rehabilitation for the upper extremity. Journal of Sport Rehabilitation 5:71–87.

Lephart, S.M., Kocher, M.S., Fu, F.H., Borsa, P.A., and C.D. Harner. 1992. Proprioception following ACL reconstruction. Journal of Sport Rehabilitation 1:188–196.

Lieber, R.L. 1992. Skeletal muscle structure and function. Implications for rehabilitation and sports medicine. Baltimore: Williams & Wilkins.

Light, K.E., Nuzik, S., Personius, W., and A. Barstrom. 1984. Low-load prolonged stretch vs. high-load brief stretch in treating knee contractures. Physical Therapy 64:330–333.

Lind, A.R. 1959. Muscle fatigue and recovery from fatigue induced by sustained contractions. Journal of Physiology (London) 147:162–171.

Livingston, L.A. 1998. The quadriceps angle; a review of the literature. Journal of Orthopaedic & Sports Physical Therapy 28: 105-109

Lofvenberg, R., Karrholm, J., Sundelin, G., and O. Ahlgren. 1995. Prolonged reaction time in patients with chronic lateral instability of the ankle. American Journal of Sports Medicine 23:414–417.

Lundin, P. 1985. A review of plyometric training. National Strength Coaches Association Journal 7: 69–74.

MacDougall, J.D., Elder, G.C.B., Sale, D.G., Moroz, J.R., and J.R. Sutton. 1980. Effect of training and immobilization on human muscle fibers. European Journal of Applied Physiology 43:25–34.

Madding, S.W., Wong, J.G., Hallum, A., and Medeiros, J.M. 1987. The effect of duration of passive stretch on hip abduction range of motion. Journal of Orthopaedic and Sports Physical Therapy.

Maitland, G.D. 1990. Vertebral manipulation. Boston: Butterworth-Heinemann.

Maitland, G.D. 1991. Peripheral manipulation. London: Butterworth-Heinemann.

Manheim, C.J. 1994. The myofascial release manual. Thorofare, NJ: Slack.

Mann, R.A. 1980. Biomechanics of walking, running, and sprinting. American Journal of Sports Medicine 8:345–350.

Markolf, K.L., Gorek, J.F., Kabo, J.M., and M.S. Shapiro. 1990. Direct measurement of resultant forces in the anterior cruciate ligament. An in vitro study performed with a new experimental technique. Journal of Bone and Joint Surgery 72A:557–567.

Martinez-Hernandez, A., and P.S. Amenta. 1990. Basic concepts in wound healing. In Sports-induced inflammation, ed. W.B. Leadbetter, J.A. Buckwalter, and S.L. Gordon. Park Ridge, IL: American Academy of Orthopaedic Surgeons.

Massie, D.L., and J.C. Spiker. 1990. Foot biomechanics and the relationship to rehabilitation of lower extremity injuries. Berryville, VA: Forum Medicum.

McDonough, A.L. and J.P. Weir. 1996. The effect of postsurgical edema of the knee joint on reflex inhibition of the quadriceps femoris. Journal of Sport Rehabilitation 5:172-182

McNair, P.J., and S.N. Stanley. 1996. Effect of passive stretching and jogging on the series elastic muscle stiffness and range of motion of the ankle joint. British Journal of Sports Medicine 30: 313–317.

McQuade, K.J., Dawson, J., and G.L. Smidt. 1998. Scapulothoracic muscle fatigue associated with alterations in scapulohumeral rhythm kinematics during maximum resistive shoulder elevation. Journal of Orthopaedics & Sports Physical Therapy 28:74-80.

McWaters, G. 1988. Deep water exercise for health and fitness. Laguna Beach, CA: Publitech Editions.

Mellman, M.F., McPherson, E.J., Dorr, L.D., and P. Kwong. 1996. Differential diagnosis of back and lower extremity problems. In The spine in sports, ed. R.G. Watkins. St. Louis: Mosby.

Melzak, R. 1973. The puzzle of pain. New York: Basic Books.

Mero, A., Komi, T.V., Korjus, T., Navarro, E., and R.J. Gregor. 1994. Body segment contributions to javelin throwing during final thrust phase. Journal of Applied Biomechanics 10:166–177.

Micheli, L.J., and C.M. Coady. 1997. Approaching hip, pelvis, and groin injuries in athletes. Biomechanics 4:22–26.

Mirzabeigi, E., Jordan, C., Gronley, J.K., Rockowitz, N.L., and J. Perry. 1999. Isolation of the vastus medialis oblique muscle during exercise. American Journal of Sports Medicine 27: 50–53.

Moll, J., and V. Wright. 1971. Normal range of spinal mobility: A clinical study. Annals of Rheumatic Diseases 30:381–386.

Montgomery, J.B., and J.R. Steadman. 1985. Rehabilitation of the injured knee. Clinics in Sports Medicine 4:333–343.

Morin, G.E., Tiberio, D., and G. Austin. 1997. The effect of upper trapezius taping on electromyographic activity in the upper and middle trapezius region. Journal of Sports Rehabilitation 6:309–318.

Moritani, T., and H.A. deVries. 1979. Neural factors versus hypertrophy in the time course of muscle strength gain. American Journal of Physical Medicine 58:115–130.

Moynes, D.R., Perry, J., Antonelli, D.J., and F.W. Jobe. 1986. Electromyography and motion analysis of the upper extremity in sports. Physical Therapy 66:1905-1911.

Muller, E.A. 1970. Influence of training and of inactivity on muscle strength. Archives in Physical Medicine and Rehabilitation 51:449–462.

National Athletic Trainers' Association Board of Directors. 1999. From the field. NATA News, March, 7.

Nirschl, R.P. 1977. Tennis elbow. Primary Care 4:367–382.

Nuber, G.W., Jobe, F.W., Perry, J., Moynes, D.R., and D. Antonelli. 1985. Fine wire electromyography analysis of muscles of the shoulder during swimming. American Journal of Sports Medicine 14: 7–11.

O'Kane, J.W. 1999. Anterior hip pain. American Family Physician 60:1687-1696.

Orchard, J.W., Fricker, P.A., Abud, A.T., and B.R. Mason. 1996. Biomechanics of iliotibial band friction syndrome in runners. American Journal of Sports Medicine 24:375–379.

Ounpuu, S. 1994. The biomechanics of walking and running. Clinics in Sports Medicine 13:843–863.

Page, P. 2003. More than meets the eye. Advance for physical therapists & PT assistants 14:47-48.

Page, P.A., Labbe, A. and R.V. Tropp. 2000. Clinical force production of Thera-bands. Journal of Orthopedic and Sports Physical Therapy 30:A47-A48.

Pappas, A.M., Zawacki, R.M., and T.J. Sullivan. 1985. Biomechanics of baseball pitching, a preliminary report. American Journal of Sports Medicine 13:216–222.

Paris, S.V., and C. Patla. 1988. E1 course notes: Extremity dysfunction and manipulation. St. Augustine, FL: Patris.

Peacock, E.E. 1965. Physiology of tendon repair. American Journal of Surgery 109:283.

Peacock, E.E. 1984. Wound repair. 3rd ed. Philadelphia: Saunders.

Perlan, R., Frank, C., and G. Fick. 1995. The effect of elastic bandages on human knee proprioception in the uninjured population. American Journal of Sports Medicine 23:251–255.

Perry, J. 1978. Normal upper extremity kinesiology. Physical Therapy 58:265–278.

Perry, J. 1983. Anatomy and biomechanics of the shoulder in throwing, swimming, gymnastics, and tennis. Clinics in Sports Medicine 2:247–270.

Perry, J. 1990. Gait analysis in sports medicine. Instructional Course Lectures 39:319–324.

Perry, J. 1992. Gait analysis—normal and pathological function. Thorofare, NJ: Slack.

Peterson, P. 1986. The grief response and injury. Athletic Training 21:312–314.

Pink, M., Perry, J., Browne, A., Scovazzo, M.L., and J. Kerrigan. 1991. The normal shoulder during freestyle swimming. American Journal of Sports Medicine 19:569–576.

Posner-Mayer, J. 1995. Swiss ball applications for orthopedic and sports medicine. Denver: Ball Dynamics International.

Powers, C.M., Maffucci, R., and S. Hampton. 1995. Rearfoot posture in subjects with patellofemoral pain. Journal of Orthopaedic and Sports Physical Therapy 22:155–160.

Pratt, K. and R. Bohannon. Effects of a 3-minutes standing stretch on ankle-dorsiflexion range of motion. Journal of sport rehabilitation 12:162-173.

Prentice, W.E. 1983. A comparison of static stretching and PNF stretching for improving hip joint flexibility. Athletic Training 18:56-59.

Ray, R. 2005. Management strategies in athletic training. 3rd ed. Champaign, IL: Human Kinetics.

Reider, B. 1996. Medial collateral ligament injuries in athletes. Sports Medicine 21:147–156.

Reilly, D.T., and M. Martens. 1972. Experimental analysis of the quadriceps muscle force and patello-femoral joint reaction force for various activities. Acta Orthopaedica Scandinavica 43:126–137.

Richardson, A.B., Jobe, F.W., and H.R. Collins. 1980. The shoulder in competitive swimming. American Journal of Sports Medicine 8:159-163.

Risberg, M.A., Holm, I., Tjomsland, O., Ljunggren, E., and A. Ekeland. 1999. Prospective study of changes in impairments and disabilities after anterior cruciate ligament reconstruction. Journal of Orthopaedic and Sports Physical Therapy 29:400–412.

Rodgers, M.M. 1988. Dynamic biomechanics of the normal foot and ankle during walking and running. Physical Therapy 68:1822–1830.

Rotella, R.J. 1985. The psychological care of the injured athlete. In Sports psychology: Psychological consideration in maximizing sport performance. Ann Arbor, MI: McNaughton & Gun.

Rovere, G.D., Clarke, T.J., Yates, C.S., and K. Burley. 1988. Retrospective comparison of taping and ankle stabilizers in preventing ankle injuries. American Journal of Sports Medicine 16:228–233.

Ryu, R.K.N., McCormick, J., Jobe, F.W., Moynes, D.R., and D.J. Antonelli. 1988. An electromyographic analysis of shoulder function in tennis players. American Journal of Sports Medicine 16:481–485.

Saal, J.S. 1987. Flexibility training. In Rehabilitation of sport injuries, ed. J.A. Saal. Philadelphia: Hanley & Belfus.

Sady, S.P., Wortman, M., and D. Blanke. 1982. Flexibility training: ballistic, static or proprioceptive neuromuscular facilitation. Archives of Physical Medicine & Rehabilitation 63:261-263.

Sahrmann, S. 2002. Diagnosis and treatment of movement impairment syndromes. St. Louis: Mosby.

Salter, R.B., Simmons, D.F., Malcom, B.W., Rumble, E.J., Macmichael, D., and N.D. Clements. 1980. The biological effect of continuous passive motion on the healing of full-thickness defects in articular cartilage. Journal of Bone and Joint Surgery 62A:1232–1251.

Saunders, J.B.deC.M., Inman, V.T., and H.D. Eberhart. 1953. The major determinants in normal and pathological gait. Journal of Bone and Joint Surgery 35-A:543-558.

Scott, G.A., Jolly, B.L., and C.E. Henning. 1986. Combined posterior incision and arthroscopic intra-articular repair of the meniscus. Journal of Bone and Joint Surgery 68A:847–861.

Seto, J.L., and C.E. Brewster. 1994. Treatment approaches following foot and ankle injury. Clinics in Sports Medicine 13:695–719.

Shelbourne, K.D., Patel, D.V., Adsit, W.S., and D.A. Porter. 1996. Rehabilitation after meniscal repair. Clinics in Sports Medicine 15:595–612.

Shellock, F.G., and Prentice, W.E. 1985. Warming-up and stretching for improved physical performance and prevention of sports-related injuries. Sports Medicine 2:267–278.

Shrier, I. and K. Gossal. 2000. Myths and truths of stretching. Individualized recommendations for healthy muscles. Physician and Sportsmedicine 28: 57-63.

Shultz, S.J., Houglum, P.A., and D.H. Perrin. 2005. Examination of Musculoskeletal Injuries 2nd ed. Champaign, IL: Human Kinetics.

Siler, B. 2000. The Pilates Body. New York: Broadway Books.

Silver, F.H., and A.I. Glasgold. 1995. Cartilage wound healing. Otolaryngologic Clinics of North America 28:847–864.

Simons, D.G. 1981. Myofascial trigger points: A need for understanding. Archives of Physical Medicine and Rehabilitation 62:97–99.

Sinacore, D.R., Bander, B.L., and A. Delitto. 1994. Recovery from a 1-minute bout of fatiguing exercise: Characteristics, reliability, and responsiveness. Physical Therapy 74:234–244.

Sitler, M., Ryan, J., Wheeler, B., McBride, J., Arciero, R., Anderson, J., and M.B. Horodyski. 1994. The efficacy of a semirigid ankle stabilizer to reduce acute ankle injuries in basketball. American Journal of Sports Medicine 22:454–461.

Somes, S., Worrell, T.W., Corey, B., and C.D. Ingersoll. 1997. Effects of patellar taping on patellar position in the open and closed kinetic chain: A preliminary study. Journal of Sport Rehabilitation 6:299–308.

Spencer, J.D., Hayes, K.C., and I.J. Alexander. 1984. Knee joint effusion and quadriceps reflex inhibition in man. Archives of Physical Medicine and Rehabilitation 65:171–177.

Stamford, B. 1985. The difference between strength and power. Physician and Sportsmedicine 13: 155.

Stanton, P., and C. Purdam. 1995. Hamstring injuries in sprinting - the role of eccentric exercise. Physiotherapy in Sport 18:6-11.

Staron, R.S., Leonardi, M.J., Karapondo, D.L., Malicky, E.S., Falkel, J.E., Hagerman, F.C., and R.S. Kikada. 1991. Strength and skeletal muscle adaptations in heavy-resistance-trained women after detraining and retraining. Journal of Applied Physiology 70:631–640.

Steadman, J.R., Forster, R.S., and J.P. Silferskiold. 1989. Rehabilitation of the knee. Clinics in Sports Medicine 8:605–627.

Stewart, K.M. 1992. Tendon injuries. In Concepts in hand rehabilitation, ed. B.G. Stanley and S.M. Tribuzi. Philadelphia: Davis.

Stone, M.H., and M.S. Conley. 1994. Bioenergetics. In Essentials of strength training and conditioning, ed. T.R. Baechle. Champaign, IL: Human Kinetics.

Stone, R.G., Frewin, P.R., and S. Gonzales. 1990. Long-term assessment of arthroscopic meniscus repair: A two- to six-year follow-up study. Arthroscopy: The Journal of Arthroscopic and Related Surgery 6:73–78.

Strasmann, T., van der Wal, J.C., Halata, Z., and J. Drukker. 1990. Functional topography and ultrastructure of periarticular mechanoreceptors in the lateral elbow region of the rat. Acta Anatomica 138:1–14.

Sullivan, M.K., DeJulia, J.J., and T.W. Worrell. 1992. Effect of pelvic position and stretching method on hamstring muscle flexibility. Medicine & Science in Sport & Exercise 24:1383-1389.

Sutherland, D.H., Kaufman, K.R., and J.R. Moitoza. 1994. Kinematics of normal human walking. In Human walking, 2nd ed., ed. J. Rose and J.G. Gamble. Baltimore: Williams & Wilkins.

Sutton, G.S., and M.R. Bartel. 1994. Soft-tissue mobilization techniques for the hand therapist. Journal of Hand Therapy 7:185–192.

Taylor, D.C., Dalton, J.D., Jr., Seaber, A.V., and W.E. Garrett, Jr. 1990. Viscoelastic properties of muscle–tendon units. The biomechanical effects of stretching. American Journal of Sports Medicine 18:300–309.

Tenuta, J.J., and R.A. Arciero. 1994. Arthroscopic evaluation of meniscal repairs. Factors that effect healing. American Journal of Sports Medicine 22:797–802.

Thein, J.M., and L.T. Brody. 1998. Aquatic-based rehabilitation and training for the elite athlete. Journal of Orthopaedic and Sports Physical Therapy 27:32–41.

Thigpen, C.M. 1983. Early management of fractures of the foot and ankle. Current Concepts in Trauma Care 6:4–8.

Tiberio, D. 1987. The effect of excessive subtalar joint pronation on patellofemoral mechanics: A theoretical model. Journal of Orthopaedic and Sports Physical Therapy 9:160–165.

Travell, J. 1976. Myofascial trigger points: Clinical view. In Advances in pain research and therapy, vol. 1, ed. J.J. Bonica and D. Albe-Fessard. New York: Raven Press.

Travell, J.G., and D.G. Simons. 1983. Myofascial pain and dysfunction. The trigger point manual. Vol. 1. Baltimore: Williams & Wilkins.

Travell, J.G., and D.G. Simons. 1992. Myofascial pain and dysfunction. The trigger point manual. Vol. 2. Baltimore: Williams & Wilkins.

Upton, A.R.M., and A.J. McComas. 1973. The double crush in nerve entrapment syndromes. Lancet 2:359–362.

Warren, C.G., Lehmann, J.K., and J.N. Koblanski. 1971. Elongation of rat tail tendon: Effect of load and temperature. Archives of Physical Medicine and Rehabilitation 52:465–474.

Warren, C.G., Lehmann, J.K., and Koblanski, J.N. 1976. Heat and stretch procedures: An evaluation using rat tail tendon. Archives of Physical Medicine and Rehabilitation 57:122–126.

Wathen, D. 1994. Load assignment. In Essentials of strength training and conditioning, ed. T.R. Baechle. Champaign, IL: Human Kinetics.

Wegener, L., Kisner, C., and D. Nichols. 1997. Static and dynamic balance responses in persons with bilateral knee osteoarthritis. Journal of Orthopaedic and Sports Physical Therapy 25:13–18.

Wells, K.F., and K. Luttgens. 1976. Kinesiology: Scientific basis of human motion. 6th ed. Philadelphia: Saunders.

Wilk, K.E., Arrigo, C., Andrews, J.R., and W.G. Clancy, Jr. 1999. Rehabilitation after anterior cruciate ligament reconstruction in the female athlete. Journal of Athletic Training 34:177–193.

Wilk, K.E., Voight, M.L., Keirns, M.A., Gambetta, V., Andrews, J.R., and C.J. Dillman. 1993. Stretch-shortening drills for the upper extremities: Theory and clinical application. Journal of Orthopaedic and Sports Physical Therapy 17:225–239.

Williams, K.R. 1985. The biomechanics of running. Exercise and Sport Sciences Reviews 13:389–441.

Wilmore, J.H., and D.L. Costill. 2004. Physiology of sport and exercise, 3rd ed. Champaign, IL: Human Kinetics.

Wilt, F. 1975. Plyometrics. What it is—how it works. Athletic Journal 55:76–90.

Winter, D.A. 1987. The biomechanics and motor control of human gait. Waterloo, ON: University of Waterloo Press.

Witvrouw, E., Sneyers, C., Roeland, L., Victor, J., and J. Bellemans. 1996. Reflex response times of vastus medialis oblique and vastus lateralis in normal subjects and in subjects with patellofemoral pain syndrome. Journal of Orthopaedic and Sports Physical Therapy 24:160–165.

Woodall, W., and J. Welsh. 1990. A biomechanical basis for rehabilitation programs involving the patellofemoral joint. Journal of Orthopaedic and Sports Physical Therapy 11:535–542.

Worrell, T.W., Corey, B.J., York, S. L., and J. Santiestaban. 1992. An analysis of supraspinatus EMG activity and shoulder isometric force development. Medicine and Science in Sport and Exercise 24:744-748

Worrell, T.W., Crisp, E., and C. LaRosa. 1998. Electromyographic reliability and analysis of selected lower extremity muscles during lateral step-up conditions. Journal of Athletic Training 33:156–162.

Worrell, T.W., Ingersoll, C.D., Bockrath-Pugliese, K., and P. Minis. 1998. Effect of patellar taping and bracing on patellar position as determined by MRI in patients with patellofemoral pain. Journal of Athletic Training 33:16–20.

Young, A., Stokes, M., and J.F. Iles. 1987. Effects of joint pathology on muscle. Clinical Orthopaedics 219:21–27.

Zinovieff, A.N. 1951. Heavy-resistance exercises. The "Oxford Technique." British Journal of Physical Medicine 14:129–132.

SUGGESTED READING

Adriani, E., Luziatelli, S., and P.P. Mariani. 1993. Medial instability of the elbow: Surgical management and rehabilitation. Journal of Sports Traumatology and Related Research 15:45–52.

Allegrucci, M., Whitney, S.L., and J.J. Irrgang. 1994. Clinical implications of secondary impingement of the shoulder in freestyle swimmers. Journal of Orthopaedic and Sports Physical Therapy 20:312–318.

Andrews, J.R., and J.A. Whiteside. 1993. Common elbow problems in the athlete. Journal of Orthopaedic and Sports Physical Therapy 17:289–295.

Andrews, J.R., and K.E. Wilk. 1994. The athlete's shoulder. New York: Churchill Livingstone.

Åstrand, P.O., and K. Rodahl. 1977. Textbook of work physiology. New York: McGraw-Hill.

Barker, C. 1988. Evaluation, treatment, and rehabilitation involving a submuscular transposition of the ulnar nerve at the elbow. Athletic Training 23:10–12.

Basmajian, J.V. 1973. Electromyographic analysis of basic movement patterns. In Exercise and Sport Sciences Reviews, vol. 1, ed. J.H. Wilmore. New York: Academic Press.

Batt, M.E. 1995. Shin splints—a review of terminology. Clinical Journal of Sports Medicine 5:53–57.

Berardi, G. 1995. Proprioceptive training following acute Achilles injury in dance. Impulse 3:200–213.

Bonci, C.M., Sloane, B., and K. Middleton. 1992. Nonsurgical/surgical rehabilitation of the unstable shoulder. Journal of Sport Rehabilitation 1:146–171.

Borsa, P.A., Lephart, S.M., Kocher, M.S., and S.P. Lephart. 1994. Functional assessment and rehabilitation of shoulder proprioception for glenohumeral instability. Journal of Sport Rehabilitation 3:84–104.

Braatz, J.H., and P.P. Gogia. 1987. The mechanics of pitching. Journal of Orthopaedic and Sports Physical Therapy 9:56–69.

Breig, A. 1978. Adverse mechanical tension in the nervous system. Stockholm: Almqvist & Wiksell.

Brewster, C., and D.R. Moynes Schwab. 1993. Rehabilitation of the shoulder following rotator cuff injury or surgery. Journal of Orthopaedic and Sports Physical Therapy 18:422–426.

Brunet, M.E., Haddad, R.J., Sanchez, J., and E. Leonard. 1984. How I manage sprained finger in athletes. Physician and Sportmedicine 12:99–108.

Burnett, W.R. 1992. Rehabilitation techniques for ligament injuries of the hand. Hand Clinics 8: 803–815.

Cibulka, M.T. 1992. The treatment of the sacroiliac joint component to low back pain: A case report. Physical Therapy 72:917–922.

Clemens, S., and B. Foss-Campbell. 1993. Rehabilitation following traumatic hand injury: Hand therapists' perspective. Part 1: Acute phase of hand rehabilitation. Plastic Surgical Nursing 13: 129–139.

Cordova, M.L., and C.W. Armstrong. 1996. Reliability of ground reaction forces during a vertical jump: Implications for functional strength assessment. Journal of Athletic Training 31:342–345.

Cornwall, M.W. 1984. Biomechanics of non contractile tissue. Physical Therapy 64:1869–1873.

Corrigan, B., and G.D. Maitland. 1989. Practical orthopaedic medicine. Boston: Butterworth.

Craeger, C.C. 1996. Therapeutic exercises using foam rollers. Berthoud, CO: Executive Physical Therapy.

Culham, E., and M. Peat. 1993. Functional anatomy of the shoulder complex. Journal of Orthopaedic and Sports Physical Therapy 18:342–350.

Daniels, L., and C. Worthingham. 1977. Therapeutic exercise for body alignment and function. Philadelphia: Saunders.

Davies, G.J., and S. Dickoff-Hoffman. 1993. Neuromuscular testing and rehabilitation of the shoulder complex. Journal of Orthopaedic and Sports Physical Therapy 18:449–458.

Denegar, C.R., E. Saliba, and S. Saliba. 2005. Therapeutic modalities for musculoskeletal injuries. 2nd ed. Champaign, IL: Human Kinetics.

Dillman, C.J., Fleisig, G.S., and J.R. Andrews. 1993. Biomechanics of pitching with emphasis upon shoulder kinematics. Journal of Orthopaedic and Sports Physical Therapy 18:402–408.

Dovelle, S., and P.K. Heeter. 1985. Early controlled mobilization following extensor tendon repair in zone V–VI of the hand: Preliminary report. Contemporary Orthopaedics 11:41–44.

Dumbelton, J.H., and J. Black. 1975. An introduction to orthopedic materials. Springfield, IL: Charles C Thomas.

Ellenbecker, T.S. 1995. Rehabilitation of shoulder and elbow injuries in tennis players. Clinics in Sports Medicine 14:87–104.

Erhard, R.E., Delitto, A., and M.T. Cibulka. 1994. Relative effectiveness of an extension program and a combined program of manipulation and flexion and extension exercises in patients with acute low back syndrome. Physical Therapy 74:1093–1100.

Evans, R.B., and D.E. Thompson. 1992. An analysis of factors that support early active short arc motion of the repaired central slip. Journal of Hand Therapy 5:187–201.

Feldenkrais, M. 1973. Body and mature behavior. New York: International Universities Press.

Feldenkrais, M. 1990. Awareness through movement. San Francisco: Harper.

Foster, D.N., and M.N. Fulton. 1991. Back pain and the exercise prescription. Clinics in Sports Medicine 10:197–209.

Frankel, V.H., and M. Nordin. 1980. Basic biomechanics of the skeletal system. Philadelphia: Lea & Febiger.

Frost, H.M. 1973. Orthopedic biomechanics. Springfield, IL: Charles C Thomas.

Gardiner, M.D. 1981. The principles of exercise therapy. London: Bell.

Greenman, P.E. 1996. Principles of manual medicine. Baltimore: Williams & Wilkins.

Grieve, G.P. 1984. Mobilisation of the spine. New York: Churchill Livingstone.

Groves, R., and D.N. Camaione. 1983. Concepts in kinesiology. Philadelphia: Saunders.

Grubbs, N. 1993. Frozen shoulder syndrome: A review of literature. Journal of Orthopaedic and Sports Physical Therapy 18:479–487.

Grundnes, O., and O. Reikeras. 1992. Blood flow and mechanical properties of healing bone. Acta Orthopaedica Scandinavica 63:487–491.

Halikis, M.N., and J. Taleisnik. 1996. Soft-tissue injuries of the wrist. Clinics in Sports Medicine 15:235–259.

Hartley-O'Brien, S.J. 1980. Six mobilization exercises for active range of hip flexion. Research Quarterly for Exercise and Sport 51:625–635.

Hillman, S.K. 2004. Introduction to athletic training. 2nd ed. Champaign, IL: Human Kinetics.

Hodges, P.W., and C.A. Richardson. 1997. Contraction of the abdominal muscles associated with movement of the lower limb. Physical Therapy 77:132–144.

Holt, L.E., Travis, T.M., and T. Okita. 1970. Comparative study of three stretching techniques. Perceptual and Motor Skills 31:661–616.

Hopkins, T.J., and A.A. White. 1993. Rehabilitation of athletes following spine injury. Clinics in Sports Medicine 12:603–618.

Hunter, J.M., Schneider, L.H., Mackin, E.J., and A.D. Callahan, eds. 1990. Rehabilitation of the hand: Surgery and therapy. St. Louis: Mosby.

Institute of Physical Art. 1991. Integrating function: The foam roll approach. Steamboat Springs, CO: Author.

Irrgang, J.J., Whitney, S.L., and E.D. Cox. 1994. Balance and proprioceptive training for rehabilitation of the lower extremity. Journal of Sport Rehabilitation 3:68–83.

Janisse, D.J. 1994. Indications and prescriptions for othoses in sports. Orthopedic Clinics of North America 25:95–107.

Jobe, F.W., and J.P. Bradley. 1989. The diagnosis and nonoperative treatment of shoulder injuries in athletes. Clinics in Sports Medicine 8:419–438.

Jobe, F.W., Moynes, D.R., and C.E. Brewster. 1987. Rehabilitation of shoulder joint instabilities. Orthopedic Clinics of North America 18:473–482.

Jobe, F.W., and G. Nuber. 1986. Throwing injuries of the elbow. Clinics in Sports Medicine 5:621–636.

Johannsen, F., Remvig, L., Kryger, P., Beck, P., Warming, S., Lybeck, K., Dreyer, V., and L.H. Larsen. 1995. Exercises for chronic low back pain: A clinical trial. Journal of Orthopaedic and Sports Physical Therapy 22:52–59.

Jones, F.P. 1978. Body awareness in actions. New York: Schocken Books.

Kapandji, I.A. 1980. The physiology of the joints. Vol. 1. Upper limb. New York: Churchill Livingstone.

Kegerreis, S. 1983. The construction and implementation of functional progressions as a component of athletic rehabilitation. Journal of Orthopaedic and Sports Physical Therapy 5:14–19.

Kegerreis, S., Malone, T., and J. McCarroll. 1984. Functional progressions: An aid to athletic rehabilitation. Physician and Sportsmedicine 12:67–71.

Kegerreis, S., and T. Wetherald. 1987. The utilization of functional progressions in the rehabilitation of injured wrestlers. Athletic Training 22:32–35.

Kendall, H.O., Kendall, F.P., and D.A. Boynton. 1970. Posture and pain. Huntington, NY: Robert E. Krieger.

Kenneally, M., Rubenach, H., and R. Elvey. 1988. The upper limb tension test: The SLR of the arm. In Physical therapy of the cervical and thoracic spine, ed. R. Grant. New York: Churchill Livingstone.

Keskula, D.R., Duncan, J.B., Davis, V.L., and P.W. Finley. 1996. Functional outcome measures for knee dysfunction assessment. Journal of Athletic Training 31:105–110.

Kleinert, H.E., and C. Verdan. 1983. Report of the committee on tendon injuries. Journal of Hand Surgery (Am) 7:794–798.

Kottke, F.J. 1982. Therapeutic exercise to maintain mobility. In Krusen's handbook of physical medicine and rehabilitation, ed. F.J. Kottke, G.K. Stillwell, and J.F. Lehmann. Philadelphia: Saunders.

Kuzmich, D. 1994. The levator scapulae: Making the con-NECK-tion. Journal of Manual and Manipulative Therapy 2:43–54.

Lattanza, L., Gray, G.W., and R.M. Kantner. 1988. Closed versus open kinetic chain measurements of subtalar joint eversion: Implications for clinical practice. Journal of Orthopaedic & Sports Physical Therapy 9:310–314

Leanderson, J., Eriksson, E., Nilsson, C., and A. Wykman. 1996. Proprioception in classical ballet dancers. A prospective study of the influence of an ankle sprain on proprioception in the ankle joint. American Journal of Sports Medicine 24:370–373.

Lee, D. 1986. Principles and practice of muscle energy and functional techniques. In Modern manual therapy of the vertebral column, ed. G. Grieves. New York: Churchill Livingstone.

Lee, D.G. 1986. "Tennis elbow": A manual therapist's perspective. Journal of Orthopaedic and Sports Physical Therapy 8:134–142.

Lee, H.W.M. 1994. Progressive muscle synergy and synchronization in movement patterns: An approach to the treatment of dynamic lumbar instability. Journal of Manual and Manipulative Therapy 2:133–142.

Leibowitz, J. 1990. The Alexander Technique. New York: Harper & Row.

Lephart, S.M., and T.J. Henry. 1995. Functional rehabilitation for the upper and lower extremity. Orthopedic Clinics of North America 26:579–592.

Lephart, S.M., Perrin, D.H., Fu, F.H., and K. Minger. 1991. Functional performance tests for the anterior cruciate ligament insufficient athlete. Athletic Training 26:44–50.

Levine, W.R. 1992. Rehabilitation techniques for ligament injuries of the wrist. Hand Clinics 8: 669–677.

Litchfield, R., Hawkins, R., Dillman, C.J., Atkins, J., and G. Hagerman. 1993. Rehabilitation for the overhead athlete. Journal of Orthopaedic and Sports Physical Therapy 18:433–442.

Livingston, L.A. 1998. The quadriceps angle; a review of the literature. Journal of Orthopaedic & Sports Physical Therapy. 28: 105-109.

Loudin, J.K., and S.L. Bell. 1996. The foot and ankle: An overview of arthrokinematics and selected joint techniques. Journal of Athletic Training 31:173–178.

Mackinnon, S.E. 1992. Double and multiple crush syndromes. Hand Clinics 8:369.

Maitland, G.D. 1990. Vertebral manipulation. Boston: Butterworth-Heinemann.

Maitland, G.D. 1991. Peripheral manipulation. Boston: Butterworth-Heinemann.

Manheim, C.J. 1994. The myofascial release manual. 2nd ed. Thorofare, NJ: Slack.

Markolf, K.L., Gorek, J.F., Kabo, J.M., and M.S. Shapiro. 1990. Direct measurement of resultant forces in the anterior cruciate ligament. An in vitro study performed with a new experimental technique. Journal of Bone and Joint Surgery 72-A:557–567

Mascaro, T.B., and L.E. Swanson. 1994. Rehabilitation of the foot and ankle. Orthopedic Clinics of North America 25:147–160.

May, E.J., Silfverskiold, K.L., and C.J. Sollerman. 1992. Controlled mobilization after flexor tendon repair in zone II: A prospective comparison of three methods. Journal of Hand Surgery 5:942–952.

McPoil, T.G. 1988. Footwear. Physical Therapy 68:1857–1865.

McQuade, K.J., and G.L. Smidt. 1998. Dynamic scapulohumeral rhythm: The effects of external resistance during elevation of the arm in the scapular plane. Journal of Orthopaedic and Sports Physical Therapy 27:125–133.

Meister, K., and J.R. Andrews. 1993. Classification and treatment of rotator cuff injuries in the overhand athlete. Journal of Orthopaedic and Sports Physical Therapy 18:413–421.

Miller, A.S., and T.M. Narson. 1995. Protocols for proprioceptive active retraining boards. Chiropractic Sports Medicine 9:52–55.

Morris, M., Jobe, F.W., Perry, J., Pink, M., and B.S. Healy. 1989. Electromyographic analysis of elbow function in tennis players. American Journal of Sports Medicine 17:241–247.

Moynes, D.R. 1983. Prevention of injury to the shoulder through exercises and therapy. Clinics in Sports Medicine 2:413–422.

Murray, M.P., Drought, A.B., and R.C. Kory. 1964. Walking patterns of normal men. Journal of Bone and Joint Surgery 46A:335–360.

Nordin, M., and V.H. Frankel. 1980. Biomechanics of collagenous tissues. In Basic biomechanics of the skeletal system, ed. V.H. Frankel and N. Nordin. Philadelphia: Lea & Febiger.

Oliver, J. 1994. Back care: An illustrated guide. Boston: Butterworth-Heinemann.

Ollivierre, C.O., and R.P. Nirschl. 1996. Tennis elbow. Current concepts of treatment and rehabilitation. Sports Medicine 22:133–139.

Pappas, A.M., Zawacki, R.M., and C.F. McCarthy. 1985. Rehabilitation of the pitching shoulder. American Journal of Sports Medicine 13:223–235.

Payne, R.M., and M. Voight. 1993. The role of the scapula. Journal of Orthopaedic and Sports Physical Therapy 18:386–391.

Pezzullo, D.J., Karas, S., and J.J. Irrgang. 1995. Functional plyometric exercises for the throwing athlete. Journal of Athletic Training 30:22–26.

Plancher, K.D., Litchfield, R., and R.J. Hawkins. 1995. Rehabilitation of the shoulder in tennis players. Clinics in Sports Medicine 14:111–137.

Rasch, P.J., ed. 1989. Kinesiology and applied anatomy. Philadelphia: Lea & Febiger.

Ray, R. 2005. Management strategies in athletic training. 3rd ed. Champaign, IL: Human Kinetics.

Reynolds, N.L., and T.W. Worrell. 1991. Chronic Achilles peritendinitis: Etiology, pathophysiology, and treatment. Journal of Orthopaedic and Sports Physical Therapy 13:171–176.

Rubin, D. 1981. Myofascial trigger point syndromes: An approach to management. Archives of Physical Medicine and Rehabilitation 62:107–110.

Safran, M.R., Caldwell, G.L., Jr., and F.H. Fu. 1994. Proprioception considerations in surgery. Journal of Sport Rehabilitation 3:105–115.

Saudek, C.E., and K.A. Palmer. 1987. Back pain revisited. Journal of Orthopaedic and Sports Physical Therapy 8:556–566.

Seto, J.L., and C.E. Brewster. 1994. Treatment approaches following foot and ankle injury. Clinics in Sports Medicine 13:695–719

Shultz, S.J., Houglum, P.A., and D.H. Perrin. 2005. Assessment of musculoskeletal injuries. 2nd ed. Champaign, IL: Human Kinetics.

Sisto, D.J., Jobe, F.W., Moynes, D.R., and D.J. Antonelli. 1987. An electromyographic analysis of the elbow in pitching. American Journal of Sports Medicine 15:260–263.

Smith, K.F. 1979. The thoracic outlet syndrome: A protocol of treatment. Journal of Orthopaedic and Sports Physical Therapy 1:89–99.

Smith, L.K., Weiss, E.L., and L.D. Lehmkuhl. 1996. Brunnstrom's clinical kinesiology. Philadelphia: Davis.

Snyder-Mackler, L., DeLuca, P.F., Williams, P.R., Eastlack, M.E., and A.R. Bartolozzi. 1994. Reflex inhibition of the quadriceps femoris muscle after injury or reconstruction of the anterior cruciate ligament. Journal of Bone and Joint Surgery 76A:555–560.

Stanish, W.D, Curwin, S. and S. Mandel. 2000. Tendinitis: Its etiology and treatment. New York: Oxford University Press.

Steinkamp, L.A., Dillingham, M.F., Markel, M.D., Hill, J.A., and K.R. Kaufman. 1993. Biomechanical considerations in patellofemoral joint rehabilitation. American Journal of Sports Medicine 21: 438–444.

Stone, J.A., Lueken, J.S., Partin, N.B., Timm, K.E., and E.J. Ryan. 1993. Closed kinetic chain rehabilitation for the glenohumeral joint. Journal of Athletic Training 28:34–37.

Stone, J.A., Partin, N.B., Lueken, J.S., Timm, K.E., and E.J. Ryan, III. 1994. Upper extremity proprioceptive training. Journal of Athletic Training 29:15–18.

Strauss, R.H., ed. 1979. Sports medicine and physiology. Philadelphia: Saunders.

Stroyan, M., and K.E. Wilk. 1993. The functional anatomy of the elbow complex. Journal of Orthopaedic and Sports Physical Therapy 17:279–288.

Tan, J.C., and M. Nordin. 1992. Role of physical therapy in the treatment of cervical disk disease. Orthopedic Clinics of North America 23:435–449.

Tanigawa, M.C. 1972. Comparison of the hold-relax procedure and passive mobilization on increasing length. Physical Therapy 52:725–735.

Thein, J.M., and L.T. Brody. 1998. Aquatic-based rehabilitation and training for the elite athlete. Journal of Orthopaedic &F Sports Physical Therapy 27:32-41.

Tippett, S.R., and M.L. Voight. 1995. Functional progressions for sport rehabilitation. Champaign, IL: Human Kinetics.

Urban, M.K. 2000. COX-2 Specific inhibitors offer improved advantages over traditional NSAIDs. Orthopedics 23:761s-764s.

Walker, J.M. 1992. The sacroiliac joint: A critical review. Physical Therapy 72:903–916.

Wallin, D., Ekblom, B., Grahn, R., and T. Nordenborg. 1985. Improvement of muscle flexibility. A comparison between two techniques. American Journal of Sports Medicine 13:263–268.

Warren, C.G., Lehmann, J.K., and Koblanski, J.N. 1971. Elongation of rat tail tendon: Effect of load and temperature. Archives of Physical Medicine and Rehabilitation 52:465–474.

Wadsworth, C.T. 1983. Clinical anatomy and mechanics of the wrist and hand. Journal of Orthopaedic and Sports Physical Therapy 4:206–216.

Watkins, R.G. 1996. The spine in sports. St. Louis: Mosby.

Wegener, L., Kisner, C., and D. Nichols. 1997. Static and dynamic balance responses in persons with bilateral knee osteoarthritis. Journal of Orthopaedic and Sports Physical Therapy 25:13–18.

Wehbe, M.A. 1996. Early motion after hand and wrist reconstruction. Hand Clinics 12:25–29.

Werner, S.L., Fleisig, G.S., Dillman, C.J., and J.R. Andrews. 1993. Biomechanics of the elbow during baseball pitching. Journal of Orthopaedic and Sports Physical Therapy 17:274–278.

Wilk, K.E., and C. Arrigo. 1993. Current concepts in the rehabilitation of the athletic shoulder. Journal of Orthopaedic and Sports Physical Therapy 18:365–378.

Wilk, K.E., C. Arrigo, and J.R. Andrews. 1993. Rehabilitation of the elbow in the throwing athlete. Journal of Orthopaedic and Sports Physical Therapy 17:305–317.

Wilk, K.E., Voight, M.L., Keirns, M.A., Gambetta, V., Andrews, J.R., and Dillman, C.J. 1993. Stretch shortening drills for the upper extremities: Theory and clinical application. Journal of Orthopaedic and Sports Physical Therapy 17:225–239.

Wilk, K.E., Arrigo, C., Andrews, J.R., and W.G. Clancy Jr., 1999. Rehabilitation after anterior cruciate ligament reconstruction in the female athlete. Journal of Athletic Training 34:177–193.

Wilk, K.E., Andrews, J.R., Clancy, Jr., W.G., Crockett, H.C., and J.W. O'Mara. 1999. Rehabilitation programs for the PCL-injured and reconstructed knee. Journal of Sport Rehabilitation. 8:333-362.

Wilkerson, G.B., and A.J. Nitz. 1994. Dynamic ankle stability: Mechanical and neuromuscular interrelationships. Journal of Sport Rehabilitation 3:43–57.

Wilmore, J.H., and D.C. Costill. 1994. Physiology of sport and exercise. Champaign, IL: Human Kinetics.

Witvrouw, E., Sneyers, C., Lysens, L., Victor, J., and J. Bellemans. 1996. Reflex response times of vastus medialis oblique and vastus lateralis in normal subjects and in subjects with patellofemoral pain syndrome. Journal of Orthopaedic and Sports Physical Therapy 24:160–165.

Wood, E.C., and P.D. Becker. 1981. Beard's massage. Philadelphia: Saunders.

Worrell, T.W., Crisp, E., and C. LaRosa. 1998. Electromyographic reliability and analysis of selected lower extremity muscles during lateral step-up conditions. Journal of Athletic Training 33:156–162.

Worrell, T.W., Ingersoll, C.D., Bockrath-Pugliese, K., and P. Minis. 1998. Effect of patellar taping and bracing on patellar position as determined by MRI in patients with patellofemoral pain. Journal of Athletic Training. 33:16–20.

Young, A., Stokes, M., and J.F. Iles. 1987. Effects of joint pathology on muscle. Clinical Orthopaedics & Related Research. 219:21–27.

Zimmerman, G.R. 1994. Carpal tunnel syndrome. Journal of Athletic Training 29:22–30.

Zmierski, T., Kegerreis, S., and J. Scarpaci. 1995. Scapular muscle strengthening. Journal of Sport Rehabilitation 4:244–252.

Index

Note: Page numbers followed by an] italicized f or t refer to the figure or table on that page, respectively.

1 RM 211, 222*f*

A
A-band 201, 202*f*, 203*f*, 204*f*
abdominal exercises 517–523
    using foam rollers 447
    using Swiss balls 438, 439
abduction, definition 141
acceleration
    definition 67, 80
    and functional activities 304
acceleration phase 357, 371, 373
accessory joint motion 95, 96, 174
acetabular labral tears 935–936
acetabulum 893
    click syndrome 932
acetylcholine 31*t*, 206
Achilles
    flexibility exercises 781–782
    rupture 802–803
    tendinitis 798–801
ACL injuries
    closed chain exercises 828
    open kinetic chain activity 828
    sprain 860–863
acromioclavicular joint
    joint mobilization 587
    sprain 636–637
actin
    and cross-bridge structure 204*f*
    and sarcomere structure 201
action potential 201, 206
action-reaction 67
active assisted range of motion (AAROM) 230
active insufficiency 76
active range of motion (AROM) 93–94, 230
    recording 138
active stretches
    elbow 664–665
    knee 844–847
    shoulder 590–593
active trigger point 165
activity perception 266–267
Actron 55*t*
adduction, definition 141
adenosine diphosphate (ADP)
    and immobilization 127
    and muscle contraction 203

adenosine triphosphate (ATP)
    and immobilization 127
    and muscle contraction 203
    and muscle fiber type 210
adhesions
    effect of massage 155
    and friction massage 157
    in hand 692
    and immobilization 128
    and joint mobilization 178
    and joint range of motion 42
    stripping technique 164
    in tendons 460
    and trigger point therapy 170
    and ultrasound 53
adhesive capsulitis (shoulder) 633–635
adrenaline 31*t*, 32*t*
Advil 55*t*
aerobic shoes 760–761
afferent nerve fibers 133
afferent nervous system
    cutaneous proprioceptive receptors 261
    and muscle contraction 202
    and proprioception 261, 262*f*
    and proprioceptive neuromuscular facilitation
        (PNF) 243
    and referred pain 184
    response to ice-stretch technique 169*f*
    response to myofascial release 161
age
    and healing process 57
    and muscle imbalances 337
    and osteoarthritis 90
    and plyometrics 283
    and range of motion 134
    and spine joint mobilization 491
agility
    about 268–272
    definition 22–23
    exercises for spine 524–525
    and functional activities 305–306
    functional exercises 311*f*, 312*f*
    and knee rehabilitation 829–830, 858–859
    lower extremity exercises 791
    and proprioception 260
agonistic muscle pattern 247
agonists
    muscle strength imbalances 159
    and proprioception 263
    and proprioceptive neuromuscular facilitation 143
    and reciprocal inhibition 142

Aleve 55*t*
Alexander technique 347–349
alignment. *See also* posture
    correcting spine lateral shift 506
    and deep-water exercise 405
    femoral neck 893
    foot 751–753
    of knee and hip due to lateral pelvic shift 363*f*
    lower extremity 331–336, 826
    muscle energy techniques 170–173
    patella 823–824, 877
    pathological 329–331
    pelvic neutral 507
    sacroiliac joint 530
    sitting 328
    spine 341*f*
    standing 327–328
    upper extremity 336
alpha efferent fibers 133
ambulation aids 896
American Academy of Orthopedic Surgeons 617
amortization phase of plyometrics 279–280
anastamosis 39*f*
anconeus 649
angiogenesis
    definition 31*t*
    and epidermal wound healing 39*f*
    during proliferation phase of healing 41
angiotensin-converting enzyme inhibitors 56
angle of pull 76
    and muscular strength 78
angular motion 75
ankle
    capsular patterns of motion 177*t*
    and gait kinematics 367, 372*f*
    goniometer placement 139*f*
    joints 745
    motions 746*f*
    during normal gait 362
    and pathological gait 376
    range of motion 136
    resting and close-packed positions 181*t*
    during running 381
ankle injuries
    Achilles rupture 802–803
    Achilles tendinitis 798–801
    dislocation 795–797
    fractures 811–813
    and gait abnormalities 376
    sprain 795–797
    tendinitis 804–805
ankle rehabilitation
    aquatic exercises 414–415
    deep tissue massage 774
    flexibility exercises 781–784
    functional activities 795
    general considerations 744–748
    hopping activities 794

joint mobilization 774–779
strengthening exercises 784–789
talocrural joint mobilization 776
treadmill exercises 793
using Swiss balls 442
annulospiral ending 133
Ansaid 55*t*
antacids, and NSAID medications 56
antagonist muscle pattern 247
antagonists
    and active stretching 141
    inhibition by group I nerve fibers 133
    muscle strength imbalances 159
    and proprioception 261
    and proprioceptive neuromuscular facilitation 143
anterior cruciate ligament. *See also* ACL injuries
    and proprioception 263
anterior horn 200*f*, 205
anterior superior iliac spine (ASIS)
    and poor posture 329
    and standing alignment 328
anterior tibialis
    during running 380*f*
    stretching 450
anteversion 332, 893
antibiotics 56
anticoagulants 56
anti-inflammatory drugs 54–56
antineoplastic drugs 56
aquatic exercise
    advantages 400–401
    contraindications 401–402
    deep-water exercise 404–405
    equipment 397–400
    indications 400
    lower extremity 411–417
    precautions 401
    program design using water's properties 402
    progression of exercise 403–404
    properties of water 393–395
    spine 406–411
    upper extremities 417–421
    using foam rollers 444
    water temperature 402
arachidonic acid
    definition 31*t*
    and kidney function 56
    and NSAID medications 55
arches of foot 747–748
    structural deformities 749
arches of hand 689*f*
Archimedes' principle 393
areolar (loose) connective tissue 125
arm. *See* upper extremity
arthritis
    and age 90
    cartilage transplantation 50
    and leg-length discrepancy 896

and recurring injuries 90
arthrokinematic motions 175
articular cartilage
    and immobilization 127
    in knee joint 822
    remobilization 128
aspirin 55t, 56
assessment
    about 17–18
    definition 88, 99
    of functional activities 102
    functional examination 303, 309–310
    lower extremity functional scale 19f
    lower extremity functional testing 315
    manual muscle testing 222–229
    and manual therapy 155
    as ongoing process 101–102
    questionnaires 18–20
    record keeping 109
    of sacroiliac joint 530–534
    tools for outcomes-based rehabilitation 18–20
    and treatment goals and plan 100–101
    vertebral artery compromise 480
assistive devices
    for aquatic exercise 397
    fitting 381
    four-point gait 384
    gait patterns 381
    and hip mechanics 896
    and hip stress reduction 897
    safety and precautions 386–387
    single support 384
    stairs 385–386
    three-point gait 383
assistive stretches
    elbow 665–666
    night splints for elbow 662
    shoulder 593–595
athletic trainers
    NATA 9
    NATA contact information 11
athletic training students 6
atrophy 127
autogenic inhibition 133
autonomic nervous system
    response to myofascial release 161
    response to trigger points 165
axon 200f

B
back
    capsular patterns of motion 177t
    Moll and Wright spinal ROM 137f
back exercises
    using foam rollers 448
    using Swiss balls 433–438
back injuries. See also sacroiliac joint; spine
    disk lesions 527–528

and double-crush syndrome 185
    facet injuries 528
    sciatica 527–528
    spondylosis, spondylolysis, spondylolisthesis 526–527
    thoracic outlet syndrome 546–549
back pain
    and bending 341f
    and body mechanics 340–342
    and muscle imbalances 337
    Roland-Morris questionnaire 20
balance 264–266
    functional exercises 310, 311
    and knee rehabilitation 829–830, 858–859
    lower extremity exercises 269–271
    and proprioception 260
    and Swiss ball exercises 427
    using foam rollers 450
balance boards 790
ballistic stretching 144–145
balls. See Swiss balls
Bankart lesion 625
BAPS board 310, 311f
    and ankle flexibility 783
    upper extremity exercises 315
barbell 237
barrier 171
barriers to movement 536
baseball, functional exercises 316f
baseball pitching 557–558
    and elbow stress 647
    Little League elbow 676–677
    mechanics and elbow injuries 647
    summation of forces 78
base of support 70
    and advanced functional activities 308
    with assistive devices 382f
    and stability 342
    and Swiss ball exercises 430f
basketball shoes 761
basophil 31t
bench press 452
beta blockers 56
Bextra 55t
biceps brachii
    muscle fibers per motor unit 201t
    pain referral 650f
    soft-tissue mobilization 649
    tendon injuries 638
biceps femoris
    action during gait cycle 372f
    and running 380
Biodex 240–242
biofeedback 565
blisters 81
blood
    erythrocyte 32t
    granular leukocytes 33t

leukocytes 34*t*
platelets 35*t*
polymorphonuclear leukocyte (PMN) 36*t*
blood clotting
    Hageman factor 33*t*
    heparin 56
    during inflammation phase of healing 38
    and NSAID medications 56
blood pressure 56
blood vessels
    angiogenesis during proliferation phase 41
    damage at time of injury 38
    and tendon injury 47
body-awareness programs
    Alexander technique 347–349
    Feldenkrais method 345–347
    Pilates method 349–351
Body Blade 615
body composition 393
body levers 72–74
body mechanics
    athletic events 343
    for clinician 344
    definition 340
    lifting 342
body-weight exercises
    ankle 787–789
    hip muscles 917–920
    lower extremity 787–789
B.O.I.N.G. 615
bone
    cell types 35*t*
    fracture and callus formation 31*t*
    healing process 50–51
    specific gravity 393
    stress fracture 130
    structural fatigue 81
    tensile strength after injury 52
bony end-feel 95
Bouhler exercises 516, 606
boutonniere deformity 735
braces
    hand 696–698
    knee 829
    and proprioception 271
brachialis
    and elbow structure 647
    pain referral 651*f*
    physiological advantage 76
    soft-tissue mobilization 649
brachial plexus
    stretch 192*f*
    tension test 187
brachioradialis
    muscle fibers per motor unit 201*t*
    soft-tissue mobilization 654
bradykinin 31*t*, 34*t*

brain and proprioception 262*f*, 263
Brannock measuring device 759, 760*r*
bug exercises 508
bunion 750
buoyancy 393, 402
    assistive devices 397
bursitis, hip 930–931

C
calcium 202, 203
callus 31*t*
capillaries 41, 43
capsular end-feel 95
capsular patterns of motion 176, 177*t*
cardinal motion 95
cardiovascular exercise
    and back injuries 479
    in water 400, 414
carpal fracture 727–728
carpal tunnel
    anatomy 690
    location in wrist 692
carpal tunnel syndrome 731–732
    as double-crush syndrome 185
carpometacarpal joint 689
    joint mobilization 707–708
    range of motion 135*t*
cartilage
    chondrocytes 45
    repair 49–50
    sounds of injured part 90–91
    transplant in knee 882–883
    types 49
    types in knee 822
Celebrex 55*t*
cell aggregation centers 40
center of buoyancy 393
center of gravity 68
    and body position changes 70*f*
    for body segments 69*t*
    and lever system 72
    pathway during gait cycle 359
    and stability 341
central nervous system
    and balance 264
    and proprioception 261, 263–264
certified athletic trainer 6
cervical lordosis 331
cervical spine
    capsular patterns of motion 177*t*
    flexibility exercises 497–501
    joint mobilization 492–493
    passive neck flexion test 186
    and shoulder injuries 567
    soft-tissue mobilization 480–486
    strengthening exercises 513–514
    thoracic outlet syndrome 546–549
chemotactic factor 31*t*

chemotactin 31*t*
chemotaxis 31*t*
    during inflammation phase of healing 40
    during proliferation phase of healing 41
chondrocytes
    and cartilage injury 50
    effect of growth factors 45
    and remobilization 128
chronic inflammation 46
circulatory system
    angiogenesis 31*t*
    capillaries 43
    capillaries and wound healing 42
    effect of massage 155
    and immobilization 126
    and tendinitis 460
    vascular permeability 40
    vasoconstriction and vasodilation during healing 38
    vertebral artery compromise 480
clavicular joint mobilization 587–588
claw toes 336*f*
clicking sound 91
clinician. *See* rehabilitation clinician
Clinoril 55*t*
closed chain activities
    definition 219–221
    elbow rehabilitation 646
    and force on patella 825
    knee rehabilitation 828
    and motions of foot 745
    for proprioception 272
close-packed joint positions 181–182
coach
    communication with 9
    as part of rehabilitation team 7
Codman's exercises 589
cohesion 394
collagen 31*t*
    arrangement at rest 131
    and bone healing process 50
    and cartilage injury 49
    in connective tissue 124–125
    cross links and mobility 126*f*
    in extracellular matrix 42
    and flexibility exercises 59
    and joint mobilization 178
    and ligament injury 46
    during proliferation phase of healing 41
    stress-strain curve 131
    and tensile strength of tissue 52
    transition during remodeling phase 43
    type and wound tensile strength 42
    and ultrasound 53
collagenase 31*t*, 42
Colles fracture 726
communication 7–9, 25
compact bone 51

comparable sign 92
compartment syndrome
    lower extremity 806–808
    role of fascia 158
compassion 8
complement system 31*t*
complexity of exercise 307–308
compliance
    encouraging patient 14
    and psychological effect of injury 24
component joint motion 174
compression stress 130
concave-convex rule 176
    elbow 648
    shoulder 581
concentric action of muscle 218–219
concentric phase of plyometrics 280
conditioning level, maintaining 472
confidence
    and advanced functional activities 309
    and functional activities 303, 305
connective tissue
    composition 124–125
    and immobilization 125–128
    mechanical properties 128–132
    in muscle 199
    periarticular 127–128
    physical properties 130–132
    remobilization 128
    slack length 131
    stretch model 129*f*
consent 11–12
conservation of energy 79
contact pressure 825
continuous passive motion machines 145
    knee rehabilitation 842
contractile elements 277
contraction phase 208
contract-relax technique 144
contracture 208
    hand 692
contraindications
    foam rollers 445
    joint mobilization 183
    massage 157
    myofascial release 165
    neural mobilization 193
    plyometrics 285
    Swiss ball exercises 430
contusions, hip 928–929
coordination 266–268
    definition 22–23
    exercises for spine 524–525
    of neuromuscular system and plyometrics 279
    and proprioception 260
    and Swiss ball exercises 427
core strength 507–512

corns 336

corticosteroids 56

Coulomb model of dry friction 130

counterforce brace 674*f*

COX-1 inhibitors 54–56

COX-2 inhibitors 54–56

coxa valga 332, 893

coxa vara 332, 893

Craig's test 893

crawl stroke mechanics 561–563

creatine 127

creatine phosphate 127

creep 81, 130, 158

crepitus 90–91

cross-bridges
    and muscle contraction 202
    structure 204*f*

cross-friction massage
    elbow 658
    for tendinitis 463

cross-training 251
    shoes 762

crunches 518

crutches. *See* assistive devices

Cybex 240–242

cycling in water 414

cyclooxegenase-1 (COX-1) inhibitors 54–56

cyclooxegenase-2 (COX-2) inhibitors 54–56

Cyriax, James 174*t*

D

DAPRE resistance training technique 252–253

Daypro 55*t*

dead-bug exercises 509

debridement
    during inflammation phase of healing 40
    and tendon injury 47

deceleration 80

deceleration phase 357
    and muscle action 371
    and muscle activity 373

deconditioning
    and muscle fatigue 209
    preventing 15–16

deep water exercises 404–405
    ambulation activities 415
    hip rehabilitation 415–416
    knee rehabilitation 417
    spine rehabilitation 410–411
    upper extremities 420–421

degenerative disk 329

dehiscence 822

delayed-onset muscle soreness 218

Delorme and Watkins strength progression 252

deltoid mobilization 579

dendrites 200*f*

depression 24

De Quervain's disease 732–733

dermatome 186

diabetes 56, 57

diagonal-plane exercises 618

diarthrodial joints 49

diclofenac 55*t*

diploma 116

discharge summary 112, 115

disease, and healing process 57

disk disruption 892

disk lesions 527–528

dislocation
    ankle 795–797
    elbow 681
    hip 893, 934–935
    patella 871–872
    peroneal tendon 798

diuretics 56

documentation. *See* record keeping

"do no harm" 13

dorsal root 200*f*

dorsiflexion
    and ankle stability 746
    definition 141, 745
    flexibility exercises 782
    and joint mobilization 776
    during running 380*f*
    strengthening exercises 785

double-crush syndrome 185

double-float phase 377

double-limb support 357

dowager's hump 331

downward rotation of scapula 141

drag 394

drug interaction 31*t*

drugs. *See* medications

dumbells 237
    for aquatic exercise 398

duration of exercise
    active stretching 141
    and lactate levels 209
    passive stretching 142

dynamic muscle activity 218–219

dynamometer 222*f*

E

eccentric action of muscle 218–219

eccentric phase of plyometrics 279

edema
    and advanced functional activities 309
    and aquatic exercise 402
    and effleurage 156
    and electrical stimulation 52
    and fibrosis 126
    of hand 692
    and healing 39, 43, 57
    and ice 52
    and initial treatment 89
    and neural injury 185

and NSAID medications 54
and quadriceps strength 826–827
as sign of inflammation 40
education, role of rehab clinician 6
efferent nerves
motor neural pathways 205
and proprioception 263
effleurage 156
elastic band. *See* rubber tubing exercises
elastic components 279
elasticity 129
and active stretching 141
and creep 81
definition 80
of muscle 208
elastic limit 81
elastin 32*t*
in connective tissue 124–125
in extracellular matrix 42
elbow
capsular patterns of motion 177*t*
goniometer placement 139*f*
joint stresses 647
range of motion 135
resting and close-packed positions 181*t*, 648
structure 647–648
elbow injuries
arthroscopy 682
dislocation 681
epicondylitis 673–676
Little League elbow 676–677
sprain 677–678
ulnar collateral ligament repair 678–679
ulnar nerve injury 679–680
elbow rehabilitation
aquatic exercise 419, 421
cross-friction massage 658
flexibility exercises 662–666
functional activities 672
general considerations 646–648
joint mobilization 658–661
plyometrics 672
soft-tissue mobilization 649–658
strengthening exercises 667–672
electrical stimulation 52
electrogoniometer 134, 136*f*
electrothermally assisted capsular shift 635–636
elevation of scapula 141
elgon 134
Elvey's test 187
empty end-feel 95
end-feel of movement 95–96
and myofascial release 160
endomysium 199
endotenon 47
endothelial cells 32*t*, 41
endurance. *See* muscular endurance

endurance limit 81, 130
energy
definition 79
sources for muscle contraction 203, 205
enzymes
collagenase 31*t*, 42
fibrinolysin 39
Hageman factor 33*t*
kallikrein 34*t*
myosin ATPase 203
plasmin 35*t*
protease 36*t*
thrombin 37*t*
epicondylitis 656, 673–676
epidermal tissue 39*f*
epimysium 199
epinephrine 32*t*
epitenon 47
epithelial cells 41
epithelial growth factors (EGF) 45
erector spinae 372*f*
erythrocyte 32*t*
and ligament injury 46
ethics 11
Etokolac 55*t*
eversion 745
definition 141
strengthening exercises 784, 785
examination
about 17–18
accessory joint motion 96
additional information 90–91
assessment 99–102
comparable sign 92
definition 88
end-feel of movement 95–96
history of injury 89
irritable injuries 92
medical history 89–90
muscular strength 96
neurological tests 97–98
observation 93
pain profile 91–92
palpation 98–99
range of motion 93–95
record keeping 102, 103–107, 112
special questions 90
special tests 96–97
subjective 89–92
and treatment 471
visual inspection 93
exercise progression. *See* progression of exercise
extension 141
extensor lag 724, 827–828
external force 66
and angle of pull 76
external rotation 141

extracellular matrix 32*t*
  and immobilization 127
  during remodeling phase of healing 43
extrafusal fibers 132, 201
extrinsic hand muscles
  flexibility exercises 713–714
  soft-tissue mobilization 699–701
exudate 32*t*

F
facet injuries 528–529
factor XII 32*t*, 40
family
  communication with 8
  as part of rehabilitation team 6–7
fascia 158–159
  and neural mobilization 184
fascicle 200*f*
fasciculus 199*f*
fast-twitch fibers 210–211
fatigue
  effects on strength and recovery 250*f*
  and muscle contraction 209
  and recovery period 213
fatigue failure 81, 130
feedback 266, 624*f*
Feiss line test 748
Feldene 55*t*
Feldenkrais method 345–347
Feldenkrais, Moshe 346
femoral nerve 894
  stretch 192*f*
femur, alignment 332*f*
fenoprofen 55*t*
fibrin 32*t*
  and immobilization 126
fibrinogen 32*t*
  during inflammation phase of healing 38
fibrinolysin 32*t*
  during inflammation phase of healing 39
fibroblast 32*t*
  and epidermal wound healing 39*f*
  during proliferation phase of healing 41–42
  during remodeling phase of healing 43
fibroblast growth factor (FGF) 45
fibrocartilage 49
fibrocyte 32*t*
fibronectin 32*t*
  during inflammation phase of healing 38
fibrosis 125, 126, 128
fingers. *See also* hand
  boutonniere deformity 735
  capsular patterns of motion 177*t*
  De Quervain's disease 732–733
  extensor tendon excursions 694*t*
  joint mobilization 708
  phalangeal fractures 728–729
  putty exercises 722–724

range of motion 135–136
  soft-tissue mobilization 656, 657, 702–704
Fitter^TM 791
fixation 72
flexibility. *See also* stretching
  and agility 268
  definition 21, 124
  and muscle imbalances 337
  and plyometrics 281
  and Swiss ball exercises 427
flexibility exercises. *See also* stretching
  cervical spine 497–501
  hamstrings 846–847, 914
  hand 711–715
  hip adductors 912
  hip extensors 914–915
  hip flexors 911
  knee rehabilitation 842–847
  lower extremity 779–782
  lumbar rotation 909
  pectorals 501
  during phases of healing 59
  piriformis 915
  quadratus lumborum 503
  quadriceps 844–846
  scalenes 500
  shoulder 588–599
  tensor fascia lata 909–910
  thoracic outlet syndrome 549*f*
  trapezius 499
  wrist 711–715
  wrist flexion and extension 714*f*
flexion 141
flexor digitorum longus 372*f*
flexor hallucis longus 372*f*
flower-spray ending 133
flow, laminar and turbulent 394
fluorimethane 167
flurbiprofen 55*t*
foam roller exercises
  about 444–445
  lower extremity rehabilitation 449–451, 859*f*
  stork stand 270*f*
  trunk exercises 445–449
  upper extremity rehabilitation 451–452
Focus on Therapeutic Outcomes (FOTO) 20
foot
  alignment 334
  arches 334, 335*f*, 747–748
  capsular patterns of motion 177*t*
  center of gravity 69*t*
  joints 746–747
  metatarsophalangeal joints 747
  midtarsal joints 746–747
  motions 745
  orthotics 753–757
  planar motions 746*f*

pronation 335*f*
resting and close-packed positions 181*t*
tarsometatarsal joints 747
toe extensors 771–772
toe flexors 773
foot flat 357
foot injuries
    fractures 811–813
    plantar fasciitis 808–809
    sesamoiditis 810
    tarsal tunnel syndrome 809–810
    turf toe 810–811
foot-pounds per second 79
foot problems
    bunion 750
    claw toes 336*f*
    corns 336
    forefoot varus and valgus 752, 753*f*
    hallux valgus 336*f*, 750
    hammertoes 336*f*
    pes cavus 749
    pes planus 749
    rearfoot varus and valgus 751
foot rehabilitation
    deep tissue massage 774
    flexibility exercises 782–783
    functional activities 795
    general considerations 744–748
    hopping activities 794
    joint mobilization 778–779
    soft-tissue mobilization 763–766
    toe strengthening exercises 787
    treadmill exercises 793
foot strike 357, 377
footwear. *See* shoes
force
    and advanced functional activities 307
    and body mechanics 342
    and class of levers 72–74
    for concentric and eccentric activities 278
    definition 66
    determining factors for muscle contraction 214–216
    and elbow injuries 648
    ground reaction forces 373–375
    and hand grips 695
    and isometric muscle activity 217*f*
    joint mobilization 581
    in manual muscle testing 224
    during manual resistance training 232
    on menisci 823
    and muscle energy technique 171–172
    and muscle strength 211
    myofascial release 160
    of overhand motions 556
    on patella 824–825
    and plyometrics 278–279
    and power 79, 280
    relationship to torque 75
    summation of 78
    and tendinitis 460
    and work 79
force arm 72
force couples 566
force deformation 130, 142
forearm, range of motion 135
form drag 394
four-point gait 384
fractures
    ankle 811–813
    hand and wrist 726–729
    hip 933–934
    knee 882
free weight exercises 236–239
    ankle 789
    Bouhler exercises 606
    elbow extension 670*f*
    elbow flexion 669*f*
    foot and ankle rehabilitation 789
    scapular retraction 603*f*
    scapular rotation 607
    shoulder abduction 610
    wrist rehabilitation 719
friction 81
    Coulomb model of dry friction 130
frictional drag 394
friction massage 157
frog-eyed patellae 332, 893
frontal plane 141
frozen shoulder 625
fulcrum 72
functional activities
    advanced exercise progression 306–308
    ankle 795
    baseball 316*f*
    basic exercise progression 305
    definition 302, 303
    elbow 672
    foot 795
    goals 303
    golf 317*f*
    hand 725
    hip 926
    knee 859–860
    lower extremity 310–312, 312*f*, 314, 795
    as part of rehabilitation process 303–305
    precautions 308–309
    shoulder 624
    softball 316*f*
    tennis 318*f*
    upper extremity 315–319
    wrist 725
functional assessment 102
functional evaluation 309–310

definition 303
lower extremity 315
upper extremity 319
Functional Independence Measure 20
functional scale 19*f*

G

GAGs. *See* glycosaminoglycan (GAGs)
gait. *See also* assistive devices
ankle motion 362
and aquatic exercise 403
center of gravity pathway 359
definition 356
ground reaction forces 373–375
and hip abductor strength 895–896
and hip stress reduction 897
kinematics 363–370, 368–370 *t*
kinetics 368*f*, 370–373
knee action 361
muscle activity 372*f*
non-weight bearing 383
normal walking speed 359
pathological 375–376
pelvic rotation 360
pelvic tilt 361
and quadriceps strength 827
shock absorption 371
walking speed 377
weight transmission 367*f*
gait control theory 169
gait cycle 357, 358*f*
gamma efferent fibers 133
gastrocnemius
action during gait cycle 372*f*
flexibility exercises 779–780
muscle fibers per motor unit 201*t*
during running 380*f*
soft-tissue mobilization 769
strengthening exercises 787–789
stretching using foam rollers 450
gastrointestinal irritation with medications 54
gate theory of pain 169
gender
Q-angle 826
and range of motion 134
genu recurvatum 332, 333*f*
genu valgus 332, 333*f*
genu varus 332, 333*f*
giant cells 46
glenohumeral joint
capsular patterns of motion 177*t*
capsular restriction 581
joint mobilization 581–586
resting and close-packed positions 181*t*
and scapular imbalance 565
soft-tissue mobilization 575–580
strengthening exercises 608–610
glenoid labral tears 632–633

gluteus maximus
action during gait cycle 372*f*
flexibility exercises 914
soft-tissue mobilization 899
gluteus medius
action during gait cycle 372*f*
flexibility exercises 914
rubber tubing exercises 921
soft-tissue mobilization 900
gluteus medius gait 376
gluteus minimus
action during gait cycle 372*f*
flexibility exercises 914
soft-tissue mobilization 901–902
glycogen
and immobilization 127
and lactate levels 209
glycoprotein 33*t*, 42, 43
glycosaminoglycan (GAGs) 33*t*
and immobilization 127
and myofascial restriction 160
during proliferation phase of healing 42
during remodeling phase of healing 43
goals 16–17
of functional exercises 303
as part of assessment 100
plyometrics 284
relationship to problems identified 100
setting with patient 25
golf
functional exercises 317*f*
mechanics and elbow injuries 647
swing mechanics 563–564
golfer's elbow 673–676
Golgi tendon organs 133–134
and ballistic stretching. *See also* stretching
and muscle energy technique 171
and plyometrics 278
and proprioception 261
Golg-Mazzoni corpuscle 262*f*
goniometer
accuracy 138
description 134
illustration of placement 139*f*
use of 137–138
gracilis 372*f*
granular leukocytes 33*t*
and chronic inflammation 46
granulation tissue 33*t*, 41
granuloma 33*t*, 46
grasshopper eye (patella) 332
gravity 66. *See also* center of gravity
and active range of motion 94
and deep-water exercise 404
line of 70
rate of acceleration 80
and weight 67

greater trochanteric bursitis 930
grief 23–24
grips 695
    strengthening exercises 721–722
grip size 675
groin strain 929
ground reaction forces 373–375, 375f, 379f
ground substance 33t
    in connective tissue 124–125
    and immobilization 126
    during proliferation phase of healing 42
growth factor 33t
    and chronic inflammation 46
    functions 44–45
    during inflammation phase of healing 38
    during proliferation phase of healing 41
growth plate fracture, hip 934
Gymnic Swiss balls 426

H
Hageman factor 33t, 40
half-life 33t
hallux valgus 750
hammertoes 336f
hamstring rehabilitation
    flexibility exercises 505, 846–847, 914
    isometric exercises 849
    non-weight-bearing isotonic exercises 850
    soft-tissue mobilization 834, 835f
    weight-bearing resistive exercises 851–856
hamstrings 836–838
    action during gait cycle 372f
    action during running 380f
    and knee action 824
    physiological advantage 77
    strain 880
hand
    arches 689f
    carpal bone arrangement 707f
    center of gravity 69t
    edema 692
    fascia and ligaments 689–690
    finger extensors 656
    finger flexors 657
    grips 695–696
    muscles 690, 691f, 692
    pulley system 690
    range of motion 135–136
    skeletal structure 689
    tendon-glide excursions 694, 695t
    tendon glide exercises 715–718
    tendon sheaths 690
    tendon zones 691f, 692–694
hand injuries
    carpal tunnel syndrome 731–732
    De Quervain's disease 732–733
    dislocations 729–730
    fractures 727–729

reflex sympathetic dystrophy 736–738
    splinting 696–698
    sprains 729–730
    tendon injuries 733–736
hand rehabilitation
    flexibility exercises 711–715
    functional activities 725
    joint mobilization 705–711
    plyometrics 725
    putty exercises 720–723
    soft-tissue mobilization 654–657, 698–704
head, center of gravity 69t
healing process
    about 30
    and advanced functional activities 309
    bone 50–51
    cartilage 49–50
    chronology of events 44t
    epidermal tissue 39f
    factors affecting 57–58
    inflammation phase 37–41
    ligaments 46–47
    medications affecting 56
    and modalities 52–53
    muscles 48–49
    and NSAID medications 54–56
    overlap of phases 41f
    phases 37, 43
    primary and secondary intention 37
    primary intention 35t
    proliferation phase 41
    remodeling phase 42–43
    role of growth factors 44–45
    and scar tissue mobility 22
    secondary intention 36t
    and tendinitis 459
    for tendons 47–48
    tensile strength 51–52
    timing of therapeutic exercise 58–59
Health Insurance Portability Accountability Act
        (HIPPA) 9
heat
    after injury 53
    and tissue elasticity 81
heel-off 357
heel strike 357
heparin 56
hiking shoes 761
hip
    alignment due to lateral pelvic shift 363f
    capsular patterns of motion 177t
    close-packed position 895
    Craig's test 893
    and gait kinematics 365, 368f
    goniometer placement 139f
    joint mechanics 895–896
    joint mobility 895

manual muscle testing 224–227, 224f, 225f
neural structures 894–895
osseous structures 893
pain referral 897
range of motion 136
resting and close-packed positions 181t
during running 380–381
stability and shoulder injuries 566–567
stabilization 895
hip adductors
    action during gait cycle 372f
    flexibility exercises 912
    manual muscle testing 226f, 227f
    soft-tissue mobilization 833, 834f
hip flexors
    muscle imbalance syndrome 927
    stretching exercises 504
hip injuries
    acetabular labral tears 935–936
    bursitis 930–931
    contusions 928–929
    dislocation 893, 934–935
    fractures 933–934
    groin strain 929
    muscle imbalance 927
    osteitis pubis 931–932
    rice krispie syndromes 932
    sprain 929
    tendinitis 931
hip pointer 928–929
hip rehabilitation
    aquatic exercises 412–413, 415–416
    flexibility exercises 908–915
    functional exercises 926
    joint mobilization 904–908
    proprioceptive exercises 926
    soft-tissue mobilization 897–903
    strengthening exercises 916–925
histamine 33t
    and inflammation 40
    and trigger points 166
    and vascular permeability 40
history of injury 89
hold-relax technique 143
Hooke's law 80–81, 130
horizontal extension 141
horizontal flexion 141
horizontal plane 141
hormones
    epinephrine 32t
    growth factor 33t
    histamine 40
    and inflammation 40
    prostaglandin (PG) 36t
    serotonin 36t
horsepower 79
humeroradial joint 648

resting and close-packed positions 181t
humeroulnar joint 181t
hyaline cartilage 49
hyaluronic acid 33t
    during proliferation phase of healing 42
hydrodynamics 394
hydrostatic pressure 394, 402
hypermobility 93, 96
    of foot 334
    and joint mobilization 581
    and muscle imbalances 338
    of spine 479
hypertrophy of tendons 460
hypomobility 93, 96
    and joint mobilization 178
    and muscle imbalances 338
    of spine 479
hysteresis 132
    and fascia 158
H-zone 202f, 204f
    and sarcomere structure 201

I
I-band 201, 202f, 203f, 204f
ibuprofen 54, 55t
ice 52
ice-and-stretch. See soft-tissue mobilization
ice-stretch technique 167–168
iliac crest, trigger points 900
iliopectineal bursitis 931
iliopsoas
    action during gait cycle 372f
    flexibility exercises 911
    snapping at hip 932
    soft-tissue mobilization 898
iliotibial band
    deep tissue massage 838
    flexibility exercises 506
    massage using foam rollers 449
    and snapping at hip 932
    syndrome 882
iliotibial (ITB) band friction syndrome 339
immobilization
    and articular cartilage 127
    changes in soft tissue 125–126
    and elbow injury 647
    and muscle tissue 126–127
    and periarticular connective tissue 127–128
    and stretching exercises 148
    and tendon repair 47–48
impingement, shoulder 627–629
inclinometer 134
individualization of treatment 14
Indocin 55t
indomethacin 55t
inertia 67
infection 57
inflammation

chronic 46
and pain profile 92
and pain type 185–186
signs 40–41
of tendons 460
inflammation phase 37–41
cellular reactions 38, 39
chemical reactions 40
and NSAID medications 54–56
tensile strength loss 52
and use of ice 52
inflares 544
infraspinatus
assistive stretches 593
soft-tissue mobilization 572
inhibition 266
initial contact 357
initial swing 357
inner ear 265
intensity of exercise
and advanced functional activities 307
and delayed-onset muscle soreness 218
and lactate levels 209
plyometrics 282
as principle of rehabilitation 14–15
and recovery period 213
internal force 66
internal rotation 141
internuncial activation 133
internuncial connecting nerve 263
interpersonal skills 5
interphalangeal (IP) joint 689
joint mobilization 710
range of motion 135–136 t
resting and close-packed positions 181t
intertarsal joint mobilization 778
intrafusal fiber 132
intrinsic hand muscles
flexibility exercises 715
soft-tissue mobilization 702–704
inversion 745
definition 141
strengthening exercises 784, 785
irritable injuries 92
ischemia 185–186
ischemic compression 169–170
ischiogluteal bursitis 931
isokinetic exercises
and compressive force on knee 825
elbow 672
knee 857–858
shoulder 616
wrist 725
isokinetic machines 240–242
isokinetic muscle activity 219
isometric exercises
ankle 784–785
cervical spine 513

elbow 667
foot 784–785
hip muscles 916–917
knee 848–849
recovery time 213
shoulder 599–601
isometric muscle activity 217–218
during manual resistance training 231
and muscle energy technique 171, 172–173
and muscle fatigue 209
and muscular strength 78
isotonic exercises
knee rehabilitation 849–850
recovery time 213
shoulder 601–607
isotonic machines 239–240
isotonic muscle activity 218–219
and muscle energy technique 171, 172

J
joint angle 214
joint mobilization 472–473
ankle 776–778
application 178–183
capsular patterns of motion 176, 177t
cervical spine 492–493
clavicular joint 587–588
close-packed positions 181–182
concave and convex rules 176
contraindications 183
cracking noise 178
definition 174
distal radioulnar joint 704–705
effects 177–178
elbow 658–661
foot 778–779
glenohumeral joint 581–586
grades of movement 178–179
hip 904–908
loose-packed positions 181–182
lumbar spine 494–497
movement diagram 180
PA (posterior-anterior) 492
patellofemoral joint 839
rules for application 182–183
sacroiliac 494–497
scapulothoracic joint 586–587
shoulder injuries 581–588
superior tibiofibular joint 838
thoracic spine 493–494
tibiofemoral joint 840–842
tibiofibular joint 774–775
types of joint motion 174, 175
joint moments 379
joint play 174
joints
accessory motion 96
adhesion formation 42

of ankle 745
arthrokinematic motions 175
braces and proprioception 271
elbow 648
flexibility. *See* flexibility
and lever system 72–74
motions during running 378–379
proprioceptive receptors 262
range of motion 21, 135–136
sounds 90–91
types and arthrokinematics 175
types of motion 174
joules per second 79
J-stroke 163
jumping. *See also* plyometrics
functional exercises 311
jump sign 165

K
kallikrein 34*t*
during inflammation phase of healing 40
Kaltenborn, Freddy 174*t*
keloid formation 42
keratinocytes 45
ketoprofen 55*t*
kinesthesia 271
and scapula stabilization 613
kinetic energy 79
kinetics, running gait 380–381
kinins 34*t*
chemical reaction during inflammation phase 40
and trigger points 166
knee
alignment 332, 333*f*
alignment due to lateral pelvic shift 363*f*
biomechanics 824–826
capsular patterns of motion 177*t*
and gait kinematics 366–367, 371*f*
goniometer placement 139*f*
joint capsule 821
ligaments 821–822
malalignment 339–340
manual muscle testing 224–227, 228*f*
meniscus structure 822–823
during normal gait 361, 362*f*
patellofemoral joint 823–824
primary and secondary restraint 822
Q-angle 826
range of motion 136
resting and close-packed positions 181*t*
during running 381
screw home mechanism 823
and sitting posture 335*f*
structure 821–824
knee injuries 872
ACL sprain 860–863
autologous-chondrocyte implantation 882–883
cartilage transplant 882–883

collateral ligament sprains 867
extensor lag 827–828
fractures 882
and gait abnormalities 376
hamstring strain 880
iliotibial band syndrome 882
meniscus 867–871
Osgood-Schlatter disease 872
osteochondritis dissecans 883–884
patella dislocations 871–872
patella plica syndrome 872
patellar tendinitis 878–879
patellar tendon rupture 879–880
patella subluxations 871–872
patellofemoral syndrome 872–878
and pathological gait 376
and postinjury strength 826–827
quadriceps contusions 881
quadriceps strain 880–881
and tibial torsion 750
knee rehabilitation
aquatic exercises 413–414, 417
bracing 829
closed kinetic chain activities 828
deep tissue massage 836–838
flexibility exercises 842–847
functional exercises 859–860
general considerations 827–830
isokinetic exercises 858
isometric exercises 848–849, 848–849
isotonic exercises (non-weight-bearing) 849–850
isotonic exercises (weight-bearing) 851–856
machine exercises 856–857
open kinetic chain activity 828
program progression 829–830
proprioceptive exercises 858–859
shear stress 829
soft-tissue mobilization 830–836
Kubler-Ross's stages of grief 23–24
kyphosis 330

L
labrocytes 34*t*
lactic acid
and muscle contracture 208
and muscle fatigue 209
in sarcoplasmic reticulum 205
laminar flow 394
latent trigger point 165
lateral collateral ligament
knee 822
sprain 867
latissimus dorsi
assistive stretches 595
soft-tissue mobilization 576
strengthening exercises 523
law of conservation of energy 79
laws of motion 66

Hooke's law 80–81
Lazarevic's test 187
legal issues
    HIPAA 9
    patient right to privacy 9
    record keeping 102
    standards of care 11
    state regulations 11
    touch as part of rehab process 12–13
leg, center of gravity 69*t*
leg length discrepancy 330
    assessment 532
    and gait 375
    and hip mechanics 896
    and sacroiliac alignment 530
Leighton flexometer 134
length-tension relationship 214–215
Leseague's test 187
leukocytes 34*t*
leukotriene 34*t*
levator scapulae 481, 573
lever arm
    and form drag 402
    length and force production 215
    and muscular strength 78
    and pulley system for resistance training 238
    and Swiss ball exercises 428*f*
levers
    about 72–73
    classes 73–74
    effects of 74
    and force 75–76
    and single support assistive devices 384
lifting technique 342
ligaments
    dehiscence 822
    hand and wrist 689–690
    healing process 46–47
    knee 821–822
    proprioceptive receptors 263
    structure 125
    tensile strength after injury 52
limbs, center of gravity 69*t*
linear motion 75
line of gravity 70
    and base of support 71*f*
line of pull 75–76
lipid 34*t*
Little League elbow 676–677
loading response 357
Lodine 55*t*
loose-packed joint positions 181–182
lordosis
    cervical spine 331
    lumbar 329
low back. *See also* sacroiliac joint
    agility and coordination exercises 524–525

    flexibility exercises 501–507
    joint mobilization 494–497
    and pelvic stabilization 507–512
    soft-tissue mobilization 487–490
    strengthening exercises 517–523
lower body
    center of gravity 69*t*
    range of motion 136
lower extremity
    alignment 331–336, 826
    center of gravity 69*t*
    functional testing 315
    injury and posture/muscle imbalances 339
    movement patterns 246*f*
    muscle action during gait 372*f*
    muscle compartments 747*f*
    neural tension tests 187
    patterns of movement 243–244
    superior tibiofibular joint 824
    tendinitis case study 464–465
    tibial torsion 750
    tibial varum 751
    tibiofibular joint mobilization 774–775
Lower Extremity Functional Scale (LEFS) 19*f*
lower extremity injuries
    Achilles rupture 802–803, 802–803
    Achilles tendinitis 798–801
    compartment syndrome 806–808
    fractures 811–813
    iliotibial (ITB) band friction syndrome 339
    peroneal tendon dislocation 798
    shin splints 805–806
    tendinitis 804–805
lower extremity rehabilitation
    aquatic exercise equipment 399
    aquatic exercises 411–417
    deep tissue massage 774
    flexibility exercises 779–782
    functional activities 795
    functional exercise progression 314*f*
    functional exercises 310–312
    functional scale 19*f*
    general considerations 744–748
    hopping activities 794
    leg pull technique 164
    plyometrics 288–295, 792
    proprioception exercises 269–271
    range of motion 135–136 *t*
    soft-tissue mobilization 767–771
    strengthening exercises 784–789
    stretching 148
    treadmill exercises 793
    using foam rollers 449–451
    using Swiss balls 440–442
lumbar lordosis 329
lumbar spine
    capsular patterns of motion 177*t*

flexibility exercises 501–507
joint mobilization 494–497
soft-tissue mobilization 487–490
strengthening exercises 517–523
lumbar support 328
lunges 521
lymphocytes 34*t*
lymph system 38, 155

M
machine exercises
foot and ankle rehabilitation 789
hip muscles 923–925
isokinetic machines 240–242
isokinetics for elbow 672
isokinetics for shoulder rehabilitation 616
isotonic machines 239–240
knee 856–857
macrophages 34*t*
and chronic inflammation 46
during proliferation phase of healing 41
Maitland, Geoffrey 174*t*
malalignment. *See* alignment
manipulation. *See* joint mobilization
manual muscle testing 96, 222–229
manual-resistance exercises 231–232
elbow 667–668
manual therapy
common principles 154
description 154
joint mobilization 173–183
massage 155–158
muscle energy techniques 170–173
myofascial release 158–165
neural mobilization 183–193
and patient assessment 155
schools of thought 174*t*
trigger points 165–170
massage 155–158
elbow 658
foot 764*f*, 774
and iliotibial (ITB) band friction syndrome 339
knee 836–838
lower extremity 774
supraspinatus 580
using foam rollers 445, 449
mast cells 34*t*
matrix 34*t*
M-bridge 202*f*, 204*f*
and sarcomere structure 201
McConnell, Jenny 875
McKenzie extension exercises 479
mechanical properties of tissue 128–132
mechanics. *See* body mechanics
mechanism of injury 89
medial collateral ligament
knee 821–822
sprain 867

medial tibial stress syndrome 805–806
median nerve
stretch 192*f*
tension test 188*f*
medical history 89–90
medical records. *See* record keeping
medications
about 53–56
and aquatic exercise 401
drug interaction 31*t*, 56
duration of action 31*t*, 53
and examination of injury 89
half-life 33*t*, 53–54
NSAIDs 54–56
over-the-counter 53
steady state 36*t*, 54
medicine-ball exercises
shoulder rehabilitation 621–623
spine rehabilitation 524
Meissner's corpuscles 205
Meloxicam 55*t*
meniscus
injuries 867–871
structure 822–823
transplant 870
Mennell, James 174*t*
metabolism
and muscle contracture 208
and myofascial restriction 160
and trigger points 166
metacarpal fractures 727–728
metacarpophalangeal (MCP) joint 689
joint mobilization 708, 710
range of motion 135*t*
resting and close-packed positions 181*t*
metatarsophalangeal joints 747
mobilization 779
turf toe 810–811
midstance 357
midswing 357
midtarsal joints 746–747
forefoot varus and valgus 752
resting and close-packed positions 181*t*
misalignment. *See* alignment
mitochondria
and immobilization 127
and muscle fiber type 210
in sarcoplasmic reticulum 205
Mobic 55*t*
mobilization. *See* joint mobilization
modalities 21
and healing process 52–53
as part of treatment plan 471
for tendinitis 462
Moll and Wright spinal ROM 137*f*
moment arm 72, 75
moment force 221

momentum 67
monocyte 34*t*
   during inflammation phase of healing 39
mononuclear phagocyte 34*t*
   and chronic inflammation 46
monosynaptic response 133
Morton's toe 900
motion of body
   descriptive terms 141
   multiplanar 304
motor neural pathways 205*f*
motor unit
   components 199
   number of muscle fibers 201*t*
   and smooth muscle contraction 205
   structure 200*f*
movement patterns 243–244
multifidus 508–509
   fiber direction 485
multi-joint muscles 76–77
muscle action
   and lever system 72–74
   line of pull 75–76
   physiological advantage 76, 77*f*
muscle activity
   during normal gait 372*f*
   during running 380*f*
   static 217–218
muscle contraction
   absolute refractory period 207
   alignment and muscle energy techniques 170–173
   all-or-none principle 206
   and alpha efferent fibers 133
   biochemical processes 201–205
   definition 217
   force production 214–216
   interaction of SEC, PEC, and contractile elements 277
   internuncial activation 133
   monosynaptic response 133–134
   and muscle structure 167*f*
   neuromuscular physiology 205–209
   refractory period 207
   speed and force production 216
   threshold stimulation 206
   and trigger points 166
muscle energy techniques 170–173
   sacroiliac joint 536–546
muscle fiber type
   description 210–211
   and force of contraction 216
   and lactate levels 209
muscle imbalance
   causes 337–338
   hip 927
   and iliotibial (ITB) band friction syndrome 339
   and patellofemoral pain syndrome 878
   and shoulder injuries 564

and tendinitis 460
   treatment 338
muscles
   active insufficiency 76
   activity gradations 230–231
   atrophy following injury 53
   fibers per motor unit 201*t*
   and gait kinetics 371
   of hand 690, 692
   healing process 48–49
   imbalances 159
   and immobilization 126–127
   length vs. tension 77*f*
   manual testing 222–229
   massage 155
   maximum force production 215
   multi-joint 76–77
   passive insufficiency 77
   pennate fiber arrangement 216
   physiological advantages 76–78
   properties 206–209
   recovery time 213
   and remobilization 128
   resting length 76
   size and force production 216
   specific gravity 393
   as stabilizers 72
   structure 167*f*, 199–201
   tensile strength after injury 52
   trigger point examination 167
muscle spasm
   and aquatic exercise 400
   and electrical stimulation 52
   and facet injuries 529
   and healing process 57
   and joint mobilization 177
   vs. muscle contracture 209
   and myofascial restriction 160
   and oscillation technique 163
   and proprioceptive neuromuscular facilitation 144
   and scoliosis 331
muscle spindle 132–133
   and ballistic stretching 144–145
   and muscle energy technique 171
   and plyometrics 278
   and proprioception 261
muscle strength. *See* strength
muscle twitch 206, 207
muscular end-feel 95
muscular endurance. *See also* endurance
   definition 22, 212
   and muscle fatigue 209
   and plyometrics 282
   relationship to strength 212–214
   and scapular imbalance 565
muscular strength. *See* strength
myoblast 35*t*
   and muscle repair 49

myofascia 159
    acute biomechanical forces 160
    nonacute biomechanical forces 159
myofascial release 158–165
    autonomic response 161
    palpation 160
    superficial to deep structures 160
    techniques 161–164
    terminology 160
myofascial trigger points. *See* trigger points
myofibrils 199*f*, 201, 277
myofibroblasts 35*t*
    during remodeling phase of healing 42
    and ultrasound 53
myogenic cells 35*t*
    and muscle repair 49
myosin 201, 204*f*
myositis ossificans 881
myotatic reflex 278
myotubes 49

N
Nabumetone 55*t*
naproxen sodium 54, 55*t*
National Athletic Trainers' Association (NATA) 9, 11
Nautilus 242
neck. *See* cervical spine
negative acceleration 80
nerve root compression
    and poor posture 329
    and scoliosis 331
nervous system
    motor neural pathways 205*f*
    neural mobilization 183–193
    and proprioception 261–263
    results of injury 185
    sensory neural pathways 205*f*
    and strength gains after injury 250
    structures in hip 894–895
neural mobilization
    afferent nervous system 184
    contraindications 193
    double-crush syndrome 185
    fascial connection 184
    and pain type 185–186
    precautions 191
    previous injury 185
    self-mobilization techniques 191, 192*f*
    susceptible sites 184
    tests 186–189
    treatment precautions 186
neurological tests 97–98
neuromuscular facilitation. *See* proprioceptive
        neuromuscular facilitation (PNF)
neuromuscular junction 200*f*, 206
neuromuscular physiology 205–209
neuromuscular system
    Golgi tendon organs 133–134

monosynaptic response 133–134
    muscle spindle 132–133
    and plyometrics 277–278
    and proprioception 260
neurotransmitters 35*t*
neutral spine 340
neutrophil 35*t*, 39
Newton-meters per second 79
Newton's laws of motion 66
nicotine 56
nociceptors 262
    and NSAID medications 54
    and referred pain 184
norepinephrine 35*t*
Norwegian test 530
NSAIDs 54–56
nuclear bag fiber 132
nuclear chain fiber 132
nutrition and healing 57

O
Ober's test 930
objective examination 92–99
    definition 88
    record keeping 109
objectives of rehabilitation 15–16
    goals 16–17
observation 93
obturator nerve 895
oculomotor system 265
open chain activities
    definition 219–221
    elbow 646
    and knee joint stress 825
    and motions of foot 745
    for proprioception 272
    for quad strength 828
    for shoulder rehabilitation 616–618
opponenes pollicis 201*t*
opposition 141
orthotics 753–757
oscillation technique 163
Osgood-Schlatter disease 872
osteitis pubis 931–932
osteoarthritis
    and age 90
    and leg-length discrepancy 896
    and meniscus repairs 868
osteoblasts 35*t*, 50
osteochondritis dissecans 883–884
    elbow 647
osteoclasts 35*t*, 50
osteocytes 35*t*
osteogenic cells 51
OTC medications 54–56
outcomes-based rehabilitation 18–20
outflares 544
overhead sports

baseball pitching 557–558
  golf 563–564
  and lower-extremity stability 566–567
  racket grip size 675
  swimming 561–563
  tennis 558–560
overpressure 95
over-the-counter medications 53
overuse injuries. *See also* tendinitis
  and chronic inflammation 46
  hand and wrist 730–731
  and timing of therapeutic exercise 60
overuse syndromes 81
ovoid joint 175
oxaprozin 55*t*
Oxford technique of strength progression 252

P
Pacinian corpuscles 205, 262*f*
pain
  and active range of motion 94
  and advanced functional activities 309
  and aquatic exercise 400
  and classification of tendinitis 462*t*
  and edema 58
  gate theory 169
  and ice 52
  and ice-stretch technique 169
  inflammation-based 185–186
  ischemic-related 185–186
  and joint mobilization 177, 180
  and NSAID medications 54
  and quadriceps strength 827
  referral chart 168*f*
  referred 184
  referred with trigger points 166
  and resistance training 251
  as sign of inflammation 40–41
  and stretching 146
  and treatment program 471
  types 185–186
pain profile 91–92
pain referral
  anconeus 649
  biceps brachii 649, 650*f*
  brachialis 649, 651*f*
  cervical disk 567
  deltoid 579
  finger extensors 656
  foot muscles 764*f*, 765–766
  gluteus maximus 899
  gluteus medius 900
  gluteus minimus 901
  groin 892
  hamstrings 834, 835*f*
  hand extrinsic muscles 699–701
  hip 892
  hip adductors 833*f*

  iliopsoas 898
  latissimus dorsi 576
  lower extremity 767–771
  pectineus 903
  pectoralis major 578
  piriformis 902
  popliteus 836*f*
  quadratus lumborum 489
  quadriceps 831
  rhomboids 575
  rotator cuff 568, 570, 571, 572
  scapular muscles 573
  serratus posterior inferior 490
  in spine 478
  supinator 653
  tensor fascia lata 836
  teres major 577
  triceps brachii 649, 652*f*
  wrist extensors 654*f*
  wrist flexors 657
palmaris longus 699
palpation 98–99
  legal issues 12–13
  and myofascial release 160
PA (posterior-anterior) 492
parallel-elastic component (PEC) 277
paraspinals 487–488
paratenon 459
parents 6–7, 8
Paris, Stanley 174*t*
Pascal's law 395
passive inefficiency 77
passive insufficiency 77
passive neck flexion test 186
passive range of motion (PROM) 94–95, 230
  recording 138
passive stretching 142–143
  and trigger point therapy 170
patella
  alignment 332, 823–824, 825
  alignment and soft tissue mobility 877
  contact pressure 825
  dislocations 871–872
  and knee biomechanics 824–825
  malalignment 339–340
  orientation 874*f*
  subluxations 871–872
  taping technique 875–876
  tendinitis 878–879
  tendon rupture 879–880
patella alta 824
patella baja 824
patella plica 872
patellofemoral joint
  contact patterns 825*f*
  mobilization 839
  resting and close-packed positions 181*t*

stress vs. range of motion 828f
syndrome 872–878
pathoneurodynamics 184
patient
communication with 8
consent for treatment 11–12
expectations 90
as part of rehabilitation team 7
psychological effect of injury 23–24
support system 25
viewing as whole person 15
PDGF growth factors 45
pectineus 903
pectorals
flexibility exercises 501
soft-tissue mobilization 575, 578
pelvic neutral 340, 507
pelvic rotation 360
pelvic tilt 329
and normal gait 361
strengthening exercises 517
pelvis
and gait kinematics 364–365
and hip movement 895–896
lateral rotation during normal gait 363
and posture 329
Penny and Giles eletrogoniometer 136f
periarticular connective tissue 127–128
perimysium 199
periosteum 47
peroneals
action during gait cycle 372f
soft-tissue mobilization 768
tendon dislocation 798
pes cavus 334, 749
pes planus 334, 749
petrissage 156
PGE1. See prostaglandin
PGE2. See prostaglandin
phagocyte
during inflammation phase of healing 39
and muscle injury 49
phospholipids 35t, 38
physician
communication with 8
as part of rehabilitation team 6
and return-to-competition 23
Physician and Sportsmedicine 501
physics
acceleration 80
angle of pull 76
body levers 72–74
center of gravity 68
creep 81
elasticity 80
energy 79
fixation 70–72

force 66–67
friction 81
gravity 66
line of pull 75–76
muscle advantages 76–78
Newton's laws of motion 67–68
power 79
resistance arm 77f
stability 70–72
strength 78
stress and strain 80–81
structural fatigue 81
torque 75
velocity 79
work 79
Physioball 429
physiological joint motion 95, 174
physiotherapy 500
Piedallus test 530
Pilates 349–351
as body-weight resistance exercise 234
piriformis
flexibility exercises 505, 915
soft-tissue mobilization 902
piroxicam 55t
pitching. See baseball pitching
planes of body 141
and foot motions 745
and gait kinematics 363
and rotator cuff exercises 567–568
and standing alignment 327
plan for treatment 101
record keeping 109
plantar fasciitis 808–809
plantar flexion 745
and ankle sprains 746
definition 141
manual muscle testing 229f
during running 380f
strengthening exercises 785–786
plasmin 35t
plasminogen activator 35t
during proliferation phase of healing 41
plastic deformation
of fascia 158
and passive stretching 142
plasticity 130
and active stretching 141
plastic range 81
platelet-derived growth factor (PDGF) 35t
platelets 35t
during inflammation phase of healing 38
platysma 201t
plica 872
plyometrics
contraindications 285
description 276

elbow 672
equipment 285–287
exercise phases 279–280
force production 278–279
hand and wrist 725
lower extremity 792
lower extremity exercises 288–295
patient readiness 280–281
precautions 285
program design 281–285
and proprioception 270, 272
shoulder 619–623
technique 284
upper extremity exercises 296–297
PNF. See proprioceptive neuromuscular facilitation (PNF)
polymorphonuclear leukocyte (PMN) 36t
during inflammation phase of healing 39
popliteus 836f
popping sound 91
posterior cruciate ligament (PCL) sprain 864–866
posterior superior iliac spine (PSIS)
and poor posture 329
and standing alignment 328
posture
definition 326
improving 338
lower extremities 331–336
pathological alignment 329–331
pelvic neutral 507
and shoulder impingement 628
and shoulder injuries 567
sitting alignment 328
standing alignment 327–328
upper extremity 336
potassium 206
potential energy 79
and elasticity 129
and plyometrics 278–279
power
and agility 268
calculating 276
definition 79, 212
and force 280
and functional activities 304–305
and plyometrics 276
pregnancy 56
pressure
and inflammation 40
and Pacinian corpuscles 205
pressure-sensitive nerve endings 42
preswing 357
priformis 927
primary ending 133
primary intention 35t, 37
principles of rehabilitation 13–14
privacy 9

professionalism 2, 9–11
progression of exercise 18
for advanced functional activities 306–308
for agility and balance 313f
aquatic exercise 403–404
plyometrics 284
stretching 147–148
progressive overload 251
progress report form 113–114
proliferation phase 41–42
prolonged stretches
elbow 662
knee rehabilitation 843–844
pronation
definition 141, 745
of foot 335f
forearm exercises 720
stretches at elbow 666f
pronator teres 699
soft-tissue mobilization 657
proprioception
agility 268–272
and aquatic exercise 403
balance 264–266
central nervous system 263–264
coordination 266–268
definition 22–23, 260
and functional activities 304
joint receptors 262
in knee joint 822
lower extremity exercises 269–271
neurophysiology 261–263
and plyometrics 281
somatosensory system 265
and timing of therapeutic exercise 59
upper extremity exercises 271–272
proprioceptive exercises
ankle 789–794
foot 789–794
hip 926
knee 858–859
lower extremity 789–794
proprioceptive neuromuscular facilitation (PNF) 132, 170
description 143–144, 242–243
lower extremity patterns 246f
patterns of movement 243–244
principles 244, 246
and scar tissue 148
shoulder rehabilitation 616
techniques 247–248
upper extremity patterns 245f
verbal cues 243
prostaglandin (PG) 36t
during inflammation phase of healing 40
and NSAID medications 54–56
and trigger points 166

protease 36t, 46
proteins
    collagen 31t
    complement system 31t
    elastin 32t
    electrical stimulation and synthesis 52
    fibrin 32t
    growth factor 44–45
proteoglycan 36t
    during proliferation phase of healing 41, 42
    and remobilization 128
protraction of scapula 141
psychological considerations 23–26
pulling technique 343
pulsed ultrasound 53
pus 40
pushing technique 343
push-ups
    and elbow stress 648
    plyometric for shoulder rehabilitation 620
    progression 233f
    using body weight 233
    using foam rollers 451
    using Swiss balls 443

Q
Q-angle 826
quadratus lumborum
    flexibility exercises 502
    massage using foam rollers 445
    soft-tissue mobilization 489
    strengthening using foam rollers 449
quadriceps
    contusions 881
    deep tissue massage 836–838
    edema and strength 826–827
    flexibility exercises 844–846
    and genu valgus 332
    injury and gait abnormalities 376
    isometric exercises 848–849
    and knee action 824
    manual muscle testing 227–228
    massage using foam rollers 449
    non-weight-bearing isotonic exercises 849–850
    during running, walking, sprinting 380f
    as shock absorbers 371
    soft-tissue mobilization 831–832
    weight-bearing resistive exercises 851–856
quadriceps gait 376
questionnaires, for assessment 18–20

R
racket grip size 675
radial deviation 141
radial flexion 689
radial nerve
    stretch 192f
    tension test 189

radiohumeral joint mobilization 660
radioulnar joint 648
    joint mobilization 661, 704–705
    resting and close-packed positions 181t
range of motion
    accuracy of measurement 138
    active 93–94, 230
    active assisted 230
    and angle of pull 75–76
    and aquatic exercise 403
    barriers to movement 536
    capsular patterns 176, 177t
    and collagen fiber failure 131
    definition 21, 124
    for different joints 135–136
    equipment for measuring 134
    goniometer placement 139f
    goniometry terminology 140
    and joint mobilization 178
    and manual muscle testing 224
    normal 134
    normal joint mobility 180–181
    passive 94–95, 230
    and patellofemoral stress injuries 825
    rearfoot 748
    recording 138
    resisted 230
    during running 380f
    using a goniometer 137–138
reciprocal-exercise equipment 923
reciprocal inhibition 142
reciprocal innervation 171
record keeping 6
    about 102
    diploma 116
    discharge summary 115
    examination form 103–107
    progress report form 113–114
    signing and dating 102
    treatment 108–110
recovery
    and goal of rehabilitation 16
    of muscle tissue 213
    plyometrics 282
rectus femoris 911
    action during gait cycle 372f
    and running 380
recurring injuries 90
referred pain. See pain referral
reflex inhibition 250
reflex sympathetic dystrophy (RSD) 165, 736–738
refractory period 172
rehabilitation clinician
    description of responsibilities 5
    interaction with team members 7–9
    interpersonal skills 5–6
    role in psychological recovery 24

rehabilitation team 4–7
Relafen 55t
relative density 393
relative refractory period 207
remobilization 128
remodeling phase 22, 42–43
repetitions vs. resistance 213–214
repetitive stress syndromes 81
resistance arm 72
    and changes in position 77f
resistance training
    cross-training 251
    elbow 667–671
    exercise progression 252–253
    free weights 236–239
    and friction 81
    isokinetic machines 240–242
    isotonic machines 239–240
    manual resistance 231–242
    Nautilus 242
    pain 251
    pre-exercise stretch 215
    progressive overload 251
    recovery period 213
    repetitions vs. resistance 213–214
    SAID principle 249
    for tendinitis 463
    using body weight 232–234
    using rubber tubing and bands 234–236
    and viscosity of muscle 208
    in water 399
resisted range of motion (RROM) 231
rest 13–14
    plyometrics 282
resting potential 206
reticulin 36t
    in connective tissue 124–125
    in extracellular matrix 42
retroversion 332, 893
return to sport
    criteria 23, 319
    and functional examination 310
reversal of antagonists techniques 248
rhomboids
    flexibility exercises 592
    soft-tissue mobilization 575
rhythmic initiation 248
rhythmic stabilization, shoulder 613–614
rice krispie syndromes 932
Roland-Morris questionnaire 20
Rolfing 158
Roman chair 522
rotational motion 75
    and line of pull 75–76
rotator cuff
    planes of exercises 567–568
    soft-tissue mobilization 568–572
    tendinitis 337, 339

traumatic injury 629–631
rotatores 485
rubber tubing exercises 234–236
    ankle 785
    glenohumeral joint 608–610
    hip 920–922
    and principle of elasticity 80
    shoulder 603–604, 617–618
Ruffini endings
    in knee joint 822
    and proprioception 262f
running
    in deep water 405
    shoes 760
    in water 414
running gait 377–381
    joint motions 378–379
    kinetics 380–381
    speed 377

S
saccule 265
sacroiliac joint
    anatomy 529–530
    dysfunction and symptoms 535t
    examination 530–534
    and hip pain 892
    joint mobilization 494–497
    muscle energy treatment 536–546
    pathology 536t
saddle joint 175
safety
    and Swiss ball exercises 429–430
    water exercise 395–396
sagittal plane 141
    and alignment of femur and tibia 332
SAID principle 249
sarcolemma 199
sarcomere
    as contractile element 277
    and muscle contraction 202f
    structure 167f, 201
sarcoplasm 199f
sarcoplasmic reticulum 202f, 205
sartorius 372f
satellite cells 36t, 48–49
scalenes
    flexibility exercises 500
    soft-tissue mobilization 483
scapula motions 141
scapular muscles 565–566
    retraction using Swiss balls 444
    soft-tissue mobilization 573
    stabilization exercises 611–616
    strengthening exercises 601–607
scapulothoracic joint
    isotonic exercises 601–607
    joint mobilization 586–587

scar tissue
and active stretching 141
and cartilage injury 49
effectiveness of stretching 148
elasticity 81
and elbow structure 647
and fascia 158–159
formation during proliferation phase 41
and friction massage 157
and healing by secondary intention 37
and healing process 30
and immobilization 126
keloid formation 42
matrix formation 160
mobility 22
and muscle injury 48–49
to neural tissue 185
prolonged stretch effectiveness 143
and range of motion 128
and recurring injuries 90
during remodeling phase of healing 42
and stretching 147
and trigger point therapy 170
sciatica 329, 527–528
sciatic nerve 894
stretch 192f
scoliosis 330–331
screw home mechanism 823
secondary intention 36t, 37
sellar joint 175
semicircular canals 265
semimembranosus
action during gait cycle 372f
and running 380
semispinalis muscles 485–486
semitendinosus 372f
sensory neural pathways 205f
series elastic component (SEC) 277
serotonin 36t
chemical reaction during inflammation phase 40
and trigger points 166
serratus anterior
soft-tissue mobilization 573
strengthening exercises 601
serratus posterior inferior 490
sesamoiditis 810
set 132
SF-16 health status tool 18
shallow water exercises
ankle rehabilitation 414–415
elbow rehabilitation 419
knee rehabilitation 413–414
lower extremity rehabilitation 411–413
shoulder rehabilitation 417–419
spine rehabilitation 406–410
shear force 130
during normal gait 373

and open kinetic chain activities 221
shin splints 805–806
shoes
for aquatic exercise 399
fit 759
and injury history 759
lacing patterns 762–763
and plyometrics 284
sport-specific 760–762
structure 758–759
wear patterns 759
short-term goals 16–17
duration 100
shoulder
dynamic restraints 624
force couples 566
golf swing mechanics 563–564
goniometer placement 139f
manual muscle testing 228, 228f
movement patterns 245f
pitching mechanics 557–558
range of motion 135, 556
stability 564
static restraints 624
swimming mechanics 561–563
tennis mechanics 558–560
shoulder injuries
acromioclavicular sprain 636–637
adhesive capsulitis 633–635
American Academy of Orthopedic Surgeons web
site 617
arm pull 580
biceps tendon injuries 638
electrothermally assisted capsular shift 635–636
frozen shoulder 625
glenoid labral tears 632–633
impingement 339, 627–629
instability 624–626
and posture 567
rotator cuff tendinitis 339
rotator cuff (traumatic injury) 629–631
thoracic outlet syndrome 546–549
and trunk/hip stability 566–567
TUBS (traumatic, unilateral, Bankart lesion,
surgery required) 625
shoulder rehabilitation 621–623
aquatic exercises 417–419, 420
Codman's exercises 589
exercise planes 568
flexibility exercises 588–599
functional activities 624
general considerations 564–568
joint mobilization 581–588
pulley exercises 599
sample goals 17
soft-tissue mobilization 568–580
strengthening exercises 599–610, 613t

wand exercises 596–598
Simons, David 165
single-leg support 357
single-support gait 384, 896
sitting alignment 328
sit-to-stand 343
   with assistive devices 386
sit-ups
   sidelying 520
   using Swiss balls 439
skin
   as *areolar* connective tissue 125
   of hand 692
   subcutaneous proprioceptive receptors 261
slow reversal-hold-relax technique 144
slow-twitch fibers 210–211
slump test 187, 188*f*
Smith's fracture 726
snapping palpation 165, 167
SOAP notes
   assessment 99–102
   discharge summary 112
   examination 103–107
   progress report form 113–114
   progress reports 112
   treatment 108–110
soccer shoes 761
sodium 206
sodium-potassium pump 206
softball 316*f*
soft end-feel 95
soft tissue approximation end-feel 95
soft-tissue mobilization 158
   cervical spine 480–490
   deltoid 579
   elbow 649–658
   finger extensors 656
   foot 763–766
   gluteus maximus 899
   gluteus medius 900
   gluteus minimus 901–902
   hamstrings 834, 835*f*
   hand 698–704
   hip adductors 833, 834*f*
   iliopsoas 898
   knee 830–836
   lumbar spine 487–490
   pectineus 903
   pectoralis major 578
   pectoralis minor 575
   piriformis 902
   popliteus 835–836
   quadriceps 831–832
   rhomboids 575
   rotator cuff muscles 568–572
   scapular muscles 573
   self-mobilization technique 491

thoracic spine 487–490
   wrist 654–657, 698–704
soleus
   action during gait cycle 372*f*
   flexibility exercises 780–781
   physiological advantage 76
   soft-tissue mobilization 770
   strengthening exercises 787–789
   stretching using foam rollers 450
somatosensory system 265
sounds of injured part 90–91, 178
spasm. *See* muscle spasm
special tests 96–97
Specific Adaptations to Imposed Demands principle
      249
specific gravity 393
speed
   and advanced functional activities 307
   and agility 268
   and velocity 79
   walking 359
   walking and running 377
   and walking in water 394
spinal cord and proprioception 263
spinal reflex 263
spine
   alignment 327–328, 341*f*
   alignment in deep-water exercise 405
   and body mechanics 340–342
   capsular patterns of motion 177*t*
   kyphosis 330*f*
   lumbar lordosis 331*f*
   pathological alignment 329–331
   range of motion 137
   scoliosis 330*f*
spine injuries. *See also* sacroiliac joint
   disk lesions 527–528
   facet injuries 528
   sciatica 527–528
   spondylosis, spondylolysis, spondylolisthesis 526–
      527
   thoracic outlet syndrome 546–549
spine rehabilitation
   agility and coordination exercises 524–525
   aquatic exercises 406–411
   flexibility exercises (cervical spine) 497–501
   flexibility exercises (thoracolumbar spine) 501–507
   general guidelines 479, 525
   joint mobilization 491–497
   soft-tissue mobilization 480–490
   stabilization exercises 507–512
   strengthening exercises 512–523
   Swiss ball exercises 431–439
spleni muscles 484
   fiber direction 485
splints
   hand 696–698

for prolonged stretching 145–146
spondylolisthesis 526–527
spondylolysis 526–527
    and hip pain 892
spondylosis 526–527
spongy bone 51
sport participation. *See* return to sport
sport-specific demands 305. *See* functional activities
sprain
    ACL (anterior cruciate ligament) 860–863
    acromioclavicular joint 636–637
    ankle 795–797
    back 525–526
    collateral ligament (knee) sprains 867
    elbow 677–678
    hip 929
    PCL (posterior cruciate ligament) 864–866
springy end-feel 95
    and myfascial release 160
sprinting 80
squats
    using foam rollers 451
    using Swiss balls 429f, 440f
squinting patellae 332, 333f, 893
stability 70–71
stabilization 72
    and functional activities 304
    and multi-joint muscles 76–77
    during normal gait 371
    and passive stretching 143
    role of hip 895
    of scapula and stretching 148
    of shoulder 564
    and stretching 147
stabilization exercises
    scapular muscles 611–616
    shoulder 611–616
stages of grief 23–24
stance, and base of support 70–71
stance phase 357
state regulations 11
static restraints, shoulder 624
steady state of drug 36t, 54
step length
    running 377
    walking 359
sternoclavicular joint mobilization 588
sternocleidomastoid 482
steroid medications 55
    corticosteroids and healing time 56
stiffness, and pain profile 92
Stone Foundation 50
straight-leg raise test 187
strain
    back 525–526
    definition 80–81, 130
    groin 929

hamstrings 880
    quadriceps 880–881
strain-counterstrain 158
strength
    and agility 268
    and balance 264–266
    of collagen vs. elastin fibers 125
    and concentric vs. eccentric muscle training 218
    definition 22, 78, 211
    examination 96
    evaluation equipment 221–222
    and functional activities 304
    gains in rehabilitation program 250f
    grades 97t
    imbalances 159
    isokinetic testing 222f
    and plyometrics 280
    and power 79
    and range of motion 21
    rates of loss and recovery 14
    relationship to muscular endurance 212–214
strengthening exercises
    and active stretching 142
    elbow 667–672
    hip 916–925
    knee (isometric) 848–849
    knee (isotonic, non-weight-bearing) 849–850
    knee (isotonic, weight-bearing) 851–856
    knee (machines) 856–857
    and phases of healing 59
    sample progression 18
    shoulder 599–610, 613t
strength training. *See* resistance training; strengthening
        exercises
stress 80–81
stress fracture
    hip 933–934
    and physical properties of bone 130
    structural fatigue of bone 81
stress-strain principles 130–131
    and tendinitis 459
stretching
    active 141–142
    assistive devices 145–146
    ballistic 144–145
    contraindications 146
    and early wound healing 42
    exercise progression 147–148
    indications 146
    and muscle contracture 208
    passive 142–143
    precautions 146–147
    proprioceptive neuromuscular facilitation 143–144
    special considerations 148–149
    and stress-strain of tissue 131
    techniques 141–146
    using Swiss balls 427

stretch model of connective tissue 129f
stretch reflex
    and plyometrics 278
    and proprioceptive neuromuscular facilitation
        (PNF) 243, 247
stride length
    and fore-aft shear force 374f
    running 377
    walking 359
stride width 359
stripping technique 164, 170
structural fatigue 81, 130
subjective examination 89–92
    definition 88
    record keeping 109
subluxations, patella 871–872
suboccipital muscles 485–486
subscapularis
    assistive stretches 594
    soft-tissue mobilization 570
subserous fascia 158
subtalar joint 745
    mobilization 777
    neutral position 748
    range of motion 136
    resting and close-packed positions 181t
sulindac 55t
summation of forces 78, 209
superior tibiofibular joint 824
    joint mobilization 838
supination
    definition 141
    of foot 745
    forearm exercises 720
    stretches at elbow 666f
supinator 653
support system 25
supraspinatus
    assistive stretches 593
    flexibility exercises 593
    friction massage 580
    soft-tissue mobilization 568–569
surface
    and assistive devices 385–386
    and plyometrics 283
    for Swiss ball exercises 429
    and tendinitis 459
    unstable for shoulder rehabilitation 620
surface tension 394
surgical repair
    of arthritic joints 49–50
    and healing process 57
    of tendon injury 48
Swedish procedure (cartilage) 50
swelling. See edema
swimming
    mechanics of shoulder motion 561–563
    muscle imbalances 337

swing phase 357
swing-through 357
Swiss ball exercises
    adding difficulty 428
    back 433–438
    Bouhler exercises 606
    contraindications 430
    hip 925
    lower extremity 440–442
    scapula stabilization 612
    squats 429f
    trunk 430–439
    upper extremity 442–444
    for upper extremity proprioception 272f
Swiss balls
    care 430
    description 426
    manufacturers 426
    safety 429–431
    sizes 430t
    versatility 426–427
sympathetic nervous system 161
synergistic muscles 133
    and proprioception 261
synovial fluid 178
synovial sheath
    and tendon injury 47
    tenosynovitis 458
    and timing of therapeutic exercise 59
synovitis 90–91

T
talocrural joint 745
    mobilization 776
    resting and close-packed positions 181t
tape, types of 566
taping
    patella 875–876
    and scapular imbalance 566
tarsal tunnel syndrome 809–810
tarsometatarsal joints 747
    mobilization 779
team. See rehabilitation team
technician 2
temperature
    and creep 130
    and hysteresis 132
    and muscle stiffness 208
    and referred pain 184
    as sign of inflammation 40
    of water for aquatic exercise 402
temporomandibular joint disorder 331
tendinitis
    Achilles tendon 798–801
    biceps 638
    classifications 462t
    definition 458
    general treatment 461–462

hip 931
    inflammatory response of tendon tissue 460
    lower-extremity case study 464–465
    patellar tendon 878–879
    and physical properties of connective tissue 130
    and recurring injuries 90
    rotator cuff 339
    sounds of injured part 90–91
    treatment phases 462–464
    upper-extremity case study 465–466
tendinosis 458
tendons
    excursions in hand 694
    healing process 47–48
    patellar tendon 823
    repair and flexibility exercises 59
    response to loads 461f
    structure 125, 458–459
    tensile strength after injury 52
    tensile strength and electrical stimulation 52
tennis
    footwear 760
    functional exercises 318f
    grip size 675
    mechanics 558–560
    mechanics and elbow injuries 647
tennis elbow 673–676
tenocyte 36t
tenosynovitis 458
tensile strength 37t, 38
    and collagen cross-linking 43
    and extracellular matrix 42
    of fascia 158
    during healing process 51–52
    of tendons 459
    of tendons and electrical stimulation 52
tension stress 130
tensor fascia lata
    action during gait cycle 372f
    flexibility exercises 909–910
    soft-tissue mobilization 836
tensor tympanii 201t
teres major
    assistive stretches 595
    soft-tissue mobilization 577
teres minor
    assistive stretches 594
    soft-tissue mobilization 571
terminal branches 200f
terminal stance 357
terminal swing 357
TGF growth factors 45
therapeutic exercise
    components 21–23
    individualization 475
    modalities 21
    outcomes-based rehabilitation 18–20

    phases 473–474
    principles of rehabilitation 13–15
    progression of program 18
    psychological consideration 23–26
    rehabilitation objectives 15–17
    timing of treatment 58–59
thigh
    center of gravity 69t
    muscles 824
thigh injuries
    iliotibial band syndrome 882
    myositis ossificans 881
    Osgood-Schlatter disease 872
    osteochondritis dissecans 883–884
thoracic outlet syndrome 330, 331, 546–549
thoracic spine
    flexibility exercises 501–507
    joint mobilization 493–494
    and shoulder injuries 567
    soft-tissue mobilization 487–490
three-point gait 383
threshold stimulation 206
thrombin 37t
thromboxane 37t
thumb
    flexibility exercises 712f
    joint mobilization 709
    range of motion 135
    soft-tissue mobilization 702
tibialis anterior
    manual muscle testing 229f
    muscle fibers per motor unit 201t
    soft-tissue mobilization 767
tibialis posterior
    action during gait cycle 372f
    soft-tissue mobilization 770–771
tibial torsion 332, 750
tibial varum 751
tibiofemoral joint
    mobilization 840–842
    resting and close-packed positions 181t
    structure 821
tibiofibular joint 824
    mobilization 774–775, 838
time, and acceleration 80
timing of rehabilitation 13–14
toe extensors 771–772
toe region 131
Tolectin 55t
tolmetin Na 55t
torque 75
    and force of muscle contraction 214
touch
    massage 155–158
    myofascial release 158–165
    and neuromuscular physiology 205
    and normal joint mobility 180–181

as part of rehabilitation process 12–13
training volume 213
transverse abdominis 508–509
transverse plane 141
transverse tubule 203*f*
trapezius
    flexibility exercises 499
    manual muscle testing 229*f*
    muscle fiber direction 485
    soft-tissue mobilization 480–481, 573
Travell, Janet 165
Trendelenburg gait 376
triceps brachii
    exercises using foam rollers 452
    pain referral 652*f*
    soft-tissue mobilization 649
    Swiss ball exercises 442
trigger points
    causes 166
    characteristics 166
    definition 165
    examination 167
    ice-stretch treatment 167–169
    ischemic compression 169–170
    and proprioceptive neuromuscular facilitation
        (PNF) 170
    snapping palpation 165
    stripping massage treatment 170
    treatment 167–170
trigger point therapy. *See* soft-tissue mobilization
tropomyosin 202, 204*f*
troponin 202, 204*f*
trunk
    extension exercise 522
    and gait kinematics 364
    lateral rotation 521
    range of motion 137
    stability and shoulder injuries 566–567
    stretching 148
trunk exercises
    using foam rollers 445–449
    using Swiss balls 430–439
T-tubules 203
    and muscle contraction 202
tubule system 203*f*
turbulent flow 394
turf toe 810–811
twitch response 167

U
ulnar collateral ligament repair 678–679
ulnar collateral ligament sprain 678
ulnar deviation 141
ulnar flexion 689
ulnar nerve
    injury 679–680
    stretch 192*f*
    tension test 189

ulnohumeral joint 648
    joint mobilization 659–660
ultimate strength 131
ultrasound treatment 53
    in children 90
upper body
    center of gravity 69*t*
    range of motion 135
upper extremities
    alignment 336
    center of gravity 69*t*
    functional examination 319
    and gait kinematics 364
    muscle length-tension relationship 215*f*
    neural tension tests 187, 189, 190*f*
    patterns of movement 243–244, 245*f*
    range of motion 135–136 *t*
    stretching techniques 148
upper extremity injuries
    rotator cuff tendinitis 339
    shoulder impingement 339
    tendinitis case study 465–466
upper extremity rehabilitation
    aquatic exercise equipment 399–400
    aquatic exercises 417–421
    arm pull technique 164
    functional exercise progression 315–319
    plyometrics 296–297
    proprioception exercises 271–272
    stretching 148
    using foam rollers 451–453
    using Swiss balls 442–444
upper-limb tension test 187, 188*f*, 189, 190*f*
upward rotation of scapula 141
utricle 265

V
vacuum click 91
valgus
    forefoot 752, 753*f*
    rearfoot 751
Valsalva maneuver 217, 231
varus
    forefoot 752, 753*f*
    rearfoot 751
vascular permeability 40
vascular tissue
    capillary formation during healing 41
    and neural injury 185
    and tendon repair 47–48
vasoconstriction
    during inflammation phase of healing 38
    and trigger points 166
vasodilator
    acetylcholine 31*t*
    bradykinin 31*t*
    and inflammation 40
    during inflammation phase of healing 38

vastus medialis (VMO)
  action during gait cycle 372f
  and extensor lag 827–228
  weakness 339–340
velocity 79
  and acceleration 80
  definition 79
  of overhand motions 556
ventral root 200f
vertebrae
  facet injuries 528–529
  and poor posture 329
vertebral artery compromise 480
vestibular system 265
Vioxx 55t
viscoelasticity 129
  of tendons 458–459
viscosity 129f
  of fluids 394
  of muscle 208
visual input
  and balance 264
  oculomotor system 265
visual inspection 93
VMO (vastus medialis oblique)
  and extensor lag 827–828
  weakness 339–340
volitional muscle activity 266
volleyball shoes 761
Voltaren 55t
volume of exercise, plyometrics 282

W
walking. See also gait
  shoes 761
  in water 414
water. See also aquatic exercise
  and proliferation phase of healing 42
  properties of 393–395
wave drag 394
Web sites
  Alexander technique 347
  American Academy of Orthopedic Surgeons 617
  cartilage transplant 49–50
  Health Insurance Portability Accountability Act
    (HIPPA) 9

National Athletic Trainers' Association (NATA) 11
  Physician and Sportsmedicine 501
  physiotherapy information 500
  Pilates method 351
weight
  and acceleration due to gravity 80
  and gravity 67
weight bearing in water 395, 396f
white blood cells 39
Williams flexion exercises 479
withdrawal reflex 41
work, definition 79
wound healing. See healing process
wringing technique 163
wrist
  capsular patterns of motion 177t
  fascia and ligaments 689–690
  range of motion 135
  resting and close-packed positions 181t
  skeletal structure 689
  tendon sheaths 690
wrist injuries
  carpal tunnel syndrome 731–732
  dislocations 729–730
  fractures 726–727
  reflex sympathetic dystrophy 736–738
  sprains 729–730
  tendon injuries 733–736
wrist rehabilitation
  flexibility exercises 711–715
  functional activities 725
  isokinetic exercises 725
  joint mobilization 705
  plyometrics 725
  soft-tissue mobilization 654–657, 698–704
  strengthening exercises 715–720
  tendon glide exercises 715–718

Z
Z-disk 202f, 203f, 204f
  and muscle contraction 202
  and sarcomere structure 201

About the Author

Peggy A. Houglum, PhD, ATC, PT, is an assistant professor at Duquesne University in Pittsburgh. She has more than 30 years of experience in rehabilitation providing patient and athlete care. Her extensive background as a certified athletic trainer and physical therapist has provided her with a unique perspective regarding rehabilitation programs that make therapeutic exercise techniques meaningful and appropriate for athletic injury treatment.

Dr. Houglum has clinical experience in a variety of settings including acute care and rehabilitation hospitals, sports medicine clinics, and athletic training facilities. She has also served as an athletic trainer with the United States Olympic Sports Festivals, Olympic Games, and World University Games.

A member of the American Physical Therapy Association's Sports Medicine Section and National Athletic Trainers' Association (NATA), Houglum is currently chair of the NATA Continuing Education Committee. She created the NATA's first formal continuing education programming in 1991. In 2002 she was named to the NATA Hall of Fame, the association's highest award, and received NATA's Most Distinguished Athletic Trainer Award in 1996. Dr. Houglum is also clinical applications editor of the *Journal of Athletic Training*. She earned her bachelor's degree in physical therapy from the University of Minnesota, master's degree in athletic training from Indiana State University, and PhD in sports medicine from the University of Virginia.